FOOD AND NUTRITION

We dedicate this edition of *Food and Nutrition* to our children and grandchildren, here and yet to come: Ingmar, Kerstin, Gustav, Oriane, Otto, Malia, Mikaela, Patrik and Eliza. May our concerted efforts ensure they will have sustainable livelihoods on a habitable planet well into the future.

We acknowledge the First Nations peoples of Australia and New Zealand and pay our respects to their elders past, present and future. We recognise their strong and unbroken connection to land and sea and that addressing and fulfilling issues around sovereignty, treaties and human rights are long overdue. The full enactment of these rights will be essential to ensure food security into the future.

We would like to thank Rebecca Borradale and David Borradale for their contributions to the conceptualisation and construction of many of the diagrams in this edition of the textbook.

FOOD AND NUTRITION

Sustainable food and health systems

4th edition

EDITED BY

Mark L. Wahlqvist and Danielle Gallegos

CONTRIBUTORS

Janis Baines
David Borradale
Janeane Dart
Leisa McCarthy
Christina McKerchar
Claire Palermo
Gayle S. Savige
Jolieke C. van der Pols
Naiyana Wattanapenpaiboon

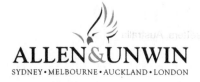

ALLEN&UNWIN
SYDNEY·MELBOURNE·AUCKLAND·LONDON

Allen & Unwin
83 Alexander Street
Crows Nest NSW 2065
Australia
Phone: (61 2) 8425 0100
Email: info@allenandunwin.com
Web: www.allenandunwin.com

 A catalogue record for this
book is available from the
National Library of Australia

ISBN 978 1 76029 610 0

Internal design by Romina Panetta
Index by Garry Cousins
Set in 10.5/13 pt Bembo by Midland Typesetters, Australia
Printed by Tien Wah Press, Singapore

10 9 8 7 6 5 4 3 2 1

CONTENTS

LIST OF FIGURES AND TABLES

The colour section is between pages 14 and 15.

FIGURES

TABLES

CONTRIBUTORS

MARK L. WAHLQVIST

{BMedSc, MB, BS, MD (Adelaide), MD (Uppsala), FRACP, FAFPHM, FAIFST, FACN, FTSE}

A graduate of Adelaide and Uppsala universities, Mark has pursued a career as an educator and clinician in medicine, public health and nutrition. He held the first Australian Chair of Human Nutrition, at Deakin University, and was Professor and Head of Medicine at Monash University and the Monash Medical Centre in Melbourne, Australia. He has held senior appointments at universities and research institutes in Australia, Sweden, Indonesia, Taiwan and mainland China. He has led scientific, academic, food safety, food-and-nutrition policy and community-based organisations. He was president of the International Union of Nutritional Sciences and editor-in-chief of the *Asia Pacific Journal of Clinical Nutrition*. His principal scientific contributions have been in socio-econutritional approaches to cross-cultural health.

DANIELLE GALLEGOS

{BSc, Grad Dip Nut & Diet, PhD, FDAA}

Danielle is Professor of Nutrition and Dietetics at Queensland University of Technology, a Fellow of the Dietitians Association of Australia and a member of the Public Health Association of Australia and the World Public Health Nutrition Association. She is currently the chair of the Council of Deans Nutrition and Dietetics, Australia and New Zealand. She has lectured in community and public health nutrition, the sociology of food, and nutrition and research methodologies. Her research focuses on families, children, food literacy and household food security. She has worked extensively in Vietnam developing nutrition and dietetics as a profession.

JANIS BAINES

{MSc Human Nutrition, MA Chemistry}

Janis is a dietary exposure expert who worked at Food Standards Australia New Zealand (FSANZ) for 24 years and continues to attend Food and Agriculture Organization/World Health Organization food safety meetings. Janis managed the 2011–2013 Australian Health Survey for the Commonwealth Department of Health. Previously, she taught nutrition at the University of New England and University of Canberra and worked as a nutritionist in Papua New Guinea.

DAVID BORRADALE

{BAppSc (Food Science), BHSc (Nut & Diet), MSc (Appl Sci Research), PhD, APD}

David is a lecturer at the Queensland University of Technology, where he has taught across the program in both nutrition science and dietetics. David's research interests include novel food technologies, potential applications of nutrigenomics and the microbiome and how they can be applied to personalised nutrition.

JANEANE DART

{BSc, Grad Dip Nut & Diet, Grad Cert Acad Pract., AdvAPD}

Janeane is a senior lecturer and researcher at Monash University and has had an extensive career as a dietitian working in Australia and the United Kingdom. Janeane has a particular interest in education and developing the art of practice for nutrition professionals, including personal development and professionalism.

LEISA McCARTHY

{BAppSc (Nutrition), M Community Nutrition, PhD}

Leisa is a Warumungu woman from the Northern Territory and public health nutritionist with over 20 years of experience working in Aboriginal health within government and the Aboriginal Community Controlled Health sectors. Leisa's research has focused on Aboriginal control and management of health research and research into Aboriginal people's experiences of nutrition and food insecurity.

CHRISTINA McKERCHAR

{BCApSc, MSc (Otago)}

Christina is of Ngāti Kahungunu, Tūhoe and Ngāti Porou descent. She trained as a nutritionist, and worked for a number of years, for Te Hotu Manawa Māori a national Māori health provider in New Zealand. She lecturers in Māori health at the University of Otago in Christchurch and is completing her PhD, titled 'Food availability for Māori children—a rights based approach'.

CLAIRE PALERMO

{BSc, MND, MPH, Grad Cert Health Prof Ed, PhD, AdvAPD}

Currently an associate professor at Monash University, Claire leads a body of research and teaching practice dedicated to the development of a workforce adequately equipped to address the complex nutrition issues facing our populations.

GAYLE S. SAVIGE

{Dip Teach, BSc, Grad Dip Dietetics, PhD}

Gayle is a former Accredited Practising Dietitian and was a Research Fellow at the School of Public Health and Preventive Medicine, Monash University.

JOLIEKE C. VAN DER POLS

{BSc, MSc, PhD, Grad Cert (Higher Education)}

Jolieke is currently an associate professor at Queensland University of Technology. She is a nutritional epidemiologist with over 20 years' experience in research into nutritional factors in the causation and prevention of chronic diseases. Special interests include cancer, obesity, digestive health, mental health and longitudinal studies.

NAIYANA WATTANAPENPAIBOON

{BSc (Pharm), MSc (Pharm), PhD}

Naiyana (also known as Tikky) is a graduate of Chulalongkorn University in Thailand and Monash University in Australia. She is a Research Fellow at the Monash Asia Initiative, Monash University, with research interests in human nutrition, ecohealth disorders and food chemistry. She has conducted cross-sectional community-based research and nutrition interventions.

{CHAPTER 1}
AN ECONUTRITION APPROACH TO HEALTH

Mark L. Wahlqvist and Danielle Gallegos

OBJECTIVES

- Describe a scientific approach to food and nutrition systems to underpin lifelong learning.
- Describe an ecological systems approach to health, human nutrition and food systems.
- Define the elements of human nutrition.

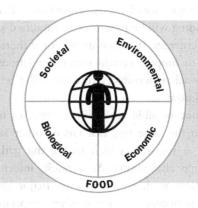

INTRODUCTION

Nutrition is fundamentally a science. It is premised on an understanding of human physiology and biochemistry and the action of nutrients and other food constituents. Nutrition scientists also need to have an appreciation of food—its chemistry and structure, and how manipulating it can change the availability, absorption and effectiveness of its inherent constituents.

The fundamental science of nutrition emerged in the 18th and 19th centuries, after the discovery of oxygen in the 18th century laid the foundations for nutritional biochemistry and an understanding of energy and nutrient metabolism. As a science, nutrition is constantly evolving. As we learn more about the human body, the expression of certain genes and general health and wellbeing as they relate to the environments we live in, we develop a more sophisticated understanding of how food and nutrition can be manipulated for improvements in health. However, improvements in health will only

be possible if we can work within social, economic and environmental frameworks that operate locally, nationally and globally.

This chapter provides an introduction to the approach taken in this textbook. Most nutrition textbooks emphasise the biological elements of nutrition. They tend to focus on body systems and the biochemical and physiological aspects of nutritional intake or lack thereof. This book views the human body as part of a complex, dynamic, constantly evolving system that integrates the environment with social, economic and biological systems. Working with individuals, communities and populations to develop new solutions to optimise the world's nutrition requires thinking about all these systems and how they interact. In this chapter, we define an ecological approach to food, human nutrition and food systems, the dimensions of human nutrition and some of its historical origins. These concepts are further elaborated in following chapters, giving you a holistic but practical guide to the dimensions of human nutrition for the future.

NUTRITION AS A SCIENCE

Scientific methods and studies are vital in helping us understand the interaction between food, food systems, the environment and health. The basic principle of any scientific inquiry is that we are uncertain about all we discover. Indeed, *the only certainty is that things are uncertain.* Therefore, experiments and studies are constantly conducted and the best recommendations, practices and policies are made based on what we currently know. There is, and always should be, an expectation that our understanding will be progressively modified as new evidence emerges. If we are unsure, or if there is no evidence to support certain recommendations, it is a professional responsibility to convey the limits of what we know.

It is not possible to conduct experiments on humans in the same way that rats or other animals are used in research, which makes the gathering of evidence challenging. As a result, information on nutrition is drawn from two major sources. The first is laboratory science, where experimental animals—and, to a lesser extent, human subjects—are used. The other main source of information is **epidemiology**—the study of nutrition and disease in populations (see Chapter 24). Epidemiology shows relationships such as an association between heart disease and high intakes of certain saturated fats, or between a higher incidence of the congenital disease spina bifida and low intakes of the B-vitamin folacin. Where such associations or predictions are found, laboratory science takes over to determine the nature of cause and effect.

Statistical analysis must also be used to determine whether a certain finding might have arisen by chance or not. Even so, knowledge that seemed firmly established may change as continuing research uncovers new information. Assessing the significance of new information can be complicated. Scientists do not necessarily agree and arguments may go on for years before finally being settled. This can lead to a public perception that experts can never agree on what people should be eating. This is further compounded by some people in the nutrition field being selective about what they believe. Sometimes their reasons are based on personal beliefs and values, or they may have a financial interest in proclaiming certain 'facts'.

The importance of qualitative research in nutrition (see Chapter 3) is increasingly recognised as we grapple with how people's beliefs, values, experiences, perceptions and behaviours relate to putting food on the table and into their mouths. This qualitative work can provide valuable data that supplement statistical analysis and increase our understanding of nutrition in action.

To ensure that individuals and populations have access to the evidence, it is imperative that nutrition professionals understand how to critically evaluate the science as well as the 'fake news'. Access to information is no longer a problem; the more difficult problem is sorting factual information from that which is biased. To become expert in this area, you will need to develop a range of professional skills (see Chapter 2) and to critically evaluate and communicate the evidence as it comes to light (see Chapter 3). What this means is that, as an individual, for your own health and that of your family, and as a health professional keeping up-to-date, critically evaluating the science as it emerges is a lifelong task.

WHAT IS AN ECOSYSTEMS APPROACH?

The ecosystems approach to human health is a strategy designed to shift our thinking from traditional, one-dimensional **biomedical** approaches towards a new transdisciplinary and integrated approach (Heasman & Lang 2015). It makes use of the conceptual idea of an **ecosystem** to examine the complex and myriad factors influencing human health concerns and seeks ways to improve human health and wellbeing through sustainable management of all components of the environment. The health of individuals, as well as that of communities, is inextricably linked to the health of biophysical, social and economic environments, and all ought to be considered together.

We can learn much from the concept of health and wellbeing as understood by Indigenous communities who have traditionally lived in a more integrated way with their natural environment. For many such communities, health encompasses not only physical health but also social, emotional and cultural wellbeing. This extends beyond the individual to the community. We are ecological creatures, intimately connected to our environment, not environmentally discrete individuals. We are connected with the **animate** environment through the food and beverages we ingest, our several **microbiomes**, our senses, our environmentally derived hormonal profiles and more. We are connected with the inanimate environment—things not considered to be alive, such as the weather—through the effects of rain and drought on agriculture and our ability to live in comfort and safety from storms, fires and other natural disasters.

The linkages between human health and ecosystems are complex, dynamic and, in some respects, political or dependent on governance; for example, a government may fail to adequately control the release of pollution into waterways. For thousands of years, ecosystems have provided humans with essential services or benefits, such as food, water, shelter and medicine. On the one hand, human health has benefited by sacrificing the 'health' of ecosystems. Examples of this include damming wild rivers, destroying wetlands, diverting water for irrigation, converting wilderness to farmland, timber removal, local extinctions of wild animals and loss of arable land for residential and commercial development. On the other hand, archaeological evidence has shown that the destruction of ecosystems has led to the downfall of civilisations (Ehrlich & Ehrlich 2013). At one and the same time, ecosystems protect against and mediate health risk and the transmission of disease. There are many settings in which ecosystems are vital for our health and need to be assessed. The most obvious are places where food is produced, processed and distributed to consumers. Other settings include the home, school and education system; the workplace and workforce with their specific characteristics and patterns, such

as shift-work; the operational healthcare system; communication and transport systems; and facilities for recreation (Wahlqvist 2014).

At the global level, the Millennium Ecosystem Assessment (www.millenniumassessment.org), launched in 2001 by a conglomerate of international organisations, involved a major assessment of human impact on the environment designed to inform decision-making and policy development. The results suggest that global ecosystems are losing their ability to provide the services that are essential for human health and wellbeing as a result of increasing human pressure. Given human dependence on ecosystems for the necessities of life (food, water, shelter), this trend is likely to continue. The Millennium Ecosystem Assessment has triggered the development of several ecosystem assessments, at global, regional and national levels, in response not only to changes in scientific understanding, but also to a changing policy landscape (Allison & Brown 2017).

Food—how we produce, prepare, share and consume it—is fundamental to our wellbeing. An ecological approach to food and nutrition recognises that food as a commodity is the conduit connecting people and planet—highlighting our dependence on environmental elements (Lang et al. 2009; Pirk et al. 2017). Humans are ecological creatures and, as such, we must see ourselves as intimately connected to our ecosystems if we are to optimise our nutritional status and health (Wahlqvist 2014).

There is a new imperative to take an ecological approach to food and nutrition. In the last 100 years, the global population has increased fourfold. While world population growth has slowed, an increase in longevity and the mobility of people has increased the stress on the food system. Accelerating climate change is altering the available material resources, while local and global economic and political developments (trade agreements, civil unrest) influence the availability of and access to food and health. The growing prevalence of nutrition-sensitive ill-health (obesity, diabetes, heart disease, allergy) and the inability to resolve micronutrient deficiencies (such as iron, vitamin A and iodine deficiencies) are a result of multiple ecosystems failure. As ecological creatures, we depend on our household, locality and community for our health status. Our **genome** is influenced by our environment and our evolution is ecological and intergenerational. For example, the emerging field of **epigenetics** indicates that what a mother eats and does during pregnancy will impact the genetics of her baby; because a female infant's eggs are created in the womb, these impacts will in turn affect these eggs and, potentially, the children they eventually become. We cannot expect that our health will be optimal unless our biology, food system, surroundings and social affairs are in harmony. For these reasons alone, our priorities, livelihoods and relationships must be environmentally attentive. Ecosystem damage and loss is the gravest threat to our health and survival. Consequently, health and nutrition professionals need to have an understanding of food systems and the dimensions of nutrition in order to optimise health now and into the future.

FOOD SYSTEMS

Food is the primary source of nutrients needed to sustain life, promote health and optimal growth and development, and assure human productivity. Foods are produced by systems that are ecologically and health relevant at every stage from production and harvest, through transport, processing, storage, sale, packaging, food preparation and to consumption (see Part 2). A safe food supply is essential for human life, and safety breaches of food systems result in loss of life (mortality) and ill-health (**morbidity**) (Chapter 5). Such systems therefore need to be governed by increasingly complex policies, procedures and regulations (chapters 6 and 7). Understanding food and its constituents is essential in order to understand the contribution individual foods and food combinations make to the dietary intake of an individual and dietary patterns of populations (Chapter 8).

Neither nutrients nor other food components have single functions or act alone. In other words, foods affect the body in a number of ways and nutrients work together to create the desired impact. Failure to understand this can lead to extrapolations from nutritional biochemistry to food products where the risk–benefit profile may be unacceptable. For example, while vitamin A is important for health, there are serious risks associated with over-supplementation or even unique ingestion in the absence of other food constituents. Generally, a biodiverse diet should provide most people with sufficient vitamin A (Wahlqvist et al. 1989) (see Chapter 8). Insofar as possible, food or food patterns, rather than food components, should be the basis of therapeutic strategies in order to maximise its broader benefits and minimise the risk (Wahlqvist 2016).

With this in mind, nutrition for health is best served by food-based guidelines. People eat food, not nutrients, and it is reasonable to look to food and food intake patterns as a way of optimising health, as long as other personal behaviours—physical activity, sleep, stress management and substance abuse (as with alcohol, tobacco and drugs, legal and illegal)—are also addressed. Consequently, most countries have established food-based guidelines to advise their populations on optimal dietary patterns for health (see Chapter 19). However, the emergence of new technologies is challenging our understanding of the fundamental question 'what is food?'. Meat grown from stem cells (cultured meat) and food produced and made via 3D-printing, which is extruded and reconstructed to look like produce, are just two examples. Quite profound questions arise for food processors, consumers and regulators about these significant changes in food culture. If present environmental pressures on the food supply increase, we may find ourselves in much greater need of food and nutrition literacy to safely, sustainably and healthfully manage our food supply (chapters 26 and 27).

WHAT IS ECONUTRITION?

The concept of '**econutrition**' is based on the synergy between food and health through ecosystems, where the integrity of these is basic to food, human and planetary sustainability (Wahlqvist et al. 2012; Wahlqvist & Specht 1998). The concept has been used in developing interdisciplinary approaches that are critical to linking the basic sciences in multiple areas to address global **'wicked' problems** such as poverty, climate change and food insecurity (Deckelbaum et al. 2006) (see also Chapter 2).

An example would be the Millennium Villages Project discussed in Chapter 29. The vicious cycles that lead to loss of nutrients, soil erosion and decreasing biodiversity are linked to environmental degradation and result in decreased food production (refer to Chapter 26). Lack of food is associated with malnutrition, illness and declining labour productivity, which exacerbates poor agricultural management. An interdisciplinary approach is needed to break these kinds of vicious cycles.

Econutrition conceptualises how we and other living things can acquire the nutrients we need to optimise our wellbeing, health and lifespan in ways that are sustainable and respectful of the animate and inanimate environment. Wahlqvist and Specht (1998) identified ways in which biodiversity might contribute to successful econutrition, which included an essential varied food supply for human health; a range of diverse food sources as security against natural disaster, climate change and pestilence; a rich source of medical compounds, many as yet unknown; ecosystem buffers against invasive plants and animals, and against pathogens and toxins; and recognising a 'spiritual' value in diversity and ecosystems with consequent mental health benefits and the feeling of 'belonging to the landscape'. Seasonality—meaning growing and consuming foods according to their natural season rather than attempting to have **seasonal produce** available all year round—can add to the diversity (or variety) and robustness of food sources. From an econutrition perspective, health problems such as malnutrition and some chronic diseases, including cardiovascular disease, diabetes and some cancers, can be solved or alleviated through local, ecologically sustainable, biodiverse food systems (Chapter 31).

THE DIMENSIONS OF ECONUTRITION

Nutrition can be divided into 'pre-swallowing' and 'post-swallowing' aspects (Crotty 1995). 'Pre-swallowing' considerations can be divided into those that deal with food production and supply, and those concerning the anthropological and sociological influences that determine what we choose to eat. The 'post-swallowing' aspects relate to the biochemistry, genetics and physiology of nutrition. In 2005, the International Union of Nutritional Sciences recommended in its 'Giessen Declaration' that nutrition science be inclusive of biomedical, societal, environmental and economic sciences (Beauman et al. 2005). In this text, we use this as a guiding framework and divide the study of human nutrition into four dimensions: biological, societal, economic and environmental. These dimensions map to the four components of ecosystems impacting on public health that are connected in multiple ways (Lang & Rayner 2012) (Figure 1.1):

- environmental: includes the physical building blocks that are needed for life, such as soil, water, energy and food
- biological: the biophysiological processes of all living things (animals, plants, microorganisms, humans)
- societal: encompasses interpersonal relationships, community, group and family traditions, and the

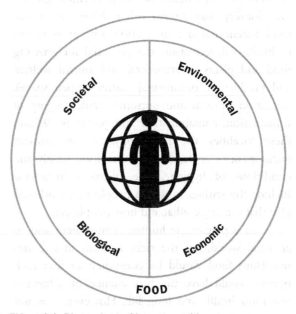

Figure 1.1: Dimensions of human nutrition

institutions that frame daily living, including laws and social arrangements
- economic: includes the role of nutrition in global and national economic growth, as well as the role of income and prices on food choice.

These dimensions will be highlighted for each chapter. Remember, however, that it is usually rare for only one dimension to be present. For example, the chapter on food systems may be identified as 'environmental', but as you read the chapter you will realise that farming practice is also a social phenomenon, that economic power is one of the main drivers and that foods are inherently biological in nature. The human and globe icons at the centre of Figure 1.1 remind us that the four dimensions—with food as the primary vehicle—are essential for human health, which is dependent on planetary health.

Environmental

The importance of environmental health has been discussed above in the context of developing and maintaining healthy ecosystems. The locality in which we are born and live is a major differentiator of wellbeing and health across population groups. Our locality may, among other things, affect our food system and our interaction with it in regard to livelihood, recreation, the potential for growing food and plants (horticultural and animal welfare and production, ornamental features, open space), migration inwards and outwards, trade, degree of urbanisation, contamination and pollution. Within these localities, the macro-physical environment encompasses climate, shelter, water, food supply and conditions of hygiene. The micro-environments include the settings in which people live, work and play that influence what and how people eat.

Food is part of the human environment and, in an ideal world, just the right amount of safe and nutritious food would be consumed so that each person would have the best chance of achieving optimum health and long life. However, it is not as simple as that. Not all available foods are equally

nutritious. The types and quality of the foods consumed can be the result of several factors:
- food-processing environments (see Chapter 5)
- government regulations regarding a safe food supply (see chapters 6 and 7)
- what foods are supplied by farmers, food manufacturers and supermarkets (see Chapter 8)
- what foods we choose to buy and eat (see chapters 25 and 28)
- the sustainability of the food system, particularly given the escalation of climate change (Chapter 26).

Biological

The biological dimension encompasses the ways in which food contributes to all bodily functions, their intergenerational transfer and their dependence on personal behaviours, socio-environmental factors and **homeostatic** mechanisms, which allow a range of food patterns to provide for optimal health across diverse contexts. This dimension describes mostly post-swallowing mechanisms.

At its fundamental level the biological dimension describes the:
- physiological bodily processes for extracting nutrients from foods (Chapter 9)
- biochemical and physiological actions of nutrients (chapters 10–18)
- consequences of too little or too much of these nutrients (chapters 10–18)
- nutritional requirements of the human body at different life stages to optimise health (chapters 20–22)
- assessment of the outward manifestation of nutritional status in individuals (Chapter 23) and populations (Chapter 24).

The biological dimensions of nutrition and their interaction with the environments in which we live have continued to evolve. Nutritional biology explores the role of nutrition in the expression of certain genes and how diet can affect gene expression in future generations (epigenetics). These innovations are leading to **nutrigenomics** and personalised nutrition, or **nutrigenetics**. It may be that, in the future, a 'reading' of a child's genome will provide insight into the dietary requirements necessary to prevent the occurrence of particular diseases, although this will depend on a number of ethical and socioeconomic issues.

The biological environment in which individuals are conceived and develop *in utero*, followed by early nurturing and breastfeeding as an infant is now recognised as vital to human health. It is now known that the health and nutrition of the mother (and probably the father) can influence the health of the child many years later as an adult, particularly with regard to diseases such as heart disease and diabetes (Barker 2007) (see Chapter 20). The microbiome—that is, the microscopic (bacteria, archaea, fungi, viruses, algae) ecosystems and the combined genetic material in our body systems (the gut, on the skin, in the respiratory and reproductive tracts and elsewhere)—is increasingly being recognised as influential for overall health. The food we eat and how it is eaten, as well as the environments we live in, all impact on the microbiota (see chapters 8, 30 and 31).

Societal

Food and eating are central to the human experience, not only providing fuel for bodies to work but also providing means to make a living and to bring people together socially. The foods we choose to grow, cook, eat and share form our identity, and ensuring their availability, access and safety is essential for human survival. We are the only species that cooks, so fuel sources and food preparation skills have affected our survival. Our membership of families, groups and communities has also characterised our food and social systems and, vice versa, our food consumption defines our membership. The societal element of nutrition science is instrumental in understanding the historical influences on the way we eat, how policy and regulations can be enacted, the influence of culture, the impact of class and poverty and the role of family and community. Food as the delivery unit for nutrients is only part of the story; as Margaret Visser notes, food has a key role in shaping and expressing identity.

Food—what is chosen from the possibilities available, how it is presented, how it is eaten, with whom and when, and how much time is allocated to cooking and eating it—is one of the means by which a society creates itself and acts out its aims and fantasies. Changing (or unchanging) food choices and presentations are part of every society's tradition and character. Food shapes us and expresses us even more definitively than our furniture or houses or utensils do. (Visser 1986, p. 12)

Food habits and nutritional outcomes are impacted by a range of social factors including where you live, how much money you earn and your education. These are called the social determinants of health (see Chapter 27). Food cultures, beliefs and cuisines have emerged over time and, in some cases, have been codified as the rules of religion or as markers of national identity (Chapter 27). Fasting, for example, is part of many religious and philosophical traditions, but may have been a societal way of achieving equity in food distribution or eking out limited supplies of certain commodities—for example, meat. Such intentions, overt or covert, may have had biological justification in terms of preferred meal patterns, or avoidance of over-consumption (propositions even now not fully tested), or respect for animal life.

Food is culturally symbolic and distinctive food habits (reflected as cuisines) persist in migrant groups longer than most characteristics. While they may undergo alignment with the host culture with time, the reverse also takes place. This is especially evident in culturally pluralistic immigrant societies like Australia, New Zealand, the USA and Canada (see Chapter 27). Indigenous populations are considered custodians of **foodways** and are instrumental in preserving biodiversity. Their health is linked to their ecosystems and the complexities of their social and economic circumstances (Kuhnlein et al. 2006). Indigenous peoples around the world continue to suffer disproportionately from poverty, racism and poor health, but they have also demonstrated extraordinary resilience in maintaining a sense of identity (that includes dietary patterns) in the face of significant, prolonged histories of colonialism and genocide (Chapter 28).

We are now creating new food cultures, although we may be unaware of doing so. Shopping and cooking confer survival advantages, but food dispensing or vending machines are now commonplace in most urban settings. The new era of the '**internet of things**' and '**Uberisation**' allows the ordering, activation of cooking and food preparation, delivery and more to be remote (Figure 1.2). Shopping, cooking and commensality (eating and drinking at the same table) are fundamental social activities. Ongoing research indicates that these activities reduce social isolation and contribute to longevity (see Chapter 28).

Economic

Nutrition as a science emerged from the understanding that well-nourished workers (and soldiers) were more productive and better able to contribute to the economic development of not only their immediate households but also the nation. Reducing hunger has been a key United Nations development goal, in recognition of the fact that human potential and endeavour are restricted when nutritional health is sub-optimal. The relationship between economics and nutrition is complex and multilayered, occurring at the macro or global level as well as at the micro or household level.

At the global level, consideration needs to be given to the influence of trade agreements. There is increasing recognition of the role trade agreements play internationally in the shaping of local food environments. Policies that emphasise greater market access to food exports and the opening of domestic markets to foreign investment have created environments that encourage the consumption of foods that promote obesity and the development of non-communicable diseases (see Chapter 25) (Ravuvu et al. 2017). A small number of transnational food companies peddle ultra-processed foods to a global consumer market. 'Big Food' is forging new markets in low and middle income countries with profit and economic gain as the primary driver (Williams & Nestle 2017). Agri-food companies have a monopoly on the development and dissemination of seeds, reducing biodiversity and limiting the ability of local farmers to build and maintain sustainable livelihoods (see Chapter 26). Global food prices are linked to the prices of individual commodities, as well as global fertiliser prices and oil prices, all of which impact on the cost of food production. Food prices have been extremely variable in the 21st century and are likely to continue to be volatile as the impacts of climate change are felt.

Consumer food choices are greatly influenced by food price and household income. Families on lower incomes tend to purchase foods that are low cost and maximise energy intake, resulting in poor diet quality. Food prices also tend to be higher in more remote areas due to difficulties associated with transport and storage (see chapters 25 and 27).

AIMS OF THIS BOOK

This textbook will enable you to explore all the dimensions of nutrition at individual, local and global levels. It will enable you to develop a lifelong appreciation of the dynamic and changing nature of nutrition science that translate into practical messages for human health. Finally, it will enable you to understand the complexity of nutrition and its interactions between food and environmental, social and economic systems, and how you can impact your own health and the health of others as you develop as a global citizen and as a health professional.

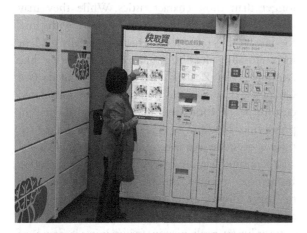

Figure 1.2: The trend towards smart phone–managed food systems: an unstaffed or 'peopleless' food and meal vending outlet in Taipei

Source: Wahlqvist (2016)

SUMMARY

- Nutrition science is constantly evolving as we build a deeper understanding of the human body and its dynamic interactions with environmental, social and economic systems.
- Experiments, quantitative and qualitative studies, epidemiology and statistical analyses are all tools used to build our understanding and knowledge of nutrition and its impact.
- An ecosystems approach understands that the health of individuals and communities is linked to the health of the biophysical, social and economic environments. An ecological approach to nutrition recognises that food as a commodity connects people and planet. Humans must see themselves as an integral part of the ecosystem across space and time.
- Econutrition is defined as the interrelationship between nutrition and human health, agriculture and food production, and environmental health, mediated by the economic and social environments. It covers pre-swallowing and post-swallowing aspects.
- Econutrition encompasses four key elements embedded within a food system:
  —environmental: includes the physical building blocks that are needed for life, such as soil, water, energy and food
  —biological: the biophysiological processes of all living things (animals, plants, microorganisms, humans)
  —societal: encompasses interpersonal relationships, community, group and family traditions, and the institutions that frame daily living, including laws and social arrangements
  —economic: includes the role of nutrition in global and national economic growth, as well as the role of income and prices on food choice.

KEY TERMS

Animate: beings which have life, including animals and plants; **inanimate** refers to objects that are not considered to be alive, such as rocks and buildings. The inanimate and animate are inextricably linked, such that there is usually reproductive capacity or life in the most apparently lifeless places.

Biomedical: describes systems that focus on the physical and medical aspects of health. They promote individual responsibility and tend to treat people in isolation from their environments.

Econutrition: the interrelationships between nutrition and human health, agriculture and food production, and environmental health, mediated by social and economic systems (Blasbalg et al. 2011).

Ecosystem: a dynamic complex web of plant, animal (including humans) and microorganism communities that interact with the non-living (material) environment and come together as a functional unit (Millennium Ecosystem Assessment Board 2003).

Epidemiology: from the Greek words *epi*, meaning on or upon, *demos*, meaning people, and *logos*, meaning the study of. Epidemiology therefore means 'the **study** of the **distribution** and **determinants** of **health-related states or events** in **specified populations**, and the **application** of this study to the control of health problem' (Last et al. 2000).

Epigenetics: the study of changes in organisms due to modification in gene expression rather than alteration of the genetic code itself.

Foodways: the cultural, social and economic practices relating to the production and consumption of food of a group of people, a region or a historical period of time.

Genome: the complete set of genes or genetic material present in a cell or organism.

Homeostasis: from the Greek *homos*, meaning similar, and *stasis*, meaning standing still, is the ability to achieve a state of equilibrium between different but interdependent groups of elements. Within the body, regulating body temperature via shivering or sweating, and the regulation of blood glucose levels, are examples of internal homeostasis.

Internet of things: the embedding of information technology into physical devices, cars, home appliances and other objects to allow greater connectivity and create efficiencies. The 'smart' home and 'smart' refrigerator would be examples.

Microbiome: the combined genetic material of microorganisms in a particular environment—for example, in the soil or in parts of the body (gut, lung, skin).

Morbidity: term used to describe a state of ill-health or diseases. For example, data may describe mortality rates (i.e. death rates) or morbidity rates (i.e. rates of disease). In clinical practice a patient may be described as having multiple morbidities, indicating that they suffer from more than one disease.

Nutrigenetics: the effects of genetic variation on nutrient requirements.

Nutrigenomics: the nutrient regulation of gene expression.

Seasonal produce: describes foods that are readily cultivated and at their best, nutritionally and in terms of taste, at particular times of the year. Consuming foods out of season involves costs to the environment in terms of cultivation, transportation and storage and is therefore not considered sustainable.

Uberisation: within an economic system, the development of platforms to mobilise under-utilised resources with low transaction costs. The term comes from 'Uber', a platform that matched those in need of a ride with those with a car. It refers to the elimination of the 'middle man', putting the provider and the customer of the service in direct contact.

Wicked problem: a social or cultural problem, such as poverty or obesity, that is difficult or impossible to solve because of:
- root causes being difficult to recognise
- incomplete, contradictory or changing requirements or knowledge
- interconnection with *other* problems
- the large number of people and opinions involved
- the problem contributing a large economic burden. (Kolko, 2012)

REFERENCES

Allison, H. & Brown, C., 2017, 'A review of recent developments in ecosystem assessment and its role in policy evolution', *Current Opinion in Environmental Sustainability*, *29*: 57–62, doi:10.1016/j.cosust.2017.11.006

Barker, D.J., 2007, 'The origins of the developmental origins theory', *Journal of Internal Medicine*, *261*(5): 412–17, doi:10.1111/j.1365-2796.2007.01809.x

Beauman, C., Cannon, G., Elmadfa, I., Glasauer, P., Hoffmann, I. et al., 2005, 'The principles, definition and dimensions of the new nutrition science', *Public Health Nutrition*, *8*(6a): 695–8, doi:10.1079/PHN2005820

Blasbalg, T.L., Wispelwey, B. & Deckelbaum, R.J., 2011, 'Econutrition and utilization of food-based approaches for nutritional health', *Food and Nutrition Bulletin*, *32*(1_Suppl): S4–S13, doi:10.1177/15648265110321S102

Crotty, P., 1995, *Good Nutrition? Fact and fashion in dietary advice*, Sydney: Allen & Unwin

Deckelbaum, R.J., Palm, C., Mutuo, P. & DeClerck, F., 2006, 'Econutrition: Implementation models from the Millennium Villages Project in Africa', *Food and Nutrition Bulletin*, 27(4): 335–42, doi:10.1177/156482650602700408

Ehrlich, P.R. & Ehrlich, A.H., 2013, 'Can a collapse of global civilization be avoided?', *Proceedings of the Royal Society B: Biological Sciences, 280*(1754), article 20122845, doi:10.1098/rspb.2012.2845

Heasman, M. & Lang, T., 2015, *Food Wars: The global battle for mouths, minds and markets*, London: Routledge

Kolko, J. 2012, 'Wicked problems: Problems worth solving', <www.wickedproblems.com.au>, accessed 14 June 2019

Kuhnlein, H., Erasmus, B., Creed-Kanashiro, H., Englberger, L., Okeke, C. et al., 2006, 'Indigenous peoples' food systems for health: Finding interventions that work', *Public Health Nutrition, 9*(8): 1013–19, doi:10.1017/PHN2006987

Lang, T., Barling, D. & Caraher, M., 2009, *Food Policy: Integrating health, environment and society*, Oxford: Oxford University Press

Lang, T. & Rayner, G., 2012, 'Ecological public health: The 21st century's big idea? An essay by Tim Lang and Geof Rayner', *BMJ, 345*: e5466, doi:10.1136/bmj.e5466

Last, J.M., Spasoff, R.A. & Harris, S.S. (eds), 2000, *Dictionary of Epidemiology*, New York, NY: Oxford University Press

Millennium Ecosystem Assessment Board, 2003, *Ecosystems and Human Well-being: A framework for assessment*, <http://pdf.wri.org/ecosystems_human_wellbeing.pdf>, accessed 15 January 2019

Pirk, C.W., Crewe, R.M. & Moritz, R.F., 2017, 'Risks and benefits of the biological interface between managed and wild bee pollinators', *Functional Ecology, 31*(1): 47–55, doi:10.1111/1365-2435.12768

Ravuvu, A., Friel, S., Thow, A.-M., Snowdon, W. & Wate, J., 2017, 'Monitoring the impact of trade agreements on national food environments: Trade imports and population nutrition risks in Fiji', *Globalization and Health, 13*(1): 33, doi:10.1186/s12992-017-0257-1

Visser, M., 1986, *Much Depends on Dinner*, London: Penguin Books

Wahlqvist, M.L., 2014, 'Ecosystem health disorders: Changing perspectives in clinical medicine and nutrition', *Asia Pacific Journal of Clinical Nutrition, 23*(1): 1–15, doi:10.6133/apjcn

—— 2016, 'Future food', *Asia Pacific Journal of Clinical Nutrition, 25*(4): 706–16, doi:10.6133/apjcn

Wahlqvist, M.L., Lo, C.S. & Myers, K.A., 1989, 'Food variety is associated with less macrovascular disease in those with type II diabetes and their healthy controls', *Journal of the American College of Nutrition, 8*(6): 515–23, doi:10.1080/07315724.1989.10720321

Wahlqvist, M.L., McKay, J., Chang, Y.-C. & Chiu, Y.-W., 2012, 'Rethinking the food security debate in Asia: Some missing ecological and health dimensions and solutions', *Food Security, 4*(4): 657–70, doi:10.1007/s12571-012-0211-2

Wahlqvist, M.L. & Specht, R.L., 1998, 'Food variety and biodiversity: Econutrition', *Asia Pacific Journal of Clinical Nutrition, 7*: 314–19

Williams, S.N. & Nestle, M., 2017, *Big Food: Critical perspectives on the global growth of the food and beverage industry*, London: Routledge

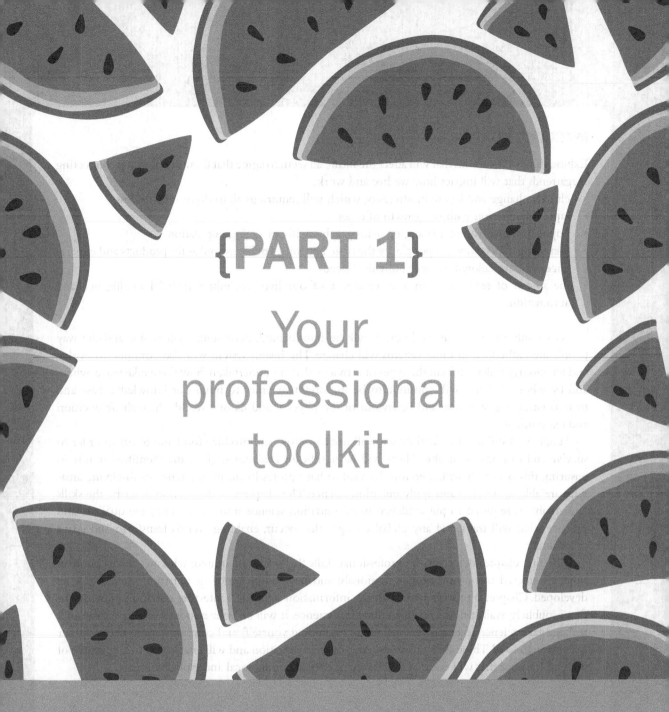

{PART 1}

Your professional toolkit

INTRODUCTION

Explorations of the trends that will affect the future all seem to agree that there are five interconnecting megatrends that will impact how we live and work:

- climate change and loss of biodiversity, which will require us all to do more with less
- rapid urbanisation with the growth of cities
- population growth but a changing demographic with an ageing population
- increasing expectations of people for the basic necessities of life as well as for products and experiences that are tailored to meet individual needs
- the spread of technology into every aspect of our lives, including artificial intelligence and automation.

As a result, the world as we know it will be transformed. Ecosystems will evolve and the way people are embedded in these systems will change. The health system will also continue to evolve and technology will transform the types of activities that are undertaken, how these take place, where and by whom. Science will continue to be important in order to build our knowledge base and to understand the structure and behaviour of the physical and natural worlds through observation and experiment.

People will still need food; they will still need to grow and produce food and to eat in order to survive and to optimise health. There will be significant challenges, given the identified trends, in ensuring this occurs. It will, therefore, be vital to have professionals from a range of discipline areas who are able to develop and apply nutrition science. The chapters in this section describe the skills and attributes required to put evidence-based nutrition science into action. They are qualities and practices that will transcend any global changes that occur, enabling you to transform and adapt accordingly.

The first chapter describes the professional skills that will be required; who are, at this point in time, considered to be nutrition professionals; and how competency in nutrition science can be developed. Chapter 3 provides you with the information needed to interpret nutrition information that is publicly available. As experts in nutrition science, it will be your responsibility to sift through real and fake science to empower individuals (including yourself) and communities to live healthier lives through food. These skills are transferable beyond nutrition and will enable you to take a path of lifelong learning that will ensure adaptability in ever-changing local and global contexts.

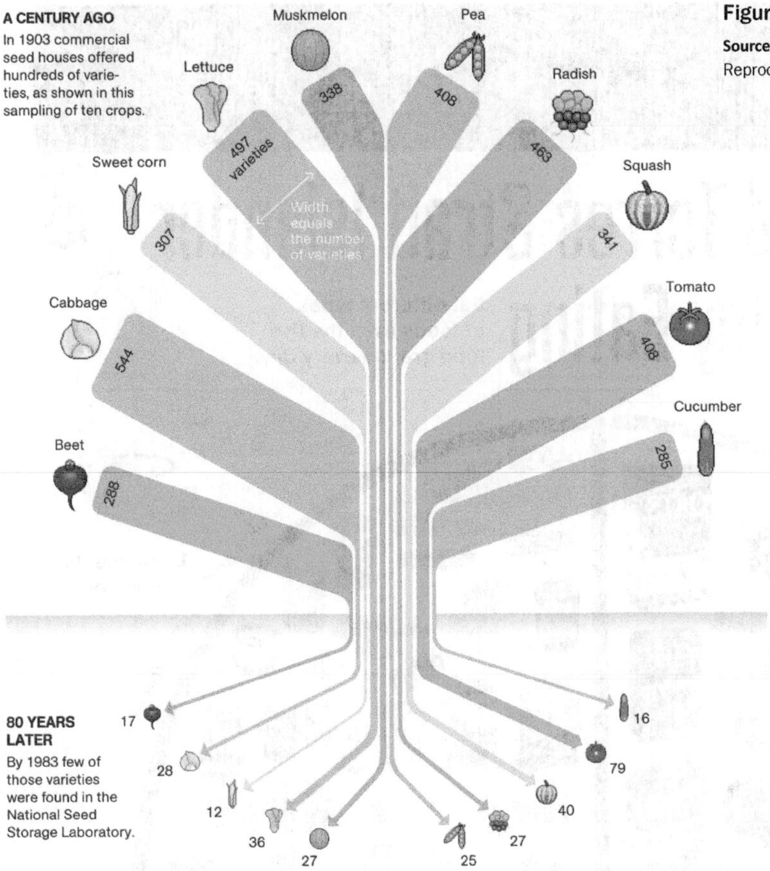

A CENTURY AGO
In 1903 commercial seed houses offered hundreds of varieties, as shown in this sampling of ten crops.

Muskmelon
Pea
Lettuce
Radish
497 varieties
338
408
463
Sweet corn
Squash
307
341
Cabbage
Tomato
544
408
Beet
Cucumber
288
285

Width equals the number of varieties

80 YEARS LATER
By 1983 few of those varieties were found in the National Seed Storage Laboratory.

17
16
28
79
12
40
36
27
27
25

Figure 4.6: Food biodiversity loss

Source: John Tomanio/National Geographic Creative. Reproduced with permission from Siebert (2011)

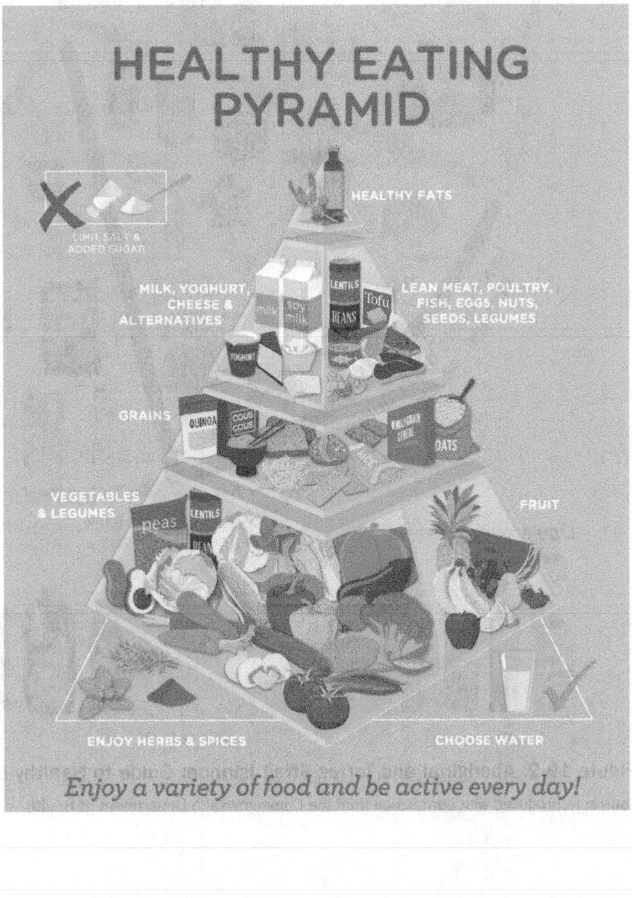

Figure 19.1: Nutrition Australia Healthy Eating Pyramid (2015)

Source: Reprinted with permission from The Australian Nutrition Foundation Inc.

HEALTHY EATING PYRAMID

HEALTHY FATS

LIMIT SALT & ADDED SUGAR

MILK, YOGHURT, CHEESE & ALTERNATIVES

LEAN MEAT, POULTRY, FISH, EGGS, NUTS, SEEDS, LEGUMES

GRAINS

VEGETABLES & LEGUMES

FRUIT

ENJOY HERBS & SPICES

CHOOSE WATER

Enjoy a variety of food and be active every day!

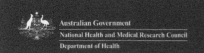

Aboriginal and Torres Strait Islander Guide to Healthy Eating

Eat different types of foods from the five food groups every day.

Drink plenty of water.

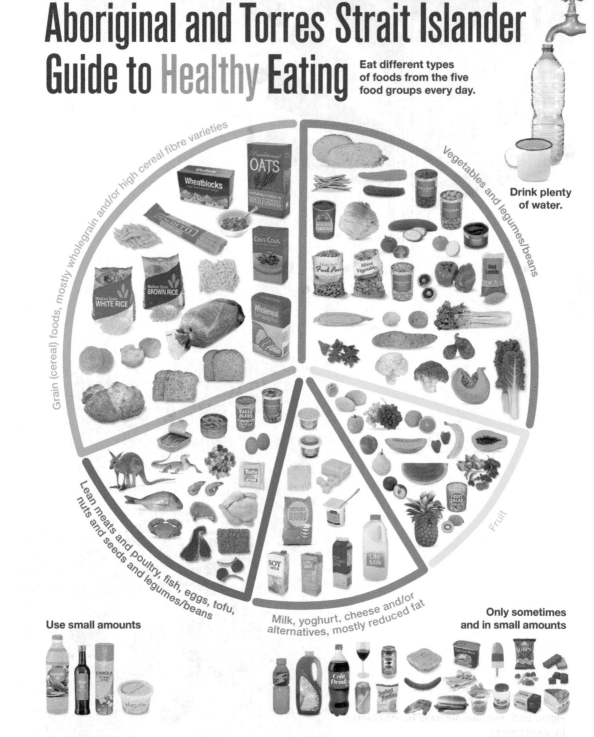

Figure 19.2: Aboriginal and Torres Strait Islander Guide to Healthy Eating

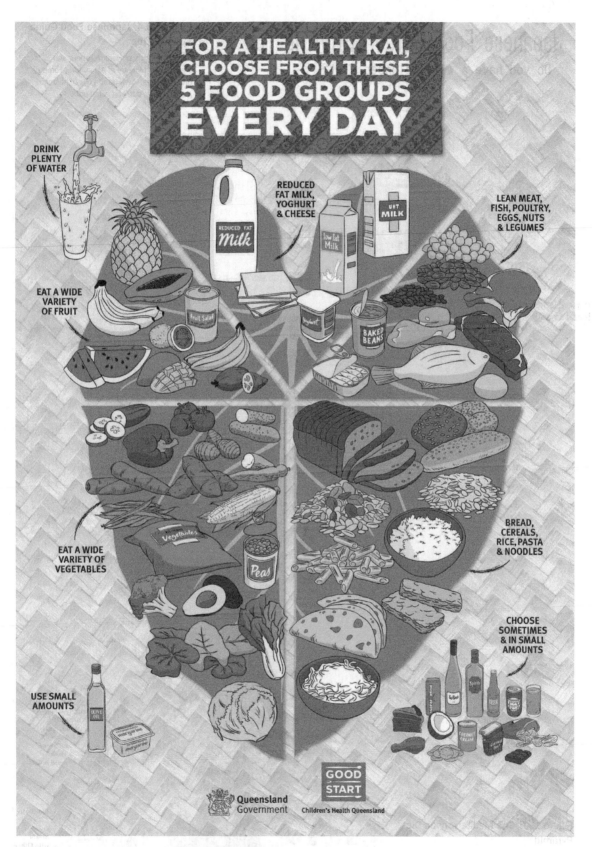

Figure 19.3: Food-based dietary guidelines for Pacific Islanders living in Queensland

Source: Reproduced with permission from The State of Queensland 2018

Japanese Food Guide Spinning Top

Do you have a well-balanced diet?

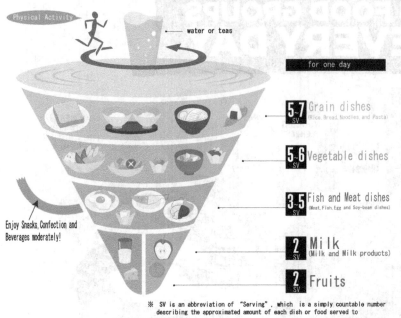

Physical Activity

water or teas

for one day

5-7 SV Grain dishes (Rice, Bread, Noodles, and Pasta)

5-6 SV Vegetable dishes

3-5 SV Fish and Meat dishes (Meat, Fish, Egg and Soy-bean dishes)

2 SV Milk (Milk and Milk products)

2 SV Fruits

Enjoy Snacks, Confection and Beverages moderately!

※ SV is an abbreviation of "Serving", which is a simply countable number describing the approximated amount of each dish or food served to one person

Figure 19.4: Japanese Food Guide Spinning Top

Source: Ministry of Health, Labour and Welfare and Ministry of Agriculture, Forestry and Fisheries, <www.maff.go.jp/j/balance_guide/b_use/pdf/eng_reiari.pdf>

Mediterranean Diet Pyramid
A contemporary approach to delicious, healthy eating

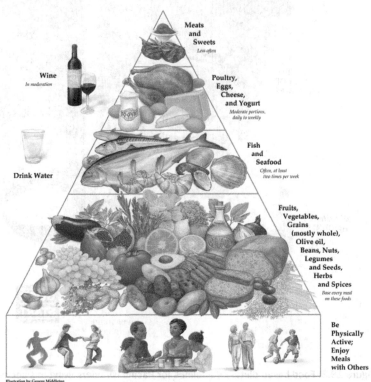

Wine
In moderation

Drink Water

Meats and Sweets
Less often

Poultry, Eggs, Cheese, and Yogurt
Moderate portions, daily to weekly

Fish and Seafood
Often, at least two times per week

Fruits, Vegetables, Grains (mostly whole), Olive oil, Beans, Nuts, Legumes and Seeds, Herbs and Spices
Base every meal on these foods

Be Physically Active; Enjoy Meals with Others

Illustration by George Middleton

© 2009 Oldways Preservation and Exchange Trust • www.oldwayspt.org/medpyramid

Figure 19.5: The Mediterranean Diet Pyramid

Source: Oldways Preservation and Exchange Trust. Reproduced with permission

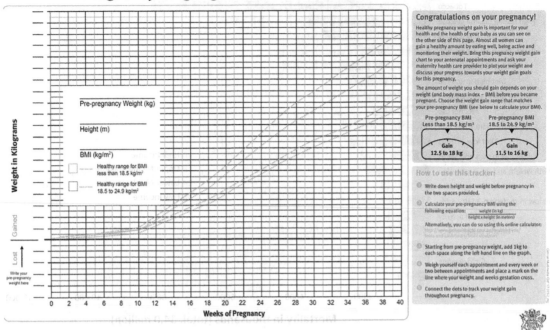

Figure 20.6: Weight gain charts for pregnancy

Source: www.health.qld.gov.au/__data/assets/pdf_file/0023/152393/antenatal_wtnorm.pdf. Reproduced with permission S. De Jersey © 2017

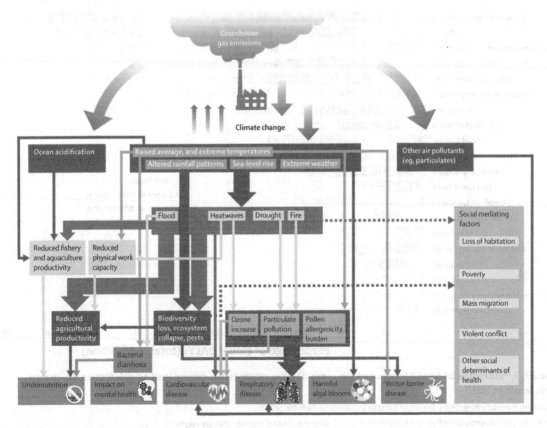

Figure 26.2: Impact of climate change on health

Source: Watts, Adger, Ayeb-Karlsson, Bai, Byass et al. (2017). Reprinted with permission from Elsevier

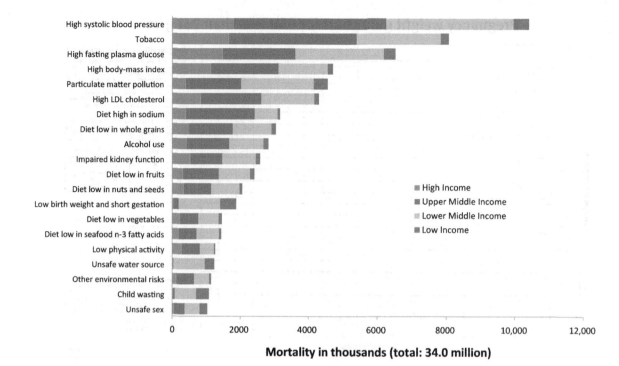

Mortality in thousands (total: 34.0 million)

Figure 29.2: Deaths attributed to twenty leading risk factors by country income level* in 2017

Source: Drawn from data from Global Burden of Disease Collaborative Network (2018)

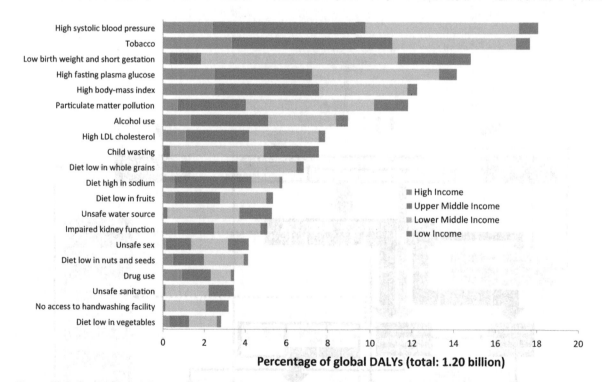

Percentage of global DALYs (total: 1.20 billion)

Figure 29.3: Percentage of disability-adjusted life years (DALYs) attributed to twenty leading risk factors, by country income level* in 2017

Source: Drawn from data from Global Burden of Disease Collaborative Network (2018)

Note: * World Bank's country classification by income level based on gross national income (GNI) per capita
High income: USD $12,235 or more   Lower middle income: USD $1006 – $3955
Upper middle income: USD $3956 – $12,235   Low income: USD $1005 or less

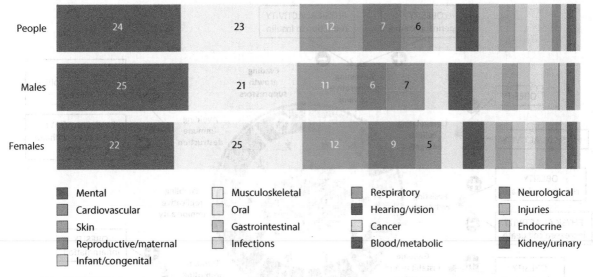

Mental | Musculoskeletal | Respiratory | Neurological
Cardiovascular | Oral | Hearing/vision | Injuries
Skin | Gastrointestinal | Cancer | Endocrine
Reproductive/maternal | Infections | Blood/metabolic | Kidney/urinary
Infant/congenital

Figure 31.2: Proportion of burden of disease among Australians in 2011

Source: AIHW (2016). © Creative Commons BY 3.0

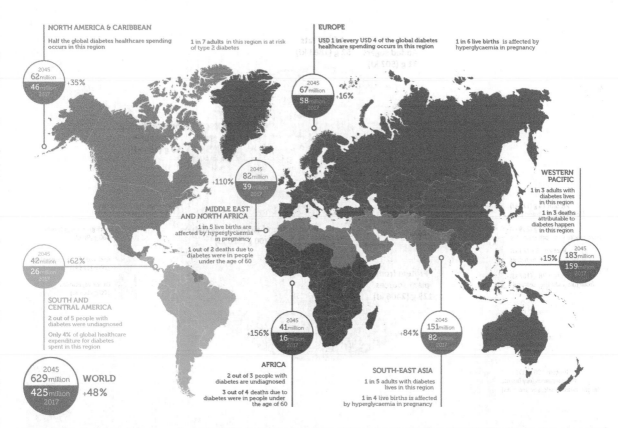

Figure 32.1: Estimated number of people with diabetes globally and by region in 2017 and 2045 (20–79 years)

Source: IDF (2017a) © 2017. Reproduced with permission from International Diabetes Federation

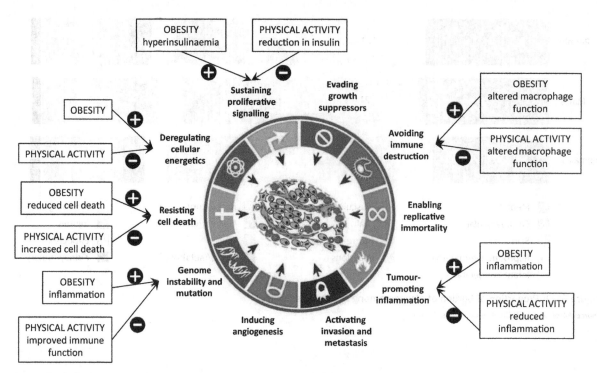

Figure 32.8: Obesity or overfatness, physical activity and the cancer-characterised phenotypic changes

Sources: Modified from Hanahan & Weinberg (2011); WCRF & AICR (2018)

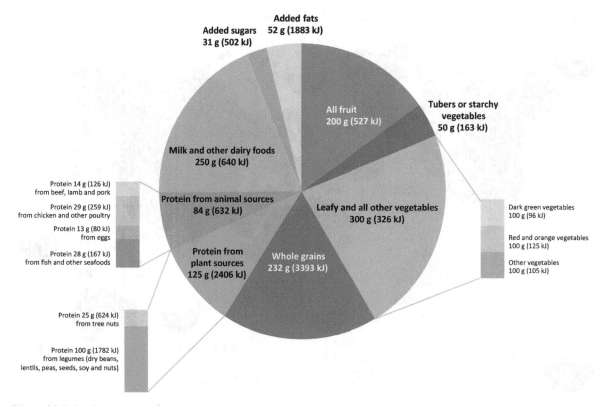

Figure 33.5: A reference model of the 'planetary health diet' for an intake of 10 MJ/day

Source: Developed from Willett et al. (2019)

{CHAPTER 2}
THE TOOLKIT FOR NUTRITION PRACTICE

Claire Palermo, Janeane Dart and Danielle Gallegos

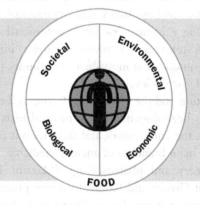

OBJECTIVES

- Define the attributes and skills required for nutrition practice.
- Apply the attributes and skills required for nutrition practice in a number of contexts.

INTRODUCTION

As described in Chapter 1, poor diets are unequivocally linked to a greater burden of illness and death than any other modifiable risk factor. The food system as a whole is connected to our health and wellbeing, and with a changing climate the threats to both environmental and nutritional health are real and growing. New health and disease patterns and crises will continue to emerge, and many of these will have nutrition factors as contributors and nutrition interventions as part of their management (Wahlqvist 2013). Such interventions will be across the continuum of care, from population approaches within communities to individual approaches within healthcare systems. Nutrition involves the broad study of food and diet, in addition to the more specific study of nutrients and other components that exist within food. Whether you are training to be a nutrition professional (nutritionist or dietitian), a clinician in another area of health, a scientist, or are just interested in food and nutrition, you

need to develop some key skills to optimise your understanding of the concepts and the scope of your influence. Improving the food consumption of individuals and populations in order to optimise health requires everybody to work together.

This chapter outlines the skills and attributes you need to develop in order to put nutrition science into action. These will be your toolkit, and activities throughout the book will link back to these in order to enable you to grow in confidence.

WHO ARE NUTRITION PROFESSIONALS?

Well-trained nutrition professionals are able to integrate foundational knowledge of human and nutrition science with detailed knowledge of diets and eating patterns, food composition and nutrient value and to apply this across different cultural and population groups in different contexts. This may include, for example, working with plant biologists to provide a whole-of-diet approach to the genetic modification of plants; developing a nutritionally adequate meal plan for a vegan athlete; designing a menu for groups living in care; developing a healthy eating program for a recently arrived migrant community; developing healthier food products; or developing and implementing regulatory approaches to improve food choices. The reality is that this knowledge takes a dedicated program of study and commitment to lifelong learning to keep abreast of the changing science. Nutrition professionals rarely work in isolation, and strong communication, collaboration and teamwork skills are essential. There is increasing evidence that inter-professional teams that work together can more effectively improve nutrition outcomes at individual, community, population and systems levels.

Nutrition and the relationship between diet and health has been documented in medical texts from as early as the 2nd century, and dietetics was one of the three main branches of ancient medicine, along with surgery and pharmacology (Mazzini 1999). In ancient Greece and Rome, food was given high importance; in particular, an individual's ability to live modestly and to control their desires (including food) was a source of pleasure (Coveney 2006). The aim was to cure illness but to also prevent ill-health. The term 'nutrition' in its various forms, at least in the English language, appears to have originated in the 15th and 16th centuries. The study of nutrition science as it is recognised in recent times emerged from the 18th century and the French chemical revolution. This occurred when the main elements

of chemistry were identified and analytical methods developed that began to extend understanding and testing of both old and new knowledge and beliefs (Carpenter 2003). Some key discoveries (such as protein digestion and the action of vitamins) occurred during the 19th and 20th centuries (Carpenter 2003) and provided the foundations for nutrition science, which continues to develop and expand today.

Table 2.1 summarises the different titles given to specified nutrition professionals. These titles can have variations in meaning and interpretation in different countries around the world. Preparing nutrition professionals with the necessary knowledge, skills, attitudes and behaviours (also termed competencies) aims to ensure they work safely and effectively to improve the nutrition of those with whom they work. Knowing what communities need and want from a nutrition professional is also an essential part of developing the nutrition workforce, and evolves over time as the health needs of the community and the social conditions in which we live change.

'Community nutrition', although a largely superseded term, has been described as public health nutrition at the local level or with smaller population reach (Hughes & Somerset 1997). Nutritionists, public health nutritionists and dietitians are all nutrition scientists.

Table 2.1 describes only those who are specifically trained in nutrition. There are a range of other professions that can impact on food systems and nutritional health (see Table 2.2). All of these professions would benefit from an increased

Table 2.1: Nutrition professional titles and their descriptions

Nutrition scientist	Nutritionist	Dietitian	Public health nutritionist
Applies the science of human or animal nutrition. It is based on biochemistry, biology and the social sciences.	Applies the science of nutrition to the feeding and education of groups and individuals for health. Nutritionists may provide individual dietary advice to people with disease under the supervision of regulated professionals (Association for Nutrition 2018).	Applies the science of nutrition to the feeding and education of groups and individuals in health and disease (Dietitians Association of Australia 2015a).	Work in the prevention of nutritionally related disease in populations and the maintenance of the nutritional health of well populations (Hughes & Somerset 1997).

Table 2.2: Professions that have the potential to influence nutrition

Health	Education	Scientists/Other
· Dietitians and nutritionists	· Health and physical education teachers	· Farmers/food producers
· Doctors		· Agronomists
· Nurses	· Early education and care teachers	· Plant biologists
· Occupational therapists	· Primary school teachers	· Lawyers
· Speech pathologists	· Home economics teachers	· Economists
· Exercise physiologists	· Science teachers	· Politicians
· Physiotherapists	· Sport coaches	· Environmental scientists
· Psychologists	· Personal trainers	· Social marketers
· Pharmacists		· Chefs

understanding of nutrition in order to integrate it into their roles (Wahlqvist & Isaksson 1983). It is vital for all those working in health to have a deeper understanding of the role of nutrition in prevention and care. However, as nutrition becomes increasingly complex, working with a nutrition professional—who has expert and in-depth knowledge and application of nutrition—will become increasingly important. Additionally, all professionals will need a more nuanced understanding of conflicts of interest that may arise with the recommendation and sale of dietary products (for example, by pharmacists).

PROFESSIONALISM

Underpinning the science and the art of nutrition practice is professionalism. Professionalism can be defined as:

• a commitment to improve and maintain skills and expertise
• engaging in effective interactions with others
• reliability
• being ethical and accountable
• taking responsibility for your practice. (Wilkinson et al. 2009)

Professionalism is a means of reassuring the public that the guidance they receive is evidence-based, safe and effective. Being professional includes being competent in your specialised knowledge, being committed to continuing to learn, taking care of yourself, and only working within the boundaries of your knowledge and skills. It also

encompasses broader aspects such as empathy, being self-aware and being able to manage your emotions in the workplace appropriately, as well as managing interpersonal relationships with clients, colleagues and others you encounter. The 'Evaluating your professionalism' box includes some questions that allow you to explore your professionalism. The 'Managing your social media' box provides another example of professionalism in action.

Competency

Key attributes of an effective nutrition workforce include its competence (Hughes 2006) to meet the health needs of the communities it is working within. Competence refers to 'the habitual and judicious use of communication, knowledge, technical skills, clinical reasoning, emotions, values, and reflection in daily practice for the benefit of the individual and community being served' (Epstein & Hundert 2002, p. 226). 'Competency is a skill and competence is the attribute of a person' (Khan & Ramachandran 2012). Competency standards provide a framework for workforce development and describe the outcomes a profession hopes to achieve in the systems in which it operates. Development of the workforce must acknowledge the multidimensional, dynamic, developmental and contextual nature of competence. For example, assessment of malnutrition in a rural region of a low-income country will require a different approach to the assessment of malnutrition in an acute tertiary hospital in a high-income country. A skilled nutrition professional knows and

EVALUATING YOUR PROFESSIONALISM

Take time to think about each question. Your responses will assist you in exploring your professionalism.

Individually
- What are your beliefs and values?
- Do you have a good sense of who you are and what you care about?
- Are you able to manage your emotions in a work setting?
- Do you take responsibility for your health and wellbeing?
- When you make a mistake do you blame others, or do you consider what you could have done differently?

Interpersonally
- Do you respect people from cultural and social backgrounds different from your own?
- Are you able to interact and communicate effectively with others from a range of contexts and cultures?
- Are you able to work with someone with a different belief system to you?
- Can you manage your emotions in a range of situations?
- Are you able to actively listen to someone with a very different opinion to yourself and begin to understand their perspective?

In the broader workplace and society
- Can you advocate to improve the nutrition for a vulnerable group in the population?
- Are you able to abide by workplace/organisation policies and rules?
- Can you work within codes of conduct and ethical practice (which may be different from organisational rules)?
- Are you able to admit when you have made a mistake and take responsibility?

Think about the scenario below and what constitutes professionalism in this case. Consider how you would manage the situation.

A student has commenced study in the first semester of a bachelor degree coming straight from secondary school. He is required to write an essay worth 30 per cent of one subject. He did not enjoy essay writing at school and so has decided not to submit this essay. He thinks he can manage a pass for the unit without this, as he has performed well on all the other assessment tasks for the subject. His lecturer emails him to ask why he has not submitted the essay but he decides to ignore the email as he doesn't really like to participate in awkward conversations. When the lecturer catches him after a tutorial he is embarrassed and, instead of listening, gets angry and storms off. In his anger he writes an email saying that the lecturer is unfairly targeting him and the date for submission was not clear enough.

Think about how this student has behaved. If you were the student how would you approach this situation? What would be a more professional approach?

MANAGING YOUR SOCIAL MEDIA PROFILE

Your social media profile will be one of your key forms of communication. It needs to portray your professionalism and credibility. You need to ensure the image you are projecting is professional and that your privacy is protected. The platforms may change over time but the principles will remain the same. Below are some tips for managing your online profile.

1. Search for yourself online. You should regularly put your name into an online search engine and social media to ensure you are being presented in a positive light. Make sure that any photos that appear are professional. If you have a similar name to another person, make sure your profile is distinguished by location or a photo.

2. Make sure your email address is professional. If you are at university you will be given a university email address but you will also have a private or a business email address. When you leave university, you may need to use a private email address. Ensure that this address is professional and conveys a professional image. For example, if your email is currently hotchick@ggmail.com then there is scope for improvement.

3. Manage your Facebook and Instagram. These are great ways to keep in contact with family and friends, or even to keep a personal diary. However, prospective employers are increasingly exploring these sites to gain an insight into individuals, so it pays to play it safe.
   • Keep your personal life off these accounts unless you are happy to manage two separate accounts (professional and personal) that are not linked.
   • Ensure your profile information is updated and correct.
   • Update your privacy settings; keep them very high for Facebook and Instagram—this will minimise the opportunity for an employer to view information.
   • Be careful when commenting on other people's posts as they may not keep their content set to private.
   • Pay attention to where you have checked in and what pages you have liked—do these reflect your values?

applies the most relevant approach, selecting one that is contextually relevant and that best meets the needs of the specific population.

Competency is not an end-point; rather, it requires continual acquisition of skills that will vary depending on the context and what you are doing. The model of skill acquisition in Figure 2.1 is useful to think about when considering the development of competencies. When you first start in a new area you are generally a novice, and so you need to be given the 'rules' or process to undertake a task. You will see that an expert is able to know 'what works' in a range of different situations. This requires not only content knowledge

but also experience and the application of critical thinking in order to be adaptable. All professionals move backwards and forwards continuously over their careers as new information becomes available or as systems develop and change. This is why it is important that you are lifelong learners knowing how to collect and critically process information that will inform your practice. This model links in with the four stages of competence (Figure 2.2); in order to be **safe to practise**, you need to be at least 'consciously incompetent'—that is, one of the characteristics of a professional is that they know the limits of their competence.

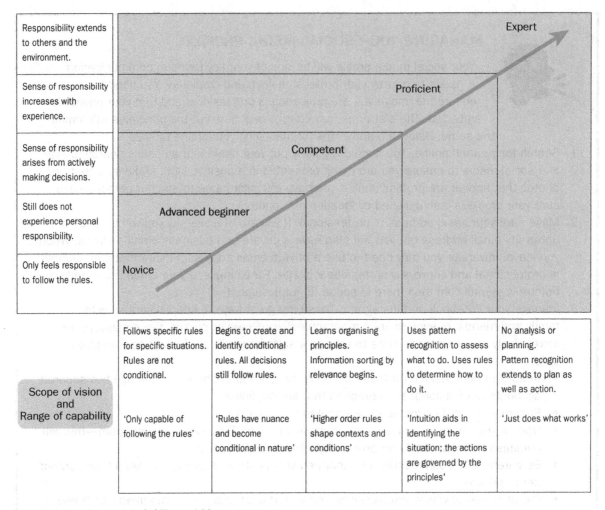

Figure 2.1: Dreyfus model of skill acquisition

Source: Cosman et al. (2017). Reprinted by permission from Springer Nature

Competency standards in nutrition

As mentioned earlier, some sectors of the nutrition workforce have codified the required standards of competence for practice. Such competency standards broadly describe requirements for the nutrition workforce to be able to use evidence-based science to improve nutritional health, work with multidisciplinary and multisectorial teams and practise professionally. Examples include:
- the National Competency Standards for Dietitians in Australia (Dietitians Association of Australia 2015b)

- the Competency Standards for Nutrition Science (Nutrition Society of Australia 2016)
- the Competency Standards for Public Health Nutrition (World Public Health Nutrition Association 2011).

YOUR PROFESSIONAL TOOLKIT

Professionals need to be equipped with a core set of attributes and skills to support their major work roles and enable them to improve nutrition and health outcomes. A conceptual model of the necessary skills

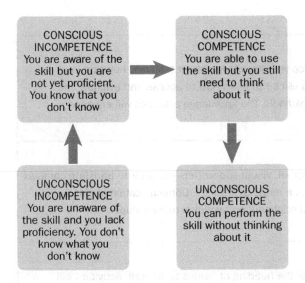

Figure 2.2: Four stages of competence

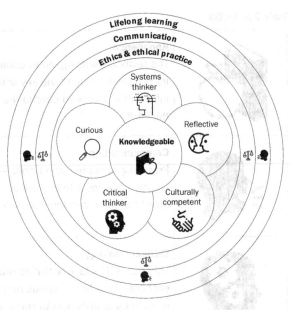

Figure 2.3: Professional toolkit

and attributes of a nutrition professional is illustrated in Figure 2.3.

Each of the skills and attributes that you will be developing is described in Table 2.3. This chapter explores each of these and highlights their application to understanding food and nutrition and to optimise health outcomes across different systems. Throughout the book, look for activities and boxes that will continue this lifelong journey.

Knowledge

Knowledge encompasses the facts, information and skills developed through education (perceiving, learning or discovering) or experience on any given subject. It refers to both theoretical and practical understandings. Knowledge helps you to filter information.

Science has contributed to knowledge through inquiry based on observable and measurable evidence according to the principles of reasoning and experimentation. It requires the formulation and testing of hypotheses via the collection of data through observation and experimentation. However, in nutrition there is an argument that some forms of knowledge (e.g. biochemical nutrient knowledge) are privileged over others (food knowledge). In some cases, food knowledge gives way to a focus

on single foods in isolation from whole diets, which are then either glorified (e.g. super foods) or vilified (e.g. processed foods) (Scrinis 2008). As discussed in Chapter 1, a range of knowledge is necessary in order to fully understand the complexity of the interaction between biological, food, environmental, social and economic systems.

Nutrition is a science and is **premised** on an understanding of a range of conceptual fields that underpin higher learning in this area, including:

- chemistry: organic and inorganic, to underpin biochemistry and the understanding of how food functions
- biochemistry: the chemicals and chemical processes that occur within human beings
- physiology: the biology of the normal functions of the body
- pathophysiology: the biology of the body in disease
- food science: the chemical and physical properties of food and how they change with processing and storage
- sociocultural dimensions: the social, cultural and personal factors that impact on food choice and eating behaviours.

Table 2.3: Toolkit

	**Knowledge** The textbook is designed to enhance your knowledge about food and nutrition in all its complexity. One of the key skills will be to learn how to access and evaluate the information you need beyond the textbook. The knowledge activities will enhance this skill.
	Communication Practising communication skills—verbal, visual and written—in order to translate complex nutrition science into actions across a range of settings. Communication is also being able to develop and maintain interdisciplinary professional relationships.
	Critical thinking This tool will include activities under the heading of 'curiosity' as well. Activities will encourage you to be curious and to collect, synthesise and critique data from a range of sources to allow you to come up with a defensible conclusion or solution.
	Reflection A key skill to develop innovative solutions that are safe. The activities will encourage you to develop your reporting, relating, reasoning and reconstructing abilities in order to inform practice.
	Cultural competency Activities in the text will integrate cultural elements to enable you to understand your own culture and to take it into consideration in practice.
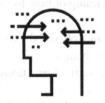	**Systems thinking** The book aims to assist in joining the dots between biological, ecological, food and social systems. You will have opportunities to explore systems thinking in order to see how all the pieces of nutrition and health fit together.
	Ethics and ethical practice Ethical practice will be integrated into activities enabling you to explore the increasingly complex ethical issues that surround nutrition and health globally and locally.

However, this type of knowledge needs to be combined with the knowledge that is brought by individuals and communities about the practicalities of their daily lives and what they believe to be true (Gallegos & Chilton 2019).

Communication

Being able to communicate to a wide variety of audiences is a key requirement for many professionals, particularly those working in health and nutrition. These audiences may be other health professionals, media, politicians, community leaders, clients or the general public. Being able to translate complex scientific principles into language that is easily understood and that enables individuals to apply this information to practical everyday food-based behaviours is a skill that needs to be learned. The way you communicate varies depending on the context and the people involved. Key attributes for a good communicator include:

- establishing rapport
- practising empathy
- **active listening**
- interpreting and responding to **non-verbal cues**
- taking a person-centred approach
- counselling skills. (Cant & Aroni 2008; Power & Lennie 2012)

Communicating in writing is also an important skill, and nutrition professionals need to develop skills in a range of genres, including reports, client notes, scientific papers, education materials, email, social media entries and blogs. Increasingly, nutrition professionals need to understand the power of story-telling and to communicate through the development of diagrams (infographics) and videos.

In this textbook there will be opportunities for you to practise your communication and translation of nutrition concepts. These will be integrated with other skills such as critical thinking.

Critical thinking

Critical thinking has been defined as gathering and seeking information, questioning and investigating, analysing, evaluating and making **inferences**, as well as problem-solving and applying theory to problems (Chan 2013). It does not mean being negative or full of criticism, but it does mean not accepting information at face value without questioning and carefully evaluating it. A good critical thinker is sceptical and curious. Chapter 3 will cover how to evaluate the reliability of nutrition information and give you a chance to practise this skill. Critical thinking is essential for professionals as it is embedded in **evidence-based practice**.

It is acknowledged that not all developing professionals possess critical thinking skills; therefore, these abilities need to be taught (Pithers & Soden 2000). Critical thinking is important for you not only as a professional but also as a global citizen. The goal of critical thinking is to enable people to live their lives as informed and engaged citizens of their local and global communities and to be able to develop a sense of social responsibility towards themselves and others (Naiditch 2013). As a professional, it is essential you deploy critical thinking in order to ensure that the most up-to-date evidence is used and communicated and that you also convey the limits of what you know. You will have access to information on nutrition from a variety of different sources and it will be essential for you to think critically in order to be able to:

- decide what counts as evidence
- select which types of evidence are the most appropriate for a given context
- determine the reliability and accuracy of the evidence and information
- sort through, select and apply the evidence.

There are six steps to critical thinking.
- Step 1: Knowledge: acquisition of knowledge enables you to identify what is being said.
- Step 2: Comprehension: understanding the material you are listening to or reading.
- Step 3: Application: applying the information to an actual situation. Problem- or case-based learning has been suggested as a method for developing this component of critical thinking (Kong et al. 2014).

- Step 4: Analysis: involves breaking down what you read or hear into its component parts, to make clear how the ideas are ordered, related or connected to other ideas.
- Step 5: Synthesis: putting together the parts you have analysed to create something original.
- Step 6: Evaluation: appraising the information to decide whether or not the argument and conclusions are supported.

The attributes of a critical thinker are:

1. Self-awareness—understands own learning and communication styles as well as culture.
2. Open-mindedness—willing to hear a range of different points to view and enjoys debating them.
3. Analytical—does not just accept things at face value but looks for properly constructed arguments that present evidence-based reasoning and formulate sound conclusions.
4. Active questioning—questions what they are reading and hearing, including the underlying assumptions and frame of reference.
5. Alert to context—looks at circumstances that may require modification of approaches.
6. Confidence—wants to seek out more to find out about ideas and insights.
7. Curious—seeks to know and understand through observation and thoughtful questioning, asks questions and looks for reasons.
8. Intellectual integrity—seeks the 'truth' through honest, robust processes even if the results are contrary to their own beliefs and assumptions.
9. Flexible—has the capacity to adapt, accommodate, modify or change thoughts, ideas and behaviours.
10. Creative—able to generate, discover or reimagine ideas and to develop alternatives.
11. Courageous—stands up for beliefs and is an advocate for themselves and others. (Adapted from Costa & Kallick 2000)

There will be a number of critical thinking skills that you will develop in—and continue to develop throughout—your professional life. These are outlined in Table 2.4. Critical thinking activities will be designed to extend your curiosity, practise synthesising information or begin developing your clinical reasoning.

Reflection and reflexivity

Implicit in the definition of being a professional is the capacity to be reflective. Reflection or reflective practice has been defined as purposeful, regular consideration of one's beliefs, values or knowledge while processing experiences to develop new understanding (Mann et al. 2009). Reflection is the ability to consider one's strengths and weaknesses in different situations in order to develop new understanding. Being able to reflect enhances your ability to deal with the complexity inherent in nutrition practice, potentially assisting in influencing choices and decisions in situations that are morally and ethically ambiguous. Being unable to reflect on your own thinking processes and actions can lead to overconfidence, which can contribute to poor practice (Wald et al. 2012).

Reflection can be broken down into four distinct steps (see 'The 4 Rs of reflection' box).

Reflexivity is the ability to use reflection and to take self-conscious and ethical actions. Building reflexivity allows professionals to act in more responsible and responsive ways. In practice, attention is also turning to the competence not only of individuals but also of interdisciplinary teams. This requires team reflexivity, which is defined as the extent to which group members can reflect upon and communicate about the group's objectives and strategies and adapt them across different contexts.

The 'Strategies for building reflexivity' box provides some ideas for building reflexive habits.

Building reflexivity as a habit will assist you in:

- extending your self-awareness and **emotional intelligence**
- developing your ability to inspire, influence and motivate others
- enhancing your ability to make informed decisions
- growing your capacity to be an innovative problem-solver

Table 2.4: Elements of critical thinking

Element	Description	Assessment
ANALYTICAL		
Evaluate evidence and its use	• Evidence can be evaluated independently of the position put forward. • The factual basis of the evidence is interrogated independently (sources/bias). • Evidence can be evaluated on the basis of how it is used, e.g. to draw a conclusion that is not supported or to extend a conclusion beyond the evidence provided.	• Evaluate evidence in larger context. • Evaluate relevance and expertise of sources. • Recognise possibilities of bias. • Evaluate relevance of evidence and how it supports the stated or implied conclusion.
Analyse and evaluate arguments	• Understand the structure of an argument and recognise the underlying assumptions.	• Identify stated and unstated premises, conclusions and intermediate steps. • Evaluate argument structure. • Distinguish valid from invalid arguments, including recognising structural flaws and holes in reasoning.
SYNTHETIC		
Understand implications and consequences	• Draw a conclusion of an argument that is not necessarily stated. • Understand implications and consequences of the argument beyond what is stated. • Infer possible results (intended or otherwise) of a course of action.	• Draw or recognise conclusions from evidence provided. • **Extrapolate** implications supported or implied.
Develop sound and valid arguments	• Be able to develop arguments that are valid (based on good reasoning) and sound (valid and based on good evidence).	• Development of valid and sound arguments.
GENERAL		
Understand causation and explanation	• Involves the consideration of evidence, implications and argument structure, as well as evaluation or argument production.	• Evaluate causal claims, including distinguishing causation from **correlation** and considering possible alternative causes or explanations.

Source: Adapted from Liu et al. (2014)

• building your ability to be compassionate and empathetic towards yourself and others.

Cultural competence

A culturally competent health professional is defined as one having a set of attitudes, skills and behaviours that allows them to work in cross–cultural situations and achieve outcomes for different groups. There are a number of different terms used in this area (see Table 2.5) but most have essentially the same principles:

• culture is defined broadly
• there is a focus on understanding self, one's own culture and relationship with others in the social world as the important first and ongoing step
• it requires consideration of power and equity issues, dominant **discourses**, the potential for harm and considerations for ethical practice.

Being culturally competent goes beyond being able to list a set of cultural foods or characteristics for particular groups, although a basic understanding

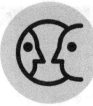

THE 4 RS OF REFLECTION

Reporting and responding
- Report what happened or what the issue or incident involved.
- Why is it relevant?
- Respond to the incident or issue by making observations, expressing your opinion, or asking questions.

Relating
- Relate or make a connection between the incident or issue and your own skills, professional experience, or discipline knowledge.
- Have I seen this before?
- Were the conditions the same or different?
- Do I have the skills and knowledge to deal with this? Explain.

Reasoning
- Highlight in detail significant factors underlying the incident or issue.
- Explain and show why they are important to an understanding of the incident or issue.
- Refer to relevant theory and literature to support your reasoning.
- Consider different perspectives. How would a knowledgeable person perceive/handle this? What are the ethics involved?

Reconstructing
- Reframe or reconstruct future practice or professional understanding.
- How would I deal with this next time?
- What might work and why? Are there different options?
- What might happen if ...?
- Are my ideas supported by theory? Can I make changes to benefit others?

Source: QUT DRAW Project (2010)

of this is essential for nutrition professionals as part of underlying knowledge (Bainbridge et al. 2015; Wilson et al. 2015). Cultural competence is based on a concept of 'culture'. This concept is often reduced to **race**, **ethnicity** or **indigeneity**, but culture is a broader concept and encompasses patterns of human behaviour that include communication, actions, beliefs, thoughts, values and institutions. Culture therefore also encompasses, for example, gender; sexuality, religion, education level, occupation, where you grew up, migration history, political views. We all have a number of cultures that may be mobilised in given contexts and define who we are and how we act. Culture is not static but constantly changing. In health, it is important to acknowledge these cultures, especially if they interrupt the ability to access health care or to manage one's own health.

A number of key attributes have been identified as exemplifying the culturally competent practitioner.
- **Reflecting on the concept of culture.** This means understanding the concept of culture, the dominant social structures in which you are working, the culture of the profession you are working in, and your own culture.

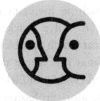

STRATEGIES FOR BUILDING REFLEXIVITY

- Build in time to be reflective.
- Journalling—some people find writing about their experiences provides a deeper understanding.
- Seek feedback—ask others about what they think is going on, what they would do in a given context.
- Move out of your comfort zone—seek out experiences that will stretch you, that enable you to experience something outside your usual sphere of activity.
- Reframing, scripting and rehearsal—conceptualising and practising different approaches.
- Work through case studies and problem-solving tasks.
- Find a mentor.
- Engage in peer learning.

Source: Schmutz & Eppich (2017)

Table 2.5: Terms used interchangeably with cultural competence

Term	Description
Cultural awareness	Highlights an understanding of individual differences and of cultures different from your own. Cultural awareness is an important starting point but it looks only at individuals, not systems, and is about building knowledge rather than changing behaviours (Bainbridge et al. 2015).
Cultural sensitivity	Still focuses on the individual—builds in reflection and starts the engagement with the lived experiences of others (NACCHO, 2011).
Cultural safety	Begins the shift away from individuals to systems. Was developed to address the ways **colonial processes** and structures shape and negatively affect Indigenous health in the dominant health systems. There is an emphasis on professional empathy and reflective practice rather than awareness of culturally specific beliefs. Shifts the focus to the people receiving care. Critics indicate that cultural safety has been reduced to creating culturally safe environments which for some is a lower benchmark, although this was not the intention.
Cultural competence	Aims to improve awareness, knowledge and skills. There is a strong focus on knowledge with self-awareness and reflexivity (Purnell 2002). However, critics are concerned that competence implies an end-point rather than an ongoing cycle of reflection in a range of different contexts. The disruption of **normative power** imbalances is implied but not explicit.
Cultural intelligence	Defined as 'an individual's capability to detect, assimilate, reason, and act on cultural cues appropriately in situations characterized by cultural diversity' (Van Dyne et al. 2012). It is commonly used in business and aligns with emotional intelligence.
Critical cultural consciousness	The development of critical consciousness involves a reflective awareness of differences in power and privilege and the inequities embedded in social relationships. The development of this type of consciousness is both through thinking and emotions/feeling and leads to engaged discourse, collaborative problem-solving, and a 'rehumanisation' of human relationships (Kumagai & Lypson 2009).

- **Practising ongoing self-reflection and critical self-awareness.** This means that there is an understanding of yourself as 'other' and as 'professional' and the power that gives you. It means having an understanding of how culture influences the way you view the world and recognising that not everybody shares that understanding.
- **Understanding that the world is socially constructed.** This requires a grounding in current affairs, politics and history. It requires an understanding of the principles of social justice and of the structures that create and recreate power imbalance and inequities.
- **Working effectively with people.** This includes ways of working and delivering information that resonate with those with whom you are working, in order to facilitate change. It is about suspending assumptions, seeking to understand the other person's perspectives (empathy) and working flexibly.
- **Communicating in a way that acknowledges culture.** This includes being able to ask the right questions in the right way, being curious and exploring diversity, and sharing some of yourself to create genuine connections.
- **Disrupting the construction of expert.** This attribute requires the understanding that you are expert in some areas (for example, nutrition science) but that the people you work with are experts in their own lives. This also requires using evidence from a variety of sources—not only scientific sources but also socially and culturally generated evidence.
- **Building a knowledge base.** This knowledge base includes a broad general knowledge that covers social determinants of health, historical influences, colonisation, migration, politics, racism, social justice, current affairs, the role of women and the philosophy of science. It also includes the basis of health beliefs, where to go to find out information and, finally, the role of food in culture, variations in what people eat, cooking practices, cultural occasions and the impact of **social constructs** and religious structures.

Systems thinker

The value of a systems approach is increasingly recognised, especially in trying to solve 'wicked' problems. This is because the point at which a problem or opportunity is identified is often not where the problem or opportunity originated (Wahlqvist 2014). In order to be an effective nutrition professional, you will need to develop your ability to be a systems thinker. A system is an 'interconnected set of elements that is coherently organised in a way that achieves something' (Wright & Meadows 2009, p. 11). Nutrition is a series of embedded systems, beginning with the body as a biological system nested in a range of other systems: political, educational, health, agricultural, food, social, housing and local. Systems thinking allows the physical, economic, social and environmental elements of nutrition to be identified and the dynamics between them defined. Taking an econutrition approach is a form of systems thinking.

Systems thinking is highly relevant to nutrition, as obesity, non-communicable diseases, malnutrition and climate change are conceptualised as complex problems that require systems thinking in order to develop solutions (Ison 2010; Richmond 1993). In nutrition, systems thinking means paying attention to the unpredictable interactions between stakeholders, sectors, disciplines and determinants of nutrition (SPRING 2015). Using a systems approach acknowledges that it is not possible to understand an issue by focusing on the individual elements; instead, attention needs to be given to how the parts interact and adapt (Friel et al. 2017).

There are a range of skills needed to be a systems thinker, but six key tools have been identified; these are described below and illustrated in Figure 2.4.

1. **Interconnectedness**—understanding that everything is connected; moving away from linear to circular models.
2. **Synthesis**—the ability to see interconnectedness. It moves beyond analysis, which is breaking things down to their elements in order to understand them individually. Synthesis is understanding the whole and the elements at the same time; that is, being able to see the trees and the forest. Synthesis is a part of critical thinking.

3. **Emergence**—understanding that larger things emerge from the sum of their parts. Different things emerge from different synergies—making systems very dynamic.

4. **Feedback loops**—recognising that as everything is interconnected, there needs to be feedback loops that reinforce or balance the outcomes. Reinforcing loops can contribute to **exponential growth** and instability; balancing feedback loops provide means for self-correction and stability.

5. **Causality**—being able to decipher and map interrelationships and how they impact on each other.

6. **Systems mapping**—the ability to map all the elements, understand how they interconnect and act. This mapping can provide insights into leverage points for influencing the system. (Acaroglu 2017)

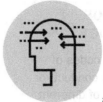

GETTING A HANDLE ON SYSTEMS THINKING

Read the following article:

Friel, S., Pescud, M., Malbon, E., Lee, A., Carter, R. et al. (2017), Using systems science to understand the determinants of inequities in healthy eating, *PLoS One*, *12*(11): e0188872.

- Summarise the key points from the article, focusing on the interactions between the systems.
- Describe the elements of systems thinking that have been used.

Ethics and ethical practice

Ethics are norms or standards of conduct that distinguish between acceptable and unacceptable behaviour. There are two types of reasoning that influence professional practice, moral and ethical. Moral reasoning is guided by personal standards of right and wrong, while ethical reasoning is guided by professional standards. All professionals are required to work ethically, using codes of conduct and ethical frameworks. These codes and frameworks are designed to protect the public and the profession of nutrition against non-evidence-based practice. Most nutrition professional societies have a code

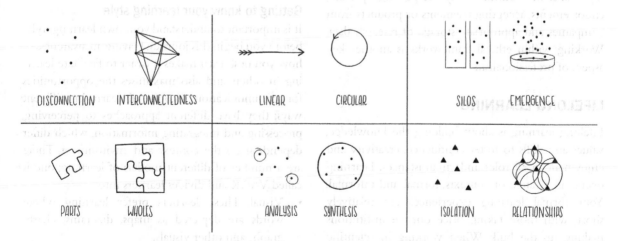

Figure 2.4: Tools of a system thinker

Source: Reproduced with permission from Disrupt Design (Acaroglu 2017)

CODES OF CONDUCT

Find the codes of ethics or conduct for a number of different nutrition organisations (this could include nutrition societies or dietitian associations). Compare and contrast the codes: what are the similarities and differences? Look at the code of ethical practice for the International Confederation of Dietetic Associations; are they similar or different?

Develop a list of components that are common across all associations.

WHAT WOULD YOU DO?

While you are studying your bachelor nutrition course, you are offered a job with a company as a salesperson for a nutritional product. This nutritional product claims to improve certain aspects of health but there is no evidence to support the claims. However, the money you are offered is good and would help relieve some of your financial pressures. The product most likely will not do any harm and it would be easy to convince people to buy it. What would you do in this instance?

of conduct or ethical guidelines that members are required to follow.

Ethical dilemmas do present themselves in the context of working in nutrition. Food and eating are very personal topics and are often attached to strong personal belief systems. Strict ethical principles apply in many areas of nutrition, including (but not limited to) consent, confidentiality, respecting privacy, endorsements, accepting payments or products from companies and appropriate storage of research data. Working within ethical frameworks is another key aspect of professionalism.

LIFELONG LEARNING

Lifelong learning is about building the knowledge, values and skills to foster confidence, creativity and enjoyment in all roles and circumstances. Learning occurs in a range of contexts, formal and informal. Your formal learning experiences are relatively short, with those taking place outside institutions making up the bulk. When working in scientific and clinical contexts where the evidence and the understanding of the evidence is fluid, and where its

application can make a difference, ensuring that you maintain currency is essential. In order for you to make every opportunity a learning opportunity, the skills outlined in the toolkit above are essential. This professional toolkit will ensure your employability in the face of rapid change and will enhance your experience of the world around you.

Getting to know your learning style

It is important to understand your own learning styles before you begin this journey. Having an awareness of how you best learn makes it easier to facilitate learning in others and also maximises the opportunities for communication. People all learn in different ways; they have different approaches to perceiving, processing and integrating information, which differ depending on the context and environment. There are a number of different models of learning; one is called VARK and divides learners into:

- **Visual.** These learners prefer learning where words are depicted as maps, diagrams, charts, graphs and other visuals.
- **Aural.** These learners learn best by listening and talking things through.

- **R**ead/Write. These learners prefer lists, notes and texts in a variety of formats.
- **K**inaesthetic learners rely on the use of experience and practice, including demonstrations, simulations, videos, case studies, practice and application. (VARK Learn Limited 2017)

Another model is Kolb's theory of experiential learning, which recognises the role that personal and social experiences play in shaping learning and that learning is a process of experience, reflection, conceptualisation and experimentation (Kolb 1984). This theory has been applied to determine an individual's preference for the four different learning phases:

- **Diverging (Reflectors).** These learners prefer to watch rather than do, tend to gather information and use imagination to solve problems. They want a lot of opportunities to read and discuss. If you are a reflective learner you need to take time to review what you have read and to think of possible questions or applications.
- **Assimilating (Theorists).** These learners need to take a concise, logical approach. They require a good clear explanation. They want handouts, additional readings, something to take away and study.
- **Converging (Pragmatists).** These learners like to solve problems and make decisions by finding solutions to questions. They want to observe and consider; they are interested in short cuts and tips to make their job easier.
- **Accommodating (Activists).** This is a 'hands-on' learning style. These learners prefer to take a practical, experiential approach. If you are an active learner you need to discuss concepts and undertake problem-solving tasks.

Most people learn using a combination of these styles. Understanding your 'natural' learning style will assist you in understanding what learning situations may challenge you and how to prepare for lifelong learning. There is no 'correct' or ideal style and we may demonstrate different preferences for learning in different contexts. The key is to develop insights into how you prefer to learn and implement strategies to maximise the opportunities for learning.

HOW DO YOU LEARN?

Look online for a quiz that will assist you in identifying your learning style. Based on your preferences, think about whether you could implement some of the following strategies.

Visual
- Develop flashcards or write notes to learn
- Use a highlighter to identify material
- Convert text into diagrams or maps
- Use mind-mapping as a technique

Auditory
- Speak new information out aloud
- Listen to lectures or podcasts
- Develop a discussion group to enable you to talk about key concepts

Read/write
- Take lots of notes
- Interpret and rewrite those notes in your own words
- Develop bullet-point lists
- Turn diagrams and representations into words

Kinaesthetic
- Learn by building a model or doing an activity
- Use role-playing as a way to consolidate new information
- Walk around when you are learning new material

SUMMARY

- Nutrition is a vast and dynamic area of science, and a wide array of career paths are available to pursue.
- Competency levels progress from novice to expert but competency requires a continual acquisition of skills. All professionals move backwards and forwards along the trajectory of competence during their careers, which is why lifelong learning is important.
- Your professional toolkit includes knowledge, communication, curiosity, critical thinking, reflexivity, cultural competence, systems thinking and ethical practice.
- Knowledge is shifting and practice changes as we learn more about different areas. Nutrition is an area that will expand and diversify into the future. Knowing your learning style and what constitutes professionalism is essential to developing your skills.
- Being flexible in your approach as a nutrition practitioner and being committed to lifelong learning and self-reflection are key to maintaining currency as a nutrition professional.

KEY TERMS

Active listening is the process of engaging with another person and understanding not only what they are saying but how they are saying it. It involves:
- paying attention
- using non-verbal cues to show you are listening
- paraphrasing to ensure you are understanding what is being said
- deferring judgement
- responding appropriately.

Colonial processes: policies and practices of power that subjugate one people (or their territory) to another.

Correlation: the tendency for two variables to increase or decrease in parallel; a connection or relationship between any two variables.

Discourse: the way(s) we think and communicate about people, things, the social organisation of society and the relationships within and between them. Discourses are embedded in and emerge out of relations of power, because institutions such as the media, politics, law, medicine and education control their formation and dissemination.

Emotional intelligence: the way you perceive, understand, express and manage your emotions when interacting with others. Attributes of emotional intelligence include thinking about your reactions; modifying your emotions; seeing situations as a challenge; praising others; apologising; and being able to conceptualise what others are feeling.

Ethnicity: refers to shared social, cultural and historical experiences stemming from common national or regional backgrounds, which make subgroups of a population different from one another. It is a social category.

Evidence-based practice: care that integrates individual clinical expertise, information from high-quality quantitative and qualitative research and the client's values and preferences.

Exponential growth: an increase in number or size at a constantly growing (rather than constant) rate.

Extrapolate: to extend an idea or application of a method or conclusion to an unknown situation.

Indigeneity: the noun of being indigenous—born or produced in a land or region.

Inference: a conclusion reached based on evidence and reasoning.

Non-verbal cues: behaviours that are forms of communication. They include postures, facial expression, gaze, gestures and tone of voice.

Normative power: power exerted on an individual by a dominant group to conform to the group's norms of behaviour.

Premise: a previous statement or proposition from which another is inferred or follows as a conclusion.

Race: categories of people who share certain inherited physical characteristics, such as colour, stature and facial features. Race can be a biological category or a social category.

Safe to practise: a practitioner is safe to practise when they recognise their professional limitations and scope of practice and seek assistance as required; engage in lifelong learning and apply best available evidence to any given situation; and work with clients to achieve positive outcomes.

Social construct: something socially constructed has been created through shared meaning between people. For example, gender—which represents ways of talking about, describing or perceiving men and women—is a social construction. Gender represents attempts by society to construct feminine and masculine identities.

REFERENCES

Acaroglu, L., 2017, 'Tools of a systems thinker', *Disruptive Design*, <https://medium.com/disruptive-design/tools-for-systems-thinkers-the-6-fundamental-concepts-of-systems-thinking–379cdac3dc6a>, accessed 17 July 2019

Association for Nutrition, 2018, *Frequently Asked Questions About Registration*, <www.associationfornutrition.org/Default.aspx?tabid=126>, accessed 18 June 2018

Bainbridge, R., McCalman, J., Clifford, A. & Tsey, K., 2015, *Cultural Competency in the Delivery of Health Services for Indigenous People* (Issue Paper No. 13), Canberra: Australian Institute of Health and Welfare, <www.aihw.gov.au/reports/indigenous-australians/cultural-competency-in-the-delivery-of-health-services-for-indigenous-people/contents/table-of-contents>, accessed 17 January 2019

Cant, R.P. & Aroni, R.A., 2008, 'Exploring dietitians' verbal and nonverbal communication skills for effective dietitian–patient communication', *Journal of Human Nutrition and Dietetics, 21*(5): 502–11, doi:10.1111/j.1365–277X.2008.00883.x

Carpenter, K., 2003, 'A short history of nutritional science Part 1 (1785–1885)', *Journal of Nutrition, 133*(3): 638–45, doi:10.1093/jn/133.3.638

Chan, Z.C.Y., 2013, 'A systematic review of critical thinking in nursing education', *Nurse Education Today, 33*(3): 236–40, doi:10.1016/j.nedt.2013.01.007

Cosman, P.H., Sirimanna, P. & Barach, P., 2017, 'Building surgical expertise through the science of continuous learning and training', in J.A. Sanchez, P. Barach, J.K. Johnson & J.P. Jacobs (eds), *Surgical Patient Care: Improving safety, quality and value*, Cham: Springer International Publishing, pp. 185–204

Costa, A.L. & Kallick, B., 2000, *Habits of Mind: A developmental series*, Alexandria, VA: Association for Supervision and Curriculum

Coveney, J., 2006, *Food, Morals and Meaning: The pleasure and anxiety of eating* (2nd edn), Oxford: Routledge

Dietitians Association of Australia, 2015a, *Definition of a Dietitian*, <https://daa.asn.au/what-dietitans-do/definition-of-a-dietitian/>, accessed 18 June 2018

—— 2015b, *National Competency Standards for Dietitians in Australia*, <https://daa.asn.au/maintaining-professional-standards/ncs/>, accessed 16 January 2019

Epstein, R.M. & Hundert, E.M., 2002, 'Defining and assessing professional competence', *JAMA, 287*(2): 226–35, doi:10.1001/jama.287.2.226

Friel, S., Pescud, M., Malbon, E., Lee, A., Carter, R. et al., 2017, 'Using systems science to understand the determinants of inequities in healthy eating', *PLoS One, 12*(11): e0188872, doi:10.1371/journal.pone.0188872

Gallegos, D. & Chilton, M., 2019, 'Re-evaluating expertise: Principles for food and nutrition security research, advocacy and solutions in high-income countries', *International Journal of Environmental Research and Public Health, 16*(4): 561, doi:10.3390/ijerph16040561

Hughes, R., 2006, 'Socioecological analysis of the determinants of national public health nutrition work force capacity: Australia as a case study', *Family and Community Health, 29*(1): 55–67, <www.ncbi.nlm.nih.gov/pubmed/16340678>, accessed 17 July 2019

Hughes, R. & Somerset, S., 1997, 'Definitions and conceptual frameworks for public health and community nutrition: A discussion paper', *Australian Journal of Nutrition and Dietetics, 54*(1): 40–5

Ison, R., 2010, *Systems Practice: How to act in a climate-change world*, London: Springer

Khan, K. & Ramachandran, S., 2012, 'Conceptual framework for performance assessment: Competency, competence and performance in the context of assessments in healthcare—Deciphering the terminology', *Medical Teacher, 34*(11): 920–8, doi:10.3109/0142159X.2012.722707

Kolb, D.A., 1984, *Experiential Learning: Experience as the source of learning and development*, New Jersey, US: Prentice Hall

Kong, L.N., Qin, B., Zhou, Y.Q., Mou, S.Y. & Gao, H.M., 2014, 'The effectiveness of problem-based learning on development of nursing students' critical thinking: A systematic review and meta-analysis', *International Journal of Nursing Studies, 51*(3): 458–69, doi:10.1016/j.ijnurstu.2013.06.009

Kumagai, A.K. & Lypson, M.L., 2009, 'Beyond cultural competence: Critical consciousness, social justice, and multicultural education', *Academic Medicine, 84*(6): 782–7, doi:10.1097/ACM.0b013e3181a42398

Liu, O.L., Frankel, L. & Roohr, K.C., 2014, 'Assessing critical thinking in higher education: Current state and directions for next-generation assessment', *ETS Research Report Series, 1*: 1–23, doi:10.1002/ets2.12009

Mann, K., Gordon, J. & MacLeod, A., 2009, 'Reflection and reflective practice in health professions education: A systematic review', *Advances in Health Sciences Education, 14*(4): 595–621, doi:10.1007/s10459-007-9090-2

Mazzini, I., 1999, 'Diet and medicine in the ancient world', in J. Flandrin & M. Montanari (eds), *Food: A culinary history*, New York, NY: Columbia University Press, pp. 141–52

NACCHO (National Aboriginal Community Controlled Health Organisation), 2011, *Creating the NACCHO Cultural Safety Training Standards and Assessment Process: A background paper*, <www.csheitc.org.au/wp-content/uploads/2015/11/CSTStandardsBackgroundPaper-NACCHO.pdf>, accessed 17 January 2019

Naiditch, F., 2013, 'A media literate approach to diversity education', *Journal of Media Literacy Education, 5*(1): 337–48, <https://digitalcommons.uri.edu/jmle/vol5/iss1/6/>, accessed 17 July 2019

Nutrition Society of Australia, 2016, *Competency Standards for Nutrition Science*, <http://nsa.asn.au/wp-content/uploads/2016/04/Competencies-in-Nutrition-Science.pdf>, accessed 15 January 2019

Pithers, R. & Soden, R., 2000, 'Critical thinking in education: A review', *Educational Research, 42*(3): 237–49, doi:10.1080/001318800440579

Power, B.T. & Lennie, S.C., 2012, 'Pre-registration dietetic students' attitudes to learning communication skills', *Journal of Human Nutrition and Dietetics, 25*(2): 189–97, doi:10.1111/j.1365–277X.2012.01226.x

Purnell, L., 2002, 'The Purnell model of cultural competence', *Journal of Transcultural Nursing, 13*(3): 193–6, doi:10.1177/10459602013003006

QUT DRAW Project, 2010, *The 4Rs Model of Reflective Thinking*, <www.citewrite.qut.edu.au/write/4Rs-for-students-page1-v1.5.pdf>, accessed 17 January 2019

Richmond, B., 1993, 'Systems thinking: Critical thinking skills for the 1990s and beyond', *System Dynamics Review, 9*(2): 113–33, doi:10.1002/sdr.4260090203

Schmutz, J. & Eppich, W., 2017, 'Promoting learning and patient care through shared reflection: A conceptual framework for team reflexivity in healthcare', *Academic Medicine, 92*(11): 1555–63, doi:10.1097/ ACM.0000000000001688

Scrinis, G., 2008, 'On the ideology of nutritionism', *Gastronomica, 8*(1): 38–48, doi:10.1525/gfc.2008.8.1.39

SPRING, 2015, *Systems Thinking and Action for Nutrition: A working paper.* Arlington, VA: <www.spring-nutrition. org/sites/default/files/publications/briefs/spring_systems_thinking_and_action_for_nutrition.pdf>, accessed 17 January 2019

Van Dyne, L., Ang, S., Ng, K.Y., Rockstuhl, T., Tan, M.L. & Koh, C., 2012, 'Sub-dimensions of the four factor model of cultural intelligence: Expanding the conceptualization and measurement of cultural intelligence', *Social and Personality Psychology Compass, 6*(4): 295–313, doi:10.1111/j.1751-9004.2012.00429.x

VARK Learn Limited, 2017, 'VARK: A guide to learning preferences', <http://vark-learn.com/>, accessed 22 July 2019

Wahlqvist, M.L., 2013, 'The clinical practice of food security', *Journal of the Australasian College of Nutritional and Environmental Medicine, 32*(1): 3–8, <https://search.informit.com.au/documentSummary;dn=367183887628 965;res=IELHEA>, accessed 17 July 2019

—— 2014, 'Ecosystem Health Disorders—Changing perspectives in clinical medicine and nutrition', *Asia Pacific Journal of Clinical Nutrition, 23*(1): 1–15, doi:10.6133/apjcn.2014.23.1.20

Wahlqvist, M.L. & Isaksson, B., 1983, 'Training in clinical nutrition: Undergraduate and postgraduate', *Lancet, 322*(8362): 1295–7, doi:10.1016/S0140–6736(83)91162–5

Wald, H., Borkan, J., Taylor, J., Anthony, D. & Reis, S., 2012, 'Fostering and evaluating reflective capacity in medical education: Developing the REFLECT rubric for assessing reflective writing', *Academic Medicine, 87*(1): 41–50, doi:10.1097/ACM.0b013e31823b55fa

Wilkinson, T., Wade, W. & Knock, D., 2009, 'A blueprint to assess professionalism: Results of a systematic review', *Academic Medicine, 84*(5): 551–8, doi:10.1097/ACM.0b013e31819fbaa2

Wilson, A.M., Mehta, K., Miller, J., Yaxley, A., Thomas, J. et al., 2015, 'Review of Indigenous health curriculum in nutrition and dietetics at one Australian university: An action research study', *The Australian Journal of Indigenous Education, 44*(1): 106–20, doi:10.1017/jie.2015.4

World Public Health Nutrition Association, 2011, *Competency Standards for the Public Health Nutrition Profession,* <https://wphna.org/our-profession/competency-standards>, accessed 16 January 2019

Wright, D. & Meadows, D.H., 2009, *Thinking in Systems: A primer* (2nd edn), Oxford: Earthscan

{CHAPTER 3}
EVALUATING THE RELIABILITY OF NUTRITION INFORMATION

Mark L. Wahlqvist

OBJECTIVES

- Explain how current nutrition information and advice is developed.
- Identify and apply methods for assessing the reliability of nutrition information in scientific papers, on the internet and social media and from nutrition 'experts'.

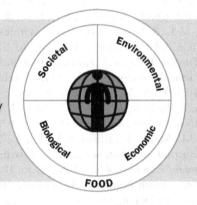

INTRODUCTION

As mentioned in previous chapters, nutrition information is constantly evolving and changing as our knowledge and understanding expand through nutrition research. Unlike the established facts and concepts in physics, maths and chemistry, nutrition research is a relatively new area of science. One of the reasons it is such an active area of research is because eating food is a complex affair, and there are limitations and confounding factors associated with dietary studies. Establishing the true food intake of individuals can be difficult, and thus the findings of dietary studies can be interpreted incorrectly or be of uncertain biological significance. For example, distinguishing cause and effect from coincidence or chance association can be quite a challenge when performing dietary studies. Findings can also be limited by incomplete knowledge of the essential

nutrient and other chemical (such as phytonutrients) composition of foods at the time of the study. Therefore, there will be varying degrees of consensus regarding particular questions in human nutrition at a particular point in time. Nonetheless, we can usually be confident that consistency in advice given is a consensus view based on the current best available evidence.

New ideas will be debated and tested. The nutrition advice given in the near future may not be the same as that offered today if new and convincing evidence emerges. For example, prior to the 1990s, nuts were not recommended for the management of heart disease due to their high fat content. In contrast, nuts are now recommended daily due to new evidence that they can, in fact, protect against heart disease and stroke. This protection may be mediated via their micronutrients (folic acid and vitamin B-6), which suppress damaging blood homocysteine levels, by their antioxidant phytonutrients, their dietary fibre and the proteins rich in the amino acid arginine.

In an informed and educated society, it should be possible to live with uncertainty and change of this kind, with the understanding that this is the nature of scientific inquiry and that we benefit from it. While some aspects of nutrition—such as the basic processes of digestion and absorption—are well known, even here new questions will arise. Many other issues are still being researched, however, and the results will either build upon or overturn findings reported in past studies. The difference in the 21st century is that now we are seeing the democratisation of knowledge. The internet and global circulation of information means that everybody can disseminate data as an 'expert' and, concurrently, that information is available to nearly everybody. This heightens the need for those with specific nutrition expertise to assist in deciphering the large volume of information available and also to improve the skills of the public in sifting through what is evidence-based rather than **anecdotal**.

This chapter will outline the approaches involved in assessing the reliability of nutrition information in scientific papers and **grey literature** on the internet and social media and from nutrition 'experts'. It will also highlight that the information from these sources should be based on the current best available evidence, which is subject to change if new evidence emerges in the future. Finally, it will explore **nutrition informatics** as a pathway for more effective, informed and individualised use of contemporary knowledge about food and health.

WHAT IS CONSIDERED EVIDENCE IN NUTRITION?

> 'We're drowning in information and starving for knowledge.'
>
> —Rutherford D. Rogers

The 21st century has seen a rapid democratisation of knowledge. That is, knowledge can be transferred quickly to a wide variety of audiences without distinction. This means that everybody can disseminate information (without knowledge) as an 'expert' and concurrently that information (without interpretation) is available to nearly everybody.

The development of technologies that make the dissemination of knowledge possible offers significant opportunities for nutrition and for empowering people to lead healthier lives. However, there are also risks. The sheer volume of information, available from a variety of sources and interpreted from a range of perspectives, means that evidence-based science can sometimes be misinterpreted, misused or not used at all. As a constantly evolving science, a balance must be struck between the conservative interpretation of solid evidence through scientific inquiry and a willingness to accept new evidence and interpretations. Wherever or however nutrition information is presented, it pays to retain a healthy cynicism and to always seek to understand the underlying science.

As a professional you should be seeking primary (unfiltered) rather than secondary (filtered), and scholarly rather than non-scholarly, sources (see Table 3.1).

When it comes to primary sources and studies there is also a hierarchy of research design. In this hierarchy the strongest evidence results from randomised controlled trials (RCT) and intervention studies. Weaker evidence results from case reports and expert opinion (see Figure 3.1 and Table 3.2).

Typically, randomised controlled trials are considered the 'gold standard' for evidence. For food and nutrition evidence, however, **double-blind** RCTs are particularly problematic. These can rarely, if ever, be contextual. They are unable to take into account the broad circumstances of eating, meals cannot be blinded, the studies are almost never representative of the population in question, and the studied characteristics are usually nutrients irrespective of dietary patterns, food structure or its sensory properties and social role (Wahlqvist 2016; Wahlqvist et al. 1999). There is also a misconception that, if a nutritional state is changeable by an intervention, this constitutes **causality**, which it does not. The actual cause may be quite different.

Table 3.1: Different sources of information

Primary	Secondary	Scholarly	Non-scholarly
• Raw data; interpretation of own work. • Data from experiments; surveys; questionnaires. • Original ideas expressed in sources such as government reports.	• Reporting another person's work or ideas. • Textbooks, articles in scientific journals that report the results of other researchers. • Reports/fact sheets.	• Written by academics, mostly published in peer-reviewed journals. • Discipline-specific. • Written by experts in the field. • Provide detail specific to those working in a similar field. • Acknowledge sources/reference. • Academic style of referencing.	• Can be written by anyone, for anybody interested in that particular topic. • Often not written by experts in the field. • Often give broader rather than more detailed information. • Written in 'layman's' terms including diet books, other popular literature. • Often not referenced.

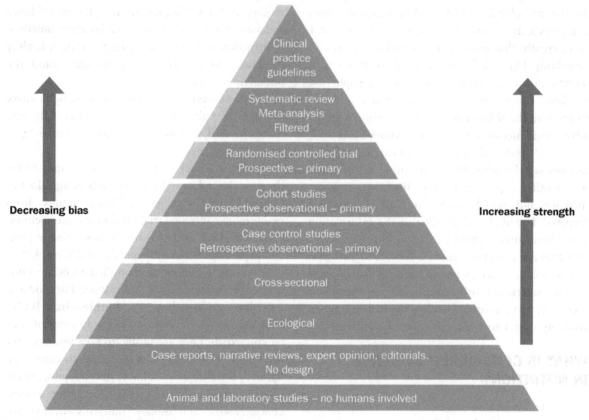

Figure 3.1: Hierarchies of evidence for research design

The next level of evidence is considered to be epidemiological or observational studies, which may be of cohorts or cases and their controls. Finally, animal experimental and cell biology studies are often valuable for the understanding of mechanisms. The strength of evidence is enhanced by the agreement of evidence from different sources, and by dose–response relationships. Science proceeds

Table 3.2: Types of research design

Type	Design	Definition
OBSERVATIONAL	Cohort	Cohort studies are sometimes called longitudinal. They follow a group of people who share common characteristics and assess whether exposure to a particular factor can lead to a particular outcome. They can be prospective (forward-looking), planned in advance and carried out over a period of time. They can also be retrospective (backward-looking), looking at data that already exist to identify risk factors for particular conditions.
	Case-control	Case-control studies compare groups of people who have a disease or outcome (cases) with groups of people who do not have the disease or outcome (controls). This study design looks back (retrospectively) to compare groups to determine the relationship between the risk factor and the disease. There is no intervention.
	Cross-sectional	Cross-sectional studies are observational and examine associations at a single point in time to assess prevalence of exposure to a risk factor or disease outcome. In these studies the risk factors and outcome are measured simultaneously, and it may therefore be difficult to determine whether the exposure preceded or followed the disease.
	Ecological or epidemiological	An ecological or epidemiological study is an observational study defined by the level at which data are analysed, namely at the population or group level, rather than individual level. They are often used to measure prevalence and incidence of disease.
EXPERIMENTAL	Clinical trial	Clinical trials use a particular type of person or group of people and follow a pre-defined intervention plan.
	Randomised controlled trial	A trial in which people are allocated by chance to receive the intervention or a control. The control may be standard practice, a placebo ('sugar pill') or nothing at all.
REVIEWS	Systematic	A type of literature review that uses a systematic approach to identifying and selecting papers, critically appraising and synthesising studies. These reviews will list the methodology so they can be repeated.
	Narrative	These are publications that describe, critically analyse and discuss the state of the science of a specific topic or theme from a particular theoretical point of view. These types of review articles tend not to list the methodological approach in detail.
	Meta-analysis	An approach that pools the results of many studies to establish statistical significance in quantitative studies and to develop a more complex analysis in qualitative studies. 'Meta' in this context means analysing the original subject but at a higher, more abstract level.

by decreasing uncertainty, but we can never be certain. To increase the level of certainty, it is more helpful to be integrative (drawing on biological, environmental, societal and economic perspectives) and to look at the overall 'portfolio' of evidence of different kinds and at different times, for the health of both human beings and the environment. Evidence should not be discounted based on its position in the hierarchy but, rather, reviewed critically and as part of a holistic body of knowledge.

It is perhaps also timely to remember that much of what we know about the actions of food and nutrition on health comes from trial and error. It has emerged as sociocultural truth before being 'proven' scientifically. Think, for example, of 'meat makes you strong' (protein, iron); 'fish is brain food' (protein, fatty acids). Another example would be the Mediterranean diet developed over time and observed to promote health and longevity. Through scientific endeavour, the unique combination of food and nutrients that impact on health have been identified.

Table 3.3: Likely differences between food/nutrition and drug trials

	Food and nutrition trial	Drug trial
Form	Complex	Simple
Compliance	Low	High
Biochemical interaction —within components —with other components	High High	Low Low
Metabolism	Complex	Simple
Bioavailability	Low	High
Measurable outcomes	Low yield	High yield
Dose response	Shallow slope (relatively low toxicity over time)	Steep slope (relatively high toxicity over time)
Side effects	Low	High
Investigator workload	High	Low
Time for study	Long	Short

Source: Wahlqvist et al. (1999)

HOW HAS EVIDENCE CHANGED OVER TIME?

As the evidence evolves, nutrition advice has changed over time. In this activity you are asked to interview an older person (over the age of 60 years) and ask them about some of the dietary advice they knew about or practised when they were younger. Contenders could be:

- Don't eat egg yolks, as they increase your cholesterol.
- Drink beer or stout while you are breastfeeding to increase your iron.
- Eat wheat bran to reduce constipation.
- Change from lard/dripping to vegetable oil.

Think about why these recommendations were made and what evidence has emerged to change the advice given.

To find a body of evidence to base decisions upon, you need to phrase your question so you can get a specific answer. You can use PICO for this:

- **[P]**atient or population. Who or what is your patient or population group?
- **[I]**ntervention or indicator. What is your intervention or indicator?
- **[C]**omparison or control. What is your comparison or control?
- **[O]**utcome. What outcome are you looking for?

For public health an **[S]** is sometimes added to reflect setting (i.e. PISCO). In other words:

In: <_____>

How does: <_____>

Compared with: <_____>

Affect: <_____>

Some examples of PICO questions include:

- In [P] overweight adults, how do [I] low glycaemic index foods compared with [C] high glycaemic index foods effect [O] weight loss?
- In [P] individuals with osteoarthritis how do [I] glucosamine supplements compared to [C] no treatment [O] improve symptoms of osteoarthritis?
- In [P] adults, how does [I] reliable access to fruit and vegetables in [S] remote areas [C] compared with little or no access to fruit and vegetables [O] impact on health?

EVALUATING TEXTS

Texts can be a range of materials. They can include scientific papers, grey literature, reports, textbooks, books written for the general public, media articles, websites, blogs, Facebook sites, Instagram pages, food products and advertisements. Regardless of the type of text, there are a number of questions you need to ask in order to be able to interpret the information they provide. These questions include:

- What sort of information is it? Is it an academic study, a media piece, an expert opinion or an anonymous website? Is it a primary source (original thinking or research) or secondary (somebody else's interpretations and evaluations)?

- Who is the author: do they have credibility? What are their qualifications?
- Does the author have any conflicts of interest? Are they receiving funding from anyone that may influence what they are writing? Are they making money through their experiences?
- Why is the text being written? Is it to gain a qualification? To extend the evidence base? To make money?
- How is the text written? Is it presented as factual? Is it presenting all sides of an argument? Is it part of a campaign? If the text is research, how well was it done?
- When was the text written? Constantly emerging evidence and changing contexts influence the veracity of what is written.
- How did you find the text? Did somebody recommend it? Did you do a systematic search? Did you just come across it?

EVALUATING SCIENTIFIC PAPERS

Scientists and healthcare professionals aspire to have their work published in 'refereed' or 'peer-reviewed' journals. This work, referred to as journal articles or papers, may be original articles, reviews or compilations of data sets as with '**meta-analyses**'. Papers published in refereed journals are subjected to critical appraisal by members of the scientific community. The paper is endorsed, usually by two or more expert referees nominated by the editorial board. Papers reporting original research usually include a detailed description of the study methods so that the study can be repeated by other workers and validated if necessary. However, other investigators may repeat the study using the same methodology and obtain different results. This would become apparent in the literature, and as a result the first published study would be cast into doubt. Thus, the scientific literature must be seen as a whole and not as a series of isolated articles. Increasingly authors are required to declare conflicts of interest and funding sources as well as ensure they have followed ethical practice (see the 'Ethical research' box).

ETHICAL RESEARCH

All research on human subjects needs to abide by ethical practice. The Declaration of Helsinki developed by the World Medical Association is considered to be the cornerstone of most ethics principles globally. Most peer-reviewed papers now require a statement about ethical practice and studies without ethical clearance are considered non-publishable. The basic principles include:

1. Do no harm.
2. Informed consent—participants need to know what the pros and cons of participating might be.
3. There should be no pressure on individuals to participate.
4. Respect individual autonomy.
5. Maintain anonymity and confidentiality.
6. Take particular care with vulnerable groups or groups where there is a power imbalance.

In Australia, the National Health and Medical Research Council provides the guidelines for ethical practice—the *National Statement on Ethical Conduct in Human Research* (NHMRC 2007). In New Zealand, the Health Research Council of New Zealand has developed the *HRC Research Ethics Guidelines* (Health Research Council of New Zealand 2017).

In recent years there has been an increase in the number of journals publishing scientific literature, as well as an increase in quasi-scientific journals. To identify a quality journal, look for:

- the impact factor of the journal—this is based on how often papers within the journal have been cited by others

- the credentials of the editorial board
- whether or not the journal is indexed in the major citation databases, such as Scopus or Web of Science
- the robustness of the peer-review process.

You can use databases such as Scimago to determine the quality of a journal in a specific discipline. If a journal is not listed, it may be because it does not represent objective scientific reporting and therefore should be treated with caution. Several food and other related industries offer information or abstracting services in nutrition to health professionals. Such information is easily obtainable and may provide a useful addition to your reference banks. However, the potential for topics, articles or authors to be biased towards supporting the interests of the industry providing the information should not be overlooked.

How do you find a scientific paper?

To find evidence you need to look through databases (see the 'Searching databases' box for tips). There are a range of databases available through university libraries or, in some cases, through professional associations. These databases can cover peer-reviewed papers in journals, dissertations (the report of a major piece of research undertaken for a higher degree), and newspaper and media articles. Table 3.4 provides examples of databases that are appropriate for nutrition.

Table 3.4: Database description

Database name	Details
CINAHL	This database is published by EBSCO and is found in the meta-databases EBSCOhost, ProQuest and Ovid. Provides indexing of the top nursing and allied health literature. Literature covers a wide range of topics including nursing, biomedicine, health sciences librarianship, alternative/complementary medicine, consumer health and 17 allied health disciplines.
Cochrane Library	This is a meta-database owned by Cochrane and published by Wiley. It consists of the Cochrane Database of Systematic Reviews, Central Register of Controlled Clinical Trials and Clinical Answers.
Google Scholar	Google Scholar is a web search engine that specifically searches scholarly literature and academic resources. Google Scholar will not contain everything that is in the library's databases. Use Google Scholar as a starting place.
Informit	This is a meta-database providing access to 100 databases with primarily Australian content. These cover business, law, engineering and public affairs (including health).
MEDLINE	MEDLINE is the US National Library of Medicine database and contains more than 25 million references to journal articles in life sciences with a focus on biomedicine. MEDLINE indexes entries with Medical Subject Headings (MeSH).
PubMed	PubMed is used to search MEDLINE and other biomedical papers. Includes open access articles and those in process.
PEN	Practice-based Evidence in Nutrition is a knowledge translation database providing access to timely, current and authoritative guidance on food and nutrition.
ProQuest	This is a meta-database comprising 40 different databases. It is multidisciplinary and will cover areas such as business, science and technology, health and medical, social sciences, arts and humanities, interdisciplinary, news, and dissertations.
PyschINFO	This database is available through EBSCOhost, ProQuest and Ovid. It is published by the American Psychological Association and covers articles published in behavioural and social sciences.
ScienceDirect	This database is published by Elsevier and provides access to scientific and medical research.
Web of Science	This is a meta-database published by Clarivate Analytics. It covers science, social science, arts and humanities citations. MEDLINE is included in this database.

SEARCHING DATABASES

This strategy applies to finding evidence for a particular topic.

Step 1: Decide on the databases to search. Will you search all databases or a targeted number?

Step 2: Devise a systematic search strategy.
- Identify key concepts for your topic.
- Brainstorm key words for each concept—using your PICO can help with this.
- Understand how the database uses combinations of key words with the use of AND, OR, NOT (see Figure 3.2).

How keywords are combined will influence what information is retrieved:
- AND limits what you retrieve—you are only getting evidence that has both keywords.
- OR expands what you retrieve.
- NOT limits and removes all evidence that contains those words.

Step 3: Combine the search terms according to the guidelines for the databases you are using.

Step 4: You may need to filter your findings. Depending on the database, you can do this by:
- year
- type of publication
- language
- human or animal research.

Depending on your search terms, you may have found a large number or a small number of publications. If very small, your search may need to be broadened; if too large, you may need to refine your search terms. The next step will be deciding which papers are relevant. After you do this, you will need to decide on the quality of the paper, using a range of available tools.

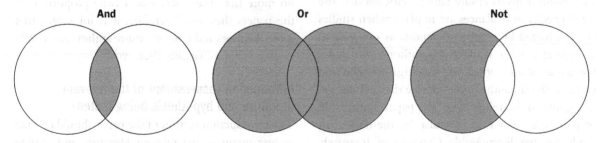

Figure 3.2: Combining keywords

Services that compile evidence systematically and with reliability are provided by organisations like the Cochrane Library and the World Cancer Research Fund (WCRF), which regularly update information to do with diet, physical activity and cancer, and related policy. The same applies to reports and guidelines from various organ- and disease-centred organisations, such as those to do with cardiovascular disease, diabetes, obesity, bone health, neurological disease and gastrointestinal disease.

EVALUATING RELIABILITY

When evaluating the reliability of nutrition information in published papers, you are looking for CARS:

- **C**redibility—author qualifications, reputability
- **A**ccuracy—currency of the evidence
- **R**easonability—transparency of methodologies
- **S**upport—use of references.

Reputable institutions

Papers published in reputable journals will usually include the name of the institution at which the research was performed. It is rare for individuals to publish scientific papers from a private or non-institutional source. There is usually strong pressure on individuals working in a reputable institution to maintain standards of integrity in their work. It is unlikely, though not impossible, that bogus research findings would be published from reputable institutions.

Reputable authors

Most studies are conducted by teams of researchers; therefore, most scientific papers are co-authored. Co-authors may be from different institutions, but the bulk of the research is usually carried out at one institution by the first or principal author. Group authorship helps to ensure authenticity, because the usual checks and balances are in place when studies are conducted by teams of scientists as opposed to a single researcher. If the group authorship includes the name of an outstanding investigator (who can often be the last author), you can use their reputation as a guide to the reliability of the paper. Authorship of papers is guided, in Australia, by the Australian Code for the Responsible Conduct of Research. This guarantees that all authors have contributed to the publication through the concept and design of the project, analysis and interpretation of the data, drafting significant parts of the work or providing critical review so as to contribute to interpretation.

Key questions: What are the author's professional and academic qualifications? Have they published on this topic before?

Funding for the study

Government funding bodies use public money to support research work. These bodies usually have a stringent refereeing and assessment system. Examples of such bodies include the highly respected National Health and Medical Research Council (NHMRC) and Australian Research Council (ARC). Non-government funding bodies, especially industry bodies such as the food and pharmaceutical industries, are not directly accountable to the government or the public for their disbursement of funds. Therefore, research funded by industry bodies must be scrutinised more carefully for possible bias or inconsistency. In addition, authors may be affiliated with a range of organisations or have accepted other funding that could potentially influence how the results are reported. These are called conflicts of interest and should be reported.

Key questions: Is the funding of the research transparent? Are all conflicts of interest stated?

PARTS OF A SCIENTIFIC PAPER

Summary or abstract

The abstract should summarise the entire paper, including the introduction, methods, results and discussion/conclusion. Due to the large volume of scientific papers published, many people will read no more than the abstract of a large proportion of the papers they see. Therefore, it is important that journal editors and referees ensure authors are strictly accurate in summarising their work.

Introduction (assessment of the relevant literature and hypothesis being tested)

The introduction section of the paper should include an assessment of the relevant literature and outline gaps in scientific knowledge. The introduction will summarise factual information about the topic area and will then go on to present an idea as a hypothesis or statement (if it is qualitative research) that the authors intend to test.

Key questions: Is the aim and research question clearly stated? Is there enough background presented to justify the research?

Study methods

As a general rule, the methods section of the paper should include sufficient detail to allow other scientists to duplicate the results. The methods used will therefore reveal the scientific rigour that has been applied to the work. The methods section should also include a description of the statistical methods used for the analysis of the results; statistical analyses help to separate meaningful observations from those that are likely to occur by chance. For qualitative papers, this section should include the theoretical underpinning, sampling and how the research and analysis was conducted.

Key questions: Is there a rationale for the chosen methods/tools? Is the method appropriate for the research question? Is there enough information on data collection, participants? Have the ethical considerations been addressed? Is there enough detail in the methods to allow replication?

Results

The results section will depend on whether the research was quantitative, qualitative or mixed methods. For quantitative research, results should always be available as numerical data in order to support the conclusions of the paper. Results should be available in such a way that primary data are either presented (for example, as tables) or can be calculated (such as from graphs). The reader needs to check for internal consistency in this section; it is important that the text describing the results is supported by the experimental data.

For qualitative data, depending on the methodology used, results should be presented clearly, the number of participants taken into consideration when presenting the results, there should be sufficient description to enable interpretation and illustrative quotes or specific incidences should support the findings.

Key questions: Were the steps involved in the data analysis explained and the strategies justified? Was the data analysis rigorous enough to substantiate the claims? Were all data taken into account? If not, why not? Are the presented results relevant to the research question? Do the tables and graphs (if any) make the data analysis clearer?

UNDERSTANDING THE STATISTICS

The probability that an event might have occurred by chance alone is expressed as a P value. It may be termed significant, $P < 0.05$ (5 per cent, i.e. that event would be expected to occur by chance not more than once in twenty repeats of the experiment), or highly significant, $P < 0.01$ (1 per cent, i.e. not more than a one in 100 occurrence by chance) or $P < 0.001$ (0.1 per cent, not more than a one in 1000 occurrence by chance).

Some papers may describe the results as being a type I or type II error. A type I error occurs when a difference between two means is deemed to be significant when it is not. A type II error is said to have occurred when the difference between two means is said to be not significant when in fact it is, though the investigator could not detect it. This often occurs if the sample size is not large enough.

When a difference is found but does not reach significance, authors may discuss it as 'a tendency' or 'trend'. This expression is useful because it enables discussion of a result that may have been statistically significant if type II errors could have been avoided. Furthermore, studies may find statistically significant differences or changes, but the authors need to address whether they are of biological significance.

Discussion and interpretation of findings

Research usually builds on previous work. It is quite unusual for a study to take a completely novel approach; therefore, most studies can usually be compared with related studies in the literature. In the discussion section of the paper, the authors usually make an assessment of how the present findings fit with those of other workers. If the study findings are contrary to those of other papers, some judgement must be exercised as to the nature of the true situation (see Table 3.5). In this case, the scientific community withholds judgement until further data are available from other research teams or laboratories. The authors should acknowledge the limitations of the present study and distinguish between factual observations and interpretation. A good discussion will clearly separate ideas from facts. A variety of phrases are used by authors to introduce ideas: *the results suggest that*; *the results tend to support*; *the results are consistent with*. Ideas are important and should be discussed, but the reader needs to be aware that they are still ideas and not facts. Reputable scientific authors are generally cautious about the interpretation of the data because they are aware that apparently minor variations in

Table 3.5: Body of evidence matrix and NHMRC grades of recommendations

Component	Excellent	Good	Satisfactory	Poor
Evidence base	One or more level I studies with a low risk of bias or several level II studies with a low risk of bias	One or two level II studies with a low risk of bias or a systematic review/several level III studies with a low risk of bias	One or two level III studies with a low risk of bias, or level I or II studies with a moderate risk of bias	Level IV studies, or level I to III studies/ systematic reviews with a high risk of bias
Consistency	All studies consistent	Most studies consistent and inconsistency may be explained	Some inconsistency reflecting genuine uncertainty around clinical question	Evidence is inconsistent
Clinical impact	Very large	Substantial	Moderate	Slight or restricted
Generalisability	Population/s studied in body of evidence are the same as the target population for the guideline	Population/s studied in body of evidence are similar to the target population for the guideline	Population/s studied in body of evidence differ to target population for guideline but it is clinically sensible to apply this evidence to target population	Population/s studied in body of evidence differ to target population and hard to judge whether it is sensible to generalise to target population
Applicability	Directly applicable to Australian healthcare context	Applicable to Australian healthcare context with few caveats	Probably applicable to Australian healthcare context with some caveats	Not applicable to Australian healthcare context

NHMRC overall grades of recommendations:
Grade A = Body of evidence can be trusted to guide practice.
Grade B = Body of evidence can be trusted to guide practice in most situations.
Grade C = Body of evidence provides some support for recommendation(s) but care should be taken in its application.
Grade D = Body of evidence is weak and recommendation must be applied with caution.
A recommendation cannot be graded A or B unless the evidence base and consistency of the evidence are both rated 'excellent' or 'good'.

Note: The components of the body of evidence listed in the table should be rated and the overall grade of the recommendation determined based on a summation of the rating for each individual component.

Source: Adapted from NHMRC (2009)

study procedures can change the significance of the results. If the claims of an author are bold and not tempered with caution, the reader should probably not accept these claims without reservation. The significance of findings or the reasons for unexpected results or inconsistencies should also be debated. The discussion usually concludes with an indication of where further work needs to be done and a hypothesis for future investigation.

Key questions: Have the results been interpreted with respect to the research question? Has other research supporting or refuting the findings been incorporated? Have the most important results been highlighted? How relevant or useful are the results to practice? Are the conclusions supported by the data?

There are a number of checklists available to assist in writing and interpreting scientific research papers. Most journals now request the submission of these checklists with the paper. These vary according to the research design. For example, PRISMA covers systematic reviews; STROBE, observational studies; CONSORT, quasi-experimental and experimental studies and COREQ qualitative studies. The following websites provide entry points to explore these checklists:

- www.equator-network.org/
- https://joannabriggs.org/ebp/critical_appraisal_tools
- https://casp-uk.net/casp-tools-checklists/

There are other comparable systems for the evaluation of evidence, such as GRADE for the Clinical Nutrition recommendations of PEN (Practice-based Evidence in Nutrition) (www.gradeworkinggroup.org/).

EVALUATING THE INTERNET

Internet use by Australians is among the highest in the world, with most households having access. The internet has become the world's greatest repository of readily accessible information. Everybody, regardless of educational, social or financial backgrounds, can now gain free access to an expanding volume of information that previously was inaccessible. Health and nutrition informatics are among the fastest-growing areas of interest on the internet.

It has been predicted that the internet will essentially change the way health and medicine are practised—one important change is that consumers will have more control. The internet connects millions of computers globally. It consists of academic, commercial, government, non-government and military networks, has no central location and is not owned by a particular entity. Established in 1992, the World Wide Web (www), is the front end of the internet, allowing people to combine text, graphics, audio and video into a rich communications medium or multimedia environment, making it more accessible and user-friendly. Emerging players however are dominating the internet and its information flow; these include rival governments, search engines like Google, social media platforms like Facebook, Instagram, YouTube (video sharing) and messaging agencies like Twitter. Advertisers and opinion-makers, whose vested interests are not always evident, are pervasive.

The large volume of health information resources available on the web has great potential to improve health. However, amidst the plethora of health- and nutritionally related websites are many that provide less-than-reliable information. Increasingly, food and nutrition information is being circulated via social media sites such as Facebook and Instagram and, given that social networking is the foremost use of the internet, the potential for the distribution of misinformation has increased. For the average consumer, sorting through this information for credibility can be daunting and the potential for harm from misleading and inaccurate health information is of concern.

The internet has been described as the largest collection of misinformation the world has ever seen. One of the biggest disadvantages is the difficulty sourcing and authenticating information. Virtually anyone can set up a website, which increases the risk of misinformation due to bias, misinterpretation or ignorance. Website authors can often hide commercial or other interests, making it more difficult for consumers to distinguish between credible and not-so-credible information. The internet brings information directly to individuals, cutting out interpretation and validation by those with an in-depth knowledge such as nutrition scientists, dietitians, nutritionists and medical practitioners. The internet increases access to information but also increases the risk of accessing unreliable or incorrect information.

The dissemination of information by the internet provides many opportunities for nutrition. Given the evolution of nutrition science, information on the internet can be updated more regularly and with greater ease. Individuals and professionals therefore expect that the information they are receiving is up-to-date and correct. The internet also provides opportunities for people who are not ambulatory, or who live in remote communities, to access nutrition and health information. Spending some time on the net before seeing a health professional may assist with improving health literacy and empowering individuals to get more from the consultation.

Website fitness check-up

In seeking out new information on the web, while at the same time attempting to separate hearsay, anecdotal reporting and quackery from authentic information, readers should ask themselves a series of questions, such as those outlined in the website fitness check-up in the 'Evaluating websites' box.

After answering these questions, individuals should have a good idea as to whether or not the website in question is credible. The domains .gov (government), .edu and .ac (education) can only be registered by government and educational institutions and reflect a higher order of authority than .com (commercial), .org (organisation) or .net (networking and commercial) sites. However, all sites need to be scrutinised equally, as all have vested interests that may impact on the information available. These should all be considered secondary sources and not used to verify or justify key arguments.

Searching for and locating information on the internet are only starting points—judging whether the information is credible may present a greater challenge. Therefore, the internet should not be used in place of doctors and health professionals. Health professionals are trained to collate, distil and apply clinical research and to manage uncertainty in clinical knowledge.

Wikipedia

Wikipedia is the most popular educational and reference destination on the web. Wikipedia is a free online encyclopaedia ('wiki' is a Hawaiian word for quick) that covers just about any topic you can think of. It is operated by the Wikipedia Foundation, a non-profit company. It has over eight million

---

EVALUATING WEBSITES

Search for ten food and nutrition websites internationally and nationally. Use the website fitness check-up below to provide a critique of each website. Come up with your top five websites for providing nutrition information to the public.

WEBSITE FITNESS CHECK-UP
Authority
Who are the contributors? The first question to ask is why did the person or organisation create the website? What is in it for them? Any medical or health advice provided and hosted should only be given by trained and qualified health professionals unless a clear statement is made that the advice offered is from a non-medically qualified individual or

organisation. Nutritionists and healthcare professionals with their appropriate credentials should be prominently displayed.

Does the website identify its publisher properly? What institution/affiliation supports the authors? Most websites have owners and/or sponsors who may have a proprietary interest in promoting a product or agenda. It should be clear from the home page or by a direct link from the home page who owns the site, with whom they are affiliated and who the significant investors are. Copyright ownership should also be indicated.

Does the website identify its sources of revenue? Is the information designed to sell you something? Any commercial sponsorship or financial support should be clearly indicated, and content should easily be distinguished from advertising.

Does the site have an advertising policy? The site should indicate if advertising is a source of funding and there should be a clear statement of the advertising policy. There should be a clear distinction between advertising and other promotional material and content.

Information about registration? Registration requirements, any necessary payment and privacy protection should be provided and easy to find.

Currency

The date of the last modification of the content must appear on the web page. All information should be updated regularly.

Do the links work? All hyperlinks on the page should be current.

Has updated research been cited? New studies are being published all the time, and even cited research that is 12 months old could be out of date.

Accuracy

Is there an editorial process, is information up-to-date and is the site efficiently managed? A description of the editorial process and method of content review should be posted on the site, as should a list of staff members and other individuals responsible for content quality. The site should be updated frequently. Generally, the most recent updates are posted. There should also be a 'search' component to access all the resource information of the website. The dates that content is posted, revised and updated should be indicated clearly, and time-sensitive content should periodically be reviewed.

Is the information balanced? Does the author present two sides of an argument, are possible biases discussed, and are the authors' and publishers' interests in the topic declared?

Does the information contain traceable references to support the evidence presented? Is the information based on sound scholarly sources? Sources of specific content should be identified clearly (i.e. author by-line, or the name of the organisation providing the content; affiliations and relevant financial disclosures for authors and content producers should be indicated clearly). The source of the information provided on the site should be explicitly mentioned and include, if possible, a hyperlink to the original source.

What links to other websites and databases are provided? There should be links to other reputable professional sources of information, such as the National Library of Medicine's MEDLINE, which holds records and abstracts of medical journals and other publications.

Sources: Health on the Net (HON) (2018); Kouris-Blazos et al. (2001); National Network of Libraries of Medicine (2018)

articles in over 200 languages. Wikipedia allows anybody, regardless of knowledge or qualification, to write and edit its pages, even anonymously, and thus has been described as a 'sum of public human knowledge'. Authors and editors must not include original research and must have a neutral point of view, make use of verifiable sources and consent to a special licence agreement that allows contributed material to be reproduced without royalties.

However, because of this submission model, there has been considerable dispute over the accuracy of some Wikipedia articles. Wikipedia has resources dedicated to resolving such issues, and usually strives to publish all sides of any argument; all submissions and edits are moderated and regulated by a staff of regular volunteers. Nevertheless, it is advisable to independently check citations and references used in these articles before relying on the information. Citing Wikipedia as a reference is usually not recommended for academics and students. Wikipedia can be a useful starting point, but is not primary or original source material and must be regarded as a secondary source of food, nutritional and health information.

EVALUATION OF SOCIAL MEDIA

Nutrition information is not only available via websites and through nutrition experts but in a variety of formats that reflect the explosion of the digital age. In evaluating information available from Twitter and Facebook, first principles apply as described above. In other words, what is the expertise of the person delivering the information, are there links to an evidence base and what authority do they have?

Mobile phone apps are a relatively new innovation and are especially prominent in the health arena. More than 197 billion apps were downloaded in 2017 and so they need careful evaluation before either using or recommending them. Considerations for determining the quality of mobile apps include:

- **Information:** quality and quantity of information, credibility (does it have a legitimate source), has it been trialled and tested in the scientific literature

- **Functionality:** easy to learn, logical, navigation
- **Aesthetics:** visual appeal, graphic design
- **Engagement:** fun, interesting, customisable, interactive, well-targeted to intended audience. (Stoyanov et al. 2015)

While aesthetics and engagement are not scientific principles they are required as part of a package to ensure that people are attracted to them and want to continue using them. This is essential if messages are to be relayed and information acted upon. They are part of the science of communication and marketing.

EVALUATION OF NUTRITION EXPERTS

So-called nutrition experts appear on radio, television and the internet, or in magazines, newspapers, blogs and shopping centres. It is worth considering how they can be evaluated.

Field of expertise

Is their field of expertise really nutrition, or is it some other unrelated field like engineering, politics or agriculture? This can be difficult to evaluate when the individual has a background in, for example, food. A knowledge of food and cooking, however, does not translate into an understanding of the science of nutrition.

Qualifications and membership

Are the 'expert's' qualifications from a recognised tertiary institution and are they specifically in human nutrition? Is the 'expert' a member of credible bodies such as the Dietitians Association of Australia, Nutrition Australia, the National Health and Medical Research Council or the Heart Foundation? Has the individual ever received research funding from reputable bodies?

Peer review and scrutiny

Is the 'expert' subject to scrutiny by qualified peers? In most fields, research conducted in universities, government-funded institutions and teaching hospitals is carried out in the presence of at least some scrutiny by junior and senior colleagues. Scientific fraud has been exposed from time to time by peers. Is the expert available for public debate and scrutiny? Credibility needs to be established over an extended period of time.

Vested interest

Does the 'expert' have a vested interest? Will they profit from the advice being given and is their advice therefore biased? Are they sponsored by a commercial company to give advice or perform research? What is the motive of the company for the sponsorship?

Frame of reference

What is the 'expert's' frame of reference? Is the advice being given because of the individual's philosophy, cultural beliefs, religion, self-interest or some other motive? Even a medical doctor or scientist may have moved to another frame of reference in the giving of advice. In other words, the professional qualifications of the expert do not necessarily guarantee that the advice will be correct and unbiased. Current nutrition information and advice in scientific papers, on the internet or by nutrition 'experts' is a consensus view based on the current best available evidence. In other words, the nutrition advice given in the future may not be the same as that offered today if new and convincing evidence emerges.

EVALUATING POPULAR DIET BOOKS

Identify the five current bestselling 'diet' books and critique the authors based on the criteria for identifying an expert. For one of these books, check the references.

- Are they up-to-date?
- Are they scholarly?
- Are they primary or secondary sources?
- How confident do you feel that the references are legitimate?

Select a proportion of the references and find them in a database. Check the quality of the reference and the strength of the evidence based on the above criteria.

- How confident do you feel about the evidence presented?
- Write a review of the book based on your findings.

Select two current nutrition blogs. Use the criteria for currency, relevance, authority, accuracy and purpose in the website section to check its 'fitness' as well as the criteria on nutrition experts. Write a short paragraph justifying your conclusions.

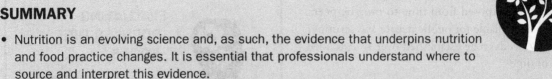

SUMMARY

- Nutrition is an evolving science and, as such, the evidence that underpins nutrition and food practice changes. It is essential that professionals understand where to source and interpret this evidence.
- There are different levels of evidence ranging from randomised controlled trials to observational studies. RCTs can be difficult to carry out in nutrition due to ethical considerations.
- Nutrition professionals need to be able to evaluate a range of sources of evidence including scientific papers, websites and social media. In addition, the number of people calling themselves nutrition 'experts' has increased, so being able to assess the background and reliability of these is becoming increasingly important.
- As information is potentially compromised by conflict of interest among its purveyors, it is important to recognise that some sources of information may be biased due to finance.
- Accessing, understanding, interpreting and communicating the science of nutrition is a key role for nutrition professionals and one that takes considerable skill.

KEY TERMS

Anecdotal: anecdotes are based on personal observation or from single case studies. For example, 'My grandfather lived to 99 years of age and ate butter and sausages every day.'

Causality: what connects one process (the cause) with another process (the effect), where the first is partly responsible for the second, and the second partly depends on the first. For example, there is a correlation between poor diet and chronic health conditions but we cannot prove that poor diet causes chronic health conditions. This is why we say that diet is a risk factor.

Double-blind: this is a study design where neither the study subjects or the researchers know which subjects are receiving the test or the control.

Grey literature: documents of many different types, in either print or electronic form, that are produced through non-commercial channels such as government, academics, business and industry. Examples of grey literature include scientific conference papers/proceedings, theses or dissertations, research reports, government publications, policy statements and issues papers, and newsletters and bulletins.

Meta-analysis: the statistical procedure for combining and systematically assessing data from previous research studies to derive conclusions about that research topic. Meta-analysis allows a consolidated and quantitative review of a large, and often complex, sometimes apparently conflicting, body of literature.

Nutrition informatics: the effective retrieval, organisation, storage and optimum use of information, data and knowledge for food and nutritionally related problem-solving and decision-making (Maunder et al. 2014).

REFERENCES

Health on the Net (HON), 2018, *The HONcode Principles,* <www.hon.ch/en/certification.html#principles>, accessed 25 August 2018

Health Research Council of New Zealand, 2017, *HRC Research Ethics Guidelines,* <www.hrc.govt.nz/resources/hrc-research-ethics-guidelines-december-2017>, accessed 22 November 2018

Kouris-Blazos, A., Setter, T.L. & Wahlqvist, M.L., 2001, 'Nutrition and health informatics', *Nutrition Research, 21*(1): 269–78, doi:10.1016/S0271–5317(00)00290–6

Maunder, K., Williams, P., Walton, K., Ferguson, M., Beck, E. & Probst, Y., 2014, 'Introduction to nutrition informatics in Australia', *Nutrition & Dietetics, 71*(4): 289–94, doi:10.1111/1747–0080.12138

National Network of Libraries of Medicine, 2018, *Evaluating Health Websites,* <https://nnlm.gov/initiatives/topics/health-websites>, accessed 25 August 2018

NHMRC, 2007, *National Statement on Ethical Conduct in Human Research,* <www.nhmrc.gov.au/book/national-statement-user-guide–0>, accessed 22 November 2018

—— 2009, *NHMRC Levels of Evidence and Grades for Recommendations for Guideline Developer,* Canberra: NHMRC, <www.nhmrc.gov.au/_files_nhmrc/file/guidelines/developers/nhmrc_levels_grades_evidence_120423.pdf>, accessed 25 August 2018

Stoyanov, S.R., Hides, L., Kavanagh, D.J., Zelenko, O., Tjondronegoro, D. & Mani, M., 2015, 'Mobile app rating scale: A new tool for assessing the quality of health mobile apps', *JMIR Mhealth and Uhealth, 3*(1): e27, doi:10.2196/mhealth.3422

Wahlqvist, M.L., 2016, 'Food structure is critical for optimal health', *Food & Function, 7*(3): 1245–50, doi:10.1039/C5FO01285F

Wahlqvist, M.L., Hsu-Hage, B.H.-H. & Lukito, W., 1999, 'Clinical trials in nutrition', *Asia Pacific Journal of Clinical Nutrition, 8*(3): 231–41, doi:10.1046/j.1440–6047.1999.00120.x

REFERENCES

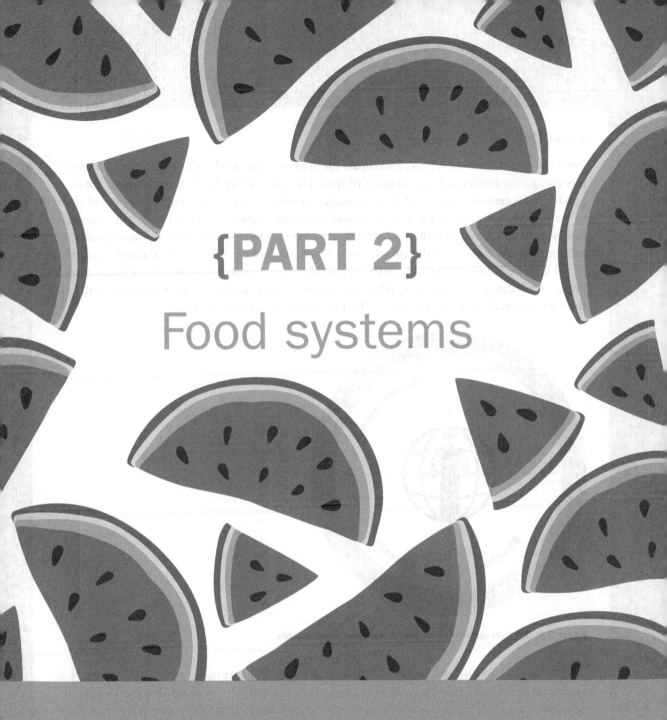

{PART 2}

Food systems

INTRODUCTION

Food systems, at their most basic, encompass the activities that involve the production, harvesting, processing, distribution and consumption of food. This view of the food system refers to a flow of goods; food is created at one point, flows through a number of steps (processing, transport and retail) to arrive at the point at which it is consumed and finally disposed (Lester 1994). It is important, however, to understand that any complete description of a food system must also incorporate the influences on the system and the consequences that stem from the flow of food through the system (Food Climate Research Network 2018). The food system is made up of multiple internal systems but has significant consequences on other systems—the environment, society, biological systems and the economy, as illustrated in Figure 2.A (Oxford Martin Programme 2018).

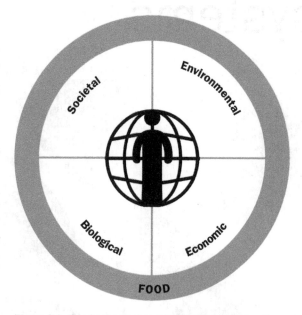

Figure 2.A: The food system interacts with multiple other systems

The food system is also highly dynamic and the flow between activities and outcomes is bidirectional; for instance, inadequate food production can lead to poor health, but the poor health of workers can result in inadequacies in food production contributing to ill-health (Hawkes & Ruel 2006). From early human cultures to modern megacities, food systems have become progressively more complex. Adding to this complexity is a future that holds many uncertain prospects for food systems, including continuing population growth, ecosystem degradation and climate change (Wahlqvist 2016). Adopting a systems-based approach offers many opportunities to face these challenges. The food system, when understood as a series of interconnected activities and outcomes embedded in a dynamic environment driven by socioecological change, allows us to better make connections, solve problems and find solutions in an inclusive and integrative way to current and future food system challenges (Termeer et al. 2018).

In these next chapters, you will gain a greater understanding of the complex system that feeds us and an appreciation that it should not be viewed in isolation from wider environmental, societal, economic and health issues. Chapter 4 provides an overview of the food system and the multiple actors involved in ensuring food moves from production to people's mouths. Chapter 5 goes into detail regarding food processing. Food processing involves the transformation of raw ingredients into food or of food into other forms and includes harvesting, transportation, sorting, cleaning, blending, drying, preserving, cooking, packing, marketing and storage of the end products. It includes small-scale food processing, large-scale food processing and beverage manufacturing and is an integral component of the food system, which also includes all agriculture that relates directly to food production.

Chapter 6 recognises the complexity of the food system and the multiple regulatory and non-regulatory approaches that ensure that individuals are able to access and consume food that is safe. It provides an overview of the food regulation system in Australia and New Zealand, including the range of potential hazards, the process of risk analysis and the monitoring that is required to ensure a safe food supply. Finally, Chapter 7 looks in more depth at microbiological risk and food safety. Food-borne illness is a significant burden on the health of populations globally. Our regulatory system ensures outbreaks are minimal; however, food safety is an integral component of food security and requires a vigilant and informed population as well as a robust regulatory system.

REFERENCES

Food Climate Research Network, 2018, *An Overview of Food System Challenges,* <www.foodsource.org. uk/chapter/1-overview-food-system-challenges>, accessed 15 December 2018

Hawkes, C. & Ruel, M., 2006, 'The links between agriculture and health: An intersectoral opportunity to improve the health and livelihoods of the poor', *Bulletin of the World Health Organization, 84*: 984–90

Lester, I.H., 1994, *Australia's Food and Nutrition*, Canberra: Australian Institute of Health and Welfare

Oxford Martin Programme, 2018, *Future of Food,* <www.futureoffood.ox.ac.uk/>, accessed 15 December 2018

Termeer, C.J., Drimie, S., Ingram, J., Pereira, L. & Whittingham, M.J., 2018, 'A diagnostic framework for food system governance arrangements: The case of South Africa', *NJAS–Wageningen Journal of Life Sciences, 84*: 85–93, doi:10.1016/j.njas.2017.08.001

Wahlqvist, M., 2016, 'Future food', *Asia Pacific Journal of Clinical Nutrition, 25*(4): 706–15, doi:10.6133/apjcn.092016.01

{CHAPTER 4}

FOOD SYSTEMS AND SECURITY

Mark L. Wahlqvist and David Borradale

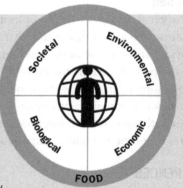

OBJECTIVES

- Define food systems in the Australian and New Zealand context.
- Describe the evolution of food systems over time.
- Identify the key components and resource implications of the food system.
- Explain the relationship between food security and food system.
- Discuss the link between food security, nutrition security and food and nutrition policy.

EVOLUTION OF THE FOOD SYSTEM

The **food system** has evolved from hunter-gatherers to the global industrialised system, and there are elements of each of these in our current system depending on the context. For example, some Indigenous communities continue to practise as hunter-gatherers; and in the modern industrialised context there is a return to foraging. The call for the development of alternative local food systems has elements of subsistence and village farming.

Hunter-gatherers

It is believed that for most of their several hundred thousand years' existence, human populations lived as hunters and gatherers. Edible parts of plants, including roots, seeds and fruits, insects, honey, and fish and animals of many kinds were collected and cooked or eaten raw. The range of foods collected was determined by the local environment and the season. Food might be plentiful at some times of the year and scarce at others; thus, humans would have been at risk of periodic famine and shortage of food for climatic or locality reasons. Population densities were also generally low, and people usually moved from area to area to find food. This nomadic way of life ensured access to a broader variety of foods, thereby reducing susceptibility to nutrient deficiencies when compared to staying in one fixed place. The diet of Aboriginal and Torres Strait Islander peoples prior to European settlement was once considered that of the hunter-gatherer (Specht et al. 2000). More recently, however, evidence suggests that Aboriginal and Torres Strait Islander peoples domesticated plants and sowed, harvested, irrigated and stored food; these behaviours are not associated with the hunter-gatherer way of life but are linked instead to subsistence farming (Pascoe 2014).

Subsistence farming

With time, nomadic hunters and gatherers settled into permanent villages and obtained their food by planting and harvesting crops. Animals, including sheep, cattle and buffalo, appear to have been domesticated after about 10,000 BC. Archaeological evidence shows the gradual evolution of crops from this period onwards. Selection of improved crops occurred as seed from the best plants was kept for planting. The food crops selected and used in different geographic areas were closely related to the environment and indigenous plants of the area. In most areas, a few crops proved to be palatable and reliable and became major sources of food energy for people living in that area. These are called **staple crops**. Table 4.1 lists some staple crops used in different parts of the world.

Village diets consisted of staple crops, to which were added other less energy-rich foods for variety, when available. The village food system depicted in Figure 4.1 included a degree of specialisation. Farmers produced food and traded their food at markets for other goods and services. Millers, for example, specialised in storing and milling grain. There are several nutritional consequences of the development of this village or peasant farming system. The range of foods was generally reduced compared with that in a hunter–gather system, but the reliability of the food supply was increased with the planting of crops. The beginnings of food processing, such as milling of grain—which increased the palatability of grains by making a flour that could be cooked—can also be observed within this system.

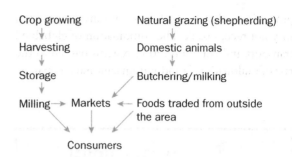

Figure 4.1: Village food system

Development of an industrialised and global food system

Permanent settlement and urbanisation, as well as technological developments in transport and agriculture, have been key drivers in the development of the current global food system. Initially, in village-type food systems, goods were transported by horse- or cattle-drawn wagons, but such transport was slow and ineffective, often not reaching its destination. As more efficient transport systems were invented, and foods were able to be transported greater distances, larger cities were able to be developed. Also essential have been key technological innovations such as canning, refrigeration and freezing that have allowed food to be stored and transported globally, allowing the current large-scale global food trade (Hueston & McLeod 2012). Increasing mechanisation of farming and improvements to crop yields through processes such as selective breeding, improved pest control and the application of fertilisers have increased food production. This system has also seen the rise of food

Table 4.1: Some staple crops in different parts of the world

Major staple crops	Favourable climate	Areas of highest production and usage
Wheat	Warm and relatively dry	USA, Canada, Australia, Mediterranean
Rice	Warm and wet, often irrigated	South China and southern Asia
Rye	Cool to cold, moderate to low rainfall	Northern Europe, Russia
Potatoes	Cool to cold, high rainfall	South America, northern Europe
Corn	Hot, high rainfall, often irrigated	USA, Central America, Africa
Sorghum	Hot, withstands dry conditions	Central Africa
Sweet potato	Tropical, moderate rainfall	Pacific Islands

processing—the original food origins of products may not recognisable. The combination of globalised transport and communication systems has led to the rise of multinational food and agricultural companies; it is estimated that just ten multinational companies control a majority of processed foods internationally (Hoffman 2013) (see the 'Multinational food companies' box).

Consequences of the global food system include; accelerated ecosystem change, increased population growth and changes in health outcomes, both adverse and favourable. In response to the growth of an industrialised and globalised food system, there is renewed focus on alternative food systems; these are described in more detail below.

THE AUSTRALIAN AND NEW ZEALAND FOOD SYSTEM

The Australian and New Zealand food systems are made up of farmers, food transporters and food manufacturers, wholesalers and retailers. The retail sector in Australia is dominated by several primary food retail chains, including Woolworths and Coles, plus many other retailers, convenience stores, fast food outlets and restaurants. In New Zealand, two primary food chains also dominate the market, with other gourmet and independent retail food chains also popular (Austrade 2018). While Australia and New Zealand are currently major food exporters, this is threatened by a range of issues including climate change. Figure 4.2 depicts the interrelationships within a modern food system and allows an appreciation of where it is vulnerable—for example, in terms of fertiliser (especially nitrogen, potassium and phosphate), water, energy and arable land.

The food system has three organisational levels:
1. primary production, concerned with the growing of plant and animal foodstuffs on farms or harvesting and foraging food—for instance, the harvesting of wild fish
2. food processing, concerned with off-farm activities employing technology to modify the primary produce into recognisable items of food (such as processing pigs into ham, or wheat into bread or ready-to-eat cereals)
3. retail food industries, responsible for the distribution and sale of food products.

MULTINATIONAL FOOD COMPANIES: WHICH COMPANIES OWN THE FOOD THAT YOU EAT?

The Big 10 refers to the ten largest food and beverage companies globally (Oxfam 2014). These companies own some of the best-known food brands, many of which are sold in Australia and New Zealand. Visit www.behindthebrands.org/ to see which companies own some of the most popular food brands, and how they score.

These **multinational food companies** have enormous influence on food systems, communities and environments worldwide, and the ethical and environmental practices of these companies are increasingly under scrutiny. The Behind the Brands website provides scores for each of these companies using a scorecard based on seven main themes, including fairness for farmers and workers and action on climate change.

Look at the foods you buy every week and determine where they are grown or manufactured and who owns the companies behind the products. How can you minimise your consumption of food produced by multinational companies? What are the risks associated with a small number of companies controlling most of the food products?

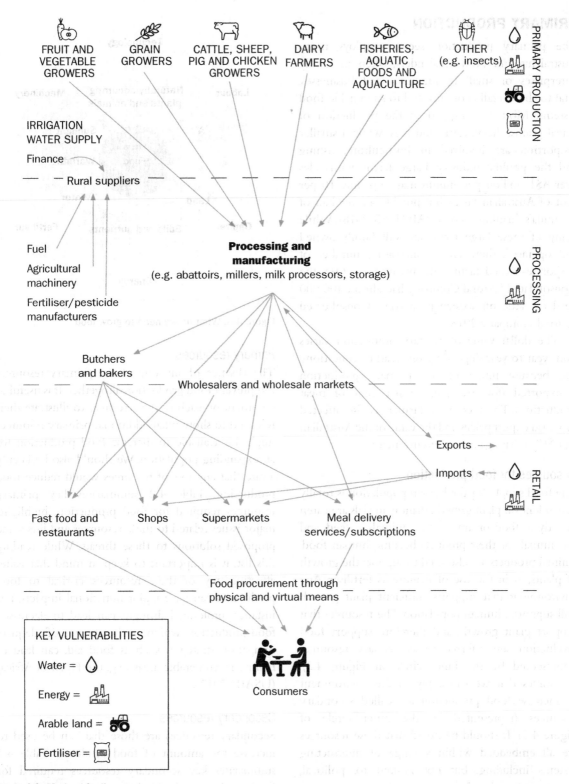

Figure 4.2: Modern food system

PRIMARY PRODUCTION

The primary production sector employs many Australians and New Zealanders, often in family enterprises or small to medium-sized businesses, vital to the overall economy and to sustainable food systems. Most are engaged in the production of cereal grains, sheep, cattle and pigs, while a smaller proportion are involved in horticulture, fishing and the poultry industry. Large farms with sales over A$1 million per annum make up only 10 per cent of Australian farms but provide almost half of Australia's farming income (ABARES 2018). While many of these large farms are still family-owned and operated, there are an increasing number of corporate-owned farms—for instance, in 2018 the Consolidated Pastoral Company had almost 400,000 head of cattle on sixteen properties (Consolidated Pastoral Company 2018).

The dollar value of primary production varies from year to year depending on weather conditions, and because much of our primary production is exported (for example, 40 per cent of meat production). The income to farmers is also affected by world export prices and the value of the Australian and NZ dollar against other currencies.

Resources for food production

The food supply for the human population is totally dependent on plant growth. Plant materials are eaten directly as food or are used by animals as feed, and the animals or their products become human food. Animal products are also used to support the growth of plants, as in the use of manure as fertiliser. Any environment that supports sufficient plant growth will support a human population. The resources that support plant growth, and therefore support food production, are referred to as primary resources (represented by the inner circle in Figure 4.3). Resources that we can apply to the environment to increase food production are called secondary resources (represented by the outer circle of Figure 4.3). It should be noted that these resources are all embedded within a range of intersecting systems including, but not limited to, political, economic, social and environmental.

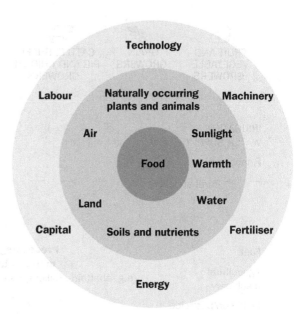

Figure 4.3: What do we need to grow food?

Primary resources

The absence of any one of the primary resources can prevent food production altogether. It is useful to comment on each of the resources to illustrate their role, and to show what additional primary resources might be available to increase food production for an expanding population. We should also be keenly aware that any loss of resources would reduce food production. Table 4.2 summarises key primary resources required for food production, highlights major issues related to these resources and lists some proposed solutions to these threats. While reading this list, it is important to keep in mind that issues affecting any of these resources critical to food production can have major nutritional impacts. For instance, prolonged drought can lead to decreased food production, which, in the absence of adequate mitigation strategies such as food aid, can lead to famine in vulnerable areas (e.g. the Horn of Africa) (USAID 2017).

Secondary resources

Secondary resources are those that can be used to increase the amount of food produced. Table 4.3 summarises key secondary resources required for food production, highlights major issues related to

Table 4.2: Primary resources required for food production

Resource	Attributes for food production	Major issues	Current and future solutions
Land	• Adequacy of physical space for growth and raising of food products. • Quality of land varies between locations.	• Population growth increasing food production demand, resulting in use of less suitable land to grow food. • Urbanisation encroaching on agricultural land.	• Increased productivity of existing land used for food production, e.g. increased use of technology such as machinery, selective breeding of crops, genetically modified foods. • Conservation of land not currently under agriculture to preserve biodiversity.
Soil and nutrients	• Provides nutrients for plants to grow, especially topsoils, which are rich in nutrients. • Amount of available nutrients in soils varies between locations.	• Erosion of topsoils by wind and rain caused by overuse, e.g. overgrazing by animals and excessive crop frequency. Also, deterioration of soils by acidification and salinisation greatly reduces capacity of soils to support plant growth.	• Implement soil conservation techniques such as contours and diversions for water and preventing overuse, e.g. by implementation of crop rotation strategies (Healthy Soils Australia 2019; Pimentel & Burgess 2013).
Water	• Required by all living organisms for survival. For plants, is essential for photosynthesis, transport of nutrients within plant, and structure and growth.	• Climate change causing increasing drought frequency. • Degradation of water quality and salinisation of freshwater resources (e.g. impact of freshwater fisheries). • Rises in water levels impacting coastal agriculture and fisheries.	• Improved irrigation systems. • Desalinisation plants. • Mitigation and adaptation strategies to climate change. • Policy to ensure water quality and safety.
Air	• Carbon dioxide is essential for plants. Incorporated into carbohydrate during photosynthesis.	• While increased carbon dioxide (such as that increased by human activities) can increase crop yield, benefits may be counteracted by climate change impacts on other areas such as water resources and increased pests and weeds.	• Mitigation and adaptation strategies to climate change.
Sunlight and warmth	• Sunlight drives photosynthesis (energy from sunlight produces a reaction in which carbon dioxide combines with hydrogen from water to form carbohydrate and other molecules that make up plants).	• Excessive warmth.	• Mitigation and adaptation strategies to climate change.
Plants and animals		• Plant and animal diseases. • Over-reliance on monocultures.	• Diversification of eating patterns. • Continued selection of animal and plants by selection breeding of desirable traits for food production. • Genetic modification. • New technologies, e.g. *in vitro* meat and 3D printing of food.

Table 4.3: Secondary resources required for food production

Resource	Attributes for food production	Major threats	Proposed current and future solutions
Labour	• Manual labour required to grow and process crops.	• Impacts to human health, e.g. malnutrition and disease impacting food productivity. • Inequity and poverty.	• Improving food security, e.g.: —food security reserves: stored foods such as grains for use when food production drops —agroecology: making the most of local land and climate to maximise food production. • Fair trade.
Machinery	• Equipment for growing, harvesting and processing foods.	• Most machinery still reliant on fossil fuels. • Expensive, especially for developing countries.	• Cost-effective and efficient machinery designs suitable for smaller farms.
Fertilisers	• Sources of plant nutrients. • May be organic (compost/manure) or chemical-based. • Provide nitrogen, potassium and phosphorus to plants—elements required by plants in the greatest amount.	• Run-off to water sources and eutrophication (water enrichment by nutrients that can result in algal blooms and death of aquatic life). • Overuse of nitrogen fertilisers contributes nitrogen oxide to the atmosphere—a potent greenhouse gas.	• Regulation and education around efficient use of fertilisers to avoid overuse.
Irrigation	• To provide sufficient water to plants/crops.	• Widely used **flood irrigation** is inefficient in water use and frequently leads to problems of salt accumulation in the soil. • Strain on water resources.	• More efficient use of water in irrigation systems—e.g. use of drip irrigation.
Pesticides, herbicides and antibiotics	• Pesticides/herbicides used to poison insect pests/weeds. Unlikely that sufficient food could be produced globally without these.	• Contamination of foodstuffs. • Impact on non-targeted species. • Development of resistance in targeted species. • Environmental contamination (e.g. soil and water).	• Use of non-chemical pest control (e.g. growing of crops more resistant to pests). • Development of more targeted, lower-toxicity chemicals. • Education on using pesticides in a more efficient and controlled manner. • Regulation (e.g. banned use of antibiotics in animal products).
Technology	• Broad term encompassing multiple advances in agriculture that can result in major increases in food production yields.	• Costs and lack of access to new technology in some regions.	• Introduction of low-cost technological solutions such as breeding of superior plants, development of herbicide-resistant crop plants, soil moisture sensors, watering to achieve maximum crop production without damage to the soil.
Energy	• Used for multiple processes in food production.	• Fossil fuels currently used throughout processes. Need to start looking at sources of renewable energy, e.g. biofuels.	• Increased use of renewables such as solar, wind, farm bio-waste to reduce impact of fossil fuels.
Capital	• Money required for the input of secondary resources (for in-depth discussion, see Chapter 25).	• Poverty and corruption. • Economic crises.	• Social responsibility for big food companies (e.g. providing more capital for small landholders and labourers). • Microfinance.

these resources and lists some proposed solutions to these threats.

FOOD PROCESSING

The food-processing industry adds further economic value to the products of agricultural production through processing operations that preserve food and increase product diversity and that therefore make healthy food more available. A major change in the food supply over the past century has been the steady increase in the use of industry-prepared foods. At the village stage of development, food was prepared for cooking within the home. This would involve grinding of grains, killing and cleaning of animals for meat, and digging or collection of vegetables and fruit. With the development of technologies, most of this food preparation has moved from the home to industry. Of course, many food industries have been in existence for 2000 years or more, including flour mills, bakeries, butcheries, dairies and wineries. Food industries appearing through the 18th and 19th centuries included specialised factories for the production of, for example, biscuits, smallgoods, canned fruits and vegetables, soups, jams and confectionery. During the 20th century, food manufacturing companies became steadily larger, taking over smaller companies and broadening their range of products. There has been a steady growth in food manufacturing using both ingredients and processes not readily available within the natural and home environments. See Chapter 19 for an explanation of how foods are categorised according to their level of processing.

The food industry is generally a free-enterprise system that depends for its existence on profitability. Any business that is not profitable cannot continue to operate, and business activities are therefore directed towards competitive advantage. New developments in the food industry (new foods, new marketing strategies) result from companies seeking a competitive advantage. Major food companies have usually grown by buying other businesses that they see have good products and are successful.

For further information on food processing, see Chapter 5.

Transport and trade in food

From the early 19th century to the present, developments in transport and trade have had a major influence on food availability and use. Effective transport widens the geographical distribution of food from its production location. Transport of food began as simple inter-village trading with foods and other goods carried by people or on pack animals or carts. Wagons drawn by horses or cattle were slow and could not travel when roads became too boggy. The development of efficient transport—first by water or railway, and later using motor transport on sealed roads—has been a major factor in the rapid growth of cities and spread of urbanisation. For a city early in the 20th century, rail and road transport could bring food from hundreds of kilometres away. With modern transport utilising containers and road, sea and air transportation, food reaches the city from all over the world. As the technologies of food transport, storage and preservation have developed, they have almost eliminated the effect of season on food availability. In the case of wealthy communities in developed countries, famine has disappeared because local drought is overcome by importing food from areas that have had good seasons. Efficient transport reduces the cost of food, since less time and labour are required to get the food from surrounding fishing grounds or farms to the market. Additionally, faster transport reduces loss by spoilage. More competition in the market (more farmers and more traders) also holds prices down. World trade in food is one of the largest trade domains, and is growing. Energy, climate and financial crises may, however, put a brake on this trend and food insecurity can follow.

RETAIL

The sector of the food system that focuses on selling food to consumers is the retail food industry. Prior to the 1950s, foods were bought from specialised food shops. These included the grocer (packaged, dry and canned foods), greengrocer (fruit and vegetables), baker, butcher, milk bar/confectionery shop. A large grocery store would have stocked many products, most being ingredients that would be used in the home to make complete meals. The composition of most of the food products was obvious to the purchaser (for example, flour, sugar, butter), thus not requiring detailed food labelling. Nutritional advice at that time was given in terms of food groups (cereals and cereal products; meats; milk and milk products; vegetables; and fruits).

During the 1960s, supermarkets began to appear in Australia and New Zealand and now most food retailing is controlled by these retailers, which are spacious, allowing room for many more food products. Food-processing companies, keen to expand their businesses, have employed food technologists to develop an ever-increasing range of new products aimed specifically at supermarkets. The forces driving the increase in variety of products include:

- the endeavour to increase sales and maximise profits by both the food manufacturer and the supermarket
- the attractiveness to consumers of products with a wider variety of tastes and textures
- a preference by consumers for foods that need less time and work to prepare.

A modern supermarket may stock around 30,000 different items (Food Marketing Institute 2017). This increase in the variety of foods on sale, along with the increased complexity of food formulations, has resulted in the composition of foods being less obvious to the consumer. Whereas food groups were generally fairly well understood, many of the more complex food products do not fit these categories and their composition is not obvious. Prepared desserts, pasta sauces, highly flavoured snack foods and toasted muesli are examples of complex manufactured foods with compositions that are not apparent from appearance or taste. As a result, ingredient lists on food labels and nutrition panels on the packaging of food products have become a necessity for the consumer who wants to know what is in the food.

If a manufacturer brings a new product to the supermarket, the supermarket can demand that the manufacturer advertise to ensure product sales. If sales are not adequate, the supermarket will decline to stock the item, which ensures that that food product will no longer be available. New products are continually being tried, with some succeeding and many failing. The key figure for the supermarket is sales and profit per unit area of shelf space, though profit margins vary across different products. Standard items, such as milk, bread and potatoes, have relatively small margins compared with 'luxury items' such as confectionery and snack foods. It is in the supermarket's interest to offer good quality and price on standard items to bring customers back and then tempt them to buy the luxury items while they are there. The layout of the supermarket is designed to achieve this. Milk, margarine, cheese, bread, meat, vegetables and fruit are dispersed around the perimeter of the supermarket while the luxury items are in the centre or placed close to the checkout to encourage impulse buying.

Technological innovations introduced by supermarkets to cut costs and improve convenience have had, and continue to have, an enormous impact on the food retail sector. One outstanding example is barcode identification of individual products and the linking of this to checkout registers and computer stock management, introduced in the early 1980s. More recently, self-service or cashier-free checkouts, which cut labour costs for supermarkets, have become common across supermarkets in Australia and New Zealand, and the automation of food retailing has been expanded even further with the introduction of automated stores, relying on advanced technology instead of human cashiers, by large multinationals such as Amazon.

There is evidence the activity of shopping is itself associated with improved life expectancy (Chang et al. 2012). This raises the possibility that the development of remote food-ordering facilities, as with online food sales, and of automated food outlets may not have the same health advantages as the more traditional food system linkages. On the other hand, these technological developments in the food system may also improve food availability and access to those who are unable to utilise more traditional food retail options

A remarkable change in Australian food habits in recent years has been the rise in eating away from home (especially for those on higher incomes), ready-to-eat meals and now eating in-home with home-delivered restaurant meals and meal delivery services (Choice 2018; Future Food 2018; Market Research Reports 2018). Also growing in importance are the use of home food-delivery services by consumers; these can include boxed meals or delivery of take-away and restaurant meals by emerging companies. Changing patterns of wealth, leisure time, cultural diversity, smart phones, food trade and fashion, and the media are probably all partly responsible for changes in food habits. The extent of the 'eating out' industry is shown by the rapid expansion in the number of restaurants over recent years. The nutritional quality of the food offered varies widely, from excellent to excessively processed, fatty and salty. The nutritional effects of dining away from home will be complex, mediated by its several pathways—biomedical, societal, environmental and economic.

Building services into foods

The increased efficiency in the growing, manufacturing and marketing of foods has resulted in food being more affordable for many people. It should be noted here that the cost of food has to be thought of in 'inflation-adjusted' terms. Data from the Australian Bureau of Statistics (ABS) Household Expenditure Survey show that, on average, Australians spent 20 per cent of earnings on food and non-alcoholic beverages in 1984, whereas in 2015–16 expenditure on food and non-alcoholic beverages was 15 per cent of earnings (ABS 2017). For low-income families the proportion spent on food and non-alcoholic beverages can be significantly higher, with research showing that to support a healthy diet, low-income families in Australia would need to be spending 20–31 per cent of household income on food and non-alcoholic beverages (Lee et al. 2016) (see Chapter 27).

HOW DOES THE SUPERMARKET INFLUENCE WHAT YOU PURCHASE?

Supermarkets control a large proportion of all global food purchases. Australia has one of the most concentrated supermarket industries in the world, with two retailers controlling the majority of purchases. Supermarkets in the first instance control what is available to purchase through choice vetting. They then employ complex choice architecture mechanisms to manipulate what customers will purchase (Thorndike 2017). Some examples include:

- putting milk at the back of store so customers need to walk past other items before purchasing
- placing nutrient-poor, energy-dense foods in end of aisle and checkout locations.

Visit a supermarket and consider the following questions.

- How often do you visit a supermarket? Do you purchase any items outside the supermarket?
- Where is the supermarket located? Is it in a convenient location?
- Where are products placed, both within the supermarket and on the shelf?
- As you make your way through the entrance, which items do you first see? Which are most accessible?
- How could you rearrange the supermarket to improve the purchase of healthier food items?

Customers do not necessarily purchase cheaper food. Convenience foods are often chosen in preference to cheaper foods that require more time to prepare. Many convenience foods require only opening the packaging, followed by heating and serving. In such cases, the consumer is choosing to pay for the convenience of having the food prepared ready for use—or, in other words, the consumer is paying for a service built into the food product.

The most recent initiative is the push to sell fully prepared meals, either hot and ready to eat or simply requiring heating and serving. Of course, ready-to-eat foods have always been available in one form or another, but the volume of ready-to-eat meals for consumption in the home is steadily increasing and supermarkets estimate that this product line is the one likely to show the fastest rise over the next few years. The chilled and frozen food sections in supermarkets are steadily expanding. For further discussion of discretionary and processed foods, see Chapter 19.

ALTERNATIVE FOOD SYSTEMS

Increasingly in Australia, in order to reconnect citizens with their food supply, there is a call for alternative food systems. These can include:

* community-supported agricultural boxes or shares—where you can buy a 'share' of a farm and in return receive a weekly box of whatever is in season
* farmer's markets—where the grower sells directly to the public within a local area
* agroecology (see Chapter 26)
* farm-to-school and farm-to-restaurant programs—which connect local food producers to schools or restaurants for food provisioning
* co-operatives—a food distribution system owned by employees or members who pay a nominal fee for joining; these can be small (a group buying produce in bulk and sharing out) or larger (e.g. employees and members owning a supermarket)
* urban agriculture initiatives and micro-entrepreneurial endeavours. (Phillips & Wharton 2015)

All of these initiatives are designed to bypass corporate agriculture, major supermarkets and multinational food providers, instead connecting with local producers and stimulating local economies (see Chapter 26 on tips for eating locally).

THE FOOD SYSTEM AND FOOD SECURITY

Food and nutrition security is defined as

> when all people at all times have physical, social and economic access to food, which is safe and consumed in sufficient quantity and quality to meet their dietary needs and food preferences, and is supported by an environment of adequate sanitation, health services and care, allowing for a healthy and active life. (FAO 2012)

Globally, there is still sufficient food to feed the human population, although its distribution and quality are commonly problematic (FAO 2018). Trade in surplus and value-added food to generate export earnings is a priority for many countries, but climate change, conflict and poor governance can rapidly change this state of affairs. A secure food supply is essential for health, as represented in dietary guidelines, reference standards, and food and nutrition policy. In many countries, nutritional health and wellbeing are not optimal: too many people suffer from malnutrition or chronic diseases associated with inadequate or poor-quality food intake. Most often, when nutritional health indicators (such as birthweight, growth development and nutrition-related wellbeing, disorder, disease or death) have improved in a country, these advances are not shared equally across the population. Figure 4.4 illustrates the pathways from food insecurity to multiple forms of malnutrition, including wasting and stunting, overweight and obesity and micronutrient deficiencies.

Food security has been defined at a number of levels: national, community, household and individual. Improved agricultural technologies introduced as part of the **'Green Revolution'** helped many countries achieve security at the national level, but

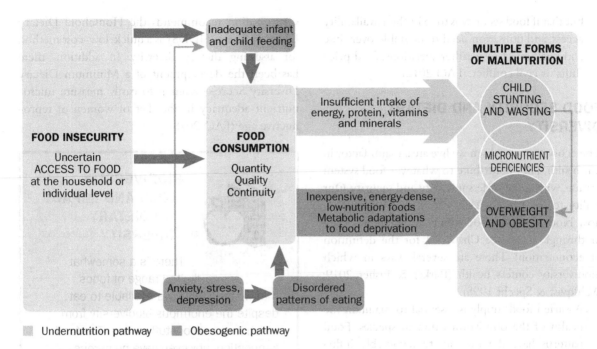

Figure 4.4: Pathways from food insecurity to malnutrition

Source: FAO (2018). Reproduced with permission

these benefits were often not distributed evenly to ensure security at the household and the individual levels (see Chapter 20). In the 21st century, regional conflict, mounting global social inequities and climate change are associated with greater food insecurity (Wahlqvist et al. 2012). While there have been previous reductions in global hunger, there have been increases indicating that progress towards eradicating hunger by 2030 is not on track (FAO 2018).

Food security has four broad dimensions (Figure 4.5). These are food safety, sufficiency, sustainability and satisfactoriness (or diversity, nutritional quality, palatability and acceptability). These align with the four pillars of food security identified by the FAO.

1. Availability: a reliable and consistent source of quality, nutritious food for an active and healthy life.
2. Access: there are economic and physical resources to put food on the table.
3. Utilisation: the intake of sufficient and safe food to meet individual physiological, sensory and

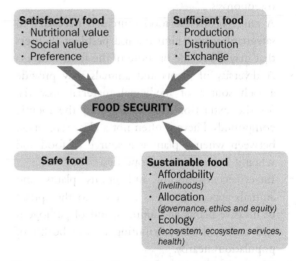

Figure 4.5: The four dimensions of food security

cultural requirements, and the physical, social and human resources to transform food into meals. It encompasses food safety but also sanitary and hygienic conditions.

4. Stability and sustainability: recognising that food insecurity can be transitory, cyclical or chronic,

but that if food security is to exist then availability, access, and utilisation need to be stable over time and not subject to weather variations, food price shifts or civil conflict. (FAO 2012)

FOOD SECURITY AND DIETARY DIVERSITY

The ecosystems in which we live are a major factor in our health. They contribute to whatever food system we use, with more or less integrity and security. Our ability to eat a biologically varied diet depends on how biodiverse our food supply is, whether locally or through trade (see Chapter 1 for the definition of econutrition). There are several ways in which biodiversity confers health (Barker & Fisher 2019; Wahlqvist & Specht 1998).

- A varied food supply is essential to maintain the health of the omnivorous human species. Food patterns have the capacity to favourably influence health on several fronts at the same time, as in cardiovascular disease, cancers, diabetes and osteoporosis.
- A range of diverse food sources is necessary to safeguard against climatic and pestilent disasters that may affect one or more of the food sources.
- A diversity of plants and animals may provide a rich source of medicinal material, essential for the extraction of undiscovered therapeutic compounds. There is often not a clear separation between when a plant is a source of food and when it has medicinal properties.
- Intact ecosystems of indigenous plants and animals appear to act as a buffer to the spread of invasive plants and animals, and of pathogens and toxins, thus contributing to the health of populations nearby.
- The 'spiritual' value of exploring the diversity of plants, animals and ecosystems in an area appear to have a beneficial effect on mental health, strengthening the feeling of 'belonging to the landscape'.

The importance of dietary diversity has been recognised and has been used as a proxy for the 'access' pillar of household food security (Hoddinott & Yohannes 2002). The Food and Agriculture Organization recommends the Household Dietary Diversity Score (HDDS) as a quick, low-cost method for assessing dietary diversity. In addition, there has been the development of a Minimum Dietary Diversity Score—Women to easily measure micronutrient adequacy in the diet of women of reproductive age (FAO 2018).

BIODIVERSITY LOSS AND IMPACT ON DIETARY DIVERSITY

There is a somewhat limited range of foods that we routinely have available to eat, despite the enormous biodiversity from which human foodstuff comes. The foods in question, however, have numerous **cultivars** which have provided alternatives in different ecological settings. Over the last 100 years or so, we have lost scores of cultivars of most plant foods and of types of animal food sources (see Figure 4.6, colour section). This loss puts the food system in a precarious state, since monocultures are more prone to crop failure with disease, pestilence or climate change.

The Slow Food Movement, an international movement that began in Italy, has developed the International Ark of Taste. This archive is of single food items as well as cultural foods that may already be extinct or on the verge of extinction. As of 2018, Australia had 63 items listed in the ark, and New Zealand had five.

Search for the Ark of Taste and explore the foods listed. Are you familiar with these foods? Can you find them where you are? What needs to happen to promote biodiversity?

DRIVERS OF FOOD SYSTEM CHANGE AND ACTION TOWARDS SUSTAINABLE AND HEALTHY FOOD SYSTEMS

Many factors are currently driving changes in food systems. These drivers of change include challenges to the food system, such as climate change (see Chapter 26) and political instability, but some drivers of change, including technology and innovations, also provide great opportunity to build sustainable and healthy food systems. Figure 4.7 shows some of the main drivers of change organised into five main categories by a panel of experts representing the UN Committee on World Food Security in 2017 (High Level Panel of Experts on Food Security and Nutrition 2017). See Chapter 26 and Chapter 30 for a discussion of the Sustainable Development Goals and the United Nations' Decade of Action on Nutrition as examples of how these drivers are being addressed.

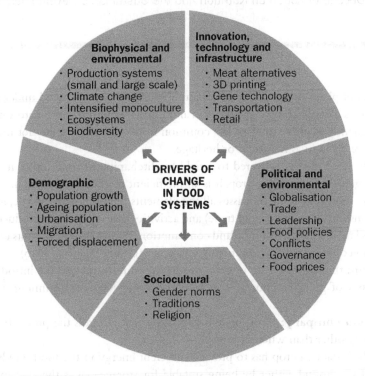

Figure 4.7: Drivers of change in food systems
Source: High Level Panel of Experts on Food Security and Nutrition (2017)

SUMMARY

- Food systems encompass all the elements and activities that relate to the production, processing, distribution and marketing, preparation and consumption of food and the outputs of these activities, including socioeconomic and environmental outputs.
- Food systems have evolved from hunter-gatherer systems to globalised industrial food systems. Food systems in Australia and New Zealand are complex and contain elements of globalised industrial, village and subsistence (alternative local systems) and hunter-gatherer (some Indigenous communities) systems.

- The contemporary food chain consists of three main organisational levels: primary production, processing and distribution, and the retail food industry. The food chain is undergoing significant changes as a result of technological innovations and changing consumer behaviour.
- Efficient, equitable food systems that are able to supply adequate food and dietary diversity sustainably to all people are an essential element for ensuring food security. Challenges to achieving this include conflict, social inequities and climate change.
- Changes in the food system include biophysical and environmental, innovation, technology and infrastructure, political and environmental, sociocultural and demographic drivers. These drivers of change and associated challenges require an international response to improve food systems, such as the UN's Decade of Action on Nutrition and the Sustainable Development Goals.

KEY TERMS

Cultivar: varieties of plants developed from a natural species and maintained under cultivation. For example, beefsteak, cherry, kumato, green zebra and roma are cultivars of tomato. Varieties that were previously frequently available and are less common now because they are not under widespread cultivation are referred to as heirloom or heritage.

Flood irrigation: water that is delivered to a field by ditch, pipe or some other means and simply flows over the ground through the crop. It is an inefficient method of irrigation.

Food system: the food system encompasses all the elements (environment, people, inputs, processes, infrastructure, institutions, markets and trade) and activities that relate to the production, processing, distribution and marketing, preparation and consumption of food and the outputs of these activities, including socioeconomic and environmental outcomes (United Nations 2015).

Green Revolution: the large increase in grain production due, in part, to the introduction of high-yielding varieties of grain to countries such as India and Mexico beginning in the mid-20th century.

Multinational food company: a corporate organisation that controls the production of food in at least one country other than where it is legally based.

Staple crop: to be a staple, a crop has to provide sufficient energy in the food supply and must also be available all year round, either by being suitable for storage—as is the case for grains, which dry easily—or by being able to be left in the ground to be dug when required—as for potatoes or sweet potatoes.

REFERENCES

ABARES, 2018, *Australian Farm Survey Results 2013–14 to 2015–16*, <https://data.gov.au/dataset/pb_afsr_p9absf20160427_11a>, accessed 29 November 2018

ABS, 2017, *Household Expenditure Survey, Australia: Summary of results, 2015–16*, <http://abs.gov.au/household-expenditure>, accessed 23 January 2019

Austrade, 2018, *Export Markets—New Zealand: Food and beverage to New Zealand*, <www.austrade.gov.au/Australian/Export/Export-markets/Countries/New-Zealand/Industries/food-and-beverage>, accessed 5 December 2018

Barker, T. & Fisher, J., 2019, 'Ecosystem health as the basis for human health', in J.M.H. Selendy (ed.), *Water and Sanitation Related Diseases and the Changing Environment*, West Sussex: John Wiley & Sons, pp. 245–70

Chang, Y.H., Chen, R.C., Wahlqvist, M.L. & Lee, M.S., 2012, 'Frequent shopping by men and women increases survival in the older Taiwanese population', *Journal of Epidemiology & Community Health, 66*(7): e20, doi:10.1136/jech.2010.126698

Choice, 2018, *Meal Delivery Services and Subscription Food Boxes,* <www.choice.com.au/food-and-drink/eating-out/fast-food/articles/gourmet-meal-delivery-services>, accessed 15 December 2018

Consolidated Pastoral Company, 2018, *About Us,* <https://pastoral.com/en>, accessed 15 December 2018

FAO, 2012, *Coming to Terms with Terminology: Food security, nutrition security,* <www.fao.org/docrep/meeting/026/MD776E.pdf>, accessed 15 December 2018

—— 2018, *State of Food and Nutrition Security in the World 2018: Building climate resilience for food and nutrition security,* <www.fao.org/3/I9553EN/i9553en.pdf>, accessed 15 December 2018

Food Marketing Institute, 2017, *Supermarket Facts,* <www.fmi.org/our-research/supermarket-facts>, accessed 23 January 2019

Future Food, 2018, *Eating Out in Australia: 2016 in review,* <http://futurefood.com.au/blog/2017/1/18/eating-out-in-australia-2016-in-review>, accessed 15 December 2018

Healthy Soils Australia, 2019, *About Us,* <www.healthysoils.com.au/about>, accessed 23 January 2019

High Level Panel of Experts on Food Security and Nutrition, 2017, *Extract from the Report 'Nutrition and Food Systems',* <www.fao.org/fileadmin/user_upload/hlpe/hlpe_documents/HLPE_S_and_R/HLPE_2017_Nutrition-and-food-systems_S_R-EN.pdf>, accessed 16 December 2018

Hoddinott, J. & Yohannes, Y., 2002, *Dietary Diversity as a Food Security Indicator* <https://ageconsearch.umn.edu/record/16474/>, accessed 23 February 2019

Hoffman, B., 2013, *Behind the Brands: Food justice and the 'Big 10' food and beverage companies,* Oxford: Oxfam

Hueston, W. & McLeod, A., 2012, 'Overview of the global food system: Changes over time/space and lessons for future food safety', in Institute of Medicine, *Improving Food Safety Through a One Health Approach: Workshop summary,* Washington DC: National Academies Press, pp. 189–98

Lee, A.J., Kane, S., Ramsey, R., Good, E. & Dick, M., 2016, 'Testing the price and affordability of healthy and current (unhealthy) diets and the potential impacts of policy change in Australia', *BMC Public Health, 16*(1): 315, doi:10.1186/s12889-016-2996-y

Market Research Reports, 2018, *Ready to Eat Food,* <www.marketresearchreports.com/ready-eat-food>, accessed 15 December 2018

Oxfam, 2014, *Behind the Brands,* <www.oxfamamerica.org/explore/stories/these-10-companies-make-a-lot-of-the-food-we-buy-heres-how-we-made-them-better/>, accessed 15 December 2018

Pascoe, B., 2014, *Dark Emu: Black Seeds—Agriculture or accident?,* Broome: Magabala Books

Phillips, R. & Wharton, C., 2015, 'Growing Livelihoods: Local food systems and community development,* London: Routledge

Pimentel, D. & Burgess, M., 2013, 'Soil erosion threatens food production', *Agriculture, 3*(3): 443–63, doi:0.3390/agriculture3030443

Siebert, C., 2011, 'Food Ark', *National Geographic,* (July): 108.

Specht, R.L., McArthur, M. & McCarthy, F.D., 2000, 'Nutrition studies (1948) of nomadic Aborigines in Arnhem Land, northern Australia', *Asia Pacific Journal of Clinical Nutrition, 9*(3): 215–23, doi:10.1046/j.1440-6047.2000.00192.x

Thorndike, A.N., 2017, 'Obesity prevention in the supermarket-choice architecture and the supplemental nutrition assistance program', *American Journal of Public Health, 107*(10): 1582, doi:10.2105/AJPH.2017.303991

United Nations, 2015, *High Level Task Force on Global Food and Nutrition Security,* <www.un.org/en/issues/food/taskforce/wg3.shtml>, accessed 14 December 2018

USAID, 2017, *Horn of Africa,* <www.usaid.gov/crisis/horn-africa>, accessed 16 December 2018

Wahlqvist, M.L., McKay, J., Chang, Y.-C. & Chiu, Y.-W., 2012, 'Rethinking the food security debate in Asia: Some missing ecological and health dimensions and solutions', *Food Security, 4*(4): 657–70, doi:10.1007/s12571-012-0211-2

Wahlqvist, M.L. & Specht, R.L., 1998, 'Food variety and biodiversity: Econutrition', *Asia Pacific Journal of Clinical Nutrition,* 7: 314–19, <http://apjcn.nhri.org.tw/server/APJCN/7/3/4/314.pdf>, accessed 23 January 2019

{CHAPTER 5}
FOOD PROCESSING

Janis Baines and David Borradale

OBJECTIVES

- Define food processing.
- Describe the importance of the food processing industry in Australia and New Zealand.
- Explain the science that underlies the behaviour of food during cooking and processing.
- Describe commonly used food preservation techniques.
- Discuss how new food processing and packaging technologies and the increased focus on sustainable food processing may influence food processing in the future.

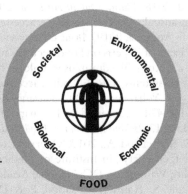

INTRODUCTION

The practice of processing food began early in history and was probably a response to food shortages. The use of fire must also have led to the discovery of new and interesting cooked flavours as well as other ways to prepare and store food. In some countries, small-scale food processing remains an important part of village economies, but in many others the Industrial Revolution from the 18th century onwards saw the development of large, centralised food-processing operations and sophisticated distribution systems as well as national and international food regulations systems.

As an integral component of the food system, food processing contributes significantly to the economic and social development of a country. In Australia in 2015, just over half a million people (522,100)

were employed in food and **agribusiness**: of these, approximately 40 per cent (206,700) were employed in food processing and manufacture and 6 per cent (33,000) in beverage and tobacco manufacture; nearly 50 per cent (251,200) in agriculture and another 5 per cent (26,900) in aquaculture or fishing, hunting and trapping and support services, with the remainder (5000) in machinery and equipment manufacture (Chaustowski & Dolman 2015).

Australia's food and agribusiness industry produced A\$53.9 billion of industry value added in 2014–15, equivalent to 3.3 per cent of total GDP (Chaustowski & Dolman 2015). Food available for consumption in Australia may be made in the country or imported; some food produced in the country is exported to other countries. Australia is a net exporter of food and agribusiness products and exports over half its agricultural produce. The value of food and agribusiness exports has grown at a rate of 6.1 per cent per annum over the past ten years (year-on-year) and was worth A$40.8 billion in 2015. The past five years have seen both an increase in the rate of growth in Australia's food and agribusiness exports as well as an increase in the sector's share of total exports. Imports of food and agribusiness products to Australia were worth A$17.1 billion in 2015 (Chaustowski & Dolman 2015).

There are different types of processing and these may result in either positive or negative health impacts for those consuming the resultant foods. Minimally processing foods does not change a food's essential structure or nutritional properties. Ultra-processed foods are predominantly the product of large-scale processing and often include ingredients that have been manufactured (see Chapter 19). There is a continuum of processing in between minimally and ultra-processed. Understanding the processes that underpin the transformation of food is essential in order to understand the implications for nutritional content.

FOOD PROCESSING METHODS

There are many traditional food-processing methods, including milling, cooking, baking, fermentation, pickling and other means of preservation; there are also some new technologies used to produce and package foods, including minimal food-processing techniques. Some of the main methods are covered in more detail in the sections below.

Minimal food-processing techniques

Minimal food-processing or preservation techniques are those that cause little change to the food's structure or nutritional properties, while giving sufficient treatment to the food to extend shelf life for the consumer beyond the limited number of days the food in its raw state would normally have. It is important to note that while changes to the food are minimised with these techniques, there may still be some minor nutrient losses. Table 5.1 summarises the main techniques.

Milling and polishing

Of the large number of processing operations and specialist food industries, milling and polishing deserve attention because they are extensively used to treat staple food items, particularly cereal grains.

Although the structures of the various cereal grains are different, there are some common features they all share (see Figure 5.1).

- **Bran**—the multilayered outer skin of the grain, which is rich in vitamins, minerals, phytonutrients and fibre.
- **Endosperm**—the food supply for the germ, which is dense in starchy carbohydrates and protein.
- **Germ**—the embryo, which contains the genetic material for a new plant, is abundant in essential fatty acids, vitamin E, B-group vitamins, minerals and phytonutrients.

The term 'whole grain' is used to describe an intact grain, flour or a food that contains all three parts of the grain. Processing grains does not necessarily produce 'refined grains' or exclude them from the Australian definition of a 'whole grain' (Grains & Legumes Nutrition Council 2018). Cereal grains may be milled and/or polished. Commercial production of wheat flour entails crushing kernels in a series of rollers (milling) and separating the fragments in a series of sieves; from these segments, either wholemeal or white flour can be produced. After milling, if all the various fractions (endosperm, bran and germ) are combined the result is wholemeal flour. White flour is obtained by excluding the branny outer layers and embryo (germ), leaving a flour enriched in starchy endosperm and depleted in dietary fibre, thiamin, plant oils and vitamin E (see chapters 16 and 17). This occurs because the distribution of nutrients is not uniform within the kernel, bran being relatively rich in dietary fibre, the germ rich in oil including vitamin E and other antioxidants, and the endosperm rich in starch. Similarly, white rice is produced by abrading (polishing) brown rice grains to remove the outer layers removing bran and germ. Cereals are used to produce a wide range of food products, including

Table 5.1: Minimal food-processing techniques

	Examples	Process	Potential impact on food
Membrane separation processes (concentrates solutions and selectively removes solutes by passing solution across a semi-permeable membrane)	Ultra-filtration	Low osmotic pressure used to remove large molecules, such as proteins and colloids; no heat applied.	Large pore sizes used may result in losses of sugars, water-soluble vitamins and amino acids where present.
	Reverse osmosis	High osmotic pressure concentrates solutions with low molecular solutes; no heat applied.	
Extraction (components removed from food at relatively low temperatures)	Supercritical fluid extraction	Substances above their critical temperature and pressure used as SCF, e.g. decaffeination of coffee, extraction of n-3 fatty acids from fish oils using carbon dioxide (critical temperature of 31.1°C).	No deleterious effect on flavour or composition, SCF not retained in end product, useful for heat-labile materials.
Encapsulation	Ingredients and/or food additives encapsulated within food matrix (Hsieh & Ofori 2007)	Encapsulation increases stability of product during thermal processing and controls the rate of release of the substance.	Reduced nutrient loss due to thermal processes, especially heat-sensitive vitamins such as thiamin, vitamin C.
Non-thermal processes	High-pressure treatment (Black et al. 2007, 2010; Ohlsson 1994)	Ruptures cell wall of microorganisms and inactivates enzymes; coagulates proteins or swells starches—may be combined with thermal processing or freezing.	Depending on the pressure applied, reversible or irreversible protein denaturation may occur.
	Electric pulse treatment	Field strengths of 10–20 kV/cm cause the rupture of cell membranes and therefore the inactivation of microorganisms—in particular, yeasts.	May help to preserve the antioxidant content of some foods such as fruit juices.
	Non-ionising radiation (Bhat et al. 2009; Hirneisen et al. 2009)	Use of radiation, e.g. ultra-violet (UV) radiation, may help to preserve the antioxidant content of fruit products, and reduce fungal load and, hence, the level of some mycotoxins in food.	

flour, bread, pastries, cakes, biscuits, breakfast cereals, pasta, noodles and savoury or sweet snacks.

Cooking foods

The colour and flavour of foods can be affected to varying degrees by cooking. For example, food boiled in water is blander and less coloured than when it is cooked in hot air (oven-baked) or hot oil (fried or roasted). The higher temperatures of roasting and baking develop appetising colours, flavours and aromas due to many factors, in particular two kinds of complex chemical reactions: **caramelisation** and **Maillard browning** (see Croxford and Stirling (2017) for more detail). The nutrient content of foods after cooking may vary from the original ingredients and between different cooking methods (FSANZ 2019).

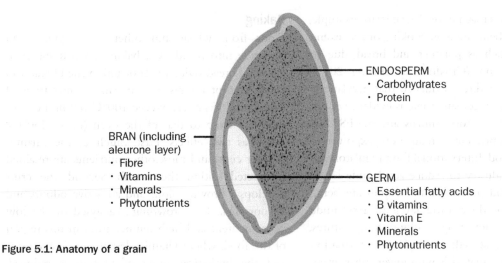

ENDOSPERM
· Carbohydrates
· Protein

BRAN (including aleurone layer)
· Fibre
· Vitamins
· Minerals
· Phytonutrients

GERM
· Essential fatty acids
· B vitamins
· Vitamin E
· Minerals
· Phytonutrients

Figure 5.1: Anatomy of a grain

WHAT IS THE DIFFERENCE BETWEEN WHOLEMEAL AND WHITE FLOUR?

Answer the following questions using the resources on the Food Standards Australia New Zealand and the Grains and Legumes Nutrition Council websites including:

- the *Australia New Zealand Food Standards Code*, Standard 2.1.1—Cereals and cereal products (Australian Government 2017a)
- the Australian Food Composition Database (previously known as NUTTAB) (FSANZ 2019)
- Grains and Legumes Nutrition Council (Grains & Legumes Nutrition Council 2019).

What is the legal definition of wholegrain flour?

How are the different flours produced?

How does production of these flours affect their nutrient content?

COMPARE AND CONTRAST NUTRIENT CONTENT OF RAW AND COOKED FOODS

Using the Australian Food Composition Database or equivalent (FSANZ 2019), compare and contrast the raw and cooked versions of the following foods. For each food, think about what your recommendation on food preparation would be to maximise the nutrient content of each food.

- carrot: raw, roasted, boiled (skin on, skin off)
- tomatoes: raw, sun-dried, tomato puree
- potatoes: raw, boiled, roasted, chips (shoestring), chips (wedges) (skin on, skin off)
- beef: raw, grilled, fried
- egg: raw, poached, fried.

Some reactions may not be desirable; for example, acrylamide may be formed on cooking or processing starchy foods, such as potatoes and bread, due to a Maillard reaction (Croxford & Stirling 2017). While there is no direct evidence that acrylamide can cause cancer in humans, there is evidence it can cause cancer in laboratory animals, and the FSANZ believes that it is prudent to reduce our exposure to acrylamide in food. International food regulators are working with industry to reduce acrylamide levels. New farming and processing techniques are being investigated to produce lower levels of acrylamide by, for example, lowering cooking temperatures, using enzymes that reduce acrylamide formation and obtaining raw materials with lower sugar levels. Genetically modified potato varieties have also been developed with low acrylamide-forming potential, and have been approved for use in Australia (FSANZ 2016a). However, reducing acrylamide in some foods, such as coffee, is difficult without changing its taste (FSANZ 2016a).

Baking

Flour from wheat and other cereal grains can be made into bread by a baking process, either as leavened bread (with yeast) or unleavened bread (no yeast). Except for biscuits, internal temperatures of baked products rarely exceed 100°C, but in the crust they rise close to that of the oven (up to 250°C). This has two effects. First, much of the thiamin (80 per cent) and most other nutrients are retained unaffected within the crumb. Second, the crust develops a brown colour and attractive odours and flavours (Maillard browning), catalysed by the low water content and high temperatures in this region of the food, where vitamin destruction is extensive and the biological value of protein is reduced. Products made with chemical leavening agents, such as baking powder (generating carbon dioxide gas), are virtually devoid of thiamin because the vitamin is unstable in the alkaline environment created by a residue of sodium carbonate.

HOW CAN I EAT LESS ACRYLAMIDE?

Acrylamide is a chemical compound used in the manufacture of polymers. In 2002 it was found to develop in food when starchy foods (such as potatoes) were heated above 120°C. Read the consumer information on acrylamide from FSANZ (www.foodstandards.gov.au/consumer/chemicals/acrylamide/pages/default.aspx) and, reflecting on your own diet, identify three ways you could reduce your consumption of acrylamide either through reducing your consumption or changing cooking practices.

Here are some tips for storing and cooking starchy foods.

- Don't store potatoes in the refrigerator or exposed to light, as this can increase the components that promote acrylamide formation.
- Soak potatoes in water for 15–30 minutes, or blanch in boiling water before frying or roasting; this reduces the components that promote acrylamide formation.
- Follow manufacturer's cooking instructions—many manufacturers have adjusted their instructions to reduce acrylamide levels in their foods.
- Cook potato products such as oven fries, hash browns and roast potatoes in a moderate oven (180–190°C) to a light golden colour only. Deep-fried chips should be cooked at a maximum of 175°C. Chunkier style chips are preferable.
- Toast bread or other foods to the lightest colour acceptable to your taste, noting that the crust will have higher levels of acrylamide.

Fermentation and pickling

Many societies have developed food processing methods that actually encourage the growth of microorganisms in order to transform a variety of plant and animal products into foods with a different taste and texture, which can sometimes be stored for longer periods than the raw materials from which they were made.

Fermentation in food processing is the process of converting carbohydrates to alcohol or organic acids using microorganisms, yeasts or bacteria, under **anaerobic** conditions. They use some of the nutrients in food for their own metabolism and growth, increasing their cell mass, and liberate the end products of their metabolism into the food (ethanol, lactic and other acids), inhibiting microbial growth. As a result, the fermented foods may have a different colour and nutrient content, altered digestibility, a sour taste if acid has been produced or an aerated (leavened) texture if gas was formed (Battcock & Azam-Ali 1998; Chadwick 2009).

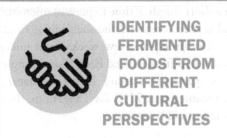

IDENTIFYING FERMENTED FOODS FROM DIFFERENT CULTURAL PERSPECTIVES

Different cultural groups have fermented foods to increase their shelf life. Identify the different bioactive products that are produced from the foods listed in a range of cultural groups. If you have not tried these, seek them out and reflect on the taste:

- cabbage
- milk
- fish
- wheat
- soybeans
- rice.

The manufacture of beverages containing ethanol (alcohol) is an ancient food-processing technique, used in early European, Greek and Roman societies. It was only relatively recently, however, that Louis Pasteur (1822–95) and others identified yeasts as being responsible for the fermentation of carbohydrate solutions from cereal grains or from grapes to produce ethanol in beer and wine respectively, as well as in many other types of beverage. The ethanol content of fermented beverages covers a wide range: from 1–3 per cent in African beers (keffir beers) to 40 per cent in spirits (such as whisky) (FSANZ 2019).

Similar processes take place in the leavening of bread (carbon dioxide produced by yeast activity), and in the preservation of sour foods with the production of lactic acid, such as sauerkraut and yoghurt. Fermentation of soybeans to produce sauces or condiments that impart a meat-like flavour was established more than 3000 years ago in China. Other widely consumed fermented foods include vinegar, olives and cheese. More localised foods prepared by fermentation may also be based on beans, grain, vegetables, fruit, honey, dairy products, fish, meat or tea. The composition of some fermented foods is controlled by the Food Standards Code; for example, beverage alcohol content, or chloroproponal (an undesirable by-product) content in naturally fermented soy sauce.

Cooking, baking, fermentation and pickling could all be described as ways of preserving food. Other methods of preserving foods to enable them to be transported or stored for longer periods of time is described below.

OTHER FOOD PRESERVATION TECHNIQUES

Food is an unstable biological material that decays as a result of **autolytic** processes, chemical oxidation and microbiological growth. Storage times vary from 1–2 days for animal and fish products to over a year for dried fruit, nuts and seeds. Since consumption rarely occurs at the time of harvest, and consumers are often geographically remote from the places of primary production on farms and at fisheries, there is a need to arrest the process of decay as soon as possible so that food can be stored and transported in good condition. There are many different processing operations used to achieve this objective, and these are described in the next section. They all have in common the creation of an environment in which the food is less susceptible to chemical or biological change and undesirable microbial growth.

The main food processing techniques used for food preservation include thermal processes, cold processing, control of the water content of the food and use of sugar, salt or other food additives (Figure 5.2).

The effects of these processes on nutrient content cannot be described in general terms, as the results can vary widely with both the food and the process involved. Nutrient losses, where they occur, usually affect the more heat-sensitive micronutrients, such as vitamin C and thiamin, as the macronutrients—fat, protein, carbohydrate and dietary fibre—are quite stable (for more information on macronutrients, see chapters 10 to 14), with the exception of polyunsaturated fat, which is vulnerable to developing unpleasant smells and tastes when exposed to oxygen. On the other hand, the concentration of foods by removal of water or other components can lead to an increase in the content of those nutrients that remain (per unit weight of the food).

High temperature methods

Heating methods include blanching, pasteurisation and sterilisation. At temperatures above about 60°C, some important changes occur in foods; contaminating microorganisms begin to lose their viability, internal enzymes become inactivated, texture can change and, at higher temperatures, cooked flavours develop.

Blanching involves immersion of the food briefly in boiling water or steam to inactivate enzymes in vegetables and reduce the level of microbial contamination. For example, blanching can be used to wilt leafy vegetables to facilitate packing in containers and as a pre-treatment to arrest undesirable changes, such as browning of peeled potatoes, before further processing.

During blanching, vegetables may lose a portion of their water-soluble vitamins (10–20 per cent of vitamin C), minerals and sugars through leaching, but these losses are only a part of the nutrient losses that may be sustained by foods that are subsequently dried, canned, boiled, fried or otherwise treated.

Pasteurisation is a relatively mild heat treatment applied for a short length of time to prevent microbial growth and is used to extend the shelf life of foods from a few days (milk) to a few weeks (fruit juice) or months (bottled fruit, canned beer). For example, milk can be pasteurised using high-temperature, short-time techniques at 72°C for 15 seconds, then rapidly cooled to kill bacteria.

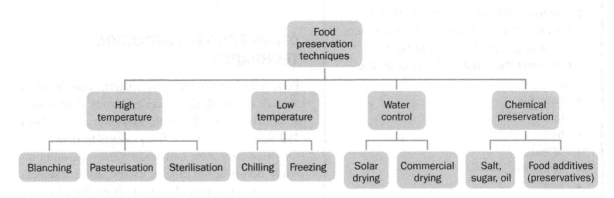

Figure 5.2: Food preservation techniques

Nutrient losses are usually small compared to other heat processes; for example, milk typically loses 25 per cent of vitamin C and 10 per cent of thiamin, vitamin B-6, B-12 and folic acid during pasteurisation.

Sterilisation uses high temperatures in excess of 100°C on foods for a sufficient duration to reduce the probability that bacteria that can cause disease (pathogenic) or their heat-resistant spores will survive to an acceptably low statistic. Under these conditions, foods are said to be commercially sterile. The best-known examples of this process are ultra-heat treatment (UHT) of liquids and canning. Milk and other liquid foods can be commercially sterilised by the use of UHT—for example, 140°C for two seconds—and can be stored in sealed cartons for several months without refrigeration. Fruit, vegetables, fish and meat may be canned, whereby food is cooked inside sealed metal containers. Processing temperatures and times are very carefully controlled and can closures monitored to ensure they are hermetically sealed to prevent recontamination (FSANZ 2018b).

The vigorous heat treatment used in canning may alter nutrient content—for example, reducing water-soluble or oxygen-labile nutrients such as B group vitamins and vitamin C as well as changing colour, flavour, aroma and texture (Rickman et al. 2007a; Rickman et al. 2007b). However, once sealed, foods treated in this way retain their nutrient content for several months, or even years, if kept in sterile containers. Not all changes are detrimental; the flavour developed in canned tomatoes, for example, is considered to be highly desirable.

Low temperature methods

Cooling methods include chilling and freezing. Cooling food to below ambient (room) temperature slows the rate of all reactions, whether chemical or biological, but although the shelf life is extended, many foods are still regarded as perishable items under these conditions.

Chilled storage employs temperatures of between −1°C and +8°C. It is used in the range −1°C to +1°C for fresh meat and fish, while milk products and baked goods such as pizza can be stored at slightly higher temperatures (0°C to +4°C). Butter, margarine and some cheeses can be held at up to +8°C.

The nutrient content of chilled foods should not be significantly reduced during storage provided the foods are not physically damaged and are consumed within the normal shelf life, although some tropical fruits do not store well.

Commercial freezing depends for its success on a rapid decline in temperature, which causes the formation of small ice crystals; although these rupture cell membranes, the damage to tissue structure is less severe than when large crystals are formed. During thawing of many frozen foods, cytoplasm (the liquid inside a cell) escapes (drips) and the original firmness and shape is lost. Frozen foods can be stored for up to a year when held at −18°C (the temperature of most domestic freezers) without undue loss of quality. Nutritional losses from freezing are usually small compared with those that occur during subsequent thawing and cooking.

Water control methods

Dehydration involves the removal of moisture from food by the application of heat. The residual water concentration is usually too low to support the growth of microbes and, providing the foods are kept dry, they can have a very long storage life.

Solar drying is extensively used in those parts of the world with abundant sunlight; traditionally, fruits, vegetables, fish and meat have been dehydrated this way. For example, many Asian open-air markets sell dried fish and dried fruits, but these can only be stored for a limited time, particularly if the atmosphere is humid.

Commercial drying may use large-scale spray, belt, fluidised bed, kiln, vacuum and hot roller driers and other methods in food factories and gives a greater degree of control over the rate and extent of water removal than solar drying. This makes it possible to manufacture a diverse range of storage stable products—for example, milk powder, infant formula, air-dried peas, freeze-dried peas, banana chips, egg powder, apple rings, potato powder and instant coffee, which are familiar items in retail outlets in most countries. These factory-made foods require specialised packaging if they are not to absorb moisture from the air and become spoiled through the growth of microbes on surfaces moistened by the hygroscopic (absorbs moisture out of the air) nature of the food.

Drying is carried out under a wide range of temperatures and conditions and it is not surprising that the nutrient losses are also very varied. Solar drying and air drying cause more nutritional damage than spray drying or freeze drying, with B group vitamins and vitamin C being most affected.

PHYSICAL PRESERVATION

Physical preservation includes packaging and storage of foods as well as techniques such as irradiation and other thermal processing.

Packaging and storage

Since wine was stored in pottery containers by people living in Mesopotamia more than 5000 years ago (Tannahill 1995), food has been packaged in one form or another. Packaging performs a multitude of functions, including prevention of contamination with microbes and undesirable chemicals, keeping foods dry or moist, acting as a barrier to light or gases, and preventing physical damage. The manufacture of food packaging is today a very large industry, producing diverse materials including glass, paper, plastics, metal foils, aluminium and steel cans, as well as composite materials of sophisticated design and engineering. Ideally, packaging should be inert both to the food and the external environment. Food businesses are responsible for ensuring the foods they sell are safe and suitable for consumption in Australia and New Zealand. All food sold must meet the requirements of the Food Acts in each Australian state and territory and in New Zealand, and Standards 1.1.1, 1.4.1, 2.6.2, 3.2.2, 4.2.1 and relevant schedules under the *Australia New Zealand Food Standards Code* (FSANZ 2018d). Careful selection of appropriate packaging materials can help ensure acceptable organoleptic (taste, texture) properties, stabilise nutrient content and ensure adequate hygiene.

The production of packaging is a relatively mature industry in Australia with limited overall growth (FSANZ 2017). A significant change since the 1990s has been the growth of the plastics sector at the expense of other materials (particularly metal cans). By international standards the Australian market is small, as the value of world packaging is estimated to be US$300 billion (PCA 2005). In 2009, 4000 billion pieces of packaging were sold globally; plastics represented 54 per cent of the global market share, followed by paper/cardboard (18 per cent), composites (11 per cent), metal (9 per cent) and glass (8 per cent) (Euromonitor International 2019).

The packaging supply chain includes a diverse range of businesses (Figure 5.3), including raw material providers, packaging manufacturers and suppliers, packaging converters, packaging importers and suppliers, food manufacturers, brand owners and retailers. Packaging is made explicitly for the products of the brand owners and the specifications of the packaging are set out by the brand owner. Retailers with private labels/home brands are the largest brand owners and are therefore a critical link in the packaging supply chain (FSANZ 2017). More novel packaging solutions are discussed in the section 'New and emerging technologies in food production'.

Food irradiation

Irradiation, which has been used to treat food since the late 1950s, provides processors with an alternative to chemical and heat treatments to reduce levels of harmful bacteria (and some viruses), alleviate pests of quarantine concern and extend the shelf life of foods. Research has shown that food irradiation is safe and effective. The process has been examined thoroughly by the World Health Organization, the United Nations Food and Agriculture Organization, the European Community Scientific Committee on Food, the US Food and Drug Administration, a United Kingdom House of Lords committee and by scientists at FSANZ. Irradiation of foods has been permitted in Australia and New Zealand since 2009. FSANZ must give permission before a food or group of foods can be irradiated under Standard 1.5.3—

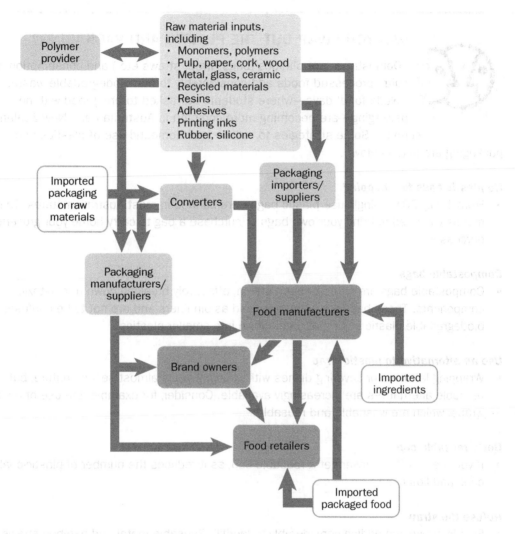

Figure 5.3: Overview of the packaging supply chain
Source: FSANZ (2017). Reproduced with permission

Irradiation of food, which lists foods permitted to be irradiated (Hyde et al. 2017; Roberts 2014).

FSANZ assessments consider:
- the technological need for the treatment
- the safety of the treatment
- effects on food composition
- any effects on the nutritional quality of the food.

FSANZ does not allow irradiation to be used to clean up food that is unsafe or unsuitable for human consumption (FSANZ 2018d). As of 2018, the following irradiated foods have been approved:

- herbs, spices and herbal infusions (under application A413)
- tropical fruits (mango, breadfruit, carambola, custard apple, litchi, longan, mangosteen, papaya and rambutan) (under application A443)
- persimmons (under application A1038)
- tomatoes and capsicums (under application A1069)
- apple, apricot, cherry, nectarine, peach, plum, honeydew, rockmelon, scallopini, strawberry, table grape, zucchini (courgette) (under application A1092)
- blueberries and raspberries (under application A1115).

CAN YOU SWAP OUT THE PLASTIC AND PACKAGING?

Domestic use of plastics (bags, wrap, straws etc.) and consumption of ultra-processed foods add considerably to non-biodegradable waste. 'Nude food' days—where students are asked to bring food with no packaging—are becoming more common in Australian and New Zealand schools. Some strategies to reduce your domestic use of plastics and packaging are listed below.

No plastic bags for shopping

- From 1 July 2018, single-use plastic bags were banned in most Australian states. This means you need to bring your own bags or purchase a bag to carry home your groceries and purchases.

Compostable bags

- Compostable bags are made of plant starch, effectively breaking down to non-toxic components. These bags are commonly sold as bin liners and are not to be confused with biodegradable plastic bags that break down into smaller plastics.

Use an alternative to plastic wrap

- Wrapping leftovers or covering dishes with plastic wrap is almost second nature, but reusable alternatives are increasingly available. Consider, for example, the use of beeswax wraps, which are washable and reusable.

Get a reusable cup

- If you are a coffee drinker get a reusable cup, as it reduces the number of plastic-coated cups and lids used.

Refuse the straw

- Plastic straws are adding considerably to landfill. Reusable metal and bamboo straws are becoming more popular (The Last Straw 2018).

The food is exposed to ionising radiation, either from gamma rays or a high-energy electron beam or powerful x-rays. Radiation is measured in kilograys (kGy). Technology allows for a precise dose to be measured. The doses permitted range from a maximum of 1 kGy for some fruits and vegetables up to 30 kGy for herbs and spices. A food that has been irradiated, or food that contains irradiated ingredients or components, must be labelled to show that the food, ingredients or components have been treated with ionising radiation (Standard 1.5.3—Irradiation of Food). If the food is not normally required to be labelled, such as fresh fruit and vegetables, then the required labelling must be displayed close to the food.

Other thermal processing techniques

Table 5.2 provides some examples of other thermal techniques used to preserve foods.

Table 5.2: Other thermal processing techniques

Examples	Process	Comments
Continuous microwaving (Fellows 2009)	Used for pasteurisation, sterilisation, drying, blanching, thawing and tempering of frozen foods and baking—microorganisms killed via thermal effect.	Variable composition of food may lead to 'hot' or 'cold' spots with variable levels of destruction and level of control.
Ohmic heating (Shiby Varghese et al. 2014)	Electric current passed through an electrically conducting food, which is converted to thermal energy with heat being distributed evenly.	Heated products can be aseptically packaged to enable the product to be shelf-stable.
Micronisation	Mid-infra-red wavelength range (1.8–3.4 micrometres) applied, usually, for less than five minutes to reduce microbial load, gelatinise starch in cereals and reduce the activity of anti-nutritional factors such as trypsin inhibitors in cereals.	

CHEMICAL PRESERVATION

Many chemical agents are added to food to create an environment unsuitable for the growth of food spoilage microorganisms—for example, salt, sugar and other food additives.

Salt has a long history of use and works by creating a high **osmotic pressure** (reducing water activity), preventing microbial cells from taking up the water they need for growth. When used at relatively high concentrations, such as in salami sausages (10 per cent salt) and brine (10 per cent salt) in bottles of olives, salt is very effective.

Sugar is used to preserve foods and also acts via osmotic pressure to reduce the water available for microbial cell growth. Examples of foods preserved by high concentrations of sugar include fruit preserves such as jams and marmalades.

Oil may be used to assist in preservation of foods but there is a risk that 'home-preserved' vegetables in oil (including garlic, sun-dried tomatoes, chilli, ginger, eggplant, capsicum and mushrooms) could support the growth of pathogenic organisms.

Chemical preservatives or food additives are generally used at much lower levels than salt or sugar because they are more toxic to cells of bacteria, yeast and moulds and thus less is needed to achieve the desired technological function of preservation. Their use is subject to strict legislative controls set out in the *Australia New Zealand Food Standards Code*, Chapters 1.1.1 and 1.3.1 (Food Additives) and Schedules 7, 8 and 14–16 (Australian Government

WHAT WOULD BE YOUR STORAGE ADVICE?

Over time, manufacturers have reduced the amount of salt and sugar used in their products. This can change the storage of particular items. What would be your advice on the storage of these products and why?

- Vegemite/Marmite
- peanut butter/salt-reduced peanut butter
- soy sauce/salt-reduced soy sauce
- jam.

2017b, 2017d). Preservatives alone do not confer long storage life and are usually employed in conjunction with the other methods, such as pasteurisation (fruit juices), dehydration (dried fruit), cooking (canned foods) and packaging (various containers and wraps).

FOOD ADDITIVES

Food additives play an important part in ensuring our food is safe and meets the needs of consumers. When added to food during processing, they may improve sensory characteristics, the stability and quality of food, including nutrient content, and/or extend shelf life (FSANZ 2016b). For a complete list of additives permitted for use in Australia and New Zealand, refer to the *Australia New Zealand Food Standards Code,* Standard 1.3.1—Food Additives (Australian Government 2017b). Some food additives have more than one use and some have restrictions on their use. Examples of the most common class names are listed below.

- **Acids/acidity regulators/alkalis** help to maintain a constant acid level in food. This is important for taste, as well as to influence how other substances in the food function. For example, an acidified food can retard the growth of some microorganisms.
- **Anti-caking agents** improve flow characteristics and reduce the tendency of individual food particles to adhere. For example, seasoning that contains an added anti-caking agent flows freely and doesn't clump together.
- **Antioxidants** retard or prevent the oxidative deterioration of foods. For example, in fats and oils, rancid flavours can develop when they are exposed to oxygen.
- **Bulking agents** contribute to the volume of the food without contributing significantly to its available energy. For example, some low-joule foods need bulking agents added to them to replace the bulk normally provided by sugar.
- **Colours** add or restore colour to foods, e.g. icing mixture is coloured to make it more attractive on cakes.
- **Emulsifiers** facilitate or prevent oil and water from separating into layers, e.g. emulsifiers may be used in margarine to prevent oil forming a layer on top of the margarine.
- **Flavour enhancers** enhance the existing taste and/or odour of a food.
- **Firming agents/stabilisers** maintain the uniform dispersion of substances in solid and semi-solid foods.
- **Foaming agents** maintain the uniform dispersion of gases in aerated foods.
- **Gelling agents** modify the texture of the food through gel formation.

- **Glazing agents** impart a coating to the external surface of the food, e.g. a wax coating on fruit to improve its appearance.
- **Humectants** reduce moisture loss in foods, e.g. glycerine may be added to icing to prevent it from drying out.
- **Preservatives** retard or prevent the deterioration of food by microorganisms and thus prevent spoilage of foods.
- **Raising agents** liberate gases, thereby increasing the volume of a food, and are often used in baked goods.
- **Sweeteners** replace the sweetness normally provided by sugars in foods without contributing significantly to their available energy.
- **Thickeners** increase the viscosity of a food, e.g. a sauce might contain a thickener to give it the desired consistency.

Food additives in most packaged food must be listed in the statement of ingredients on the label by their class name followed by the name of the food additive or the food additive number—for example, Colour (Caramel I) or Colour (150a). Most flavourings (or flavours) do not need to be named or identified by a food additive number and can be labelled by their class name only (for more about additive labelling, see FSANZ 2016d).

Applications can be made to FSANZ to extend the range of use of existing food additives or for new additives. This requires sufficient information to be submitted in the application to enable FSANZ to assess the additive's technological function and benefits as well as potential health and safety risks, as specified in the FSANZ Application Handbook (see Chapter 6) (FSANZ 2016c).

FOOD MODIFICATIONS AND NOVEL FOODS

One of the advantages of the food processing system is that it has been able to develop a range of modified foods to meet specific needs. Major developments are summarised in Table 5.3. These foods are specifically formulated to meet a particular dietary requirement,

FOOD ADDITIVES AND HYPERACTIVITY IN CHILDREN

In the late 1970s early 1980s, Ben Feingold hypothesised that hyperactive behaviour and associated learning difficulties in children were linked to the consumption of food additives (in particular, artificial colours and flavours) and salicylates. Most of the studies linking food additive consumption were based on small numbers and were poorly designed. However, a UK study that was randomised, double-blind and placebo-controlled tested the effects of the preservative sodium benzoate and six artificial food colourings on hyperactivity in 153 preschoolers. The colours studied were tartrazine (102), quinoline yellow (104), sunset yellow FCF (110), carmoisine (122), ponceau 4R (124) and allura red AC (129). The study concluded that consumption of these additives could explain about 10 per cent of the behavioural difference between a child with attention deficit hyperactivity disorder (ADHD) and one without the disorder (Schab & Trinh 2004). These colours are typically found in ultra-processed foods (soft drink, lollies, cheese snacks) and consumption should therefore be minimised as these foods are typically energy dense and nutrient poor.

The European Union has put a warning on foods containing six colouring agents that it says may cause hyperactivity in children. The Food and Drug Administration in the USA has not indicated a link between artificial food colours and hyperactivity in children. FSANZ has assessed the consumption of colouring agents among children and has found very low consumption, with even the highest consumers well within the Acceptable Daily Intake and found that a ban is not warranted (FSANZ 2012).

Using your skills in searching scientific literature, determine the current evidence on food colouring agents and hyperactivity disorder. Based on this evidence, write a letter to FSANZ as to whether there should or should not be a review of permitted colouring in the Australian and New Zealand food supply.

---

such as gluten-free foods for people with coeliac disease, low-energy foods for people consuming reduced-energy diets, carbohydrate-modified foods for people with diabetes and lactose-free foods for people with lactose intolerance. Public health policies aim to improve the health of citizens and reduce the risk of disease. The *Australian Dietary Guidelines* list measures for consumers to adopt to improve their health and lower their risk of developing chronic diseases (NHMRC 2013). For example, the guidelines advise the consumption of a diet that is moderate in total fat and, in particular, low in saturated fat.

The food-processing industry has developed foods with either an increased or reduced level of biologically active components with the aim of increasing the choice for consumers, enabling them to follow dietary guidelines to improve health and/or reduce the risk of diet-related disease (see Table 5.3). The *Australia New Zealand Food Standards Code* permits certain **nutrition content** and **health claims** to be made on individual food products, providing certain compositional requirements are met (Standard 1.2.7—Nutrition, health and related claims) (Australian Government 2018).

Foods that are developed to offer consumers a choice when selecting an appropriate diet must retain their appeal or they will not be consumed. The need for a low or reduced fat content, for example, requires developing foods that retain their organoleptic and physical properties, and therefore their appeal. Replacing sugar with intense sweeteners

Table 5.3: Modified foods

	Examples	Process	Food Standards Code
Fortification of food with additional nutrients to replace losses from processing or to achieve equivalence to counterpart food (WHO & FAO 2006)	Thiamin in wheat flour for breadmaking (replacement of processing losses). Vitamin D in margarine (equivalent level to that found in butter).	Add additional nutrients during processing.	Specific food standards: Standard 2.2.1—Cereal and cereal products: Wheat flour that is sold as suitable for making bread to which this section applies . . . must contain no less than 6.4 mg/kg thiamin. Standard 2.4.2—Edible oil spreads: A food that is sold as a 'table' edible oil spread . . . or margarine . . . must contain no less than 55 µg/kg of vitamin D.
Fortification of food with additional nutrients: mandatory or voluntary addition of nutrients (WHO & FAO 2006)	Range of vitamins and minerals may be added to all breakfast cereals (12 permitted); vitamin D to breakfast cereals meeting set nutrition criteria. Mandatory addition of folic acid to flour for bread making and iodine to salt used in bread.	Add additional nutrients during processing.	Voluntary addition requirements: Standard 1.3.2—Vitamins and minerals; with Schedule 17—Vitamins and minerals; with reference to Standard 1.2.7—Nutrition, health and related claims Standard 1.2.8—Nutrition Information Requirements, and Schedules 11–13. Mandatory iodine and folic acid requirements: Standard 1.2.1—Cereal and cereal products.
Reduced-fat foods	Reduced-fat cheese, milk, yoghurts.	Use ingredients low or reduced in fat or add other ingredients to replace the functional roles of fat (fat replacers generally aim to mimic the mouthfeel and texture of fat).	Standard 1.2.8—Nutrition information requirements: Low-fat foods must contain less than 3 g fat per 100 g or less than 1.5 g fat per 100 g. Reduced fat foods must have a reduction of at least 25 per cent of the total fat content compared with the same quantity of the reference food and an absolute reduction of at least 3 g fat per 100 g of food (or a reduction of 1.5 g fat per 100 g of liquid food).
Low-energy foods	Low-energy drinks, e.g. diet cola drinks.	Substitute lower-energy ingredients for higher-energy ingredients (e.g. intense sweeteners may replace sugar).	Standard 1.2.7—Nutrition, health and related claims: Required to contain no greater than 170 kJ per 100 g of solid or semi-solid food and a maximum of 80 kJ per 100 mL for beverages and liquid foods.

	Examples	Process	Food Standards Code
Carbohydrate-modified foods	Boiled sweets, chocolate for people with diabetes.	Replace sugars (monosaccharides and disaccharides) with sugar alcohols or polyols.	Standard 1.3.1—Food Additives
Gluten-free or low-gluten foods	Gluten-free flour, pasta, noodles, cakes.	Gluten-free foods can be formulated by using cereal grains where gluten has been removed or by substituting other non-gluten-containing cereals for wheat, barley, oats, rye and triticale, e.g. rice, corn (maize), buckwheat or legumes (such as soybeans).	Standard 1.2.7 Free: The food must not contain – (a) detectable gluten; or (b) oats or their products; or (c) cereals containing gluten that have been malted, or their products Low: The food contains no more than 20 mg gluten per 100 g of the food.
Lactose-free foods	Lactose-free milk, yoghurt, cheese, dairy desserts.	Products are formulated using ingredients that are lactose-free such as soy protein isolates and/or ingredients where lactose has been wholly or partially removed.	Standard 1.2.7 The food contains no detectable lactose.
'Probiotics' (viable microorganisms that benefit health by improving the intestinal microbial balance) and 'prebiotic' foods (used to promote the growth of good bacteria)	Fermented dairy products such as yoghurt, lassi.	Foods with probiotics must contain living microorganisms in appreciable numbers at the end of the product's shelf life. The choice of strain of microorganism is important to avoid removal of micronutrients from the food, production of adverse components such as vasoactive amine, opportunistic lactic acid bacterial pathogens.	No formal definitions for terms 'probiotics' and 'prebiotics' in the Food Standards Code.
Formulated caffeinated beverages (contain caffeine and have the purpose of enhancing mental performance)	Sports drinks.	Flavoured non-alcoholic beverages to which other substances (carbohydrates, amino acids, vitamins) may be added as well as caffeine during processing.	Standard 2.6.4—Formulated caffeinated beverages 'must contain no less than 145 mg/L and no more than 320 mg/L of caffeine in total, from any source . . . and may contain a listed substance' (see Schedule 26).
Special purpose foods	Infant formula, infant foods, formulated meal supplements, foods for special medical purposes.	Foods formulated for specific groups.	Standards 2.9.1 to 2.9.6, Schedule 29.

may provide equivalent sweetness but care must be taken to find other modifying agents to replace the technical function of sugars in these foods as required. Sugar(s) may also function as a preservative (by lowering water activity) in foods, caramelise baked goods, absorb moisture to delay staling and texturise the crumb in baked goods, provide bulk and volume and act as a **substrate** for fermentation.

Novel foods are foods that do not have history of use of human consumption in a given country, such as Australia or New Zealand. Non-traditional foods are foods that may be used elsewhere in the world but not in the country of interest. In most countries novel and non-traditional foods are subject to a pre-market assessment, to review health and safety issues, prior to approval for use as a food or food ingredient. Approved foods are listed in the *Australia New Zealand Food Standard Code*, with conditions of use given; examples include phytosterols, phytostanols and their esters, which can be added to edible oil spreads, breakfast cereals or yoghurt to reduce consumers' blood cholesterol, and the use of novel sugars D-tagatose and trehalose to replace sugars and other carbohydrates (see Standard 1.5.1—Novel foods, Schedule 25) (Australian Government 2017c).

NEW AND EMERGING TECHNOLOGIES IN FOOD PRODUCTION

Recent improvements in traditional forms of food processing have included the production of traditional and new food ingredients and components from biotechnology, and the development of improved packaging materials (WHO 2005). Recent developments in food technologies have enabled the production of some foods with improved nutritional value, organoleptic properties, convenience and lower cost. Advances in the food industry also include efforts to develop sustainable agricultural practices and to develop environmentally friendly packaging materials while still retaining the essential characteristics of the food and ensuring that it is microbiologically and chemically safe (see Figure 5.4).

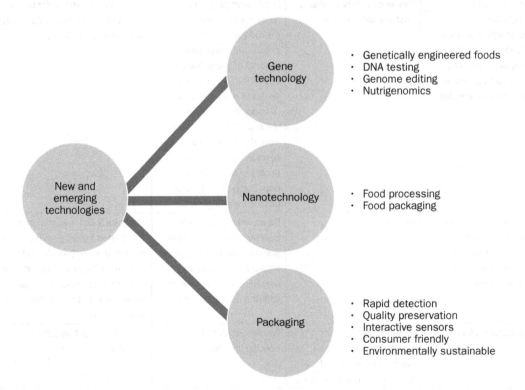

Figure 5.4: New and emerging technologies

Gene technology

'Gene technology' is the name given to a range of activities concerned with understanding gene expression, taking advantage of natural genetic variation, modifying genes and transferring genes to new hosts. Genes are found in all living organisms and are passed on from one generation to the next. They are the coded instructions an organism uses to make proteins, and it is these proteins that make up the structures and perform the functions of living things (CSIRO 2015).

People have been manipulating the genetic make-up of plants and animals for countless generations. This is referred to as traditional cross-breeding and involves selecting plants and animals with the most desirable characteristics (e.g. disease resistance, high yield, good meat quality) for breeding the next generation. Current techniques use new ways of identifying particular characteristics and transferring them between living organisms. For example, it is now possible to make a copy of a particular gene from the cells of a plant, animal or microbe, and insert the copy into the cells of another organism to give a desired characteristic. It is also possible to silence a gene using RNA interference, a way of reducing or switching off the activity of genes which now enables scientists around the world to target specific gene activity (CSIRO 2015). Emerging technologies such as genome editing which modifies genomes of organisms, are also now available (FSANZ 2018c). The actual process of genetic modification is done mainly using one of two techniques: 'agrobacterium-mediated transformation' and 'biolistic transformation'. An example of agrobacterium-mediated transformation is provided in Figure 5.5.

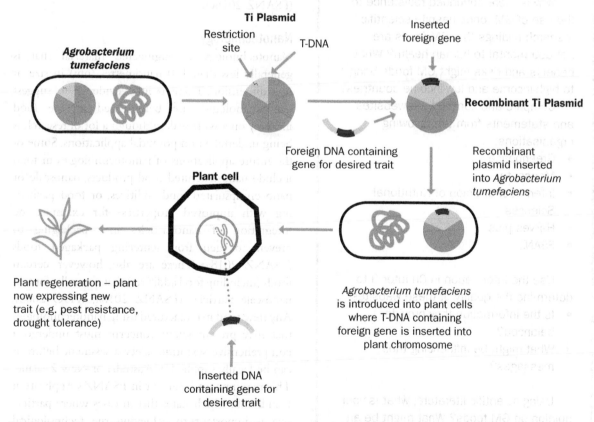

Note: Restriction site = short DNA sequences recognised by a restriction enzyme where foreign genetic material is inserted; Plasmid = small circular DNA separate from the chromosomal DNA; T-DNA = transfer DNA, DNA from plasmid that can be transferred to a plant; Ti plasmid = tumour-inducing plasmid

Figure 5.5: Agrobacterium-mediated transformation

Foods derived from genetically modified organisms are called genetically modified or 'GM' foods. All of the GM foods approved so far in Australia and New Zealand are from GM plants— for example, corn plants with a gene that makes them resistant to insect attack, or soybeans with a modified fatty acid content that makes the oil better suited for frying.

In Australia, the Office of the Gene Technology Regulator oversees the development and environmental release of GM organisms under the *Gene Technology Act 2000* (Australian Government 2016). In New Zealand, similar functions are undertaken by the Environmental Protection Authority (Environmental Protection Authority of New Zealand 2019) under the *Hazardous Substances and New Organisms Act 1996*. GM foods are regulated under Standard 1.5.2—Food produced using gene technology, in the *Food Standards Code* (Australian Government 2019). Approved GM foods are listed in Schedule 26 of the *Food Standards Code*. Anyone seeking to amend the Code to include a new GM food is required to make an application to FSANZ (FSANZ 2016c).

WHY IS THE DEVELOPMENT OF GM FOODS SO CONTROVERSIAL?

This is an example of systems thinking as it involves the intersection of agricultural, environmental, marketing and biological systems.

Why is there continued resistance to the use of GM foods despite scientific research findings that GM foods are not detrimental to human health? What benefits and risks might GM foods bring to high-income and low-income countries?

Compare and contrast the websites and statements from the following organisations:
- Greenpeace
- Monsanto
- International Union of Nutritional Sciences
- Harvestplus
- FSANZ.

Use the information in Chapter 3 to determine the quality of these websites.
- Is the information they provide balanced?
- What might be influencing their messages?

Using scientific literature, what is your opinion on GM foods? What might be an alternative to GM foods?

Nanotechnology

Nanotechnology is engineered material that is generally less than 100 nanometres (nm) in size in one dimension. There is little evidence to suggest nanotechnologies are being used in the food industry on a wide scale, although a lot of research is being undertaken on potential applications. Some of the future applications of nanotechnologies in food include nanostructured food products, nanoscale or nano-encapsulated food additives, or food packaging with improved properties—for example, the integration of nanoparticles into packaging to prevent oxygen from entering packaged foods (FSANZ 2018a). There are also, however, certain foods (including food additives) that naturally contain nanoscale particles (FSANZ 2018a; WHO 2005). Any new food manufactured using nanotechnologies that may present safety concerns must undergo a comprehensive scientific safety assessment before it can be legally supplied in Australia or New Zealand. This requirement is set out in FSANZ's Application Handbook, which states that in cases where particle size is important to achieving the technological function, or may relate to a difference in toxicity, information must be provided on particle size, size distribution, and morphology, as well as any size-dependent properties (FSANZ 2016c).

Food-based applications for nanotechnology might include the potential enhanced bioavailability of nutrients; less use of fat; improvement in stability, consistency, taste and texture; and traceability and security of food products (Chaudhry et al. 2008; Drew & Hagen 2016; Hannon et al. 2015). Table 5.4 lists potential applications of nanoparticles.

Packaging
Vacuum and modified atmosphere packaging
Vacuum packaging involves placing the product in a plastic or aluminium foil pouch and withdrawing most of the air prior to sealing (0.3 to 3 per cent may remain). *Sous-vide* is a processing technique where food is vacuum-packed then heated (usually pasteurised) to extend shelf life while maintaining organoleptic qualities. Products are vacuum-packed prior to pasteurisation, giving an improved shelf life under refrigerated conditions (less than 3°C).

Modified atmosphere packaging (MAP) relies on altering the composition of gases in contact with the food within the package by replacing air with a single gas or mixture of gases, combined with low temperature storage (less than 3°C). Increasing the concentration of carbon dioxide (up to 10 per cent) inhibits the growth of bacteria and fungi. Typically, concentrations of carbon dioxide of 20–100 per cent are used in MAP. Depending on the type of food being stored, oxygen concentrations may be nil or very low, excepting MAP of fresh red meats where oxygen is important in maintaining a 'fresh' red colour. Nitrogen is often used to displace oxygen. The aim of MAP is to exclude oxygen and retain the moisture content of the food, as well as to inhibit the growth of **aerobic** microorganisms. Facultative anaerobic bacteria such as *Clostridia* and *Enterobacteriaceae* (for example, *E. coli*, *Salmonella*) are less affected by MAP than aerobic microorganisms. Under anaerobic conditions, control of anaerobic pathogens requires particular attention to the water activity and pH of the product, and to storage temperature. The Hazard

Table 5.4: Potential applications for nanoparticles in foods and food packaging

Potential use	Example
Improve the bioavailability of nutrients	Nanomaterials used to encapsulate vitamins, colours and other food additives.
Reduced fat products	Texture and consistency mimics the creaminess of higher fat products.
Improvements in product stability and consistency	Altering the colour, flavour, texture, consistency.
Improved sensory qualities and appearance	Developing new tastes and sensations in the mouth.
Water filters	To remove pathogenic bacteria and viruses.
Packaging materials	Improved flexibility, biodegradable packaging materials with improved mechanical properties, improved gas barrier properties, improved temperature and moisture stability (e.g. nanoclays).
'Active' packaging that improves food safety and quality	Incorporation of anti-microbial nanoparticles (for example, nanosilver to reduce microbial growth on packaging surface) or oxygen-scavenging nanoparticles.
'Smart' packaging incorporating nanosensors to monitor and report the condition of the food	Detection of leaks for foods packed under vacuum or inert atmosphere, indications of time–temperature variations such as freeze–thaw–freeze, rapid detection of bacteria or viruses.
'Smart' packaging materials containing nanobarcodes within the printing inks or coatings	Product traceability and authenticity.

Analysis and Critical Control Points (HACCP) system (see Chapter 7) is important in ensuring that attention to temperature control, for example, is maintained (see Stewart 2013).

Packaging materials commonly used for MAP of fruits and vegetables are flexible plastic films, typically PVC, polyethylene, polypropylene and polystyrene. Films with varying permeability to oxygen, carbon dioxide and water vapour are used for different applications. The choice of a flexible packaging material depends on the recommended storage temperature of the final product, the relative humidity within the package, the respiration rate of the produce and the effect, if any, of light on the contents (for example, potatoes need to be packed in opaque films to prevent solanine (the poisonous substance in green potatoes) development). Vacuum-packing and MAP reduce oxidative rancidity and are therefore useful for products prone to rancidity, such as high-fat foods.

Active packaging

In active packaging, materials are added to modify the composition of gases during storage. Oxygen scavengers (absorbers) present in the food package reduce the level of oxygen in the headspace (the space between the top of the food and the packaging material). Ionic iron (Fe^{2+}) is often used, and is oxidised to Fe^{3+}. Reducing the level of oxygen in the headspace reduces the growth of aerobic microorganisms and delays the development of oxidative rancidity. Another example of active packaging is the use of ethylene scavengers in films produced for packaging fruits and vegetables. As fruits and vegetables ripen, they release the ripening-stimulating hormone ethylene; by scavenging the ethylene, the ripening process is delayed, thereby increasing the shelf life. Other potential applications include incorporating ascorbic acid or vitamin E (vitamin antioxidants) into packaging films to retard the oxidation of food components (Brody et al. 2008). Another form of active packaging are films made from chitosan which may be generated from recycling crustacean shells. Chitosan coating protects fresh vegetables and fruits from fungal degradation possibly by acting as a barrier between the nutrients contained in the produce and microorganisms (Appendini & Hotchkiss 2002).

WHAT IS 3D PRINTED FOOD?

3D printing, also referred to as additive manufacturing, refers to the process whereby specialised computer programs direct a printer to build a 3D object. 3D objects are created by melting plastic or other material and building the desired design by laying down consecutive material layers. This technology has also been extended to food manufacturing, using a similar principle to standard 3D printers but with plastic being replaced by food ingredients such as sugar, chocolate and dough. Food particles in a semi-liquefied form are layered consecutively from syringes or nozzles onto a platform to 'build' a processed food (Lam et al. 2002).

So, what food products can be produced by these specialised printers? Common uses include the production of highly intricate chocolate designs, pasta and even printed pizza; the main limitation is that food must be in the form of a paste to be printed (Sun et al. 2015). A range of 3D food printers are now available for home and commercial use, but typically (as of 2019) these are very expensive. Overcoming consumer attitudes may be a key challenge (Lupton & Turner 2018).

Edible coatings

Edible coatings for foods may be made from films of proteins, waxes or polysaccharides. The coatings protect the food from external oxygen, minimise loss of water vapour (moisture) and volatile components, and may also reduce microbial contamination. Applications are likely for products that are dry, frozen and semi-moist, and fresh and minimally processed fruits and vegetables (Lin & Zhao 2007).

Biodegradable food packaging

New developments in food packaging in Australia and New Zealand include the introduction of environmentally friendly biodegradable packaging materials to reduce waste. An example is packaging trays made from cotton residue, rice straw and residue from palm production.

Self-heating packaging

Recent developments include the inclusion of calcium or magnesium oxide and water to generate exothermic (heat-producing) reactions within the food package. The heating device occupies approximately half of the total package volume and has applications including plastic coffee cans, military rations and on-the-go meals (Brody et al. 2008).

SUMMARY

- Food processing describes the transformation of raw ingredients using mechanical and/or chemical methods to change or preserve food. The food and beverage processing and manufacturing sector is a key employer and economic resource in Australia and New Zealand.
- Processing of foods dramatically increases the variety of food products available—for example, from wheat, processing can produce cereal flakes, breads, cakes, biscuits and pasta. Changes from processing, however, can come at a cost, with reduced or modified nutritional content of processed foods compared to the original foods or food ingredients.
- The main methods used for food preservation can be classified as high temperature, cold temperature, control of water content, chemical and physical preservation methods. The impact of preservation on the nutrient content and sensory characteristics of foods depends on the type of food and technique of preservation.
- Chemical additives have important roles in ensuring food safety and improving the characteristics of processed foods. Common reasons for using additives are to extend the shelf life and safety of food, enhance sensory characteristics and improve quality and stability.
- New and emerging food production technologies may produce foods with higher nutritional values, enhanced organoleptic properties, improved convenience and/or lower cost. Many of these technologies are controversial, with consumers having concerns around safety and environmental impact. Minimal processing techniques such as ohmic heating promise extended shelf life for foods while retaining the natural organoleptic and nutritional qualities of foods.
- Packaging of food has been used for thousands of years. A wide variety of packaging materials are used today to protect food from physical damage and biological and chemical contamination. Advanced packaging includes vacuum and modified air packaging, while active and smart packaging use materials that dynamically alter gas composition and inhibit microbial growth.

KEY TERMS

Aerobic: refers to presence of oxygen; in particular the growth of bacteria and yeasts in the presence of oxygen

Agribusiness: the group of industries dealing with agricultural produce and services required in farming. Includes agrichemicals, breeding, production, distribution, machinery, seed supply and marketing.

Anaerobic: refers to the absence of oxygen; in particular, the growth of bacteria and yeasts in the absence of oxygen.

Autolytic: known as self-digestion, refers to the destruction of a cell through the action of its own enzymes.

Caramelisation: the oxidation of sugar as a result of cooking for both sweet and savoury foods, resulting in a nutty flavour and brown colour.

Health claim: a claim that states, suggests or implies that a food or a property of food has, or may have, a health effect (Australian Government 2018). A health effect means an effect on the human body, including an effect on one or more of the following:
- biochemical process outcome
- physiological process or outcome
- functional process or outcome
- growth and development
- physical performance
- mental performance
- a disease, disorder or condition.

Maillard browning: a chemical reaction between amino acids and reducing sugars that gives browned food its distinctive flavour.

Nutrition content claim: a claim that is about the presence or absence of a biologically active substance; dietary fibre; energy; minerals; potassium; protein; carbohydrate; fat; the components of any one of protein, carbohydrate or fat; salt; sodium; or vitamins, or a claim that is about glycaemic index or glycaemic load.

Osmotic pressure: the pressure created when water passes across a membrane from a more concentrated solvent (or a more dilute solution) to a less concentrated solvent (or a more concentrated solution), for example, when you have a cucumber in brine and the water from inside the cells of the cucumber crosses the cell membrane into the surrounding brine.

Substrate: a substance (also called a reactant) that reacts with a reagent or another substance to generate a product.

ACKNOWLEDGEMENT

This chapter has been modified and updated from those written by Gwynn Jones, Louise Lennard, Janis Baines and Ingrid R.E. Rutishauser, which appeared in the third edition of *Food and Nutrition*.

REFERENCES

Appendini, P. & Hotchkiss, J.H., 2002, 'Review of antimicrobial food packaging', *Innovative Food Science & Emerging Technologies, 3*(2): 113–26, doi:10.1016/S1466-8564(02)00012-7

Australian Government. 2016, *Gene Technology Act 2000*, <www.legislation.gov.au/Details/C2016C00792>, accessed 23 January 2019

—— 2017a, *Cereals and Cereal Products* (Standard 2.1.1), <www.foodstandards.gov.au/code/Pages/default.aspx>, accessed 23 January 2019

—— 2017b, *Food Additives* (Standard 1.3.1), <www.legislation.gov.au/Series/F2015L00396>, accessed 22 January 2019

—— 2017c, *Novel Foods* (Standard 1.5.1), <www.legislation.gov.au/Details/F2017C00324>, accessed 22 January 2019

—— 2017d, *Structure of the Code and General Provisions*, <www.legislation.gov.au/Series/F2015L00383>, accessed 22 January 2019

—— 2018, *Nutrition, Health and Related Claims* (Standard 1.2.7), <www.legislation.gov.au/Details/F2018C00942>, accessed 14 July 2019

—— 2019, *Food Produced Using Gene Technology* (1.5.2), <www.legislation.gov.au/Details/F2019C00131>, accessed 14 July 2019

Battcock, M. & Azam-Ali, S., 1998, *Fermented Fruits and Vegetables: A Global Perspective* (FAO Agricultural Services Bulletin No. 134), <www.fao.org/docrep/x0560e/x0560e07.htm>, accessed 22 January 2019

Bhat, R., Rai, R.V. & Karim, A.A., 2009, 'Mycotoxins in food and feed: Present status and future concerns', *Comprehensive Reviews in Food and Feed: Present Status and Future Concerns, 9*(1): 57–81, doi:10.1111/j.1541-4337.2009.00094.x

Black, E.P., Hirneisen, K.A., Hoover, D.G. & Kniel, K.E., 2010, 'Fate of Escherichia coli O157:H7 in ground beef following high-pressure processing and freezing', *Journal of Applied Microbiology, 108*(4): 1352–60, doi:10.1111/j.1365-2672.2009.04532.x

Black, E.P., Setlow, P., Hocking, A.D., Stewart, C.M., Kelly, A.L. & Hoover, D.G., 2007, 'Response of spores to high-pressure processing', *Comprehensive Reviews in Food Science and Food Safety, 6*: 103–19, doi:10.1111/j.1541-4337.2007.00021.x

Brody, A.L., Bugusu, B., Han, J.H., Sand, C.K. & McHugh, T.H., 2008, 'Scientific status summary: Innovative food packaging solutions', *Journal of Food Science, 73*(8): R107–16, doi:10.1111/j.1750-3841.2008.00933.x

Chadwick, J., 2009, *The Beginner's Guide to Preserving Food At Home: Easy instructions for canning, freezing, drying, brining, and root cellaring your favorite fruits, herbs and vegetables* (3rd edn), Massachusetts, MA: Storey Publishing

Chaudhry, Q., Scotter, M., Blackburn, J., Ross, B., Boxall, A. et al., 2008, 'Applications and implications of nanotechnologies for the food sector', *Food Additives and Contaminants, 25*(3): 241–58, doi:10.1080/02652030701744538

Chaustowski, R. & Dolman, S., 2015, *Australia's Food and Agribusiness Sector – Data Profile*, Canberra: Commonwealth of Australia, <https://archive.industry.gov.au/industry/IndustrySectors/FoodManufacturingIndustry/Documents/Food-and-Agribusiness-Data-Pack.pdf>, accessed 21 February 2019

Croxford, S. & Stirling, E., 2017, *Understanding the Science of Food: From molecules to mouthfeel*, Crows Nest: Allen & Unwin

CSIRO, 2015, *Overview of Gene Technology Research at CSIRO*, <www.csiro.au/en/Research/Farming-food/Innovation-and-technology-for-the-future/Gene-technology/Overview>, accessed 19 June 2018

Drew, R. & Hagen, T., 2016, *Nanotechnologies in Food Packaging: An exploratory appraisal of safety and regulation*, <www.foodstandards.gov.au/publications/Pages/Nanotechnologies-in-Food-Packaging-an-Exploratory-Appraisal-of-Safety-and-Regulation.aspx>, accessed 22 January 2019

Environmental Protection Authority of New Zealand, 2019, *Environmental Protection Authority / Te Mana Rauhi Taiao*, <www.epa.govt.nz/>, accessed 19 June 2018

Euromonitor International, 2019, *Packaging*, <www.euromonitor.com/packaging>, accessed 19 June 2018

Fellows, P.J., 2009, *Food Processing Technology: Principles and practice* (3rd edn), Sawston: Woodhead Publishing

FSANZ, 2012, *Supplementary Food Colours Report*, <www.foodstandards.gov.au/science/surveillance/pages/supplementaryfoodcol5571.aspx>, accessed 19 June 2018

—— 2016a, *Acrylamide and Food*, <www.foodstandards.gov.au/consumer/chemicals/acrylamide/pages/default.aspx>, accessed 18 June 2018

—— 2016b, *Additives*, <www.foodstandards.gov.au/consumer/additives/additiveoverview/Pages/default.aspx>, accessed 19 June 2018

—— 2016c, *Application Handbook* <www.foodstandards.gov.au/code/changes/Documents/Application%20 Handbook%20as%20at%201%20March%202016.pdf>, accessed 22 January 2019

—— 2016d, *Food Additive Labelling*, <www.foodstandards.gov.au/consumer/labelling/Pages/Labelling-of-food-additives.aspx>, accessed 19 June 2018

—— 2017, *Chemical Migration From Packaging Into Food* (P1034), <www.foodstandards.gov.au/code/proposals/ Pages/P1034ChemicalMigrationfromPackagingintoFood.aspx>, accessed 22 January 2019

—— 2018a, *Completed ISFR Food Surveys*, <www.foodstandards.gov.au/science/surveillance/Pages/isccomponent1. aspx>, accessed 19 June 2018

—— 2018b, *Evaluation Report Series*, <www.foodstandards.gov.au/science/Pages/Evaluation-report-series.aspx>, accessed 18 June 2018

—— 2018c, *Food Derived Using New Breeding Techniques: Review*, <www.foodstandards.gov.au/consumer/gmfood/ Pages/Review-of-new-breeding-technologies-.aspx>, accessed 18 June 2018

—— 2018d, *Food Standards Code*, <www.foodstandards.gov.au/code/Pages/default.aspx>, accessed 23 January 2019

—— 2019, *The Australian Food Composition Database*, <www.foodstandards.gov.au/science/monitoringnutrients/ afcd/Pages/default.aspx>, accessed 18 February 2019

Grains & Legumes Nutrition Council, 2018, *Whole Grains*, <www.glnc.org.au/grains/grains-and-nutrition/ wholegrains/>, accessed 18 June 2018

—— 2019, *Types of Grains*, <www.glnc.org.au/grains/types-of-grains/>, accessed 24 January 2019

Hannon, J.C., Kerry, J., Cruz-Romero, M., Morris, M. & Cummins, E., 2015, 'Advances and challenges for the use of engineered nanoparticles in food contact materials', *Trends in Food Science and Technology, 43*(1): 43–62, doi:10.1016/j.tifs.2015.01.008

Hirneisen, K.A., Black, E.P., Cascarino, J.L., Fino, V.R., Hoover, D.G. & Kniel, K.E., 2009, 'Viral inactivation in foods: A review of traditional and novel food-processing technologies', *Comprehensive Reviews in Food Science and Food Safety, 9*(1): 3–20, doi:10.1111/j.1541-4337.2009.00092.x

Hsieh, Y.H. & Ofori, J.A., 2007, 'Innovations in food technology for health', *Asia Pacific Journal of Clinical Nutrition, 16*(Supp. 1): 65–73, doi:10.6133/apjcn.2007.16.s1.13

Hyde, M.L., Larter, C., Fields, B. & Stanley, G., 2017, 'FSANZ risk assessment of phytosanitary food irradiation of selected fruits and vegetables', *Journal of Nutrition & Intermediary Metabolism, 8*: 102–3, doi:10.1016/ j.jnim.2017.04.160

Lam, C.X.F., Mo, X.M., Teoh, S.H. & Hutmacher, D.W., 2002, 'Scaffold development using 3D printing with a starch-based polymer', *Materials Science and Engineering: C, 20*(1): 49–56, doi:10.1016/S0928-4931(02)00012-7

Lin, D. & Zhao, Y., 2007, 'Innovations in the development and application of edible coatings for fresh and minimally processed fruits and vegetables', *Comprehensive Reviews in Food Science and Food Safety, 6*(3): 60–75, doi:10.1111/ j.1541-4337.2007.00018.x

Lupton, D. & Turner, B., 2018, '"I can't get past the fact that it is printed": Consumer attitudes to 3D printed food', *Food, Culture & Society, 21*(3): 402–18, doi:10.1080/15528014.2018.1451044

NHMRC, 2013, *Australian Dietary Guidelines* (N55), <www.nhmrc.gov.au/guidelines-publications/n55>, accessed 21 February 2019

Ohlsson, T., 1994, 'Minimal processing-preservation methods of the future: An overview', *Trends in Food Science & Technology, 5*(11): 341–4, doi:10.1016/0924-2244(94)90210-0

PCA, 2005, *Australian Packaging: Issues and trends* (Issues Paper 18), <www.pca.org.au/application/files/4314/ 3795/7882/00499.pdf>, accessed 22 January 2019

Rickman, J.C., Barrett, D.M. & Bruhn, C.M., 2007a, 'Nutritional comparison of fresh, frozen and canned fruits and vegetables, Part 1: Vitamins C and B and phenolic compounds', *Journal of the Science of Food and Agriculture, 87*(6): 930–44, doi:10.1002/jsfa.2825

Rickman, J.C., Bruhn, C.M. & Barrett, D.M., 2007b, 'Nutritional comparison of fresh, frozen and canned fruits and vegetables, Part 2: Vitamin A and carotenoids, vitamin E, minerals and fiber', *Journal of the Science of Food and Agriculture, 87*(7): 1185–96, doi:10.1002/jsfa.2824

Roberts, P.B., 2014, 'Food irradiation is safe: Half a century of studies', *Radiation Physics and Chemistry, 105*: 78–82, doi:10.1016/j.radphyschem.2014.05.016

Schab, D.W. & Trinh, N.H., 2004, 'Do artificial food colors promote hyperactivity in children with hyperactive syndromes? A meta-analysis of double-blind placebo-controlled trials', *Journal of Developmental and Behavioral Pediatrics, 25*(6): 423–34, doi:10.1097/00004703-200412000-00007

Shiby Varghese, K., Pandey, M.C., Radhakrishna, K. & Bawa, A.S., 2014, 'Technology, applications and modelling of ohmic heating: A review', *Journal of Food Science and Technology, 51*(10): 2304–17, doi:10.1007/s13197-012-0710-3

Stewart, M., 2013, *The seven principles of HACCP*, <www.foodsafety.com.au/blog/the-seven-principles-of-haccp>, accessed 22 January 2019

Sun, J., Peng, Z., Zhou, W., Fuh, J.Y.H., Hong, G.S. & Chiu, A., 2015, 'A review on 3D printing for customized food fabrication', *Procedia Manufacturing, 1*: 308–19, doi:10.1016/j.promfg.2015.09.057

Tannahill, R., 1995, *Food in History* (revised edn), New York, NY: Broadway Books

The Last Straw, 2018, *The Last Straw,* <www.laststraw.com.au/>, accessed 19 June 2018

WHO, 2005, *Modern Food Biotechnology, Human Health and Development: An evidence-based study*, <www.who.int/iris/handle/10665/43195>, accessed 22 January 2019

WHO & FAO, 2006, *Guidelines on Food Fortification with Micronutrients*, <www.who.int/nutrition/publications/micronutrients/9241594012/en/>, accessed 22 January 2019

{CHAPTER 6}
FOOD SAFETY: REGULATION, RISK ANALYSIS AND FOOD CHEMICALS

Janis Baines and David Borradale

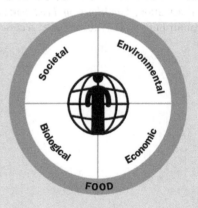

INTRODUCTION

The food system is a complex interconnection between a range of systems and involving a multitude of actors and stakeholders. As such, it requires the intersection of multiple regulatory and non-regulatory approaches to ensure that individuals are able to access and consume food that is safe. Unsafe food, whether due to adulteration (accidental or deliberate), microbiological action or other factors, is responsible for high levels of illness, reducing the ability to work and leading, in some cases, to death. Safe food is an essential element and measurable outcome of food security. Regulations and frameworks are essential and exist to assist in protecting people from failures of the food system, from 'paddock to plate'. Figure 6.1 provides a summary of the food production chain in which regulatory and non-regulatory mechanisms exist.

This chapter will focus on the regulatory and non-regulatory approaches related to ensuring food is uncontaminated or safe for consumption. Chapter 26 focuses on broader threats to the sustainability of the food system, such as climate change and reduced biodiversity.

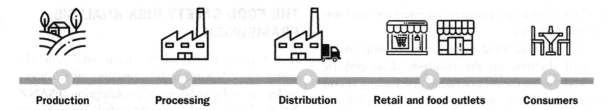

| Production | Processing | Distribution | Retail and food outlets | Consumers |

Figure 6.1: Food production chain (paddock to plate)

THE FOOD REGULATION SETTING IN AUSTRALIA AND NEW ZEALAND

Australia has a long history of food regulation, with the first legislation passed in the colony of New South Wales in 1838 (*Adulteration of Bread Act 1838*). From 1905 onwards the states of Australia passed various pure food acts, which from the 1950s were often voluntarily adopted from standards developed by the National Health and Medical Research Council (NHMRC). A Model Food Act was adopted in 1980 to provide uniformity across the country, with the idea that uniform standards (based on the NHMRC standards) and food hygiene regulations would follow. In 1991, the National Food Authority (NFA) was established in Australia under the *National Food Authority Act 1991* to develop and administer a Food Standards Code. In New Zealand, a similar process had occurred with establishment of a national *Food Act 1981,* amended in 2014 (MPI 2016). These developments were linked with the establishment of the **Codex Alimentarius** Commission in 1962, a joint FAO/WHO food standards program that aimed to facilitate world trade by setting international food standards that could be adopted by member countries (FAO/WHO 2018).

In 1996 a joint agency of the Australian and New Zealand governments was established, the Australia New Zealand Food Authority (ANZFA); however, the joint *Australia New Zealand Food Standards Code* did not come into full effect until 2002 (Australian Government 2016). Under the arrangement each country retains its own food safety standards and maximum residue level standards for agricultural and veterinary chemicals. There are also some other differences—for example, in country of origin labelling standards and in mandatory fortification standards, as New Zealand does not have a mandatory fortification standard for thiamin and folic acid in flour for breadmaking. In mid-2002, ANZFA was renamed as Food Standards Australia New Zealand (FSANZ) under the *FSANZ Act 1991*, with a new additional responsibility for primary production and processing standards (Australia only).

The roles and responsibilities in the current intergovernmental agreement are described in Figure 6.2. FSANZ is a partner in the food regulation system with Australian federal, state, territory and New Zealand governments, with a role in developing and administering food standards (FSANZ 2018a). The *FSANZ ACT 1991* (Section 18) (Australian Government 2016) outlines core objectives to be achieved when developing food standards: protecting public health and safety, providing adequate information on food to enable consumers to make informed choices and preventing misleading and deceptive conduct. It also directs FSANZ to use an evidence-based approach, achieve consistency between domestic and international food standards (for example, Codex standards) and promote fair trade. Over the years, the NFA, ANZFA and FSANZ all worked to a board of external part-time members, comprising qualified people with interests related to food regulation (such as in public health, food science, human nutrition, consumer affairs, food allergy, medical science, microbiology, food safety, biotechnology, veterinary science, primary food production, the food industry, small business, and international trade) and representatives from the NHMRC and government. The FSANZ Board reviews the draft standards prepared by agency staff against the FSANZ Act objectives prior to public consultation and approves a final version to be presented to government ministers for decision (FSANZ 2018d).

A joint ministerial council (the Forum) makes a final decision on the standards developed by FSANZ, while the New Zealand government (Food Regulation 2018) and Australian states and territories implement and enforce the standards. The Forum has general oversight of the implementation of standards and can adopt, amend or reject them and ask FSANZ to review them or create new ones. The Forum also develops food regulatory policy and policy guidelines that FSANZ must have regard to when setting food standards. It is assisted by the Food Regulation Standing Committee and the Implementation Subcommittee for Food Regulation, which draw members from government regulatory departments and agencies in both countries (Food Regulation 2018).

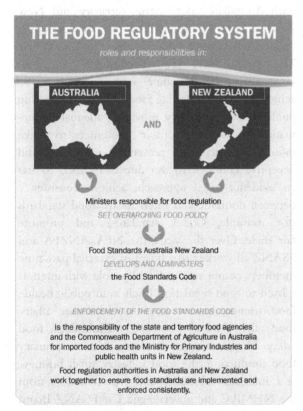

Figure 6.2: The food regulatory system in Australia and New Zealand

Source: FSANZ (2018e). Reproduced with permission

THE FOOD SAFETY RISK ANALYSIS FRAMEWORK

In the context of food, the term 'safe' generally means there is a reasonable certainty of no harm under normal conditions of consumption (FSANZ 2013). This means that under normal circumstances and levels of exposure to the components in the food, the probability that eating it will produce an adverse outcome is very low. In order to assess this risk, the World Health Organization (WHO) and the United Nations Food and Agriculture Organization (FAO) developed a framework for food safety risk analysis to be used when setting Codex food standards (see Figure 6.3). This framework is also used in setting joint Australian and New Zealand standards.

RISK ASSESSMENT

The science-based phase of the risk analysis framework includes four steps:

1. Hazard identification—identifying the hazard and its potential adverse health effects.
2. Hazard characterisation—identifying the nature and severity of the adverse health effects and determining whether the effects differ depending on the level of exposure.
3. Exposure assessment—determining the level of exposure/intake from the diet and other sources.

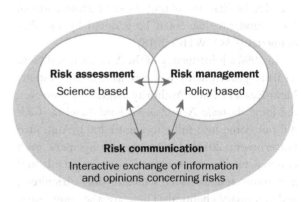

Figure 6.3: Codex risk analysis framework

Source: FAO/WHO (1995); FSANZ (2013). Reproduced with permission

4. Risk characterisation—integrating the information from the hazard and exposure assessments to determine the likelihood and severity of an adverse effect occurring in any given population.

To determine the level of risk, the different sources of evidence are assessed by food regulatory agencies and a relative weighting given to each source; an example is given in Figure 6.4. In this figure, the bigger the circle the more weighting the evidence receives.

However, consumers may not always perceive the level of risk to be the same as the actual risk level as assessed by scientists, so risks may be ranked differently by each group. Ranking may also vary for different population groups within one country or between countries (Covello & Sandman 2001).

What are potential hazards?

The first step is to identify potential hazards in food, such as microbiological or physical substances, food chemicals (additives, contaminants, pesticides or veterinary drug residues, naturally occurring toxicants or nutrients) or ingredients (novel foods or ingredients, genetically modified ingredients) with the potential to cause an adverse effect. New technologies can also potentially lead to a new or increased risk in food—although, as discussed in Chapter 5, some may also provide a health benefit to the consumer (see Table 6.1). There is a potential for overlap in these categories—for example, a dietary macrocomponent could also be novel food; a nanoscale material could be a food additive or a processing aid or a nano-encapsulated nutrient (see Chapter 5 for more information on nanotechnology).

The main chemicals found in food that may lead to potential health risks are food additives, contaminants, pesticides and veterinary drug residues, naturally occurring toxicants and, in some cases, nutrients. Of these, food additives are intentionally added to foods, while pesticides and veterinary drugs are used in agriculture and animal husbandry to achieve good quality produce and may result in traces of the

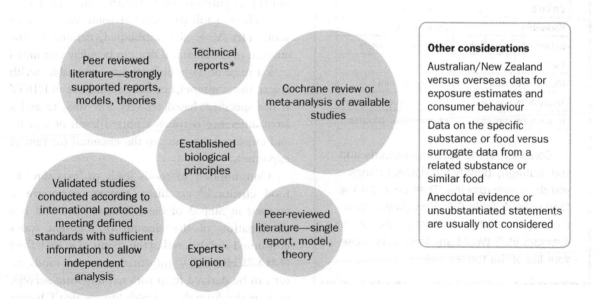

Other considerations

Australian/New Zealand versus overseas data for exposure estimates and consumer behaviour

Data on the specific substance or food versus surrogate data from a related substance or similar food

Anecdotal evidence or unsubstantiated statements are usually not considered

Note: * May include company-generated reports, reports from other food regulatory agencies, non-peer reviewed abstracts, etc.

Figure 6.4: Different sources of evidence used by FSANZ and relative weighting

Source: FSANZ (2013). Reproduced with permission

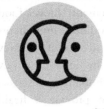

RISK PERCEPTION

Risk perception is the subjective judgement that people make about the characteristics and severity of a risk:

Perceived risk = hazard + outrage

A hazard is defined as a potential for harm or an adverse effect. Outrage has more individual responses and can be culturally determined. Outrage factors for safe and risky behaviour are outlined below (Covello & Sandman 2001).

'Safe'	'Risky'
Voluntary	Coerced
Natural	Industrial
Familiar	Exotic
Not memorable	Memorable
Not dreaded	Dreaded
Chronic	Catastrophic
Knowable	Unknowable
Individually controlled	Controlled by others
Fair	Unfair
Morally irrelevant	Morally relevant
Trustworthy sources	Untrustworthy sources
Responsive process	Unresponsive process

Considering the potential hazards and your outrage, identify the riskiest things you do in everyday life. Then consider the food risks in Table 6.1. How do you rank them against other risks we encounter in everyday life? Would any food risks make your list of the top ten risks?

chemicals in the final food. Contaminants are not intentionally added to foods but may be introduced to a food via the environment, either due to natural occurrence or from human activity. Nutrients may occur naturally or be added to a food for a health benefit.

The 16th-century scientist Paracelsus (1493–1541) recognised that 'all substances are poisons [and that] the right dose differentiates a poison and remedy'. The task of food regulators is to assess or characterise the potential risks of the different chemicals found in foods to those who consume them and determine what level is determined to be safe in the food, given the known patterns of consumption in any population (FAO/WHO 2009; FSANZ 2013). Risk assessment is the first step of risk analysis for food chemicals.

Once the first two steps of risk assessment, Step 1 (hazard identification) and Step 2 (hazard characterisation), are completed, a **health-based guidance value** (HBGV) may be set for the food chemical (FAO/WHO 2009; FSANZ 2013) (see Table 6.2). Toxicological studies on animals are often used as the basis for HBGVs, with safety or uncertainty factors applied to take account of differences between effects of the chemical on animals compared to humans and differences in sensitivity among the human population; such factors may also reflect the lack of a full data set. For some chemicals an acute HBGV is also established, defined as the amount of the chemical that can be safely consumed over a meal or 24 hours without appreciable health risk to the consumer. For some substances an HBGV is not specified, based on very low toxicity and a large difference between reported levels of toxicity and estimated exposure to the chemical (margin of exposure).

Consumption of foods leads to 'exposure' to food chemicals' via diet. **Dietary exposure** is assessed in Step 3 of the risk assessment and is a combination of the amount of different foods consumed and the level of the chemical in each food (FAO/WHO 2009). Information on the foods we eat can be derived from national nutrition surveys, such as the Australian Health Survey (see Chapter 24) or the New Zealand Nutrition Surveys (ABS 2016; MOH 2011). Information on the levels of all the food chemicals can be found by analysis (for

Table 6.1: Agents or factors in food that could contribute to risk/benefits

Chemicals	Microbiological agents (see Chapter 7)	Physical factors[†]
Environmental contaminants	Bacteria (infectious and toxin-producing)	Metals
Food additives and processing aids	Protozoa and helminths	Glass
Naturally occurring toxicants	Viruses	Stones
Agricultural and veterinary (agvet) chemicals	Moulds	Plastics
Packaging materials	Prions	Wood
Allergens		Bone and bone fragments
Nanoscale materials*		
Nutritive substances*		
Dietary macrocomponents*		
Novel food ingredients (may be whole foods)*		
Genetically modified ingredients with enhanced nutritional profile*		

Notes: * Can contribute to health benefit as well as risk; [†] Refers to actual objects (foreign bodies) contaminating foods

Source: Adapted from FSANZ (2013)

Table 6.2: Health-based guidance values (HBGVs) for food chemicals

Food chemical	HBGV (long term)	HBGV (short term)
Food additive	Acceptable Daily Intake (ADI)	
Pesticide or veterinary drug residue	Acceptable Daily Intake (ADI)	Acute Reference dose
Contaminant	Provisional tolerable daily, weekly or monthly intake	
Nutrient	Nutrient Reference Value (NRV)	

example, through the Australian Total Diet Study and New Zealand Total Diet Study), from food manufacturers (food additives, nutrients) or from agricultural trial data (agvet chemical residues), from national residues surveys in Australia or New Zealand (agvet chemical residues, contaminants) or ad hoc surveys; see the monitoring section below for further information (Department of Agriculture and Water Resources 2018b; FSANZ 2011; MPI 2018a, 2018b).

In Step 4, the estimated dietary exposure is compared with the relevant HBGV to determine the level of risk for the populations studied. Risk assessors also need to know if there is likely to be exposure to the same chemical through a different route—for example, via air or skin—as the combined exposure from all routes may increase the total burden on the body.

The potential risks posed by food chemicals are managed in different ways because of the nature of the chemical and the reasons they are found in food.

RISK MANAGEMENT

The risk management process used by Codex and FSANZ is the policy-based part of the overall risk analysis and is common to many regulatory agencies. It essentially involves four stages: (a) preliminary activities that identify the issue, establish risk management goals and develop risk assessment questions; (b) risk management option formulation; (c) implementation of the decision; and (d) monitoring and evaluation of the effectiveness of the risk management measure(s) taken, as outlined in Figure 6.5 (FAO/WHO 1997; FSANZ 2013).

RISK COMMUNICATION

Essential to the whole risk analysis process is risk communication, both between risk assessors and risk managers within an agency and with external interested parties, often termed 'stakeholders', which may include governments (state or territory, international), other agencies and research institutions, the food industry (production, manufacture and

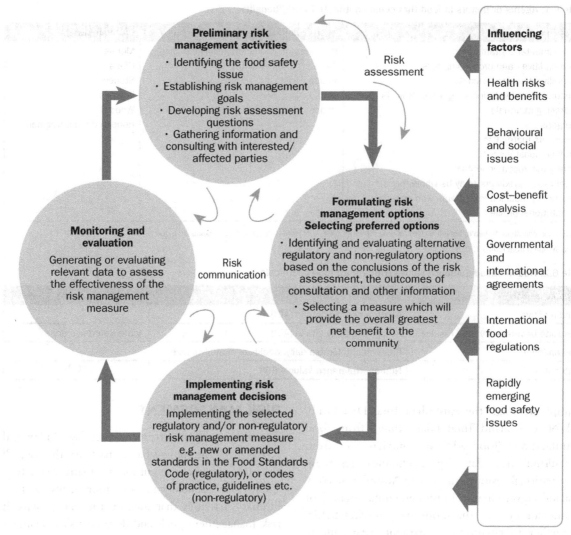

Figure 6.5: Components of risk management of food-related health risks
Source: FSANZ (2013). Reproduced with permission

retail), consumers and public health professionals. Communication strategies at FSANZ are developed according to four levels of risk combinations, based on scientific risk (as determined by regulatory agencies such as FSANZ) and perceived risk (as seen by the community); see Table 6.3 (FSANZ 2013).

Following identification of the food health and safety issues and development of the risk assessment question to be answered, possible risk management options are developed and evaluated (FSANZ 2013). Regulatory measures include:

- food standards that restrict levels of a food chemical or microbiological agent in specific foods or food groups or prohibit the sale of foods for retail sale that are high-risk
- food-labelling standards (mandatory warning and advisory statements, other requirements).

Non-regulatory measures include:
- codes of practice
- guidelines/protocols
- consumer information/advice.

Table 6.3: Communication strategies

Level	Risk combination	Communication strategy	Communication vehicle
1	LOW risk—LOW perceived risk	Passive	Direct notification to interested and affected parties; for example, proposed use of a processing aid (minor food component not intended to be present in final food).
2	LOW risk—HIGH perceived risk	Responsive	Media releases, proactive media liaison, provision of updates, social media; for example, aspartame (intense sweetener) use in food.
3	HIGH risk—LOW perceived risk	Educative	Education campaign to alert an otherwise unaware community, web-based materials, social media; for example, advice on mercury content of fish and consumption levels for pregnant women.
4	HIGH risk—HIGH perceived risk	Proactive	Early media release, media liaison, release of information and advice, social media; for example, BSE (mad cow disease), hepatitis A virus in frozen berries.

Source: Adapted from FSANZ (2013) risk management options

A combination of regulatory and non-regulatory measures may be employed, particularly when many parts of the food system are involved. For example, to manage the potential risk of consuming fish that contains mercury, Standard 1.4.1—Contaminants and Natural Toxicants of the *Australia New Zealand Food Standards Code* sets maximum levels for mercury in fish and seafood offered for sale, but advice is also given by FSANZ on its website on how much fish of different species certain population groups can eat each week, particularly vulnerable groups such as pregnant women and young children (see Chapter 20) (FSANZ 2011). A graduated risk analysis approach might be taken in some cases to ensure that the resources (FSANZ, enforcement agencies and food industry) applied are proportional to the risks being managed—for example, processing aids (such as yeast enzyme) which are not present in the final food are not regulated to the same degree as some other food additives (FSANZ 2018e).

Non-regulatory measures alone, such as industry codes of practice or guidelines, might be used when the assessed risk to public health and safety is considered low and development of a standard is not warranted. In all cases, communication via websites and social media on potential risk for the general public is important.

NAVIGATING THE FOOD STANDARDS CODE

Find the following foods in the Food Standards Code and use the code to write a definition for:
- ice cream (what would 'ice cream' not meeting this definition be called?)
- fruit juice (what would 'fruit juice' not meeting this definition be called?)
- meat pie
- sausage.

THE *AUSTRALIA NEW ZEALAND FOOD STANDARDS CODE*

The *Australia New Zealand Food Standards Code* has five main sections, as outlined in Figure 6.6 (FSANZ 2018a). There is additional information on the FSANZ website including user guides, factsheets for consumers and small business on a large number of topics, information on making nutrition-related health claims and a guide to Chapter 3, 'Food safety standards (Australia only)' (FSANZ 2016a; 2016b).

Australia New Zealand Food Standards Code

Chapter 1 Introduction and standards that apply to all foods

1.1—Preliminary

1.2—Labelling and other information requirements

1.3—Substances added to food (e.g. food additives, vitamins & minerals, processing aids)

1.4—Contaminants and residues (e.g. contaminants, natural toxicants, agvet chemicals, prohibited and restricted plants & fungi)

1.5—Food requiring pre-market clearance (e.g. novel foods, foods produced using gene technology, irradiation of foods)

1.6—Microbiological limits and processing requirements

Chapter 2 Food Standards

2.1—Cereals

2.2—Meat, eggs and fish

2.3—Fruits and vegetables

2.4—Edible oils

2.5—Dairy products

2.6—Non-alcoholic beverages

2.7—Alcoholic beverages

2.8—Sugars and honey

2.9—Special purpose foods (e.g. infant formula)

2.10—Standards for other foods

Chapter 3 Food safety standards (Australia only)

3.1—Preliminary

3.2—Food safety requirements

3.3—Food safety programs for service to vulnerable people

Chapter 4 Primary production and processing standards (Australia only)

4.1—Preliminary provisions

4.2—Product standards (e.g. seafood, poultry meat, meat, dairy products, egg and egg products, seed sprouts)

4.5—Wine production requirements

Schedules 1–29

Figure 6.6: Structure of the *Australia New Zealand Food Standards Code*

Source: FSANZ (2018e). Reproduced with permission

SPECIFIC FOOD CHEMICALS: RELATED HEALTH RISKS AND THEIR MANAGEMENT

Food additives and processing aids

The reasons for the addition of food additives to food during the processing and preparation of food products are covered in Chapter 5. To assess their safety, extensive testing of food additives is required, including animal studies and human studies if they are available. Food regulatory agencies undertake risk assessments before new additives or extensions of use for existing additives are permitted in Australia and New Zealand under Standard 1.3.1—Food additives (Australian Government 2017). In the risk assessment, a country may set an HBGV or adopt international values from the Joint FAO/WHO Expert Committee on Food Additives (JECFA), usually an Acceptable Daily Intake (FAO/WHO 2018).

As food additives and processing aids are intentionally added to foods, the amount permitted to be added is controlled by setting **maximum permitted levels (MPLs)** in nominated foods or allowing use at **good manufacturing practice (GMP)** levels in the *Australia New Zealand Food Standards Code* (Standard 1.3.1—Food additives, and Schedules 7, 8, 14–16; Standard 1.3.3—Processing aids, and Schedule 18). The MPLs are determined through the risk-assessment process such that the level for each food assigned an MPL is considered safe given its HBGV, where one is established, and known consumption patterns in Australia and New Zealand of all foods likely to contain the additive. In some cases, the added and free sugars database prepared by FSANZ in 2016 as part of the 2011–13 Australian Health Survey has been used to assess potential uses of other added intense and bulk sweeteners and to determine major sources of added sugars (ABS 2016).

Contaminants

Contaminants are substances that are not intentionally added to food but may be present as a result of production, manufacture, processing, preparation, treatment, packaging, transport or holding of food or as a result of environmental contamination. The presence and concentration of contaminants in food are therefore less predictable than other food chemicals, and often less information is available for risk assessors to use (Crossley & Baines 2014). Metals such as arsenic, mercury, cadmium, lead and tin and other chemicals such as methanol and aflatoxins may contaminate food. Occasionally, chemical contamination can result from tampering or deliberate addition to foods—for example, the addition of melamine to milk in China in 2007–2008 (Wen et al. 2016; WHO 2008).

In a risk assessment for a contaminant, a country may set an HBGV, but more commonly international values from the JECFA are used, along with information on food consumption patterns and food chemical concentrations in each country (FAO/WHO 2018). Many countries have monitoring programs to provide information on current levels of contaminants in food (Crossley & Baines 2014). Raw produce and/or food available for consumption may be analysed; for examples, see the Australian Total Diet Study and the New Zealand Total Diet Study (FSANZ 2017b; MPI 2018b) (see the section 'Monitoring chemicals and nutrient content in food' below).

Levels of contaminants in food are hard to manage and it is not possible or desirable to set standards for the thousands of chemicals that may inadvertently enter the food supply or be added through criminal activity. **Maximum levels (MLs)** for contaminants and natural toxicants are set in standards only where they serve an effective risk-management function, are based on a scientific risk assessment and usually only for those foods that make a significant contribution to total dietary exposure to the chemical (Abbott et al. 2003). MLs are set at the lowest possible levels, following the 'as low as is reasonably achievable' principle (FAO/WHO 2009), such that levels permitted ensure consumers are protected without removing the food completely from the food supply; an example is setting MLs for the natural toxicant hydrocyanic acid in cassava products. However, there are some foods that are prohibited or restricted in Standard 1.4.4—Prohibited and restricted plants and fungi, Schedules 23 and 24, due to their chemical content.

Some contaminants may be managed at the source as well as by setting food standards as part of a wider risk management program. An example of this is cadmium, an element occurring in soil, rocks, plants, water and animals (i.e. ubiquitous in the environment) that can accumulate in humans and at high levels poses a health risk. The level of cadmium in potatoes, for example, is managed at source by implementing a range of measures such as using low-cadmium fertilisers, low-chlorine irrigation water, adding organic matter to the soil, sourcing potatoes for commercial products from areas known to have low cadmium soils where possible, and providing educational materials (see Figure 6.7, CRCSLM/CSIRO 1999). In the Food Standards Code, MLs are set for cadmium for a limited number of foods that are estimated to contribute less than 5 per cent to dietary exposure: roots and tubers such as potatoes, leafy vegetables, chocolate and cocoa products, peanuts, molluscs, salt, rice, wheat, meat, kidney and liver (cattle, sheep, pig) (*Australia New Zealand Food Standards Code*, Schedule 19).

Natural toxicants in food

Naturally occurring toxicants are normal components of foods but in some circumstances can be hazardous to health, often when large amounts of the major food source are consumed. Sometimes a toxin is present as a naturally occurring pesticide to ward off insect attack or to protect the plant from spoilage; sometimes they form when the food is damaged (see Table 6.4 for some commonly occurring natural toxicants in food). The toxicological effect on humans of each natural toxicant varies and, as with other contaminants, a country may set an HBGV or use international values from JECFA in a risk assessment for a natural toxicant. The levels of some natural toxicants permitted in some foods offered for sale are limited, for example, in Australia and New Zealand under Standard 1.4.1—Contaminants and natural toxicants, Schedule 19; the level of caffeine and alcohol in products is regulated elsewhere in the Food Standards Code (FSANZ 2018e). For some

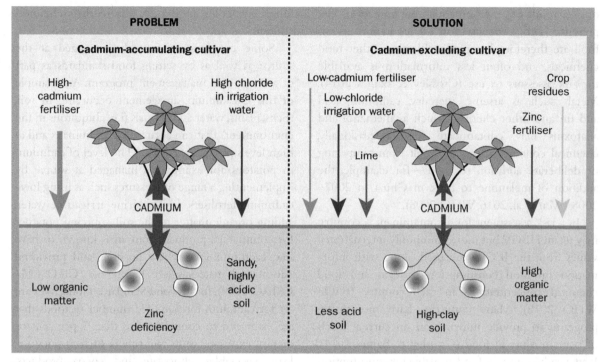

Figure 6.7: Managing cadmium in potatoes

Source: CRCSLM/CSIRO (1999). Reproduced with permission

contaminants and natural toxins there are additional food safety risk management measures, such as labelling requirements in Chapter 1 of the *Australia New Zealand Food Standards Code*. For example, there are required labelling directions for the preparation of cassava and bamboo shoots to prevent acute cyanide intoxication from inadequately prepared foods.

Pesticide and veterinary drug residues

Agricultural and veterinary (agvet) chemicals are intentionally used on animals and plants to control pests and diseases so that high-quality food is produced and food losses are reduced; however, in some cases residues from these chemicals may remain in the final food. Many food producers use pesticides and veterinary drugs on a regular basis, while others use them rarely. The Australian Pesticides and Veterinary Medicines Authority (APVMA) and New Zealand Ministry for Primary Industries (MPI) assess the safety of agvet chemical use in each country and determine appropriate patterns of use

for the application of each chemical. Potential health risks posed by agvet chemical residues are managed by setting **maximum residue limits** (MRLs) for specific chemical/food combinations in food standards (Standard 1.4.2). The MRLs for Australia are automatically adopted into the Schedule 20 of the *Australia New Zealand Food Standards Code* once determined by the APVMA. FSANZ also sets extraneous residue limits for agvet chemicals no longer in use in Schedule 21 (Australia only). In New Zealand, MRLs for agricultural compounds are published in a food notice under the 2014 *Food Act* (MPI 2016).

FSANZ has a harmonisation program for imported foods because agricultural practices may be different in other countries, resulting in agvet chemical residues being found in imported foods that are not permitted for domestic use. FSANZ generally prepares one MRL proposal each year after calling for requests to vary Schedule 20 to permit residues in imported foods. These requests to harmonise with

Table 6.4: Some naturally occurring toxicants and their food sources

Food component	Major food source
Agaric acid*	Mushrooms Alcoholic beverages
Berberine*	Alcoholic beverages
Caffeine[†]	Coffee, tea, cocoa, cola-type beverages
Erucic acid*	Edible oils
Favism-causing compounds	Broad beans (*Vicia faba*)
Furans	Thermally processed foods, such as coffee, canned and jarred foods including baby foods, soups and sauces; lower levels in other foods, including products from vegetables, meat, milk and cereals
Glycoalkaloids	Potatoes
Hydrocyanic acid, total*	Cassava, some varieties of lima bean, apricot kernels, bitter almonds, apple seeds, bamboo shoots
Histamine*	Fish and fish products
Lectins (haemagglutinins)	Many species of legume
Nitrate/nitrite	Cabbage, celery, lettuce, spinach
Oxalates	Rhubarb, spinach, tea
Oestrogens	Apples, carrots, cabbage, rice, soy beans, vegetable oils, wheat
Phytates	Cereal grains, some legumes
Protease inhibitors	Many species of legume
Pyrrolizidine alkaloids	Grains, honey, milk, offal and eggs, comfrey, some herbs
Quinine*	Mixed alcoholic drinks, tonic drinks, bitter drinks and quinine drinks Wine-based drinks and reduced-alcohol wines
Tutin*	Honey

Notes: * Maximum levels set in *Australia New Zealand Food Standards Code*, Standard 1.4.2—Contaminants and natural toxicants, Schedule 19 (FSANZ 2018e); [†] There are no maximum levels for naturally occurring caffeine. Maximum caffeine levels are set for the addition of caffeine to foods: in cola-type soft drinks (Schedule 15—Substances that may be used as food additives) and energy drinks (Standard 2.6.—Formulated caffeinated beverages), where the maximum level includes any contribution from guarana; Schedule 9—Mandatory advisory statements, also requires an advisory statement indicating a product contains caffeine/guarana and Standard 1.2.4—Information requirements, requires listing of added caffeine in the statement of ingredients (FSANZ 2018e)

a relevant Codex MRL or an MRL established in another country undergo a strict risk assessment process before new MRLs are considered. The MRL proposal may also include MRLs (or deletions of MRLs) requested by the APVMA as a result of a review of an older chemical that has been in use for some time. There is no formal harmonisation system in New Zealand. Foods imported into New Zealand may comply with the relevant NZ MRLs, international standards (Codex MRLs including a default value of 0.1 mg/kg where no MRL is set), or, for food imported from Australia, with Australian MRLs.

Each agvet chemical product permitted for sale by the APVMA or the New Zealand MPI has safety and use directions that are designed to protect people, animals, crops, the environment and trade interests. The APVMA and MPI provide details of HBGVs used in their risk assessments, which include work health and safety assessments as well as dietary exposure assessments (AVPMA 2018; MPI 2016). Enforcement agencies use MRLs to help monitor whether an agvet chemical has been used as directed to control pests and diseases in food production. Differences in climate, soil and other growing conditions may mean the use patterns for the same agvet chemical are different in Australia and New Zealand, and MRLs may be different.

Nutrients

Nutrients occur naturally in foods but may also be added for specific purposes. Codex defines fortification as 'the addition of one or more essential nutrients to a food, whether or not it is normally contained in the food, for the purpose of preventing or correcting a demonstrated deficiency of one or more nutrients in the population or specific population groups' (FAO/WHO 2018). Addition of nutrients may:

- replace nutrients lost in processing (restoration)
- make one product equivalent to another similar one (equivalence)
- add nutrients for a known health benefit (fortification).

NATURAL TOXICANTS IN FISH AND SHELLFISH

A range of microbial toxins produced by different algae (tiny plants) may be found in a number of environments and can be eaten by fish and shellfish; although not toxic to the fish or shellfish, they are toxic to humans when consumed and may cause poisoning. These toxins include dinoflagellates and cyanobacteria. Ichthyosarcotoxism means poisoning by consumption of fish whose flesh or organs contain toxic substances, the main manifestations are ciguatera, tetradotoxism, clupeotoxism and scombroid poisoning.

Ciguatera toxin is the most common and tends to accumulate in large predatory fish (weighing over two kilograms), such as the barracuda and other carnivorous reef fish, because they eat other fish that consume toxin-producing algae, in this case dinoflagellates (Friedman et al. 2008).

Poisonous seafood neither looks nor tastes different from uncontaminated seafood, and cooking and other treatments of shellfish do not destroy the toxins. Costly monitoring programs are needed in shellfish and finfish farming areas to check for toxic algae in the water and, whenever these are present, regular tests for toxins in associated seafood products are required (Sanders 2003). However, there are no regulatory tests in common use.

It is not possible to predict if a fish will be hazardous to the consumer; hence, diagnosis for someone who is unwell is usually based on clinical presentation and dietary history of the person presenting for treatment. In Australia, Spanish mackerel has been the fish that has most often caused ciguatera poisoning, and it is more common in fish procured from seas off northern Queensland and the Northern Territory (Food Safety Information Council 2019; NSW Food Authority 2017). With high numbers of people originating from the Pacific Islands living in Australia and New Zealand, it is important to consider where people have visited or have obtained fish for consumption. Cases in New Zealand, for example, have resulted from the consumption of eel originating from Samoa (Armstrong et al. 2016).

Read the following article and identify four key strategies for reducing the risk of ciguatera poisoning.

- Friedman, M.A. et al., 2017, 'An updated review of ciguatera fish poisoning: Clinical, epidemiological, environmental, and public health management', *Marine Drugs, 15*(3): 72.

In risk assessments undertaken prior to permitting the addition of nutrients to food, the potential for inadequate and excessive intakes to occur is assessed, with estimated nutrient intakes compared to HBGVs for nutrients to characterise the risk (Baines et al. 2011). In Australia and New Zealand, HBGVs or nutrient reference values (NRVs) were set in 2006, with some fluoride and sodium values updated in 2017 (NHMRC 2006; 2017a; 2017b). For assessments of nutrient inadequacy for a population or population subgroup, the Estimated Average Requirement (EAR) or Adequate Intake (AI) are the appropriate NRVs to use; for assessment of nutrient excess, the upper level of intake (UL) is used. Recommended Dietary Intakes (RDIs) should only be used in individual assessments.

Any potential risks associated with permitting nutrients to be added to foods are managed by setting minimum and/or maximum levels in food standards, with information on content managed by setting labelling requirements for mandatory nutrition information panels and establishing rules for making nutrition and health claims on food labels or on advertising material. The permitted levels are based on a risk assessment and set such that consumers are not likely to exceed the UL, where one is assigned to a nutrient.

In the *Australia New Zealand Food Standards Code*, the addition of vitamins and minerals to foods is covered for both Australian and New Zealand by a number of standards, described in Table 6.5.

Labelling provisions aim to provide nutrition information to consumers to enable them to make an informed choice when purchasing food and, with health education programs, form part of a wider risk-management program to manage public health risks and chronic disease, such as the increasing prevalence of obesity and diabetes.

Voluntary nutrition labelling schemes that provide additional information on the nutrient content of foods—for example, the health star rating system and the glycaemic index (see Chapter 12)—are also permitted if executed in accordance with Code labelling requirements.

NOVEL, GENETICALLY MODIFIED AND IRRADIATED FOODS

For some categories of foods or food processes, pre-market approval is required by FSANZ before permissions for use are given under the Code, particularly where the technology used is new or emerging (see Chapter 5). Applications are required to FSANZ for novel foods, genetically modified foods and for new food uses of irradiation before they can be introduced to the food supply, and conditions may be applied to that use (Standard 1.5.1—Novel foods, Standard 1.5.2—Food produced using gene technology, Standard 1.5.3—Irradiation of food).

For example, novel food applications are subject to a pre-market safety assessment, which includes a review of public health and safety considerations having regard to:

- the potential for adverse effects in human
- the composition or structure of the food
- the process by which the food has been prepared
- the source from which it is derived
- patterns and levels of consumption of the food
- any other relevant matters.

Table 6.5: Standards covering the addition of nutrients to food

Standard	Schedule
1.2.7—Nutrition, health and related claims	Schedule 4—Nutrition, health and related claims Schedule 5—Nutrient profile scoring method Schedule 6—Required elements of a systematic review
1.2.8—Nutrition Information requirements	Schedule 11—Calculation of values for nutrition information panel Schedule 12—Nutrition information panels Schedule 13—Nutrition information panels required for small packages
1.3.1—Food additives	Schedule 14—Technical purposes performed by substances used as food additives Schedule 15—Substances that may be used as food additives Schedule 16—Types of substances that may be used as food additives
1.3.2—Vitamins and minerals	Schedule 17—Vitamins and minerals
Chapter 2 Food standards	Requirements for specific foods or food groups e.g. mandatory iodine, folic acid and thiamin fortification requirements in Standard 2.1.1—Cereals and cereal products, vitamin and mineral content of infant formula in Standard 2.9.1—Infant formula products and Schedule 29

Source: FSANZ (2018a)

Moving a food component from a whole food to a concentrated extract means it is then considered to be a novel food. It also means the risk of potentially adverse effects increases, and extracts may be converted to pharmacological agents with all of the risks associated. The framework provided by FSANZ allows for assessment of these risks. In the event that these novel foods are more pharmacological in their action, the Therapeutic Goods Administration would also be involved in their assessment.

In Australia and New Zealand, novel foods and novel food ingredients are regulated under Standard 1.5.1—Novel Foods in the Food Standards Code—with permitted novel foods listed in Schedule 25—and may have composition limits or labelling associated with their use. A novel food cannot be sold as food or used as a food ingredient unless it is listed in the Standard. Examples are phytosterols (see Chapter 18), phytostanols and their **esters**, which can be added to edible oil spreads, breakfast cereals or yoghurt; D-tagatose and trehalose, which may be used to replace sugar and other carbohydrates; and permitted sources of docosahexaenoic acid (DHA), which may be added to infant formula products, according to Standard 2.9.1.

A 'non-traditional food' or 'novel food' is defined in clause 1 of Standard 1.5.1 as:

- a food that does not have a history of human consumption in Australia or New Zealand; or
- a substance derived from a food, where that substance does not have a history of human consumption in Australia or New Zealand other than as a component of that food; or
- any other substance, where that substance, or the source from which it is derived, does not have a history of human consumption as a food in Australia or New Zealand.

FOOD ALLERGENS

Food allergens are a group of substances that are regulated in the *Australia New Zealand Food Standards Code* through mandatory labelling to manage potential food safety risks. The presence of food allergens or substances listed in Standard 1.2.3 and Schedule 9

WHAT ARE THE BENEFITS AND POTENTIAL RISKS OF EATING FISH?

Fish is a very important part of a healthy diet. Fish and other seafood are the major sources of healthful long-chain n-3 fats in our diets and are also rich in other nutrients such as vitamin D, iodine and selenium, high in protein, and low in saturated fat. Advice for a healthy diet is to eat at least two serves of fish a week.

However, fish and other seafood may also contain other chemicals that pose potential risks for consumers. For example, mercury may accumulate in fish at the top of the food chain (shark, marlin, swordfish, some tuna species) and in some long-living fish (e.g. orange roughy), so restricted consumption is recommended for some population groups, such as pregnant women. In some environments, fish may also contain residues from pesticides due to run-off from farms into local waterways or veterinary drug chemicals (e.g. growth hormones, antibiotics) if farmed rather than fresh-caught, as well as other industrial chemicals such as dioxins and polychlorinated biphenyls (PCBs).

Investigate a range of websites including FSANZ, the US Environmental Protection Agency, the UK Food Standards Agency and the FAO.

- What population groups may need to restrict consumption of some fish species because of its mercury content? Why?
- Why might the advice on consuming fish vary from country to country?

must be declared on the food label for health and safety reasons, or information made available on request at food service outlets. There are a few labelling exemptions for certain highly refined foods.

MONITORING CHEMICALS AND NUTRIENT CONTENT IN FOOD

There are some state and national programs that take representative samples of different foods available for sale and test for food chemical content, the extent of these programs being limited by resources allocated to plan and implement them, report on outcomes and formulate a response to the findings. The FSANZ Implementation Subcommittee for Food Regulation (ISFR) organises coordinated food surveys with an annual plan that cover the Australian states and territories and New Zealand. Examples of coordinated surveys include a 2015 survey of hydrocyanic acid content in a number of foods, a 2014 survey of the trans fatty acid content of Australian and New Zealand foods and a 2014 survey of inorganic arsenic in seaweed and seaweed products (FSANZ 2018a).

National residue and contaminant surveys

Both Australia and New Zealand have ongoing monitoring programs for agvet chemical residues and contaminants in the food supply. These surveys generally test raw agricultural produce at the farm gate or at the point of sale. Results on the food chemical content of the foods surveyed are published and may be compared with maximum levels permitted in food standards.

The Australian National Residue Survey (Department of Agriculture and Water Resources 2018b) is an important part of the overall risk management system for agvet chemical residues and contaminants in Australia and aims to support primary producers and agricultural industries by confirming Australia's status as a clean food producer, both for domestic and export markets. The National Residue Survey was started in the 1960s to test produce intended for export against requirements in the *Australia New Zealand Food Standards Code* for maximum

levels (MPLs for residues, MLs for contaminants), so the focus was on cereal, dairy and meat products; however, the list has since been expanded to cover other animals and plants.

The New Zealand Food Residues Survey Programme (MPI 2018a), formerly called the Food Residue Surveillance Programme, was established in 2003 to monitor pesticide residues and contaminants in domestically produced and imported food and to collect baseline data on food chemical content to determine if good agricultural practice was being followed. Testing against requirements in the New Zealand *Food Act 2014* (MRLs for residues) or the *Australia New Zealand Food Standards Code* (MLs for contaminants) is reported.

Total diet studies

Total diet studies differ from the national residue and contaminant surveys described above in several ways:

- foods are selected to form a representative sample of major food groups that make up the diet in each country
- individual samples of a single food from different areas of the country may be composited before analysis
- foods are prepared 'ready for consumption' before analysis (e.g. meat is dry-cooked)
- a dietary exposure assessment is reported for each chemical surveyed
- a risk characterisation is undertaken where relevant HBGVs exist.

Information obtained from total diet studies over time can inform the development and review of food standards to ensure that food eaten by the average person in a population continues to be safe. The methodology for total diet studies for planning, implementing and reporting on the results is well documented (Abbey et al. 2013).

The Australian Total Diet Study (ATDS) (FSANZ 2017b) is undertaken by FSANZ as part of the ISFR-coordinated survey plan. The NHMRC conducted the first total diet survey (known as the Australian Market Basket Survey) in 1970 (Abbey et al. 2013). The ATDS is conducted every two to

SHOULD AUSTRALIANS AND NEW ZEALANDERS BE WORRIED ABOUT CHEMICALS AND HEAVY METALS IN THEIR FOOD?

Many people are concerned about the level of chemical residues and heavy metals in the food supply. Based on your understanding of monitoring of these materials in the Australian and New Zealand food supplies, do you think Australians and New Zealanders have cause for concern? Write a paragraph explaining your opinion. What would be your response regarding hormones in the Australian or New Zealand food supply?

three years, resources permitting. The sampling and analysis of foods usually take place in one year, and the report writing and planning for the next survey take place in the following year(s). Traditionally, agvet chemical residues and contaminants (heavy metals, mycotoxins) are studied; however, food additives and nutrients may be included.

The New Zealand Total Diet Study was first established in 1974 and is currently undertaken by the MPI every five years (MPI 2018b). It aims to assess New Zealanders' exposure to certain agricultural compounds, contaminant elements and nutrients from a range of foods consumed in a typical diet (Vannoort 2013). The inclusion of a standard list of chemicals and nutrients—for example, iodine and selenium—enables a trend analysis to be reported.

Food composition monitoring

Many countries have national food composition programs that track changes in macro- and micro-nutrient composition over time in key foods and provide valuable data for nutrient risk assessments. Published food composition tables may be for reference or developed specifically for use in national nutrition surveys. In Australia, FSANZ currently publishes the Australian Food Composition Database (FSANZ 2019), a reference data set, and AUSNUT, the data set used in the 2011–2013 Australian Health Survey (FSANZ 2016a); in New Zealand, the Department of Health with the New Zealand Institute for Plant and Food Research supports similar data sets (NZIPFR & MOH 2018).

Ad hoc surveys

Other surveys may be undertaken as the need arises—for example, if a particular hazard is identified in a food incident, if there is a lack of information for a specific risk assessment or in response to an issue reported overseas where the current risk status in Australia or New Zealand is unknown. These may be undertaken as part of the ISFR-coordinated survey plan or by an individual agency. Recent FSANZ surveys include added colours in foods, heavy metals in canned fruit and scheduled pharmaceuticals in foods intended to promote weight loss (FSANZ 2016a; 2018a; 2018b).

Imported foods monitoring

The Department of Agriculture and Water Resources inspects imported food to check that it meets Australian public health and safety requirements and to ensure it complies with the *Australia New Zealand Food Standards Code* (Department of Agriculture and Water Resources 2018a). Foods that are assessed as being high-risk will be inspected more frequently than those that are low-risk. The risk list is based on advice from FSANZ, which takes an evidence-based approach to determine if foods present a food safety risk (FSANZ 2017a). Potentially hazardous foods may be included in the list. Biosecurity restrictions also exist on food such as meat, fruit, eggs, vegetables and dairy products from certain countries. The New Zealand MPI has a similar role.

Under the Trans-Tasman Mutual Recognition Arrangement (*TTMRA Act 1997*), foods imported to Australia from New Zealand are accepted without testing and vice versa.

In addition to routine testing of imported foods, the Australian Department of Agriculture and Water Resources and New Zealand MPI may conduct additional surveys to inform future risk assessments; these can sometimes be undertaken as part of the ISFR–coordinated food survey plan (see above).

FOOD RECALLS

A food may need to be removed from the food supply because routine monitoring by the food industry has identified a problem, because enforcement agencies have identified a problem from a survey or investigation of an incident or, on occasion, because overseas countries have notified a problem with foods that may be imported into Australia or New Zealand. A food recall is action taken to remove unsafe food from distribution, sale and consumption. All food businesses must be able to quickly remove food from the marketplace to protect public health and safety. FSANZ coordinates and monitors food recalls in Australia (FSANZ 2018c); in New Zealand, food recalls are coordinated by the MPI (MPI 2018c). Common problems are undeclared allergens, microbial spoilage, physical contamination (e.g. metal, glass, plastic fragments), incorrect labelling and food chemical content over permitted levels.

EVALUATION OF FOOD MANAGEMENT MEASURES

A formal evaluation of the impact of a food management approach determines how well the risk management measures are working by comparing intended aims or objectives with actual outcomes pre- and post-implementation. Monitoring programs that collect data on the food supply are a critical part of risk management systems (see Figure 6.4) and provide feedback on how effective risk management measures have been, as well as data for future risk assessments. Total diet studies may also form part of an evaluation of how well food standards are working for various food chemicals. In cases where the results of a food survey indicate further risk management measures may be needed, enforcement action may be taken by regulatory agencies if a standard has not been followed, amendments to a food standard may be considered and/or other risk management measures may be taken. Most food businesses throughout the food chain have internal monitoring and quality

TRACKING FOR FOOD RECALLS

Traceability is the ability to track any food through all stages of production, processing and distribution (including importation and at retail). Traceability should mean that movements can be traced one step backwards and one step forwards at any point in the supply chain.

To ensure that, in the event of a food safety incident, they are able to effectively recall a product, food manufacturers must be able to keep records including:

- name and address (and other contact details) of suppliers and a description of products or inputs supplied (raw materials, additives, other ingredients, packaging)
- name and address (and other contact details) of customers and a description of the product supplied to them
- date of transaction or delivery
- batch or lot identification (or other markings)
- volume or quantity of product supplied or received
- any other relevant production records.

assurance programs to ensure their products are of good quality and safe for consumption in accordance with food standard and other requirements; however, small businesses may not have the resources to run comprehensive programs.

FSANZ conducted several evaluations following the restructure of the *Australia New Zealand Food Standards Code* from 2000 onwards (FSANZ 2018b). For example, the 2004 intense sweetener survey checked if sweeteners such as aspartame were being used in Australia and New Zealand in line with the new food additives standard and that estimated dietary exposures were not exceeding relevant HBGVs (FSANZ 2004). The MPLs for one sweetener, cyclamate, were later reduced (FSANZ 2007).

An important evaluation recently undertaken by the Food Regulation Standing Committee and the Australian Health Ministers' Advisory Council in three stages from 2013 to 2017 assessed whether the mandatory iodine and folic acid fortification standard had been successful in meeting its public health objectives.

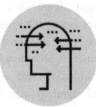

BIOFORTIFICATION VERSUS FORTIFICATION

In Australia, a number of foods are fortified in order to improve the delivery of micronutrients, such as thiamin, iodine and folate. These have reduced the incidence of a range of conditions that emerged as a result of deficiencies. Fortification is, however, controversial and **biofortification** is seen as an effective alternative. Both require complex cross-system approaches.

Explore the peer-reviewed literature to answer the following questions.

- Why do you think mandatory fortification is controversial?
- What are the alternatives?
- When might biofortification be feasible or more appropriate?
- What systems and actors are involved in each strategy?
- Do a SWOT (Strengths, Weaknesses, Opportunities and Threats) analysis of fortification and its alternatives.

Here are some articles to get you started:

- Akhtar, S., Anjum, F.M. & Anjum, M.A., 2011, 'Micronutrient fortification of wheat flour: Recent development and strategies', *Food Research International, 44*(3): 652–9
- Saltzman, A. et al., 2013, 'Biofortification: Progress toward a more nourishing future', *Global Food Security, 2*(1): 9–17
- Scrinis, G., 2016, 'Reformulation, fortification and functionalization: Big Food corporations' nutritional engineering and marketing strategies', *Journal of Peasant Studies, 43*(1): 17–37
- Sinclair, M.I. et al., 2000, 'Risk science and communication issues and challenges for food: An Australian perspective', *Asia Pacific Journal of Clinical Nutrition, 9*(4): 318–21
- Wahlqvist, M.L., 2008, 'National food fortification: A dialogue with reference to Asia: Policy in evolution', *Asia Pacific Journal of Clinical Nutrition, 17*(S1): 24–9

SUMMARY

- Food Standards Australia and New Zealand (FSANZ) is a joint agency of the Australian and New Zealand governments whose role is to develop and administer food standards via the *Australia New Zealand Food Standards Code*.
- Managing risk in the food system primarily involves four stages: preliminary activities that identify the issue, establishing risk management goals and developing risk assessment questions; risk management options formulation; implementation of the decision; and, monitoring and evaluation of the effectiveness of the risk management measure(s) taken.
- Enforcement of the Food Standards Code is the responsibility of state and territory food agencies, with national responsibility for imported foods via the Commonwealth Department of Agriculture and Water Resources in Australia and Ministry for Primary Industries in New Zealand.
- Chemicals present in foods can be intentionally added to food, as with food additives and processing aids, residues in food from chemicals intentionally used on animals and plants to control pests and diseases (agricultural and veterinary chemicals), or present as contaminants.
- Effective monitoring programs are a key component of risk management systems and are essential to managing food-related health risks. Monitoring allows action to be taken in cases where regulations and standards are not followed appropriately. In Australia and New Zealand, ongoing food monitoring programs include the National Residue Survey (Australia), New Zealand Food Residues Survey Programme and total diet surveys in both countries.
- Tracking changes in the macro- and micronutrient composition of foods is also an important aspect of monitoring systems—for example, in Australia with AUSNUT and the Australian Food Composition data sets.

KEY TERMS

Biofortification: the process of improving the nutritional value of foods during crop growth, rather than adding in nutrients post–harvest during the processing of food.

Codex Alimentarius ('Codex'): the international code for food standards and provides international food standards, guidelines and codes of practice to contribute to the safety, quality and fairness of the international food trade. The Codex includes provisions in respect of food hygiene, food additives, residues of pesticides and veterinary drugs, contaminants, labelling and presentation, methods of analysis and sampling, and import and export inspection and certification. Codex standards are recognised by the World Trade Organization (WTO). They are not imposed on member countries but, as a WTO member, Australia is obliged, where possible, to harmonise its domestic regulations with Codex standards. FSANZ takes Codex standards into account when developing and revising domestic food standards.

Dietary exposure to food chemical = amount food consumed × level of chemical in food.

Ester: an organic compound made by replacing the hydrogen of an acid by an alkyl or other organic group. Many naturally occurring fats and essential oils are esters of fatty acids.

Good Manufacturing Practice (GMP): a set of practices required in order to ensure that products are consistently produced and controlled to the quality standards appropriate to their intended use and as required by the product specification. GMP covers all aspects of production from the starting materials, premises and equipment to the training and personal hygiene of staff. The main purpose of GMP is always to prevent harm from occurring to the end user.

Health-based guidance values (HBGVs): used by government agencies such as the Department of Health to indicate the amount of a chemical in drinking water or food that can be consumed regularly without significant risk to health.

Maximum level (ML): the highest amount of a specified contaminant or natural toxicant that is permitted to be present in a nominated food.

Maximum permitted level (MPL): the highest amount of a food additive or processing aid that is permitted to be present in a nominated food for sale as a result of use in accordance with Good Manufacturing Practice.

Maximum residue limit (MRL): the highest amount of an agricultural or veterinary (agvet) chemical residue that is legally allowed in a food product for sale, whether it is produced domestically or imported.

Perceived risk: the uncertainty consumers associate with a product—for example, the uncertainty a consumer feels about the safety of a new food product

ACKNOWLEDGEMENT

This chapter has been modified and updated from those written by Gwynn Jones, Louise Lennard, Janis Baines and Ingrid R.E. Rutishauser, which appeared in the third edition of *Food and Nutrition*.

REFERENCES

Abbey, J.L., Baines, J., Laajoki, L. & Hambridge, T., 2013, 'Australia's experience: Total Diet Surveys', in G. Moy & R.W. Vannoort (eds), *Total Diet Studies*, New York, NY: Springer Science, pp. 211–17

Abbott, P., Baines, J., Fox, P., Graf, L., Kelly, L. et al., 2003, 'Review of the regulations for contaminants and natural toxicants', *Food Control*, 14(6): 383–9, doi:10.1016/S0956-7135(03)00040-9

ABS, 2016, *Australian Health Survey: Consumption of food groups from the Australian Dietary Guidelines, 2011–12*, <www.abs.gov.au/AUSSTATS/abs@.nsf/Latestproducts/4364.0.55.012Glossary02011-12>, accessed 22 November 2018

Akhtar, S., Anjum, F.M. & Anjum, M.A., 2011, 'Micronutrient fortification of wheat flour: Recent development and strategies', *Food Research International*, 44(3): 652–9, doi:10.1016/j.foodres.2010.12.033

Armstrong, P., Murray, P., Nesdale, A. & Peckler, B., 2016, 'Ciguatera fish poisoning', *New Zealand Medical Journal*, 129(1444): 113–16, <www.ncbi.nlm.nih.gov/pubmed/27806035>, accessed 15 July 2019

Australian Government, 2016, *Food Standards Australia New Zealand Act 1991*, <www.legislation.gov.au/Series/F2015L00383>, accessed 22 January 2019

—— 2017, *Food Additives* (Standard 1.3.1), <www.legislation.gov.au/Series/F2015L00396>, accessed 22 January 2019

AVPMA, 2018, *Health-based Guidance Values*, <https://apvma.gov.au/node/26581>, accessed 18 June 2018

Baines, J., Cunningham, J., Leemhuis, C., Hambridge, T. & Mackerras, D., 2011, 'Risk assessment to underpin food regulatory decisions: An example of public health nutritional epidemiology', *Nutrients*, 3(1): 164–85, doi:10.3390/nu3010164

Covello, V. & Sandman, P.M., 2001, 'Risk communication: Evolution and revolution', in A. Wolbarst (ed.), *Solutions to an Environment in Peril*, Baltimore, MD: Johns Hopkins University Press, pp. 164–78

CRCSLM/CSIRO, 1999, *Managing Cadmium in Potatoes for Quality Produce*, <www.cadmium-management.org.au/documents/Managing_Cd_in_potatoes_brochure.pdf>, accessed 25 January 2019

Crossley, S.J. & Baines, J., 2014, 'Public health measures: Monitoring of contaminants', in Y. Motarjemi (ed.), *Encyclopedia of Food Safety*, Waltham: Academic Press, pp. 55–61

Department of Agriculture and Water Resources, 2018a, *Imported Food Inspection Scheme*, <www.agriculture.gov.au/import/goods/food/inspection-compliance/inspection-scheme>, accessed 24 January 2019

—— 2018b, *National Residue Survey*, <www.agriculture.gov.au/ag-farm-food/food/nrs/>, accessed 24 January 2019

FAO/WHO, 1995, *Report of the Joint FAO/WHO Expert Consultation on Application of Risk Analysis to Food Standards Issues*, <www.fao.org/docrep/008/ae922e/ae922e00.htm>, accessed 25 January 2019

—— 1997, *Report of the Joint FAO/WHO Expert Consultation on Risk Management and Food Safety*, <www.fao.org/3/a-w4982e.pdf>, accessed 25 January 2019

—— 2009, *Environmental Health Criteria (EHC): 240 Principles and Methods for Risk Assessment of Chemicals in Foods*, <www.who.int/foodsafety/publications/chemical-food/en/>, accessed 25 January 2019

—— 2018, *Codex Alimentarius: International Food Standards*, <www.fao.org/fao-who-codexalimentarius/codex-texts/list-standards/en/>, accessed 25 January 2019

Food Regulation, 2018, *Australian and New Zealand Ministerial Forum on Food Regulation*, <http://foodregulation.gov.au/internet/fr/publishing.nsf/Content/Forum>, accessed 24 January 2019

Food Safety Information Council, 2019, *Natural Toxins in Foods*, <http://foodsafety.asn.au/natural-toxins-in-food/>, accessed 24 January 2019

Friedman, M.A., Fernandez, M., Backer, L.C., Dickey, R.W., Bernstein, J. et al., 2017, 'An updated review of ciguatera fish poisoning: Clinical, epidemiological, environmental, and public health management', *Marine Drugs*, 15(3): 72, doi:10.3390/md15030072

Friedman, M.A., Fleming, L.E., Fernandez, M., Bienfang, P., Schrank, K. et al., 2008, 'Ciguatera fish poisoning: Treatment, prevention and management', *Marine Drugs*, 6(3): 456–79, doi:10.3390/md20080022

FSANZ, 2004, *Intense Sweeteners Survey* <www.foodstandards.gov.au/publications/pages/evaluationreportseries/intensesweetenerssurveymarch2004/Default.aspx>, accessed 22 January 2019

—— 2007, *Final Assessment Report: Proposal P287*, <www.foodstandards.gov.au/code/proposals/documents/P287_FAR_Cyclamate_Review_FINAL.pdf>, accessed 22 January 2019

—— 2011, *Mercury in Fish*, <www.foodstandards.gov.au/consumer/chemicals/mercury/Pages/default.aspx>, accessed 25 January 2019

—— 2013, *Risk Analysis in Food Regulation*, <www.foodstandards.gov.au/publications/riskanalysisfoodregulation/Pages/default.aspx>, accessed 18 June 2018

—— 2016a, *Monitoring Nutrients in our Food Supply*, <www.foodstandards.gov.au/science/monitoringnutrients/Pages/default.aspx>, accessed 25 January 2019

—— 2016b, *Safe Food Australia: A guide to food safety requirements*, <www.foodstandards.gov.au/publications/Pages/safefoodaustralia3rd16.aspx>, accessed 18 June 2018

—— 2017a, *Advice on Imported Food*, <www.foodstandards.gov.au/consumer/importedfoods/Pages/FSANZ-advice-on-imported-food.aspx>, accessed 19 June 2018

—— 2017b, *Total Diet Survey*, <www.foodstandards.gov.au/science/surveillance/Pages/australiantotaldiets1914.aspx>, accessed 25 January 2019

—— 2018a, *Completed ISFR Food Surveys*, <www.foodstandards.gov.au/science/surveillance/Pages/isccomponent1.aspx>, accessed 19 June 2018

—— 2018b, *Evaluation Report Series*, <www.foodstandards.gov.au/science/Pages/Evaluation-report-series.aspx>, accessed 18 June 2018

—— 2018c, *Food Recalls*, <www.foodstandards.gov.au/industry/foodrecalls/Pages/default.aspx>, accessed 18 June 2018

—— 2018d, *Food Standards Australia New Zealand Board*, <www.foodstandards.gov.au/about/board/Pages/default.aspx>, accessed 19 June 2018

—— 2018e, *Food Standards Code*, <www.foodstandards.gov.au/code/Pages/default.aspx>, accessed 23 January 2019

—— 2019, *The Australian Food Composition Database,* <www.foodstandards.gov.au/science/monitoringnutrients/afcd/Pages/default.aspx>, accessed 18 February 2019

MOH, 2011, *Nutrition Survey,* <www.health.govt.nz/nz-health-statistics/national-collections-and-surveys/surveys/past-surveys/nutrition-survey>, accessed 25 January 2019

MPI, 2016, *Food Act 2014,* <www.mpi.govt.nz/food-safety/food-act-2014/>, accessed 25 January 2019

—— 2018a, *Food Residues Survey Programme,* <www.mpi.govt.nz/food-safety/food-monitoring-and-surveillance/food-residues-survey-programme/>, accessed 25 January 2019

—— 2018b, *New Zealand Total Diet Survey,* <www.mpi.govt.nz/food-safety/food-monitoring-and-surveillance/new-zealand-total-diet-study/>, accessed 25 January 2019

—— 2018c, *Recalled Food Products,* <www.mpi.govt.nz/food-safety/food-recalls/recalled-food-products/>, accessed 25 January 2019

NHMRC, 2006, *Nutrient Reference Values for Australia and New Zealand,* <https://nhmrc.gov.au/sites/default/files/images/nutrient-refererence-dietary-intakes.pdf >, accessed 28 November 2018

—— 2017a, *Australian and New Zealand Nutrient Reference Values for Sodium,* <www.nrv.gov.au/sites/default/files/content/resources/2017%20ANZ%20NRVs%20for%20Sodium%20%28containing%20recommendations%29.pdf>, accessed 24 January 2019

—— 2017b, *NHMRC Public Statement: Water Fluoridation and Human Health in Australia,* <https://nhmrc.gov.au/about-us/publications/2017-public-statement-water-fluoridation-and-human-health>, accessed 24 January 2019

NSW Food Authority, 2017, *Ciguatera Poisoning,* <https://foodauthority.nsw.gov.au/_Documents/retailfactsheets/ciguatera_poisoning.pdf>, accessed 24 January 2019

NZIPFR & MOH, 2018, *New Zealand Food Composition Database,* <www.foodcomposition.co.nz/>, accessed 25 January 2019

Saltzman, A., Birol, E., Bouis, H.E., Boy, E., De Moura, F.F. et al., 2013, 'Biofortification: Progress toward a more nourishing future', *Global Food Security, 2*(1): 9–17, doi:10.1016/j.gfs.2012.12.003

Sanders, T.A., 2003, 'Food safety and risk assessment: Naturally occurring potential toxicants and anti-nutritive compounds in plant foods', *Forum of Nutrition, 56*: 407–9

Scrinis, G., 2016, 'Reformulation, fortification and functionalization: Big Food corporations' nutritional engineering and marketing strategies', *Journal of Peasant Studies, 43*(1): 17–37, doi:10.1080/03066150.2015.1101455

Sinclair, M.I., Savige, G.S., Dalais, F.S. & Wahlqvist, M.L., 2000, 'Risk science and communication issues and challenges for food: An Australian perspective', *Asia Pacific Journal of Clinical Nutrition, 9*(4): 318–21, doi:10.1046/j.1440-6047.2000.00200.x

Vannoort, R.W., 2013, 'New Zealand's experience: Total Diet Surveys', in G. Moy & R.W. Vannoort (eds), *Total Diet Studies,* New York, NY: Springer Science, pp. 357–71

Wahlqvist, M.L., 2008, 'National food fortification: A dialogue with reference to Asia: Policy in evolution', *Asia Pacific Journal of Clinical Nutrition, 17*(S1): 24–9, doi:10.6133/apjcn.2008.17.s1.06

Wen, J.-G., Liu, X.-J., Wang, Z.-M., Li, T.-F. & Wahlqvist, M.L., 2016, 'Melamine-contaminated milk formula and its impact on children', *Asia Pacific Journal of Clinical Nutrition, 25*(4): 697–705, doi:10.6133/apjcn.072016.01

WHO, 2008, *Expert Meeting to Review Toxicological Aspects of Melamine and Cyanuric Acid,* <www.who.int/foodsafety/fs_management/conclusions_recommendations.pdf>, accessed 25 January 2019

{CHAPTER 7}
FOOD SAFETY: MICROBIOLOGICAL RISKS

Janis Baines and David Borradale

OBJECTIVES

- Explain the role of factors that affect microbial growth and survival.
- Identify important microorganisms responsible for foodborne illness.
- Demonstrate an understanding of the importance of food safety programs, such as HACCP, in reducing the risk of foodborne illness.
- Classify potentially hazardous foods and describe the key food hygiene and handling requirements to minimise risk of foodborne illness.

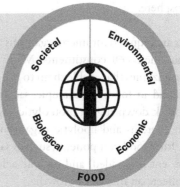

INTRODUCTION

While microbes are an essential element in the production of many foods, such as yeasts in beer and lactic acid-producing bacteria in yoghurt, food can also provide an environment for the growth of pathogenic (or disease-causing) microbes. Foodborne illness due to microbial contamination of food is a significant health burden worldwide; however, the risk of illness is significantly reduced with a basic knowledge of the factors influencing microbial growth and by following some simple steps for the storage, preparation and handling of food. Health professionals, including nutritionists, play an essential role in educating the public about potentially hazardous foods and how to reduce the risk of foodborne illnesses caused by microbiological agents.

ASSESSMENT OF MICROBIOLOGICAL RISK

Assessments of the risk of exposure to the microbiological hazards take account of the ability of the pathogen to grow, survive or be inactivated in a food. The risk analyst needs information on the level of the organism (hazard), the prevalence (how often it occurs in a population), the frequency, the amount of the food consumed, the population consuming the food and the severity of the illness (FSANZ 2013).

For some microbiological hazards, some of this information may not be available and mathematical models are needed to predict the growth, inactivation and survival of an organism throughout the food chain ('paddock to plate').

Microbial growth and food

The most important factors affecting the ability of microorganisms to survive, grow or multiply in foods are:

- available nutrients
- moisture (available water)
- time and temperature
- pH level
- gas atmosphere.

Nutrients are required for microorganisms to grow and maintain their cell constituents. Many species have specific enzymes that enable them to use specific substrates found in food; for example, saccharolytic organisms break down sugars, proteolytic organisms break down proteins and lipolytic organisms break down fats. Other food components, such as salt (both naturally present and added) and organic acids, have inhibitory effects on microbial growth.

Moisture is required by microorganisms to grow. The amount available for use is in the form of 'free' water (i.e. not bound in the **food matrix**), expressed as water activity (a_w or A_w). This is determined by measuring the relative humidity of the vapour in the air over the solution or substance (a water activity or a_w of 0.75 is equal to a relative humidity of 75 per cent). Each species has a maximum, optimum and minimum a_w for growth; in general, bacteria require a higher a_w than yeasts, which require a higher a_w than moulds. Minimum water activity for growth ranges from an a_w of 0.61 for xerophilic (dry-loving) fungi to 0.90 for most bacteria.

Time and *temperature* are critical to the ability of microorganisms to grow, as microorganisms can reproduce rapidly under optimal temperature conditions; rates of generation depend on species and conditions. For example, bacteria from the genus *Campylobacter* spp. grow between 30 and 45°C; at 32°C, the *C. jejuni* species doubles in six hours.

Campylobacter spp. can survive at lower temperatures, but it is destroyed when treated at temperatures above 55–60°C for a few minutes (FSANZ 2017a). Organisms are also classified according to the temperature range they need to grow; psychrophiles are low-temperature organisms, mesophiles are medium-temperature organisms and thermopiles are high-temperature organisms. Due to the diversity of microorganisms, survival is highly organism-dependent; for instance, *Salmonella* has been observed to survive on frozen fruit stored at −20°C for six months (Strawn & Danyluk 2010).

The *pH* of the environment markedly affects microbial growth and activity, with each microorganism having a maximum, optimum and minimum pH for growth. Most bacteria prefer low-acid conditions (pH 6–8); yeasts prefer more acid environments (pH 4.5–6) while moulds can tolerate acid conditions (pH 3–4). Due to the significance of the microbial relationship with pH conditions, foods are classified as acid foods (pH<4.5) or low-acid foods (pH >4.5). The pH range is different for fruits (pH 1.8–9.7), vegetables (4.2–7.3), meats (5.1–6.4), fish and shellfish (5.5–7.0), bread (5.4), milk (6.3–6.5) and eggs (7.0–9.0 for egg whites but 6.4 for egg yolk).

Gas atmosphere affects microbial activity, particularly oxygen and carbon dioxide, with microorganisms classified according to their gaseous requirements for growth. Moulds are entirely aerobic (requiring oxygen for growth); some yeasts are facultative anaerobes (i.e. they can grow in the presence or absence of oxygen) but most are also aerobes. Microorganisms vary widely in their tolerance to carbon dioxide, with the growth of some organisms completely suppressed in a carbon dioxide atmosphere, a characteristic that is utilised in modified-atmosphere packaging of foods (see Chapter 5). Another example of how atmospheric composition affects microbial activity is in low-oxygen environments, such as those found in bottled, canned or vacuum-packed foods that have been inadequately processed, as these environments favour the growth of anaerobic bacteria such as *Clostridium botulinum*.

Other factors may also influence the viability of microorganisms, such as the oxidation-reduction (redox) potential of the food, natural inhibitors present in the food, other stresses (including physical stresses) and interaction between factors.

FOODBORNE DISEASE

Foodborne disease is a significant cause of morbidity and mortality across the globe and the increased internationalisation of food production and distribution means pathogens associated with food know no borders (FSANZ 2017a). Information on the burden of foodborne diseases can inform policy-makers and assist in allocating appropriate resources for food safety control and intervention efforts.

The main causes of foodborne illness are:
• bacteria (infections, toxin production)
• viruses
• parasites, including protozoa
• mycotoxins
• cyanobacterial toxins
• prions.

A 2015 report prepared by the WHO Foodborne Disease Burden Epidemiology Reference Group, provided the first estimates of global foodborne disease incidence, mortality, and disease burden in terms of disability-adjusted life years (DALYs). The most frequent causes of foodborne illness were diarrhoeal disease agents, particularly norovirus and *Campylobacter*. Other major causes of foodborne deaths were *Salmonella typhi, Taenia solium,* hepatitis A virus, and aflatoxin. Although a limited range of organisms are responsible for the majority of foodborne disease, their potential survival, growth and toxin production, and therefore their pathogenicity, is dependent to a significant extent on the food structure in which they are present (FSANZ 2017a).

In 2000, Australia improved national surveillance of gastrointestinal and foodborne illness by adapting the US Centers for Disease Control and Prevention's FoodNet model of active surveillance (Angulo et al.

2008). An annual OzFoodNet Report summarises the incidence of diseases potentially transmitted by food in Australia and details outbreaks associated with food in 2011 (OzFoodNet 2012). OzFoodNet sites reported almost 31,000 notifications of nine diseases or conditions that may be transmitted by food. The most commonly notified infections were *Campylobacter* followed by *Salmonella*. The most frequently notified *Salmonella* serotype was *S. typhimurium*, accounting for 48 per cent of all Salmonella notifications (OzFoodNet 2012). Similar annual reports are available for New Zealand for 2016 (MPI 2017), where *Campylobacter* was also the organism of most concern.

Figure 7.1 shows the notification rate per 100,000 population for *Salmonella* in Australia by year of diagnosis. There is slight upward trend, from a low of 31.4 per 100,000 population in 1996 to a high of 54.3 per 100,000 population in 2011. The period from 2008 to 2010 shows the most rapid increase in rates (OzFoodNet 2012).

Estimates of changes in the burden of foodborne disease over time in Australia, from circa 2000 to 2010, are given by Kirk et al. (2014) based on incidence, hospitalisations and deaths attributed to food, with approximately 25 per cent of gastroenteritis cases caused by contaminated food. The number of cases and incidence rates decreased between 2000 and 2010 from 4.3 million (a rate of 224,000 per million population) to 4.1 million (186,000 per million population). However, in both periods cases of salmonellosis and campylobacteriosis were the leading causes of hospitalisations, while *Listeria monocytogenes* and *Salmonella* spp. infections were the leading causes of deaths (Kirk et al. 2014).

PATHOGENS RESPONSIBLE FOR FOODBORNE ILLNESS

This section provides an overview of the main classes of pathogens responsible for causing foodborne illness in humans. For further detail on specific foodborne pathogens, see the online technical series *Agents of Foodborne Illness* by FSANZ (FSANZ 2017a).

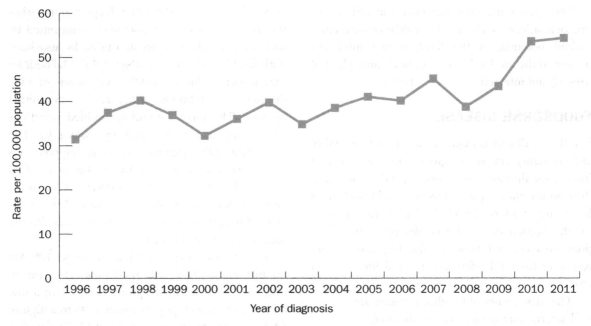

Figure 7.1: Notification rate for salmonellosis in Australia, by year of diagnosis

Source: OzFoodNet (2012). Reproduced by permission

Bacteria

There are two ways bacteria can cause foodborne illness: bacterial infections and bacterial produced toxins.

Bacterial infections

Bacterial infections are due to microorganisms that invade the **mucosa** of the human gut where, depending on their numbers, they cause severe, mild or subclinical symptoms. Apart from the symptoms of acute food poisoning, the sufferer may experience chronic after-effects, including malabsorption (for example, from *Salmonella* spp., *Shigella* spp.), Guillain–Barré syndrome (*Campylobacter jejuni*) or autoimmune diseases such as reactive arthritis. Table 7.1 lists some of the important pathogenic bacteria responsible for foodborne infections (FSANZ 2017a).

Some information on the three most important bacterial infections causing foodborne illness in Australia and New Zealand is given below.

Salmonella spp. are bacteria that cause salmonellosis, a common form of foodborne illness in humans. Outcomes from exposure to *Salmonella* spp. can range from mild symptoms to severe disease and can be fatal (FSANZ 2017a).

Infections caused by *Salmonella* spp. fall into two major groups: typhoid and paratyphoid fevers caused by *Salmonella typhi* and *S. paratyphi* A, B and C; and enteric infections caused by any one of the approximately 2000 *Salmonella* species (Kirk et al. 2014).

Salmonella spp. are carried by a range of domestic and wild animals and birds and the presence of any species of *Salmonella* in a foodstuff ready for human consumption is viewed as a potential health hazard. The production of *Salmonella*-free animal products is very difficult, particularly in large-scale poultry processing. For safety, all raw poultry and raw egg products should be treated as though they may contain *Salmonella*. Outbreaks of *S. enteriditis* may be due to infection of the laying hen's reproductive organs, which means the contents of an egg within its intact shell may not be sterile. Consumption of raw eggs should be avoided, especially by certain individuals such as the elderly, infants and those who are immunocompromised.

Table 7.1: Bacteria that cause infections

Organism	Most common occurrence in food	Symptoms
1. *Salmonella typhi* 2. *Salmonella paratyphi* A, B, C 3. *Salmonella* spp.	1 and 2 in water, raw milk 3 in meat, poultry, eggs, milk, desiccated coconut	1: Typhoid fever, septicaemia, enlarged spleen, fever, delirium, peritonitis, possible death within 8–20 days. 2: Paratyphoid fever: fever, gastroenteritis. 3: Diarrhoea, vomiting, abdominal cramps, fever, chills, prostration within 6–48 hours.
Aeromonas spp.	Water, shellfish, vegetables including lettuce, chilled foods	Watery diarrhoea or loose stools with blood and mucus, septicaemia in immunocompromised individuals or those with certain cancers; usually lasts 1–7 days; symptoms occur 28–48 hours after exposure.
Campylobacter spp.	Poultry, meat, raw shellfish, raw milk, mushrooms	Watery diarrhoea, severe abdominal pain, high fever, malaise within 1–11 days, reactive arthritis; Guillain–Barré syndrome may develop later.
E. coli (enterohaemorrhagic strains)	Undercooked meat (e.g. ground beef, hamburgers, mettwurst), raw milk, lettuce, alfalfa sprouts	Bloody diarrhoea (haemorrhagic colitis), renal failure and anaemia, haemolytic uraemic syndrome, thrombotic thrombocytopaenic purpura; within 1–8 days, death can occur.
Listeria monocytogenes	Soft cheeses (e.g. brie, camembert, ricotta), paté, smoked fish and seafoods, cold meat products, ready-to-eat peeled prawns, soft-serve ice cream, dips, pre-prepared salads, unpasteurised dairy products, cold cooked diced chicken, ham, salami	Meningitis, septicaemia, endocarditis, pregnant women may experience flu-like symptoms, fever, headache, premature labour, miscarriage/stillbirths; abscesses in liver, spleen, lung, kidney, brain within 1–90 days; significant mortality.
Shigella spp.	Water, faecally contaminated food, imported baby corn	Dysentery, severe abdominal pain, fever, vomiting, diarrhoea with blood and mucus, dehydration within 1–7 days.
Vibrio cholerae	Fish, raw shellfish, vegetables, water	Profuse diarrhoea, dehydration, within 1–3 days, significant mortality.

Campylobacter spp. are bacteria that cause the gastro-intestinal disease campylobacteriosis, with symptoms that can mimic appendicitis. Most cases of campylobacteriosis are not fatal. Infection with *Campylobacter* spp. has also been associated with Guillain–Barré syndrome, which results in progressive muscle weakness or paralysis. *Campylobacter* spp. are widespread in nature and are present in the intestine of many wild and domestic animals and birds (FSANZ 2017a). Evidence to date suggests that the main source of infection in humans is via raw milk, raw or undercooked poultry, or cross-contamination from poultry to other foodstuffs eaten without further cooking.

Listeria monocytogenes is a bacterium that causes listeriosis, a disease that can have severe consequences for particular groups of the population. It can cause miscarriages in pregnant women, illness in newborn babies and be fatal in immunocompromised individuals and the elderly. In healthy people, listeriosis generally only causes a mild form of illness. *L. monocytogenes* can be found throughout the environment. It has been isolated from domestic and wild animals, birds, soil, vegetation, fodder, water and from floors, drains and wet areas of food processing factories (FSANZ 2017a).

L. monocytogenes has the ability to grow over a wide temperature range (−1.5° to 45°C, with the optimal temperature being 30–37°C) and is tolerant to high salt concentrations (10 per cent). Temperatures above 50°C are lethal to *L. monocytogenes*. Dairy foods—including cheese, raw unpasteurised milk and ice-cream products—have been implicated in many outbreaks of human listeriosis, but cases have also been reported from consumption of deli and ready-to-eat meats, salad, fish and smoked fish, and, recently in Australia, rockmelons (FSANZ 2017a).

Bacterial produced toxins

Some bacteria cause human disease as a result of their ability to produce a toxin (Table 7.2). Of these, the botulinum toxins are the most poisonous substances known; it is estimated that approximately 10^{-8} g (0.01 micrograms) will kill an adult human. This form of foodborne illness is unusual in that the symptoms are neurological, not gastric. Foods that have been incorrectly home-processed—usually canned low-acid vegetables, smoked or pickled fish or meat, or high-moisture cheeses—predominate as a cause of botulism. Infant botulism may occur during the first six months of age. Ingested botulinum spores may germinate and release toxins inside the infant's intestine. Honey is suspected of being the vehicle for *C. botulinum* spores. It is, therefore, prudent not to give honey to infants aged under one year. Botulinum toxins can be deactivated by heating at 80°C for ten minutes.

Viruses

Viruses found in food may be passed on to humans; see Table 7.3 for commonly reported viruses that have caused foodborne-illness, often associated with symptoms of diarrhoea and vomiting. In 2015, there was a lot of media interest in Australia in cases of hepatitis A linked to consumption of imported frozen ready-to-eat berries. Hepatitis A affects the liver and is a disease caused by the hepatitis virus. Unlike hepatitis B and C, it does not cause chronic (long-lasting) liver disease. In most hepatitis A cases, a person's immune system will clear the infection and the liver will completely heal. The most common sources of contamination are food grown in contaminated water; produce picked or packed by a person infected with hepatitis A; and, produce washed in contaminated water. The virus can survive for several hours outside of the body and can persist on people's hands and in food. It is resistant to heating and freezing. Australia introduced new requirements for frozen berries being imported from all countries (FSANZ 2015).

Table 7.2: Bacteria that produce toxins

Organism	Most common occurrence in food	Symptoms
Clostridium botulinum	Low-acid home-canned or home-bottled fruit and vegetables, sushi (raw fish), home-preserved pork and sausage, inadequately processed canned food, honey.	Vomiting, constipation, abdominal cramps, double vision, difficulty swallowing, dry mouth, disturbed speech, cardiac and respiratory failure within 12–48 hours; significant mortality.
Staphylococcus aureus	Ham, cold meat, poultry, some salads (e.g. potato, egg, macaroni, tuna) custard and cream-filled bakery products.	Nausea, vomiting, abdominal cramps, diarrhoea within 1–6 hours; duration 1–2 days.
Clostridium perfringens	Beef, pork, poultry, gravies slowly cooled after cooking.	Abdominal cramps, diarrhoea, weakness within 8–24 hours.
Bacillus cereus	1: Proteinaceous foods (meat and meat products), vegetables, soups, sauces, puddings, spicy foods, dairy foods.	Profuse watery diarrhoea, abdominal pain without vomiting (resembling *Clostridium perfringens* poisoning) within 8–16 hours; duration 12–24 hours.
	2: Farinaceous foods (e.g. cooked rice, pasta, noodles, porridge).	Vomiting, nausea (resembling *Staphylococcus aureus* poisoning) within 1–5 hours; duration 6–24 hours.

Table 7.3: Viruses associated with foodborne illness

Organism	Most common occurrence in food	Symptoms
Hepatitis A	Water, raw shellfish, milk, salads, sandwiches, fruit, pastries; also found in frozen berries	Fever, anorexia, nausea, vomiting, weakness, jaundice, enlarged liver, lethargy, chronic liver damage within 2–6 weeks; many infected people, particularly children under the age of five, do not show any symptoms.
Rotaviruses	Water	Fever, vomiting, dehydration, severe watery diarrhoea within 1–3 days; duration 5–7 days.
Noroviruses	Raw oysters, orange juice, salad vegetables	Severe (projectile) vomiting, diarrhoea, nausea, abdominal cramps, myalgia within 15–50 hours.
Hepatitis E	Faecally contaminated food	Jaundice, anorexia, enlarged liver, abdominal pain and tenderness, nausea, vomiting, fever within 40 days.

AVIAN INFLUENZA (BIRD FLU): WHY DOES IT CONCERN HUMAN POPULATIONS?

There are three types of influenza viruses: A, B, and C. Influenza A viruses infect humans and many different animals. Influenza B viruses only circulate among humans and cause seasonal epidemics. Influenza C viruses can infect both humans and pigs, but infections are generally mild and are rarely reported.

Depending on the origin host, influenza A viruses can be classified as avian influenza, swine influenza or other types of animal influenza viruses. Wild birds commonly 'host' avian influenza A, which can be passed on to domestic birds (ducks, chickens) through direct contact with infected waterfowl or other infected poultry, or through contact with surfaces that have been contaminated with the viruses. All of these animal influenza type A viruses are distinct from human influenza viruses and do not easily transmit between humans.

However, infections with avian and **zoonotic** influenza viruses have been reported in humans and are primarily acquired through direct contact with infected animals or contaminated environments.

In 1997, human infections with the HPAI A(H5N1) virus were reported during an outbreak in poultry in the Hong Kong region. Since 2003, this avian virus has spread from Asia to Europe and Africa and has become entrenched in poultry populations in some countries. In 2013, human infections with the LPAI A(H7N9) virus were reported in China. Outbreaks have resulted in millions of poultry infections and slaughter of poultry flocks, several hundred human cases and many human deaths.

Up to August 2015 no infections had been reported in Australia, but travellers may be susceptible abroad. Although a number of species of wild waterfowl (wading birds) do migrate to Australia, they are not the normal hosts or spreaders of avian influenza found elsewhere in the world.

Sources: Centers for Disease Control and Prevention (2017); Department of Agriculture and Water Resources (2017); Department of Health (2018); WHO (2017)

Other causes of foodborne illness
Protozoa

While bacteria and viruses receive much of the attention as causes of foodborne illness another important cause of foodborne illness includes some species of protozoa; single-celled microscopic animals of a group of phyla from the kingdom Protista. An example of a pathogenic protozoan transmitted via both food and water is *Giardia lamblia*, the cause of giardiasis, a condition associated with severe diarrhoea and, in some cases, malabsorption and dehydration, if the condition continues over weeks. Another protozoan infection caused by *Cryptosporidium parvum* can be life-threatening in severely immunocompromised patients, such as AIDS patients. The spores of both *Cryptosporidium* and *Giardia* are commonly found in water and are particularly resistant to the concentrations of chlorine normally present in drinking water. However, boiling water rapidly for one minute will destroy spores. Information on common foodborne protozoa that can cause illness, sources and symptoms of infection is provided in Table 7.4.

Mycotoxins

Mycotoxins are a structurally diverse group of metabolites of filamentous fungi or moulds with a range of toxic effects that also cause foodborne illness. Most mycotoxins are produced by moulds growing on grains or other low-moisture plant foods and feeds, with the rate of growth depending on the substrate, temperature and water activity (Semple et al. 2011). They can also be found in milk and milk products, as well as in certain tissues of animals that have been fed contaminated feed.

Aflatoxins are a highly **hepatotoxic** and carcinogenic example of a mycotoxin produced by *Aspergillus* spp. moulds. Commonly associated with peanuts and tree nuts, they can also accumulate in corn, cereals, soybeans, dried fruits, spices and maize (Semple et al. 2011). Control methods, such as low temperature storage and control of moisture levels post-harvest, are important to reduce aflatoxin contamination; however, concerns exist over aflatoxin levels in imported foods such as peanuts and pistachios (FSANZ 2017a).

THE AUSTRALIAN FOOD SAFETY STANDARDS AND THE PREVENTION OF FOODBORNE ILLNESS

Australian businesses are required to produce food that is safe to eat under the Food Safety Standards to minimise the risk of foodborne illness and food spoilage, while businesses in New Zealand are required to comply with the *Food Act 2014* (FSANZ 2016b; MPI 2016). Chapter 3—Food Safety Standards (Australia only) in the *Australia New Zealand Food Standards Code* covers food safety programs (Standard 3.2.1), food safety practices and general requirements (Standard 3.2.2), food premises and equipment (Standard 3.2.3) and food safety plans for food service to vulnerable persons (those in acute care hospitals, psychiatric hospitals, nursing homes for the aged, hospices, establishments for chemotherapy and renal dialysis and childcare centres) (Standard 3.3.1) (FSANZ 2018b). FSANZ also publishes *Safe Food Australia*, a guide to food safety requirements to assist food businesses in implementing these standards, and a

Table 7.4: Protozoa organisms

Organism	Most common occurrence in food	Symptoms
Entamoeba histolytica	Water, fruit, vegetables	Dysentery, abscess formation in liver, lungs or brain
Giardia lamblia	Water, vegetables	Explosive diarrhoea, abdominal cramps, flatulence, nausea, malaise
Toxoplasma gondii	Pork, lamb, other meats, vegetables	Swollen lymph nodes, intermittent fever, anorexia, high lymphocyte count
Cryptosporidium parvum	Water	Profuse watery diarrhoea, abdominal pain, vomiting, fever

WHAT CAUSES BOVINE SPONGIFORM ENCEPHALOPATHY (BSE)?

Bovine spongiform encephalopathy (BSE), commonly known as mad cow disease, is a fatal neurodegenerative disease of cattle. It is caused by proteinaceous infectious particles known as prions. Prions are small, abnormal, distorted proteins containing 231 amino acids, found in the cell membrane of brain cells. While the prions are not 'alive', the infective prion has an abnormal conformation (three-dimensional shape) that, when in contact with normal brain cell protein, causes the latter to change shape, with loss of protein functionality. BSE is a good example of why a systems approach and an understanding of the interconnectedness of those systems is essential. BSE is the only transmissible spongiform encephalopathy of animals that is known to be infectious to humans through the consumption of contaminated meat. The human form of the disease is known as variant Creutzfeldt-Jakob disease (vCJD) (FSANZ 2017b).

There is strong evidence to show that vCJD is caused by ingestion of BSE infective material. Classic BSE prions from affected cows and vCJD prions from the brains of infected humans produce the same lesions in mice. The biochemical properties of BSE prions from cattle and vCJD prions from humans are indistinguishable. Iatrogenic (diseases or conditions caused by medical intervention) transmission of vCJD has occurred via blood transfusions and through growth hormone preparation and corneal or dura mater grafts (Simmons et al. 2018). This is why when you donate blood in Australia or New Zealand you are asked if you lived in the UK (in New Zealand this is extended to France and the Republic of Ireland) for a total of six months or more between 1 January 1980 and 31 December 1996, which coincides with the peak outbreak.

A twofold difference was seen between the prevalence of vCJD in the north versus the south of the UK. Contemporaneous National Dietary Surveys showed that consumption of mechanically recovered beef products (e.g. hamburgers) was much higher in the north of the UK. Mechanically recovered beef is more likely to be contaminated with infective material, and recovery of beef by this method is no longer permitted for human foodstuffs in Europe (FSANZ 2017b). Since BSE was identified as a major risk to human health in 1996, Australia and New Zealand have had comprehensive arrangements in place to protect consumers from BSE-contaminated food.

compendium of microbiological criteria (FSANZ 2016a; 2016b).

The Chapter 4 Primary Production and Processing Standards (Australia only), in the *Australia New Zealand Food Standards Code* covers the first part of the food chain and includes general provisions including requirements for food safety management statements (Standard 4.1.1), standards for seafood (Standard 4.2.1), poultry meat (Standard 4.2.2), meat (Standard 4.2.3), dairy products (Standard 4.2.4), eggs and egg products (Standard 4.2.5), seed sprouts (Standard 4.2.6) and wine (Standard 4.5.1). There may also be relevant Australian standards for production of certain foods that need to be met by the food industry (Standards Australia 2018).

Food safety programs

A food safety program is a written document indicating how a food business will control the food safety hazards associated with the food-handling activities of the business. Only certain high-risk food businesses are required to have food safety programs; for example, businesses that serve or process potentially hazardous food for service to vulnerable people, or seafood businesses that engage in the primary production or processing of, or manufacturing activities concerning, bivalve molluscs. Businesses producing manufactured and fermented meats are required to develop a food safety management system in accordance with Standard 4.2.2—Poultry Meat and Standard 4.2.3—Meat. The requirement for food businesses is to implement a food safety plan using Hazard Analysis and Critical Control Points (HACCP) principles.

Potentially hazardous foods

In Standard 3.2.2, potentially hazardous food is defined as 'food that has to be kept at certain temperatures to minimise the growth of any pathogenic microorganisms that may be present in the food or to prevent the formation of toxins in the food.

Potentially hazardous foods are also referred to as 'temperature control for safety foods' (FSANZ 2016b).

Potentially hazardous foods have certain characteristics that support the growth of pathogenic microorganisms or the production of toxins. Factors affecting microbial growth include the nutrients, moisture, acidity (pH) and gas atmosphere of the food. If the combination of these factors creates a favourable environment and the food is not kept under temperature control, microorganisms can grow and form toxins. If the levels of pathogenic microorganisms or toxins reach unsafe levels, foodborne illness may result (FSANZ 2016b). Examples of foods that are normally considered potentially hazardous include:

- raw and cooked meat/poultry or foods containing raw or cooked meat/poultry; for example, burgers, curries, kebabs, paté and meat pies
- foods containing eggs (cooked or raw), beans, nuts or other protein-rich food; for example, batter, mousse, quiche and tofu

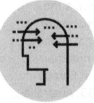

WHAT IS HACCP?

The Hazard Analysis and Critical Control Point (HACCP) system is used by the food industry at all stages (growing, harvesting, distributing, processing and preparation of food) to ensure that food processes are designed to eradicate and control specific food hazards, including the presence and/or growth of pathogenic microorganisms.

HACCP originated in the United States in the 1960s during development of foods for the space program. The advantages of HACCP include focusing control effort and resources on the critical steps in the process, monitoring the process by the use of quick and reliable parameters, and having results available for immediate action. FSANZ reported that the application of principles of HACCP has resulted in lower levels of pathogenic microorganisms present in foods.

Visit the websites of the Australian Institute of Food Safety (www.foodsafety.com.au/blog/the-seven-principles-of-haccp) and the Codex Alimentarius Commission (www.fao.org/docrep/005/Y1579E/y1579e03.htm) and answer the following questions.

- What are the seven steps involved in the HACCP?
- Where in the healthcare system would you see HACCP implemented?
- What other systems are linked to HACCP?

- dairy products and foods containing dairy products; for example, milk, dairy-based desserts, bakery products filled with fresh cream or with fresh custard (yoghurt is not included here as it is an acidified product)
- seafood (excluding live seafood) and foods containing seafood; for example, sushi
- sprouted seeds; for example, of beans and alfalfa
- prepared fruits and vegetables; for example, cut melons, salads and unpasteurised juices
- cooked rice and both fresh and cooked pasta
- foods that contain any of the above foods; for example, sandwiches, pizzas and rice rolls.

Many of the products listed above require refrigerated storage to prevent food spoilage or achieve the stated shelf life (see Chapter 5). Some types of food listed will not be considered potentially hazardous if they have been processed in certain ways—for example, if they contain certain preservatives (e.g. nitrites, sulphites) or have been commercially sterilised. Other foods may have been processed in a way that minimises microbial growth (e.g. dried, salted, acidified). Food processing techniques are discussed in more detail in Chapter 5.

If a food does not contain pathogens or does not support the growth of a pathogen or toxin production, then it is not potentially hazardous. Some foods (e.g. foods that are naturally acidic) do not support pathogen growth in their natural state because their intrinsic properties create an unfavourable environment (FSANZ 2016b).

Examples of food types considered to be not potentially hazardous include (FSANZ 2016b):

- biscuits and crackers
- bottled marinades
- bottled pasta sauces
- bottled salsas
- confectionary
- dried fruit
- dry goods
- fermented dried meats
- fruit cakes
- fruit juices
- hard cheeses
- honey and jam
- nuts in the shell
- peanut butter
- pickles
- plain breads and bread rolls
- plain cakes
- raw whole fruit and vegetables
- salad dressings
- sauces—Asian/soy, ketchup style
- salted dried meats
- unopened canned foods
- yoghurts.

Food hygiene and handling

Food hygiene and handling requirements are covered in the *Food Act 2014* for New Zealand and in Chapter 3 of the *Australia New Zealand Food Standards Code* for Australia, with guidance provided by Safe Food Australia (2018), and involve four essential elements:

1. cleaning and sanitising of food preparation areas and equipment
2. personal cleanliness, including effective hand-washing
3. time and temperature control of food
4. avoidance of cross-contamination. (FSANZ 2016b, 2018b)

Cleaning and sanitising

The term 'sanitation' means creating and maintaining hygienic and healthful conditions; it is derived from the Latin word *sanitas*, meaning 'health'. Effective cleaning to minimise contamination of food with microorganisms requires several steps, including pre-cleaning, washing, rinsing and sanitising. The importance of improving post-harvest water quality for washing fresh produce is seen in outbreaks of illness after consumption of fresh fruits and vegetables, including rockmelon, papaya and alfalfa sprouts (Angulo et al. 2008).

Different cleaning compounds are used for specific purposes in commercial applications; for example, alkalis dissolve protein, acids dissolve mineral scale and detergents emulsify grease. Depending on the types of microorganisms expected to be present in a particular food-handling premises, various sanitisers can be chosen—for example, iodine-based sanitisers are effective for viruses, while other sanitisers are useful for destroying *Listeria* species.

Personal cleanliness

Certain procedures need to be followed to minimise contamination of food by food handlers, which is particularly important if preparing food for vulnerable groups, including the young, elderly or immunocompromised.

- *People must not handle food if they are suffering from certain illnesses and conditions* (for example vomiting, diarrhoea, fever, jaundice, any discharge from the nose or eye, or any infected skin lesion; food handlers must legally be excluded from preparing food for sale if they suspect or are known to be suffering (or carriers) of hepatitis A, *Shigella* spp., *Salmonella typhi* or enterohaemorrhagic *E. coli*, or other gastrointestinal illnesses).

- *Adequate handwashing* involves washing hands with running warm water and soap for twenty seconds before drying them completely using single-use disposable paper towels or by using an air dryer or a combination of both methods. It is imperative that food handlers use a specially designated sink for handwashing (see the WHO or the Australian Institute of Food Safety guidelines for more information and specific steps).

- *Other personal hygiene procedures* may be used, such as wearing clean outer clothing while food is being prepared and removing it when the food handler visits the toilet. Food handlers are required to avoid contaminating food or surfaces that come into contact with food unnecessarily— for example, by handling cutlery by the handles and holding clean glasses by the base or stems only. Gloves can be useful, provided hands are adequately washed prior to wearing them and they are used for a single purpose only.

Temperature control

Most foodborne microorganisms will not grow below 5°C or above 60°C. For this reason, potentially hazardous foods (see section above) most at risk of causing food poisoning should always be stored outside this temperature range to minimise microbial growth (Figure 7.2).

Temperature control involves appropriate storage, such as chilling and freezing; effective processing techniques, including cooking and pasteurisation; and awareness of the importance of time when holding food at particular temperatures (see Chapter 5). However, some microorganisms may grow in foods

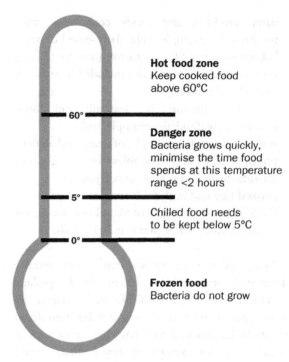

Hot food zone
Keep cooked food above 60°C

Danger zone
Bacteria grows quickly, minimise the time food spends at this temperature range <2 hours

Chilled food needs to be kept below 5°C

Frozen food
Bacteria do not grow

Figure 7.2: Danger zones for temperature and food

stored between −1°C and 5°C, including *Listeria monocytogenes*, *Yersinia enterocolitica*, some types of *Clostridium botulinum* and *Aeromonas hydrophila*. Pregnant women are advised to avoid foods likely to contain *L. monocytogenes* if the foods have been stored between −1°C and 5°C (FSANZ 2017c).

The Food Safety Standards (Chapter 3 of the Code) specify that potentially hazardous foods must be stored, displayed, transported and, where possible, prepared at safe temperatures. We can also use time, rather than temperature, to keep food safe. Ready-to-eat potentially hazardous food may be kept between 5°C and 60°C for varying times. The 2-hour/4-hour guide is used to assist food handlers including consumers to decide what to do with food that has been left for some time between these temperatures (FSANZ 2016b, 2017a):

- Food that has been subject to temperatures between 5°C and 60°C for a total of less than two hours must be refrigerated or used immediately.

- Food that has been subject to temperatures between 5°C and 60°C for a total of more than two hours but less than four hours must be used immediately.
- Food subjected to temperatures between 5°C and 60°C for more than four hours in total must be discarded.

When cooling foods after cooking, such as casseroles, food should be put into shallow, covered containers to ensure rapid cooling. It is also important to avoid conditions that support the growth of pathogenic organisms while food is being thawed. While the centre of a block of frozen food is frozen, bacteria on the outer, thawed surfaces can multiply rapidly if the food is thawed above 5°C. Food such as chicken or raw fish can be safely thawed in a refrigerator (on the bottom shelf to avoid dripping onto ready-to-eat food) or, alternatively, foods can be thawed in a microwave; in the latter case, the thawing time is usually of short duration.

The WHO has developed the 'Five Keys to Safer Food' program to promote safe food-handling behaviours and educate all food handlers, including consumers, with tools that are easy to adopt and adapt (Table 7.5). The WHO's food hygiene message is spread using posters in multiple languages, as well as training materials and videos (WHO 2018). To ensure the same understanding is reflected in practice along the full food production chain, the WHO has developed additional Five Keys materials directed to rural people who grow fruits, vegetables and aquaculture fish for their own use or for sale on local markets. The WHO's objective is to target those who usually do not have access to food safety education despite the important role they play in producing safe food for their communities (e.g. rural women).

Preventing cross-contamination

Many reported outbreaks of foodborne disease have been attributed to cross-contamination of pathogens from one food or surface to a ready-to-eat food (or surface in contact with the latter). Simple but important measures to avoid cross-contamination include storing raw and ready-to-eat food separately. If a single refrigerator is used to store both raw and ready-to-eat foods, raw foods such as meats, poultry, fish and eggs should be covered and stored below foods that will not be cooked further (e.g. in a drawer at the base of the fridge). Other simple but effective measures include using separate utensils, chopping boards and equipment for preparing raw and ready-to-eat foods.

Developing a food safety culture

A growing area of interest in protecting and promoting food safety is the development of a food safety culture within a business; this is reflected in how everyone (owners, managers, employees) thinks and acts in their daily job to make sure that the food they make or serve is safe (Figure 7.3). It is about taking

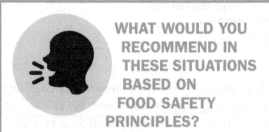

WHAT WOULD YOU RECOMMEND IN THESE SITUATIONS BASED ON FOOD SAFETY PRINCIPLES?

- An aged care facility wants to start serving eggnog containing raw eggs to residents. What is your recommendation and rationale?
- A childcare service mistakenly defrosted more chicken breasts than needed. They defrosted fully on the bench. What is your recommendation and rationale for using the defrosted chicken?
- A large quantity of rice has been cooked for a fete tomorrow. What is your recommendation and rationale for how the rice should be stored until required?
- Develop a simple communication strategy for the most appropriate action to take for each scenario.

Table 7.5: The WHO's Five Keys to Safer Food Programme

Message	Main points
Keep clean	• Wash your hands before handling food and during food preparation. • Wash your hands after going to the toilet. • Wash and sanitise all surfaces and equipment used for food preparation. • Protect kitchen areas and food from insects, pests and other animals.
Separate raw and cooked	• Separate raw meat, poultry and seafood from other foods. • Use separate equipment and utensils such as knives and cutting boards for handling foods.
Cook thoroughly	• Cook food thoroughly, especially meat, poultry, eggs and seafood. • Bring foods like soups and stews to boiling to make sure that they have reached 70°C. For meat and poultry, make sure that juices are clear, not pink. Ideally, use a thermometer. • Reheat cooked food thoroughly.
Keep food at a safe temperature	• Do not leave cooked food at room temperature for more than two hours. • Refrigerate all cooked and perishable food promptly (preferably below 5°C). • Keep cooked food piping hot (more than 60°C) prior to serving. • Do not store food too long, even in the refrigerator. • Do not thaw frozen food at room temperature.
Use safe water and raw materials	• Use safe water or treat it to make it safe. • Select fresh and wholesome foods. • Choose foods processed for safety, such as pasteurised milk. • Wash fruits and vegetables, especially if eaten raw. • Do not use food beyond its expiry date.

Source: WHO (2018)

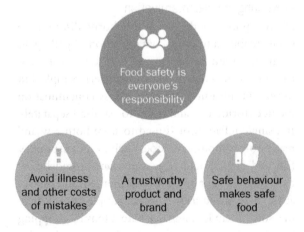

Figure 7.3: Food safety culture
Source: FSANZ (2018a)

pride in producing safe food every time, recognising that a good quality product must be safe to eat. Food safety is a top priority for all food businesses (FSANZ 2018a).

A strong food safety culture comes from people understanding the importance of making food safe and committing to doing whatever it takes, every time. It starts at the top but needs everyone's support across the business. First you need to know about your business, identify and make changes to improve the culture and then follow through to see how you are going (FSANZ 2018a).

SUMMARY

- Microorganisms are reliant on a variety of factors for survival and growth; some of the main factors relevant to food are time, nutrient availability, moisture, temperature, pH and gas atmosphere for growth. Microorganisms have a wide range of growth requirements and knowledge of these requirements is important to control microbial growth in food to reduce food spoilage and possible food illness.
- While many microorganisms are important in food production (e.g. for beer and yoghurt), others are a major cause of foodborne illness. Major microbial pathogens include bacteria, viruses and protozoa. Toxins produced by bacteria and moulds can also be a major source of foodborne illness.
- Microbiological risks are managed with a combination of regulatory (food standards) and non-regulatory approaches, including education on personal hygiene practices and reducing risks of cross-contamination. Food safety programs are essential for businesses that process or serve potentially hazardous foods, with the HACCP system used throughout all stages of the food chain to control specific food hazards, such as pathogenic microorganisms.
- Food hygiene and handling requirements are particularly important for food businesses and in the home to reduce microbiological risks. They involve four essential elements: cleaning and sanitising, personal cleanliness, temperature control and preventing cross-contamination.

KEY TERMS

Food matrix: refers to the support architecture or the structure of food resulting from various physical and chemical interactions between the compounds present in the food, giving it its form, thickness, density, hardness, porosity, colour and crystallinity.

Hepatotoxic: refers to compounds that are damaging to liver cells (hepatocytes).

Mucosa: one or more layers of epithelial cells that line the internal surface of organs, e.g. the small and large intestine.

Temperature control for safety foods: foods that have to be kept at certain temperatures to minimise the growth of any pathogenic microorganisms.

Zoonotic: Infectious diseases that are spread between animals and humans.

ACKNOWLEDGEMENT

This chapter has been modified and updated from those written by Gwynn Jones, Louise Lennard, Janis Baines and Ingrid R.E. Rutishauser, which appeared in the third edition of *Food and Nutrition*.

REFERENCES

Angulo, F.J., Kirk, M.D., McKay, I., Hall, G.V., Dalton, C.B. et al., 2008, 'Foodborne disease in Australia: The OzFoodNet experience', *Clinical Infectious Diseases,* 47(3), pp. 392–400, doi:10.1086/589861

Centers for Disease Control and Prevention, 2017, *Avian Influenza in Birds,* <www.cdc.gov/flu/avianflu/avian-in-birds.htm>, accessed 25 January 2019

Department of Agriculture and Water Resources, 2017, *Avian Influenza or Bird Flu,* <www.agriculture.gov.au/pests-diseases-weeds/animal/avian-influenza?wasRedirectedByModule=true>, accessed 24 January 2019

Department of Health, 2018, *Avian Influenza or Bird Flu,* <www.health.gov.au/avian_influenza>, accessed 25 January 2019

FSANZ, 2013, *Risk Analysis in Food Regulation,* <www.foodstandards.gov.au/publications/riskanalysisfoodregulation/Pages/default.aspx>, accessed 18 June 2018

—— 2015, *FSANZ Advice on Hepatitis A and Imported Ready-to-eat Berries,* <www.foodstandards.gov.au/consumer/safety/Pages/FSANZ-advice-on-hepatitis-A-and-imported-ready-to-eat-berries.aspx>, accessed 25 January 2019

—— 2016a, *Compendium of Microbiological Criteria* <www.foodstandards.gov.au/publications/Pages/Compendium-of-Microbiological-Criteria-for-Food.aspx>, accessed 22 January 2019

—— 2016b, *Safe Food Australia: A Guide to Food Safety Requirements,* <www.foodstandards.gov.au/publications/Pages/safefoodaustralia3rd16.aspx>, accessed 18 June 2018

—— 2017a, *Agents of Foodborne Illness,* <www.foodstandards.gov.au/publications/Pages/agentsoffoodborneill5155.aspx.>, accessed 25 January 2019

—— 2017b, *Bovine Spongiform Encephalopathy (BSE),* <www.foodstandards.gov.au/industry/bse/Pages/default.aspx>, accessed 18 June 2018

—— 2017c, *Pregnancy and Healthy Eating,* <www.foodstandards.gov.au/consumer/generalissues/pregnancy/pages/default.aspx>, accessed 19 June 2018

—— 2018a, *Food Safety Culture,* <www.foodstandards.gov.au/foodsafety/culture/Pages/default.aspx>, accessed 19 June 2018

—— 2018b, *Food Standards Code,* <www.foodstandards.gov.au/code/Pages/default.aspx>, accessed 23 January 2019

Kirk, M., Ford, L., Glass, K. & Hall, G., 2014, 'Foodborne illness, Australia, circa 2000 and circa 2010', *Emerging infectious diseases, 20*(11): 1857–64, doi:10.3201/eid2011.131315

MPI, 2016, *Food Act 2014,* <www.mpi.govt.nz/food-safety/food-act-2014/>, accessed 25 January 2019

—— 2017, *Foodborne Disease in New Zealand 2016,* <www.foodsafety.govt.nz/science-risk/human-health-surveillance/foodborne-disease-annual-reports.htm>, accessed 25 January 2019

OzFoodNet, 2012, *Monitoring the Incidence and Causes of Diseases Potentially Transmitted by Food in Australia: Annual report of the OzFoodNet Network, 2011,* <www.health.gov.au/internet/main/publishing.nsf/Content/cda-cdi3902g.htm>, accessed 25 January 2019

Safe Food Australia, 2018, *About Us,* <www.safefoodaustralia.com.au/>, accessed 25 January 2019

Semple, R.L., Frio, A.S., Hicks, P.A. & Lozare, J.V., 2011, *Mycotoxin Prevention and Control in Foodgrains: A Collaborative publication of the UNDP/FAO Regional Network Inter-Country Cooperation on Preharvest Technology and Quality Control of Foodgrains (REGNET) and the ASEAN Grain Postharvest Programme,* <www.fao.org/docrep/x5036e/x5036E00.htm>, accessed 25 January 2019

Simmons, M., Ru, G., Casalone, C., Iulini, B., Cassar, C. & Seuberlich, T., 2018, 'DISCONTOOLS: Identifying gaps in controlling Bovine Spongiform Encephalopathy', *Transboundary and Emerging Diseases, 65*(S1): 9–21, doi:10.1111/tbed.12671

Standards Australia, 2018, *About Us,* <www.standards.org.au/>, accessed 25 January 2019

Strawn, L.K. & Danyluk, M.D., 2010, 'Fate of Escherichia coli O157:H7 and Salmonella on fresh and frozen cut pineapples', *Journal of Food Protection, 73*(3): 418–24, doi:10.4315/0362-028x-73.3.418

WHO, 2017, *Influenza (Avian and Other Zoonotic),* <www.who.int/en/news-room/fact-sheets/detail/influenza-(avian-and-other-zoonotic)>, accessed 24 January 2019

—— 2018, *The Five Keys to Safer Food Programme,* <www.who.int/foodsafety/consumer/5keys/en/>, accessed 25 January 2019

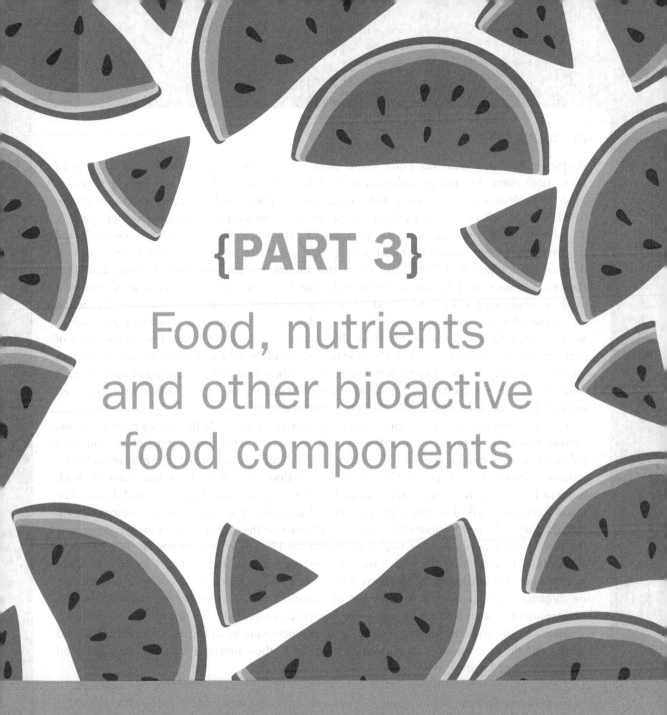

{PART 3}

Food, nutrients and other bioactive food components

INTRODUCTION

People eat food, not nutrients. Food is also eaten for a whole range of reasons (pleasure, social interaction) other than just physiological survival. What is eaten and not eaten from the array of foods available is a matter of social and cultural norms. These foods are categorised into groups based on similar characteristics. Each food group provides unique and overlapping nutrient profiles. To be able to effectively advocate for nutritional health within biological, social, economic and food systems, a deep understanding of the types of foods that constitute a diet is essential. Our diets are predominantly derived from plants and animals but may also include fungi and algae. Bacteria, although not a food in their own right, may be consumed as a component of fermented foods. Similarly, yeast and moulds are added to particular foods to enhance texture and flavour and are consumed indirectly as a result of this process. It is vitally important as a nutrition professional to understand the complexity of the foods that provide nutrients for health. The combination of nutrients and how they are delivered (the food matrix) are likely to be as important as the constituent bioactive compounds. The chapters in this section contribute to our understanding of the biological dimensions of econutrition. However, in exploring the social and cultural uses of different foods, and alcohol, the social and economic dimensions are also considered.

Chapter 8 provides a comprehensive guide to each group of foods: the nutrients they contain, current trends in consumption, benefits and risks associated with their consumption, and their cultural and social significance. After consumption, foods are digested within the human body; this process is described in Chapter 9. The process of digestion breaks food down into nutrients. Each nutrient has specific functions within the body and is thus implicated in health and disease. The macronutrients, so called because they are required in the body in large amounts, are protein, fat, carbohydrate and water. Chapters 10, 11, 12 and 14 describe the classification of these components, the body's requirements, and the role of each. Chapter 13 explores the conversion of protein, fat and carbohydrate to meet the body's need for energy. Alcohol, discussed in Chapter 15, is not strictly a nutrient but has nutritive effects within the body, contributing to energy intake. Due to its ubiquitous consumption, it is important to consider the impact of alcohol on body systems. Micronutrients (vitamins, minerals and other bioactive compounds) are needed in much smaller quantities by the body but are essential for optimal functioning of all organs. Chapters 16, 17 and 18 describe the biochemistry and physiological actions of these nutrients and other bioactive food components (see Figure 3.A).

Finally, all the science is distilled into food-based dietary guidance to provide assistance to individuals and communities regarding the amounts and combinations of foods required to deliver the optimal nutrient profile. Chapter 19 explains how scientific information about foods and their nutrients is translated into food-based dietary guidance systems to assist people in consuming healthier diets.

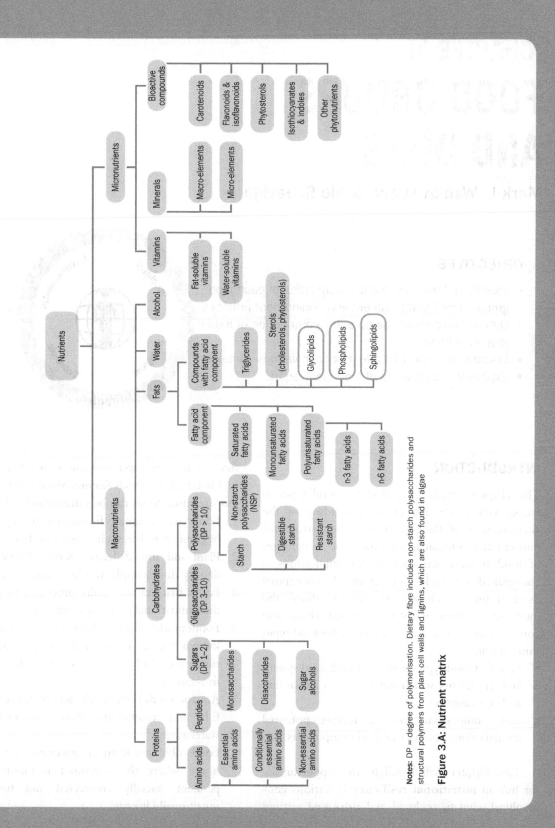

Notes: DP = degree of polymerisation. Dietary fibre includes non-starch polysaccharides and structural polymers from plant cell walls and lignins, which are also found in algae

Figure 3.A: Nutrient matrix

141

{CHAPTER 8}
FOOD GROUPS AND DIETS

Mark L. Wahlqvist and Gayle S. Savige

OBJECTIVES

- Identify and describe the characteristics of each food group (including the nutrient and non-nutrient profiles).
- Outline and discuss the potential contribution of food groups to health.
- Discuss the important role of food in various contexts.
- Explain the importance of food biodiversity.

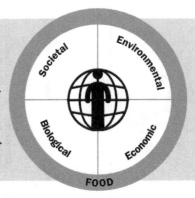

INTRODUCTION

This chapter introduces each of the food types to enable you to develop an understanding of the characteristics of these foods and their structural, nutrient and non-nutrient profiles. The recognition of food systems and their health implications is encouraged for each food group. A conceptual diagram for this chapter (Figure 8.1) shows the interconnectedness of foods, their acquisition and consumption. As you consider each of the food types think about:

- how that food type sits in the overall food system and the factors which determine its availability and consumption
- their composition and the relative potential contributions of bioactive food components.

This chapter will highlight the opportunities for human **nutritional resilience** in various geographical, climatic, cultural and urbanised settings through the consumption of a biodiverse diet in which highly nutritious foods feature. More nutritious and less hazardous foods can be summarised as follows:

1. Foods whose innate function is to support the beginnings of life, such as eggs, seeds and nuts.
2. Plant and animal-derived foods of low energy density (for example, whole grains, lean meats).
3. Foods that are minimally processed to preserve their nutritional properties and ensure their safety.
4. Foods produced and delivered from a food system known for its integrity (uncontaminated and sustainable) and proximity to nature (for example, free-range).
5. Aquatic foods such as salt- and freshwater plants, fish and crustaceans from uncontaminated waterways.
6. Foods obtained from environments outside the home where the consumer is mobile, independent, socially connected and food and nutritionally literate.

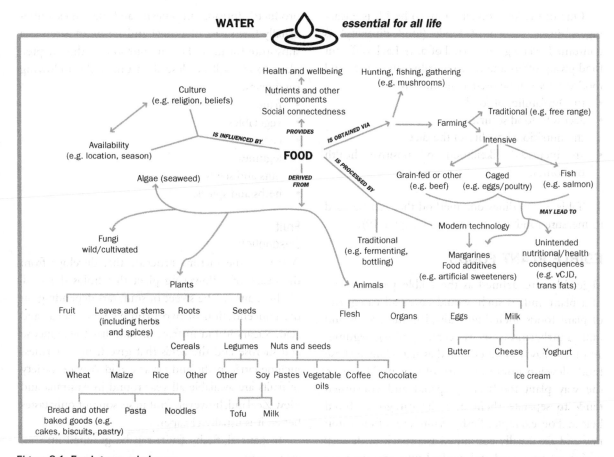

Figure 8.1: Food group mind map

FOOD GROUP MIND MAPPING

Mind mapping is a good way to brainstorm about a topic without worrying about structure. It allows you to construct a visualisation. It starts with the central concept and moves to ideas and then sub-ideas, all interlinked. Mind maps can assist with developing ideas and with recalling information. They work particularly well if you are a visual learner.

Take a particular food item and develop a mind map that covers all the aspects of that food you can think of, including its production, transport and consumption. Think about how that food type sits in the overall food system and the factors that determine its availability and consumption. Remember to include the physical and nutrient attributes of the food, as well as the social and cultural perspectives. Discuss your mind map with another student. What things were similar? What things were different? Discuss your food items and see if you can extend your mind map in any way. Re-do the mind map after reading this chapter.

One of the key contributions to health is ensuring a diverse range of foods (food diversity) is consumed over a given period of time. Each different food group offers a unique contribution to diet, and food variety can be used as an indicator of:
• the availability of food
• access to food security
• the nutritional quality of the diet
• an increased likelihood of positive health outcomes.

Table 8.1 outlines one method that can be used to measure food variety (see also Chapter 19).

EDIBLE PLANT FOODS

Vegetables are defined as the edible part or parts of a plant and, as such, would cover all categories of plant foods, including fruits, legumes, seeds and nuts. Furthermore, seeds (cereal grains), legumes and nuts may also be classified as fruits, since these foods develop from the ovary of a plant. However, the way plant foods are prepared and consumed tends to separate them into the categories listed below. For example, fleshy fruits are often eaten raw and are usually consumed as a snack or dessert; grains are processed and cooked into various food

products (bread, noodles); and legumes/pulses usually form part of a meal and are often eaten as a substitute for meat. For the purpose of this chapter, plant foods will be described under the following categories:
• fruit
• vegetables
• cereals
• legumes
• nuts and seeds
• herbs and spices.

Fruit
Description
A fruit is the mature structure that develops from the ovary of a flowering plant that holds the seed. Fleshy fruits can be sweet or sour/tart depending on the concentration of two main elements, sugar and acid. Sugars found in fruit include fructose, glucose and sucrose and the acids that give fruit its tartness include citric, malic and tartaric acid. A wide variety of fruits are available all year round in Australia and New Zealand; however, fruit in season not only tastes better, it is usually cheaper.

In general, fleshy fruits can be grouped into six categories:

Table 8.1: Food variety checklist

Biologically distinct food groups	Score	Biologically distinct food groups	Score
1 Eggs (all variety)		6 Fish (saltwater)	
Dairy		7 Fish (freshwater)	
2 Milk, ice cream, cheese, yoghurt (without live culture)		8 Roe (caviar, dip—taramasalata)	
Live cultures		9 Shellfish and mollusc (e.g. mussels, oysters, squid, scallops)	
3 Yoghurt (with live culture, e.g. acidophilus, bifidobacteria)		10 Crustaceans (e.g. prawns, lobster, crab, shrimps)	
Yeast/Yeast extract		**Meat**	
4 Brewer's yeast, Vegemite		11 Lamb, beef, veal	
Fish (including canned)		12 Pork (excluding ham and bacon)	
5 Fatty fish (tuna, anchovies, salmon, kipper, sardines, herring, mackerel, pilchards)		13 Poultry (e.g. chicken, duck, turkey)	
		14 Game (e.g. quail, wild duck, pigeon)	
		15 Game (e.g. kangaroo, rabbit)	

Biologically distinct food groups	Score	Biologically distinct food groups	Score
16 Liver		36 Flowers (broccoli, cauliflower)	
17 Brain		37 Stalks (celery, asparagus)	
18 All other organ meats		38 Onion (spring onion, garlic, leeks)	
Legumes (including canned)		39 Tomatoes, okra	
19 Peas (fresh, dried, split peas); chickpeas (dried, roasted); beans (haricot, kidney, lima, broad); lentils (red, brown, green); soy products (tofu, milk)		40 Beans (green, snow peas)	
		41 Leafy greens (spinach, cabbage, silverbeet, endive, kale, chicory, parsley, lettuce)	
Cereals		42 Peppers (capsicum, chillies)	
20 Wheat (bread, pasta, ready-to-eat)		43 Marrow-like (zucchini, squash, cucumber, turnip, eggplant, swede, pumpkin)	
21 Corn (includes ready-to-eat)			
22 Barley (includes ready-to-eat)		44 Fungi (e.g. mushrooms)	
23 Oats (includes ready-to-eat)		45 Herbs/spices	
24 Rye (includes ready-to-eat)		**Nuts and seeds**	
25 Rice (includes ready-to-eat)		46 Almond, cashew, chestnut, coconut, hazelnut, peanuts, peanut butter, pecan, pine nut, pistachio, walnut, pumpkin seed, linseed, sesame seed, tahini, hommus, sunflower seed	
26 All other grains and cereals (e.g. buckwheat, millet, quinoa, sago, semolina, tapioca, triticale)			
Fats and oils			
27 Oils		**Chocolate**	
28 Hard/soft spreads		47 Dark	
Beverages		**Fruit**	
29 Water (including mineral)		48 Stone (nectarine, peach, cherries, plum, apricot, avocado, olive, prune)	
30 Non-alcoholic (tea, coffee, cocoa) and alcoholic (wine, beer, spirits)			
Fermented foods		49 Pome (apple, pear, nashi)	
31 Miso, tempeh, soy sauce		50 Berries (raspberry, strawberries)	
32 Sauerkraut		51 Grapes (including raisins, sultanas)	
33 All other variety		52 Bananas	
Sugar		53 Citrus (orange, lemon)	
34 Honey (in its pure form), maple syrup, honey ants		54 Melon (honeydew, watermelon)	
Vegetables (including canned, frozen)		55 Tropical (mango, pineapple, guava, jackfruit, lychee, papaya, star fruit)	
35 Root (potato, carrot, sweet potatoes, beetroot, parsnip, bamboo shoots, ginger, radish, water chestnut)		56 Other (kiwi, date, passionfruit)	
		Total weekly variety score	

Scoring: Score 1 point for each food category eaten over the last week. The maximum score for this checklist would be 56.

Grains and cereals: Wheat includes wholemeal or white bread, ready-to-eat cereals such as Weet-Bix, Bran Flakes.

Serving size: Quantities smaller than 1–2 tablespoons (except for fats, oils, Vegemite, chilli, herbs, spices) would not be eaten in sufficient quantity to rate a score (e.g. slice of tomato in a hamburger).

Source: Savige et al. (1997)

- citrus (e.g. oranges, lemons, grapefruits, limes)
- drupes (e.g. stone fruits such as cherries, apricots, plums, peaches)
- pomes (e.g. apples, pears, quince, loquats)
- tropical (e.g. mangoes, pineapples, papayas, lychees)
- berries (e.g. strawberries, raspberries, blueberries, blackberries, mulberries)
- melons (e.g. rockmelon, watermelon, honeydew).

The consumption of fruits may be as a piece, a puree, a jam or juice, preserved or canned, dried or fermented. They can be eaten alone, with meals or as a snack, or mixed with other basic food commodities, such as breakfast cereals, breads, yoghurt, ice cream, nuts and meats. The form in which fruit is consumed is highly relevant to its physiological effects and health risk profile. For example, while whole fruit may protect against chronic conditions, other forms, such as juice, may increase the risk (see chapters 30, 31 and 32).

Nutritional qualities

Fruits provide dietary fibre and various vitamins, minerals and phytonutrients. They mostly comprise simple carbohydrates, making them a source of energy, usually with little fat or protein. There are fatty fruits, however, which include avocadoes, cacao, olives, coconuts and palm fruit (used in various ways by different cultures as the unrefined fruit flesh, and not necessarily as the refined oil). Citrus fruits are often sources of vitamin C, bananas are a source of vitamin B-6 and mangoes are a source of β-carotene, the precursor of vitamin A. Fruit contains very little sodium and most fruits are high in potassium, resulting in a high potassium-to-sodium ratio. A diet with a high potassium-to-sodium ratio can help protect against high blood pressure and possibly other health problems, including hearing impairment. Having a banana a day makes a ready improvement in vitamin B-6 and potassium intakes.

Berries, like nuts, have a special place in both the earliest and most contemporary of human diets as items which can be collected and eaten with little if any preparation. Many kinds—strawberries, blackberries, blueberries, raspberries, wolfberries, lingonberries, cranberries and more—are found in cold and temperate zones and serve to round out dietary patterns, with benefits for immune function, neuroprotection and dampening inflammation. Like all food commodities with such physiological attributes, it is likely that they operate, in part, through the gut microbiome. Bioactive compounds in berries of particular interest are anthocyanins, which may execute some of the functions found with regular berry intakes (Battino et al. 2009). In other climatic settings, other foods—such as grapes, plums and cherries—can fulfil the roles that berries serve (Castañeda-Ovando et al. 2012) (Figure 8.2).

The popular saying that 'an apple a day keeps the doctor away' may have merit given apples' structural and phytonutrient profile and the related potential health benefits. Apples, like other fruits, contain myriad different chemicals giving each fruit its unique colour, odour and flavour. They have the distinction of being one of three foods found to be protective against cardiovascular disease in a Netherlands study, the others being tea and onions (Hertog et al. 1993).

Health benefits/risks

Perhaps one of the most important health benefits of eating fruit is that fruit is an excellent source of dietary fibre, which contributes to gut function and integrity. Low fruit intake is associated with an increased risk of all-cause mortality, cardiovascular disease and cancer; intakes lower than 500 g per day probably contribute to 5.6 million premature deaths globally (Aune et al. 2017). The current Australian and New Zealand recommendation is for adults to consume the equivalent of two pieces of fruit per day.

Cultural/traditional significance and uses

Once ripe, most fresh fruits have a fairly short shelf life, as the sugars found in fruit are readily fermented by microorganisms. The earliest of food cultures fermented fruit to produce alcoholic beverages, such as cider from apples and wine from grapes (see Chapter 15). Sugar also acts as a preservative and has been added to heated fruit to produce fruit preserves

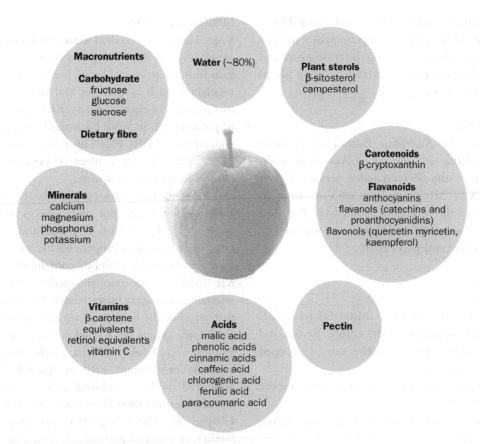

Figure 8.2: Some of the nutrients and bioactive compounds found in an apple
Source: Lisa Valder/iStock (apple).

WHAT ARE FODMAPS?

FODMAPs (fermentable oligo-, di- and monosaccharides and polyols) are short-chain carbohydrates that are poorly absorbed in the small intestine. They include short-chain oligosaccharide polymers of fructose (fructans) and galacto-oligosaccharides (stachyose, raffinose), disaccharides (lactose), monosaccharides (fructose), and sugar alcohols (polyols) such as sorbitol, mannitol, xylitol and maltitol. FODMAPs are naturally present in food and the human diet, and their restriction appears to improve symptom control in people with irritable bowel syndrome (IBS) and other functional gastrointestinal disorders. There is emerging research that the FODMAP diet may be an effective therapy in the management of IBS symptoms. This does not present a cure but is a suggested dietary approach to improve symptoms and quality of life. Of concern is that FODMAPs avoidance requires a reduced intake of a number of micronutrients and other healthful bioactives. Another risk of a FODMAPs exclusion diet is that avoidance of oligosaccharides may lead to reduced consumption of beans and legumes, which have been shown to increase life expectancy and reduce the burden of so-called chronic diseases, such as diabetes.

(bottled/canned), jams, jellies and crystallised/candied fruit. Other methods of preservation include drying and freezing. Controlling the atmosphere and vacuum-sealing are used to extend the shelf life of fresh produce (see Chapter 5).

Current trends

In 2011–12, the Australian Bureau of Statistics (ABS) found that around half of Australian adults failed to meet the recommended serves of fruit each day (ABS 2016). Of those who ate fruit on the day before the interview, apples were the most commonly consumed fruit (23 per cent) followed by bananas (18 per cent) (ABS 2016).

Vegetables
Description

Vegetables are derived from many different parts of plants and contribute to the colour, flavour and texture of many dishes. Vegetables can be grouped into three categories:

- edible underground parts, such as roots, tubers, and bulbs
- edible aboveground parts, such as stems, leaves, and flowers
- edible fruits and seeds, such as pumpkin and corn.

Nutritional qualities

Vegetables are an excellent source of dietary fibre and are usually a better source of vitamins and minerals than fruit. Most vegetables are low in fat, and starchy vegetables (such as potatoes and tubers) provide a useful source of energy. However, the energy content of potatoes can increase by around sevenfold when cooked in fat (Table 8.2). This not only substantially increases the energy content of potatoes but also reduces its nutritional density.

Cruciferous vegetables (such as broccoli, cabbage and cauliflower) are not only sources of vitamins (such as C, E, K and folate), minerals and carotenoids but also of bioactive components like glucosinolates. Glucosinolates are sulphur-containing chemicals responsible for the pungent quality of cruciferous vegetables and, when broken down, form compounds that are thought to protect against certain cancers. Dark leafy greens are a good source of β-carotene, vitamin C and folate. Lutein, a carotenoid present in dark leafy greens such as spinach, has been associated with a reduced risk of age-related macular degeneration (Eisenhauer et al. 2017) (see Chapter 22). There is growing evidence, too, that lutein is neuroprotective and may slow down declines in cognitive function. A nutritionally secure diet will

Table 8.2: Effect of adding fat on the energy (kJ) content of 100 g of potatoes

Steamed or boiled with no added fat (~0.1 g fat)
(~260 kJ)
Mashed with 1½ tablespoons of regular milk & teaspoon butter (~5.0 g fat)
(~494 kJ)
Dry-baked then served with tablespoon of sour cream (~7.5 g fat)
(~588 kJ)
Chips (~8.0 g fat)
(~1175 kJ)
Crisps (~34.0 fat)
(~2230 kJ)

Source: Values obtained from the Australian Food Composition Database (formerly the Nutrient Tables, or NUTTAB) (FSANZ 2019). The database contains data on 1534 foods available in Australia and up to 256 nutrients per food.

be biodiverse and obtain these food components from other sources as well. Lutein is found in berries like wolfberry (much championed in Chinese food and medicinal culture in a dried form known as goji); the yellow colour in eggs, depending on what the hens eat; and corn, depending on cultivar.

Eating ten serves of fruit and vegetables a day (where a serve is equivalent to 80 g) is known to reduce the risk of cardiovascular disease and premature death by 28 per cent and 31 per cent respectively (Aune et al. 2017). Vegetables associated with the greatest benefits include green leafy vegetables, cruciferous vegetables and other green and yellow vegetables (such as green beans, carrots and capsicums). These benefits are seen irrespective of serum cholesterol or lipid status.

Health benefits/risks

In general, a diet that is rich in vegetables (and fruits) can enhance our health and wellbeing. The regular consumption of fruits and vegetables can lower blood pressure, reduce the risk of cardiovascular disease and protect against some types of cancer (Aune et al. 2017). The current recommendation is for Australians and New Zealanders to consume five serves of vegetable per day, equating to approximately 400 g (also recommended by the World Cancer Research Fund and the World Health Organization) (WCRF/AICR 2018).

Cultural/traditional significance/uses

Potato and cassava are major food staples globally. Cabbage is eaten by many cultures and is often consumed as a fermented vegetable, especially in Korea (kimchi) and Eastern Europe (sauerkraut). Onions have been used in cooking for centuries to add flavour to other foods and as a main ingredient (e.g. roasted or pickled). The pungent quality of onions, garlic and leeks is related to their volatile sulphur compounds.

Current trends

Most Australians do not eat enough vegetables to meet the Australian Dietary Guidelines. The Australian Bureau of Statistics (ABS) survey (2016)

WHAT IS CASSAVA?

Cassava is a root vegetable that is very easy to grow and is the third largest contributor to carbohydrate consumption (after rice and maize) in tropical regions. Both the tuber and the leaves are consumed. Its primary contribution to diets is as a source of energy and **resistant starch**. Cassava cannot be consumed in its raw state as it contains cyanogenic glycosides, which can release cyanide into the body after consumption. To ensure cassava is safe for consumption it should be peeled, soaked and cooked. Eating in combination with protein can also assist. Most commonly consumed forms of cassava include:

- Australia/UK/Asia: tapioca, dessert, bubble tea
- Brazil: farofa—a toasted cassava flour mixture used as an accompaniment to a variety of dishes
- Africa: fufu is a staple food—a thick paste/dough that is used as a carbohydrate accompaniment to stews.

has estimated that only 6.8 per cent of the population consume the recommended number of serves. Potatoes remain the most popular vegetable (consumed by 31 per cent of the survey population) followed by tomatoes (18 per cent), leafy vegetables (mainly lettuce) (17 per cent) and carrots (14 per cent).

The ABS also found that between 1995 and 2011–12, the Average Daily Intake of serves from the vegetables (including legumes/beans) group fell by 10 per cent (from 3.8 serves to 3.4 serves per 10,000 kJ). This decline was relatively uniform across the major vegetable groups. For example, the

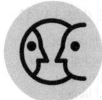

WHAT IS A SERVE?

The Australian Guide to Healthy Eating indicates that a serve of vegetable is equivalent to:

- ½ cup cooked green or orange vegetables
- 1 cup of green leafy or raw salad vegetables
- ½ medium potato
- 1 medium tomato.

Over the next three days, choose three different meals and evaluate the serves of vegetable they contain for one person. Include:

- a mixed dish like a stew, curry or pasta dish
- a separated dish such as roast meat with vegetables, or chicken and vegetables
- a hamburger or sandwich that includes salad.

You may want to cook or prepare these dishes and see how many vegetables are used.

Report on what you found and relate this to how easy or difficult it would be to increase vegetable serves for another person. What do you need to know in order to encourage increased consumption of vegetables? Can five serves of vegetable be readily consumed in a single meal, or across three meals a day?

proportion of starchy vegetables accounted for 22 per cent in 1995 and 21 per cent in 2011–12, with green and brassica vegetables showing the same proportions (i.e. 22 per cent in 1995 and 21 per cent in 2011–12) (ABS 2016).

Cereals

Description

Cereals are the edible grains or seeds of grasses belonging to the Poaceae family. Around the world, cereals such as maize (corn), rice and wheat are important staples. Other varieties of cereals include barley, oats, rye, triticale (a wheat–rye hybrid), millet, bulgur and sorghum. Grains not belonging to the Poaceae family include quinoa, amaranth and buckwheat.

Nutritional qualities

Wholegrain cereals are composed of three edible layers: the bran (outer layer), endosperm (middle layer) and germ (inner layer) (see Chapter 5). The outer layer provides all of the fibre as well as B vitamins, minerals (such as magnesium, iron and zinc), phytochemicals and some protein. The middle layer is mostly made up of carbohydrate (starch) and some protein. The inner layer includes B vitamins, unsaturated fats, vitamin E, minerals and phytochemicals.

Whole grains that are cracked, crushed or flaked will retain their nutritional quality as long as the bran, endosperm and germ are retained in the same proportions as the intact grain. Refining cereals to remove both the bran and germ layers results in a loss of fibre, vitamins, minerals and phytonutrients. For example, when wheat is milled to make white flour, only the grain's endosperm (middle layer) remains; therefore, white flour must be 'enriched' to restore some of the vitamins and minerals lost during the milling process.

Health benefits/risks

The regular consumption of whole grains is linked to a lower risk of cardiovascular disease and may help to reduce the risk of type 2 diabetes. On the other hand, diets high in refined grains are associated with a higher risk of obesity, type 2 diabetes and cancer (see Part 7).

Cultural/traditional significance and uses

The cultivation of cereals has led to a great diversity of foods across various cultures. Leavened bread (derived from wheat) is commonly consumed across the world; flat bread such as pita (wheat) is eaten throughout the Middle East; tacos and tortillas (maize) are dominant foods in Latin America. Pasta (wheat) is a staple food of traditional Italian cuisine and noodles (wheat and rice) are eaten throughout Asia. Wheat and basmati rice are important staples of the Indian diet and a typical Japanese meal consists of a bowl of rice (gohan).

Current trends

The vast majority of Australians eat from the cereal food group every day, with bread being the most common type of cereal consumed. The Australian

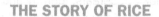

THE STORY OF RICE

Rice is an important food crop throughout the world and a major staple among many Asian countries. However, during processing (milling and polishing) to make white rice, important nutrients such as thiamin are lost. White rice has a different flavour and texture to brown rice, and it stores better and keeps longer when the bran and germ are removed. Beriberi, a neurological disease resulting from vitamin B-1 deficiency, used to be common throughout Southeast Asia until its connection with white rice was established (see Chapter 16). Enriching white rice with vitamin B-1 has reduced the incidence of the disease. White rice is enriched in two ways. Prior to milling, the rice is steamed under pressure in order to transfer all the vitamins and minerals from the bran layers into the kernel. The rice is then dried and milled. Rice that has already been milled can be submersed in a vitamin and mineral bath to coat the grains. Once coated, they are dried.

Dietary Guidelines emphasise the importance of whole grains (and/or high-fibre cereal varieties) and recommend these cereals account for at least one-third of cereal consumption. However, although approximately one-third of all cereal foods consumed by Australians were wholegrain/high fibre, the 2011–12 ABS survey found the balance of regular bread consumption favoured white bread (58 per cent), followed by mixed grain (18 per cent) and wholemeal varieties (18 per cent) (ABS 2016). Ancient grains, such as amaranth and freekeh, are also becoming more popular.

Legumes
Description

Legumes (or pulses) are the edible seeds of pods derived from plants that belong to the Leguminosae family and include beans, peas, lentils, chickpeas, lupins, soybeans and peanuts. Legumes have a symbiotic relationship with bacteria (*Rhizobium*) whereby the bacteria absorb nutrients from the host plant and fix nitrogen that can be used by the plant. Australia is the world's largest exporter of chickpeas and sweet lupins (Kouris-Blazos & Belski 2016).

Nutritional qualities

Legumes are an excellent source of dietary fibre, protein and carbohydrate. Almost all legumes are low in fat except for soybeans and peanuts. They are a valuable source of B vitamins as well as iron, zinc, calcium, magnesium and phosphorus. However, the bioavailability of iron and zinc from legumes is lower than from meat and the calcium in legumes is less readily absorbed compared to dairy foods. There is ongoing research to increase the bioavailability of iron in these items, given their widespread production and consumption.

Health benefits/risks

Legumes are part of many healthy food habits, including the Mediterranean, Japanese and South Asian diets, as well as vegetarian diets. These dried pulses are high in dietary fibre, which not only helps to promote gut health but also may help to lower blood cholesterol. They have a low glycaemic index and so

THE CONTRIBUTION OF BREAKFAST CEREALS

Ready-to-eat breakfast cereals are a commonly consumed source of grains in the Australian and New Zealand diets and are available in a variety of forms. Flaked products from wheat and maize are made by cooking coarsely ground endosperm of crushed grains in a sugar syrup under pressure. The cooked pieces are partially dried, rolled into flakes and toasted at a high temperature (>220°C). As a result, the starch is gelatinised, sugars are caramelised, and the dry product has a very long shelf life if protected against moisture. Granular, puffed and shredded cereal products can all be manufactured by combinations of cooking in water and drying processes. The manufacture of potato crisps, corn chips and expanded cereal shapes made with oil and flavourings usually involves frying or baking. These treatments may destroy more than 90 per cent of the thiamin and other vitamins present in the raw cereal ingredients. The *Australia New Zealand Food Standards Code* permits the addition of vitamins and minerals such as thiamin, folic acid, riboflavin, niacin and iron.

Visit a supermarket and select ten ready-to-eat breakfast cereals. Identify and provide an account of key nutrients in breakfast cereals and a ranking of the cereals based on these nutrients. Identify and provide a rationale for which cereals you would recommend for:

- a pregnant woman
- an adolescent elite athlete
- an adult with hypertension.

are useful in preventing as well as managing diabetes. Legumes also contain a variety of phytonutrients that may protect against other chronic diseases, including heart disease and cancer. Soybeans are best known for their phytoestrogens, known as isoflavones. Legumes are high in oligosaccharides, which are physiologically and metabolically advantageous, although they may aggravate symptoms associated with irritable bowel syndrome (see Chapter 12 and the 'What are FODMAPs?' box earlier in this chapter). All types of legumes, across various food cultures, have been shown to confer relative longevity, with as little as one or two servings per week (Chang et al. 2012; Darmadi–Blackberry et al. 2004).

Cultural/traditional significance and uses

Legumes are an important part of traditional diets around the world and are often eaten with cereal grains as part of a meal. Examples include corn and beans (North and South America), rice and soybeans (Japan) and lentils (Indian sub–continent).

BUSTING LEGUME MYTHS: TRUE OR FALSE?

Legumes are not a regular part of the Australian or New Zealand diet, although they feature heavily in the diets of other cultures. Two common beliefs about legumes are:

1. soybeans make breasts grow in men
2. beans increase flatulence.

Look for evidence that supports or refutes these beliefs. Using that evidence, develop a two-minute talk that explains the facts to a lay audience and that will encourage their consumption of legumes.

Tofu (bean curd) is an important food component in East Asian and Southeast Asian cuisines. The Chinese were the first to produce tofu, a process that requires soaking, crushing, boiling and straining soybeans to make soy milk. The soy milk is then coagulated to produce curds that are pressed into soft white blocks (tofu). A variety of products are made from fermented soybeans, such as natto, tempeh and miso. Miso is made from a fermented soybean paste that is commonly used in making miso soup.

Current trends
The latest survey by the ABS found the proportion of adults consuming legumes on the day prior to the survey was only 4.7 per cent, and although legume intake did not decline between 1995 and 2011–12, the regular consumption of legumes still remains very low in Australia (ABS 2016). Insofar as sustainable agriculture is concerned, they are one of the most important and under-utilised crops (Foyer et al. 2016). Legumes are important during both crop growth and after harvest. The inherent ability of legumes to fix atmospheric nitrogen helps to keep usable nitrogen in the soil, which reduces the need for nitrogen fertilisers. Legume crops also release organic matter into the soil, which improves soil fertility, structure and water retention.

Nuts and seeds
Description
Nuts are dry, single-seeded fruits that are enclosed in a hard shell and a protective husk. When nuts are ready to eat, the hard shell must be forcibly removed. Nut crops grown in Australia include almonds, cashews, chestnuts, hazelnuts, macadamias, peanuts (which are a legume and not a true nut), pecans, pistachios and walnuts.

Most seeds come from fruits that lack an inedible hard shell, although the seed itself has a protective coating or husk. Some seeds are eaten with the husk intact while others have this removed prior to eating. For instance, sesame seeds can be eaten with or without the husk. Commonly consumed seeds include chia, caraway, fennel, flaxseed, poppy, pumpkin, sunflower and sesame.

Nutritional qualities
Nuts and seeds are an excellent source of fibre, protein, fat, vitamins and minerals and, although relatively high in energy, are nutrient dense. The type of fat predominantly comprises monounsaturated and polyunsaturated fats (Table 8.3) and the quality of the protein is enhanced if consumed with cereals and legumes. Nuts and seeds are a very good source of vitamin E, a nutrient that functions as an antioxidant.

Health benefits/risks
Evidence suggests that regular consumption of nuts does not appear to have an adverse effect on body weight. Eating nuts is likely to enhance satiety and reduce the cravings for less healthy foods. Furthermore, regular nut consumption (about a handful most days), particularly of walnuts and almonds, appears to reduce the risk of cardiovascular disease. The properties responsible for the cardio-protective effect of nuts are likely to be related to their nutrient (including fatty acid profile) and phytonutrient profile (such as phytosterols).

Certain nuts and seeds may cause an adverse reaction in susceptible individuals. Australia has one of the highest rates of nut allergies in children in the world, resulting in the banning of nuts in many schools throughout Australia.

Cultural/traditional significance and uses
Shelled nuts are eaten whole or ground to make flour or a paste (such as tahini—a sesame seed paste widely used in the Middle East). They are also used for oil and sometimes powdered to thicken foods.

Nuts and seeds are commonly consumed as snacks or as an ingredient in foods such as breads, biscuits, cakes, health bars and breakfast cereals (such as muesli). Nuts and seeds are also used to manufacture butters and edible oils. In recent years, almond milk and a range of other nut milks have become very popular as a milk substitute, especially for those with allergies to soy and cow's milks.

Current trends
Data from the ABS indicate that nuts and seeds made an increasing, albeit small, contribution to

Table 8.3: Fatty acid profiles of selected nuts

Nut	Total fat	Total SFA		Total MUFA		Total PUFA		ALA	
	g	g	%*	g	%	g	%	g	%
Almond	50.5	3.8	7.9	30.7	63.5	12.8	26.6	0.0	0.0
Brazil nut	68.5	14.8	22.6	21.8	33.3	29.0	44.3	0.0	0.0
Cashew nut	49.2	8.4	17.8	31.1	66.2	7.6	16.1	0.1	0.2
Hazelnut	61.4	2.7	4.6	48.8	83.1	7.2	12.2	0.1	0.2
Macadamia nut	74.0	10.0	14.2	59.6	84.3	1.1	1.6	0.2	0.3
Pecan	71.9	4.5	6.6	39.3	57.2	25.0	36.3	0.6	0.9
Pine nut	70.0	4.2	6.3	23.0	34.3	39.9	59.7	0.2	0.3
Pistachio	50.6	5.8	12.0	26.7	55.2	16.1	33.4	0.3	0.7
Walnut	69.2	4.4	6.7	12.1	18.3	49.6	75.0	6.3	9.5

Notes: * % of total fatty acids; SFA = saturated fatty acids; MUFA = monounsaturated fatty acids; PUFA = polyunsaturated fatty acids; ALA = α-linolenic acid

Source: FSANZ (2019)

FOOD FAD OR SUPERFOOD: CHIA SEEDS

Chia is the seed of *Salvia hispanica*, native to southern Mexico and Guatemala. It was first used by the Aztecs and is described as a pseudo-cereal—a non-grass plant whose seed can be ground into a flour.

Nutritionally, the chia seed has a high content of n-3 fatty acids, is a source of fibre, is 20 per cent protein (but contains no gluten) and is a source of calcium (631 mg/100 g), magnesium (335 mg/100 g) and iron (7.7 mg/100 g) (Ullah et al. 2016). The biggest producers of chia in Australia are in the Ord Valley in the East Kimberley region of Western Australia.

Given its nutritional profile chia could be effective in reducing the risk of cardiovascular disease, but there are currently few studies on the health benefits of consuming chia seeds.

Based on your reading of peer-reviewed literature, write a blog post about the benefits of chia. Find a healthy recipe and use the Australian Food Composition Database to analyse its nutritional content.

diet between 1995 and 2011–12. Over this period, consumption of nuts and seeds increased from 0.14 to 0.24 serves per 10,000 kJ (ABS 2016).

Herbs and spices
Description
Spices and herbs are parts of a plant that add flavour and colour to any dish. Spices can come from the roots, rhizomes, stems, leaves, bark, flowers, fruits and seeds of a plant, while herbs are usually thought of as non-woody plants.

Nutritional qualities
Most herbs and spices are usually consumed in small amounts compared to other plant foods, so their contribution to our nutrient intake is also small. A few herbs, such as basil and parsley, are eaten in larger quantities. Parsley is a source of β–carotene

and other carotenoids such as lutein and zeaxanthin. Fresh parsley also contains folic acid, vitamin K, vitamin C and potassium, as well as phytonutrients such as flavonoids and antioxidants.

Health benefits/risks

Culinary herbs and spices contribute to health either directly or indirectly. The intake of nutrients and other biologically active compounds of most herbs and spices will be small, reflecting the quantity consumed, but these small amounts may be biologically consequential. The contribution herbs and spices make to the flavour and aroma of food also enhances the enjoyment of eating, which may in itself benefit health. Flavour and aroma can help to stimulate poor appetites and may also stimulate other physiological and neurological pathways/functions important in health.

Large doses or concentrations of herbs and spices, isolates or extracts may have health benefits, but they may also have useful properties as used in food preparation or combination. For instance, turmeric in sufficient quantities—or one of its bioactive components, curcumin—may be anti-inflammatory or neuroprotective. However, intact and in the amounts traditionally used in cooking it can also have measurable effects on cognition in vulnerable individuals (Lee et al. 2014; Small et al. 2018). A similar situation appears to apply for cinnamon (Wahlqvist et al. 2016). The Lamiaceae family of culinary herbs, including mint, rosemary and oregano, seems to be anti-inflammatory and generally healthful in the human diet (Opara & Chohan 2014). Herbs that have travelled with human migration, food and beverage consumption include mint and basil, which suggests their biological relevance.

Cultural/traditional significance and uses

Herbs and spices often give dishes their cultural nuances, distinguishing between regions, countries and localities. For example, lemongrass and coriander are a feature of Thai cuisine, while classic French cooking includes tarragon, chives, thyme, rosemary, bay leaves, chervil, parsley and nutmeg. Herbs were once used to disguise the unpleasant odours of foods

TURMERIC—IS IT ETHICAL?

Traditionally, herbs and spices have been consumed in small quantities, so consuming large amounts may also be a risk to health. However, they potentially offer a marketing opportunity for businesses. Turmeric is a current example of a spice the active ingredient of which, curcumin, has been identified as an anti-inflammatory agent. However, consumption of large amounts may increase cancer risk.

Access the peer-reviewed literature identify the:
- benefits and risks of consumption
- safe levels of consumption.

Review commonly available products and determine the amounts that could be consumed. You could choose, for example, a turmeric latte, turmeric complementary medicines or other products. Do they contain the active ingredient in quantities that could have a therapeutic benefit? Do they contain the active ingredient in levels that are safe? What happens when an individual is consuming more than one item containing turmeric?

Develop a five-minute talk on your findings and the ethics of selling these products.

that were stored during the winter months, when many fresh foods were unattainable. When eastern spices appeared in Europe, their stronger aroma made these spices very desirable and they were much sought after.

COMMON HERBS AND SPICES

Common herbs
basil
bay leaves
chives
coriander
dill
fennel
marjoram
mint
oregano
parsley
rosemary
sage
tarragon
thyme

Common spices derived from seeds
allspice
angelica
anise
annatto
black cumin
black pepper
brown mustard
caraway
cardamom
cayenne pepper
celery seed
coriander
cumin
dill
fennel
fenugreek
juniper berries
lovage
mace

mustard
myrtle
nutmeg
paprika
pepper
pimento
Sichuan pepper
star anise
tabasco pepper
tamarind
vanilla
white mustard
white pepper

Common spices derived from roots, stems, bark, leaves or flowers
curry leaf
fennel
field mint

French tarragon
garden nasturtium
ginger
hops
horseradish
hyssop
lemon verbena
lemongrass
liquorice
makrut lime
mint
oregano
peppermint
rue
saffron
sage
spearmint
turmeric
wasabi
wormwood
zedoary

Current trends

Today the range and availability of herbs and spices is extensive, as our appetite for both a variety of and mixture of cuisines continues to grow. Common spices and herbs are listed in the box above.

EDIBLE ANIMAL FOODS

An animal food typically describes all the edible parts of an animal, such as muscle, fat, internal organs, blood and integument (skin, membrane). It also includes any edible by-products such as milk and eggs. The bones of an animal, although not usually eaten (with the exception of insects and some fish) are sometimes cooked with the meat attached (to enhance flavour) or boiled to produce stock. The following section describes animal foods under the following categories:

- fish and shellfish
- meat
- milk and milk products
- eggs
- insects.

Fish and shellfish
Description

Fish and shellfish found in either fresh water (rivers, lakes) or salt water (oceans) have been an important part of the human diet for millennia. Most fish have bony skeletons, except for sharks where the skeleton is primarily of cartilage. Shellfish have an exoskeleton and can be categorised into molluscs (oysters, mussels, scallops, abalone, squid, octopus) or crustaceans (prawns, crabs, lobsters, crayfish, yabbies, scampi).

Nutritional qualities

Fish and shellfish are high in protein and low in carbohydrate. The fat content varies depending on the type of fish. In general, cold-water fish are much oilier than fish from tropical/subtropical waters. Oily fish, including salmon, sardines and tuna, are good sources of long-chain polyunsaturated n-3 fatty acids (EPA and DHA), which are associated with health benefits. Saltwater fish and shellfish are an excellent source of iodine.

Health benefits/risks

The regular consumption of saltwater fish can help protect against iodine deficiency, and oily fish containing a high concentration of n-3 fatty acids may help to reduce the risk of arrhythmias, decrease triglyceride levels and hinder the progression of atherosclerotic plaques. Reducing the risk of dementia and age-related macular degeneration might also be linked to the intake of n-3 fatty acids.

Some fish, such as those that are higher up the food chain (like sharks) are more likely to contain higher concentrations of methylmercury than other fish, so eating large quantities of these fish may pose a risk to health, especially for the unborn child (FSANZ 2004).

Cultural/traditional significance and uses

Fresh fish is usually cooked before it is consumed, but in some cultures it is eaten raw. In Japan this is sashimi; in France it is in the form of tartare; in South America, cerviche is fish cured with citrus juice. Fish can be dried, pickled, cured or smoked as a means of preservation.

Current trends

Aquaculture is increasing around Australia as the demand for fish grows. While aquaculture may help to preserve natural fish stocks, fish farmed in this way may not deliver the same benefits. For instance, farmed salmon are often fed a synthetic pigment known as astaxanthin to ensure their flesh has a similar pink appearance to wild salmon. Salmon caught in their natural habitat obtain their pink colour from the astaxanthin that occurs naturally in the crustaceans that the salmon eat. On the other hand, fish caught in the wild may be subject to certain pollutants; for instance the detection of pharmaceuticals and microplastics in aquatic ecosystems worldwide is on the rise (Scott et al. 2016; Lusher et al. 2017). There are some concerns around the sustainability of some aquaculture, related to the feed used, the effluent produced and the ethics of production (Hollingsworth 2018).

In Australia, although fish consumption is still low compared to meat and poultry, it is increasing. The ABS found the number of serves of fish and seafood (per 10,000 kJ) rose from 0.13 to 0.21 between 1995 and 2011–12 (ABS 2016).

Meat
Description

Our earliest ancestors were hunter-gatherers, so animal foods—especially meat—formed an important part of their diet. Meat is the flesh of an animal that is eaten for food and includes both muscle and organs. Today most of the muscle meat or organ meat that is eaten comes from domesticated animals, but game (i.e. wild) meats also make a small contribution.

Nutritional qualities

Meat is an important source of protein, iron, zinc and niacin equivalents. Organ meats such as liver and kidney have a greater concentration of iron, zinc and niacin equivalents than muscle meats and also contain greater amounts of cholesterol. Liver and kidney also contain a significant amount of vitamins A, B-12 and folate. Liver is also a good source of vitamin C.

The bioavailability of iron and zinc from meat is superior to plant foods. Phytate and fibre found in plant foods can bind with iron and zinc, inhibiting their absorption. Red meats, such as beef and lamb, also have higher concentrations of iron and zinc compared to white meats, such as poultry.

The protein in meat is considered to be of high nutritional quality because it contains all the essential amino acids required for human health.

Farming practices can affect the nutritional quality of meat. The fat in beef from grain-fed animals tends to be marbled whereas the fat in 'free-range'

OFFAL

Offal is the name given to the internal organs of animals. Eating the internal organs of animals has gone out of fashion among many Australians and New Zealanders; however, items such as liver, kidneys, tripe and sweetbreads were once commonly eaten. There is a movement called 'head to tail' eating which encourages the consumption of the whole animal in an effort to decrease waste and enhance respect for the animal.

Sausage casings can be made using animal intestines or manufactured from cellulose, collagen or synthetic materials.

- What are the advantages of using natural sausage casings over manufactured casings?
- Haggis is a traditional Scottish dish. What is haggis and how is it made?
- What foods or dishes made from internal organs were once commonly eaten in Australia and New Zealand?
- What are some dishes based on internal organs still consumed among some cultural groups living in Australia and New Zealand?

grass-fed animals forms a margin around the meat, making it easier to remove to produce leaner cuts of meat. The composition of fat between domesticated animals and those captured from their native habitat (game) also differs. In general, game meats are very lean, contain less saturated fat and are higher in polyunsaturated fats, especially omega-3 fatty acids.

Health benefits/risks
Lean meat is a nutrient-dense food which can help to protect against iron deficiency. Cancer is the main health risk associated with meat intake and the risk is usually related to the quantity, cooking methods (i.e. high temperatures result in the formation of nitrates associated with blackening) and type of meat consumed. In 2017, the World Cancer Research Fund concluded that although red meat probably caused colorectal cancer, processed meats almost certainly do, since the risk of colorectal cancer increased as the consumption of processed meats increased (WCRF/AICR 2018). Furthermore, recent research found that regular consumers of meat (including chicken) whose preference was for well-done/charred meat cooked at high temperatures (grilled or barbecued) appeared to be at increased risk of type 2 diabetes compared to consumers who preferred their meat lightly browned and used lower-temperature cooking methods such as stir-frying, boiling or steaming (Liu et al. 2018). The Australian Dietary Guidelines, although recognising the nutritional value of lean meat, recommend that red meat consumption should be limited to no more than 455 g per week and that the meat should be lean and unprocessed.

Meat production is also a major source of greenhouse gas emissions, uses significant water resources and contributes to land degradation (Godfray et al. 2018). Consequently, meat consumption needs to be considered with respect to environmental health as well as human health (see Chapter 26).

Cultural/traditional significance and uses
The kinds of animals used for food is often related to culture. For example, eating horse or dog is unacceptable to the vast majority of Australians and it is unlawful to sell these animals for human consumption; however, these animals are eaten by other cultures.

Eating native animals in Australia can be divisive. Kangaroo populations are at pest levels in some parts of the country and their control has led to the increasing availability of kangaroo in the Australian diet. However, parts of the population associate kangaroo with pet food, or with eating a part of the coat of arms, and therefore see it as undesirable.

In the early days of settlement it was common for more native animals to be consumed (for example, possum, dugong or emu). Many other native animals are protected from slaughter; however, Australian Aboriginal and Torres Strait Islander populations are able to hunt these animals for food as part of their traditional customs.

Religion also plays an important role in determining which meats can be consumed. For instance, observant Jews and Muslims will not eat pork and will only eat meat that has been **kosher** and **halal** certified respectively.

Current trends
According to the ABS, in 2011–12 Australians ate an average of 565 g of red meat (including higher-fat and processed varieties) each week (ABS 2016). This is well in excess of the maximum amount suggested by the Australian Dietary Guidelines. Furthermore, between 1995 and 2011–12, the consumption of lean red meat increased from 0.77 to 0.81 serves per 10,000 kJ (ABS 2016). However, despite this increase, the consumption of lean red meat as a share of the overall food group (comprising lean meat and poultry, fish, eggs, tofu, nuts and seeds and legumes/beans) has dropped, from 49 per cent in 1995 to 38 per cent in 2011–12 (ABS 2016). While the consumption of all the other foods in this group has increased over this time, the largest increase comes from poultry (from 22 per cent in 1995 to 29 per cent in 2011–12) (ABS 2016).

Milk and milk products
Description
Milk and its products are consumed by many cultures around the world. Milk—which is obtained from the mammary glands of cows, sheep, goats, buffalo, camels and yaks—is a beverage and can be fermented prior to consumption. It is also added to hot beverages such as tea, coffee or chocolate drinks (see section on beverages).

Milk products include butter, cream, yoghurt and cheese. Cream forms at the top of milk when it has been left to stand. If this is skimmed off and agitated it will become butter. Yoghurt forms when warm milk is fermented using selected strains of acid-producing bacteria that will coagulate the milk into a firm curd. Cheese is made by the coagulation of casein (milk protein). The resulting curd can then be treated in a variety of ways to produce the specific flavour, colour and texture of different cheeses.

Nutritional qualities
The diet of newborn mammals (including humans) consists entirely of milk; therefore, milk is an important source of nutrients needed for growth and development. However, the composition of milk varies according to its source. For example, human milk contains casein and whey proteins in a ratio of 40:60 respectively, while in cow's milk the ratio of casein to whey proteins is 80:20.

Milk, yoghurt and cheese are excellent sources of high-quality protein and calcium. These dairy foods are also useful sources of phosphorous, magnesium, iodine, vitamin A, riboflavin and vitamin B-12 but are a poor source of vitamin C and iron.

Health benefits/risks
Dairy foods are considered important in bone development and the prevention of osteoporosis. However, many other factors play an important role in bone health, including physical activity, vitamin D and other nutrients including vitamin K, vitamin C, magnesium, potassium and zinc. Other biologically active compounds in foods may also affect bone health.

The Dietary Approaches to Stop Hypertension (DASH) study (see Chapter 33) showed that a diet high in fruit, vegetables and low-fat dairy products was successful in lowering blood pressure (Appel et al. 1997). This reduction in blood pressure was further enhanced when sodium intakes were less than 100 millimoles per day. When these dietary characteristics are seen in various food culture settings, similar outcomes are found and extend to cardiovascular complications like stroke (Huang et al. 2014).

The regular consumption of milk appears to lower the risk of colon cancer but a high intake of dairy foods may increase the risk of prostate cancer.

In terms of cardiovascular disease, the intake of dairy foods (full-fat) appears to neither increase nor decrease the risk (Guo et al. 2017).

Cultural/traditional significance and uses

Lactose is the main sugar found in milk and is digested by the enzyme lactase. Lactase is abundant in the lining of the gut in early childhood but declines with age. However, some population groups remain lactose tolerant as adults and so dairy foods make an important contribution to the diets of many different populations. According to the FAO, milk in its liquid form is the most widely consumed dairy product globally.

There are a range of fermented milks consumed around the world. Some of the differences found in fermented milks will depend on the culture used and the source of milk. Kumiss, a carbonated milk drink that is widely consumed in Central Asia, is traditionally made from raw mare's milk. Dadiah is a traditional fermented milk of Indonesia that is made from raw buffalo milk, and kefir is a fermented milk beverage that is thought to have originated in Russia and Central Asia. As research interest in the gut microbiome and its relationship to health expands, the promotion of probiotic cultures in yoghurts and fermented milks is likely to gain traction among the health-conscious sectors of the Australian population.

Cheese, unlike milk, contains little or no lactose since most of it is lost during processing (discarded with the whey) and any remaining lactose is fermented by bacteria and moulds. There are numerous varieties of cheeses: soft, semi-hard, hard, ripened and unripened. The type of cheese depends on processing methods and, in some cases, the types of moulds used. For example, common types of cheese include blue vein, where a *Penicillium* mould culture is added to milk at start of the cheese-making process; curd cheeses, such as feta and labneh; stretched curd cheese—cheese with a soft elastic texture that melts easily when heated, such as mozzarella; hard cheeses, such as cheddar and parmesan; and fresh unripened cheeses, such as cottage, ricotta and cream cheese.

WHAT CHEESE IS THAT?

Explore the following types of cheese; where are they from and how are they used?

- haloumi
- gorgonzola
- havarti
- Limburger
- quark
- Caerphilly
- roquefort

The consumption of cheese is found in many regions of the world but has not been part of the traditional cuisines of most Southeast and East Asian countries. In France, cheese is eaten with fresh bread only (never biscuits) and at the end of a meal, before dessert. In Australia, cheese is used as an ingredient for many dishes (savoury or sweet) and is often eaten with wine and dry biscuits prior to or after a meal. A cheese toastie or cheese and biscuits are popular snacks or light meals.

Current trends

In the 2011–12 Australian Health Survey, around two-thirds of the population consumed milk. Of the milk consumed, 58 per cent was added to breakfast cereals, 23 per cent was added to a beverage (tea/coffee) and 18 per cent was consumed on its own. Cheese and yoghurt were consumed by 32 per cent and 16 per cent of the population respectively while frozen dairy foods (mainly ice cream) were consumed by 15 per cent of the population (ABS 2016). However, it should be noted that the survey under-represents those Australians from backgrounds that do not routinely eat dairy produce.

Eggs

Description

An egg is the roundish reproductive body laid by an animal. Eggs produced commercially in Australia may be classified as **cage**, **barn-laid** or **free-range** eggs. The size of the air pocket at the blunt end of an egg is an indicator of its freshness; the smaller the air space, the fresher the egg. As a result, fresh eggs will sink when placed in water.

Nutritional qualities

Eggs are an excellent source of high-quality protein and a good source of vitamin B-12, niacin equivalents, riboflavin, folate, retinol equivalents and vitamin E. They are also a useful source of iron, zinc, selenium and the carotenoids lutein and zeaxanthin (important in eye health). Free-range hens that are able to forage for greens, insects and worms produce eggs that are good sources of n-3 fatty acids. There is no difference in the nutritional quality of brown- or white-shelled eggs, as eggshell colour relates only to the breed of hen.

Health benefits/risks

In the past, the high cholesterol content of eggs was thought to adversely affect blood cholesterol, a risk factor for cardiovascular disease. However, research has shown that saturated fat and trans fats are the main substrates used by the liver to manufacture cholesterol (not dietary cholesterol). Eggs are low in saturated fat and the presence of phospholipids in eggs appears to inhibit the absorption of cholesterol. The Heart Foundation recommends up to seven eggs a week as part of a healthy diet.

For the elderly, the nutritional characteristics and low cost of eggs makes them a valuable source of protein. However, the protein found in egg white seems to be the main culprit in those affected with egg food allergies. Apart from food allergies, eggs seem to cause few health issues. However, the consumption of raw eggs in foods like mayonnaise can lead to food poisoning if the eggs are contaminated with harmful bacteria such as *Salmonella*.

Cultural/traditional significance and uses

Eggs are a very versatile food and make an important contribution to the diets of many people. They can be eaten whole (boiled, scrambled, poached) or as an ingredient in a wide range of recipes, such as sauces, custards, dressings, cakes, desserts and savoury dishes (omelette, frittata). Their versatility in recipes is due

to three important characteristics. An egg white (albumin) can form stable foams (as in meringues); its yolk can stabilise fat in water emulsions (such as mayonnaise); and when egg protein is heated it can thicken liquids to make custards and sauces.

Current trends

According to the national nutrition surveys, egg consumption increased slightly between 1995 and 2011–12. Over this time period, for adults aged 19 years and over, the median daily consumption of eggs rose from 50 g to 58 g and consumption of products containing mainly eggs from 128 g to 138 g (ABS 1999; 2016).

Insects

Description

The eating of insects (entomophagy) contributes to the diets of many cultures around the world. Of all the animal groups, insects are the most diverse. As adults, these small animals have an exoskeleton comprised of chitin, a segmented body divided into a head, thorax and abdomen, three pairs of jointed legs and (in most species) two pairs of wings. The majority of insect species have a four-stage life-cycle; egg, larva, pupa and adult. Each of these stages may serve as a food.

Nutritional qualities

Insects are a source of protein, fat and carbohydrate as well as various vitamins and minerals. Protein quality includes essential amino acids. Fat quality largely depends on what insects have been feeding on, but reports indicate high levels of n-3 and n-6 fatty acids. However, to date there is a lack of comprehensive nutrient composition and digestibility data (Roos 2018).

Health benefits/risks

The amount of protein, fats and micronutrients derived from insects makes an important contribution to the health and food security of many populations around the world.

Insects that are eaten as part of a traditional diet have been consumed over a long period and are therefore unlikely to pose a risk to health. Any potential risks associated with insect consumption are perhaps greater if insects are farmed on a mass scale, harvested from areas affected by pollution or introduced into populations where insects have not been part of the food culture.

Cultural/traditional significance and uses

Edible insects can be cooked using a variety of methods, including frying, roasting, stewing, steaming and boiling.

Insects are eaten by many cultures around the world. Indigenous Australians ate a variety of insects, especially in desert regions where the witchetty grub was an important staple. In addition to being an important food source, many Aboriginal people consider witchetty grubs a delicacy that can be eaten either raw or cooked. Insects are also a feature of many regional Chinese diets. Several ethnic groups in Indonesia eat insects including grasshoppers, crickets and termites, as well as the larvae of the sago palm weevil and bee (Nirmala & Pramono 2017). Deep-fried grasshoppers, crickets, bee larvae, silkworms, ant eggs and termites can be found in many traditional markets of Thailand. Wasps, a delicacy in Japan, are embedded in the food culture, with a traditional festival held annually to celebrate their consumption.

Current trends

Insects are under heightened consideration due to their low ecological footprint during production. Edible insect products, such as insect flour, are becoming increasingly popular around the world.

ROLE OF EDIBLE INSECTS

For more than a decade, the Food and Agriculture Organization (FAO) has been investigating the role of edible insects in human consumption. They are potentially a highly sustainable source of protein and could assist in resolving food insecurity. The FAO estimates that around 1900 species of insects are consumed worldwide, with beetles being the most commonly eaten insect.

- Conduct a quick survey of your peers to determine which members (if any) have intentionally eaten insects.
- What are the potential barriers to eating insects? How might these be overcome?
- How might insects help to address the problem of food insecurity?
- How will the consumption of insects contribute to the sustainability of the food supply?
- Edible insect products are becoming increasingly popular around the world. What insect products are available in Australia?
- Does FSANZ have a regulation for selling insects/insect products for consumption?

Based on the information you find, decide if you are pro or anti insect consumption. Develop a three-minute talk to state your case.

Resources to assist you include:

- Food and Agriculture Organization, 2018, *Insects for Food and Feed*, <www.fao.org/edible-insects/en/>
- BugMe: Entomophagy Nutrition Consulting Services, 2018, *About Us*, <www.bugme.com.au/about/>.

OTHER FOODS

The following section describes foods that fall under the following categories:

- fats and oils derived from plants and animals
- edible fungi and algae
- beverages
- chocolate.

Fats and oils (plant and animal)
Description
Fats and oils are derived from a variety of plants and animals. Animal fats include butter (from milk), suet (from meat fat found around the kidneys/internal organs of cattle, sheep and pigs), lard (clarified pig suet) and dripping (from roast meat). Oils are extracted from plants via pressing or through chemical processing and include canola, olive, peanut, safflower, sunflower, sesame and coconut oil. Fats and oils collected or extracted from various foods offer a concentrated source of fat which is usually used as a spread, in frying or as an ingredient in baked goods and salad dressings. Eating foods that are not processed (such as whole nuts and seeds) will still provide a dietary source of fats and oils but in much smaller quantities. Eating oily fish will provide a useful source of n-3 fatty acids, but oil extracted from fish enables these to be consumed in much larger (medicinal) quantities.

The chemical structure of most edible fats and oils consist of combinations of fatty acids with glycerol. Slight differences in these combinations give rise to the various forms and functions of fats and oils. Saturated fats are solid at room temperature; while most saturated fat comes from animal sources, plant sources include cooking margarine, coconut oil (copha) and palm oil. Fats that are liquid at room temperature are extracted from vegetables, nuts, seeds and fish. In general, these fats are usually classified as monounsaturated and polyunsaturated fats. Oils that are predominantly composed of monounsaturated fats include olive oil, peanut oil and canola oil. Polyunsaturated fats include n-3 and n-6 fatty acids, which are essential for health and can only be obtained from dietary sources. Fats that are good sources of n-3 fatty acids include fish oil, flaxseed oil and soybean oil. n-6 fatty acids are found in vegetable oils such as safflower, soybean, sunflower and corn oils.

Nutritional qualities
Fats and oils are energy dense and a vehicle for fat-soluble vitamins A, D, E and K. Vitamins A and D are found in animal fats and are often added to margarines. The nutritional profile of fats and oils diminishes with processing. For instance, when oils are processed without high heat or chemical solvents, their desirable qualities (vitamin E and polyphenols) are preserved. Refining, heating and light not only degrade the phenol content of oils but also shorten their shelf life.

Health benefits/risks
Some fats appear to be beneficial to health, especially cardiovascular health. Polyunsaturated fats (n-3 and n-6 fats) also seem to protect against cardiovascular disease. The benefits of n-3 fats appear to be related to their effect of lowering blood triglyceride levels and blood pressure. n-6 fats also appear to protect against heart disease if used to replace the dietary intake of saturated and trans fats.

Diets high in saturated fats are less desirable, as these fats can adversely affect cholesterol levels. However, trans fats generated from **hydrogenated vegetable oils** are the most harmful to health.

Trans fats are associated with an increased risk of cardiovascular disease and other chronic conditions. These fats are found in many processed foods, especially deep-fried foods, cakes and biscuits, and pies and pastries. Trans fats are rare in unprocessed foods but can be found in very small amounts in beef, lamb, and dairy foods (see Chapter 11).

Since fats and oils are sourced from a wide variety of plants (and, to lesser extent, animals), consuming a range of fats and oils is likely to deliver greater health benefits than relying on one type of fat or oil. Furthermore, consuming fats and oils that have undergone minimal processing (without high heat or chemical solvents) and before their use-by-date will help to provide the chemicals (polyphenols) thought to be responsible for the health benefits. Storing fats and oils away from light and heat will also preserve their phenol content.

Cultural/traditional significance and uses

Traditionally, fats and oils have been used not only to facilitate cooking but also to enhance the palatability of food. Frying enables foods to be cooked at a higher temperature and contributes to their flavour and texture.

The type of oil used within a particular cultural context appears to depend on what was available; for example, olives are native to the Mediterranean and consequently olive oil is used extensively; coconut is abundant in the tropics and coconut oil, milk and cream are widely used; in parts of Africa groundnuts (peanuts) are utilised for their oil while in other parts palm oil, which is also high in vitamin A, is used.

Current trends

The most recent ABS survey found around half (46 per cent) of the Australian population consumed fats and oils, mostly in sandwiches or on bread/baked products (85 per cent) or added to vegetables or salads (9 per cent). The overall consumption of unsaturated spreads and oils has remained fairly constant over recent years (at 2.3 serves per 10,000 kJ), but the amount sourced from unsaturated spreads (i.e. margarine) has declined from 42 per cent in 1995 to 17 per cent in 2011–12. Over this same period, increases in the contribution from unsaturated oils (from 40 per cent to 54 per cent) and nuts (from 18 per cent to 30 per cent) have matched the reduction in unsaturated spreads (ABS 2016).

Edible fungi and algae
Description

Edible fungi include mushrooms, yeasts and moulds. Fungi are commonly considered to be plants because of their long culinary use but, unlike plants, they grow without roots, stems or leaves and do not contain chlorophyll. Fungi have spores, similar to pollen or seeds, which spread or travel by wind. They depend on oxygen, typically live in dark, damp environments and obtain nourishment from dead organic matter.

There are many varieties of mushrooms which can be found growing in the wild or cultivated (usually in dark atmosphere-controlled rooms). Mushrooms safe for eating include the button, cap, flat, portobello, cremini, shiitake, oyster, enoki, maitake, matsutake, porcini, straw, morel and chanterelle and the highly prized truffle. Seaweeds are large types of red, green or brown algae. Algae has always been an important food source throughout Asia and its popularity as a nutritious food is growing globally.

Nutritional qualities

Fungi are an excellent source of fibre, vitamins (vitamin D when exposed to light, riboflavin, niacin) and minerals (potassium, selenium and chromium).

Seaweed is rich in vitamins, minerals and many other nutrients. Seaweed is obtained from sea water so it has a very high sodium content. However, it may be an important source of iodine and has potential for addressing iodine deficiency disorders in some regions where iodised salt is less acceptable due to its links to hypertension.

Cultural/traditional significance/uses

For many years mushrooms (fresh and dried) have been used across the globe in different food cultures for their ability to add flavour, colour and nutrients without adding sodium or fat. Mushrooms have been used in Japanese and Chinese cuisines from very early times and have been popular in French, Italian, German and Russian cooking for centuries.

Many wild species of mushroom, such as the common death cap mushroom, are toxic and, if consumed, can lead to illness, paralysis and even death. It is recommended that wild mushrooms be purchased from a reliable source or an experienced forager. Novices should avoid doing their own foraging.

Moulds are added to some cheeses in order to develop certain characteristics in taste and texture; for example, blue cheeses (stilton), soft ripened cheeses (camembert, brie) and rind-washed cheeses. Moulds are also used to ripen the surfaces of sausages and to extend their shelf life.

Yeasts are used in the production of bread and alcohol. Yeast extracts are also used to manufacture Vegemite (a popular Australian spread).

The Japanese have eaten seaweed for centuries. It is an important ingredient in many Japanese dishes such as miso soup, sushi and onigiri (Japanese rice balls).

Current trends
Mushrooms are popular in vegan and vegetarian diets, often described as having a 'meaty' flavour and providing a fairly good protein content. A variety of seaweeds such as kombu, nori and wakame are growing in popularity.

Beverages
Description
The range of beverages is wide and usually culturally specific. As a provider of fluid, the essential nutrient of life, water, is a fundamental requirement. Water needs to be readily and freely available as well as **potable**—microbiologically and chemically safe and contaminant-free. Despite plumbing and water treatment, potable water is still not readily available for at least one-third of the world's population (WHO/UNICEF 2017). Even this situation is precarious, as the contamination of waterways has made some 60 per cent of fresh water non-potable and unsuitable for irrigation. The failure to keep excretory waste from mixing with fresh water further compromises water supplies. For these reasons, hot beverages, in which water is boiled for infusion or other forms of flavouring, are widespread.

Soup consumption often serves as a surrogate for beverages and has the advantage of being nutritious. A major trend is for meals such as breakfast to be liquefied, but this means that foods such as grains and legumes, whose health-giving properties are partly located in food structure and physico-chemistry, no longer provide these benefits (Wahlqvist 2016). Where there is chewing difficulty or a need for tube-feeding, long-term survival is unavoidably compromised since food structure cannot equate with natural foodstuffs, but innovative technology can partly provide the required characteristics, as

with viscosity or fermentability (Lee et al. 2010). In addition, the trend towards beverage-based meals in Western food culture is a serious threat to the role of sufficient food structure in food intake patterns.

As with other dietary items, a variety of beverages will increase the range of potential benefits and reduce any risks. For a discussion of alcohol and sugar-sweetened beverages, see chapters 12 and 15.

Tea (infusion of *Camellia sinensis*) is the most commonly consumed beverage after water. Herbal infused beverages such as mint-based teas are common across North Africa and throughout the Middle East. Coffee, which originated in Ethiopia, is a traditional beverage in many parts of the world, including Europe and the Americas.

Nutritional qualities
Coffee and tea contain traces of vitamins and minerals and are important sources of flavonoids and other antioxidants that have potential health benefits. Tea contains catechins, epicatechins, quercetin, kaempferol and myricetin (all flavonoids) as well as caffeine. A number of health benefits have been ascribed to tea infused from *C. sinensis* whether in black, green, or oolong forms. However, the flavonoid concentration found in tea diminishes with oxidation, a process that contributes to the colour of tea. The degree of oxidation that occurs after harvesting is lowest during the production of green tea and highest with the processing of black tea.

Coffee contains an antioxidant called chlorogenic acid and unfiltered coffee contains cafestol and kahweol, two oily substances known as diterpenes. The importance of these substances for health is not yet clearly understood.

Cultural/traditional significance and uses
Tea plays an important role in Chinese and Japanese society and is served with every meal. Outside the home, teahouses are popular meeting places. Tea is also a strong cultural feature in other countries, including India, Russia, Morocco, Egypt, Turkey, England and France.

Coffee has been an important beverage for many cultures. As a commodity it is emerging as a

BENEFITS OF TEA AND COFFEE

Consumption of tea and coffee is significant in Australia and New Zealand and they are claimed to provide significant health benefits. As a nutrition practitioner, however, you need to ensure that the evidence matches the claims.

For this activity you need to answer the following questions.

- What are the health benefits of drinking tea and coffee? What could be the side effects?
- How much caffeine will cause adverse health effects? How does this relate to number of cups of tea or coffee?
- Are there any medical conditions in which the consumption of tea or coffee is contraindicated?

To get you started, a number of review articles are listed below. Remember, going back to the original empirical evidence is important.

- Grosso, G. et al., 2017, 'Coffee, caffeine, and health outcomes: An umbrella review', *Annual Review of Nutrition, 37*(1): 131–56
- Hayat, K. et al., 2015, 'Tea and its consumption: Benefits and risks', *Critical Reviews in Food Science and Nutrition, 55*(7): 939–54
- Poole, R. et al., 2017, 'Coffee consumption and health: Umbrella review of meta-analyses of multiple health outcomes', *BMJ, 359*: j5024.
- Vuong, Q.V., 2014, 'Epidemiological evidence linking tea consumption to human health: A review', *Critical Reviews in Food Science and Nutrition, 54*(4): 523–36.

significant symbol of ethical consumption, with consideration given to fair trade production (especially in low-income countries) as well as to elite considerations, such as variations in flavour due to origin and roasting techniques (Tucker 2017).

Current trends

The 2011–12 ABS survey found that around half (46 per cent) of the Australian population consumed coffee (including coffee substitutes), while just over one-third (38 per cent) drank tea (ABS 2016).

Chocolate

Description

Chocolate/cocoa derives from a fatty fruit, cacao, with a long mystical usage among pre-Columbian Americans. The cacao beans are fermented, shelled, roasted and milled to produce a cocoa paste, which undergoes further processing to form chocolate.

Nutritional qualities

Cocoa is a source of vitamin E, potassium, phosphorous and magnesium as well as naturally occurring antioxidants such as procyanidins and flavonoids (epicatechin). It also contains the compounds theobromine and caffeine.

The phytochemistry of chocolate, including flavonoids and methylxanthines, suggests it may have favourable effects on the skin and brain and benefits for insulin sensitivity, inflammation and cardiovascular health, depending on how it is processed (Grassi et al. 2008; Sokolov et al. 2013).

Cultural/traditional significance and uses

Although a traditional food and beverage in meso-America, it is now extensively commercialised as a discretionary food and beverage item globally.

Current trends

In 2011–12, the most popular type of confectionary eaten by Australians was chocolate (or a chocolate-based confectionary). Seventeen per cent of those surveyed reported consuming chocolate (ABS 2014).

SUMMARY

- Our food is predominantly derived from plants and animals but may also include fungi and algae.
- The nutritional and other biologically active components of food vary both within and between food groups. However, each food group tends to supply different components, so the more varied the diet the more likely all food factors contributing to health will be met.
- The variety available within and between food groups provides an abundance of flavours, colours, textures and tastes that adds interest and pleasure to eating.
- The food we eat and how it is prepared and cooked are influenced by many factors, including culture, beliefs and the food supply.
- Traditional food habits that promote health include incorporating plenty of vegetables, fruits, nuts, seeds, legumes, whole grains and fish, with smaller amounts of lean meat, eggs and dairy, while avoiding processed meat, refined grains, refined oils, foods with added sugars and other highly processed foods.
- The processing of foods can improve food security, food availability and provide greater food choice. The processing of foods can also enhance food safety and extend shelf life. However, the nutritional value of highly processed foods are compromised and this can have a negative impact on our health.

KEY TERMS

Barn-laid eggs: eggs produced by hens that are not kept in cages but instead are able to move throughout large sheds. All barns have nest boxes, but not all barns have perches or litter. Birds are usually de-beaked and kept in high-density conditions.

Cage eggs: eggs produced by hens kept in small confined cages where they have access to food and water but are unable to move around. The cage egg industry is a classic example of factory farming.

Free-range eggs: the current Australian Consumer Law (Free Range Egg Labelling) Information Standard 2017 stipulates that eggs can only be labelled as free-range if hens had access to an outdoor area during daylight hours, were able to roam and forage in this area and there were 10,000 or fewer hens in the area. However, some egg producers voluntarily have no more than 1500 hens in an area, which is considered more humane.

Halal: an Arabic word meaning lawful or permitted. In reference to food, all food is considered halal unless prohibited in the Qur'an. Food not permitted is termed haram. Meat should come from animals slaughtered according to Islamic law.

Hydrogenated vegetable oil: vegetable oil that has been heated to a high temperature and had hydrogen added to it, essentially making it saturated. The process allows the liquid oil to cool as a solid. Hydrogenated vegetable oils are found in a variety of processed foods such as biscuits, cakes, pastries, potato chips and fast foods.

Kosher: food that is considered lawful (kashrut) according to the Old Testament in Judaism. Foods not considered lawful are termed treif. All meat must come from animals slaughtered according to Jewish law.

Nutritional resilience: resilience is the ability to recover quickly from a threat or difficulties. Having reliable food systems, understanding how to put nutrition into action by preparing food and meals (food literacy), and being well-nourished at all stages of life assists in protecting diet quality when there are changes to economic, social and life-stage conditions.

Potable: safe to drink, i.e. non-contaminated. Non-potable therefore means unsafe to drink.

Resistant starch: starch that passes undigested through the small intestine and is fermented by bacteria in the colon. The short-chain fatty acids resulting from fermentation assist in maintaining the integrity of colonic cells.

REFERENCES

ABS, 1999, *National Nutrition Survey: Foods eaten, Australia, 1995,* <www.abs.gov.au/AUSSTATS/abs@.nsf/Details Page/4804.01995?OpenDocument>, accessed 23 October 2018

—— 2014, *Australian Health Survey: Nutrition first results—food and nutrients, 2011–12,* <www.abs.gov.au/AUSSTATS/abs@.nsf/Lookup/4364.0.55.007Main+Features12011-12>, accessed 23 October 2018

—— 2016, *Australian Health Survey: Consumption of food groups from the Australian Dietary Guidelines, 2011–12,* <www.abs.gov.au/AUSSTATS/abs@.nsf/DetailsPage/4364.0.55.0122011-12?OpenDocument>, accessed 22 November 2018

Appel, L.J., Moore, T.J., Obarzanek, E., Vollmer, W.M., Svetkey, L.P. et al., 1997, 'A clinical trial of the effects of dietary patterns on blood pressure', *New England Journal of Medicine, 336*(16): 1117–24, doi:10.1056/nejm199704173361601

Aune, D., Giovannucci, E., Boffetta, P., Fadnes, L.T., Keum, N. et al., 2017, 'Fruit and vegetable intake and the risk of cardiovascular disease, total cancer and all-cause mortality—a systematic review and dose-response meta-analysis of prospective studies', *International Journal of Epidemiology, 46*(3): 1029–56, doi:10.1093/ije/dyw319

Battino, M., Beekwilder, J., Denoyes-Rothan, B., Laimer, M., McDougall, G.J. & Mezzetti, B., 2009, 'Bioactive compounds in berries relevant to human health', *Nutrition Reviews, 67*(s1): S145–50, doi:10.1111/j.1753-4887.2009.00178.x

BugMe, 2018, *About Us,* <www.bugme.com.au/about/>, accessed 22 January 2019

Castañeda-Ovando, A., Sedo, O., Havel, J., Pacheco, L., Galán-Vidal, C.A. & Contreras López, E., 2012, 'Identification of anthocyanins in red grape, plum and capulin by MALDI-ToF MS', *Journal of the Mexican Chemical Society, 56*(4): 378–83, <www.scielo.org.mx/scielo.php?pid=S1870-249X2012000400004&script=sci_arttext>, accessed 21 January 2019

Chang, W.C., Wahlqvist, M.L., Chang, H.Y., Hsu, C.C., Lee, M.S. et al., 2012, 'A bean-free diet increases the risk of all-cause mortality among Taiwanese women: The role of the metabolic syndrome', *Public Health Nutrition, 15*(4): 663–72, doi:10.1017/S1368980011002151

Darmadi-Blackberry, I., Wahlqvist, M.L., Kouris-Blazos, A., Steen, B., Lukito, W. et al., 2004, 'Legumes: The most important dietary predictor of survival in older people of different ethnicities', *Asia Pacific Journal of Clinical Nutrition, 13*(2): 217–20, <http://apjcn.nhri.org.tw/SERVER/MarkWpapers/Papers/Papers 2004/P330.pdf>, accessed 21 January 2019

Eisenhauer, B., Natoli, S., Liew, G. & Flood, V.M., 2017, 'Lutein and zeaxanthin—food sources, bioavailability and dietary variety in age-related macular degeneration protection', *Nutrients, 9*(2): 120, doi:10.3390/nu9020120

FAO, 2018, *Insects for Food and Feed,* <www.fao.org/edible-insects/en/ >, accessed 22 January 2019

Foyer, C.H., Lam, H.-M., Nguyen, H.T., Siddique, K.H., Varshney, R.K. et al., 2016, 'Neglecting legumes has compromised human health and sustainable food production', *Nature Plants, 2*(8): 16112, doi:10.1038/nplants.2016.112

FSANZ, 2004, *Mercury in Fish,* <www.foodstandards.gov.au/publications/Documents/mercury%20in%20fish%20-%20further%20info.pdf>, accessed 23 October 2018

—— 2019, *The Australian Food Composition Database*, <www.foodstandards.gov.au/science/monitoringnutrients/afcd/Pages/default.aspx>, accessed 18 February 2019

Godfray, H.C.J., Aveyard, P., Garnett, T., Hall, J.W., Key, T.J. et al., 2018, 'Meat consumption, health, and the environment', *Science, 361*(6399): eaam5324, doi:10.1126/science.aam5324

Grassi, D., Desideri, G., Necozione, S., Lippi, C., Casale, R. et al., 2008, 'Blood pressure is reduced and insulin sensitivity increased in glucose-intolerant, hypertensive subjects after 15 days of consuming high-polyphenol dark chocolate', *Journal of Nutrition, 138*(9): 1671–6, doi:10.1093/jn/138.9.1671

Grosso, G., Godos, J., Galvano, F. & Giovannucci, E.L., 2017, 'Coffee, caffeine, and health outcomes: An umbrella review', *Annual Review of Nutrition, 37*(1): 131–56, doi:10.1146/annurev-nutr-071816-064941

Guo, J., Astrup, A., Lovegrove, J.A., Gijsbers, L., Givens, D.I. & Soedamah-Muthu, S.S., 2017, 'Milk and dairy consumption and risk of cardiovascular diseases and all-cause mortality: Dose–response meta-analysis of prospective cohort studies', *American Journal of Epidemiology, 32*(4): 269–87, doi:10.1007/s10654-017-0243-1

Hayat, K., Iqbal, H., Malik, U., Bilal, U. & Mushtaq, S., 2015, 'Tea and its consumption: Benefits and risks', *Critical Reviews in Food Science and Nutrition, 55*(7): 939–54, doi:10.1080/10408398.2012.678949

Hertog, M.G., Feskens, E.J., Kromhout, D., Hollman, P.C.H. & Katan, M.B., 1993, 'Dietary antioxidant flavonoids and risk of coronary heart disease: The Zutphen Elderly Study', *Lancet, 342*(8878): 1007–11, doi:10.1016/0140-6736(93)92876-U

Hollingsworth, A., 2018, 'Sustainable diets: The gulf between management strategies and the nutritional demand for fish', in W. Leal Filho (ed.), *Handbook of Sustainability Science and Research*, Cham: Springer International Publishing, pp. 711–25

Huang, L.-Y., Wahlqvist, M.L., Huan, Y.-C. & Lee, M.-S., 2014, 'Optimal dairy intake is predicated on total, cardiovascular, and stroke mortalities in a Taiwanese cohort', *Journal of the American College of Nutrition, 33*(6): 426–36, doi:10.1080/07315724.2013.875328

Kouris-Blazos, A. & Belski, R., 2016, 'Health benefits of legumes and pulses with a focus on Australian sweet lupins', *Asia Pacific Journal of Clinical Nutrition, 25*(1): 1–17, doi:10.6133/apjcn.2016.25.1.23

Lee, M.-S., Wahlqvist, M.L., Chou, Y.-C., Fang, W.-H., Lee, J.-T. et al., 2014, 'Turmeric improves post-prandial working memory in pre-diabetes independent of insulin', *Asia Pacific Journal of Clinical Nutrition, 23*(4): 581–91, doi:10.6133/apjcn.2014.23.4.24

Lee, M.S., Huang, Y.C. & Wahlqvist, M.L., 2010, 'Chewing ability in conjunction with food intake and energy status in later life affects survival in Taiwanese with the metabolic syndrome', *Journal of the American Geriatrics Society, 58*(6): 1072–80, doi:10.1111/j.1532-5415.2010.02870.x

Liu, G., Zong, G., Wu, K., Hu, Y., Li, Y. et al., 2018, 'Meat cooking methods and risk of type 2 diabetes: Results from three prospective cohort studies', *Diabetes Care, 41*(5): 1049–60, doi:10.2337/dc17-1992

Lusher, A., Hollman, P. & Mendoza-Hill, J., 2017, 'Microplastics in fisheries and aquaculture: Status of knowledge on their occurrence and implications for aquatic organisms and food safety', *FAO Fisheries and Aquaculture Technical Paper*, 615, <www.fao.org/3/a-i7677e.pdf>, accessed 17 July 2019

Nirmala, I.R. & Pramono, M.S., 2017, 'Sago worms as a nutritious traditional and alternative food for rural children in Southeast Sulawesi, Indonesia', *Asia Pacific Journal of Clinical Nutrition, 26*(Supp): S40–49, <https://search.informit.com.au/documentSummary;dn=915902145956756;res=IELAPA>, accessed 22 January 2019

Opara, E.I. & Chohan, M., 2014, 'Culinary herbs and spices: Their bioactive properties, the contribution of polyphenols and the challenges in deducing their true health benefits', *International Journal of Molecular Sciences, 15*(10): 19183–202, doi:10.3390/ijms151019183

Poole, R., Kennedy, O.J., Roderick, P., Fallowfield, J.A., Hayes, P.C. & Parkes, J., 2017, 'Coffee consumption and health: Umbrella review of meta-analyses of multiple health outcomes', *BMJ, 359*: j5024, doi:10.1136/bmj.j5024

Roos, N., 2018, 'Insects and human nutrition', in A. Halloran, R. Flore, P. Vantomme & N. Roos (eds), *Edible Insects in Sustainable Food Systems*, Cham: Springer, pp. 83–91

Savige, G.S., Hsu-Hage, B. & Wahlqvist, M.L., 1997, 'Food variety as nutritional therapy', *Current Therapeutics*, March: 57–67

Scott, W.C., Du, B., Haddad, S.P., Breed, C.S., Saari, G.N. et al., 2016, 'Predicted and observed therapeutic dose exceedances of ionizable pharmaceuticals in fish plasma from urban coastal systems', *Environmental Toxicology and Chemistry, 35*(4): 983–95, doi:10.1002/etc.3236

Small, G.W., Siddarth, P., Li, Z., Miller, K.J., Ercoli, L. et al., 2018, 'Memory and brain amyloid and tau effects of a bioavailable form of curcumin in non-demented adults: A double-blind, placebo-controlled 18-month trial', *American Journal of Geriatric Psychiatry, 26*(3): 266–77, doi:10.1016/j.jagp.2017.10.010

Sokolov, A.N., Pavlova, M.A., Klosterhalfen, S. & Enck, P., 2013, 'Chocolate and the brain: Neurobiological impact of cocoa flavanols on cognition and behavior', *Neuroscience & Biobehavioral Reviews, 37*(10, Part 2): 2445–53, doi:10.1016/j.neubiorev.2013.06.013

Tucker, C.M., 2017, *Coffee Culture: Local experiences, global connections*, London: Routledge

Ullah, R., Nadeem, M., Khalique, A., Imran, M., Mehmood, S. et al., 2016, 'Nutritional and therapeutic perspectives of Chia (Salvia hispanica L.): A review', *Journal of Food Science and Technology, 53*(4): 1750–8, doi:10.1007/s13197-015-1967-0

Vuong, Q.V., 2014, 'Epidemiological evidence linking tea consumption to human health: A review', *Critical Reviews in Food Science and Nutrition, 54*(4): 523–36, doi:10.1080/10408398.2011.594184

Wahlqvist, M.L., 2016, 'Future food', *Asia Pacific Journal of Clinical Nutrition 25*(4): 706–16, doi:10.6133/apjcn.092016.01

Wahlqvist, M.L., Lee, M.-S., Lee, J.-T., Hsu, C.-C., Chou, Y.-C. et al., 2016, 'Cinnamon users with prediabetes have a better fasting working memory: A cross-sectional function study', *Nutrition Research, 36*(4): 305–10, doi:10.1016/j.nutres.2015.12.005

WCRF/AICR, 2018, *Diet, Nutrition, Physical Activity and Cancer: A global perspective*, <www.wcrf.org/dietandcancer/resources-and-toolkit>, accessed 22 November 2018

WHO/UNICEF, 2017, *Progress on Drinking Water, Sanitation and Hygiene: 2017 update and SDG baselines*, <www.un.org/africarenewal/sites/www.un.org.africarenewal/files/JMP-2017-report-launch-version_0.pdf>, accessed 24 May 2019

{CHAPTER 9}
FOOD DIGESTION

Mark L. Wahlqvist and Naiyana Wattanapenpaiboon

OBJECTIVES

- Describe the process of digestion.
- Explain the roles of the specialised areas of the gastrointestinal tract, together with associated specialised organs, in digestion.
- Summarise the role of physical, hormonal and neural pathways in determining appetite and satiety.

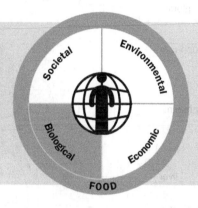

DIGESTION OF FOOD

The digestive system is the pathway through which food is taken into the body and converted to base substances to ensure the body's ongoing optimal functioning before eliminating anything not required. In the human digestive system, the component parts of the gastrointestinal tract are the mouth, oesophagus, stomach, small intestine (including the duodenum, jejunum and ileum), large intestine (including the caecum, colon and rectum) and anus (Figure 9.1).

Digestion begins before food enters the system. The 'cephalic phase' is the phase of gastric secretion before food enters the stomach. It results from the sensory aspects of food, such as its sight, smell and taste. These aspects can influence eating behaviours. In this phase, the anticipation of food prepares the body for the digestion, absorption and use of nutrients in food.

Food enters the mouth and mechanical digestion of the food, especially hard foods, starts with the action of chewing. Chewing reduces the risk of choking by breaking food up into smaller pieces, moistens food with saliva to aid swallowing, facilitates taste and smell, and aids the access of digestive **enzymes**. Saliva contains an amylase enzyme that breaks down starch molecules, producing maltose. Saliva also helps to clean the teeth and reduces dental caries (tooth decay). It contains calcium and phosphate ions and tends to repair eroded tooth enamel by enabling the re-deposition of calcium phosphate in the enamel. After food is chewed and swallowed, it then travels down the oesophagus and into the stomach by the action of **peristalsis**.

The stomach

The stomach has four main functions: storage of food, secretion of enzymes, secretion of acid and mixing. The smooth muscle of the upper level of the stomach relaxes as food is eaten, thus providing storage space for the meal. Gastric juice is made up of hydrochloric acid, digestive enzymes, mucus and bicarbonates. Hydrochloric acid is secreted by parietal cells and creates an acidic environment (pH 1–2). The digestive enzymes are secreted from glands, predominantly in the middle third of the stomach. Pepsin, a proteolytic enzyme (starting protein digestion), is secreted by specialised cells (chief cells) and is active in acidic conditions. Mucus

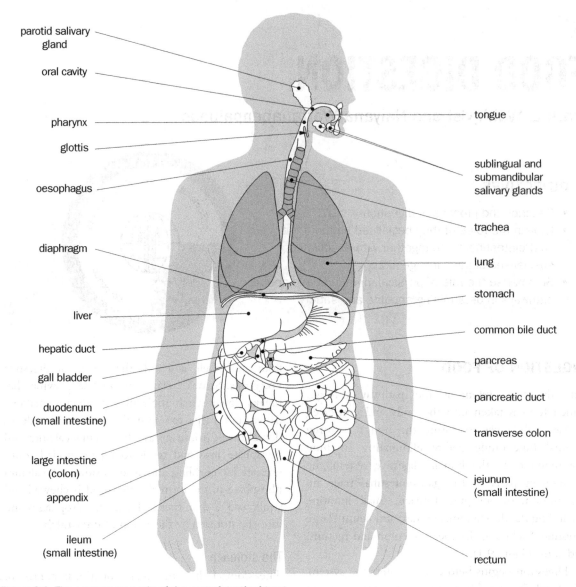

Figure 9.1: The component parts of the gastrointestinal tract

is secreted by goblet cells and acts as a shield against the damaging effects of pepsin and hydrochloric acid. Gastric acid secretion is stimulated in response to the sight and smell of food, the stretching of the stomach following eating and by particular food molecules, such as proteins and amino acids.

Mixing food with digestive secretions in the stomach effectively liquefies it to the consistency of a gruel or thick soup, and this is aided by peristaltic waves of muscle contraction. Neither water nor nutrients are absorbed in any significant quantity from the stomach. As it leaves the stomach, the 'chyme' (the mixture of partially digested food and digestive secretions) has an acidic pH, usually 2.0 or slightly less. The liquid consistency of the chyme as it enters the small intestine enables easier penetration by the digesting enzymes and easier absorption of the nutrients once they are released from the food.

The small intestine

As the chyme enters the duodenum (the first part of the small intestine, connecting the stomach with the jejunum), the acidity of the stomach is neutralised by bicarbonate secreted in bile from the liver, as well as in pancreatic secretions and the fluid from small glands embedded in the mucosa of the duodenal epithelium. The smooth muscle of the intestine continues the peristaltic contractions, which both mix the food and propel it along the intestine. As the chyme passes through the small intestine, digestion continues. The small intestine has a number of structures that effectively increase the surface area in contact with the food material (Figure 9.2).

The inside surface of the internal layer (mucosa) is covered with finger-shaped or tongue-shaped extensions, 1–1.5 mm high, called villi. Each villus is covered with epithelial cells (enterocytes), which absorb nutrients from the channel inside the small intestine (the **lumen**), and each has a capillary blood supply that carries away nutrients after they are absorbed from the intestine.

In addition, the enterocytes on the villi have a specialised outer membrane made up of many fine, finger-like projections of the cell membrane. These projections or microvilli, sometimes referred to as the 'brush border', carry the transport proteins that transfer nutrients from the gut lumen to the interior of the cells. The internal surface structures of the small intestine, including the circular folds, the villi and the microvilli, all increase the surface area available for contact with food molecules. This large surface area—calculated to be about 300 m² for the human intestine—facilitates rapid absorption of nutrients

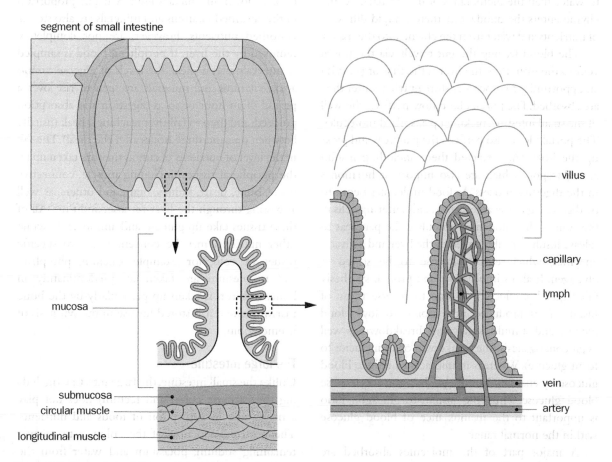

segment of small intestine

mucosa

submucosa
circular muscle
longitudinal muscle

villus

capillary

lymph

vein

artery

Figure 9.2: The surface of the small intestine

ROLE OF THE GASTROINTESTINAL MUCOSA

Read the following articles and summarise the mechanisms and role of gastrointestinal permeability.
- Samadi, N., Klems, M. & Untersmayr, E., 2018, 'The role of gastrointestinal permeability in food allergy', *Annals of Allergy, Asthma & Immunology, 121*(2): 168–73
- Schumann, M. et al., 'Celiac disease: Role of the epithelial barrier', *Cellular and Molecular Gastroenterology and Hepatology, 3*(2): 150–62
- Van Spaendonk, H. et al., 2017, 'Regulation of intestinal permeability: The role of proteases', *World Journal of Gastroenterology, 23*(12): 2106–23.

from the chyme. The epithelial membranes of the duodenum and jejunum are much more permeable to water than the membranes of the stomach. As the chyme enters the duodenum, there is rapid diffusion of nutrients and water from the chyme into the tissues.

The blood leaving the gut travels via the portal vein to the liver; thus, the liver is the first organ with an opportunity to process or store nutrients after they are absorbed. The portal blood flow perfuses the wall of the small intestine, picking up absorbed molecules. The portal blood also perfuses the pancreas and picks up the hormones secreted there, including insulin and glucagon, which are two important hormones in the digestive process. As food molecules begin to be digested, glucose and amino acids entering cells in the wall of the duodenum stimulate the pancreas to release insulin. Insulin travels to the liver and activates enzymes, which enable glucose to be stored as glycogen. It also stimulates fat and protein synthesis. Glucagon has effects that tend to reverse those of insulin. It is produced in response to low blood glucose and stimulates glycogen breakdown as well as gluconeogenesis (the breakdown of amino acids to form glucose). Whereas insulin acts to reduce blood glucose by enabling its storage, glucagon acts to raise blood glucose. Thus, the insulin-to-glucagon ratio is important to the maintenance of blood glucose within the normal range.

A major part of the molecules absorbed are removed in the first pass of the blood through the liver. Sugars are stored as glycogen or converted into fat, while amino acids are built into protein, or broken down and metabolised. A major proportion of the absorbed vitamins and minerals are also stored. Absorbed nutrients, however, are not completely removed by the liver. If peripheral blood is sampled at intervals after a meal, the levels of glucose, amino acids, vitamins and minerals are seen to rise over a period of an hour or so as digestion and absorption proceed, and then to fall after reaching a peak (usually between one and three hours after the meal). The fall in the level of nutrients occurs as they are taken up by the peripheral tissues, including muscle, connective tissue, bone, heart, kidney, brain and others, as well as passing through the liver for a second time. All of these tissues take up glucose and amino acids, while other nutrients may be concentrated into specific tissues or cells; for example, calcium, phosphate and magnesium are taken up predominantly in bone, and iron is taken up particularly by the bone marrow, where it is stored for use in the synthesis of haemoglobin.

The large intestine

Unlike the small intestine, the large intestine (including the caecum, colon and rectum) does not play a major role in absorption of foods and nutrients. The principal function of the colon is to recover remaining sodium, potassium and water from the residual chyme entering from the small intestine.

Normally, about one litre of chyme enters the colon in a day, with a maximum rate of inflow of 6–8 mL/min. Sodium and chloride are actively absorbed from the colon. Reabsorption of sodium and chloride ions (Na^+ and Cl^-) from the lumen lowers the osmotic pressure of the colonic contents and leads to net diffusion of water from the colon contents back into the tissues. The water content of faeces is normally about 50 per cent, and water loss in the faeces is usually in the range 100–250 mL/day.

Symbiosis with gut microorganisms

The colon is also the site in which microorganism-aided (largely bacterial) fermentation of unabsorbed material occurs. The colon normally contains a large number of microorganisms of many types—mostly bacteria, but also protozoa, fungi and viruses (see also Chapter 30). The bulk of the content of the colon is anaerobic (i.e. lacking oxygen), and in such environment only limited metabolism of carbohydrate by bacteria is possible. The microorganisms in the colon obtain energy principally by breaking down (fermenting) dietary fibre, which includes cellulose, pectin, gums, lignin and other polymers. A large proportion of the mucus secreted by the intestine is also broken down.

The end products of fermentation are **short-chain fatty acids (SCFAs)**, chiefly acetic, propionic and butyric acids. The SCFAs are absorbed by diffusion. Once absorbed, the fatty acids, in the presence of oxygen, can be used as a source of energy by the body's metabolism. Metabolism of absorbed SCFAs may supply about 5 per cent of the total energy requirement of the body. It is now thought that the inclusion of adequate fermentable dietary fibre is important to the maintenance of a healthy colon.

Gas in the gut (flatus)

Fermentation of dietary fibre in the colon, particularly in the caecum, produces gas (mostly hydrogen and carbon dioxide), as well as SCFAs. Most of the carbon dioxide is reabsorbed back into the body. If only small amounts of gas are produced, most of it can be absorbed; however, if the amount is larger,

WHAT IS NORMAL FLATULENCE?

Evacuation of gas from the large bowel has significant individual variation. A study on ten healthy volunteers who were fitted with a rectal catheter for 24 hours and who ate a normal diet plus 200 g of baked beans indicated gas production from 476 to 1491 mL (median 705 mL). Men and women produced equivalent amounts. Gas production peaked post-meal (Tomlin et al. 1991). Consumption of legumes purportedly increases flatulence but these claims may be exaggerated (Winham & Hutchins 2011). If we are trying to increase the consumption of plant-based diets, it will be important to address bodily functions without embarrassment.

Keep a flatulence and food diary for a week. Identify if any foods increase flatulence or change the odour of flatulence. Were there any occasions where this became socially difficult to manage? Discuss with a partner what your advice would be to a client who wanted to reduce the volume of flatulence. Does your advice comply with current dietary guidelines?

it is lost as flatus. Some foods, such as legumes, are well known for their association with flatus. This is because these foods contain sufficient indigestible but fermentable carbohydrate to act as a substrate for bacterial gas production (see Chapter 13). Flatus gas may be particularly noticeable if vegetables containing a significant amount of sulphur compounds have been eaten. This is not because of excessive gas, but because a portion of the sulphur is metabolised to mercaptans, compounds to which the human sense of smell is particularly sensitive.

Vitamin synthesis in the gut

With such large numbers of microorganisms in the colon, it is not surprising that a large number of organic molecules are synthesised. Among these are a number of vitamins, including vitamin K, vitamin B-12, folate, biotin, pantothenate, and others. The colon, however, does not have specific vitamin transport proteins in the epithelial cells. Only molecules that are small and have a significant degree of lipid solubility, such as vitamin K and biotin, are absorbed from the colon. Vitamin B-12 and folate are apparently not absorbed to a significant extent; if they were, deficiencies of these vitamins would not occur. Exactly what vitamins we obtain from the gut flora is uncertain.

Transit time of food through the gut

The interval between eating food materials and the time when the food residues are discharged from the body as faeces varies widely depending on individual characteristics and the diet consumed, and may vary day to day. The time food and its residues take to pass through the stomach and small intestine can range from four to eleven hours (the average is six to eight hours), and it could remain up to 70 hours (the average is 40 hours) in the large intestine before being excreted. The sum of these two figures is 'gut transit time'. Where a coarse diet high in fibre is eaten, transit times are short (24 hours or less) because of the bulk of the food residue that passes through. Where a highly refined diet is consumed—as is common in industrialised countries, such as Australia—dietary fibre intakes are low and only a small amount of residue enters the colon each day. As a result, there is not enough material to push the colonic contents onwards. Transit times are commonly two to three days, and for some individuals can be as long as six to ten days, or even longer. Ideally, the gut transit time should be about 12–48 hours. If food passes through too fast, there will not be enough time for nutrients to be absorbed; if it passes through much slower, there is ample time for removal of osmotically active small molecules and removal of the major part of the water. The faecal residue then tends to become dry,

dark and hard, which makes evacuation of faeces more difficult and is a major cause of constipation.

The transit time through the colon appears to affect gut bacteria's metabolism. Generally, intestinal bacteria prefer to digest dietary carbohydrates. As the food residue moves more slowly, it is more completely fermented by bacterial activity. When the carbohydrates are depleted, however, the bacteria start to break down other nutrients, such as proteins. Research shows that the longer food takes to pass through the colon, the more harmful bacterial degradation products (such as ammonia and sulphur compounds) are produced in the colon (Conlon & Bird 2015). It is postulated that these products may be associated with the development of various diseases, including colorectal cancer, chronic renal disease and autism (Roager et al. 2016).

DIGESTION OF MACRONUTRIENTS

The digestion of macronutrients is summarised in Figure 9.3 and is described in more detail in subsequent chapters on fat, protein and carbohydrate (chapters 10–12).

ADAPTABILITY OF THE DIGESTIVE SYSTEM

The structure and function of the digestive system are able to adapt, to an extent, to handle different types of diets. The relative amounts of the different pancreatic enzymes can change over several days in response to a marked change in the relative quantities of carbohydrate, fat and protein in the diet. The amount of bile salts produced by the liver can also be increased as fat in the diet is increased. The amount of the various liver enzymes required for metabolising food molecules delivered through the portal blood to the liver can also change in response to the amount and type of food molecules being digested. It makes little difference to the digestive system whether fruit salad or chops and eggs are eaten at breakfast. The body can exist equally well on six meals a day or on a single meal. If the diet changes markedly in macronutrient composition, there may be temporary intestinal discomfort. This could occur if there is a

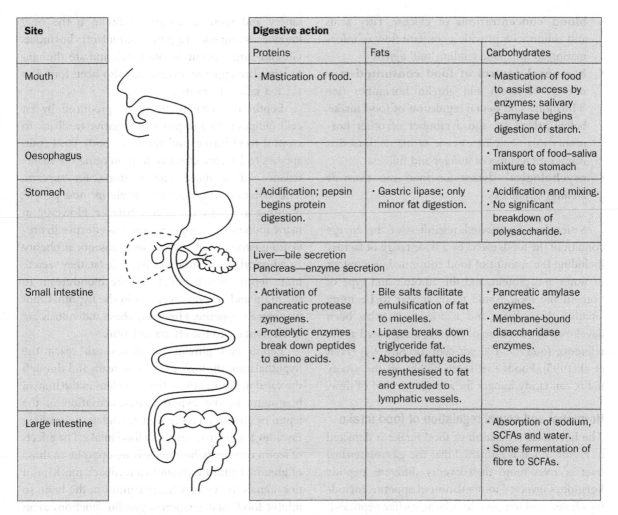

Site	Digestive action		
	Proteins	Fats	Carbohydrates
Mouth	• Mastication of food.		• Mastication of food to assist access by enzymes; salivary β-amylase begins digestion of starch.
Oesophagus			• Transport of food–saliva mixture to stomach
Stomach	• Acidification; pepsin begins protein digestion.	• Gastric lipase; only minor fat digestion.	• Acidification and mixing. • No significant breakdown of polysaccharide.
	Liver—bile secretion Pancreas—enzyme secretion		
Small intestine	• Activation of pancreatic protease zymogens. • Proteolytic enzymes break down peptides to amino acids.	• Bile salts facilitate emulsification of fat to micelles. • Lipase breaks down triglyceride fat. • Absorbed fatty acids resynthesised to fat and extruded to lymphatic vessels.	• Pancreatic amylase enzymes. • Membrane-bound disaccharidase enzymes.
Large intestine			• Absorption of sodium, SCFAs and water. • Some fermentation of fibre to SCFAs.

Figure 9.3: Summary of digestion processes for proteins, fats and carbohydrates

change from, say, a low-fat to high-fat diet, or a low-carbohydrate diet to one containing a high content of unrefined carbohydrate, but it will resolve as the body's enzyme systems and gut microbiota adjust to the new diet. In this sense the digestive system is a true system, with built-in feedback and adaptive strategies.

SATIETY AND APPETITE

Satiety is a feeling of not wanting to eat more; the appetite is satisfied and there are generally feelings of fullness. Appetite is a pleasant sensation in anticipation of eating. In a subjective sense, food intake is regulated by appetite and satiety. The initial sensation of satiety is pleasant and comfortable, but if food continues to be eaten it becomes less and less pleasant, evolving eventually to bloatedness and nausea.

Satiety, or the feeling of fullness, and its absence help control the amount of food people eat. If we feel 'full' all the time we may not eat as much as we need. If we never feel full then we may eat more than we need. The feeling of fullness or satiety is both physiological and psychological (Plata-Salamán 1991; Read 2007) and includes:

• **gastric distension**—stretch receptors operate along the vagus nerve, activating the hunger centre

- **blood concentrations** of glucose, fatty acids and amino acids provide a constant flow of information to the brain, sending 'full' signals
- **hormonal control of food consumption**—releases of leptin and ghrelin hormones (see 'Hormonal and neural regulation of food intake' below); there are also a number of other hormones in a complex cascade of interactions that impact on feelings of hunger and fullness
- **psychological desire** for food can override feelings of fullness.

Satiety can be affected, regardless of the energy content of the foods eaten, by a wide range of factors, including the amount of food consumed, its content of water and protein, and the amount and type of fibre in the food. Some foods appear to be more satiating than others, and a satiety index has been developed as a measure of fullness, using bread as the reference food (i.e. 100 per cent) (Figure 9.4) (Holt et al. 1995). Foods that score highly on the satiety index can satisfy hunger for a longer period of time.

Hormonal and neural regulation of food intake

The hormonal regulation of food intake is depicted in Figure 9.5. It is estimated that the gastrointestinal tract secretes more than twenty different peptide hormones involved in regulation of appetite, including cholecystokinin, ghrelin, glucagon-like peptide-1, peptide YY and amylin. For most of these peptides, the presence of protein, fat and/or carbohydrate in the gut stimulates their release, resulting in increased

satiety and reduced appetite. Ghrelin is the only known orexigenic (appetite stimulant) hormone. Ghrelin surges occur before meals and are thought to stimulate appetite. Insulin has also been found to act as a satiety hormone.

Leptin is a protein hormone produced by fat cells (adipocytes) and provides negative feedback to control food intake, and therefore body fat. Leptin appears to be very effective in promoting the maintenance of adequate energy stores for survival. This system can operate effectively in most people, resulting in long-term energy balance. However, in many individuals it appears to be less effective in preventing excess energy stores and consequent obesity. As adipocytes gain more triglyceride fat, they secrete more leptin, which travels via the bloodstream to the brain and acts on receptors in the hypothalamus to suppress appetite. However, obese individuals are often resistant to the effects of leptin.

Leptin and ghrelin hormones can reach the hypothalamus through the bloodstream and through the vagal nerve and the solitary nucleus in the human brainstem. In the hypothalamus, activation of the leptin or ghrelin receptor initiates different signalling cascades, leading to changes in food intake. The effects of leptin on energy homeostasis are opposite to those of ghrelin; leptin functions as a feedback mechanism that signals to key regulatory centres in the brain to inhibit food intake, whereas ghrelin functions as an appetite-stimulatory signal. It has been hypothesised that the satiety-inducing effects of leptin include the suppression of ghrelin secretion.

FEELING 'FULL'

Maintain a satiety diary for a week. Note down when you feel hungry and when you feel 'full'. When did you experience these feelings and how did you know? Note down anything that may explain these feelings. For example:
'Saturday evening meal: felt full after one slice of pizza: this was after consuming three glasses of soft drink, stomach felt full of gas, not able to eat much.'
Using your own diary, think about translating this to other people. In what circumstances may people overeat? In what circumstances might they eat less?

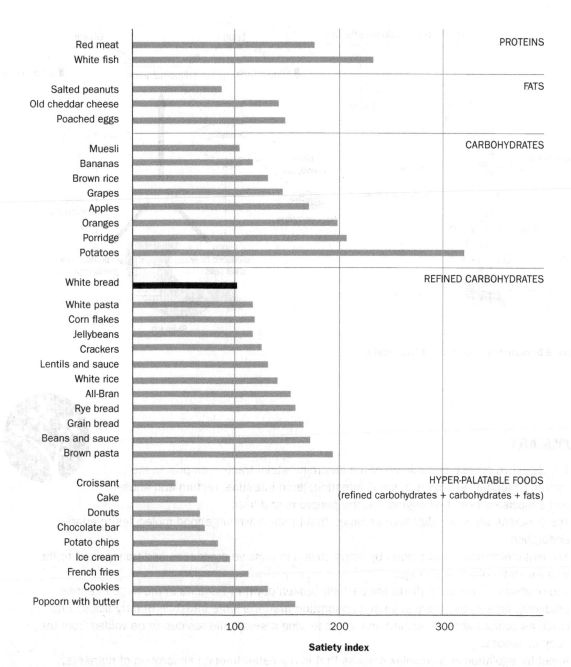

Figure 9.4: Satiety (fullness) index of different foods* based on the average degree of fullness experienced over two hours

Note: * White bread as a reference food (satiety index = 100%)

Source: Holt et al. (1995). Reprinted by permission from Springer

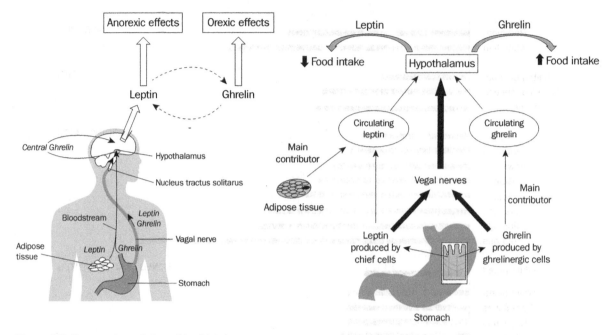

Figure 9.5: Hormonal regulation of food intake

SUMMARY

- The digestive system is made up of the gastrointestinal tract—comprising the mouth, oesophagus, stomach, small intestine, large intestine, rectum and anus—and associated digestive organs, i.e. the pancreas and liver.
- The pancreas produces digestive enzymes that break down large food molecules to enable absorption.
- Nutrient molecules are absorbed by both active and passive processes and transported to the liver for metabolism or storage.
- The unabsorbed residues (fibre) are partially broken down by bacteria in the large intestine, producing fatty acids. There is limited absorption from the large intestine of fatty acids, ions (such as sodium and potassium) and water, leaving a semi-solid residue to be voided from the body as faeces.
- Appetite regulation is a complex process that is regulated through absorption of nutrients, metabolic processes, gastrointestinal mechanisms that convey signals to the central nervous system, neuronal mechanisms and psychological factors.

KEY TERMS

Enzymes: biological catalysts, made up of protein and often including a metal atom such as iron or zinc. Enzymes enable the metabolic reaction to occur at body temperature. They react with specific substrates to produce specific products.

Lumen: the inner open space or cavity in a tubular organ, such as the intestine or an artery.

Peristalsis: the rhythmic contraction of muscles that begins in the oesophagus and continues along the wall of the stomach and the rest of the gastrointestinal tract. As food enters the oesophagus, muscles behind the food contract, pushing it forward, while the muscles in front of the food relax, keeping the food moving in one direction.

Satiety: the feeling of not wanting to eat more, generally accompanied by feelings of fullness.

Short-chain fatty acids (SCFAs): fatty acids with two to six carbon atoms. Acetic, propionic and butyric acids contain two, three and four carbon atoms respectively (see Chapter 11).

ACKNOWLEDGEMENT

This chapter has been modified and updated from the 'Digestion of food' chapter written by Jonathan M. Hodgson which appeared in the third edition of *Food and Nutrition*.

REFERENCES

Conlon, M.A. & Bird, A.R., 2015, 'The impact of diet and lifestyle on gut microbiota and human health', *Nutrients*, 7(1): 17–44, doi:10.3390/nu7010017

Holt, S.H.A., Brand Miller, J.C., Petocz, P. & Farmakalidis, E., 1995, 'A satiety index of common foods', *European Journal of Clinical Nutrition*, 49: 675–90, <www.ncbi.nlm.nih.gov/pubmed/7498104>, accessed 1 June 2019

Plata-Salamán, C.R., 1991, 'Regulation of hunger and satiety in man', *Digestive Diseases* 9(5): 253–68, doi:10.1159/000171310

Read, N.W., 2007, 'Role of gastrointestinal factors in hunger and satiety in man', *Proceedings of the Nutrition Society*, 51(1): 7–11, doi:10.1079/PNS19920004

Roager, H.M., Hansen, L.B.S., Bahl, M.I., Frandsen, H.L., Carvalho, V. et al., 2016, 'Colonic transit time is related to bacterial metabolism and mucosal turnover in the gut', *Nature Microbiology*, 1(16093): 1–9, doi:10.1038/nmicrobiol.2016.93

Samadi, N., Klems, M. & Untersmayr, E., 2018, 'The role of gastrointestinal permeability in food allergy', *Annals of Allergy, Asthma & Immunology*, 121(2): 168–73, doi:10.1016/j.anai.2018.05.010

Schumann, M., Siegmund, B., Schulzke, J.D. & Fromm, M., 2017, 'Celiac disease: Role of the epithelial barrier', *Cellular and Molecular Gastroenterology and Hepatology*, 3(2): 150–62, doi:10.1016/j.jcmgh.2016.12.006

Tomlin, J., Lewis, C. & Read, N.W., 1991, 'Investigation of normal flatus production in healthy volunteers', *Gut*, 32(6): 665–9, doi:10.1136/gut.32.6.665

Van Spaendonk, H., Ceuleers, H., Witters, L., Patteet, E., Joossens, J. et al., 2017, 'Regulation of intestinal permeability: The role of proteases', *World Journal of Gastroenterology*, 23(12): 2106–23, doi:10.3748/wjg.v23.i12.2106

Winham, D.M. & Hutchins, A.M., 2011, 'Perceptions of flatulence from bean consumption among adults in 3 feeding studies', *Nutrition Journal*, 10(1): 128, doi:10.1186/1475-2891-10-128

{CHAPTER 10}
MACRONUTRIENTS: PROTEINS

Mark L. Wahlqvist and Naiyana Wattanapenpaiboon

OBJECTIVES

- Explain the classification systems for proteins and their distribution in food.
- Describe the body's requirement for protein and the protein content of various foods.
- Explain the role of protein in the body.
- Describe how the quality of protein can be assessed.

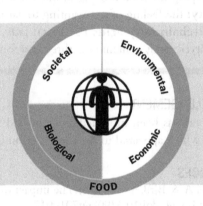

STRUCTURE OF PROTEINS IN THE BODY

Proteins are made up of chains of amino acids. There are twenty common amino acids that make up most proteins. Figure 10.1 shows the general chemical structure of amino acids, using leucine as the example. The amino acids have a basic amino ($-NH_2$) group and an acidic carboxyl ($-COOH$) group in common, and differing side chains. The chemical structures lysine, methionine, tryptophan and cysteine are also shown. The amino acids are linked by peptide bonds to form polypeptide chains. These chains are wound together like a loose ball of thread to form the three-dimensional structure of protein. The final shape of the protein is dependent on the order of amino acids in the protein. The structure is stabilised by hydrogen and/or disulphide bonds between adjacent units.

There are three groups of amino acids. The first comprises those that are indispensable or essential. These must be supplied in the diet, either because they cannot be synthesised in the body or because they cannot be synthesised at a sufficient rate to meet the body's requirements. The second group includes those that can be made within the body; these are termed dispensable or non–essential. The third group is referred to as conditionally essential amino acids. These are usually not essential, but they cannot be produced in sufficient quantities in time of increased requirements (such as those associated with injury, illness or stress). Table 10.1 lists these three groups of amino acids.

The dispensable amino acids can be synthesised by the attachment of an amino group ($-NH_2$) to a metabolic intermediate in one of the metabolic pathways. Figure 10.2 shows the pathways through which synthesis of dispensable amino acids can occur. In a normal diet there may be sufficient amounts of all the dispensable amino acids, and there may be no net synthesis of these amino acids. A diet must contain sufficient metabolisable nitrogen to allow synthesis of the many nitrogen-containing compounds in the body. This nitrogen requirement may be met by transfer of nitrogen from dispensable

(a) Amino acids (example: leucine)

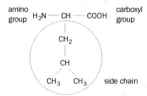

(b) Four important amino acids

methionine

lysine

cysteine

tryptophan

(c) Peptide chain: amino acids joined in specific order

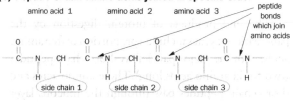

Figure 10.1: Chemical structures for amino acids and a peptide chain

Table 10.1: List of amino acids according to their essentiality in humans

Indispensable (essential)	Dispensable (non-essential)	Conditionally essential
Histidine	Alanine	Arginine
Isoleucine	Asparagine	Cysteine (synthesised from methionine)
Leucine	Aspartic acid	
Lysine	Glutamic acid	Glutamine
Methionine		Glycine
Phenylalanine		Proline
Threonine		Serine
Tryptophan		Tyrosine (synthesised
Valine		from phenylalanine)

amino acids, or nitrogen from the breakdown of excess indispensable amino acids, or from other nitrogen-containing compounds.

The sulphur amino acids, methionine and cysteine, are commonly grouped together because cysteine can be formed from methionine. Methionine and cysteine are both present in the diet. The consumption of dietary cysteine will reduce the total requirement for methionine by up to 30 per cent. Similarly, the aromatic amino acids, phenylalanine and tyrosine, are grouped together because tyrosine can be formed from phenylalanine, and tyrosine can reduce up to 50 per cent of the requirement for phenylalanine. Histidine is clearly required by infants and children, but the requirement for adults is less certain. It is regarded as indispensable, although the requirement for it is probably small.

Mixed diets should provide adequate amounts of indispensable amino acids; however, for those following vegetarian diets protein sources require more thought (see the section below).

DIGESTION OF PROTEIN

Protein digestion begins in the stomach, where pepsin secreted by the chief cells and hydrochloric acid secreted by parietal cells begin protein breakdown. Proteolytic activity in the stomach is not critical to adequate protein digestion, since more powerful proteolytic enzymes produced by the pancreas are capable of achieving complete digestion of most dietary proteins in the gut. These proteolytic enzymes include trypsin, chymotrypsin, elastase, aminopeptidase and carboxypeptidase (Table 10.2). These enzymes are potentially hazardous as, when activated, they are quite capable of digesting the pancreas itself. To avoid this problem, the enzymes are secreted as inactive precursors (zymogens), given the names trypsinogen, chymotrypsinogen, proelastase, proaminopeptidase and procarboxypeptidase.

The zymogens can safely be synthesised and secreted by the cells of the pancreas, and are not activated until they reach the lumen of the gut. The activation mechanism involves the action of enterocrinin, a proteolytic enzyme produced by specialised

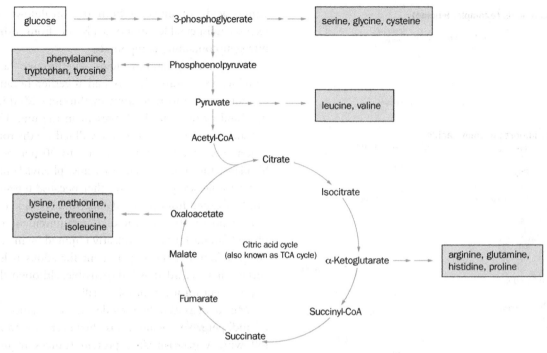

Note: Cysteine can be produced from methionine, and tyrosine from phenylalanine

Figure 10.2: General route of synthesis of some dispensable and some conditionally essential amino acids

Table 10.2: Pancreatic enzymes

Enzyme type	Substrate → Product(s)	
Carbohydrase		
Amylase	Starch	→ Maltose
Proteases		
Trypsin	Protein	→ Peptides
Chymotrypsin	Protein	→ Peptides
Elastase	Elastin	→ Peptides
Carboxypeptidase	Peptides	→ Amino acids
Aminopeptidase	Peptides	→ Amino acids
Lipase		
Lipase	Triglyceride	→ Fatty acid + 2 monoglycerides

cells in the epithelium of the gut. Enteropeptidase enzyme removes a section of peptide chain from the trypsinogen molecule, exposing the active site and activating its proteolytic activity. Thereafter, trypsin is able to activate other trypsinogen molecules and the other proteolytic enzymes through its own proteolytic activity.

The end products of protein digestion by the pancreatic enzymes include a proportion of free amino acids, with the major part left as short-chain peptides (two to six amino acids long). These amino acids and short-chain peptides pass through the mucous layer overlying the villi and come into contact with the brush border membrane, in which are embedded transport proteins for the uptake of amino acids into the epithelial cells. The brush border membrane also holds peptidase enzymes on its external membrane, in a manner similar to the disaccharidase enzymes (see Chapter 12). A proportion of the short-chain peptides are converted to single amino acids through **hydrolysis**. Active transport proteins for the amino acids are in close proximity to the peptidase enzymes.

While most dietary protein is digested and absorbed in the small intestine, the excess proteins—together with peptides that escape absorption—enter the large intestine and are fermented by the abundant microbes that colonise the gastrointestinal tract. Fermentation of protein can generate many nitrogenous compounds, such as ammonia, amines and ammonium salts. These products can form toxic substrates that are detrimental to health (see also Chapter 30).

Uptake of whole proteins

The activities of the pancreatic proteolytic enzymes result in most protein being digested. Nevertheless, a small proportion of protein does escape digestion and very small amounts of whole proteins can be absorbed into the body. There are two main types of absorption of whole proteins. First, in newborn infants there is a period of several days after birth during which whole proteins tend to be absorbed, probably by **pinocytosis**. This process enables delivery of whole antibodies from maternal milk into the bloodstream of the infant. It is thought that the delivery of proteins other than from maternal milk to the neonate during this period may predispose the infant to allergic reactions, such as milk–protein allergy, but the evidence is not yet complete.

The second type of whole protein uptake occurs in all individuals and involves the uptake of minute amounts of intact proteins. As a result of the presence of these proteins, predisposed individuals may develop allergic reactions to foods such as cow's milk, fish, peanuts, strawberries and so on.

FUNCTION OF PROTEINS IN THE BODY

Proteins make up a large part of the machinery of the living body and have a number of functions (Table 10.3). The shape of proteins is critical to their particular biological functions (i.e. as enzymes, transport proteins or antibodies). These functions depend on the presence of a binding site on the surface of the particular protein. These proteins bind or react with just one or a very few molecules because of the near-perfect fit of the substrate molecule into the binding site.

The fact that the shape of the protein, including its substrate-specific binding site, is dependent on a specific amino acid sequence explains why the supply of all of the indispensable amino acids in the diet is critical to survival. This also explains why a genetic difference resulting in minor changes to the amino acid sequence of a protein can have dramatic effects on health.

Relationship of protein and energy supply

The carbon skeletons of amino acids can be metabolised and oxidised to yield energy; as a result, there is a close relationship between protein status and energy supply. A continued supply of energy is critical to survival. If an individual is starved, body protein as well as dietary protein will be used as an energy source. The amino acids, instead of being reincorporated into new protein, are **deaminated** (amino ($-NH_2$) group removed) and diverted into glucose production, a process called gluconeogenesis. Body protein is effectively the major store of glucose in the body and, in illness or starvation, body protein tends to be used up, resulting in the wasting of muscles and other tissues.

Table 10.3: Summarised major functions of proteins in the body

Protein	Function(s)
Part of cell membranes	To enable selective transport into and out of cells.
Enzymes	To enable chemical reactions and direct metabolic pathways.
Special proteins in blood	• *Haemoglobin*: to carry oxygen from the lungs to other tissues. • *Albumin*: to contribute to osmotic pressure, controlling water balance to the cells. • *Metal-binding proteins, such as transferrin and ceruloplasmin*: to carry iron and copper, respectively, in the blood to relevant tissues.
Contractile protein in muscle	To enable muscle contraction and movement.
Antibodies	To bind and assist removal of foreign proteins, viruses and bacteria.
Nucleoproteins	To stabilise the structure of nucleic acids (DNA and RNA).

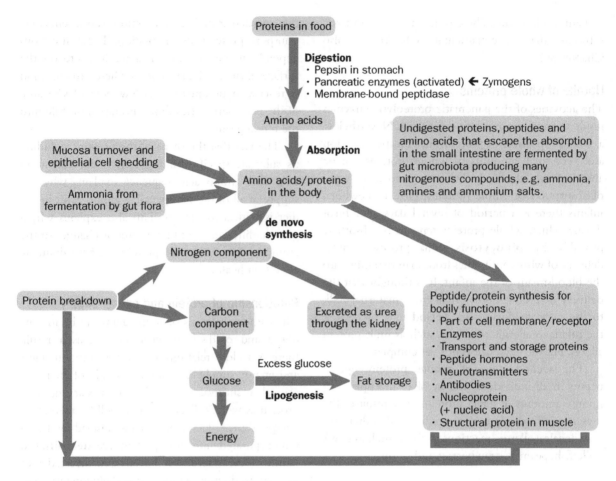

Figure 10.3: Fate of proteins in food after ingestion

The term 'protein–energy malnutrition' (PEM) is used to describe the condition in which there is a deficiency of energy and/or protein in the diet. Children affected by marasmus, a chronic shortage of both protein and energy, lose much of their lean tissues and appear to be little more than skin and bone. Dietary protein will not counteract this process unless dietary energy is first increased to a level that meets energy needs. Fat, whether body fat or dietary fat, will also not stop protein wastage because some tissues—such as the brain and red blood cells—have an obligatory requirement for glucose and while the major part of protein (amino acids) can be metabolised to produce glucose, **triglyceride** fats can provide only a very small amount of glucose derived from the glycerol component. As a consequence, a person

who has adequate fat stores may suffer a significant loss of muscle and other protein tissue if starved over more than a few days. 'Kwashiorkor' is a condition observed in children who have received sufficient food energy but insufficient protein. In this situation, the loss of protein tissue can be masked by body fat and also by oedema—fluid retention (usually a distended abdomen)—as a result of insufficient plasma protein.

PROTEIN SYNTHESIS AND TURNOVER

Proteins in the body are not retained for life; they are continually being broken down and replaced. Protein turnover is the balance between protein synthesis and protein degradation, and it is a continuous process.

Breakdown and resynthesis allow the body to regulate the amount of an enzyme or other proteins. Some proteins, such as certain enzymes, are turned over quickly and may have half-lives as short as a few hours. The proteins with the slowest turnover rate are those of the connective tissues that hold the body together. Connective proteins include elastin and collagen in tissues such as tendons, the muscle sheath and the non-mineral part of bone. These proteins are turned over slowly, with half-lives of about a year.

The breakdown process is accomplished by intracellular enzymes that hydrolyse peptide bonds, releasing free amino acids. These amino acids are added to the pool of amino acids, both in tissues and those being transported in the blood. They are available for resynthesis into new protein. Total protein turnover amounts to 250–350 g/day, and is substantially more than the normal daily protein intake, which is usually in the range 80–110 g/day. Daily protein intake is therefore 'topping up' the amino acid pool within the body.

Regulation of protein synthesis and breakdown

The processes of protein breakdown and synthesis are separately regulated by hormonal and neural mechanisms. In the post-absorptive state, which is when no meal has recently been eaten, the rate of body protein breakdown exceeds synthesis and there is a net fall in body protein. Following the next meal, absorption of amino acids leads to a rise in amino acid concentration in the blood and tissue fluid and, through the action of insulin and other hormones, protein synthesis is stimulated, amino acids are taken up and there is a net rise in body protein. There is a small diurnal (happening during the day) fluctuation in total body protein and a small fluctuation according to meal pattern.

During growth in children, the rate of synthesis outstrips breakdown—in fact, both synthesis and breakdown (turnover) of protein are faster in children. In infants, about 30 per cent of protein synthesis goes into growth, whereas in toddlers the growth component falls to about 10 per cent of total synthesis. Since there is usually no net gain of protein tissue in the adult, except if pregnant or

recovering from illness or injury, all new protein is part of general protein turnover.

Amino acid supply for protein synthesis

Proteins are synthesised in the cytoplasm of cells in all tissues. The sequence of amino acids is coded in DNA and is translated into messenger RNA, which leaves the cell nucleus and joins with ribosomes that then bind transfer RNA units carrying the amino acids specified by the messenger code. Each amino acid is bound by a peptide bond to the growing polypeptide chain on the ribosome. The completed polypeptide chain is released and spontaneously winds up on itself to assume its three-dimensional structure. Synthesis of the peptide chain can only progress on the ribosome if all twenty amino acids are available. The dispensable amino acids can be synthesised if required but the indispensable amino acids can only come into the body as part of dietary protein. A total lack of any one of the indispensable amino acids in the diet does not actually stop protein synthesis altogether, because protein turnover also provides a source of indispensable amino acids. However, it does lead to a slowdown in protein synthesis and a loss of body protein, particularly that of muscle. The body can survive a severe reduction in many, if not most, of the protein tissues in the body.

While amino acids are efficiently recycled within the body, there is also a demand for indispensable amino acids for other metabolic purposes. For example, methionine is needed for methylation reactions (e.g. in converting folic acid to a useable form), tyrosine for the synthesis of thyroid hormones, histidine for the formation of histamine, tryptophan for tryptamine, and so on. Even when dietary protein intake is low, there is continued excretion of breakdown products of the indispensable amino acids. It is the replacement of this obligatory consumption of the indispensable amino acids that is the basis of the requirement for a dietary source of indispensable amino acids.

Under normal circumstances, dietary supply of protein (amino acids) is in excess of requirements and the excess amino acids must be broken down and excreted. This occurs through deamination.

Waste nitrogen is converted into urea in the liver and excreted through the kidneys into the urine. A proportion of the nitrogen is excreted as the ammonium ion in urine as part of a mechanism to adjust acid–base balance.

Nitrogen is also lost in faeces; this is mostly in the form of protein in the gut bacteria. Epithelial cells shed into the gut (as well as the various secretions) contain nitrogen, and that which is not digested and reabsorbed will be taken up by gut microbiota. A considerable amount of the urea (about 20 per cent) circulating in the blood diffuses into the bowel and is split by bacterial urease into ammonia, most of which is reabsorbed. A proportion of the ammonia is taken up and incorporated into bacterial protein. It has been suggested that indispensable amino acids synthesised by gut bacteria and released into the gut lumen may be absorbed and incorporated into body protein (Diether & Willing 2019). A small amount of nitrogen is also lost from the body in sweat, and as hair and shed skin cells.

HUMAN PROTEIN REQUIREMENT AND NITROGEN BALANCE

According to a report by the World Health Organization, UN Food and Agriculture Organization and the United Nations University (UNU), estimates of the nutritional requirements for protein are defined as the lowest level of dietary protein intake that will balance the losses of nitrogen from the body, and thus maintain the body protein mass (assumed to be at a desirable level) in persons at energy balance with modest levels of physical activity and any special needs for growth, reproduction and lactation (WHO/FAO/UNU Expert Consultation 2007). However, it is not easy to measure total body protein, and therefore not easy to determine whether the body is gaining or losing protein.

Since most of the nitrogen in the body is in protein, it is possible to gain an indirect measure of body protein changes by a study of nitrogen balance (N-balance)—that is, by measuring the rates of nitrogen uptake and excretion to determine the net gain or loss of protein. Protein in food is most easily measured in terms of its nitrogen content. Protein and amino acids contain, on average, about 16 per cent nitrogen. It is a fairly simple chemical procedure to measure the amount of nitrogen in food, and multiplying this value by 6.25 gives a reasonable approximation of dietary protein. Nitrogen output from the body can be determined by collecting urine and faeces and chemically analysing these for nitrogen. If more nitrogen is entering the body in the form of protein than is leaving in the form of waste nitrogen in urine and faeces, the body is said to be in positive N-balance. A growing child is in positive N-balance. A negative N-balance would occur in an illness in which a person loses weight and loses muscle protein as part of that weight loss.

In practice, N-balance studies are complex and expensive. Volunteer subjects must live in a special unit called a metabolic ward for at least two weeks. During this time, they are fed a special diet that provides sufficient energy to maintain body weight and in which the test protein makes up virtually all of the protein in the diet. At the same time, all of the urine and faeces of each person must be collected and analysed so that nitrogen balance can be determined. For accurate studies, even hair combings and shower water must be collected and analysed, because small amounts of nitrogen are lost in sweat and in shed hair and skin cells.

The balance of protein quantity and quality

Human protein requirements and the nutritional quality of proteins are closely related. Protein requirement is, in fact, a requirement for indispensable amino acids. The nutritional quality of a dietary protein depends on how closely the ratio of indispensable amino acids in the food protein matches human requirements. If a food protein is rich in indispensable amino acids, and the relative amounts of the different amino acids closely match human requirements, the protein will have a high nutritional quality. The indispensable amino acid patterns of whole egg or milk proteins are often used as models against which other proteins are compared. The minimum daily requirement for protein is usually expressed as the daily requirement for a high-quality protein such as egg, milk or meat. For proteins of lower nutritional quality, more will be required in order to meet the daily requirement for indispensable amino acids.

Measuring protein requirement

Accurate measurement of protein requirement is quite difficult. As stated above, protein requirement is defined as the minimum amount of high-quality protein that must be consumed to maintain nitrogen balance. In N-balance studies, the initial diet fed has only a low level of protein and all subjects will be in negative N-balance—that is, the daily intake of protein nitrogen is insufficient to maintain body protein and there is a daily net loss of nitrogen. At intervals of several days, the protein in the diet is increased in steps and a nitrogen balance determined for each stepped increase. With each increase in dietary protein, the N-balance becomes less negative until a balance point is reached at which the intake of nitrogen in dietary protein is just sufficient to balance the daily loss. The protein intake at this point gives a measure of the minimum daily requirement for protein in terms of that particular protein. If the

experiment was repeated with a protein of lower nutritional quality, more of the protein would be required.

Adaptation to low protein intake is possible. For example, Millward et al. (2000) have shown that adaptation to low intakes of lysine does occur, and that this is probably important in populations of low-income countries heavily dependent on cereal proteins. Very low protein intakes bring about a reduction in body weight and cell mass. The rates of protein synthesis and breakdown both decline. Indispensable amino acids are more efficiently recycled and N-balance can be re-established after some time at a lower protein intake.

It is thought that the definition of protein requirement as the minimum intake of high-quality protein required to just maintain N-balance may not be the ideal. The requirement might be better defined instead as the level of protein or indispensable amino acid intake that will maintain optimum health. The optimum requirement would ideally be determined by functional criteria such as maintenance of good health, optimum growth and resistance to disease. In practice, however, this is extremely difficult, because these criteria cannot be addressed independently of other factors in foods and diet.

Table 10.4 summarises the requirements of indispensable amino acids as estimated by the WHO/FAO/UNU (WHO/FAO/UNU Expert Consultation 2007). The pattern of indispensable amino acid requirements is important because it is the basis for estimating protein quality.

RECOMMENDED INTAKES FOR PROTEIN AND OPTIMAL PROTEIN INTAKES

The Estimated Average Requirement (EAR) and Recommended Dietary Intake (RDI) values for protein intake in Australia and New Zealand were published in 2006 (NHMRC 2006) (see Chapter 19 for definitions). There may be a difference between an intake that meets requirements and one that is optimal for health. In practice, establishing an optimum protein intake is more difficult than

---

PROTEIN AND AMINO ACID REQUIREMENTS AND THEIR INTAKE RECOMMENDATIONS

Read sections 4, 7, 8 and 9 of the report of a Joint WHO/FAO/UNU Expert Consultation on Protein and Amino Acid Requirements in Human Nutrition (WHO/FAO/UNU Expert Consultation 2007).

Based on this report summarise how:
- protein and amino acid requirements in humans are assessed
- the current intake recommendations are derived.

Table 10.4: Estimates of indispensable amino acid requirements for infants, children, adolescents and adults

Amino acid	0.5 y	1–2 y	3–10 y	11–14 y	15–18 y	Adults (> 18 y)
Amino acid requirements (mg/kg per day)*						
Histidine	22	15	12	12	11	10
Isoleucine	36	27	23	22	21	20
Leucine	73	54	44	44	42	39
Lysine	64	45	35	35	33	30
Methionine + cysteine	31	22	18	17	16	15
Phenylalanine + tyrosine	59	40	30	30	28	25
Threonine	34	23	18	18	17	15
Tryptophan	9.5	6.4	4.8	4.8	4.5	4.0
Valine	49	36	29	29	28	26
Amino acid requirements (mg/g protein requirements)†						
Histidine	20	18	16	16	16	15
Isoleucine	32	31	31	30	30	30
Leucine	66	63	61	60	60	59
Lysine	57	52	48	48	47	45
Methionine + cysteine	28	26	24	23	23	22
Phenylalanine + tyrosine	52	46	41	41	40	30
Threonine	31	27	25	25	24	23
Tryptophan	8.5	7.4	6.6	6.5	6.3	6
Valine	43	42	40	40	40	39

Notes: * Amino acid requirements are calculated as the sum of amino acids needed for maintenance and growth
† Average nitrogen requirement of 105 mg nitrogen/kg per day (0.66 g protein/kg per day)

Source: WHO/FAO/UNU Expert Consultation (2007)

establishing an average requirement and an RDI. In healthy individuals, the optimum protein intake is likely to differ according to life stage and gender group. Furthermore, establishing optimum intakes cannot be done in isolation from other aspects of diet and personal behaviours or circumstances; for example, protein requirements may be elevated in individuals experiencing inflammation as a result of disease processes or healing after injury (see Part 7).

In most high-income countries, including Australia and New Zealand, the average adult consumes protein (at about 18–19 per cent of total energy) well in excess of the RDI, so protein deficiency is rare. Despite this, it has been suggested that higher-protein diets have a number of benefits, including

DETERMINING PROTEIN REQUIREMENTS

Locate the EAR and RDI for protein on the Nutrient Reference Value website (www.nrv.gov.au/). Determine the protein requirements of the following:
- a 10-year-old girl weighing 33 kg
- a 16-year-old boy weighing 60 kg
- a 30-year-old woman weighing 63 kg
- a 50-year-old man weighing 78 kg
- an 85-year-old woman weighing 59 kg.

reducing risk factors for heart disease. For example, there is evidence that a higher protein intake can lower blood pressure (Mente et al. 2017). On the other hand, there are population data showing protein intake (principally animal protein) is associated with increased risk of chronic kidney disease (Haring et al. 2017). In addition, vegetarian diets—which are generally lower in protein—are often associated with better health (Dinu et al. 2017). This may be linked to factors other than the protein itself. For example, diets high in red meat—and, more particularly, processed meats—are consistently associated with increased risk of chronic diseases, colorectal cancer in particular (Schulze et al. 2018; WCRF/AICR 2018). Thus, as long as protein intake meets requirements, good health may be compatible with a range of protein intakes. The food source of protein may have a much larger bearing on health than the total protein intake.

PROTEINS IN FOOD AND THEIR NUTRITIONAL QUALITY

Most of the foods we eat contribute some protein to the diet. It is the major component of lean meat, fish and egg white. Cereals contribute intermediate amounts of protein and fruits and vegetables much less. The amino acids of protein can be metabolised to yield 17 kJ of energy per gram of protein, and it is useful to list protein as a percentage of energy in the food.

The nutritional quality of dietary proteins depends on two factors: how well their content of indispensable amino acids matches the requirements of the human body, and the digestibility of the protein. A food protein with a high nutritional quality thus contains indispensable amino acids that closely match human requirements and also has high digestibility. The proteins of animal products have a high nutritional quality, whereas those of plant foods tend to be lower. The relative overall nutritional quality of protein depends on the food or meal from which it comes (e.g. plant- or animal-based) and how that affects amino acid and peptide bioavailability, digestibility, gut microbiomics and ultimate metabolism (see also Chapter 30).

A similar effect occurs when a relatively small amount of high-quality animal protein is added to a lower protein quality plant food. Milk added to a corn-based breakfast cereal, for example, adds lysine to the lysine-deficient corn protein, thereby increasing the overall protein quality. The complementary nature of protein mixtures is one reason for the advantages of a well-mixed diet.

Assessment of protein quality

As the world's population increases rapidly, and against the constraints of limited land, water and food resources, it is important to be able to define accurately the amount and quality of protein required to meet human nutritional needs. To match dietary supply with human protein needs is vital to supporting the health and wellbeing of human populations. Protein quality is estimated using a number of techniques: these are outlined in Table 10.5.

Table 10.5: Protein quality estimation

Technique	Equation	Description
Net Protein Estimation	NPU = [protein N in food – faecal N – urinary N]/protein N in food.	Defined as proportion of dietary protein retained in the body. Determined via animal (rat) models using a test protein equivalent to 10 per cent of energy. The amount of food consumed is recorded and all urine and faeces are collected and analysed for nitrogen. The efficiency of retention of the dietary protein, NPU, can then be calculated.

Technique	Equation	Description
Chemical estimation: Amino Acid Score (AAS)	AAS = milligrams of the most limiting amino acid in the protein relative to human requirement/number of milligrams of the same amino acid in a reference protein (whole egg) or a reference amino acid mixture representing maximum nutritional quality.	For example, the amino acid in shortest supply in relation to requirement in wheat flour protein is lysine (26 mg/g protein), whereas the lysine content of whole-egg protein is 70 mg/g. Thus, the Amino Acid Score with reference to whole-egg protein is (26/70) × 100 = 37. Chemically derived measures are cheaper and quicker than biological measures. However, while the measurement of AAS is relatively simple, it must not be assumed that the quality of the test protein is strictly proportional to the numerical value obtained. This is because deficiencies of different essential amino acids do not necessarily have equivalent effects. The capacity of humans to adapt to low intakes of lysine probably results in cereal proteins having a nutritional quality that is not as low as the Amino Acid Score noted above would suggest (Millward et al. 2000).
Digestible Indispensable Amino Acid Score (DIAAS)	DIAAS % = 100 × [(mg of digestible dietary indispensable amino acid in 1 g of the dietary protein)/(mg of the same dietary indispensable amino acid in 1 g of the reference protein)].	Measures the actual capacity of the protein to satisfy the amino acid needs using corrections for amino acid digestibility (determined at the end of the small intestine) and availability. An FAO Expert Consultation on dietary protein quality evaluation in human nutrition has recommended the use of the DIAAS as a means of assessing the protein quality of individual protein food sources and dietary mixtures (FAO 2013). The FAO Expert Consultation also recommends the use of breastmilk's amino acid pattern as a reference amino acid pattern for infants (0–6 months) and provides reference amino acid scoring patterns for preschool-age children and for older children, adolescents and adults.

VEGETARIAN DIETS

Many of the world's people are vegetarian, eating little or no meat. Many are vegetarian for cultural or religious reasons or simply because meat, milk, eggs or fish are expensive or difficult to obtain. Since many, if not most, of these people are healthy, a vegetarian diet is apparently adequate. There has also been an increasing focus, even in countries without a cultural or religious history of vegetarianism, on plant-based diets from an environmental sustainability perspective.

In response to an American Heart Association statement that 'Although plant proteins form a large part of the human diet, most are deficient in one or more essential amino acids and are therefore regarded as incomplete proteins', Dr John McDougall (2002) has argued that 'Plant foods have a complete amino acid composition'.

Read the paper by McDougall:

- McDougall, J., 2002, 'Plant foods have a complete amino acid composition', *Circulation*, *105*: e197.

Identify the appropriate use of grains and legumes in vegetarian diets for a complementary amino acid profile. Apply this information to identify the best combination of complementary proteins for Alice, a 23-year-old vegan who has the following dietary pattern. What would be your advice for Alice regarding her protein intake?

BREAKFAST
- Fruit salad
- Oat milk coffee

LUNCH
- Salad sandwich

AFTERNOON TEA
- Handful of almonds and raisins

EVENING MEAL
- Rice or pasta with vegetables (usually a combination of broccoli, beans, carrots and onion)

SUMMARY

- Protein in the body in enzymes, muscle and connective tissues is constantly being broken down and renewed.
- Protein digestion occurs in the stomach and small intestine, where various proteolytic enzymes break down food proteins into polypeptides that are then further broken down by peptidase enzymes into short-chain peptides and amino acids.
- Dietary protein is digested to yield both indispensable (essential) and dispensable (non-essential) amino acids.
- Absorbed amino acids top up the body's pool of amino acids for protein synthesis—excess amino acids are broken down to yield energy (17 kJ/g) and the waste nitrogen is excreted as urea and ammonia.
- Protein deficiency leads to loss of body protein, as amino acids released during protein turnover are used in the synthesis of key metabolites and for energy.
- The nutritional quality of dietary proteins depends on their content of indispensable amino acids. The inclusion of a variety of proteins in the diet will do much to ensure adequate quality because of complementary effects.
- Human amino acid and protein requirements have been determined using nitrogen balance and feeding studies.

KEY TERMS

Deamination: the removal of an amino group from a molecule. Deamination is used to break down amino acids for energy. The amino group is removed from the amino acid and converted to ammonia. The rest of the amino acid is made up of mostly carbon and hydrogen, and is recycled or oxidised for energy.

Hydrolysis: a chemical reaction in which water molecules are used to break one or more chemical bonds of a particular substance, such as peptides or triglycerides.

Pinocytosis: the mechanism by which a cell absorbs small particles outside the cell and brings them inside. During this process, the cell surrounds particles and then 'pinches off' part of its membrane to enclose the particles within vesicles, which are small spheres of the membrane.

Triglyceride: a class of fats or lipids that are the combination of fatty acids and glycerol.

ACKNOWLEDGEMENT

This chapter has been modified and updated from the 'Protein' chapter written by Jonathan M. Hodgson which appeared in the third edition of *Food and Nutrition*.

REFERENCES

Diether, N.E. and Willing, B.P., 2019, 'Microbial fermentation of dietary protein: An important factor in diet–microbe–host interaction', *Microorganisms*, 7(1): 19, doi:10.3390/microorganisms7010019

Dinu, M., Abbate, R., Gensini, G.F., Casini, A. & Sofi, F., 2017, 'Vegetarian, vegan diets and multiple health outcomes: A systematic review with meta-analysis of observational studies', *Critical Reviews in Food Science and Nutrition*, 57(17): 3640–9, doi:10.1080/10408398.2016.1138447

FAO, 2013, *Dietary Protein Quality Evaluation in Human Nutrition*, <www.fao.org/ag/humannutrition/35978-02317b979a686a57aa4593304ffc17f06.pdf>, accessed 22 November 2018

Haring, B., Selvin, E., Liang, M., Coresh, J., Grams, M.E. et al., 2017, 'Dietary protein sources and risk for incident chronic kidney disease: Results from the Atherosclerosis Risk in Communities (ARIC) study', *Journal of Renal Nutrition*, 27(4): 233–42, doi:10.1053/j.jrn.2016.11.004

McDougall, J., 2002, 'Plant foods have a complete amino acid composition', *Circulation*, 105(25): e197–e197, doi:10.1161/01.CIR.0000018905.97677.1F

Mente, A., Dehghan, M., Rangarajan, S., McQueen, M., Dagenais, G. et al., 2017, 'Association of dietary nutrients with blood lipids and blood pressure in 18 countries: A cross-sectional analysis from the PURE study', *Lancet Diabetes & Endocrinology*, 5(10): 774–87, doi:10.1016/S2213-8587(17)30283-8

Millward, D.J., Fereday, A., Gibson, N.R. & Pacy, P.J., 2000, 'Human adult amino acid requirements: [1-13C]leucine balance evaluation of the efficiency of utilization and apparent requirements for wheat protein and lysine compared with those for milk protein in healthy adults', *American Journal of Clinical Nutrition*, 72(1): 112–21, doi:10.1093/ajcn/72.1.112

NHMRC, 2006, *Nutrition Reference Values for Australia and New Zealand*, <https://nhmrc.gov.au/sites/default/files/images/nutrient-refererence-dietary-intakes.pdf>, accessed 22 November 2018

Schulze, M.B., Martínez-González, M.A., Fung, T.T., Lichtenstein, A.H. & Forouhi, N.G., 2018, 'Food based dietary patterns and chronic disease prevention', *BMJ*, 361: k2396, doi:10.1136/bmj.k2396

WCRF/AICR, 2018, *Diet, Nutrition, Physical Activity and Cancer: A global perspective*, <www.wcrf.org/dietandcancer/resources-and-toolkit>, accessed 22 November 2018

WHO/FAO/UNU Expert Consultation, 2007, *Protein and Amino Acid Requirements in Human Nutrition*, <https://apps.who.int/iris/bitstream/handle/10665/43411>, accessed 22 November 2018

{CHAPTER 11}
MACRONUTRIENTS: FATS

Mark L. Wahlqvist and Naiyana Wattanapenpaiboon

OBJECTIVES

- Explain the classification systems for fats, their structural features and their distribution in food.
- Describe the body's requirement for fat and the fat content of various foods.
- Summarise the process of fat digestion in the gastrointestinal tract.
- Explain the role of fat in the body and the rationale underlying fat intake recommendations.

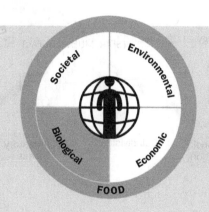

CLASSIFICATION OF FATS

Fats or lipids are a diverse group of chemical compounds, characterised by the fact that they are insoluble in water. Fats in foods occur in the greatest quantity as triglycerides (or triacylglycerols). Triglycerides are one of five classes of lipids that contain fatty acids:

1. Triglycerides are combinations of fatty acids with glycerol. Recognisable as the fats (solids) and oils (liquids) of our food supply, they serve as reserves of energy stored in adipose (fat) tissue in animals and in the seeds of some plants.
2. Glycolipids are fatty acids in combination with sugars. Occurring in small amounts, they are associated with cell surfaces in animals and with cell membranes in plants. Some sphingolipids contain sugar components.

3. Phospholipids contain fatty acids chemically linked with glycerol and phosphorus. As well as being important structural components of animal cell membranes, they also supply fatty acid precursors for the synthesis of **eicosanoids**, which are potent controllers of many physiological processes.
4. Sphingolipids are important components of brain tissues and the central nervous system of animals. They consist of fatty acids in combination with long-chain amines. They include the **ceramides**, **gangliosides** and **cerebrosides**.
5. Sterols often occur in combination with fatty acids as sterol esters. Cholesterol, the principal human sterol, has a structural role in cell membranes and is a precursor of steroid hormones, vitamin D and various fat-emulsifying agents in bile.

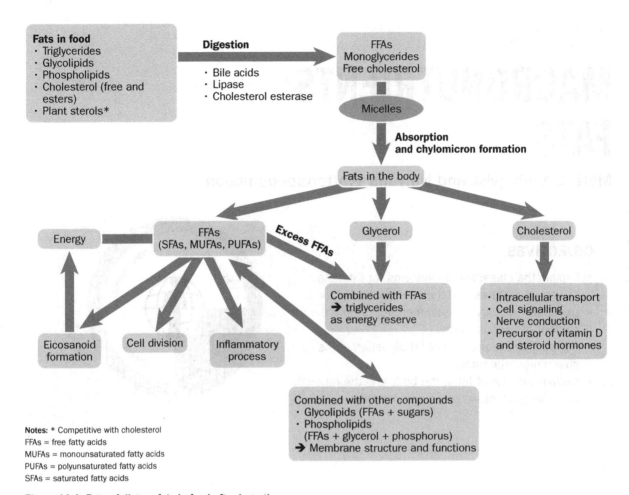

Notes: * Competitive with cholesterol
FFAs = free fatty acids
MUFAs = monounsaturated fatty acids
PUFAs = polyunsaturated fatty acids
SFAs = saturated fatty acids

Figure 11.1: Fate of dietary fats in food after ingestion

COMMON FATTY ACIDS, THEIR STRUCTURES AND NAMES

More than 40 different fatty acids occur in nature and many others are produced during processing of fats in the manufacture of margarines, shortenings, salad dressings and frying oil. Most natural fatty acids comprise linear hydrocarbon chains from two to more than 80 carbon atoms in length, with those occurring most commonly having 16, 18, 20 or 22 carbons. However, they all have a carboxyl (–COOH) group at one end and usually a methyl (–CH$_3$) group at the other (Figure 11.2).

Individual fatty acids can be named in a number of different ways. The common name is often based on the source of the original discovery; for instance,

palmitic acid, lauric acid and myristic acid were first isolated from plants of the Palmae, Lauraceae and Myristiceae families respectively. Then there is the formal chemical name, which is often long; however, there is a shorthand abbreviation which is easier to understand, as shown in Table 11.1. The length of the hydrocarbon chain is given by the number before the colon (:), and the number of double bonds by the number after the colon. The double bond is a point of unsaturation. Depending on the number

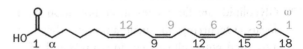

Figure 11.2: Chemical structure of a stearidonic acid (C18:4 n-3 or C18:4 ω-3)

Table 11.1: Chemical structure of some fatty acids

Common name	Chemical structure	Biochemical abbreviation	Chemical abbreviation
SATURATED FATTY ACIDS (SFAs)			
Short-chain fatty acids (up to 5 carbons)			
Propionic	CH_3CH_2COOH	C2:0	C2:0
Butyric	$CH_3(CH_2)_2COOH$	C4:0	C4:0
Medium-chain (6–12 carbons) and long-chain (13–21 carbons) fatty acids			
Capric	$CH_3(CH_2)_8COOH$	C10:0	C10:0
Myristic	$CH_3(CH_2)_{12}COOH$	C14:0	C14:0
Palmitic	$CH_3(CH_2)_{14}COOH$	C16:0	C16:0
Stearic	$CH_3(CH_2)_{16}COOH$	C18:0	C18:0
MONOUNSATURATED FATTY ACIDS (MUFAs)			
Oleic	$CH_3(CH_2)_7\textbf{CH=CH}(CH_2)_7COOH$	C18:1 n-9	C18:1$^{\Delta 9}$
Elaidic	$CH_3(CH_2)_7\textbf{CH=CH}(CH_2)_7COOH$ (*trans* isomer of oleic acid)	C18:1 n-9	C18:1$^{\Delta 9}$
Erucic	$CH_3(CH_2)_7\textbf{CH=CH}(CH_2)_{11}COOH$	C22:1 n-9	C22:1$^{\Delta 13}$
POLYUNSATURATED FATTY ACIDS (PUFAs)			
Linoleic (LA)	$CH_3(CH_2)_4\textbf{CH=CH}CH_2\textbf{CH=CH}(CH_2)_7COOH$	C18:2 n-6	C18:2$^{\Delta 9,12}$
α-linolenic (ALA)	$CH_3CH_2\textbf{CH=CH}CH_2\textbf{CH=CH}CH_2\textbf{CH=CH}(CH_2)_7COOH$	C18:3 n-3	C18:3$^{\Delta 9,12,15}$
Arachidonic (AA)	$CH_3(CH_2)_4\textbf{CH=CH}CH_2\textbf{CH=CH}CH_2\textbf{CH=CH}CH_2\textbf{CH=CH}(CH_2)_3COOH$	C20:4 n-6	C20:4$^{\Delta 5,8,11,14}$
Eicosapentaenoic acid (EPA)	$CH_3CH_2\textbf{CH=CH}CH_2\textbf{CH=CH}CH_2\textbf{CH=CH}CH_2\textbf{CH=CH}CH_2\textbf{CH=CH}(CH_2)_3COOH$	C20:5 n-3	C20:5$^{\Delta 5,8,11,14,17}$
Docosahexaenoic acid (DHA)	$CH_3CH_2\textbf{CH=CH}CH_2\textbf{CH=CH}CH_2\textbf{CH=CH}CH_2\textbf{CH=CH}CH_2\textbf{CH=CH}CH_2\textbf{CH=CH}(CH_2)_2COOH$	C22:6 n-3	C22:6$^{\Delta 4,7,10,13,16,19}$

of double bonds in its chemical structure, a fatty acid can be **saturated** (with no double bond) or **unsaturated** (with at least one double bond). Unsaturated fatty acids may have one or more points of unsaturation; hence they may be monounsaturated or polyunsaturated.

Chemists describe the position of the double bonds in the hydrocarbon chain by counting from the acid end of the molecule, as indicated by the use of a delta, Δ. The 'Δ' is the Greek letter 'delta', which translates into 'D' (for double bond) in the Roman alphabet. Biochemists describe the position of the double bonds in the hydrocarbon chain by counting from the methyl end as indicated by the letter n, the symbol ω or the word 'omega', and only the position of the first double bond is given. Omega (ω) is the last letter in the Greek alphabet, and is therefore used to indicate the 'last' carbon atom in the fatty acid

chain. For example, the abbreviation of stearidonic acid, C18:4 n–3 or C18:4 ω–3, indicates an 18–carbon chain with four double bonds, and with the first double bond in the third position from the methyl (-CH$_3$) end. The second double bond is in the sixth position counting from the methyl end, but this is not indicated. In general, the position of second and subsequent double bonds is not described because their positions can be assumed from the fact that they are usually spaced three carbons apart, a consequence of the biosynthetic mechanisms that operate in plant tissues. The important biological properties of unsaturated fatty acids are more easily described using biochemical nomenclature; therefore, this system is employed here.

Naturally occurring unsaturated acids fall into three major groups or families, the n-3 (ω-3, or omega-3), n-6 (ω-6, omega-6) and n-9 (ω-9, omega-9) acids. Animals, including humans, are unable to synthesise α-linolenic (ALA, C18:3 n-3) and linoleic acid (LA, C18:2 n-6), which are the parent n-3 and n-6 polyunsaturated fatty acids and are widely distributed in plant oils. They can be chain elongated and desaturated to produce longer chain n-3 and n-6 fatty acids (Figure 11.3). However, the conversion of ALA to longer-chain n-3 fatty acids,

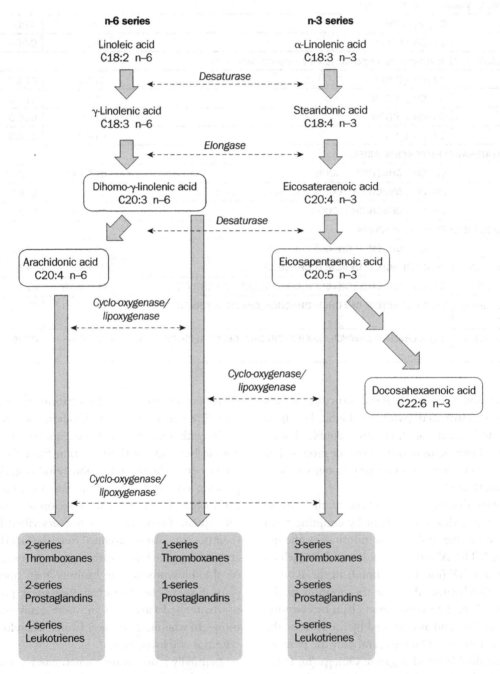

Figure 11.3: Essential fatty acid production and metabolism to form eicosanoids—at each step, the n-3 and n-6 cascades compete for the enzymes

such as eicosapentaenoic acid (EPA, C20:5 n–3) and docosahexaenoic acid (DHA, C22:6 n–3), is limited in humans. ALA, LA, EPA and DHA are required for vital functions in the body and so are referred to as '**essential fatty acids**'; as such, they need to be derived from the foods in the diet. Saturated fatty acids (SFAs) and monounsaturated fatty acids (MUFAs) can be manufactured by all mammalian cells using dietary carbohydrate, protein or fat as the starting material.

THE BIOLOGICAL ROLES OF FATTY ACIDS

Fatty acids are involved in a number of diverse and important biological processes, summarised in Figure 11.4. Unsaturated fatty acids play an important role in maintaining membrane fluidity and structure. In a number of membrane-mediated processes, dietary n–3 and n–6 fatty acids influence the rate of cell division, the immune response and tumour growth. In the skin, LA is found in long-chain ceramides, which form an impermeable water barrier.

Polyunsaturated n–3 and n–6 fatty acids exert an extensive metabolic control in human physiology through their role as precursors of eicosanoids. Eicosanoids are signalling molecules derived from 20-carbon polyunsaturated fatty acids (PUFAs), and include thromboxanes, prostaglandins, prostacyclins and leukotrienes (Figure 11.3). They help regulate a wide variety of physiological processes including those involved in inflammation, blood clotting, vascular tone and immunity. They can also act as messengers in the central nervous system.

Most diets provide enough essential fatty acids to meet metabolic requirements (about 2 g/day). The n–3 and n–6 fatty acids in the diet (mainly 18-carbon such as C18:2 and C18:3, together with small amounts of C20:4 and others) are digested, absorbed, transported and stored in many different tissues. A proportion is stored in cell membranes in the form of phospholipids. When stimulated, cell membranes release fatty acids and they can be transformed by a series of enzymes into eicosanoids. Diet can affect the levels of these eicosanoids.

Dietary fatty acids that are not either used for the synthesis of eicosanoids or stored as fat droplets in adipose tissues are oxidised to produce metabolic energy. Fat is a very energy-dense substrate, its oxidation yielding 37.7 kJ/g, about twice as much as from the same weight of carbohydrate or protein. In fact, the storage of excess dietary energy can only occur to any significant extent as body fat (adipose tissue) because humans have a limited capacity to store carbohydrate (glycogen in the liver and skeletal muscles) and protein (for example, increased muscle mass). Therefore, over-consumption of food leads to an increase in body fatness.

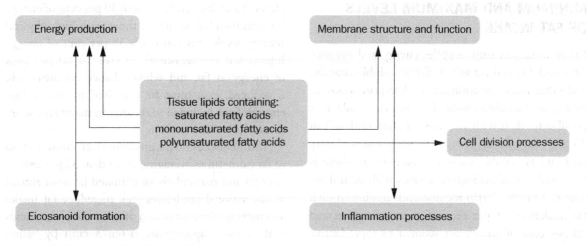

Figure 11.4: Biological roles of fatty acids

WHY IS THE RATIO OF N-6 TO N-3 PUFAS IN THE DIET IMPORTANT?

The conversion of n-6 and n-3 PUFAs to longer-chain PUFA derivatives occurs via a sequential process of desaturation and elongation using the same desaturase and elongase enzymes. This creates a competition between the two series of fatty acids for the activity of the key and rate-limiting enzymes. It follows that the consumption of one type of fatty acids in large quantities will saturate the enzyme and thus restrict the metabolic production of other types of eicosanoids. For example, the n-6 fatty acids (such as linoleic and arachidonic acid) give rise to 2-series eicosanoids, some of which promote blood clotting and some inflammation, whereas n-3 fatty acids give rise to 3-series eicosanoids that have opposing properties to the 2-series eicosanoids.

A diet rich in eicosapentaenoic acid (EPA) and docosahexaenoic acid (DHA) (both n-3 fatty acids), such as that of traditional Greenland Inuit people who eat whale and seal meat, results in reduced clotting of the blood and reduced risk of coronary thrombosis and heart attack. However, the fat in many Western diets is considered to be too rich in linoleic acid (n-6), which makes up much of polyunsaturated margarines and fat in other processed foods. High levels of linoleic acid have been associated with increased inflammation and risk of some cancers (Jandacek 2017).

Current advice to Australian consumers is to try to achieve a better balance of tissue eicosanoids by eating more of the foods rich in n-3 fatty acids, such as fish and other seafood and green leafy vegetables. While the ratio of n-6 to n-3 PUFAs is important, there are no specific recommendations for the ratio; however, there are separate recommendations for n-3 and n-6 PUFAs (FAO 2010). Some experts propose that there should be separate recommendations for plant (18:3) and marine (20:5, 22:5, 22:6) n-3 fatty acids (de Deckere et al. 1998).

MINIMUM AND MAXIMUM LEVELS OF FAT INTAKE

Fat in foods not only supplies energy and essential fatty acids but is also a vehicle for fat-soluble vitamins and other bioactive compounds. Adequate amounts of fat are therefore essential to health. While it is possible for diets with very low fat content (less than 15 per cent of total energy) to meet essential fatty acid and fat-soluble vitamin requirements, there is increased risk of inadequate intakes with such diets. The FAO (FAO 2010) recommends minimum total fat intakes of 15 per cent of energy for men and 20 per cent of energy for women of reproductive age. For most individuals with sedentary or moderate physical activity, a maximum of 30 per cent of energy is recommended, while for those with high physical activity levels, this can reach 35 per cent of energy. Infants fed on breastmilk receive 50–60 per cent of energy as fat, and when reliance on breastmilk is reduced, care must be exercised to ensure that enough fat is included in the diet to maintain energy density (see Chapter 21).

In affluent countries, given the over-consumption of fat (sometimes averaging more than 35 per cent of energy) and particularly of saturated fat from animal foods, national guidelines seek to reduce fat intake and increase the proportion of unsaturated fatty acids with a more appropriate n-6:n-3 ratio by eating more leafy vegetables, fish and legumes.

LIPIDS IN THE FOOD SUPPLY

The most abundant lipid in the human food supply is triglycerides (from fats and oils). Different foods provide different amounts of fat with characteristic fatty acid compositions (Table 11.2). In general, the adipose tissue of domesticated animals (fatty meat), bovine milk and milk products (cheese, butter, ghee) contains relatively large amounts of saturated fatty acids, particularly palmitic, and large amounts of oleic acid, together with very little n-6 and virtually no n-3 PUFAs. However, the lean tissue (muscle) of domesticated animals can be an important source of long-chain n-3 (EPA and DHA) and n-6 (arachidonic acid). Human milk fat and bovine milk fat are quite different, in that the latter comprises more short-chain saturated fatty acids while the former contains significant amounts of essential PUFAs. Marine fish such as mackerel, salmon and sardine are excellent sources of EPA and DHA.

Dietary lipids from plant sources are usually more unsaturated. There are exceptions, however; fatty acids in palm oil are nearly 50 per cent saturated and in coconut oil more than 90 per cent saturated. Two PUFAs, linoleic (C18:2 n-6, LA) and α-linolenic

Table 11.2: Fatty acid content of selected foods, fats and oils (%)

Fatty acid*	Animal origin					Plant origin							
	Butter	Lard	Beef fat	Salmon	Trout	Coconut oil	Palm oil	Olive oil	Canola oil	Corn oil	Peanut oil	Soybean oil	Sunflower oil
4:0	3												
6:0	2												
8:0						8							
10:0	3					7							
12:0	4					48							
14:0	12	2	3	3	4	16							
16:0	26	27	27	11	18	9	44	10	4	13	13	10	8
16:1 n-7	3	4	11	5									
18:0	11	11	7	4	4	2	4	2	2	3	3	4	3
18:1 n-9	28	44	48	25	21	7	40	78	56	31	38	23	15
18:2 n-6	2	11	2	5	6	2	10	7	26	52	41	51	73
18:3 n-3				5	6			1	10	1		7	0.5
18:4 n-3				2	3								
20:0													0.5
20:4 n-3					1								
20:4 n-6				5	4								
20:5 n-3				5	7								
22:4 n-6				2									
22:5 n-3				5	2								
22:5 n-6				2									
22:6 n-3				17	9								

Note: * See Table 11.1 for common names

Sources: Crawford et al. (1989); Gunstone (1996); Khor et al. (1990); Töpfer et al. (1995)

(C18:3 n–3, ALA) acids, occur in large proportions in most vegetable oils. ALA is present in high concentrations in some seeds and nuts, although its presence in normal diets is much lower than that of LA. With the advent of genetic engineering, it is now possible to modify the genes in plants that encode for the synthesis of fatty acids. Such developments have caused, and are continuing to cause, shifts in the fatty acid content of the food supply.

A further consideration is the food source of the fats and oils in the diet. Recommendations for a healthy diet take into account not only the fatty acid composition of a food but also the content of other potentially beneficial components. Essential fatty acid requirements may be reached with highly processed fats and oils in the diet. However, a varied diet containing whole foods rich in essential fatty acids increases the likelihood of receiving other essential nutrients in adequate amounts. This is one rationale behind the important dietary guideline 'to enjoy a wide variety of nutritious foods'. Intact sources of fat in the human diet, such as fish, seeds, nuts, whole grains and lean meats, are generally regarded as healthy choices. Minimally processed

HUMAN EVOLUTION AND DIET

Much of the debate concerning the role of dietary fat as a causative factor in the high incidence of heart disease in affluent countries centres on the concept of a 'protective' or 'prudent' diet. It is postulated that diet-related heart disease is a recent event in human history and that for over five million years humankind has evolved on a diet (the protective diet) quite unlike that which many of us now consume, and to which the human metabolism is unsuited. There is evidence to support this view from the fossil record and from recent research findings in nutritional science, medicine and comparative physiology.

The Palaeolithic diet is a hunter-gatherer diet thought to have been eaten by humans in the Old Stone Age, which occupied nearly all the last two million years of human evolutionary experience. This diet consisted of what 'man the hunter' could hunt, backed up by what 'woman the forager' could forage. Apparently, pre-agricultural humans ate wild game, fish, uncultivated plant foods and, when available, honey. There were no dairy products, oils, salt, processed foods, or foods without nutrient value. It has become a popular fad diet that is marketed by a range of high-profile personalities.

Read the following articles on the Palaeolithic diet:

Cordain, L. et al., 2000, 'Plant-animal subsistence ratios and macronutrient energy estimations in worldwide hunter-gatherer diets', *American Journal of Clinical Nutrition*, 71(3): 682–92

Eaton, S.B. & Konner, M., 1985, 'Paleolithic nutrition', *New England Journal of Medicine*, 312(5): 283–9

Konner, M. & Eaton, S.B., 2010, 'Paleolithic nutrition: Twenty-five years later', *Nutrition in Clinical Practice*, 25(6): 594–602.

- Identify the key differences between the Palaeolithic diet and the modern diet.
- What are the primary differences in fat intake?
- What contribution would this make to morbidity and mortality?
- What would be your key messages regarding consuming a Palaeolithic diet today?

oils, including 'cold-pressed' and 'extra virgin', are also often regarded as healthier choices.

n-3 Fatty acids

The important dietary n-3 fatty acids in humans are ALA (C18:3 n-3), EPA (C20:5 n-3) and DHA (C22:6 n-3). For much of human evolution, diets have been rich in n-3 fatty acids from plants and seafood. Over recent decades, there has been considerable interest in these fatty acids, mainly due to convincing evidence for a range of health benefits with increases in intake from low background levels. Most of the benefits are due to the long-chain n-3 fatty acids, including EPA and DHA. Fish (fish oil) are the richest source of EPA and DHA, although the levels of EPA and DHA vary considerably between species. Despite widespread knowledge of the benefits of fish and long-chain n-3 fatty acids, intakes in many populations remain low. Current recommendations are to eat at least two serves of fish each week. As this can be difficult—and is potentially unsustainable (see Chapter 26)—many people have turned to fish oil supplements, which have been shown to have many of the same health benefits as eating fish (Kris-Etherton et al. 2002). However, edible fish stocks and aquaculture are increasingly contaminated with microplastic, which has endocrine disruptor characteristics (see also Chapter 29), and this raises concerns about fish consumption. The long-term solution to optimising the intake of these essential fatty acids may not be promoting fish intake but, rather, genetic modification of plant species, resulting in the production of long-chain n-3 fatty acids in grains or seeds (Ursin 2003). This would result in a more widespread distribution of long-chain n-3 fatty acids in the food supply.

Cholesterol

Cholesterol is the principal sterol synthesised by animals. It is an essential constituent of mammalian cell membranes, where it is required for cell membrane fluidity. Cholesterol is involved in intracellular transport, cell signalling and nerve conduction, and is the precursor molecule for vitamin D and the steroid hormones such as oestrogen and testosterone. High levels of cholesterol in the circulation are associated with increased risk of heart disease. While dietary cholesterol can contribute to circulating levels, they are determined largely by *in vivo* production and recycling within the body. Fatty acid intake, especially of saturated fat and trans fat, plays a more important part in determining blood cholesterol than intake of cholesterol itself. In the diet, cholesterol is derived from animal foods, and major dietary sources include cheese, egg yolks, beef, pork and poultry.

Trans fatty acids

With industrialisation, societies consume more processed food, including chemically modified fats. In order to make natural oils more suitable as specialised food ingredients, such as pastry shortening, margarine or salad dressings, they are subjected to a variety of industrial processes that change their physical, chemical and biological properties. From a nutritional point of view, the most significant of these is **hydrogenation**, whereby the unsaturated fatty acids in oils are changed into saturated fatty acids.

Making polyunsaturated fats more saturated protects them against oxidation and therefore prolongs shelf life. It also changes the texture of foods by making liquid oil more solid, as in margarine or shortening. Hydrogenation is rarely carried out to the extent that all the unsaturated fatty acids become saturated. It appears that some of the double bonds that remain after the process change their configuration (from the naturally occurring *cis* form to a *trans* form) and their position in the carbon chain (Figure 11.5). Trans fatty acids (TFAs) from hydrogenated vegetable or fish oils have been shown to increase LDL (low-density lipoprotein) cholesterol and may decrease HDL (high-density lipoprotein) cholesterol concentrations in the blood, thus increasing the risk of heart disease. The magnitude of their detrimental effects on heart disease appears to be greater than for saturated fatty acids (FSANZ 2017).

The most common dietary sources of trans and positional isomers of unsaturated fatty acids are margarines and shortenings made from hydrogenated vegetable or fish oils. Meat and milk of **ruminant**

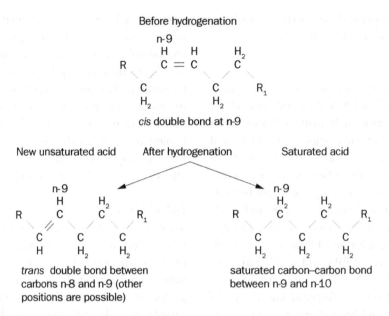

Note: R and R₁ represent those parts of fatty acid molecules not shown here

Figure 11.5: The effect of partial hydrogenation on a double bond in an unsaturated fat

animals contain similar, although not identical, TFA isomers as a result of bacterial fermentation in their rumen, but at relatively low levels (about 5 per cent of the total). There are differences in chemical composition between TFAs derived from hydrogenation of vegetable oils (so-called **industrial TFAs**) and ruminant-derived TFAs, and these differences may influence bioactivity. For example, unlike industrial TFAs, there is little evidence that ruminant-derived TFAs have detrimental health effects (Gebauer et al. 2011). However, one could argue that the failure to observe the adverse health effects of **ruminant TFAs** may be due to their relatively much lower dietary intake, compared to that of industrial TFAs. Modifications of commercial fats and changes in consumer choices have probably led to a decline in intake of industrial TFAs in many European countries and, as a result, the intake of ruminant TFAs has exceeded the intake of industrial TFAs (Craig-Schmidt 2006).

The WHO recommends that no more than 1 per cent of our daily energy intake should come from TFAs (Uauy et al. 2009). Dietary intakes of TFAs vary considerably from country to country; the consumption of these fatty acids has decreased in recent years in many industrialised societies, due to changes in processing techniques. In 2007, FSANZ conducted a review of TFAs in the food supply and found that Australians obtained on average 0.5 per cent—and New Zealanders 0.6 per cent—of energy intake from TFAs (Uauy et al. 2009). While these levels are well below the WHO recommendation, if consumption of SFAs and TFAs is combined, the results—about 12 per cent for Australian adults (ABS 2015) and 13 per cent for New Zealanders (MOH 2012)—exceed the recommendation of no more than 10 per cent of daily energy intake. Reductions of these fatty acid intakes are sought due to their detrimental effects on health.

DIGESTION AND ABSORPTION OF FAT

Fat digestion is a slower process than digestion of protein or carbohydrate. Fat is the last component of the meal to be removed from the small intestine; this contributes to its satiety effect. Bile from the liver and gall bladder has an important role in fat digestion.

The first stage of the fat digestion process is the solubilisation of fat in the small intestine. From its storage organ, the gall bladder, about 1–1.5 L of bile is secreted daily in response to the stimulus of food in the duodenum and the stomach. Bile salts act as detergents, enabling the emulsification of dietary fats into primary **micelles**, which are small droplets, 0.5–1 μm in diameter. This exposes a large surface area of fat to the water phase of the mixture. This is a particular advantage in the digestion of fats because lipase, the pancreatic enzyme responsible for the hydrolytic cleavage of triglyceride fats, can act only at the water–lipid interface.

By emulsifying fats, bile salts have a major effect in speeding up the digestive process. In the absence of bile salts, fat is poorly digested and tends to pass into the colon, leading to the production of pale, fatty, bulky, offensive stools (steatorrhoea). As well as having a role in digestion, bile also provides an important route of excretion of compounds with a low water solubility from the body via the liver. Such compounds include a variety of drugs, bilirubin and cholesterol. The bile is also the main route of excretion of metals such as copper.

Lipase action

Pancreatic lipase preferentially hydrolyses the two outermost ester bonds of triglyceride fats, producing free fatty acids and 2-monoglycerides (one fatty acid remains at the C2-position of glycerol), which are then absorbed by diffusion through the lipoprotein membrane of the epithelial cells. This is a fairly slow process, so complete digestion and absorption of fats normally take many hours. The absorption takes place mostly in the ileum, the lower half of the small intestine (see Chapter 9). This is not because the cell membranes in the upper part of the intestine are impermeable to fatty acids but because the chyme moves quite rapidly through the upper small intestine. However, after the bulk of the food molecules and water have been absorbed, the small amount of residue, rich in digested fat, moves much more slowly through the ileum. This slower movement allows time for adequate uptake by diffusion. Free fatty acids and 2-monoglycerides, once absorbed, are resynthesised into triglyceride fats and secreted into the lymphatic drainage to enter the bloodstream via the sub-clavicle vein.

SUMMARY

- There are five classes of lipids: triacylglycerols or triglycerides; glycolipids; phospholipids; sphingolipids; and sterols (e.g. cholesterol). Each has specific functions within the human body.
- Fatty acids can be classified as saturated or unsaturated based on the number of double bonds in the structure. Lipids contain fatty acids that function as sources of dietary energy, as precursors of molecules controlling important physiological processes and as structural components of many tissues.
- Fats perform important biological roles in the body, including as integral components of a variety of active compounds that help regulate physiological processes including inflammation, blood clotting and immunity; cell membrane structure and fluidity; in membrane-mediated functions related to cell division and tumour growth; maintenance of skin integrity; as vehicles for fat soluble vitamins; and energy production.
- The proportions of saturated, monounsaturated and polyunsaturated fatty acids in the diet are important determinants of health and disease.

- Processing can change the fatty acid composition of ingredients in manufactured foods.
- The minimum requirement for fat is 15 per cent of energy for men and 20 per cent of energy for women of reproductive age. For most individuals an intake of 30 per cent of energy is recommended, with most of this being from unsaturated sources. Current dietary recommendations in affluent countries are to decrease overall fat intake, decrease the proportion of saturated fat and increase mono- and n-3 polyunsaturated fatty acids.
- The safest advice for fat consumption would be to have it from a variety of relatively unrefined plant sources, like seeds and nuts, and from free-living animal sources including fish, mindful of environmental contamination.

KEY TERMS

Ceramides: waxy lipid molecules found in the layers of cell membranes. They are an active ingredient in skin-care products.

Cerebrosides: a class of glycosphingolipid found in the myelin sheath of nerves.

Eicosanoids: signalling molecules made by the enzymatic or non-enzymatic oxidation of 20-carbon polyunsaturated fatty acids such as arachidonic and eicosapentaenoic acids. They include thromboxanes, prostaglandins and leukotrienes.

Essential fatty acids: fatty acids that are required for vital functions in the body and must be obtained from food because they cannot be synthesised in the body.

Gangliosides: sialic acid–containing glycosphingolipids found in high concentrations on the surface of cell membranes, particularly in grey cell matter.

Hydrogenation: a chemical process in which hydrogen gas is bubbled through a liquid oil in the presence of a catalyst forcing unsaturated fatty acids to accept additional hydrogen atoms and thus become saturated.

Industrial TFAs: trans fatty acids produced by hydrogenation of unsaturated oils.

Micelles: lipid molecules that arrange themselves in a spherical form in aqueous solutions. The amphipathic nature of fatty acids (i.e. containing both hydrophilic and hydrophobic regions) allows them to form a micelle. The hydrophilic regions (or polar head groups) usually face to the water and form the surface of micelles, and the hydrophobic tails are inside and away from the water.

Ruminant animal: animals such as cattle, sheep, goats and deer, which bring up fermented ingesta (known as cud) from the first of their stomachs (the rumen) and chew it again. 'Rumination' is the process of rechewing the cud to further break down plant matter and stimulate digestion.

Ruminant TFAs: trans fatty acids produced naturally by ruminant animals.

Saturated: in organic chemistry, a saturated compound has no double or triple bonds in its chemical structure. All the carbon atoms are joined by single bonds and therefore cannot be combined with any additional atoms or radicals.

Unsaturated: in an unsaturated compound, two or more of the carbon atoms are joined by a double or triple bond and therefore can be combined with additional atoms or radicals.

ACKNOWLEDGEMENT

This chapter has been modified and updated from the 'Fats' chapter written by Gwynn P. Jones and Jonathan M. Hodgson which appeared in the third edition of *Food and Nutrition*.

REFERENCES

ABS, 2015, *Australian Health Survey: Usual nutrient intakes, 2011–12*, <www.abs.gov.au/ausstats/abs@.nsf/Lookup/by%20Subject/4364.0.55.008~2011-12~Main%20Features~Key%20findings~100>, accessed 22 November 2018

Cordain, L., Miller, J.B., Eaton, S.B., Mann, N., Holt, S.H.A. & Speth, J.D., 2000, 'Plant–animal subsistence ratios and macronutrient energy estimations in worldwide hunter-gatherer diets', *American Journal of Clinical Nutrition*, 71(3): 682–92, doi:10.1093/ajcn/71.3.682

Craig-Schmidt, M.C., 2006, 'World-wide consumption of trans fatty acids', *Atherosclerosis Supplements*, 7(2): 1–4, doi:10.1016/j.atherosclerosissup.2006.04.001

Crawford, M., Doyle, W., Drury, P., Ghebremeskel, K., Harbige, L. et al., 1989, 'The food chain for n-6 and n-3 fatty acids with special reference to animal products', in C. Galli & A. Simopoulos (eds), *Dietary ω3 and ω6 Fatty Acids: Biological effects and nutrition essentiality*, New York, NY: Springer, pp. 5–19

de Deckere, E.A., Korver, O., Verschuren, P.M. & Katan, M.B., 1998, 'Health aspects of fish and n-3 polyunsaturated fatty acids from plant and marine origin', *European Journal of Clinical Nutrition*, 52: 749–53, doi: 10.1007/978-1-59259-226-5_13

Eaton, S.B. & Konner, M., 1985, 'Paleolithic nutrition: A consideration of its nature and current implications', *New England Journal of Medicine*, 312(5): 283–9, doi:10.1056/NEJM198501313120505

FAO, 2010, *Fats and Fatty Acids in Human Nutrition*, <http://foris.fao.org/preview/25553-0ece4cb94ac52f9a25af77ca5cfba7a8c.pdf>, accessed 22 November 2018

FSANZ, 2017, *Trans Fatty Acids*, <www.foodstandards.gov.au/consumer/nutrition/transfat/Pages/default.aspx>, accessed 23 March 2018

Gebauer, S.K., Chardigny, J.-M., Jakobsen, M.U., Lamarche, B., Lock, A.L. et al., 2011, 'Effects of ruminant trans fatty acids on cardiovascular disease and cancer: A comprehensive review of epidemiological, clinical, and mechanistic studies', *Advances in Nutrition*, 2(4): 332–54, doi:10.3945/an.111.000521

Gunstone, F.D., 1996, 'Fatty acids—nomenclature, structure, isolation and structure determination, biosynthesis and chemical synthesis', in F.D. Gunstone, *Fatty Acid and Lipid Chemistry*, Boston, MA: Springer, pp. 1–34

Jandacek, R.J., 2017, 'Linoleic acid: A nutritional quandary', *Healthcare*, 5(2): 25, doi:10.3390/healthcare5020025

Khor, G.K., Tee, E.S. & Kandiah, M., 1990, 'Patterns of food production and consumption in the ASEAN region', *World Review of Nutrition and Dietetics*, 61: 1–40, doi:10.1159/000417525

Konner, M. & Eaton, S.B., 2010, 'Paleolithic nutrition: Twenty-five years later', *Nutrition in Clinical Practice*, 25(6): 594–602, doi:10.1177/0884533610385702

Kris-Etherton, P.M., Harris, W.S. & Appel, L.J., 2002, 'Fish consumption, fish oil, omega-3 fatty acids, and cardiovascular disease', *Circulation*, 106(21): 2747–57, doi:10.1161/01.CIR.0000038493.65177.94

MOH, 2012, *A Focus on Nutrition: Key findings from the 2008/09 NZ Adult Nutrition Survey*, <www.health.govt.nz/publication/focus-nutrition-key-findings-2008-09-nz-adult-nutrition-survey>, accessed 20 January 2019

Töpfer, R., Martini, N. & Schell, J., 1995, 'Modification of plant lipid synthesis', *Science*, 268(5211): 681–6, doi:10.1126/science.268.5211.681

Uauy, R., Aro, A., Clarke, R., Ghafoorunissa, R., L'Abbé, M. et al., 2009, 'WHO Scientific Update on *trans* fatty acids: Summary and conclusions', *European Journal of Clinical Nutrition*, 63: S68–S75, doi:10.1038/ejcn.2009.15

Ursin, V.M., 2003, 'Modification of plant lipids for human health: Development of functional land-based omega-3 fatty acids', *Journal of Nutrition*, 133(12): 4271–4, doi:10.1093/jn/133.12.4271

CHAPTER 12

MACRONUTRIENTS: CARBOHYDRATES

Mark L. Wahlqvist and Naiyana Wattanapenpaiboon

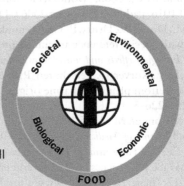

OBJECTIVES

- Describe a classification system for carbohydrates and recognise their distribution in food.
- Explain carbohydrate digestion in the body.
- Describe the body's requirement for carbohydrate and the carbohydrate content of various foods.
- Summarise the physiological effects of fibre in the small and large intestine.
- Describe the significance of glycaemic index and glycaemic load.

FORMS OF DIETARY CARBOHYDRATES

Most foods, in their natural state, contain a wide range of different carbohydrates; however, one or two specific carbohydrates often occur in greater amounts than others. In deciding how to classify dietary carbohydrates, the major challenge is that the classification needs to reflect both their various chemical categories and their significance in physiology and health. A classification based purely on chemistry does not allow a ready translation into nutritional terms, since each of the major classes of carbohydrate has a variety of physiological effects. For nutritional purposes, the WHO and FAO have jointly recommended a classification scheme for dietary carbohydrates with functional relevance, which was updated in 2007 (Cummings & Stephen 2007; WHO/FAO 1998). These are outlined in Table 12.1.

The term 'sugars' is conventionally used to describe the mono- and disaccharides; in contrast, the term '**sugar**' is used to describe purified sucrose, as are the terms 'refined sugar' and 'added sugar'. The term '**complex carbohydrate**' is generally used to describe either starch alone or the combination of all polysaccharides, and therefore distinguish sugars from other carbohydrates. It was used to encourage consumption of what were considered to be healthy foods, such as wholegrain cereals, but becomes meaningless when used to describe fruit and vegetables, which are low in starch. Furthermore, it is now realised that starch, which is by any definition a complex carbohydrate, is metabolically variable, with some forms being rapidly absorbed and having a high glycaemic index (see below for an explanation) and some being resistant to digestion. The term 'complex carbohydrate' has encompassed, at various times, starch, dietary fibre and non-digestible

Table 12.1: Classification of major dietary carbohydrates

Group (degree of polymerisation, DP)	Subgroup	Components
Sugars (DP 1–2)	Monosaccharides	Glucose, galactose, fructose
	Disaccharides	Sucrose, lactose
	Polyols (sugar alcohols)	Sorbitol, mannitol
Oligosaccharides (DP 3–9)	Malto-oligosaccharides (α-glucans) (principally those occurring from starch hydrolysis)	Maltodextrins
	Other oligosaccharides (non α-glucans)	α-Galactosides (e.g. raffinose, stachyose) Fructo-oligosaccharides, inulin
Polysaccharides (DP >9)	Starch (α-glucans)	Amylose, amylopectin, modified starches
	Non-starch polysaccharides	Cellulose, hemicellulose, pectins, hydrocolloids

oligosaccharides. It is better to discuss carbohydrate components by using their common chemical names rather than referring to them as complex or simple.

From a physiological point of view, it is the contribution food carbohydrates make to dietary energy that is their most important feature (see Chapter 13). They do this by supplying glucose into the bloodstream and through fermentation by bacteria in the large intestine. The fate of carbohydrates after ingestion is outlined in Figure 12.1.

RESISTANT (FERMENTED) CARBOHYDRATES

The major classes of resistant carbohydrates are the non-starch polysaccharides, including dietary fibre, resistant starch and resistant short–chain (oligo-saccharides) carbohydrates.

Non-starch polysaccharides

A great deal of the plant material that resists digestion in human diets originates from the cell walls in the tissues of fruits, vegetables and cereal grains. A microscopic analysis of plant foodstuffs reveals tissues made up of cells with rigid cell walls. The major chemical components of these cell walls are the carbohydrates cellulose (a glucose polymer of the β-glucan type; a polymer is a string of chemically bonded single molecules); hemicellulose (mixed polymers containing large amounts of the sugars xylose, arabinose, mannose and galactose chemically bonded together in varying arrangements); and pectic substances (polymers of the sugar acid galacturonic acid and its derivatives). Also associated with the cell walls are proteins and, occasionally, small amounts of lignin (a highly insoluble organic polymer that is not carbohydrate in nature). To differentiate cell wall carbohydrates from starch, they, together with other non-starchy storage carbohydrates found in a few plant seeds used as foods, are collectively called non-starch polysaccharides (NSP) (Table 12.2). Plant cell walls are diverse in shape and vary in composition. They provide physical strength to plant tissues, performing a support function that in animals is provided by bones, and they are chiefly responsible for the texture of vegetable foods.

Dietary fibre

There is no single definition of 'dietary fibre', but the term was originally used to describe 'the skeletal remains of plant cells that are resistant to digestion by enzymes of man' (Trowell 1972, p. 138). This, however, is not an exact description of any carbohydrate in the diet but is more a physiological concept. The use of the term has caused many difficulties over the years because of controversies regarding definition. While there is no universal agreement on terminology, the following definition of dietary fibre has been accepted by FSANZ (Standard 1.2.8) for the purposes of describing food components that can be claimed as dietary fibre on food labels.

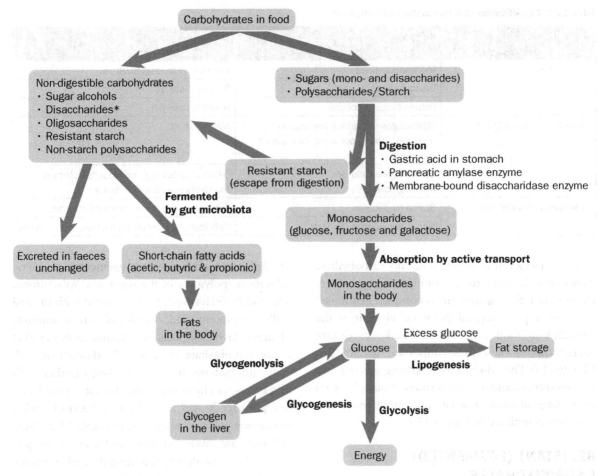

Note: * Lactose in non-lactase persistent people

Figure 12.1: Fate of carbohydrates in food after ingestion

Dietary fibre means that fraction of the edible parts of plants or their extracts, or synthetic analogues that: are resistant to the digestion and absorption in the small intestine, usually with complete or partial fermentation in the large intestine; and promote one or more of the following beneficial physiological effects: laxation, reduction in blood cholesterol, modulation of blood glucose; and includes polysaccharides or oligosaccharides that have a degree of **polymerisation** greater than 2; and **lignins**. (FSANZ 2016)

It is important to note that this definition emphasises the fact that dietary fibre has several distinctive features. These relate to its biological origins (from plants), its chemical composition (largely carbohydrate), its physiological effects (both local in the gut and systemic in the blood) and its ability to serve as a substrate for the growth of microorganisms, especially those residing in the large intestine. Omitted from this definition, however, is another important attribute: the contribution fibre makes to the physical form of foods. The indigestible box-like cell walls in plant tissues can inhibit the release of cell contents during passage through the small intestine. The tissues of many plant foods, although disrupted by chewing, contain enough intact cell structure to slow the release of cell cytoplasm containing sugars, starch and other nutrients. In the case of whole apples

Table 12.2: Chemical composition of non-starch polysaccharides (NSP) and other dietary fibre components

Dietary fibre components	Principal sugars that comprise the polymers (food source)	Observed properties of purified fibres in the gut
NON-STARCH POLYSACCHARIDES (NSPs)		
Cellulose	Unbranched polymer of glucose (all plant foods). Chains are packed into orderly arrays of microcrystals with some amorphous regions	Insoluble in water, resistant to fermentation by gut microbiota. Has little effect on faecal bulking and no effect on cholesterol excretion
Hemicelluloses (several types of polymers occur)	Mainly arabinose and xylose (cereal cell walls, e.g. wheat)	Largely insoluble in water, not extensively fermented, binds water and causes faecal bulking, i.e. is laxative
	Mainly glucuronic acid, glucose and xylose (cell walls of fruits and vegetables)	Soluble and extensively fermented; not laxative
	β-glucan (cereal cell walls, e.g. oats, barley)	Soluble, form viscous solutions, interfere with metabolism of lipids, lower serum cholesterol
Pectic substances	Mainly rhamnose and galacturonic acid (fruits and vegetable cell walls)	Soluble in water producing viscous solutions, interfere with metabolism of lipids, lower serum cholesterol
OTHER FIBRE COMPONENTS		
Lignin	An organic polymer but not a carbohydrate (small amounts eaten mainly via cereals)	May be associated with reduced risk of colon cancer

fed to volunteer subjects, the uptake of glucose into the blood was found to be ten times slower than it was from apple juice, and the whole apples also promoted a greater feeling of satiety (Haber et al. 1977). Similar observations have been made with glucose absorbed during digestion of wholegrain starchy cereals. The slower release and absorption of glucose is thought to produce more appropriate metabolic responses—for example, by the hormone insulin, resulting in better control of blood glucose levels.

Physiological differences in function attributable to the shape and size of food pieces are also evident in the large intestine. It is well known that coarse wheat bran is laxative, whereas finely ground wheat bran is constipating, and that it is the shape and size of the particles that are the functional attribute (Lewis & Heaton 1999). Dietary fibre from cereals, fruits and vegetables differs in its chemical composition as well as its physiological effects; therefore, it is not surprising that attempts to define it are complex.

It has been recommended that the use of the term 'dietary fibre' be gradually phased out or abandoned in scientific discussions because it has no

useful meaning. At a meeting of experts convened by the WHO/FAO, the following definition of fibre was proposed: 'dietary fibre consists of intrinsic plant cell wall polysaccharides' and should be more clearly linked to health (Cummings & Stephen 2007). There is now abundant research linking a higher intake of dietary fibre with reduced risk of chronic diseases. However, research has also shown that fibre is one of several interacting features of diets that may be protective against chronic diseases, and that the amount of fibre in a diet is a useful marker of many of these factors. Research has investigated potential benefits of resistant starch on chronic diseases including colon cancer, type 2 diabetes and heart disease. Current knowledge suggests that resistant starch in the diet may assist in the prevention and management of these conditions.

Soluble and insoluble fibre

In the early chemistry of non-starch polysaccharides, it was found that their **fractional extraction** could be controlled by changing the pH of solutions, and the terms 'soluble fibre' and 'insoluble fibre' were subsequently coined.

THE DIETARY FIBRE HYPOTHESIS

'Fibre' is now recognised as a key dietary factor that affects health, but this has not always been the case. Our knowledge about what fibre is and how it impacts health is continually evolving as new evidence emerges. Denis Parsons Burkitt (1911–1993) was an Irish surgeon who made two major contributions to medical science, one of which was the finding that colorectal cancer risk was high among people who ate a very low amount of fibre.

Read the following article to discover how fibre was identified to have an influence on health.

- Cummings, J.H. & Engineer, A., 2018, 'Denis Burkitt and the origins of the dietary fibre hypothesis', *Nutrition Research Reviews*, 31(1): 1–15.

Although the separation of soluble and insoluble fractions is not chemically very distinct, being dependent on the conditions of extraction, these terms proved very useful in the initial understanding of the physiological properties of fibre. The chemical separation allowed a simple division into those fibres that principally affected glucose and lipid absorption from the small intestine (soluble) and those that were slowly and incompletely fermented and had more pronounced effects on bowel habit (insoluble). However, the physiological differences are not, in fact, so distinct, with much insoluble fibre being rapidly and completely fermented and not all soluble fibre having effects on glucose and lipid absorption.

The absolute amount and relative proportions of plant cell wall material vary with the biological origins of the food, degree of maturity and extent of food processing. The tissues in leafy and root vegetables have thin-walled cells with a low concentration of NSP, typically 2–3 g per 100 g fresh weight. These foods have a high water content and lignin is virtually absent unless the vegetables are old and woody in texture. Cooking vegetables solubilises a significant proportion of the NSP. In their dry, mature form, legumes such as beans and peas have levels of cell wall polysaccharides comparable with cereal grains, but these are diluted during soaking and cooking in water. In wholegrain cereals, the concentration of NSP is much higher (9–17 per cent) than in most other foods, and they have different properties: they are much less soluble, able to bind relatively large amounts of water and are associated with measurable amounts of lignin. Like legumes, their concentration is reduced by the addition of water during food preparation—for example, from 12 per cent NSP in wholemeal wheat flour (10 per cent water) down to 8 per cent NSP in wholemeal bread (40 per cent water).

Fruits have the highest water content, and hence are lowest in cell wall components (from 0.6 per cent NSP in grapes to 3.6 per cent NSP in blackcurrants, with most having about 1 per cent NSP). Although they have thin cell walls, some have sufficiently high concentrations of pectic substances to form gels in products like jam when large amounts of sucrose are added. Such gels are unlikely to occur in the human gut as a result of consuming fresh fruit. While the seeds of some fruits (passionfruit, pomegranates and blackberries) are highly lignified, lignin itself forms a very small part of diets compared with NSP.

Some Asian cultures include significant amounts of algae (such as brown seaweed) and fungi (such as mushrooms) in their cuisine. Japanese seaweed dishes such as nori (*Pyropia tenera*), hiziki (*Hizikia fusiformis*) and wakame (*Undaria pinnatifida*) are rich sources of cell wall polysaccharides (35–50 per cent in the edible portion). More than two-thirds of this is soluble and contains considerable amounts of alginic acid, quite unlike the cell walls of terrestrial plants. Alginic acid is a polymer of D-mannuronic acid, an acidic derivative of the sugar mannose. In Australian and New Zealand diets, small amounts of these polysaccharides are used as food thickeners in processed foods.

The concentration of NSP is highest in the outer layers of plant foods; presumably it performs a protective function for the central storage tissue (endosperm), where most of the starch and protein is found. Discarding the peel from vegetables or the bran from milled cereals significantly lowers NSP content and changes food composition. For example, wholemeal or 100 per cent extraction flour consists of ground whole-wheat grains, whereas white flour is made up of only 75 per cent of the original grain—with the 25 per cent that is discarded during the extraction process including most of the NSP-rich bran layers. There appears to be a preference in many societies for foods with a low content of NSP, as evidenced by the popularity of white bread, polished rice and wheat noodles. These 'refined' foods are staples for many individuals who, if they become more affluent, also choose to eat more fat—dietary changes that are thought to predispose to diseases of affluence.

Resistant starch

Starch was historically considered as a digestible polysaccharide, but it has been shown that a significant portion is not digested in the small intestine and passes into the colon, where it forms a substrate for bacterial fermentation. This starch is called resistant starch (RS), and most nutritionists consider that it should be classified as a component of dietary fibre. It is described as the sum of starch and products of starch degradation that, on average, are not absorbed in the small intestine of healthy individuals and reach the large intestine.

The major classes of resistant carbohydrates are NSP (including dietary fibre), RS and resistant short-chain (oligosaccharides) carbohydrates. One of the major developments in our understanding of the importance of carbohydrates for health is the discovery of RS, which is defined as starch and starch degradation products not absorbed in the small intestine of healthy humans (Englyst & Cummings 1990). The main forms of RS are physically enclosed starch (i.e. within intact cell structures), some raw

starch granules and retrograded amylose. In a starchy food, the proportions of amylose and amylopectin are variable and can be altered by plant breeding. High-amylose corn starch and high-amylopectin (waxy) corn starch have been available for a long time and display quite different functional as well as nutritional properties. High-amylose starches require higher temperatures for gelatinisation and are more prone to retrograde and to form amylose–lipid complexes. Such properties can be utilised in the formulation of foods with low glycaemic index (see below for an explanation) and/or high RS content. Physical modifications of starches include pre-gelatinisation and partial hydrolysis (dextrinisation). Chemical modification comprises mainly the introduction of side groups and cross-linking or oxidation. These modifications may be used to decrease viscosity, to improve gel stability, mouthfeel, appearance and texture, and to increase resistance for heat treatment. Some modified starches may be partly resistant to digestion in the small intestine, thereby adding to resistant starch.

There are three main reasons for the incomplete digestion of starch, and these mostly relate to physical and chemical characteristics of food rather than to differences in the digestive physiology of individuals.

1. Some starch may be physically trapped inside intact cells of plant tissues, as in the coarsely ground cereal ingredients of foods like muesli and wholegrain bread. This starch is therefore inaccessible because digestive amylases are unable to penetrate or break down the cellulose cell walls.

2. Starch is stored in cells in the form of tightly packed granules, which may be particularly insoluble, and therefore indigestible, unless solubilised by thorough cooking in the presence of water. Resistant starch of this kind is found in raw potatoes and uncooked green bananas. Cooking starchy foods at temperatures greater than 70–80°C disrupts the granule structure, resulting in solubilisation of starch molecules (gelatinisation) and increased digestibility. Plant geneticists have developed varieties of maize containing starch granules with a high content of

amylose that does not gelatinise during baking, and this largely indigestible starch is used as a 'fibre' ingredient of white high-'fibre' breads and some high-'fibre' breakfast cereals.

3. Starchy foods that are cooled after cooking cause a portion of the gelatinised starch to become highly insoluble, and hence indigestible. This is called retrograded starch and is found in bread, cold cooked potatoes, cold boiled rice and so on. This is likely to be the major RS component of diets in Australia and New Zealand and it is not surprising that some starchy foods contain more resistant starch than they do NSP.

Analytical methods to measure this in foods have proved difficult to develop, and there are no protocols which are universally accepted. Thus, there are no reliable population estimates of RS intakes in Australia and New Zealand, although values of about 6 g/day per capita are considered likely. This is eaten in conjunction with 20–25 g/day of NSP. So we eat more NSP than RS, but there are many people in the world consuming diets that are very high in carbohydrate and low in fibre (such as diets with polished rice as a staple). These people probably eat more RS than NSP.

Resistant short-chain carbohydrates/non-digestible oligosaccharides

Foods contain a variety of indigestible carbohydrate components other than NSP (including dietary fibre) and RS. The raffinose group of galacto-oligosaccharides (raffinose DP 3, stachyose DP 4 and verbascose DP 5) are widely distributed in plants, occurring in significant quantities (about 1–8 per cent) in the mature seeds of legumes (beans, lentils, chickpeas, soy beans etc.). They are called flatus factors because they cause gas production (mainly carbon dioxide, hydrogen and methane) in the colon, arising from fermentation by resident bacteria. For example, studies have shown that gas production on basal (bean-free) diets can rise from 16 mL to 190 mL per hour when beans are introduced. In some people, these gases can remain trapped in tonically contracted segments of the colon, giving rise to severe pain (see Chapter 9). The galacto-oligosaccharide content of foods can be reduced by food preparation methods such as soaking in water or inoculating with edible fungi, techniques extensively used in traditional Asian cooking in the preparation of food such as tempeh.

Another group of non-digestible oligosaccharides are the fructo-oligosaccharides, found in small amounts in cereals, artichokes and onions. Intakes of these in typical Australian diets have been low up to the present day, but this might change in future as they are now appearing in relatively larger amounts as ingredients of processed foods. Industrially extracted from chicory roots, these non-digestible oligosaccharides are used either to replace fat in reduced-fat foods—especially yoghurt, confectionery and margarines—or as ingredients of functional foods. In the latter application, their consumption is claimed to deliver specific health benefits quite separate from the provision of nutrients or dietary energy. Fructo-oligosaccharides stimulate the growth of specific bacteria (for example, of the genus *Bifidobacteria*) in the colon, and this is claimed to be associated with health benefits such as improved laxation and enhanced calcium absorption. Accordingly, fructo-oligosaccharides fit the definition of dietary fibre given earlier and can be claimed as such on food labels (NHMRC 2006). On the other hand, members of the raffinose group do not fit the definition of dietary fibre because the evidence for beneficial physiological effects is not conclusive and they cannot be claimed as components of dietary fibre. Non-digestible oligosaccharides that serve to stimulate the growth of gut bacteria beneficial to human health (probiotic bacteria) are called prebiotic food ingredients.

OTHER UNDIGESTED FOOD COMPONENTS

Associated with the cell walls of plant foods are a group of compounds collectively called phytates. Occurring at levels of less than 1 per cent in cereals, legumes, vegetables, fruits and nuts, these phosphate-rich compounds form insoluble salts with the essential minerals iron, calcium and zinc, thus

THE IMPACT OF PHYTATE ON MINERAL ABSORPTION

You have been asked to identify the impact of plant-based diets on mineral absorption. Explore the literature on foods high in phytate and their impact on mineral absorption in different contexts. What are your conclusions and recommendations?

Some articles to get you started include:

- Al Hasan, S.M. et al., 2016, 'Dietary phytate intake inhibits the bioavailability of iron and calcium in the diets of pregnant women in rural Bangladesh: A cross-sectional study', *BMC Nutrition*, 2(1): 24
- Gibson, R.S., Raboy, V. & King, J.C., 2018, 'Implications of phytate in plant-based foods for iron and zinc bioavailability, setting dietary requirements, and formulating programs and policies', *Nutrition Reviews*, 76(11): 793–804
- Grases, F., Prieto, R.M. & Costa-Bauza, A., 2017, 'Dietary phytate and interactions with mineral nutrients', in O.M. Gutiérrez, K. Kalantar-Zadeh & R. Mehrotra (eds), *Clinical Aspects of Natural and Added Phosphorus in Foods*, New York, NY: Springer, pp. 175–83.

preventing their absorption from the intestine. It has been shown that the consumption of wholemeal cereals and legumes in diets that contain very little meat can lead to deficiencies of zinc and impaired iron balance. This is an example of an unusual circumstance where high–fibre diets are detrimental to consumer health.

In cereals, the bulk of phytates are found in the germ (maize) or outer layers (rice and wheat) of the grain. Consequently, wholemeal foods contain the highest levels and vegetarians consume from three to ten times more phytates than omnivorous people. Phytates are affected by processing, and there also appears to be an adaptive response to the levels of minerals in diets that affects phytate breakdown *in vivo*. It should be remembered, however, that not only phytates but also fibre, NSP, oxalic acid and polyphenolic compounds have been implicated as factors impairing the absorption of minerals from diets. Polyol sweeteners that escape digestion in the small intestine are not normally considered by nutritionists to constitute a component of dietary fibre. Some protein of dietary origin is also indigestible and enters the colon (3–9 g/day in a typical Australian diet); however, the fermentation products include ammonia, indoles and phenols,

and these can be toxic to human cells. This explains why the definition of dietary fibre is confined to undigested carbohydrate components, because fibre's properties, both in the intestine and systemically via its fermentation products, are considered protective against disease.

FOOD SOURCES OF CARBOHYDRATES

Dry cereal grains like wheat, corn and rice are rich in starch (20–85 per cent), contain up to 15 per cent of NSP, and have small amounts of fructo-oligosaccharides as well as small quantities of free sugars. Dry leguminous seeds like soy beans, beans and peas contain starch (55–65 per cent), NSP (3–15 per cent) and galacto–oligosaccharides (2–8 per cent), as well as small quantities of free sugars. Some root vegetables and tubers, such as potatoes and cassava, also contain large amounts of starch (20–25 per cent), but usually the amounts of NSP are low (about 1 per cent). Leafy vegetables contain only small amounts of starch and NSP, together with about 5 per cent sugars. It is only fruit (5–15 per cent), milk (6 per cent) and honey (74 per cent) that contain large amounts of sugars, but they contain little or no starch or NSP.

In contrast to natural foods, processed foods frequently contain added sugars to satisfy consumer demand for sweetness—for example, fruit yoghurt (15–18 per cent sugars), biscuits (35 per cent sugars) and milk chocolate (56 per cent sugars). The added sugar is often sucrose. In most cases, food processing by peeling or milling and/or adding sucrose reduces the diversity of the naturally occurring carbohydrates, substantially diminishing the levels of NSP as a result. A Joint FAO/WHO Expert Consultation on Carbohydrates in Human Nutrition has agreed that free sugars—that is, all monosaccharides and disaccharides added to foods—may have different physiological consequences from sugars naturally present within intact cell walls (Mann et al. 2007).

Polyols are another group of carbohydrate-like molecules derived from sugars that occur naturally in pears and other fruits. Unlike sugars, which are rapidly absorbed during digestion, most polyols are only slowly absorbed from the small intestine, so that much of what is consumed—depending on dose and type—passes into the colon, where it is fermented. Industrially, polyols are manufactured for use in processed foods where sweetness is required but in circumstances where the consumer needs to restrict consumption of dietary sugars, such as in diabetic subjects. Thus polyols (e.g. sorbitol, xylitol, mannitol) are extensively used in carbohydrate-modified jams, confectionery, chewing gum and so on.

A Joint FAO/WHO Expert Consultation on Carbohydrates in Human Nutrition recommends that the total carbohydrate in an individual food item be measured as the sum of individual carbohydrates (WHO/FAO 1998). However, rather than list a series of different carbohydrates, which would be a lengthy and expensive exercise, the carbohydrate content

SUGAR BY ANY OTHER NAME

In helping people to understand the hidden sugars that may be in foods, you need to be familiar with the different names that may be used for 'sugar' in the ingredient list of a food product. It is important to distinguish between products (e.g. fruit) that have a high natural sugar content and those with added sugar. Under the Food Standards Code, nutrition content claims and health claims about sugar must meet certain criteria. For example, for a claim of 'low sugar', the food must not contain more than 2.5 g of sugar per 100 mL of liquid food or 5 g per 100 g of solid food. For a 'reduced sugar' claim, the food must contain at least 25 per cent less sugar than the comparison food. There are also criteria in the Code for 'x per cent sugar-free', 'no added sugar' and 'unsweetened' claims.

Read the ingredient labels of the following products:

- fruit yoghurt
- sweet biscuit
- tomato sauce
- jube lolly
- highly coloured breakfast cereal
- muesli bar.

Identify all the types of sugar each product contains. Develop a list of sugar and its alternative names.

What would be your primary message for an individual who was trying to be healthy regarding their sugar intake?

FODMAP DIETS

FODMAPs, described in Chapter 8, are short-chain carbohydrates that are poorly absorbed in the small intestine. These carbohydrates are handled in the gut in a dose–response fashion. For example, fructose, an important fruit sugar, is tolerable for most people on usual and healthy diets containing fruit. When consumed in isolation from food, as a pure sugar, it is less tolerable. Further, as the dose increases above a certain threshold, so also do the symptoms. This does not constitute a disorder or disease but, rather, a question of sensible ways of eating. The consumption of FODMAPs, as part of relatively intact food, also requires a lower insulin response to dietary carbohydrate, because of preferable small and large intestinal physiology.

It is now recognised that while unstructured fruit juice increases the risk of diabetes, fruit, containing sugars, decreases the risk of diabetes. It is not only this physiological aspect of FODMAPs which is important to appreciate, but also the fact that the survival of these carbohydrates beyond the small intestine to the large intestine for fermentation by the gut microbiome is increasingly recognised as conducive to health. The role of FODMAPs in large intestinal physiology, especially mucosal integrity and hepatic function through the delivery of short-chain fatty acids in the portal circulation to the liver, represents a major macronutrient function.

Particular vegetables, such as onion and garlic, may contribute to the symptoms of irritable bowel syndrome (IBS) in susceptible individuals. However, the regular consumption of vegetables may also help alleviate the symptoms of IBS and prevent other digestive problems. Like fruit, vegetables are a good source of dietary fibre, especially insoluble fibre. Insoluble fibre absorbs water and expands as it passes through the digestive system, which can relieve or prevent constipation and may protect against diverticulitis.

Look for peer-reviewed journal articles on the effectiveness of following a FODMAP diet. Write a summary addressing the following questions.
- How effective are they in reducing gastrointestinal symptoms?
- Are they nutritionally balanced in the long term?
- Would you recommend FODMAP diets to anyone and, if so, who and under what conditions?

References:
Fedewa, A. & Rao, S.S., 2014, 'Dietary fructose intolerance, fructan intolerance and FODMAPs', *Current Gastroenterology Reports*, *16*(1): 370
Staudacher, H.M. & Whelan, K., 2017, 'The low FODMAP diet: Recent advances in understanding its mechanisms and efficacy in IBS', *Gut*, *66*(8): 1517–27
Whelan, K. et al., 2018, 'The low FODMAP diet in the management of irritable bowel syndrome: An evidence-based review of FODMAP restriction, reintroduction and personalisation in clinical practice', *Journal of Human Nutrition and Dietetics*, *31*(2): 239–55

for a food is expressed as 'available carbohydrate by difference'. This is to be 'calculated by subtracting from 100, the average quantity in the food, expressed as a percentage, of the following substances: water; protein; fat; dietary fibre; ash; alcohol; if quantified or added to the food—any other unavailable carbohydrate; and a substance listed' (FSANZ 2016, Schedule 11). In other words, the carbohydrate content of a food is what is left over after all the other (non-carbohydrate) constituents have been removed. The main disadvantages of this approach are that it does not adequately describe the carbohydrate in relation to its nutritional relevance, and it may provide an inaccurate estimate.

DIGESTION OF CARBOHYDRATE

The major carbohydrates in our diet are starch and the disaccharides sucrose and lactose (milk sugar). The monosaccharides glucose and fructose can also provide a significant contribution to total carbohydrate intake. Starch is made up of glucose polymers (long chains of glucose units joined together). Pancreatic amylase hydrolyses every second glucose–glucose bond in amylose to liberate maltose, a disaccharide (2-glucose unit sugar). The disaccharide sugars in the gut lumen diffuse through the mucous layer to the outer, microvillous (brush border) membrane of the villous epithelial cells (enterocytes). The cells carry disaccharidase enzymes on the exterior membrane surface (Table 12.3) and also have transmembrane transport proteins in close proximity. The monosaccharides released are transported across the cell membrane to the interior of the enterocytes by either active transport or diffusion.

Lactase persistence and lactose intolerance

Almost all infants produce lactase enzyme and can digest the lactose in their mother's milk, except in rare instances where the gut is inflamed by severe infection (such as viral or bacterial infection), in which case lactase activity may fall to a low level. As young children mature, most switch off the lactase gene expression and lose their intestinal lactase activity.

Table 12.3: Disaccharidase enzymes in disaccharide digestion

Disaccharidase enzyme	Substrate	→	Product(s)
Maltase (glucoamylase)	Maltase	→	glucose + glucose (1→4 bond)
Isomaltase (α-dextrinase)	Isomaltose	→	glucose + glucose (1→6 bond)
	Dextrins	→	glucose and maltose
Sucrase	Sucrose	→	glucose + fructose
	Maltose	→	glucose + glucose (1→4 bond)
	Isomaltose	→	glucose + glucose (1→6 bond)
Lactase	Lactose	→	glucose + galactose

When this occurs, lactose from milk products will be transported through the gut without being absorbed and may cause lactose intolerance symptoms, such as flatus, gas, bloating, cramps, diarrhoea and, rarely, vomiting. It is estimated that only about 35 per cent of the human population has an adequate persistence of lactase activity. Lactase activity appears to reach a maximum in late pregnancy but declines after 2–3 years of age and reaches a stable low level at age 5–10 years (lactase non-persistence). However, lactose-free or lactase-supplemented foods are not necessary for lactase-deficient people or lactose non-persisters. There is a wide variability of symptoms in lactase-deficient people, according to the amount of lactose ingested and the ability to digest it. Generally, foods with a high fat content and high concentration of soluble compounds decrease gastric emptying and reduce the severity of symptoms induced by lactose (Hurduc et al. 2017). A meta-analysis indicated that almost all lactose intolerants tolerated 12 g of lactose in one intake and approximately 18 g of lactose spread over the day (Corgneau et al. 2017). In fact, as lactose is not digested in the small intestine, it may favourably alter the colonic microbiota and enhance innate gut immunity in not only early but also later life, through synergistic action with other carbohydrates or short-chain fatty acids (SCFAs).

An advantage in being a lactose non-persister may be that it imposes a physiological ceiling on lactose and, therefore, dairy excess (Lukito et al. 2015).

CARBOHYDRATES AS SOURCES OF DIETARY ENERGY (DIGESTED AND/OR FERMENTED)

Carbohydrates are the principal energy source in the diets of most people and have a special role to play in energy metabolism and homoeostasis. Despite this, the energy values of some carbohydrates continue to be debated. For certain carbohydrates, the discrepancies between combustible energy, digestible energy, metabolisable energy (ME) and net metabolisable energy (NME) may be considerable (see Figure 12.2).

The three most important food crops in the world are rice, wheat and corn. These are staples of diets in many countries. Starch and sugars in these crops provide 50–75 per cent of energy in the diets of the world's population, more than that provided by fats or proteins. The actual amount of energy depends on the quantity of food consumed, its composition and the efficiency of carbohydrate digestion. About 89 per cent of carbohydrate in Western diets is digested, possibly less in diets where starchy foods are staples. This is metabolisable or glycaemic carbohydrate, and it supplies the body with 17 kJ of energy for every gram absorbed.

Not all carbohydrate is digested and absorbed. In defining the role that carbohydrate plays in metabolism, it is important to recognise that the site, rate and extent of carbohydrate digestion in and absorption from the gut is key to understanding the many roles that this group of chemically related compounds and their metabolic products play in the body. However, even the concept of digestibility has different meanings. Digestion occurs in the small (upper) bowel, while fermentation occurs in the large (lower) bowel. Although both processes result in the breakdown of food and absorption of energy-yielding substrates, the term 'digestibility' is reserved for events occurring in the upper gut. However, in the discussion of the energy value of foods, digestibility is defined as the proportion of **combustible energy** that is absorbed over the entire length of the gastrointestinal tract.

For the sake of determining energy values of carbohydrate that are of practical use, and of ascribing health benefits to individual classes of them, some coherence needs to be brought to the use of the terms 'digestible', 'digestion' and 'digestibility', and to integrating the whole of the gut process into the equation of energy balance.

Some of the polyols, some of the oligosaccharides, some starch and all of the NSP in diets pass through the small intestine and into the colon. They may be fermented in the colon by resident bacteria, resulting in the production of more bacterial cells, water, carbon dioxide and SCFAs such as acetic, propionic and butyric acids. However, some of the undigested carbohydrate may be excreted unchanged in the faeces. It has been estimated that typical Western diets provide 20–76 g of undigested carbohydrate each day; the question that then arises is, how much energy do we obtain from this? The answer depends on the extent of fermentation and how much of the bacterial SCFAs are taken up by cells lining the colon for use as fuels by human

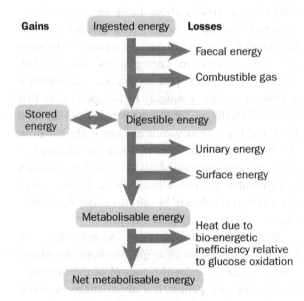

Figure 12.2: The flow of energy through the body
Source: Elia & Cummings (2007)

cells. For Australians consuming diets that provide no more than about 70 g undigested carbohydrate per day, the average energy supplied is estimated to be 8.4 kJ/g. This is described as the non-glycaemic contribution of carbohydrate to dietary energy. When foods are labelled for their energy content, both the glycaemic and non-glycaemic portions of the carbohydrate components need to be measured and appropriate factors applied (see Chapter 13). The Food Standards Code (FSANZ 2016) assigns an energy factor value of 17 kJ/g for glycaemic carbohydrate (called 'carbohydrate excluding unavailable carbohydrate' in the Code) and 8 kJ/g for non-glycaemic carbohydrate ingredients (called 'unavailable carbohydrate including dietary fibre' in the Code).

The role of carbohydrate as a regulator of appetite and energy expenditure is a subject for intensive study, propelled by the rise in obesity in many countries. Carbohydrate is generally more satiating than fat, but less satiating than protein (Chambers et al. 2015). However, studies of eating behaviour indicate that appetite regulation does not unconditionally depend on the oxidation of one nutrient and argues against the operation of a simple carbohydrate oxidation or storage model of feeding behaviour to the exclusion of other macronutrients (Mann et al. 2007). The control of appetite operates through a system with many redundancies and does not rely overwhelmingly on one or two major factors, such as energy density or on a specific macronutrient. Rather it depends on multiple factors that can interact, compensate or override each other, depending on environmental exposures and their duration. These include sensory factors, diet composition and variety of available food items, eating environment and individual subject characteristics, such as age, habitual dietary intake and prior social conditioning. It has been difficult to establish the relative importance of these factors, which are likely to differ with the environmental setting. In the light of this evidence, the role of different types of carbohydrates in eating behaviour might not be expected to have large effects on long-term energy homeostasis, and intervention studies are generally consistent with this view.

OLIGOSACCHARIDES AND GUT MICROBIOTA

Carbohydrates that reach the large bowel enter a very different type of metabolism, determined by the anaerobic microbiota of this organ, and in so doing exert an important influence on its function. However, uncertainty remains regarding the exact amounts and types of carbohydrate that reach the caecum (the first part of the large bowel) and are available for fermentation. This is largely because of the difficulties of studying this area of the gut and of variations in food processing, stage of maturity at which plant foods are eaten, post-harvest changes, day-to-day fluctuations in food intake and individual differences in gut function. It is estimated that the amounts of non-starch polysaccharides, resistant starch, non-alpha-glucan oligosaccharides, polyols and lactose that reach the large bowel are between 20 g and 40 g/day in countries with industrialised diets high in processed foods. They could reach 50 g/day where traditional staples are largely cereals or diets are high in fruit and/or vegetables (Mann et al. 2007).

GLYCAEMIC INDEX AND GLYCAEMIC LOAD

Following a meal, carbohydrates are digested and absorbed, causing a rise in blood glucose concentrations that achieves a maximum at about 30 minutes and then returns to fasting levels after 90–180 minutes. A graphical plot of glucose concentration against time gives a roughly bell-shaped curve that reflects both the rate of glucose supply from digested food and the rate at which glucose is cleared from the blood. Carbohydrates in foods are digested at different rates, and individuals have varying capacities to metabolise glucose following a meal. The sum of these factors is reflected by the area under the blood–glucose–time curve (Figure 12.3).

People with diabetes, for example, have an impaired capacity to clear glucose from the blood, a process that is under the control of the hormone insulin. For such people, it is important to eat foods that liberate glucose slowly during digestion to produce 'flatter' blood glucose curves (i.e. the peak

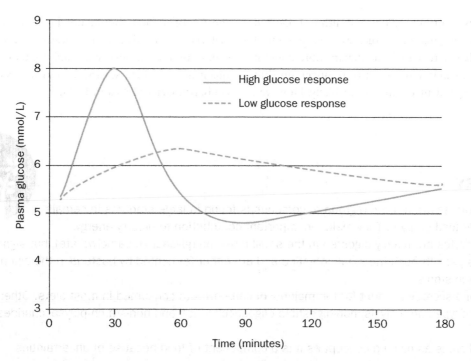

Figure 12.3: Typical blood glucose responses to high and low-GI foods

levels of glucose are not as high). These foods can be identified by comparing areas under the blood glucose curves obtained under standard conditions. Average values from a number of people are calculated, the result being the '**glycaemic index**' (GI) of the food.

The GI of a food is defined as the area under the two-hour blood glucose response curve following the ingestion of a fixed portion of carbohydrate, usually 50 g. The area under the curve of the test food is divided by the area under the curve of the standard, which is either glucose or white bread (giving two different values), multiplied by 100. Bread is a reference food and is used as a means of classifying other carbohydrate-containing foods in physiological and metabolic terms, rather than solely on chemical measures.

The average GI value is calculated from data collected in ten human subjects. It is essential that both the standard and test food contain an equal amount of available carbohydrate. The result gives a relative ranking for each tested food. Typical GI values are 30–50 for beans and lentils, 50–70 for

pasta and 70–100 for breads. Foods with large amounts of sugars have higher values than foods with large amounts of starch. In any individual, the height of the maximum glucose concentration and the rate of return to the fasting value varies due to a number of factors: the nature of the food; the method of processing; the physiological capacity of the individual to digest, absorb and metabolise carbohydrate; and the speed and viscosity of the food undergoing digestion as it passes through the absorptive sites of the intestine.

The GI can be used to guide food choices, particularly when similar carbohydrate-containing foods are being considered. For example, the GI of different types of bread can vary considerably, resulting in different '**glycaemic loads**' (GL).

Although there are many limitations to the concepts of GI and GL, they are widely regarded as being helpful for making healthy food choices. The GI and GL values of nearly 1300 food items have been compiled from documented and undocumented verified sources (Brand Miller 2018; Foster-Powell et al. 2002). The idea that low GI foods and low GL diets contribute to better health is supported by results of population studies as well as clinical trials. The degree to which the dietary fibre content of foods contributes to benefits is uncertain, but benefits independent of fibre seem likely. However, the GI of a food should not be used as the only criteria for food choice, because some low GI foods are also energy-dense and contain substantial quantities of added sugars, fat and undesirable fatty acids, primarily SFAs and TFAs.

SUMMARY

- Carbohydrates are a diverse group of compounds found in large amounts in cereals and other food staples. They make an important contribution to dietary energy.
- Carbohydrates are mainly digested in the small intestine (glycaemic carbohydrate), but significant amounts pass through the small intestine and are either fermented by bacteria in the colon or excreted in stools.
- Starch and sucrose account for the majority of carbohydrate consumed in most diets. Other important types are polyols, non-digestible oligosaccharides and non-starch polysaccharides (NSP).
- Dietary fibre is as much a concept as it is a component of food because of uncertainties surrounding the way in which it should be defined.
- The two principal components of dietary fibre are cell wall polysaccharides (NSP) from cereals, fruit and vegetables, and undigested (resistant) starch from a variety of different foods.
- Although it has well-defined chemical and physical characteristics, the effects of dietary fibre on health may not be as important as previously thought. Epidemiological evidence suggests it is not fibre alone that is protective against disease. Instead, that protection—where it occurs—is also conferred by a range of other food components found in fibre-rich foods and diets.

KEY TERMS

Combustible energy: total energy released when a substance undergoes complete combustion with oxygen.

Complex carbohydrate: a carbohydrate composed of a large number of monosaccharide building blocks such as glucose molecules.

Fractional extraction: a process of separating one or more solutes using a series of solvents with varying degrees of solubility.

Glycaemic index (GI): a scale used to rank carbohydrates in foods according to their effect on blood glucose levels. It measures how much and how fast or slow the rise of blood glucose is when a food is consumed.

Glycaemic load (GL): The GL is calculated as the quantity of carbohydrate in grams of a food or diet, multiplied by its GI and divided by 100. While the GI is valuable in planning diets for those with diabetes, where it is desirable to keep the blood glucose as low as possible through the consumption of foods with low GI, the concept of GL is helpful for those with diabetes in managing blood glucose concentrations.

Lignin: a complex polymer of phenylpropane units that form the structural materials of cell walls, especially in wood and bark. Of the polymers found in plant cell walls, lignin is the only one that is not composed of sugar monomers.

Polymerisation: a chemical reaction in which two or more identical molecules (called monomers) combine to form a larger molecule (called a polymer). The degree of polymerisation is the number of monomeric units in a polymer molecule.

'Sugar': the generic name for sweet-tasting carbohydrates. The body breaks down carbohydrates into simple sugars such as glucose. Several different sugars occur naturally in some foods such as fruit and dairy products.

ACKNOWLEDGEMENT

This chapter has been modified and updated from the 'Carbohydrates' chapter written by Gwynn P. Jones and Jonathan M. Hodgson which appeared in the third edition of *Food and Nutrition*.

REFERENCES

Al Hasan, S.M., Hassan, M., Saha, S., Islam, M., Billah, M. & Islam, S., 2016, 'Dietary phytate intake inhibits the bioavailability of iron and calcium in the diets of pregnant women in rural Bangladesh: A cross-sectional study', *BMC Nutrition, 2*(1): 24, doi:10.1186/s40795-016-0064-8

Brand Miller, J.C., 2018, 'The International Glycaemic Index Database', <https://researchdata.ands.org.au/international-glycemic-index-gi-database/11115>, accessed 22 November 2018

Chambers, L., McCrickerd, K. & Yeomans, M.R., 2015, 'Optimising foods for satiety', *Trends in Food Science & Technology, 41*(2): 149–60, doi:10.1016/j.tifs.2014.10.007

Corgneau, M., Scher, J., Ritie-Pertusa, L., Le, D.t.l., Petit, J. et al., 2017, 'Recent advances on lactose intolerance: Tolerance thresholds and currently available answers', *Critical Reviews in Food Science and Nutrition, 57*(15): 3344–56, doi:10.1080/10408398.2015.1123671

Cummings, J.H. & Engineer, A., 2018, 'Denis Burkitt and the origins of the dietary fibre hypothesis', *Nutrition Research Reviews, 31*(1): 1–15, doi:10.1017/S0954422417000117

Cummings, J.H. & Stephen, A.M., 2007, 'Carbohydrate terminology and classification', *European Journal of Clinical Nutrition, 61*: S5–S18, doi:10.1038/sj.ejcn.1602936

Elia, M. & Cummings, J.H., 2007, 'Physiological aspects of energy metabolism and gastrointestinal effects of carbohydrates', *European Journal of Clinical Nutrition, 61*: S40–S74, doi:10.1038/sj.ejcn.1602938

Englyst, H.N. & Cummings, J.H., 1990, 'Non-starch polysaccharides (dietary fiber) and resistant starch', in I. Furda & C.J. Brine (eds), *New Developments in Dietary Fiber: Physiological, physicochemical, and analytical aspects*, New York and London: Plenum Press, pp. 205–25

Fedewa, A. & Rao, S.S.C., 2014, 'Dietary fructose intolerance, fructan intolerance and FODMAPs', *Current Gastroenterology Reports, 16*(1): 370, doi:10.1007/s11894-013-0370-0

Foster-Powell, K., Holt, S.H.A. & Brand-Miller, J.C., 2002, 'International table of glycemic index and glycemic load values', *American Journal of Clinical Nutrition, 76*(1): 5–56, doi:10.1093/ajcn/76.1.5

FSANZ, 2016, *Food Standards Code*, <www.foodstandards.gov.au/code/Pages/default.aspx>, accessed 22 November 2018

Gibson, R.S., Raboy, V. & King, J.C., 2018, 'Implications of phytate in plant-based foods for iron and zinc bioavailability, setting dietary requirements, and formulating programs and policies', *Nutrition Reviews, 76*(11): 793–804, doi:10.1093/nutrit/nuy028

Grases, F., Prieto, R.M. & Costa-Bauza, A., 2017, 'Dietary phytate and interactions with mineral nutrients', in O.M. Gutiérrez, K. Kalantar-Zadeh & R. Mehrotra (eds), *Clinical Aspects of Natural and Added Phosphorus in Foods*, New York, NY: Springer, pp. 175–83

Haber, G.B., Heaton, K.W., Murphy, D. & Burroughs, L.F., 1977, 'Depletion and disruption of dietary fibre: Effects on satiety, plasma-glucose, and serum-insulin', *Lancet, 310*(8040): 679–82, doi:10.1016/S0140-6736(77)90494-9

Hurduc, V., Bordei, L., Plesca, V. & Plesca, D.A., 2017, 'OC-30 Lactose intolerance: New aspects of an old problem', *Archives of Disease in Childhood, 102*(Suppl 2): A11, doi:10.1136/archdischild-2017-313273.30

Lewis, S.J. & Heaton, K.W., 1999, 'Roughage revisited (the effect on intestinal function of inert plastic particles of different sizes and shape)', *Digestive Diseases and Sciences, 44*(4): 744–8, doi:10.1023/a:1026613909403

Lukito, W., Malik, S.G., Surono, I.S. & Wahlqvist, M.L., 2015, 'From "lactose intolerance" to "lactose nutrition"', *Asia Pacific Journal of Clinical Nutrition, 24*(S1): s1–s8, doi:10.6133/apjcn.2015.24.s1.01

Mann, J., Cummings, J.H., Englyst, H.N., Key, T., Liu, S. et al., 2007, 'FAO/WHO scientific update on carbohydrates in human nutrition: Conclusions', *European Journal of Clinical Nutrition, 61*: S132–7, doi:10.1038/sj.ejcn.1602943

NHMRC, 2006, *Nutrition Reference Values for Australia and New Zealand*, Canberra: <https://nhmrc.gov.au/sites/default/files/images/nutrient-refererence-dietary-intakes.pdf>, accessed 22 November 2018

Staudacher, H.M. & Whelan, K., 2017, 'The low FODMAP diet: Recent advances in understanding its mechanisms and efficacy in IBS', *Gut, 66*(8): 1517–27, doi:10.1136/gutjnl-2017-313750

Trowell, H., 1972, 'Crude fibre, dietary fibre and atherosclerosis', *Atherosclerosis, 16*(1): 138–40, doi:10.1016/0021-9150(72)90017-2

Whelan, K., Martin, L., Staudacher, H. & Lomer, M., 2018, 'The low FODMAP diet in the management of irritable bowel syndrome: An evidence-based review of FODMAP restriction, reintroduction and personalisation in clinical practice', *Journal of Human Nutrition and Dietetics, 31*(2): 239–55, doi:10.1111/jhn.12530

WHO/FAO, 1998, *Carbohydrates in Human Nutrition*, <www.who.int/nutrition/publications/nutrientrequirements/9251041148/en/>, accessed 22 November 2018

{CHAPTER 13}
MACRONUTRIENTS: FOOD ENERGY

Mark L. Wahlqvist and Naiyana Wattanapenpaiboon

OBJECTIVES

- Describe how food is converted into energy in the body.
- Explain how energy requirements are determined.
- Summarise the impact of food, physical activity and illness on energy expenditure and requirements.
- Calculate the proportional energy contribution made by different macronutrients.
- Describe the energy density of a variety of foods.
- Summarise the physiological mechanisms of energy deprivation.

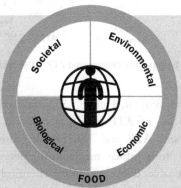

FOOD

INTRODUCTION

Living organisms require energy to maintain life. Energy is obtained by oxidation of fuels, which include carbohydrates, fats, proteins and alcohol. The oxidation process is complex, involving a large number of enzyme-mediated steps. In the case of carbohydrate being a substrate, starch—which is the major carbohydrate consumed—is broken down to the sugar glucose; this is then oxidised to carbon dioxide and water.

glucose + oxygen ➔ carbon dioxide + water + energy
$C_6H_{12}O_6$ + O_2 ➔ $6CO_2$ + $6H_2O$

Most of the energy released by this oxidation is obtained from the oxidation of hydrogen to water. This is a 'coupled' reaction, in which oxidation of hydrogen is coupled by an enzyme to the phosphorylation of adenosine diphosphate (ADP). An inorganic phosphate group (HPO_4^{2-}—abbreviated P_i) is added to adenosine diphosphate (ADP) to form adenosine triphosphate (ATP) (Figure 13.1). ATP is a large molecule that functions as an energy carrier within the cell. The oxidation of hydrogen is a 'downhill' reaction—that is, it occurs easily with the release of a relatively large amount of energy. This can be demonstrated by lighting a hydrogen gas flame; it burns readily, releasing energy as heat. The formation of ATP is an 'uphill' reaction, which means it does not occur spontaneously because, for the reaction to proceed, energy must be put in. An enzyme called ATP synthase is able to couple these two reactions together. The downhill oxidation of hydrogen is used to drive the uphill synthesis of ATP, similar to charging a battery.

ATP is subsequently used to drive other energy-requiring processes in the cell. Such processes include protein synthesis for growth or muscle contraction

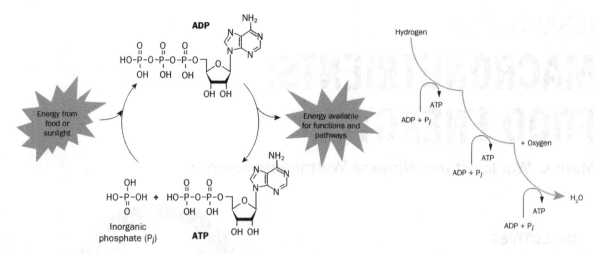

Figure 13.1: Energy metabolism and ATP/ADP cycle

to enable movement. Figure 13.2 summarises the overall process of ATP production from glucose oxidation and ATP use for muscle movement. In muscles, to produce mechanical energy, 'ATP hydrolysis' enables the release of the chemical energy that has been stored in ATP. The product is ADP and P_i, and ADP can be further hydrolysed to give energy, adenosine monophosphate and another P_i. ATP hydrolysis is considered to be the final link between the energy derived from food energy sources and metabolic functions, such as muscle contraction, and the biosynthetic and homeostatic processes necessary to maintain life.

UNITS OF ENERGY

Energy (or work) is expressed in the SI (System International) *joule* unit. The joule is a small unit and, for convenience, food energy is more often expressed in *kilojoules* (kJ, 1000 joules) or megajoules (MJ, 1,000,000 joules). An older unit, the calorie—which

is defined as the amount of energy required to raise the temperature of one gram of water by one degree Celsius—is still widely used. Again, the *kilocalorie* (kcal, 1000 calories) is a more convenient size. The term 'Calorie' (with a capital C) is sometimes used when referring to a kilocalorie but, to avoid confusion, the more accurate term kilocalorie (kcal) is preferred. One kcal is equal to 4.18 kJ.

FUELS FOR ENERGY

The energy available to the body from the enzymatic oxidative reaction of a macronutrient or other fuels can be determined simply by burning an amount of the latter in oxygen and measuring the heat energy released using an instrument called a bomb calorimeter. This instrument consists of a steel cylinder into which a small sample of food—about 1 g—is placed. High-pressure oxygen is introduced from a cylinder and the food sample ignited by a wire heated with an electric current. The food

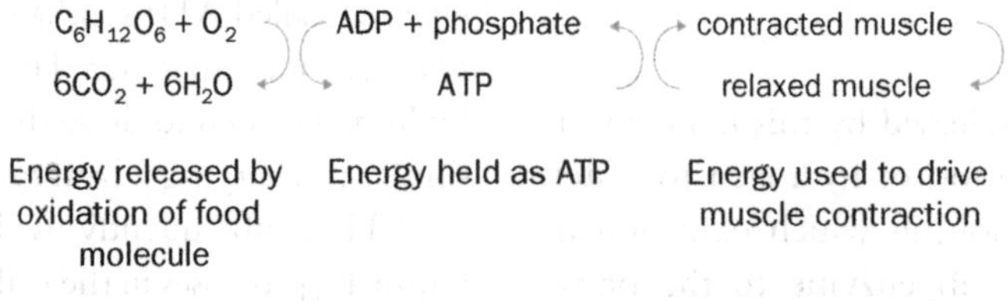

$$C_6H_{12}O_6 + O_2 \qquad ADP + phosphate \qquad contracted\ muscle$$
$$6CO_2 + 6H_2O \qquad ATP \qquad relaxed\ muscle$$

Energy released by oxidation of food molecule   Energy held as ATP   Energy used to drive muscle contraction

Figure 13.2: Energy production from glucose oxidation and energy use for muscle contraction

burns readily in the oxygen and the heat given off is measured by the rise in temperature of the steel cylinder.

The energy available to the human body, or net energy, is in fact slightly less than the gross energy, or that released by combustion in the bomb calorimeter. There are two reasons for this. The first is the efficiency of digestion and absorption. Digestion and absorption are efficient processes, but not 100 per cent efficient; small amounts of the macronutrients are lost in the faeces. The efficiency of digestion and absorption of carbohydrate is normally close to 99 per cent, of fat about 95 per cent and of protein 92 per cent. The second reason, which relates particularly to protein, is that the end products of metabolism are not the same as the end products of combustion. The end products of metabolism of protein are mainly urea with some ammonia and smaller amounts of other nitrogenous compounds, all of which are excreted through the kidney in the urine. For protein, the gross energy is 23 kJ/g, while the net energy is 17 kJ/g.

The generally accepted values for energy from macronutrients were determined via bomb calorimetry and defined as energy available in usual 'Western' diets (Table 13.1). These values are sometimes referred to as the Atwater factors after the American chemist Wilbur Atwater, who developed a system in the 19th century for allocating energy values to foods. The system uses a single energy value (factor) for each of the main groups of energy nutrients (protein, fat and carbohydrate), regardless of the food in which it is found. The energy values (based on the average

heats of combustion of each group and corrected for losses in digestion, absorption and urinary excretion of urea), or the Atwater general factors, are 17 kJ/g (4.0 kcal/g) for protein, 37 kJ/g (9.0 kcal/g) for fat and 17 kJ/g (4.0 kcal/g) for carbohydrates. The system also includes a rounded energy value for alcohol of 29 kJ/g (7.0 kcal/g). Partly because of its simplicity, the Atwater general factor system is still widely used today to estimate the net metabolisable energy of typically consumed foods.

However, these values are not necessarily exact, particularly when it comes to carbohydrate. The value for starch is close to 17 kJ/g and for glucose and sucrose 16 kJ/g. Not all carbohydrate is digestible by pancreatic enzymes. Various cell wall components (unavailable carbohydrate or dietary fibre—see Chapter 12) escape digestion in the small intestine and move into the large intestine, where they may be fermented by gut bacteria to produce organic acids that can be absorbed and metabolised for energy. Thus, dietary fibre is usually given an average energy value of 8 kJ/g. The overall availability of energy is less if the food comes as a bulky vegetarian diet because, for food items such as whole grains and undercooked vegetables, the digestive enzymes have less ready access to the food molecules and more consequently escape digestion, ultimately being lost in the faeces.

The Atwater factors refer to metabolisable energy values; however, only the net energy value is available for body maintenance, exercise, growth, weight gain or, in the case of mothers, milk production. For example, the net energy value for protein is approximately 14 kJ/g, significantly less than the 17 kJ/g Atwater factor. The difference is explained by the thermogenesis, or the thermic effect, of feeding, which is the increase in energy expenditure associated with consuming, digesting and assimilating food. In the case of meeting human energy requirements, it cannot be assumed that the energy of thermogenesis is necessarily wasted. One of the requirements of the body is sufficient energy to maintain body temperature, and if environmental temperature is lowered, food energy intake will be increased. The energy of thermogenesis is meeting

Table 13.1: Energy yield of major food macromolecules

Food macromolecules	Gross energy* (kJ/g)	Net energy† (kJ/g)
Carbohydrate	17	16
Sugar	17	16
Fat	39	37
Protein	23	17
Alcohol	29	27

Notes: * Amount of gross energy as measured with a bomb calorimeter;
† Amount of net energy available for metabolism

CALCULATING THE AMOUNT OF ENERGY CONSUMED

Calculate the amount of energy consumed via fat, protein and carbohydrate in kJ and as a percentage of the total for the following cases.

- John Jones is consuming a total of 10,200 kJ with 80 g fat and 120 g protein and remainder from carbohydrates. What is the total amount of energy from each of these sources?
- Thuy Nguyen is consuming 60 g fat, 80 g protein and 220 g of carbohydrate. What is her total energy intake and the percentage contribution from each energy source?
- Philip Cantellini is consuming 9000 kJ, of which 10 per cent is from alcohol. How much alcohol is he consuming? How does this convert to standard drinks?

A note about decimal places. When dietary intake values of both macro- and micronutrients are calculated a variety of sources are used, including an individual's recall of their diet, food composition tables, energy yield data and other sources. These all have inherent error. Consequently, information cannot be reported with any degree of accuracy. Therefore, reporting on dietary intake data of energy, macronutrients and micronutrients should generally be in whole numbers and not include any decimal places.

---

the need of temperature maintenance. However, in terms of supporting growth or adding to body fat, it is net energy value that is relevant.

The Atwater factor for fat is 37 kJ/g, whereas the energy theoretically available should vary between approximately 39.7 kJ/g for a saturated fat and 36 kJ/g for a highly unsaturated fat. However, biological assays of the net energy values for fats show that energy in highly saturated fat (beef fat, tallow, 31 kJ/g) is poorly available compared with pig fat (lard, 35 kJ/g), which is less saturated, and corn oil (38 kJ/g), which is highly unsaturated. This difference is explained mostly by the fact that SFAs—stearic and palmitic (18:0 and 16:0)—are absorbed from the intestine at only 80 per cent of the efficiency of the unsaturated fatty acids. Despite these differences, for most studies on usual Western diets, the present Atwater factors are regarded as satisfactory.

ENERGY EXPENDITURE

Energy expenditure is continuous but the rate varies throughout the day. Metabolic rate measured at the lowest rate of energy expenditure, usually after at least eight hours of rest and ten hours after the last meal, is referred to as **basal metabolic rate** (BMR). When resting—for example, sitting in a comfortable chair—the metabolic rate will be close to BMR; energy expenditure measured at rest but not under the specific conditions of BMR is usually referred to as resting metabolic rate.

DETERMINANTS OF BASAL METABOLIC RATE (BMR)

BMR values are usually in the range of 3–6 kJ/minute. A number of important factors determining BMR are listed below.

- Body size: larger bodies have more metabolising tissue and a higher BMR.
- Sex: on average, women tend to be smaller than men and therefore have a lower BMR.
- Body fat: fat tissue has a low metabolic rate because most of the fat cell (adipocyte) is taken up by a central oil globule. Bodies with a higher proportion of fat therefore have a lower BMR. A lean person of 70 kg would have a higher BMR than a 70 kg person with more body fat.

Women tend to have more body fat than men, and this is an additional reason why women, in general, have lower BMR values than men.

- Fasting: prolonged fasting or starvation can reduce BMR by up to 15 per cent. Spontaneous activity is also reduced, achieving a further 15 per cent reduction in energy expenditure. These two combine to reduce energy usage, and to conserve life.
- Hormonal and nervous controls: metabolic rate is controlled by the nervous and hormonal systems. The thyroid hormones, for example, play a key role; a person with an over-active thyroid has a raised metabolic rate.
- Infection or illness: severe infection, illness or injury commonly increases BMR. The rise in metabolic rate increases energy needs and may lead to more rapid weight loss in those who are ill.
- Certain substances: substances such as caffeine in coffee, nicotine (smoking tobacco) or drugs (prescription or illicit) raise metabolic rate slightly.

Estimating basal metabolic rate

A number of empirical equations have been developed for the estimation of basal or resting energy expenditure. Factors such as age, sex, height, weight and body surface area can be incorporated into such prediction equations. Analysis of the many experimental measurements of metabolic rate has shown that basal metabolic rate can be predicted as accurately from a set of simple equations incorporating sex, age and weight as it can from more complex equations.

There are over 30 different equations available for use to calculate resting energy expenditure (see Table 13.2). These prediction equations are not highly accurate, but they provide a useful estimate. In statistical terms, two-thirds of the predictions fall within about 8–10 per cent of the values measured for individuals. This is sufficiently accurate for the equations to be a useful basis for the estimation of energy requirements. The FAO/WHO have used the Schofield equations in their (FAO/WHO/UNU Expert Consultation 2001; Schofield 1985).

It should be noted that predictive equations are not considered accurate for individuals who are acutely and critically unwell.

However, the predictive equations have a number of limitations.

- They are based on subjects who are not representative of the same populations.
- Most are based on subjects in industrialised countries where energy expenditure is influenced by modern technology, school environments, sedentary pastimes and mechanised transport.
- Most are undertaken in temperate rather than tropical environments (resting metabolic rate is thought to be 5–20 per cent higher in tropical climates).
- They are not necessarily accurate for individuals due to inter- and intra-individual variation.
- Most require the use of injury factors, which have limited evidence. (Reeves & Capra 2003)

A much simpler and quicker way to estimate energy requirements is to use the ratio method. Requirements for energy are based on available evidence and expressed as amounts per kg of body weight. For non-hypermetabolic adults, energy requirements are in the range 100–125 kJ/kg. The requirements would go up to 125–145 kJ/kg for patients who are moderately hypermetabolic (e.g. post-surgery, infection, head injury), and to 145–160 kJ/kg for patients with hypermetabolic conditions (e.g. liver disease, burns to more than 20 per cent of the body).

While the predictive equations and the ratio method provide a useful starting point, the emphasis should be on regular reviewing and reassessment, considering changes to treatment goals, clinical conditions, biochemical and anthropometric parameters (see Chapter 23).

Energy expenditure with growth and development

BMR is higher in infants and children due to two factors: the energy demand of growth and the energy demand for maintenance of body temperature at 37°C, due to more rapid heat loss.

Table 13.2: Examples of predictive equations for resting energy expenditure

Equations	Units	Factors used in calculation	REE predictive equations
Harris Benedict 1919	kcal/d	Sex, WT (kg), HT (cm), age (y)	M: WT × 13.7516 + HT × 5.0033 – age × 6.755 + 66.473 F: WT × 9.5634 + HT × 1.8496 – age × 4.6756 + 655.0955
Harris Benedict 1984	kcal/d	Sex, WT (kg), HT (cm), age (y)	M: WT × 13.397 + HT × 4.799 – age × 5.677+ 88.362 F: WT × 9.247 + HT × 3.098 – age × 4.33 + 477.593
Mifflin et al.	kcal/d	Sex (M: 1; F:0), WT (kg), HT (cm)	9.99 × WT + 6.2 × HT – 4.92 × age + 166 × sex – 161
Mifflin et al. (BC)	kcal/d	FFM (kg)	19.7 × FFM + 413
World Schofield (age)	MJ/d	Sex WT (kg), age (y)	M: age 18–30y: 0.063 × WT + 2.896 M: age 30–60y: 0.048 × WT + 3.653 M: age ≥60y: 0.049 × WT + 2.459 F: age 18–30y: 0.062 × WT + 2.036 F: age 30–60y: 0.034 × WT + 3.538 F: age ≥60y: 0.038 × WT + 2.755
Schofield (WT, HT, age)	MJ/d	Sex, WT (kg), HT (m), age (y)	M: age 18–30y: 0.063 × WT – 0.042 × HT + 2.953 M: age 30–60y: 0.048 × WT – 0.011 × HT + 3.67 M: age ≥60y: 0.038 × WT + 4.068 × HT – 3.491 F: age 18–30y: 0.057 × WT + 1.148 × HT + 0.411 F: age 30–60y: 0.034 × WT + 0.006 × HT + 3.53 F: age ≥60y: 0.033 × WT + 1.917 × HT + 0.074
FAO (age)	kcal/d	Sex, WT (kg), age (y)	M: age 18–30y: 15.3 × WT + 679 M: age 30–60y: 11.6 × WT + 879 M: age ≥60y: 13.5 × WT + 487 F: age 18–30y: 14.7 × WT + 496 F: age 30–60y: 8.7 × WT + 829 F: age ≥60y: 10.5 × WT – 596
FAO (WT, HT, age)	kcal/d	Sex, WT (kg), HT (m), age (y)	M: age 18–30y: 15.4 × WT – 27 × HT + 717 M: age 30–60y: 11.3 × WT – 16 × HT + 901 M: age ≥60y: 8.8 × WT + 1128 × HT – 1071 F: age 18–30y: 13.3 × WT + 334 × HT + 35 F: age 30–60y: 8.7 × WT – 25 × HT + 865 F: age ≥60y: 9.2 × WT + 637 × HT + 302
Henry (age)	MJ/d	Sex, WT (kg), age (y)	M: age 18–30y: 0.0669 × WT + 2.28 M: age 30–60y: 0.0592 × WT + 2.48 M: age ≥60y: 0.0563 × WT + 2.15 F: age 18–30y: 0.0546 × WT + 2.33 F: age 30–60y: 0.0407 × WT + 2.9 F: age ≥60y: 0.0424 × WT + 2.38
Henry (WT, HT, age)	MJ/d	Sex, WT (kg), HT (m), age (y)	M: age 18–30y: 0.06 × WT + 1.31 × HT + 0.473 M: age 30–60y: 0.0476 × WT + 2.26 × HT – 0.574 M: age ≥60y: 0.0478 × WT + 2.26 × HT – 1.07 F: age 18–30y: 0.0433 × WT + 2.57 × HT – 1.18 F: age 30–60y: 0.0342 × WT + 2.1 × HT – 0.0486 F: age ≥60y: 0.0356 × WT + 1.76 × HT + 0.0448

Notes: WT = weight; HT = height; BC = body composition

Source: Jésus et al. (2015)

WHAT ARE YOUR ENERGY REQUIREMENTS?

Using your own details, height, weight, age and sex and the equations listed above in Table 13.2, as well as the ratio method, calculate your energy requirements.

- What are your maximum and minimum energy requirements?
- What has contributed to the variation?
- Which method was the easiest to calculate?

Growth involves more rapid protein turnover and, because protein synthesis and more rapid protein turnover require energy, total energy demand is increased. Total food energy intake, which reflects total energy expenditure, rises steeply with growth through early childhood and then more steadily in adulthood (Figure 13.3). BMR, which accounts for about half of total energy expenditure, also rises; the difference between BMR and total energy expenditure is accounted for mostly by physical activity and, to a small extent, the thermogenic effect of food. When energy intake and BMR are expressed on a per kilogram body weight basis, the rates of total energy utilisation and BMR are highest just after birth and fall gradually to maturity (see Chapter 21).

Thermic effect of food

The metabolic rate of a person at rest rises after eating. The thermic effect of food is this increase in energy expenditure associated with the energy cost of absorption and metabolism of food. This can be quite noticeable: one might feel cold before a meal, but comfortably warm afterwards. The extent of the increase is usually in the range 2–3 per cent up to 25–30 per cent, and varies with the size of the meal and the types of foods eaten. Dietary fat is very easy to process and raises metabolic rate least; carbohydrates have an intermediate effect; and protein has a much larger effect. The rate of metabolism begins to rise soon after eating commences and peaks two to three hours later. The thermic effect of food is the result of the many energy-requiring processes associated with eating, digesting and metabolising components of food. These include the work of peristalsis, synthesis and secretion of digestive enzymes, active transport of ions, sugars, amino acids, synthesis of amino acids into protein and excretory processes. In the overall energy balance of the body, the thermogenic effect of food adds 5–10 per cent to the total energy requirement.

The thermic effect of food is an important factor influencing energy balance and, ultimately, the development and maintenance of overweight and obesity. The thermic effect of food appears to be reduced with obesity, and this is related to the degree of insulin resistance. A higher protein intake increases thermogenesis. In addition to the well-described effect of protein on increasing satiety, it has been suggested that partially replacing refined carbohydrate in the diet with protein sources low in saturated fat could enhance weight loss (Hu 2005). The long-term impact of higher protein diets on energy balance in the setting of unrestricted diets remains uncertain. Many studies have assessed the medium-term (six months to two years) effects on weight loss, and maintenance of weight loss, in overweight individuals of diets with differing proportions of protein, carbohydrate and/or fat (Naude et al. 2014; Sacks et al. 2009). Higher-protein diets have not consistently produced better weight loss outcomes. In the setting of overweight and obesity, the focus remains on reducing energy intake and increasing energy expenditure with exercise, rather than any particular proportions of protein, fat or carbohydrate in the diet.

Water can also have a thermic effect and alter energy balance, albeit having no intrinsic energy value. This may be mediated via its effects on the autonomic nervous system through sympathetic activation (Boschmann et al. 2003).

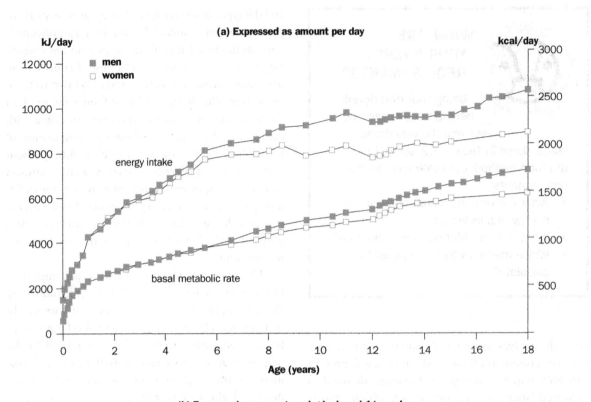

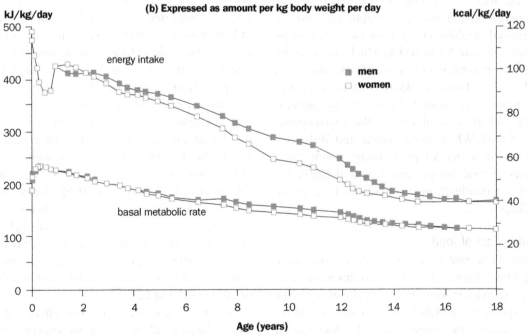

Figure 13.3: Total energy intake and basal metabolic rate from birth to adolescence

Source: Schutz & Jequier (1994)

Energy expenditure in physical work or exercise

The most variable component of total energy expenditure is physical work or exercise. Some individuals expend very little energy and are largely sedentary. As a result, their total energy expenditure is not greater than 1.2–1.4 times BMR. For those engaged in active sport or heavy physical work, total energy expenditure for the day may be more than two times BMR. Energy expenditure in work or exercise can be expressed as kilojoules per minute or a multiple of BMR.

Both BMR and energy expenditure in activities involving body movement tend to be proportional to body weight. Thus, a person with a high body weight has a relatively high BMR because of the larger amount of muscle (lean tissue) required to carry the larger body. In addition, this person has a higher rate of energy expenditure in movement activities, such as walking, sports and most physical work. The converse is true for a person of light weight. When rates of energy expenditure in physical activity for the light person and the heavy person are expressed as multiples of BMR, it is found that the difference in BMR is proportional to the

differences in energy expenditure in activity (see also Chapter 30). It is therefore convenient to categorise the rates of energy expenditure for different activities as multiples of BMR, thus avoiding any necessity to adjust the rate of energy expenditure for the body weight of the individual. Table 13.3 gives rates of energy expenditure for a range of common activities.

Note that for heavy industrial work the energy expenditure might be five times BMR, but the average energy expenditure for the day may be nearer two times BMR. This is because, first, the work period is seldom longer than about eight hours a day and, second, during that eight hours' work, the worker would normally take regular rests.

Measuring and calculating energy expenditure

When exercise or work is undertaken, the metabolic rate rises steeply as energy is used by muscles. The rates of energy expenditure of the individual organs also vary: nervous tissue, including the brain, tends to have an even rate of energy use, while the liver—the major centre of metabolism—has a relatively high rate of energy use, and this is increased after meals when absorbed nutrients are being processed. The energy

Table 13.3: Rates of energy expenditure in activities expressed as multiples of BMR

Activity level	Rate of energy expenditure	
	x BMR	**(range)**
BMR	1	
Resting, sitting or lying	1.2	1.1–1.3
Very light sitting handwork, playing cards, writing, talking, driving, standing with some moving around	1.5	1.3–2.0
Light (no obvious effect on comfort or breathing) strolling around, standing bench work, cooking, weaving, light cleaning or gardening	2.5	2–3
Moderate (stimulation of deeper breathing) light industrial or farm work, laying bricks, carpentry, dancing, tennis, walking with a 10 kg load, digging garden	3.5	3–4
Heavy (sweating if warm, breathing heavy, activity usually not continuous, intermittent rest) digging, chopping wood, industrial work, shovelling, loading, pushing wheelbarrow, jogging steadily, football, netball (average over game)	5.0	4–6
Very heavy (breathing laboured, sweating freely, unable to continue for more than a few minutes unless physically very fit) running, active football, swimming fast	7.0	6–8

Source: FAO/WHO/UNU Expert Consultation (1985)

expenditure of the muscles makes up only 20 per cent or so of the total energy expenditure at rest, but during strenuous exercise the rate of energy expenditure of the muscles may go up 50-fold or more. Methods for measuring energy expenditure are described in Table 13.4.

RECOMMENDED INTAKES FOR FOOD ENERGY

Estimation of 'safe and adequate' intakes for food energy are based on basal metabolism, plus an allowance for physical activity. These estimates are adequate for groups; however, if energy requirement is to be calculated for an individual, BMR would need to be measured because individual BMR values may vary by up to 20 per cent.

For children aged one to ten, there is little information on the types, duration and energy cost of activities, so the estimate of a safe and adequate intake of energy has been based on measured food energy intakes of healthy children plus a 5 per cent additional allowance for 'desirable' levels of physical activity. Since the introduction of the doubly labelled water technique for measuring energy expenditure, it has been possible to measure the total energy expenditure of infants and children, revealing that energy allowances previously based on estimates of intakes had overestimated requirements of children less than seven years by about 20 per cent, but allowances for older children were reasonably accurate.

From birth to ten years, the energy allowance estimations do not distinguish between girls and boys, but from eleven years there are separate allowances for boys and girls to allow for the different ages of onset of puberty and diverging activity patterns. There are significant differences in the age of onset of puberty of individual boys and girls, and there is a marked increase in energy requirement with the rapid increase in height and weight during pubertal growth. It should be emphasised, therefore, that the 'safe and adequate intakes' are a guide for population groups and cannot be applied to individuals.

Regulation of food energy intakes

The mechanisms that regulate food energy intake to meet demand are extremely complex. They involve neural connections (gut to brain and within the brain) and a variety of hormones, and they include negative feedback. The hypothalamus in the lower-central area of the brain is critical in the control of food intake. It mediates the regulation of short-term (within meal, next meal and over one to two days) and long-term (weeks to months) intake.

Table 13.4: Methods for measuring energy expenditure

Direct calorimetry	Measures heat generated. The subject is placed in a special chamber fitted with heat sensors to allow accurate measurement of heat released. Method cannot be used for ordinary activities. Expensive.
Indirect calorimetry	Measures oxidation of energy via either rate of oxygen uptake or carbon dioxide output. Subject has hood placed over head so that all the air breathed out is collected. The volume of air expired is measured and its concentration of oxygen determined. Since the concentration of oxygen in air is known, the amount of oxygen taken out of the air can be calculated.
Doubly labelled water	Based on the premise that after a dose of doubly labelled water, which contains 'heavy' hydrogen (^{2}H, deuterium) and heavy oxygen (^{18}O), the two isotopes equilibrate with total body water and then are eliminated differentially from the body. Over a period of two to three weeks after the oral administration of doubly labelled water, deuterium (^{2}H) leaves the body as the water of urine and sweat, and heavy oxygen (^{18}O) leaves as water (H_2O) and carbon dioxide (CO_2) in exhaled breath. The production of carbon dioxide can be calculated by subtracting ^{2}H elimination from ^{18}O elimination. Measurement of the ^{2}H and ^{18}O remaining in the body at the end of the experimental period allows calculation of the total carbon dioxide production over this period, and therefore of energy metabolism. Most accurate but expensive.

The interface between physical, neural and hormonal mechanisms is described in Chapter 9.

Even less is known about the long-term control of food energy intake. The existence of a long-term control is demonstrated by the observation that in a person who diets to lose weight or loses weight as a result of illness, body weight is usually regained over a period of months or years until the body fat is approximately the same or greater than before the loss of weight. This long-term control of the body energy reserve stored as triglyceride fat appears to be under the control of a hormone called leptin. The discovery of leptin appeared to be the long sought-after peripheral signal pathway from adipose tissue to the brain involved in energy balance (see also Chapter 9).

Most individuals maintain approximately constant weight, and therefore food energy intake is equal to energy expenditure. In the course of a single day, there is little correlation between energy intake and expenditure, but there is a high correlation over a four-day period. It is therefore apparent that food energy intake is regulated to cope with the demands of basal metabolism and physical activity. In a controlled environment, when energy intake is restricted, resting metabolic rate appears to be reduced and the energy expended in activity is less. However, this regulation is probably of relatively minor importance in regulating energy balance in individuals having a normal free intake of food.

It is difficult to be specific about the feelings that lead to cessation of eating. Much of the short-term control of food intake is mediated by habit and custom—for example, we might eat breakfast because we usually eat breakfast, not because we feel noticeably hungry at that time. Meals tend to have a usual structure and a usual size, and meals tend to end when the usual amount has been eaten rather than because we cannot eat any more. Food choice and meal pattern tend to be set by family experience and cultural environment.

Energy density in food

'Energy density' is the amount of energy per gram of food. Table 13.5 gives the amount of food energy

Table 13.5: Food energy content of a range of common foods

Food	Energy (kJ/g)	Food	Energy (kJ/g)
Salad oil, fat	37	Fish, steamed	7
Butter, margarine	30	Rice, boiled	5.2
Peanuts, roasted	24	Spaghetti, cooked	5
Chocolate	23	Peas, boiled	4.4
Biscuit, choc-coated	22	Ice cream (/mL)	3.8
Potato crisps	21	Banana	3.4
Biscuit, sweet	20	Potato, boiled	3.2
Toffee	18	Milk, whole	2.8
Cheese, tasty	17	Grapes	2.7
Cornflakes	15.5	Milk, 2% fat	2.3
Fruit cake	14	Yoghurt, natural	2.2
Sugar candy	14	Soft drink	2
Cheese, processed	13	Apple	2
Bread, toasted	12.5	Orange	1.5
Honey	12	Milk, skimmed	1.4
Jam	11	Carrots, boiled	0.8
Bread, white	10	Pumpkin, boiled	0.65
Bread, wholemeal	9	Tomato	0.6
Steak, lean and fat, grilled	9	Lettuce, mushrooms	0.5
Avocado	9	Cauliflower, boiled	0.4

in 40 common foods. It is important to see the wide range of energy content from the highest-energy foods to the lowest. Lower energy density foods provide less energy per gram of food. The two factors that are most important in determining the energy content of a food are water content and fat content. Low energy density foods include foods with a high water content, such as soups and stews, foods like pasta and rice that absorb water during cooking, and foods that are naturally high in water, such as fruit and vegetables. Fibre in foods like wholegrains and potatoes with skin can also help to reduce energy density. Most dried foods have a moderately high energy content, which is reduced when the food is rehydrated by cooking in water.

ENERGY-DENSE VERSUS NUTRIENT-DENSE FOODS

Certain foods are high in energy and low in nutrients (energy-dense/nutrient-poor foods) while others are nutrient-dense. Nutrient density refers to the amount of nutrient a food contains per a unit of energy it provides. Nutrient-dense foods are foods that are high in nutrients but relatively low in energy. Examples of nutrient-dense foods include fruit and vegetables, whole grains, low-fat milk products, lean meat, eggs, beans and nuts. Foods or beverages with 'empty calories' or described as energy-dense/nutrient-poor are those that provide food energy but little or no other nutritional value. They contain primarily sugar, fats or oils, or alcohol.

Develop a list of foods that are energy-dense but nutrient-poor.

- What is the primary contributor to the energy in these foods?
- Why do you think people prefer foods high in fat?
- What would be your response to somebody who said that fats are not good for health and they all need to be avoided?

High energy density foods tend to include foods that are high in fat and have a low water content—for example, biscuits and confectionery, crisps, peanuts, butter and cheese. Foods that are pure fats (fat and oil) provide about 37 kJ in each gram, while those with the lowest energy content, salad vegetables, have only one-hundredth of this value (0.3 kJ/g to 0.4 kJ/g). All of the foods providing 20 kJ or more per gram have a relatively high fat content and a low water content, while the salad vegetables have almost no fat (less than 0.5 per cent) and water contents in excess of 90 per cent. Evidence suggests that diets with a low energy density can help people maintain a healthy body weight.

FASTING AND STARVATION

Fasting and starvation both are states of abstinence from food. The main differences between the two are the purpose and length of time of that abstinence. In both cases, the physiological changes that take place help the body adapt to the nutrient deficit. Fasting is typically performed for a defined period of time for a particular purpose, such as a religious practice, in preparation for a medical procedure or to 'cleanse' the body. While fasting is generally a safe practice, it can be harmful if prolonged. Starvation can be an undesired consequence of lack of access to food or as the result of an eating disorder.

At rest, and when fasting, the body obtains about half its energy from oxidation of fat, and half from oxidation of glucose. Individual organs differ in their substrate usage: the central nervous system, such as the brain, normally uses almost entirely glucose; red blood cells use only glucose; and muscle, at low energy expenditure, uses predominantly fatty acids but uses more glucose as the rate of energy output rises. Glucose is also required in small amounts for the formation of metabolic intermediates in tissues.

Approximately 4 g of glucose are present in the blood at all times. In fasted individuals, blood glucose is maintained constant at this level at the expense of glycogen stores in the cells of the muscle and liver tissues. In response to the decline in blood glucose, glycogen is broken down to glucose via 'glycogenolysis', which is regulated by glucagon and insulin. In a normal 70 kg adult, the liver can store about 100–120 g of glycogen and the skeletal muscle can store roughly 400 g of glycogen. These glycogen stores can be used up after about a 24-hour fasting period.

If the fasting continues beyond two days, a major metabolic adjustment begins. The blood level of insulin drops and the levels of glucagon and noradrenaline rise. At this time, there is an up-regulation of **gluconeogenesis**, lipolysis and ketogenesis. The reduction of insulin secretion results in increased lipolysis and release of amino acids from muscle tissues. The body then engages in 'gluconeogenesis' to convert amino acids and glycerol into glucose for metabolism, and for the brain, which does not utilise ketone bodies to cover energy requirements at that time. After prolonged fasting, the body begins to degrade its own skeletal muscle. To keep the brain functioning, gluconeogenesis continues to generate glucose, but glucogenic amino acids—primarily alanine—are required. Muscle is the main supplier of amino acids in the short term, but in a prolonged fast all tissues lose protein and cell mass, becoming smaller and weaker. During a fast, it is possible to spare body protein by feeding a small amount of carbohydrate to suppress gluconeogenesis; however, feeding a small amount of high-quality protein is much more effective in preventing body protein loss.

The main source of energy during prolonged starvation, however, is derived from triglycerides. Compared to the 8000 kJ of stored glycogen, lipid fuels are much richer in energy content, and a normal 70 kg adult stores, mainly in adipose tissue, over 400,000 kJ of triglycerides. Triglycerides are broken down to fatty acids via lipolysis, and the remaining glycerol enters gluconeogenesis. However, fatty acids by themselves cannot be used as a direct fuel source. They must first undergo oxidation in the mitochondria (mostly of skeletal muscle, cardiac muscle, and liver cells), and the resulting acetyl coenzyme A enters the **tricarboxylic acid (TCA) cycle** and undergoes oxidative phosphorylation to produce ATP. Triglycerides with long-chain fatty acids cannot cross into brain cells due to their hydrophobicity. They must be converted in the liver into short-chain fatty acids and ketone bodies through ketogenesis. The resulting ketone bodies contain both hydrophobic and hydrophilic elements, and can then be transported into the brain (and muscles) and broken down into acetyl coenzyme A for use in the TCA cycle.

Ketones are exported from the liver and the level of ketones in the blood rises; ketone excretion

RAPID WEIGHT LOSS—WHAT IS YOUR RESPONSE?

A friend of yours who is slightly overweight has been trying out a range of diets for the last six months. She is just telling you how wonderful the lemon detox diet has been and that she has lost 4 kg in the last week but asks your opinion.

Determine the physiological basis of this weight loss. With a partner, role-play your response and recommendations.

through the kidney results in an increase in the osmotic concentration of the urine, thereby causing an increase in urinary volume (diuretic effect). The relatively steep fall in body weight in the initial few days of a fast is due in large part to the combined effects of rapid gluconeogenesis and the diuretic effect of ketone excretion. The energy equivalent of weight loss in this period is low because weight loss consists substantially of water. It is commonly observed in 'dieting' that initial weight loss is rapid, but this weight loss is mostly water and often misleads the dieter into thinking that effective loss of fat is being achieved.

The full metabolic adjustment to long-term starvation takes 4–10 days, and during this period the body makes further adjustments, principally to conserve body protein and to reduce both metabolic rate and activity in order to preserve energy. For reasons that are not entirely clear (presumably a hormonal control mechanism), the muscles stop using ketones after a prolonged starvation. This results in a rise of the blood ketones, which then enables ketones to diffuse inwards across the blood–brain barrier and to replace a major proportion of the glucose as an energy source for the central nervous system. Use of ketones by the brain spares glucose, leading to a reduction in the rate of gluconeogenesis, thereby reducing the rate of breakdown of body protein.

Conservation of body protein is of key importance in survival during starvation. Fat provides the main energy reserve in the body because of its high energy density. For individuals with normal body composition, this represents two to three months' energy store. The first requirement of the body is water, and without water survival will be no longer than one to three days. After water, vitamin and mineral supply is at least as important as energy, and deficits of sodium, potassium, vitamin C, folate and thiamin are likely to adversely affect survival. If water is provided, together with vitamin and mineral supplements, survival is much longer.

Refeeding a starved person must be done with great care. If starvation has been prolonged, all body organs and tissues, including the gut, are weakened. Fewer digestive enzymes and transport proteins are present and the gut cannot handle normal volumes of food. With a sudden return to normal food intake, malabsorption is likely to occur, resulting in diarrhoea and acidosis due to a loss of potassium along with magnesium and phosphate, as induced selective nutrient deficiencies because of increased need during refeeding. The phosphate deficiency (hypophosphataemia) can lead to inability to produce ATP and functional failure of cells such as red blood cells. Together with dehydration and electrolyte imbalance, the weakened state can rapidly be fatal. While the refeeding syndrome is rarely a cause of death in tertiary care hospitals (Matthews et al. 2017), it remains a concern where health care is less readily available.

SUMMARY

- Energy is required to maintain life and is obtained by the oxidation of the macronutrients—carbohydrates, fat and, to a lesser extent, protein.
- Energy density in food varies from 37 kJ/g for pure fat down to a hundredth of that value for some vegetables, which are high in water and fibre.
- Rate of energy expenditure is conveniently measured by measuring the rate of oxygen uptake.
- The major components of energy expenditure are basal metabolism plus energy expended in physical activity.
- Energy requirement can be predicted by the use of a range of equations to estimate basal metabolism, to which is added an allowance for physical activity.
- Energy balance is maintained by feedback controls which regulate appetite.

KEY TERMS

Adenosine diphosphate (ADP): a nucleotide, comprising adenine, ribose and two phosphate groups, that functions in the transfer of energy during the catabolism of glucose. ADP, along with energy, is a result of dephosphorylation of ATP or the removal of an inorganic phosphate (P_i) group. ADP can also be converted back to ATP for energy storage. Cycling between ADP and ATP during cellular respiration gives cells the energy needed to carry out cellular activities.

Adenosine triphosphate (ATP): the main carrier of energy that is used for all cellular activities. It comprises adenine, ribose and three phosphate groups. When ATP is converted to ADP, energy is released. In addition to being used as an energy source, ATP is used in signal transduction pathways for cell communication and is also incorporated into DNA during DNA synthesis.

Basal metabolic rate (BMR): metabolic rate measured at the lowest rate of energy expenditure, usually after at least eight hours of rest and ten hours after the last meal.

Gluconeogenesis: the synthesis of glucose from non-carbohydrate substrates, such as lactate, pyruvate, glycerol and the carbon skeleton of glucogenic amino acids.

Tricarboxylic acid (TCA) cycle: also known as the Krebs cycle or the citric acid cycle (CAC)—a series of chemical reactions that release stored energy through the oxidation of acetyl coenzyme A derived from carbohydrates, fats and proteins into chemical energy in the form of ATP and carbon dioxide.

ACKNOWLEDGEMENT

This chapter has been modified and updated from the 'Food energy and energy expenditure' chapter written by Jonathan M. Hodgson which appeared in the third edition of *Food and Nutrition*.

REFERENCES

Boschmann, M., Steiniger, J., Hille, U., Tank, J., Adams, F. et al., 2003, 'Water-induced thermogenesis', *Journal of Clinical Endocrinology & Metabolism, 88*(12): 6015–19, doi:10.1210/jc.2003-030780

FAO/WHO/UNU Expert Consultation, 1985, *Energy and protein requirements: Report of a Joint FAO/WHO/UNU Expert Consultation, World Health Organization,* <https://apps.who.int/iris/handle/10665/39527>, accessed 1 June 2019

FAO/WHO/UNU Expert Consultation, 2001, *Human Energy Requirements,* <www.fao.org/3/a-y5686e.pdf>, accessed 22 November 2018

Hu, F.B., 2005, 'Protein, body weight, and cardiovascular health', *American Journal of Clinical Nutrition, 82*(1): 242S–247S, doi:10.1093/ajcn/82.1.242S

Jésus, P., Achamrah, N., Grigioni, S., Charles, J., Rimbert, A. et al., 2015, 'Validity of predictive equations for resting energy expenditure according to the body mass index in a population of 1726 patients followed in a Nutrition Unit', *Clinical Nutrition, 34*(3): 529–35, doi:10.1016/j.clnu.2014.06.009

Matthews, K.L., Capra, S.M. & Palmer, M.A., 2017, 'Throw caution to the wind: Is refeeding syndrome really a cause of death in acute care?', *European Journal of Clinical Nutrition, 72*: 93–8, doi:10.1038/ejcn.2017.124

Naude, C.E., Schoonees, A., Senekal, M., Young, T., Garner, P. & Volmink, J., 2014, 'Low carbohydrate versus isoenergetic balanced diets for reducing weight and cardiovascular risk: A systematic review and meta-analysis', *PloS One, 9*(7): e100652, doi:10.1371/journal.pone.0100652

Reeves, M.M. & Capra, S., 2003, 'Variation in the application of methods used for predicting energy requirements in acutely ill adult patients: A survey of practice', *European Journal of Clinical Nutrition, 57*: 1530–5, doi:10.1038/sj.ejcn.1601721

Sacks, F.M., Bray, G.A., Carey, V.J., Smith, S.R., Ryan, D.H. et al., 2009, 'Comparison of weight-loss diets with different compositions of fat, protein, and carbohydrates', *New England Journal of Medicine, 360*(9): 859–73, doi:10.1056/NEJMoa0804748

Schofield, W.N., 1985, 'Predicting basal metabolic rate, new standards and review of previous work', *Human Nutrition, Clinical Nutrition, 39*: 5–41 <www.ncbi.nlm.nih.gov/pubmed/4044297>, accessed 1 June 2019

Schutz, Y. & Jequier, E., 1994, 'Energy needs: Assessment and requirements', in M.E. Shils, J.A. Olsen & M. Shike (eds), *Modern Nutrition and Health and Disease* (8th edn), Philadelphia PA: Lea and Febiger, pp. 101–11

{CHAPTER 14}
MACRONUTRIENTS: WATER

Mark L. Wahlqvist and Naiyana Wattanapenpaiboon

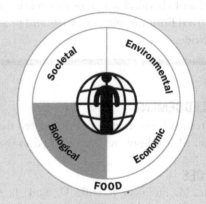

FOOD

OBJECTIVES

- Describe how water is distributed in the body. Describe how the movement of water within the body is controlled by osmotic gradients across cell membranes.
- Summarise the metabolism and functions of water in the body.
- List the physiological requirements and recommendations for water indicated by thirst, and to describe the causes of dehydration.

WATER CONTENT OF THE BODY

Water is the most important component of the human organism, which no doubt stems from our evolutionary origins in an aquatic environment. It has unusual chemical and physical properties, with a powerful solvent capacity, and acts as a medium for the myriad biochemical reactions, physiological processes and anatomical structures that support life. The water content of a developing fetus in the first few weeks after conception is approximately 93–95 per cent by weight. At birth, water comprises about 72 per cent of an infant's body mass, falling to 60 per cent a few days later (explaining some of the initial weight loss in newborns; see Chapter 21), the same proportion as is found on average in an adult male, whereas adult females have on average slightly smaller water content at 51 per cent.

The distribution of water in human tissues is not uniform, comprising 15 per cent of teeth, 20 per cent of bone, 20–30 per cent in adipose tissue, 70 per cent in muscle and 90 per cent of blood plasma. In order to understand how water is translocated and retained within the body, it is useful to consider it as occupying two main fluid compartments: that contained within cells (intracellular water) and that outside cells (extracellular water) (Table 14.1). The **intracellular fluid (ICF)** compartment includes all fluid enclosed in cells by their plasma membranes, while the **extracellular fluid (ECF)** compartment includes interstitial fluid, which is a thin layer of fluid surrounding tissue cells, the fluid portion of blood (plasma), and other fluids in small amounts such as fluid in the eye, joint capsules and the central nervous system (Figure 14.1). The whole (total body water) is contained within the body's external boundaries of skin, lungs and gastrointestinal tract.

Table 14.1: Distribution of water in the tissues of an adult male

	Amount in g/kg body weight	% total body water
Blood plasma	41	7
Interstitial lymph	121	20
Dense connective tissue and cartilage	41	7
Bone water	41	7
Transcellular water	15	2.5
Intraluminal gut water	8.4	1.4
Total extracellular water	260	43
Total intracellular water	340	47
Total body water	600	100

Source: International Commission on Radiological Protection (1975)

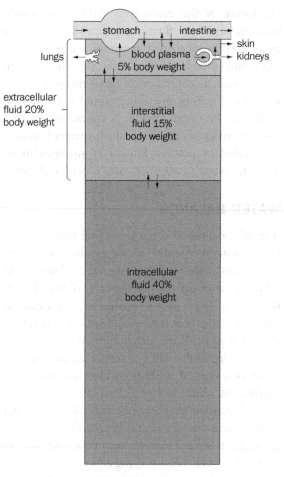

Figure 14.1: Body fluid compartments
Source: Gamble, in Rolls & Rolls (1982)

MOVEMENT OF WATER IN THE BODY AND TISSUE ELECTROLYTES

Water, just like other constituents of living tissue, is in a state of dynamic equilibrium. Approximately 5–10 per cent of total body water is turned over each day under normal circumstances. It is continually absorbed from the gut, excreted in urine by the kidneys, lost from lungs as vapour in expired air and moved about within and between the cells of all tissues, and some of it is excreted in faeces.

If this movement of water is to be achieved, it follows that it must traverse numerous membranes at the boundaries of cells. Cell membranes are permeable to water, which moves across from one side to the other, always in the direction of the fluid with the higher concentration of dissolved electrolytes (electrically charged dissolved substances such as sodium and potassium). This process is called osmosis, and water is said to have flowed across an osmotic gradient (from a lower to a higher concentration of electrolytes); in doing so, it traverses the membrane. Solutes (dissolved substances) that contribute to the osmotic gradient in body fluids are principally the ions potassium (K^+), sodium (Na^+), chloride (Cl^-), phosphate (HPO_4^{2-}), bicarbonate (HCO_3^-), ionic

forms of protein and, to a lesser extent, ions of calcium (Ca^{2+}) and magnesium (Mg^{2+}). The amount of solutes contributing to an osmotic gradient can indirectly be measured by experiment and the results expressed in terms of a unit called the *osmole* (Osm). The body has developed elaborate homeostatic mechanisms to regulate both the amount of water and the amount of solutes in fluids, maintaining their concentration and osmotic concentration within the range required for normal function.

Thus, the water and electrolyte content of tissues are closely interrelated, and an imbalance in one will affect the other. While most fluids contain concentrations of electrolytes producing about 300 mOsm/L (for example, 280–292 mOsm/L for blood plasma), the nature of the electrolytes differs significantly between different fluids. Osmotic gradients are maintained by specialised structures and processes in cell membranes, for if there were no differences in the osmotic concentration of tissue fluids on either side of cell membranes, water would not flow and could not be transported in a controlled manner. The selectivity of cell membrane for water transport is provided by proteins known as **aquaporins** or 'pores for water' (see 'Other water functions', below).

WATER BALANCE

A healthy individual at rest is in water balance—that is, the amounts of water lost are exactly balanced by the amounts consumed by eating and drinking. About 60 per cent of daily water intake is obtained from fluid drinks, 30 per cent is supplied in solid foods and a further 10 per cent is produced within cells, largely as a result of oxidative metabolism. As a result, each day a 70 kg adult might be expected to consume about two litres of water from food and drink and produce an additional 150–250 mL of metabolic water, depending on metabolic rate. However, water requirements can vary markedly according to level of physical activity and temperature of the environment in which an individual is living and working.

Human skin is permeable to water, which diffuses to the surface and evaporates. Humidification of air in the passageways of the lungs is another source of water loss; the escaping vapour can be noticed in cold weather when it condenses from exhaled air. Losses through skin and lungs are collectively called 'insensible water loss' because, under cool conditions and at rest, there is no awareness that they occur. The majority (60 per cent) of resting daily water loss occurs from the kidneys, which excrete 50–60 mL/ hour, and additional small amounts (5 per cent) are excreted in faeces. However, during exercise, there is an increased need to lose heat by evaporation. Water loss from sweat becomes more important and the output from the kidneys is reduced to conserved water. In summary, in agreeable climatic conditions, obligatory urine volume is about 600 mL/day and usually about 0.8–2 L; 800 mL from airways

and skin; and 100 mL in faeces. That means some 1.7–2.9 L/day must be matched by fluid and food water intake and metabolic water production.

Electrolyte and water balance

As with water, there is an obligatory loss of electrolytes in faeces, urine and perspiration, and these losses are replaced by absorption from food and drink to maintain a constant body composition. Deficiencies and excesses of electrolytes are rare on most diets because they are widely distributed in foods, effectively absorbed and surplus amounts are rapidly excreted. Faecal losses of electrolytes are usually small, as are those excreted in perspiration while at rest. The kidneys are chiefly responsible for regulating the body content of electrolytes, which is achieved through the control of urine output and concentration. Both perspiration and urine are produced by filtration of blood plasma. As well as being a vehicle for the regulation of tissue electrolyte concentrations, urine is required for the elimination of metabolic end products such as urea, uric acid and creatinine, which also contribute to the osmotic potential of blood plasma and urine. The regulation of osmotic gradients is controlled by the membranes of cells that make up various kidney tissues, which actively alter electrolyte concentrations. Through these processes, the kidney alters both the solute concentration and volume of blood plasma and urine.

Water content in urine is under the control of vasopressin hormone, which is released from the pituitary gland into the blood in response to small differences in the osmotic concentration of plasma. If dietary water is restricted, then urine volume is reduced and more concentrated urine is produced. The smallest amount of urine that can be produced depends upon the degree to which it can be concentrated, which in adults is about five times the osmotic concentration of plasma. If salt excretion or urea production is high then the minimum urine volume is increased. However, under most circumstances water intake is not restricted and since electrolytes are readily available in the diet, urine output in an individual is primarily determined by the frequency and amounts of water consumed.

THIRST AND DEHYDRATION

Losses of 2.5 per cent of body water can be tolerated without any adverse symptoms. A dry sensation of the mouth, or thirst, is triggered by physiological factors, including an increase in osmotic concentration of tissue fluids, reduced blood volume and cellular dehydration, which cause an individual to search for and consume water. This consumption rapidly abolishes thirst, an effect that occurs before there is time for body fluids to become fully hydrated, so the thirst mechanism must involve more than just changes to osmotic concentration and volume. Losing more than 2.5 per cent of body water can cause significant impairment of function, and a 20 per cent loss could result in death.

The most common causes of dehydration are excessive loss of sweat, prolonged diarrhoea and excessive urine production. Infants are more at risk than adults from dehydration because they have a larger surface area relative to body volume and a higher metabolic rate, so water losses through lungs and skin are relatively greater for their body weight. Additionally, the infant kidney cannot concentrate urine to the same extent as an adult and therefore requires a greater volume of urine to be produced. Diarrhoea resulting from gastrointestinal infections is a frequent cause of dehydration in infants, particularly in developing countries. This is often fatal but can effectively be prevented by oral rehydration solutions containing sodium chloride and glucose, resulting in a much more rapid uptake of water from the gut than if water alone or water with sodium chloride alone were given. In later life, thirst is often impaired (see also Chapter 22).

How much water do we need?

Most of us are familiar with the recommendation to 'drink at least eight glasses of water a day'. The amount equates to approximately two litres of water. This recommendation is often accompanied by a reminder stating that the recommendation refers to only water, and the amount specified is on top of fluid intake from other fluid sources such as tea, coffee, milk, fruit juices, soft drinks and alcohol, and from food sources. When food is metabolised, water is also produced.

It is estimated that, on average, healthy adults with a sedentary lifestyle should drink 1.5 L/day of water, in some form of liquid (Jéquier & Constant 2009); therefore, the eight glasses recommendation is likely to result in excessive fluid intake. While there is little or no evidence that water and/or fluid intake in excess of requirements has any health benefits, it is important to note that fluid requirements should not be based on minimal intake, as this could lead to deficit, particularly in situations of high ambient temperature or humidity, or higher physical activity. It is also often stated that by the time a person is thirsty, they are already dehydrated. Again, there is no

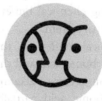

THE COLOUR OF URINE

Various states of dehydration can be ascertained via the concentration of urine. Concentration is identified by colour.

Using the chart located at Kidney Health Australia (kidney.org.au/your-kidneys/prevent/drink-water-instead) or Kidney Health New Zealand (www.kidneys.co.nz/), keep a 'wee diary' for seven days, documenting the colour of your wee, the ambient temperature and your activity level (noting if this was inside or outside activity).

- Keep a record of your fluid intake, including those fluids that hydrate and those that dehydrate (alcohol and caffeinated beverages).
- What changes should you make to your fluid intake?
- Do you need to adjust your fluid intake according to the temperature or your activity?

evidence to support this assertion; on the contrary, thirst is usually elicited well before dehydration.

As there remains little evidence to support the notion that we should 'drink at least eight glasses of water a day', we should take a broader view of water intake to include drinking fluid intake—that is, not all fluid intake need be in the form of water.

ACID–BASE BALANCE

The proper balance between the acids and alkalis, or bases, in the ECF is crucial for the normal physiology of the body and cellular metabolism.

The maintenance of acid–base balance is to keep the body fluids mildly alkaline (pH 7.32–7.42 for ECF, and pH 7.1 for cells), as the alkalinity is essential for muscle, heart and nerve cells. The body normally responds very effectively to disruptions in acid or base production, using chemical buffers, the respiratory system and the renal system.

The most abundant chemical buffer in the ECF consists of a solution of carbonic acid and the bicarbonate salt. When there is an excess of alkaline OH^- ions in the solution, carbonic acid partially neutralises them by forming bicarbonate ion and water. Similarly an excess of acid H^+ ions is partially neutralised by the bicarbonate component of the buffer solution to form carbonic acid, which is a relatively weaker acid. Other mechanisms include excretion of carbon dioxide by the lungs (about 13,000 mmol/day), which removes carbonic acid (volatile acid), and, by the kidneys, excretion of non-volatile acids, such as lactate, phosphate, sulphate and acetoacetate, or regeneration of alkali bicarbonate.

Metabolic processes generate both volatile and non-volatile acids. Volatile acid is removed through respiration as carbon dioxide, whereas non-volatile acid (H^+) must be excreted by the kidney in the form of ammonium and titratable acid. The difference between endogenous acid production and the input of alkali absorbed in the gastrointestinal tract is the net endogenous acid production, and represents the total amount of non-volatile acid that must be excreted to maintain daily acid–base balance. The three commonly reported sources of endogenous

acid production are the metabolism of sulphur amino acids (methionine and cysteine), the metabolism or ingestion of organic acids, and the metabolism of phosphate esters or dietary phosphoproteins. A diet rich in acidogenic foods, such as meat, fish and cheese, but low in alkaline foods, such as fruit and vegetables, can induce endogenous acid production. High dietary acid load has been associated with an unfavourable profile of risk factors for type 2 diabetes and CVD and with adverse effects on bone health.

Acid–base imbalance occurs when the blood pH shifts out of the normal range for any reason. However, to specify the cause of the disturbance, it is recommended that the terms 'acidosis' and 'alkalosis' be used with either 'respiratory' (indicating a change in the partial pressure of carbon dioxide), or 'metabolic' (indicating a change in the bicarbonate concentration of the ECF). Metabolic acidosis is usually associated with impaired renal acid excretion; respiratory acidosis with a reduced respiratory rate causing carbon dioxide retention. Metabolic alkalosis is uncommon, while respiratory alkalosis from hyperventilation is quite common.

OTHER WATER FUNCTIONS

There are structurally different forms of liquid water (as opposed to frozen and vaporised). These may play a role in protein folding and how it affects, for example, brain function, cognition and neurodegeneration (Maestro et al. 2016). According to Bartik (2015), water can be considered an integral part of biological macromolecules. The interaction of water (either through its hydrophobic or hydrophilic effects) is a significant factor in several biochemical processes, including protein folding, nucleic acid stability and molecular binding. Thus, the living world can be regarded as an 'equal partnership between proteins, nucleic acids and water' (Bartik 2015). Aquaporins are membrane proteins that transport water and also small solutes. They are found in various fluid and non-fluid transporting tissues. The transport of water as well as solutes, like glycerol, by aquaporins, raises the possibility of various water-function relationships yet to be understood (Verkman 2005).

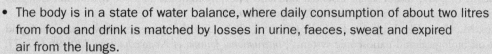

SUMMARY

- The body is in a state of water balance, where daily consumption of about two litres from food and drink is matched by losses in urine, faeces, sweat and expired air from the lungs.
- The water content of tissues is intimately connected to their content of solutes, particularly the electrolytes sodium, potassium and chloride.
- The most important organ in maintaining the volume and osmotic strength of body fluids is the kidney, which directly controls water and electrolytes in blood plasma and urine and indirectly all other fluids.
- Dietary intakes of electrolytes are usually adequate to meet the body's needs, and its water requirements are satisfied by an appropriate response to thirst.
- Dehydration caused by excessive sweating, excessive urine production or severe diarrhoea can have serious physiological consequences; children are more at risk than adults.
- Fluid requirements can be derived from a variety of sources, such as water, tea, coffee, milk and fruit juices, as well as solid foods. Drinking 'at least eight glasses of water a day' is not necessary if fluid requirements are being met from other beverages.

KEY TERMS

Aquaporins: the proteins in cell membranes that help to transport water between cells.

Intracellular fluid (ICF): the fluid inside the cells. ICF contains water and dissolved electrolytes and proteins. Potassium, magnesium, and phosphate are the three most common electrolytes in the ICF.

Extracellular fluid (ECF): all body fluid outside the cells. ECF comprises approximately 20 per cent of total body weight, and includes interstitial fluid, blood plasma, cerebrospinal fluid, lymph and fluid in the eye, bone and dense connective tissue.

Osmotic concentration (also known as osmolarity): a measure of the amount of a solute that contributes to the osmotic pressure in one litre of a chemical solution. It is usually used in situations where the osmotic pressure of the solution is important, and expressed in a unit known as osmoles per litre (Osm/L) or milliosmoles per litre (mOsm/L).

ACKNOWLEDGEMENT

This chapter has been modified and updated from the 'Water' chapter written by Gwynn P. Jones and Jonathan M. Hodgson which appeared in the third edition of *Food and Nutrition*.

REFERENCES

Bartik, K., 2015, *The role of water in the structure and function of biological macromolecules*, <www.exobiologie.fr/index.php/vulgarisation/chimie-vulgarisation/the-role-of-water-in-the-structure-and-function-of-biological-macromolecules/>, accessed 15 April 2018

Gamble, J.L., 1954, 'Chemical anatomy, physiology and pathology of extracellular fluid' (6th edn), Boston: Harvard University Press, in B.J. Rolls and E.T. Rolls (eds), 1982, *Thirst*, Cambridge University Press: Cambridge, pp. 10–22

International Commission on Radiological Protection, 1975, *Report of the Task Group on Reference Man*, Oxford: Pergamon Press

Jéquier, E. & Constant, F., 2009, 'Water as an essential nutrient: The physiological basis of hydration', *European Journal of Clinical Nutrition, 64*: 115–23, doi:10.1038/ejcn.2009.111

Maestro, L., Marqués, M., Camarillo, E., Jaque, D., Solé, J.G. et al., 2016, 'On the existence of two states in liquid water: Impact on biological and nanoscopic systems', *International Journal of Nanotechnology, 13*(8-9): 667–77, doi:10.1504/IJNT.2016.079670

Verkman, A.S., 2005, 'More than just water channels: Unexpected cellular roles of aquaporins', *Journal of Cell Science, 118*(15): 3225–32, doi:10.1242/jcs.02519

{CHAPTER 15}
ALCOHOL

Mark L. Wahlqvist and Naiyana Wattanapenpaiboon

OBJECTIVES

- Describe the use of alcohol and its fate in the human body.
- Understand the physiological effects of alcohol on body systems and its adverse health consequences.
- Discuss strategies to reduce harmful use of alcohol.

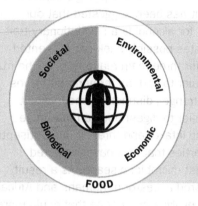

INTRODUCTION

Our body acquires nutrients from food for growth, maintenance and repair of tissues. We use carbohydrates, protein and fats, which are energy-yielding nutrients, to fuel all these activities. Another substance that contributes to energy is alcohol. However, alcohol is not considered a nutrient because it can interfere with the body's growth, maintenance and repair. The main alcohol of nutritional significance is ethanol (C_2H_5OH). One gram of ethanol generates 29.3 kJ (7 kcal) of energy.

Ethanol is produced by enzymatic fermentation of starches and sugars in the absence of oxygen gas. The specific enzymes are provided by certain yeasts, particularly *Saccharomyces*. Different societies use different sources of starches and sugars to make alcoholic beverages. High content of sugar in grapes makes them an excellent substrate for fermentation to produce ethanol. Other sources of sugar and starch include apples (to make cider), grains (beer, whisky, gin, vodka and sake) and sugarcane (rum). Before starch in these sources can ferment to ethanol, it has to be broken down to its constituent glucose. Beers are produced by malting the starch in barley, while starch in rice is hydrolysed by an amylase enzyme from a mould, *Aspergillus oryzae*, to yield glucose.

ALCOHOL CONSUMPTION

Ethanol is normally not consumed pure but in the form of alcoholic beverages. Different alcoholic beverages contain different amounts of ethanol; average beer contains about 4–5 per cent ethanol by volume, average wine contains 10 per cent, and spirits (whisky, gin, vodka, brandy) 40 per cent. A 'standard drink' is a unit of measurement of ethanol in alcoholic beverages consumed. This unit varies in different countries. In Australia and New Zealand, a standard drink provides 10 g of ethanol (equivalent to 12.5 mL) (MOH 2018; NHMRC 2009). For example, a standard drink of an average wine (12 per cent alcohol) would correspond to 100 mL. As alcohol is a liquid, its content is often expressed in volume such as millilitres (mL), and the alcohol content in beverages is then expressed by volume; for example, 1% v/v means 1 mL alcohol per 100 mL of beverage.

People use alcohol for a wide range of reasons and in different social and cultural contexts. Alcohol

HISTORY OF ALCOHOL

There are indications that humans have a long history of preparing and enjoying alcohol. In fact, it has been suggested that our taste for alcohol is an evolutionary trait. Primates possibly seek out fermented fruit for three main reasons: one, the fruit is easier to find, as fermentation gives it a stronger, distinctive smell; two, it is easier to digest and can maximise caloric intake; and three, it has antiseptic properties that may have protected against microbial disease. As a result, a shared ancestor of humans and African apes evolved an enzyme that could more rapidly digest the alcohol in fermented fruit.

In human history the earliest indications of alcohol preparation come after the domestication of barley, wheat and rice in 8000 BC. The earliest evidence of alcoholic beverages, at Jiahu, China, was a cocktail made of rice, hawthorn berries, honey, and wild grapes in 7000 BC, although a potato brew may have been produced in Chile as early as 13,000 BC and a palm wine in parts of Africa and Asia as early as 16,000 BC. Grapes were domesticated in 6000 BC and evidence of wine in the area now known as Iran came soon after.

Source: Curry (2017)

place in Australian and New Zealand culture and is consumed on a wide range of social occasions. In 2014–2015, 81 per cent of Australians aged 18 years and over had consumed alcohol in the past year. About 11 per cent reported that they never consumed alcohol and a further 8.2 per cent had consumed alcohol twelve months ago or longer (ABS 2015). Report of the apparent consumption of alcohol for the period 2016–2017 indicates that 9.4 L of pure alcohol (ethanol) was available for consumption for every person in Australia aged 15 years and over, the lowest level since 1961–1962 (ABS 2018).

Even though the sale of alcohol is prohibited to those under 18 years of age, a significant number of adolescents consume the substance. It has no nutritional value (empty calories) and may disrupt eating habits. In young people, it can lead to possible brain damage and other alcohol-related harms such as injury, violence and self-harm. The Australian Guidelines to Reduce Health Risks from Drinking Alcohol (NHMRC 2009) recommend that children under 15 years of age should not drink and that those aged 15–17 years delay the initiation of drinking for as long as possible. Results from the 2014–2015 National Health Survey suggest the latter recommendation may be gaining some traction, since the proportion of 15- to 17-year-olds abstaining from alcohol increased from 49.1 per cent in 2011–2012 to 66.2 per cent in 2014–2015 (ABS 2015).

ABSORPTION AND METABOLISM OF ALCOHOL

Alcohol is readily absorbed unchanged from the stomach and the jejunum. The rate of absorption can vary, depending on a number of factors. For example, food in the stomach, especially food high in fat or protein, can delay alcohol absorption and blunt the peak blood alcohol. Once absorbed, alcohol is then distributed in the total body water compartment. The lungs excrete a predictable portion of alcohol, and this has been used as the basis of the 'breathalyser' test for estimating blood alcohol content (BAC) from a breath sample.

can be a source of pleasure and, in small amounts, may have beneficial effects for some people. In other religious or cultural circles, wine and spirits may have special significance (for example, communion wine) and in some festivals alcohol may be used to attain 'higher states'. Alcohol occupies a significant

Most consumed alcohol is metabolised in the liver, but a small amount may be metabolised as it passes through the stomach wall. In humans, there are three possible pathways for alcohol metabolism. The major pathway in most people involves the alcohol dehydrogenase (ADH) enzyme, which is a zinc-containing enzyme in the cytoplasm of the liver. In long-term heavy drinkers, alcohol is predominantly metabolised in the microsomal ethanol oxidising system (MEOS) pathway. In both ADH and MEOS pathways, ethanol is converted to acetaldehyde, which is further metabolised to acetate by acetaldehyde dehydrogenase (Figure 15.1). Acetate is then shuttled to the peripheral tissues and used as a source of energy. The conversion of ethanol to acetaldehyde in a third minor pathway involves the catalase enzyme.

On average, a healthy person can metabolise about 5 g/hour of alcohol, but the rate can vary between individuals, being influenced by factors such as gender, ethnicity, lean body mass, pattern of previous alcohol consumption, drugs and dietary factors. Women tend to have a greater increase in blood alcohol in response to alcohol intake. This is because they often have a lower weight, a lower percentage of total body water, smaller liver—and so metabolise alcohol slower—and less ADH enzyme in the stomach mucosa.

A hangover is a combination of unpleasant symptoms following the consumption of alcohol. Hangovers can last for several hours or for more

> ## BLOOD ALCOHOL LEGAL LIMIT 0.05—WHAT DOES IT MEAN?
>
> Australia has strict laws about drinking alcohol and driving. The legal limit for driving is set at 0.05 blood alcohol concentration (BAC), which means 0.05 g alcohol/100 mL blood. Learners and probationary licence-holders must have a 0.00 BAC.
>
> On average, a 60 kg person has about 40 L of body fluid. The 10 g of alcohol from one standard drink is diluted in the body water, giving a peak concentration of 0.025g/100 mL in the blood and in the rest of body water. As the amount of body fluid is proportional to body weight, in general, a person's BAC could increase by 0.01 for men and 0.03 for women for each standard drink.

than 24 hours. The typical symptoms include headache, dry mouth, drowsiness, gastrointestinal distress such as vomiting, nausea, absence of hunger and hyper-excitability. The causes of a hangover are not fully understood but several pathophysiological changes are known to be involved, including the

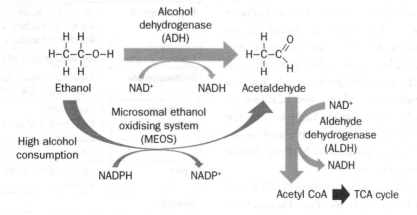

Figure 15.1: Alcohol metabolism

accumulation of acetaldehyde, decreased availability of glucose, dehydration and hormonal alterations of the cytokine pathways. Alcohol beverages contain ingredients called congeners, which could be flavouring additives or by-products of fermentation or ageing process, that, to some extent, can aggravate hangover effects.

ALCOHOL CONSUMPTION AND ADVERSE HEALTH CONSEQUENCES

Alcohol consumption is evidently a risk factor for many disorders and chronic diseases (Table 15.1). Health problems from alcohol usually arise in the form of acute and chronic conditions. A conceptual model of alcohol consumption as a risk factor for chronic diseases and conditions suggests that two separate, but related, measures of alcohol consumption— overall volume of alcohol consumption and patterns of drinking—are responsible for most of the causal impact of alcohol on the burden of chronic diseases. The type or quality of alcoholic beverages may also influence mortality and morbidity from chronic diseases, but with a much lesser extent, compared to the other two factors (Shield et al. 2013).

Compromised nutritional status

Excessive consumption of alcohol affects nutritional status in a number of ways. Primary malnutrition is be associated with alcohol. Although small amounts of alcohol stimulate the appetite, large amounts could reduce the appetite for food. The relatively high energy content of alcohol means that it displaces other sources of energy and consequently many essential nutrients in the diet. Gastrointestinal and metabolic complications caused by heavy alcohol intake, particularly liver dysfunction, can lead to secondary malnutrition. Other complications of excessive alcohol consumption include chronic gastritis, gastric or duodenal ulcers, and acute hepatitis; all of these complications have significant impact on nutritional status.

Deficiencies of fat-soluble vitamins A, D, E and K can be caused by excessive alcohol consumption. Their intakes may be low or the absorption reduced

Table 15.1: Some disorders and chronic diseases associated with alcohol consumption

System or health status affected	Chronic diseases or disorders
Cardiovascular	• Elevated blood pressure and hypertension • Stroke • Heart disease except myocardial infarction • Cardiac dysrhythmia (abnormal heartbeat) • Aortic aneurysm (enlargement of the aorta)
Gastrointestinal	• Impaired digestion and malabsorption • Gastritis (inflammation of stomach) • Pancreatitis • Fatty liver • Hepatitis • Cirrhosis and liver failure
Musculo-skeletal	• Myopathy • Cardiomyopathy • Increased bone loss and osteoporosis
Cancers	• Increased risk for cancer at various sites including the mouth, nasopharynx, oesophagus, colon and rectum, liver, larynx, and breast (in women)
Neurological	• Acute intoxication ('drunkenness') • Neuropathy (nerve damage) • Brain damage • Wernicke's encephalopathy • Impaired cognitive function and dementia • Degeneration of nervous system • Polyneuropathy
Psychological	• Withdrawal state with delirium • Mental and behavioural disorders • Psychotic disorders
Endocrinological	• Impaired control of blood glucose
Immunological	• Impaired immune function • Increased risk for infections
Nutritional status	• Malnutrition • Deficiencies of vitamins and minerals • Obesity
Injury	• Increased risk of work and road accidents
Mortality	

Source: Shield et al. (2013)

because of fat malabsorption. The metabolism and/or storage of the vitamins can be altered by alcohol-induced tissue injury. As vitamin A (retinol) shares some metabolic pathways with alcohol, its metabolism is adversely affected. Heavy drinkers with **cirrhosis** may develop night-blindness due to vitamin A deficiency. Bone density can also be decreased and the incidence of fractures increased due to reduced vitamin D intake and absorption and/or reduced formation of the 25-OH vitamin D in the liver. Problems with calcium metabolism may also occur as alcohol increases urinary calcium loss. Reduced synthesis of vitamin K by gut bacteria and the effects of liver damage may result in deficiency of the vitamin K-dependent clotting factors that are produced in the liver. Bleeding and bruising are likely to occur.

Excessive alcohol intake leads to the deficiencies of certain water-soluble vitamins (B, C and folate). Intake of foods containing some of these vitamins, particularly fruit and vegetables, may be low, and absorption and utilisation may be reduced. It is estimated that about half of malnourished heavy drinkers have low levels of water-soluble vitamins, particularly of folate and vitamin B-6. Folate metabolism is commonly impaired in heavy drinkers, and megaloblastic anaemia may be seen.

Depleted or deficient status of some minerals results from low intakes, reduced absorption and increased urinary excretion. Plasma magnesium and zinc can be subnormal in heavy drinkers. Magnesium wasting from the kidney is also common. Body potassium is reduced, possibly due to vomiting, diarrhoea, urinary losses from diuretics or increased levels of the hormone aldosterone. Iron deficiency may occur due to poor intestinal absorption or bleeding from the gastrointestinal tract.

Alcohol can also cause dehydration, as it affects the hypothalamus by reducing antidiuretic hormone release. This results in polyuria and may cause dehydration, especially after concentrated alcoholic drinks. Table 15.2 summarises the detrimental effects of alcohol on nutritional status.

Liver disease

Alcohol can cause liver damage in three stages: fatty liver (steatosis) caused by increased triglyceride synthesis in the liver cells; alcoholic hepatitis (inflammation of liver); and alcoholic cirrhosis, which may be associated with chronic alcoholism. In cirrhosis, the pattern of cells in the liver becomes deranged due to cell death and fibrosis, and acetaldehyde may stimulate collagen synthesis. Damage to the liver, as in alcohol hepatitis and liver cirrhosis, are associated

Table 15.2: Possible detrimental effects of alcohol on nutritional status

Effect	Results/Consequences
Displacement of normal food	Reduced food intake
Loss of appetite	Reduced food intake
Mucosal damage and impairment of mucosal enzymes	Impaired digestion and malabsorption
Impaired bile and pancreatic enzyme secretion	Impaired digestion and malabsorption
Altered gastrointestinal motility	Impaired digestion and malabsorption
Decreased synthesis of transport proteins	Impaired transport in the circulation
Reduced supplies and/or activities of enzymes and cofactors	Impaired activation of substrates required in metabolic processes
Increased metabolic rate	Increased requirements
Increased losses/waste	Increased excretion in bile and urine Increased faecal losses
Reduced storage	Alcoholic myopathy, sarcopenia, cachexia

with marked nutritional problems, largely due to the interruption of normal metabolic and synthetic process of the organ. When the damage becomes more severe, the liver may become unable to perform its usual functions. These include the metabolism of amino acids, glucose and fat, storage of glycogen, synthesis of protein including albumin and the clotting factors, and the metabolism and clearance of bilirubin. A heavy drinker with advanced cirrhosis can suffer from marked protein energy malnutrition, muscle wasting and oedema.

It is worth noting that not all cases of chronic hepatitis and cirrhosis are caused by alcohol excess; some are caused by the hepatitis virus. However, the most common cause of liver cirrhosis is prolonged excessive alcohol intake. A close relationship and possible interaction is observed between alcohol intake and hepatitis C infection. The risk of hepatocellular carcinoma in someone with cirrhosis is much increased with hepatitis C infection and heavy alcohol consumption.

Wernicke–Korsakoff syndrome

Alcohol induces specific changes of thiamin metabolism in the central nervous system, producing the typical clinical symptoms of Wernicke–Korsakoff syndrome (WKS). Heavy drinkers who consume large amounts of alcohol and stop eating for a long period of time are at risk of WKS due to acute thiamin deficiency resulting from low intakes, impaired absorption and storage, and reduced activation of the vitamin. Wernicke's encephalopathy is characterised by confusion, abnormalities such as nystagmus (jerky eye movements) and eye muscle paralysis, and unsteadiness. Irreversible structural lesions in the brain are found in patients with this condition. The symptoms can be treated with large doses of thiamin injection, but recovery may be slow and incomplete. Also, the patients may be left with Korsakoff's syndrome, which is characterised by a loss of recent memory, the inability to recall what has recently happened and confabulation (making up stories to cover up the lost memory). WKS has become uncommon in Australia since the implementation of mandatory addition of thiamin to

wheat flour for making bread in 1991 (Harper et al. 1998; Ma & Truswell 1995).

Fetal alcohol syndrome

Fetal abnormalities, as a result of **teratogenic** effects of alcohol, may be seen in women who drink alcohol heavily in the first few weeks or months of pregnancy, and, in some cases, before the women even know they are pregnant.

Children with fetal alcohol syndrome (FAS) show pre- and postnatal growth retardation, central nervous system dysfunction, decreased infant mental and motor development and other congenital abnormalities, caused by exposure to alcohol *in utero*. Rates of FAS are unacceptably high: for every 10,000 people in the general population globally, 15 will have FAS. Ten per cent of women globally, and 25 per cent of women in Europe, drink alcohol while pregnant (Popova et al. 2017).

Women of reproductive age should be aware that there is no safe amount of alcohol to drink while pregnant, no safe time to drink during pregnancy and no safe kind of alcohol drink. In view of the irreversible lifelong effects of alcohol during pregnancy on the unborn child, the NHMRC recommends complete abstinence from alcohol while pregnant as the safest option (NHMRC 2009).

GLOBAL STRATEGY TO REDUCE HARMFUL USE OF ALCOHOL

According to the WHO global status report on alcohol and health, alcohol consumption was related to an estimated three million deaths worldwide in 2016, representing 5.3 per cent of all deaths (WHO 2018). Different disease and injury outcomes are attributable to alcohol at various degrees. Alcohol accounted for 5.1 per cent of the global burden of disease and injury, as measured in disability-adjusted life years (DALYs), with alcohol-related liver disease in particular a major factor.

Recognising the close links between alcohol drinking, adverse health consequences and socio-economic development, the WHO released a global strategy to reduce the harmful use of alcohol

(WHO 2010). The term 'harmful use' is defined as drinking that causes detrimental health and social consequences for the drinker, the people around the drinker and society at large, as well as the patterns of drinking associated with increased risk of adverse health outcomes.

In Australia, as in many countries, alcohol is responsible for a considerable burden of death, disease and injury. It was estimated that 4.6 per cent of the total burden of disease and injury in 2011 was attributable to alcohol use. The major causes of the burden included injuries (34 per cent of the burden: 10 per cent road traffic, 8 per cent suicide and self-inflicted harm and 3 per cent homicide and violence), cancers (17 per cent) and stroke (3 per cent) (AIHW 2018b).

The NHMRC released the Australian Guidelines to Reduce Health Risks from Drinking Alcohol in 2009, with one of the objectives being to assist Australians in making informed decisions about their drinking habits. The guidelines address alcohol consumption for adults, children, adolescents and pregnant women (NHMRC 2009). These guidelines are currently under review, with final revised guidelines expected in the first half of 2020.

The Australian Institute of Health and Welfare has reported that fewer Australians are drinking alcohol at risky levels. The proportion of people aged 14 and over who are consuming on average more than two standard drinks per day decreased from 18.2 per cent in 2013 to 17.1 per cent in 2016. One in three (36 per cent) of Australians aged 14 and over consume more than four standard drinks in one sitting. Between 2010 and 2016, the proportion of people who drank, on average, more than two standard drinks per day dropped from 20 per cent to 17 per cent (AIHW 2018a).

SAFE AND ETHICAL CONSUMPTION OF ALCOHOL

Alcohol can be considered a food and a drug. Its consumption is governed by legislation but it is also an integral part of social and cultural practice. Using the safe drinking guidelines and reflecting on your own social and cultural background, what would be the public health response to the following scenarios? What are your own thoughts?

1. Mary is trying to fall pregnant. She is currently consuming a minimum of five standard drinks every weekend.
2. Jane is pregnant. She thinks it is okay to have a glass of wine with dinner every weekend.
3. Phyllis is breastfeeding. She consumes a gin and tonic every night after the last feed of her baby.
4. The Scarpetti family are originally from Italy. On special occasions all of the children are given a small glass of red wine to have with dinner.
5. The Jones family have teenagers. They purchase alcohol for their 16-year-old son for weekend parties.
6. Bob does not drink during the week but consumes the equivalent of 24 cans of beer and two bottles of spirits over a weekend, while his partner consumes a half a bottle of wine every night with dinner.
7. James is the designated driver for the evening but he doesn't want to miss out on all the fun. He has estimated he can consume a beer an hour and stay under the legal blood alcohol limit.

ALCOHOL CONSUMPTION AND ITS EFFECTS ON HEALTH: WHAT WOULD YOU RECOMMEND?

Light to moderate alcohol consumption is actively promoted to prevent disease, in particular cardiovascular disease. Red wine consumption, in particular, as part of the Mediterranean diet, is promoted for its health benefits and impact on longevity.

Using the following literature, and any additional literature you may find, summarise and synthesise the key points. Once you have done this, taking into consideration the Australian/New Zealand and global guidelines for alcohol consumption, what would be your recommendation for alcohol consumption to reduce the risk of chronic conditions?

- Hassing, L.B., 2018, 'Light alcohol consumption does not protect cognitive function: A longitudinal prospective study', *Frontiers in Aging Neuroscience*, *10*: 81
- Stockwell, T. et al., 2018, 'Underestimation of alcohol consumption in cohort studies and implications for alcohol's contribution to the global burden of disease', *Addiction*, *113*(12): 2245–9
- Wood, A.M. et al., 2018, 'Risk thresholds for alcohol consumption: Combined analysis of individual-participant data for 599 912 current drinkers in 83 prospective studies', *Lancet*, *391*(10129): 1513–23
- Zhao, J. et al., 2017, 'Alcohol consumption and mortality from coronary heart disease: An updated meta-analysis of cohort studies', *Journal of Studies on Alcohol and Drugs*, *78*(3): 375–86.

A large study involving nearly 600,000 drinkers suggests that about 100 g alcohol per week (about 5–6 Australian standard drinks per week) is the threshold for lowest risk of all-cause mortality (Wood et al. 2018). This threshold appears to be lower than the maximum level the NMRC suggested of 140 g alcohol per week, and it seems lower than the recommended limit in the USA, Italy, Portugal and Spain. Furthermore, the researchers discovered a linear relationship between alcohol consumption and risks for stroke, heart disease (excluding myocardial infarction) and death from other types of CVDs. The findings are remarkably similar for men and women, but this begs the question about pregnancy and the fetal alcohol syndrome and the clear association between alcohol consumption and breast cancer. More cautionary advice for women, and especially when pregnancy is possible, is required than the

proposed threshold would suggest. The same might be said for men with associated cancer risk factors like smoking, physical inactivity and obesity.

Scientific evidence suggests that any potential health benefits from consuming alcohol have probably been overestimated. The benefits appear to relate to middle-aged or older people and only occur with low levels of alcohol intake of about half a standard drink per day, which is within the Guidelines level. Obviously, the Guidelines do not encourage people to take up drinking for health benefits. The regulatory environments around alcohol consumption are relatively weak in Australia and New Zealand. The wine, beer and hospitality industries are substantial contributors to national employment and economics. Questions need to be asked about the influence of 'big alcohol' and its influence on research and regulatory approaches (Hawkins et al. 2018).

SUMMARY

- Alcohol provides food energy but no other nutritional value.
- The use of alcohol is a social and sometimes cultural activity in many countries.
- Alcohol has physiological effects on a number of body systems and may affect nutritional status in a number of ways.
- Excessive intake of alcohol leads to serious health problems, and can also have detrimental social consequences.

KEY TERMS

Cirrhosis: a condition in which the liver is irreversibly scarred. It is a progressive condition that develops slowly over many years, and if it is allowed to continue, the accumulation of scar tissue can eventually stop liver function.

Teratogenic: of a chemical or agent, disturbing the development of the embryo or fetus, and causing a congenital malformation (a birth defect), growth retardation, delayed mental development or other congenital disorders without any structural malformations.

REFERENCES

ABS, 2015, *National Health Survey: First Results, 2014–15,* <www.abs.gov.au/ausstats/abs@.nsf/Lookup/by%20Subject/4364.0.55.001~2014-15~Main%20Features~Alcohol%20consumption~25>, accessed 22 November 2018

—— 2018, *Apparent Consumption of Alcohol Australia, 2016–2017,* <www.abs.gov.au/AUSSTATS/abs@.nsf/Lookup/4307.0.55.001Main+Features12016-17?OpenDocument>, accessed 22 November 2018

AIHW, 2018a, *Alcohol, Tobacco and Other Drugs in Australia,* <www.aihw.gov.au/reports/alcohol/alcohol-tobacco-other-drugs-australia/contents/introduction>, accessed 24 November 2018

—— 2018b, *Impact of Alcohol and Illicit Drug Use on the Burden of Disease and Injury in Australia: Australian Burden of Disease Study 2011,* <www.aihw.gov.au/reports/burden-of-disease/impact-alcohol-illicit-drug-use-on-burden-disease/formats>, accessed 22 November 2018

Curry, A., 2017, 'A 9,000-year love affair', *National Geographic, 231*(2): 31–53, <www.nationalgeographic.com/magazine/2017/02/alcohol-discovery-addiction-booze-human-culture/>, accessed 19 January 2019

Harper, C.G., Sheedy, D.L., Lara, A.I., Garrick, T.M., Hilton, J.M. & Raisanen, J., 1998, 'Prevalence of Wernicke-Korsakoff syndrome in Australia: Has thiamine fortification made a difference?', *Medical Journal of Australia, 168*(11): 542–5, <www.ncbi.nlm.nih.gov/pmc/articles/PMC3391549/>, accessed 24 November 2018

Hassing, L.B., 2018, 'Light alcohol consumption does not protect cognitive function: A longitudinal prospective study', *Frontiers in Aging Neuroscience, 10*: 81, doi:10.3389/fnagi.2018.00081

Hawkins, B., Holden, C., Eckhardt, J. & Lee, K., 2018, 'Reassessing policy paradigms: A comparison of the global tobacco and alcohol industries', *Global Public Health, 13*(1): 1–19, doi:10.1080/17441692.2016.1161815

Ma, J.J. & Truswell, A.S., 1995, 'Wernicke–Korsakoff syndrome in Sydney hospitals: Before and after thiamine enrichment of flour', *Medical Journal of Australia, 163*(10): 531–4, doi:10.5694/j.1326-5377.1995.tb124721.x

MOH, 2018, *Alcohol,* <www.health.govt.nz/your-health/healthy-living/addictions/alcohol-and-drug-abuse/alcohol>, accessed 22 November 2018

NHMRC, 2009, *Australian Guidelines to Reduce Health Risks from Drinking Alcohol,* <https://nhmrc.gov.au/about-us/publications/australian-guidelines-reduce-health-risks-drinking-alcohol>, accessed 22 November 2018

Popova, S., Lange, S., Probst, C., Gmel, G. & Rehm, J., 2017, 'Estimation of national, regional, and global prevalence of alcohol use during pregnancy and fetal alcohol syndrome: A systematic review and meta-analysis', *Lancet Global Health, 5*(3): e290–9, doi:10.1016/S2214-109X(17)30021-9

Shield, K.D., Parry, C. & Rehm, J., 2013, 'Chronic diseases and conditions related to alcohol use', *Alcohol Research: Current Reviews, 35*(2): 155–73, <www.ncbi.nlm.nih.gov/pmc/articles/PMC3908707/>, accessed 24 November 2018

Stockwell, T., Zhao, J., Sherk, A., Rehm, J., Shield, K. & Naimi, T., 2018, 'Underestimation of alcohol consumption in cohort studies and implications for alcohol's contribution to the global burden of disease', *Addiction, 113*(12): 2245–9, doi:10.1111/add.14392

WHO, 2010, *Global Strategy to Reduce the Harmful Use of Alcohol,* <www.who.int/substance_abuse/activities/gsrhua/en/>, accessed 22 November 2018

—— 2018, *Global Status Report on Alcohol and Health 2018,* <www.who.int/substance_abuse/publications/global_alcohol_report/en/>, accessed 22 November 2018

Wood, A.M., Kaptoge, S., Butterworth, A.S., Willeit, P., Warnakula, S. et al., 2018, 'Risk thresholds for alcohol consumption: Combined analysis of individual-participant data for 599 912 current drinkers in 83 prospective studies', *Lancet, 391*(10129): 1513–23, doi:10.1016/S0140-6736(18)30134-X

Zhao, J., Stockwell, T., Roemer, A., Naimi, T. & Chikritzhs, T., 2017, 'Alcohol consumption and mortality from coronary heart disease: An updated meta-analysis of cohort studies', *Journal of Studies on Alcohol and Drugs, 78*(3): 375–86, doi:10.15288/jsad.2017.78.375

{CHAPTER 16}
MICRONUTRIENTS:
VITAMINS

Mark L. Wahlqvist and Naiyana Wattanapenpaiboon

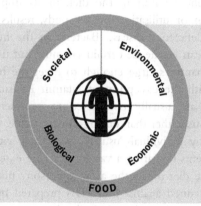

OBJECTIVES

- Describe the historical and contemporary bases for the designation 'vitamins' for a class of essential nutrients.
- Recognise the importance of various vitamins in bodily functions, and identify their toxicities.
- Identify food sources of fat-soluble and water-soluble vitamins.

INTRODUCTION

Vitamins, along with minerals, are conventionally the two types of **micronutrients**. Both are important for optimised physical and mental functions, as well as in the prevention and treatment of various conditions and disorders. Lack of micronutrients can lead to stunted growth in children and increased risk for various diseases in adulthood. Without the adequate and, ideally, food-based consumption of micronutrients, people can suffer from diseases such as xerophthalmia (dry eyes—involving conjunctiva and cornea) and blindness (lack of vitamin A), rickets (lack of vitamin D), scurvy (lack of vitamin C), and osteoporosis (lack of calcium, vitamin D, vitamin K, phytonutrients and other food components, in conjunction with too much sodium). Interestingly, there have been few population-based longitudinal studies of socioeconomically advantaged individuals evaluating the association between micronutrients and survival (Huang et al. 2012).

WHAT ARE VITAMINS?

'A vitamin is a substance that makes you ill if you don't eat it.'

—Albert Szent-Gyorgyi, Nobel Prize in Physiology or Medicine, 1937

Vitamins (vital amines) and their metabolites are essential for a large number of physiological processes, playing important role(s) in various functions as hormones and antioxidants, as regulators of tissue growth and differentiation, in embryonic development and in metabolism, among others. For an organic compound to be considered a vitamin, it must be required in the diet to prevent a deficiency disease (such as scurvy, rickets or beriberi). Each of the fourteen known vitamins has specific and vital functions in the cell and tissues of the body, so that one vitamin cannot replace or act for another. However, some functions, such as antioxidation, may overlap with other compounds or exist among vitamins. The lack or deficiency of one vitamin can also interfere with the function of another, and consumption of excessive amounts of one vitamin can lead to imbalances.

The body needs only small amounts of each vitamin each day, measured in milligrams or micrograms, to sustain normal metabolic processes. Vitamins cannot be synthesised by the body (except vitamin D, which can be made in the skin with adequate exposure to sunlight), and the continued lack of one vitamin in the diet, or its improper absorption or utilisation by the body, results in a vitamin deficiency disease. Bacteria in the human intestine can synthesise certain vitamins, but usually not in quantities large enough to meet the body's needs, with the exception of vitamin K; bacteria, however, are usually considered to represent an **exogenous**, rather than **endogenous**, source.

Healthy individuals usually meet their vitamin requirements by eating a varied diet. The extent to which the diet meets the average person's needs is often measured against the RDIs prepared by the NHMRC in Australia or similar bodies in other countries (see Chapter 19). Vitamin deficiency diseases are rare in industrialised societies such as Australia or New Zealand, but whether vitamin status is optimal is vigorously debated. Subclinical deficiency represents a state of 'nutritional risk' but is hard to measure; whether it impairs overall health is uncertain. Primary deficiency states due to dietary inadequacies are probably less common than secondary deficiency states, which may be induced by some other factor or disease in the face of an apparently adequate dietary intake. In the Asia-Pacific region, however, people and communities with vitamin A, thiamin (B-1), riboflavin (B-2), vitamin D and folate deficiency are still to be found. The possibility of an excessive and potentially harmful intake of certain vitamins has also been identified with the consumption of large doses of certain vitamins by some individuals. Such a condition is referred to as hypervitaminosis.

VITAMIN CLASSIFICATION

Vitamins are usually classified according to their solubility in either fat or water. Fat-soluble vitamins are A, D, E and K, and water-soluble vitamins include the B-complex vitamins and vitamin C. Vitamins B-6 and B-12 are two of the best-known B-complex vitamins. Vitamins also may be classified according to their function in the body. For example, some of the B-complex vitamins (thiamin, riboflavin, niacin, B-6, pantothenic acid and biotin) function as **coenzymes** in many and varied metabolic reactions involving the release of energy for cellular activity; vitamin B-12 and folate are involved in the synthesis of DNA; and others are antioxidants (vitamins A, C and E).

As vitamins were discovered, they were designated by letters assigned in alphabetical order. After they had been chemically identified, it became apparent that the vitamins were not single compounds but mixtures of compounds. For example, several different compounds, all with vitamin A activity, have been isolated. In the case of vitamin B, numerical subscripts were added to distinguish between individual vitamins as they were discovered (vitamin B-1, B-2, B-6, and so on). Many vitamins exist in food in several different forms, some of which (precursors and **provitamins**) require conversion into vitamin active compounds in the body before they can function. Some vitamins may not be completely available for absorption from the human gut, and therefore have reduced bioavailability. The term 'biological activity', when applied to a nutrient, takes into account factors that may affect its absorption and utilisation, and is therefore a measure of the nutritional effectiveness of the particular nutrient.

FAT-SOLUBLE VITAMINS

Fat-soluble vitamins are present in a wide variety of foods. They are not easily destroyed by usual cooking methods, and they do not dissolve into cooking water. The mechanism of digestion and absorption follows a similar pathway to that for the dietary fats, and any condition that hinders the function of the intestine or interferes in any way with fat absorption, such as malabsorption syndrome, will also limit the absorption of fat-soluble vitamins. They tend to accumulate within the body and are not needed on a daily basis. Also because they can be stored—mainly in the liver—the clinical symptoms of deficiency develop more slowly than for water-soluble vitamins. If taken in excessive amounts, some fat-soluble vitamins accumulate in the body and may produce undesirable toxic effects.

Vitamin A

Vitamin A is the generic description for at least seven different active forms (including retinol, retinal, retinoic acid and retinyl ester). It is present in food in two main forms: preformed vitamin A (the vitamin itself) and, more commonly, provitamin A carotenoids, which are dietary precursors of retinol (Figure 16.1). Preformed vitamin A is found almost exclusively in animal sources, usually in association with fats in foods such as dairy products and liver. Food derived from animals provides compounds that are converted to retinol in the intestine. Most of the provitamin A in a mixed diet is supplied in the form of carotenoids, mainly in deep yellow- and green-coloured plants. Only 50 of approximately 600 carotenoids found in nature are converted into vitamin A. The most important and best-known of these carotenoids is β-carotene, which can be split by an enzyme to release retinal (oxidised retinol) in the intestine and liver. β-carotene is most abundant in food and possesses the highest vitamin A activity of the carotenoids. However, it is less efficiently utilised by the body than is preformed vitamin A, partly due to the lower absorption of carotenoids, which is affected by the presence or absence of other components in the diet, such as dietary fat and protein, and by bile salts. The release of carotenoids from foods can be affected by the matrix of foods eaten; however, processing of food, such as cutting up and cooking, improves availability and thus absorption of carotenoids from foods. Some studies show improved absorption of carotenoids with increased fat intake, but the data are not consistent.

To take into account not only the absorption of carotenoids, but also the degree of conversion to retinol, vitamin A intakes or requirements are generally expressed in terms of retinol equivalents (RE). One RE is defined as the biological activity associated with one microgram of all-*trans* retinol. There has been discussion in the literature about the conversion factors from mixed vegetable diets, given lowest bioavailability is reported for leafy green vegetables and raw carrots, and highest for fruit/tuber diets (de Pee et al. 1995; Schweiggert & Carle 2017). Where green leafy vegetables or fruits are more prominent than in the usual diet, adjustment to higher or lower conversion factors could be considered. For example, in the USA, where fruit constitutes a larger portion of the diet, the Institute of Medicine suggests the use of retinol activity equivalent (RAE) factors for their dietary reference intakes. The conversion factors for retinol equivalents shown in Table 16.1 align more with sources of carotenoids in the Australian and New Zealand diets.

Retinol is needed for the visual process and one of the earliest signs of vitamin A deficiency is a failure to see in dim light, or night blindness. The function of retinal (oxidised retinol produced in the retina) in black-and-white (dim light) vision is as a component of rhodopsin (visual purple), which is bleached to visual yellow by contact with light arriving at the retina (Figure 16.2). This reaction triggers an electrical impulse that is conducted through the optic nerve to the brain; this signal is recognised as part of a visual image. Rhodopsin is regenerated so that the process can be repeated.

In the blood, retinol-binding protein (RBP), a protein produced by the liver, combines with retinol and carries it to tissues as the RBP-retinol complex. The amount of circulating retinol is set by the amount of RBP. Any dysfunction of the liver, such as protein energy malnutrition or alcoholic liver disease, can affect vitamin A status. Night blindness can also be seen with zinc deficiency, because zinc is required in the synthesis process of RBP and the conversion of retinol to retinal.

Apart from its role in visual function, vitamin A plays a part in other basic physiological processes, such as growth, reproduction, immunity and epithelial tissue maintenance. It is essential throughout the entire lifespan, but particularly critical

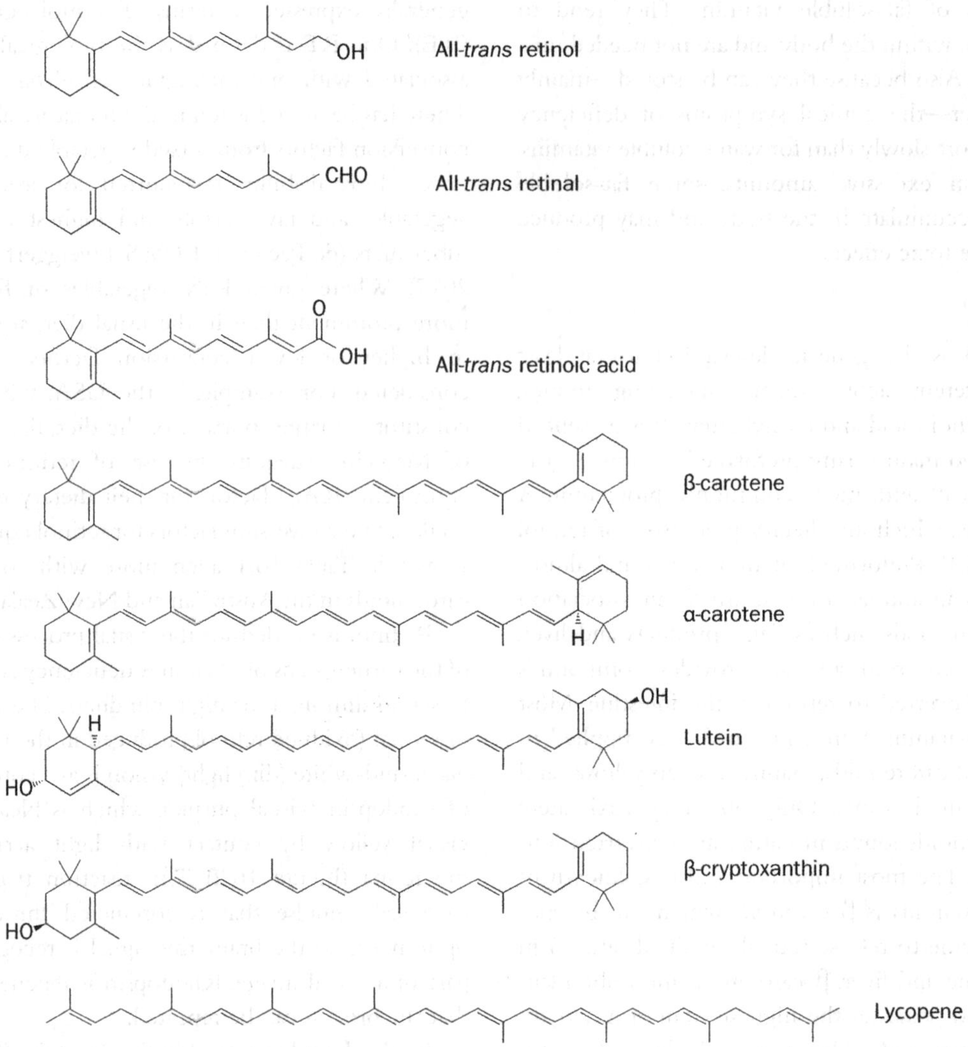

All-*trans* retinol

All-*trans* retinal

All-*trans* retinoic acid

β-carotene

α-carotene

Lutein

β-cryptoxanthin

Lycopene

Figure 16.1: Chemical structures of vitamin A-related compounds

Table 16.1: Calculation and conversion factors for retinol equivalents

µg Retinol Equivalent (RE) = µg Retinol + (µg β-carotene)/6 + (µg other provitamin A carotenoids)/12

1 µg RE   = 1 µg of all-*trans* retinol
          = 6 µg all-*trans* β-carotene
          = 12 µg of α-carotene, β-cryptoxanthin and other provitamin A carotenoids

Retinol activity equivalents (RAE) used by the US Institute of Medicine.
1 µg RAE = 1 µg of all-*trans* retinol
          = 2 µg all-*trans* β-carotene from supplements
          = 12 µg all-*trans* β-carotene from food
          = 24 µg of α-carotene, β-cryptoxanthin and other provitamin A carotenoids from food

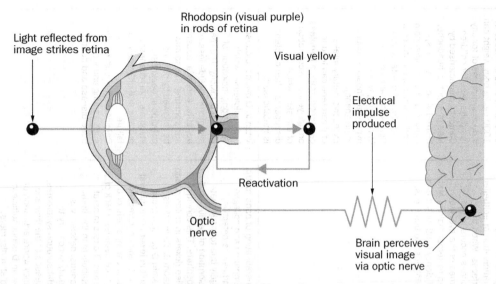

Figure 16.2: Function of vitamin A, in the retinal form as a component of rhodopsin, in the visual cycle in the retina of the eye

during periods in which cells proliferate rapidly and differentiate, such as pregnancy and early childhood. Each form of vitamin A performs specific tasks. Retinol is the major transport and storage form of the vitamin. It is required for the integrity of epithelial cells throughout the body and supports reproduction. Retinal, the oxidised form, is required by the eye to change light to neural signals for vision, and is also an intermediate in the oxidative conversion of retinol to retinoic acid. Retinoic acid is required to maintain differentiation of the cornea and conjunctiva, preventing xerophthalmia, as well as for photoreceptor rod and cone cells in the retina. It acts as an intracellular hormone and binds with a receptor to form a complex that can bind to DNA to act as a modulator of gene expression, controlling mRNA synthesis. It is thus involved in cell differentiation, growth and embryonic development, and this explains why vitamin A taken in excessive and repeated doses can be hazardous, especially during pregnancy. Excess vitamin A is both toxic and teratogenic (producing birth malformation) (Table 16.2).

Vitamin A is believed to be important for resistance to infection. Mortality from infections is high in communities where vitamin A deficiency is found, and vitamin A supplementation reduces mortality. However, inconclusive results of reduced incidence of infectious episodes have been gathered from prophylactic vitamin A supplementation trials. As a tentative resolution of apparent mortality-morbidity paradox, it is postulated that the specific intensity and lethality of infections is aggravated in the child with marginal vitamin A status (Solomons 2012).

Vitamin A deficiency remains one of the world's major nutritional problems (see also Chapter 29). Fortunately, progress is being made towards its eradication in Asia. Clinical deficiency of vitamin A is virtually never seen in Australia. Vitamin A is retained in the body more extensively than most other vitamins, and the average amount stored, mostly in the liver, can satisfy the normal requirement for between one and two years. Toxicity from excessive and prolonged intakes of vitamin A, usually in the form of supplements, is rare, but has been reported both in adults and children owing to the mistaken belief that large amounts are beneficial and safe.

Vitamin D

Vitamin D could be classified as a hormone, rather than as a vitamin. It can be produced by the body

Table 16.2: Functions, Nutrient Reference Values, food sources, deficiency and toxicity of fat-soluble vitamins

Functions	Nutrient Reference Values*	Food sources	Deficiency	Toxicity
Vitamin A • Vitamin A specially related to the retinal form plays a role in the visual cycle. • Vitamin A in the retinoic acid form plays an important role in gene transcription. • Vitamin A in the retinoic acid form appears to maintain normal skin health by switching on genes and differentiating keratinocytes (immature skin cells) into mature epidermal cells.	**Recommended Dietary Intake (RDI) as retinol equivalents** **Children** 1–3 yrs — 300 µg/day 4–8 yrs — 400 µg/day **Boys** 9–13 yrs — 600 µg/day 14–18 yrs — 900 µg/day **Girls** 9–13 yrs — 600 µg/day 14–18 yrs — 700 µg/day **Adults (19+ yrs)** Men — 900 µg/day Women — 700 µg/day **Pregnancy (19+ yrs)** — 800 µg/day **Lactation (19+ yrs)** — 1,100 µg/day	**Preformed vitamin A (retinol)** **High** Lamb liver, fried **Medium** Fish, cooked Egg yolk **Low** Chicken, cooked **Provitamin A (β-carotene equivalents)** **High** Sweet potato, cooked Carrot **Medium** Spinach Kale **Low** Bread Potato (nil)	• Night blindness. • Keratinisation of epithelial surfaces. When this process occurs in the cornea of the eye, it can lead to xerophthalmia and if deficiency continues it can rapidly lead to blindness.	• Chronic intakes in excess of 1000 µg/kg body weight can induce symptoms of toxicity in adults, less for children. • Clinically characterised by loss of appetite, headache, blurred vision, hair loss, muscle and abdominal pain and weakness, drowsiness, and altered mental status. • Congenital abnormalities in offspring when hypervitaminosis A occurs in pregnancy. • Excessive dietary intake of β-carotene can lead to carotenodermia, a harmless orange-yellow discolouration of the skin, which disappears when carotene is metabolised.
Vitamin D • Maintains normal blood levels of calcium and phosphate, which are in turn needed for the normal mineralisation of bone, muscle contraction, nerve conduction and general cellular function in all cells of the body. • Calcitriol regulates the transcription of a number of vitamin D-dependent genes which code for calcium-transporting proteins and bone matrix proteins. • Modulates the transcription of cell cycle proteins, which decrease cell proliferation and increase cell differentiation of a number of specialised cells of the body, e.g. osteoclastic precursors, enterocyte, keratinocytes. • Functions to activate the innate and dampen the adaptive immune systems.	**Adequate Intake (AI)** **Children** 1–3 yrs — 5 µg/day 4–8 yrs — 5 µg/day **Boys** 9–13 yrs — 5 µg/day 14–18 yrs — 5 µg/day **Girls** 9–13 yrs — 5 µg/day 14–18 yrs — 5 µg/day **Adults** 19–30 yrs — 5 µg/day 31–50 yrs — 5 µg/day 51–70 yrs — 10 µg/day >70 yrs — 15 µg/day **Pregnancy (19+ yrs)** — 5 µg/day **Lactation (19+ yrs)** — 5 µg/day	**High** Cod liver oil **Medium** Margarine **Low** Egg yolk Butter Cheese Milk	• Mineralisation of bone matrix and collagen synthesis is defective, largely due to inadequate absorption of calcium and phosphate. This condition is called rickets in children, and osteomalacia in adults. • Vitamin D deficiency can result in lower bone mineral density and an increased risk of osteoporosis or bone fracture because a lack of vitamin D alters mineral metabolism in the body. • In adults, deficiency is usually secondary to malabsorption syndromes, diseases of the liver and kidney where activation of vitamin D is not sufficient, and skin disorders.	• Vitamin D overdose causes hypercalcaemia, which is a strong indication of vitamin D toxicity. The main symptoms include loss of appetite, anorexia, nausea, and vomiting. These may be followed by polyuria, polydipsia, weakness, insomnia, nervousness, pruritus and ultimately renal failure. • Calcification of soft tissues such as lung and kidney, bone disease and death.

Functions	Nutrient Reference Values*	Food sources	Deficiency	Toxicity
Vitamin E • Protects lipids and prevents the oxidation of polyunsaturated fatty acids. • As an antioxidant, acts as a free radical scavenger, disabling the production of damaging free radicals in tissues. As it is fat-soluble, it is incorporated into cell membranes, which protects them from oxidative damage.	*Adequate Intake (AI) as α-tocopherol equivalents* **Children** 1–3 yrs 5 mg/day 4–8 yrs 6 mg/day **Boys** 9–13 yrs 9 mg/day 14–18 yrs 10 mg/day **Girls** 9–13 yrs 8 mg/day 14–18 yrs 8 mg/day **Adults (19+ yrs)** Men 10 mg/day Women 7 mg/day **Pregnancy (19+ yrs)** 7 mg/day **Lactation (19+ yrs)** 11 mg/day	**High** Wheat germ oil Vegetable oil **Medium** Peanut oil Olive oil Nuts, seeds, wholegrains **Low** Milk	• Deficiency has not been reported in Australian adults but may occur in malabsorption syndromes such as cystic fibrosis. • Low-birthweight infants given formula feeds low in vitamin E. They may develop a form of haemolytic anaemia associated with low blood vitamin E.	• Relatively non-toxic, though some adverse effects have been observed with daily intake of 300 mg of synthetic α-tocopherol. • Symptoms include severe influenza, malaise, fatigue and gut disturbances. • An unbalanced ratio of vitamin E and K may lead to impairment of blood coagulation in humans.
Vitamin K • Clotting of blood 1. Involved in the synthesis of certain blood-clotting factors in the liver (clotting factors II, VII, IX and X are vitamin K-dependent proteins). 2. Through the action of these clotting factors, vitamin K may influence calcium metabolism in various parts of the body. • Maintaining healthy bones 1. Enables the protein osteocalcin to bind to calcium, which subsequently helps to form bone matrix. 2. Works with vitamin D to facilitate the function of osteoblasts (bone-building cells) and inhibit the production of osteoclasts (bone-breakdown cells). • Facilitating cell growth: Gas6 is a protein important for regulating cell growth, proliferation and preventing cell death. Its functions are dependent on vitamin K.	*Adequate Intake (AI)* **Children** 1–3 yrs 25 µg/day 4–8 yrs 35 µg/day **Boys** 9–13 yrs 45 µg/day 14–18 yrs 55 µg/day **Girls** 9–13 yrs 45 µg/day 14–18 yrs 55 µg/day **Adults (19+ yrs)** Men 70 µg/day Women 60 µg/day **Pregnancy (19+ yrs)** 60 µg/day **Lactation (19+ yrs)** 60 µg/day	**High** Spinach Cabbage **Medium** Wheat bran green beans **Low** Oranges Apples	• Cases of diet-induced deficiency are rare but may be associated with lipid malabsorption such as in cystic fibrosis or coeliac disease. • Vitamin K deficiency causes a bleeding tendency through a lack of activity of the procoagulant proteins.	• No adverse effects are associated with vitamin K consumption as food or supplements. • Potentially toxic if given in large doses over a prolonged period of time.

Note: * Usual intake at or above Adequate Intake (AI) or Recommended Dietary Intake (RDI) level has a low probability of inadequacy

Sources: Briggs & Wahlqvist (1988); NHMRC (2006)

VITAMIN A CONTROVERSY

Read the following articles:

Mason, J.B. et al. 2018, 'Should universal distribution of high dose vitamin A to children cease?', *BMJ*, 360: k927

Fisker, A.B. & Greiner, T., 2017, 'High dose vitamin A capsules—rusty bullets?', *World Nutrition*, 8(1): 52–61

- Based on the evidence provided in these articles, should high-dose vitamin A supplementation continue?
- Is it ethical to continue without understanding whether such supplementation is doing more harm than good?
- What could be the alternatives to high-dose vitamin A supplementation?

Present your findings to a group of your peers. Make sure you provide a rationale for your opinions.

or obtained preformed in the diet; it is therefore not an essential dietary factor, and not technically a vitamin. Like a hormone, it is carried by the bloodstream from its site of production to act elsewhere. Of the several natural forms of vitamin D, the two most important for humans are vitamin D2 (ergocalciferol, plant origin) and vitamin D3 (cholecalciferol, animal origin) (Figure 16.3). Both of these vitamins are formed by the UV irradiation of ergosterol (provitamin D2) found in yeasts and fungi, and 7-dehydrocholesterol (provitamin D3), which is synthesised from cholesterol in the liver and then transported to the skin. The amount of cholecalciferol or vitamin D3 synthesis in skin is determined by the length and intensity of exposure to sunlight and the amount of melanin (colour pigment) in the skin. Vitamin D formed in the skin is then transported to the liver, where it is converted to calcidiol (25-hydroxy cholecalciferol; 25-OH vitamin D). The active form of vitamin D, calcitriol (1,25-dihydroxy cholecalciferol; 1,25-OH vitamin D), is formed from calcidiol in the kidneys.

Calcitriol acts in a similar manner to steroid hormones, and it is one of three hormones that normally act together to control calcium and phosphorus balance; the other two are parathyroid hormone (PTH) and calcitonin. Vitamin D raises blood concentrations of these minerals by stimulating their absorption in the small intestine, their reabsorption in the kidney, and their withdrawal from the bones into the blood (Figure 16.4). The formation of calcitriol is strictly controlled according to the body's calcium needs. The main controlling factors are the existing level of calcitriol itself and the blood parathyroid hormone, calcium and phosphorus.

Although there is no consensus on optimal levels of 25-OH vitamin D, the major circulating form in the plasma, a concentration of 30 ng/mL (75 nmol/L) or greater can be considered to indicate sufficient vitamin D. In the population, vitamin D status is generally maintained by exposure to sunlight. Vitamin D levels are determined by the quantity of sun exposure one receives; hence they can be used as a surrogate measurement of sun exposure. People who receive adequate exposure to sunlight do not need additional dietary vitamin D. However, older people can be at risk of vitamin D deficiency even with exposure to UV light because their skin contains less of the starting material, 7-dehydrocholesterol. There is also a risk of vitamin D deficiency in infants living in cold climates, especially during the winter months, and this can cause rickets. The bones fail to calcify normally, causing growth retardation and skeletal

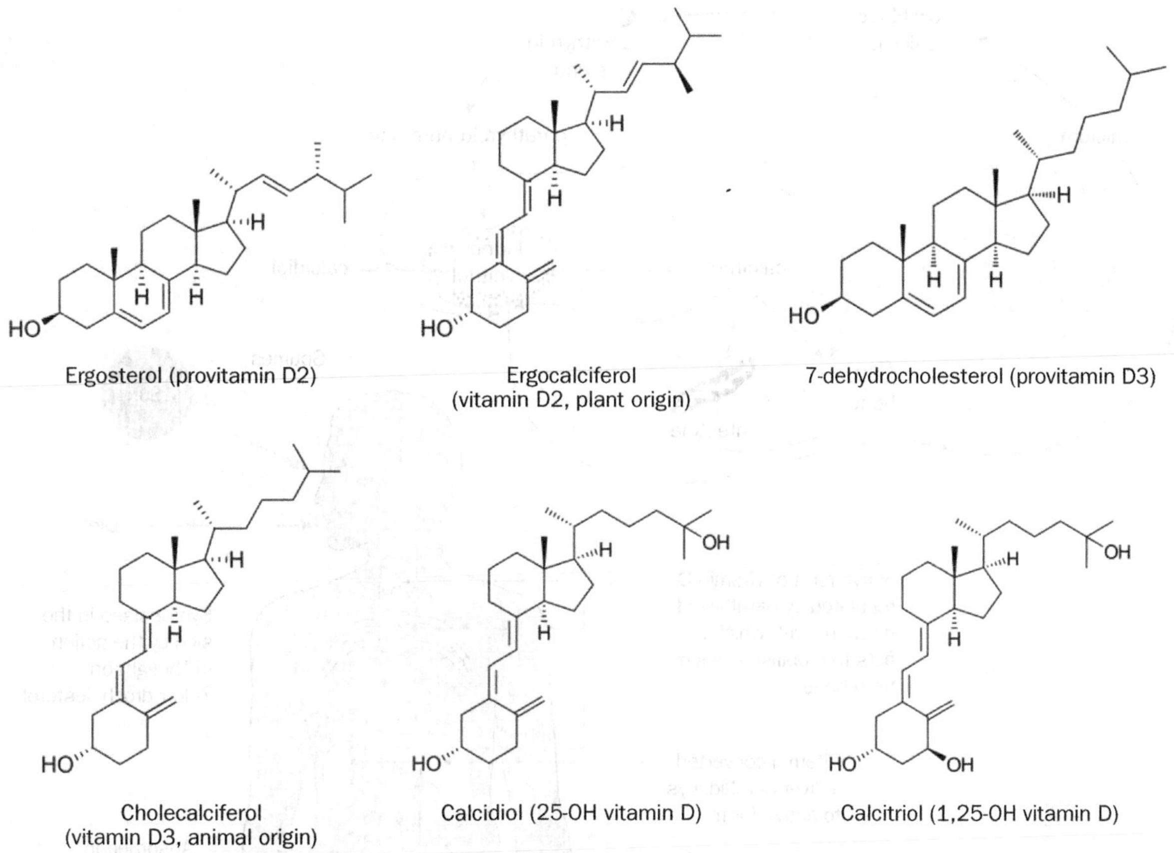

Ergosterol (provitamin D2)

Ergocalciferol
(vitamin D2, plant origin)

7-dehydrocholesterol (provitamin D3)

Cholecalciferol
(vitamin D3, animal origin)

Calcidiol (25-OH vitamin D)

Calcitriol (1,25-OH vitamin D)

Figure 16.3: Chemical structure of vitamin D-related compounds

abnormalities. The bones become so weak that they bend when they have to support the body's weight. The elderly, particularly those institutionalised for long periods, and people who wear clothes that limit sunlight exposure are also at risk of osteomalacia, the adult form of rickets. Conversely, too much sunlight exposure can increase actinic damage and risk for skin cancer. Figure 16.5 shows how protective foods might minimise actinic damage, and subsequently protect against vitamin D-related disorders.

Vitamin D intoxication is observed when blood concentrations of 25–OH vitamin D are greater than 150 ng/mL (374 nmol/L). People living near the equator who are exposed to sunlight without sun protection have robust levels of 25–OH vitamin D, above 30 ng/mL. However, vitamin D deficiency is common even in the sunniest areas when most of

the skin is shielded from sunlight. It is increasingly recognised that a significant number of Australians and New Zealanders may have less than optimal 25–OH vitamin D status; however, limited published information is available about the prevalence of vitamin D deficiency in Australia.

Due to the fact that vitamin D can be obtained from the diet and made in the skin by exposure to sunlight, it is difficult to estimate adequate dietary intake for the general population. Only a few natural food sources of vitamin D are known to exist; small amounts are found in fatty fish, butter, eggs and fortified foods such as margarine (Table 16.2). Mushrooms contain high amount of ergosterol (provitamin D2), and they can be a good dietary source of vitamin D2 if exposed to UV light. From a nutritional perspective, ergocalciferol (vitamin D2)

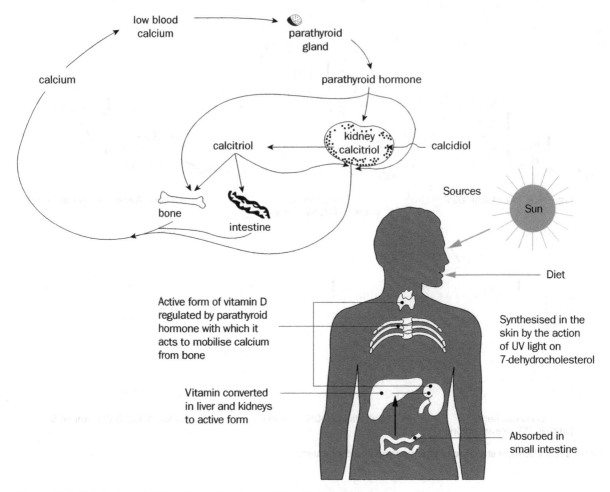

Figure 16.4: Metabolism of vitamin D and its role in calcium homeostasis

and cholecalciferol (vitamin D3) are metabolised similarly in humans, are equal in potency and can be considered equivalent.

Interest has focused on other cellular actions of calcitriol. The discovery that most tissues and cells in the body have a specific vitamin D receptor, and that several possess the enzymatic capability to convert the primary circulating form of vitamin D (calcidiol, 25-OH vitamin D) to the active form, calcitriol (1,25-OH vitamin D), has provided new insights into the function of this vitamin (Norman & Bouillon 2010). There has been a remarkable increase in our understanding of many biological actions that result from vitamin D acting through calcitriol in collaboration with its cognate vitamin D receptor.

Other physiological systems where vitamin D and its receptor generate biological responses include the muscle, the pancreas, cardiovascular and immune systems (Table 16.3). Not only can presumption of vitamin D function in most cells help to explain some of the abnormalities in vitamin D deficiency, but these abnormalities may also help to identify whether calcitriol plays a general role in all cells. Muscular weakness and susceptibility to infections in rickets or osteomalacia may reflect regulatory roles of calcitriol in the muscles and the immune systems. It has now been proposed that vitamin D is also important for insulin and prolactin secretion, stress responses and cell differentiation (Norman & Bouillon 2010).

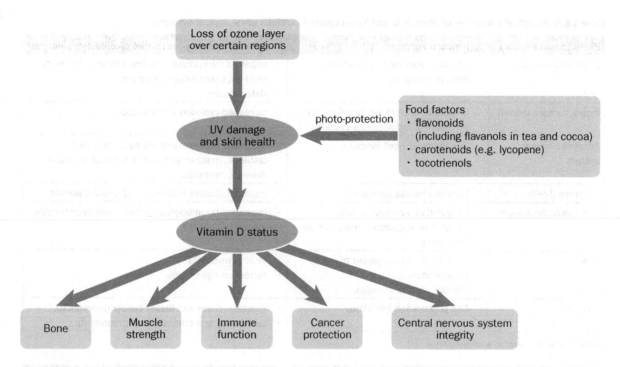

Figure 16.5: Consequences of excessive sun exposure and the possible role of phytonutrients in protecting against vitamin D deficiency-related disorders
Source: Wahlqvist & Lee (2007)

SUN EXPOSURE: HOW MUCH IS ENOUGH?

Some groups in Australia are at higher risk of vitamin D deficiency.
These include people who:

- are institutionalised and do not get sun exposure regularly
- have cultural or religious practices that mean most of their skin is covered
- have dark skins and limited exposure to sunlight
- are obese.

When the UV index is above three, as it is during summer, just a couple of minutes in the sun on most days will be adequate. When the UV index is below three, as it is in autumn and winter in southern parts of Australia, spending time outdoors in the middle of the day with some skin uncovered should ensure adequate vitamin D production. People with dark skins need to spend longer in the sun.

For people who are obese, lower vitamin D may reflect a volumetric dilution effect and whole body stores could be adequate (Walsh et al. 2017).

Table 16.3: Biological responses of vitamin D and its receptors in various physiological systems

Physiological systems	Biological responses	Vitamin D deficiency-associated disorders or diseases
Calcium homeostasis	• Intestinal absorption of calcium. • Bone remodelling.	• Impaired mineralisation of bone matrix: rickets in children, osteomalacia in adults. • Osteoporosis.
Innate immune system	• Stimulate macrophage function and synthesis of antimicrobial peptides.	• Increased prevalence of infection.
Adaptive immune system	• Dendritic and T-cell function.	• Increased autoimmune disease, e.g. type 1 diabetes, multiple sclerosis, inflammatory bowel disease, psoriasis.
Pancreas β-cells	• Facilitate insulin secretion.	• Impaired glucose tolerance and type 2 diabetes.
Cardiovascular system	• Coagulation, fibrinolysis, renin-angiotensin regulation, heart muscle functioning.	• Increased thrombogenesis, high renin hypertension, increased CVD risk.
Muscle	• Promote the development of normal skeletal muscle. • Improve muscle strength.	• Muscle myopathy. • Increased risk of falls.
All cells	• Cell proliferation inhibition.	• Prostate, colon and breast cancer (prevention). • Leukaemia and other cancers (treatment).

Source: Modified from Norman & Bouillon (2010)

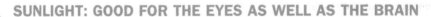

SUNLIGHT: GOOD FOR THE EYES AS WELL AS THE BRAIN

In addition to its healthy effect on our skin, sunlight also provides another positive benefit. The human eye contains photosensitive cells in its retina, with connections directly to the pituitary gland in the brain. Stimulation of these important cells comes from sunlight, in particular, the blue unseen spectrum. A study in 2008 states that, 'these photoreceptors play a vital role in human physiology and health' (Turner & Mainster 2008: 1439). The effects do not occur only in the brain, but in the whole body.

Photosensitive cells in the eye also directly affect the brain's hypothalamus region, which controls our biological clock. This influences our circadian rhythm, important not just for jet lag but also for normal sleep patterns, hormone regulation, increased reaction time and behaviour. Most cells in the body have an important cyclic pattern when working optimally, so potentially almost any area of the body can falter without adequate sun stimulation. Turner and Mainster state that, 'circadian disturbances can have significant physiological and psychological consequences' (2008: 1439). This also includes 'increasing risk of disease', as the authors state and as numerous other studies show, including cancer, diabetes and heart disease.

Vitamin E

Vitamin E is the major lipid–soluble antioxidant in the cell antioxidant defence system and is exclusively obtained from the diet. Vitamin E occurs naturally in at least eight different forms: four tocopherol and four tocotrienol forms. All forms consist of two carbon rings joined together and a 16–carbon side chain, with no double bond in the case of tocopherols and three double bonds in the case of tocotrienols (Figure 16.6). The number and position of the methyl

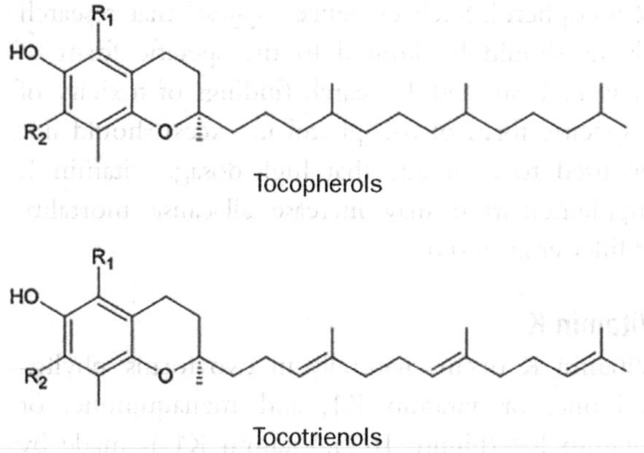

	R1	R2
α-forms:	CH_3	CH_3
β-forms:	CH_3	H
γ-forms:	H	CH_3
δ-forms:	H	H

Figure 16.6: Molecular structure of vitamin E

groups on the carbon ring differentiate one form from another (α-, β-, γ- and δ-). The compound *d*-α tocopherol is the most widely distributed and has the highest biological activity.

For dietary purposes, vitamin E activity is expressed as α-tocopherol equivalents (α-TE), where a α-TE is the activity of 1 mg *d*-α-tocopherol. To estimate the α-TE of a mixed diet containing natural forms of vitamin E, the amount in milligrams of β-tocopherol should be multiplied by 0.5, γ-tocopherol by 0.1, and α-tocotrienol by 0.3 (WHO/FAO 2004). Another way of calculating the total vitamin E activity of a varied diet is to multiply the α-tocopherol amount in milligrams by 1.2 (this accounts for the other tocopherols present). This calculation gives an approximation of total vitamin E activity expressed as 'milligrams of α-TE', but is not a complete statement about the vitamin E content.

The richest dietary sources of vitamin E are the commercially available vegetable oils. These are also the richest sources of polyunsaturated fatty acids (PUFAs), which vitamin E protects from oxidative breakdown. Nuts are the next best source, while almost all vegetables and meats have small amounts (Table 16.2). Absorption of vitamin E from the intestine depends on adequate pancreatic function, biliary secretion and micelle formation. Conditions for absorption are like those for dietary fats—that is, efficient emulsification, solubilisation within mixed bile salt micelles, uptake by enterocytes, and secretion into the circulation via the lymphatic system.

The major biological role of vitamin E is to protect PUFAs and other components of cell membranes and low-density lipoprotein (LDL) from oxidation by free radicals. The oxidative modification of LDL, which carries cholesterol to the tissues, appears to play an important part in the process of atherosclerosis. Oxidised LDL is taken up more readily than native LDL by macrophages to create foam cells. Vitamin E can inhibit the oxidative modification of LDL both *in vitro* and *in vivo*. Long-term sub-optimal vitamin E intake allows the accumulation of oxidative damage. One could propose that vitamin E supplements in excess of daily requirements could decrease the risk of chronic disease, particularly CVDs. Observational studies, including the Nurses' Health Study and Health Professionals Follow-Up Study, reported 20–40 per cent reductions in coronary heart disease risk among individuals who took vitamin E supplements for at least two years (Rimm et al. 1993; Stampfer et al. 1993). However, many vitamin E supplementation studies, such as the GISSI Prevention Trial and the Heart Outcomes Prevention Evaluation (HOPE) trial, failed to show the benefit of vitamin E in preventing heart attacks or deaths from heart disease among individuals with heart disease or those at high risk for it (GISSI-Prevenzione Investigators 1999; Yusuf et al. 2000). In fact, when the HOPE trial was extended for another four years, researchers found that study volunteers who took vitamin E had a higher risk of heart failure (Lonn et al. 2005).

Most prospective epidemiological studies suggest that vitamin E intake is in itself not related to overall risk of cancer, but that low serum vitamin E, particularly when coupled with low serum selenium, may increase the risk of some cancers, namely lung and cervical cancers. There is no justification for recommending extremely high doses as preventive or therapeutic measures.

The requirement for vitamin E in the body is difficult to estimate, since it is influenced by the amount and type of fat in the diet—that is, a high PUFA intake increases the vitamin E requirement. However, since foods that are good sources of PUFA are also generally good sources of vitamin E, the intake of the vitamin automatically increases as the intake of unsaturated oils increases. Historically, humans obtained most of their fat from unrefined sources like seeds (grains and nuts) and lean land animals, fish or other aqua-food. It seems almost impossible to induce a clinical deficiency of vitamin E through the consumption of a vitamin E deficient diet. However, the problem may arise with extensive refining of edible oils and fats. Furthermore, most of the vitamin E in PUFA oils is committed (depending on the degree of refinement of the oil) and little may be available for other metabolic functions. One advantage of a monounsaturated fat source (such as peanuts or olives) may be that it has less of a requirement for vitamin E to protect it against oxidation. Evidence of vitamin E deficiency is sometimes seen in intestinal malabsorption syndromes and in low-birthweight infants whose blood levels are low for the first month or so of life due to poor placental transfer. Because these conditions are rare, however, it is assumed that under normal circumstances enough vitamin E is supplied by the normal diet and that there is no need for a supplement (Table 16.2).

All four tocopherols and four tocotrienols share close structural similarity and hence comparable antioxidant efficacy. Apparently members of the vitamin E family with comparable antioxidant properties exhibit contrasting biological effects; this indicates that vitamin E molecules have functions independent of their antioxidant properties. Studies of the biological functions of vitamin E indicate that members in the vitamin E family possess biological functions often not shared by other family members. For example, α-tocotrienol possesses numerous functions that are not shared by α-tocopherol. α-Tocotrienol and δ-tocotrienol have emerged as vitamin E molecules with functions in health and disease that are clearly distinct from that of α-tocopherol. Such evidence suggests that research claims should be limited to the specific form of vitamin E studied. Research findings of toxicity of a specific form of tocopherol in excess should not be used to conclude that high-dosage vitamin E supplementation may increase all-cause mortality (Miller et al. 2005).

Vitamin K

Vitamin K occurs naturally in two forms: phylloquinone, or vitamin K1, and menaquinone, or vitamin K2 (Figure 16.7). Vitamin K1 is made by plants and is found in highest amounts in green leafy vegetables, soybeans and wheat bran. Fruit and most animal products contain little vitamin K1. Intestinal bacteria can convert vitamin K1 into vitamin K2. The bacteria typically lengthen the isoprenoid side chain of vitamin K2 to produce a range of vitamin K2 subtypes, most notably the MK-7 to MK-11 homologues. All forms of K2 other than MK-4 can only be produced by bacteria, which use these forms in anaerobic respiration. The MK-7 and other bacterially derived forms of vitamin K2 exhibit vitamin K activity in animals. It is estimated that approximately half of the vitamin K needed by the body can be obtained from the gut microbiota, while the remainder can be obtained from the diet. The third form of vitamin K is menadione, or vitamin K3, is a synthetic product and is used as a source of vitamin K in a wide range of animal feeds. One of the menaquinones, MK-4, is not a common product of bacterial synthesis but is synthesised from phylloquinone with menadione as an intermediate.

The human body needs vitamin K for a post-translational modification of certain proteins that are essential for blood coagulation and which the body also needs for controlling binding of calcium in bones and other tissues. The function of vitamin K in the animal cell is to add a carboxylic acid functional group to a glutamate (Glu) amino acid residue in a protein, to form a γ-carboxyglutamate (Gla) residue, resulting in the 'Gla protein'. The presence of two carboxylic acid groups on the same carbon in the Gla residue allows it to chelate calcium ions. The binding of calcium ions in this way very often triggers the

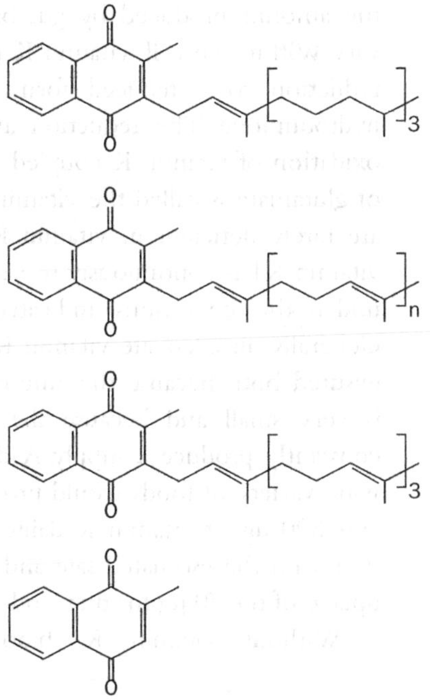

Phylloquinone (vitamin K1)

Menaquinone-n (vitamin K2)

Menaquinone-4

Menadione (vitamin K3)

Figure 16.7: Chemical structure of vitamin K-related compounds

VITAMIN K2: IS IT BETTER THAN VITAMIN K1 FOR HEART HEALTH?

Vitamin K, in either K1 or K2 form, is necessary for the formation of certain proteins required for many physiological functions, especially blood clotting and bone remodelling (see Table 16.4). Due to their differences in absorption and transport to tissues throughout the body, vitamin K1 and K2 could have profoundly different effects on the overall health.

In addition to blood clotting and bone health, vitamin K appears to play an important role in preventing heart disease by reducing calcium deposits in the vascular smooth muscle cells of arteries (Shea et al. 2009). These calcium deposits can lead to a reduction of vessel elasticity and subsequently to arterial stiffness. This arterial calcification can occur in addition to the formation of atherosclerotic plaques and is an independent predictor of cardiovascular disease (see also Chapter 33).

Observational studies have suggested that vitamin K2 is better than K1 at reducing calcium deposits in the coronary artery (Beulens et al. 2009; Gast et al. 2009). Furthermore, clinical evidence supports the notion that vitamin K2 MK-7 subtype reduces, and even reverses, arterial calcification (Knapen et al. 2015). However, further research is needed to confirm the therapeutic potential of vitamin K2.

In the meantime, it is important to focus on getting enough of both vitamin K1 and K2, such as including green leafy vegetables (for K1) and incorporating fermented foods (for K2) into the diet.

function or binding of Gla protein enzymes, such as the so-called vitamin K–dependent clotting factors. The vitamin K–related modification of the proteins allows them to bind calcium ions, which they cannot do otherwise. Some Gla-containing proteins or Gla proteins in humans have been characterised to the level of primary structure. These include blood coagulation factors II (prothrombin), VII, IX, and X, anticoagulant proteins C and S, osteocalcin (bone Gla protein) and the calcification-inhibiting matrix Gla protein (Table 16.4). The functions of these proteins have not been fully explored. In all cases in which their function is known, the presence of the Gla residues in these proteins appears to be essential for functional activity.

A Recommended Dietary Intake of vitamin K has generally not been available, because it is difficult to establish the amount required from food since the amount produced by gut bacteria is likely to vary. Within the cell, vitamin K undergoes electron reduction to a reduced form called vitamin K hydroquinone. The reduction and subsequent re-oxidation of vitamin K coupled with carboxylation of glutamate is called the vitamin K cycle. Humans are rarely deficient in vitamin K because, in part, vitamin K1 is continuously recycled in cells (except under the conditions indicated in Table 16.2). Generally, an adequate vitamin K status is probably ensured both because the amount the body needs is very small and because the intestinal bacteria constantly produce a supply. A diet consisting of a wide variety of foods would provide approximately 300–500 µg of vitamin K daily, and this compares well with the estimated safe and adequate range of uptake of 60–70 µg for men and women.

Without vitamin K, blood coagulation is

Table 16.4: Some vitamin K-dependent proteins and their roles in physiological functions

Organ or system	Protein type	Role(s) in physiological functions
Blood coagulation	Prothrombin	Procoagulant: to transform into thrombin (Factor II) Platelet aggregation Angiogenesis Atherosclerosis and inflammation Tumour growth and metastasis Cell survival Chemotaxis
	Factors VII, IX and X	Procoagulants: Components of the tissue factor pathway, in which prothrombin is activated to thrombin
	Protein C	Anticoagulant Anti-inflammatory action Anti-apoptotic actions
	Protein S	Anticoagulant Anti-inflammatory action Anti-apoptotic actions Phagocytosis of apoptotic cells Mitogenesis of vascular smooth muscle cells Neuronal protection
	Protein Z	Anticoagulant
Bone	Osteocalcin	Regulator of bone formation
	Matrix Gla protein	Inhibitor of calcification
	Protein S	(undetermined)
Others	Gas6 (Growth arrest-specific 6)	Cell differentiation, proliferation, adhesion and chemotaxis Phagocytosis and protection from apoptosis

Source: Modified from Ferland (2012)

seriously impaired and uncontrolled bleeding occurs. Symptoms of vitamin K deficiency include anaemia, bruising, nose bleeds, bleeding of the gums, and, in women, heavy menstrual bleeding. Clinical research indicates that deficiency of vitamin K2 may weaken bones, potentially leading to osteoporosis (Huang et al. 2015), and may promote calcification of arteries and other soft tissues (Knapen et al. 2015).

Newborn infants could be at an increased risk of deficiency. Other populations with an increased prevalence of vitamin K deficiency include those who suffer from liver damage or disease (such as heavy drinkers), cystic fibrosis or inflammatory bowel diseases, or who have recently had abdominal surgeries. Secondary vitamin K deficiency can occur in people with bulimia, those on stringent diets and those taking anticoagulants. Warfarin and other 4-hydroxycoumarins block the reconversion of vitamin K, resulting in decreased concentrations of vitamin K and vitamin K hydroquinone in tissues and, subsequently, the production of clotting factors with inadequate Gla. Without Gla on the amino termini of these factors, they no longer bind stably to the blood vessel endothelium and cannot activate clotting to allow formation of a clot during tissue injury. As it is impossible to predict what dose of warfarin will give the desired degree of clotting suppression, warfarin treatment must be carefully monitored to avoid overdose. It is also recognised that functions of vitamin K other than in coagulation, such as in bone, arteries, and other tissues, are affected by warfarin; for example, arterial calcification increases. As menadione, the synthetic form of vitamin K, may be toxic by interfering with the function of glutathione, it is no longer used to treat vitamin K deficiency.

WATER-SOLUBLE VITAMINS

Fat-soluble vitamins are present in a wide variety of foods. They are easily destroyed or washed out during food storage or preparation. Proper storage and preparation of food can minimise vitamin loss. Water-soluble vitamins are easily lost through bodily fluids, so they need to be replenished every day (Figure 16.8).

Thiamin

Thiamin or vitamin B-1 is widely distributed, but present only in relatively small amounts, in a large variety of animal and vegetable sources. The richest food sources of thiamin are yeast and yeast extract (for example, Vegemite), but they are usually consumed in small amounts.

The principal role of thiamin in the body is to work as a coenzyme in reactions that release energy from carbohydrates and trap it in the energy-laden compound ATP. The daily thiamin requirement, therefore, is proportional to the amount of energy consumed, particularly from carbohydrate sources. The Recommended Dietary Intake is usually expressed in terms of energy intake—that is, 0.1 mg/1000 kJ for all age groups. Storage of thiamin in the body is limited because it is water-soluble; this leads to a constant requirement for the vitamin and, compared with fat-soluble vitamins, relatively short periods of deprivation will lead to deficiency. There are bacteria in the large intestine with the ability to synthesise thiamin but its absorption into the body is minimal. In Australia, the population most likely to develop a thiamin deficiency is those who chronically drink alcohol to excess (a regular daily intake of at least 40 g alcohol) and who eat little or no food for extended periods of time; such people may develop Wernicke–Korsakoff syndrome (WKS) (see Chapter 15). Since the introduction of mandatory fortification of Australian bread with thiamin in 1991, WKS has become very uncommon. Where rice is a staple and not parboiled, thiamin deficiency is also a risk. Thiamin is removed during the refining process of cereal products, so its restoration to bread and cereals is permitted in Australia to ensure that daily requirements are met.

Riboflavin

Riboflavin or vitamin B-2 is found in small amounts in a wide variety of animal and vegetable food sources. The most important in the Australian diet are milk and dairy products, and fortified breads and cereals. Other good sources include breakfast cereals, organ meats and nuts (Table 16.5). Most of

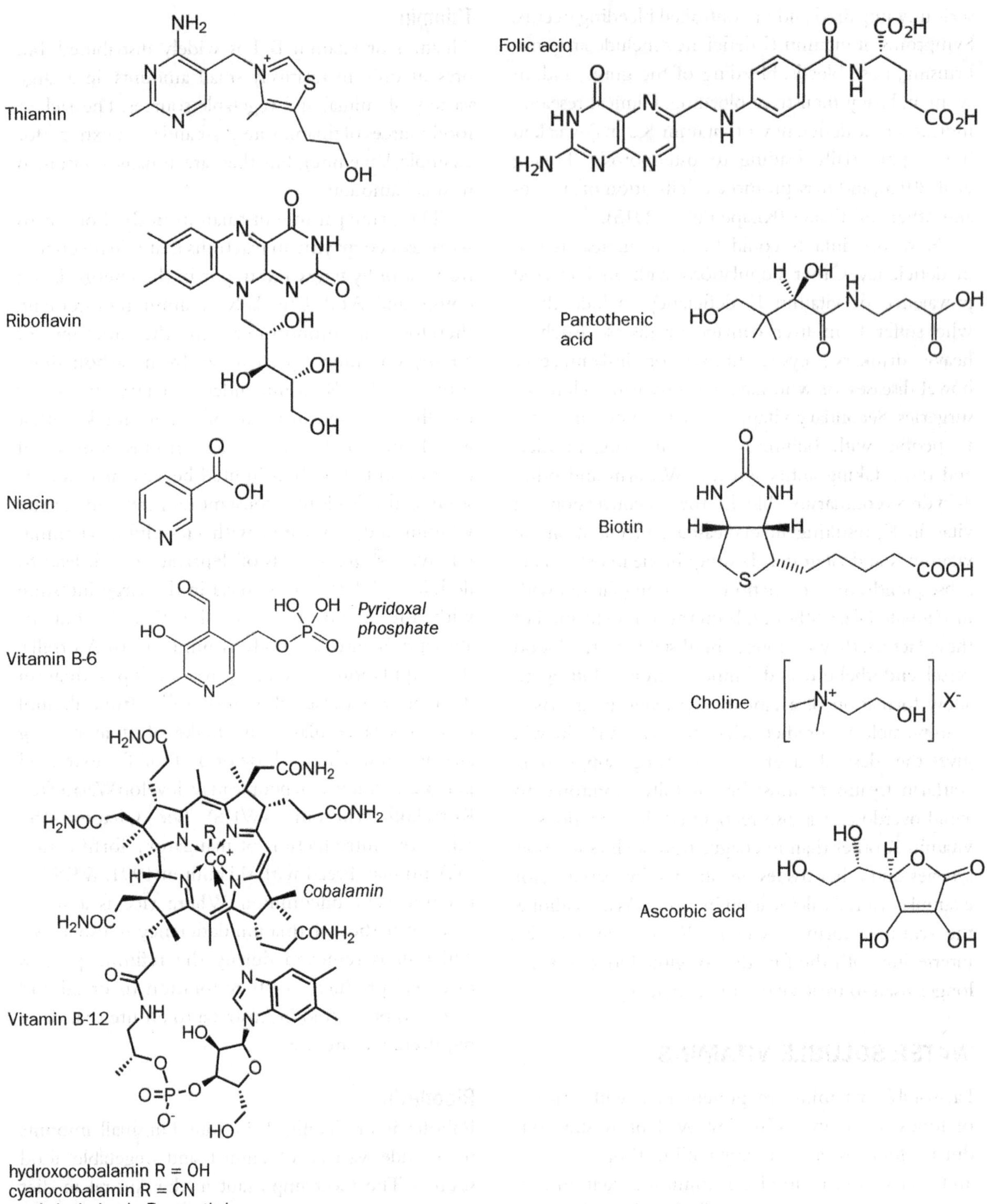

Thiamin

Riboflavin

Niacin

Vitamin B-6 / Pyridoxal phosphate

Vitamin B-12 / Cobalamin

hydroxocobalamin R = OH
cyanocobalamin R = CN
methylcobalamin R = methyl
adenosylcobalamin R = 5′-deoxyl adenosyl

Folic acid

Pantothenic acid

Biotin

Choline

Ascorbic acid

Figure 16.8: Chemical structures of water-soluble vitamins

Table 16.5: Functions, Nutrient Reference Values, food sources, deficiency and toxicity of water-soluble vitamins

Functions	Nutrient Reference Values*	Food sources	Deficiency	Toxicity

Thiamin (vitamin B-1)
· Coenzyme for major decarboxylation steps in carbohydrate metabolism.
· Coenzyme for catabolism of branched-chain amino acids.
	Recommended Dietary Intake (RDI)
	Children
	1–3 yrs 0.5 mg/day
	4–8 yrs 0.6 mg/day
	Boys
	9–13 yrs 0.9 mg/day
	14–18 yrs 1.2 mg/day
	Girls
	9–13 yrs 0.9 mg/day
	14–18 yrs 1.1 mg/day
	
	Adults (19+ yrs)
	Men 1.2 mg/day
	Women 1.1 mg/day
	Pregnancy (19+ yrs)
	  1.4 mg/day
	Lactation (19+ yrs)
	  1.4 mg/day
		· Whole grains, meat, fish and yeast.
		· Thiamin is readily destroyed by heat.
			· Beriberi.
			· Wernicke–Korsakoff syndrome.
				· No reports of toxicity from consumption of excess thiamin in food.
				· Large doses administered intravenously can cause anaphylaxis and death.

Riboflavin (vitamin B-2)
· Part of flavoproteins in the oxidation chain in mitochondria.
· Cofactors for several enzymes.
	Recommended Dietary Intake (RDI)
	Children
	1–3 yrs 0.5 mg/day
	4–8 yrs 0.6 mg/day
	Boys
	9–13 yrs 0.9 mg/day
	14–18 yrs 1.3 mg/day
	Girls
	9–13 yrs 0.9 mg/day
	14–18 yrs 1.1 mg/day
	Men
	19–70 yrs 1.3 mg/day
	>70 yrs 1.6 mg/day
	Women
	19–70 yrs 1.1 mg/day
	>70 yrs 1.3 mg/day
	Pregnancy (19+ yrs)
	  1.4 mg/day
	Lactation (19+ yrs)
	  1.6 mg/day
		· Milk and milk products
		· Eggs
		· Liver, kidney
		· Yeast extracts
		· Fortified breakfast cereals
			· Glossitis, angular stomatitis.	· Large doses taken orally appear safe.

Functions	Nutrient Reference Values*	Food sources	Deficiency	Toxicity
Niacin (vitamin B-3) • Part of coenzymes acting as hydrogen receptor in the electron chain during oxidative phosphorylation in the mitochondria.	**Recommended Dietary Intake (RDI) of niacin (as niacin equivalents)** **Children** 1–3 yrs — 6 mg/day 4–8 yrs — 8 mg/day **Boys** 9–13 yrs — 12 mg/day 14–18 yrs — 16 mg/day **Girls** 9–13 yrs — 12 mg/day 14–18 yrs — 14 mg/day **Adults (19+ yrs)** Men — 16 mg/day Women — 14 mg/day **Pregnancy (19+ yrs)** — 18 mg/day **Lactation (19+ yrs)** — 17 mg/day	• Dairy • Meat • Cereals and grain products • Vegetables	• Pellagra.	• Nicotinic acid (but not nicotinamide) produces cutaneous flushing from histamine release. • At very large doses (200 × RDI), side effects including gastric irritation, impaired glucose tolerance and disturbed liver function tests can occur.
Vitamin B-6 • Part of major coenzyme, pyridoxal 5'-phosphate (PLP), which is required in all the reactions involved in amino acid metabolism. • Associated with the enzyme in the muscle, which releases glucose from glycogen stores.	**Recommended Dietary Intake (RDI)** **Children** 1–3 yrs — 0.5 mg/day 4–8 yrs — 0.6 mg/day **Boys** 9–13 yrs — 1.0 mg/day 14–18 yrs — 1.3 mg/day **Girls** 9–13 yrs — 1.0 mg/day 14–18 yrs — 1.2 mg/day **Men** 19–50 yrs — 1.3 mg/day >50 yrs — 1.7 mg/day **Women** 19–50 yrs — 1.3 mg/day >50 yrs — 1.5 mg/day **Pregnancy (19+ yrs)** — 1.9 mg/day **Lactation (19+ yrs)** — 2.0 mg/day	• Meat • Egg yolk • Cereals and grain products • Vegetables • Fruits	• Weakness, peripheral neuropathy, dermatitis, cheilosis and glossitis, anaemia and impaired immunity.	• Large doses (133 × RDI) of pyridoxine are associated with sensory neuropathy.

Functions	Nutrient Reference Values*	Food sources	Deficiency	Toxicity
Vitamin B-12 (cobalamin) • Required for the synthesis of fatty acids in myelin, and, in conjunction with folate, for DNA and RNA synthesis. • Acts indirectly on red blood cell formation through the activation of folate coenzymes.	**Recommended Dietary Intake (RDI) of vitamin B-12** **Children** 1–3 yrs 0.9 µg/day 4–8 yrs 1.2 µg/day **Boys & girls** 9–13 yrs 1.8 µg/day 14–18 yrs 2.4 µg/day **Adults (19+ yrs)** Men 2.4 µg/day Women 2.4 µg/day **Pregnancy (19+ yrs)** 2.6 µg/day **Lactation (19+ yrs)** 2.8 µg/day	• Liver • Shellfish • Fish • Meat • Eggs • Milk and milk products • Bacterially fermented food	• Pernicious anaemia. • Neurological dysfunction.	• No evidence that the current levels of intake from foods and supplements represent a health risk.
Folate (vitamin B-9) • Coenzyme in single-carbon transfers in the metabolism of nucleotides and amino acids. • Folic acid supplements reduce the risk of neural tube defects.	**Recommended Dietary Intake (RDI) (as dietary folate equivalents)** **Children** 1–3 yrs 150 µg/day 4–8 yrs 200 µg/day **Boys & girls** 9–13 yrs 300 µg/day 14–18 yrs 400 µg/day **Adults (19+ yrs)** Men 400 µg/day Women 400 µg/day **Pregnancy (19+ yrs)** 600 µg/day **Lactation (19+ yrs)** 500 µg/day	• Leafy vegetables • Liver, kidney • Fortified breakfast cereals	• Macrocytic anaemia. • Weakness, fatigue, irritability and palpitations.	• High supplemental intake of folic acid is related to adverse neurological effects in people with vitamin B-12 deficiency as it can precipitate or exacerbate the B-12 deficiency.

Functions	Nutrient Reference Values*		Food sources	Deficiency	Toxicity
Pantothenic acid (vitamin B-5) · Component of coenzyme A and phosphopanteheine, both of which are involved in lipid metabolism.	**Adequate Intake (AI)** **Children** 1–3 yrs 4–8 yrs **Boys** 9–13 yrs 14–18 yrs **Girls** 9–13 yrs 14–18 yrs **Adults (19+ yrs)** Men Women **Pregnancy (19+ yrs)** **Lactation (19+ yrs)**	3.5 mg/day 4.0 mg/day 5.0 mg/day 6.0 mg/day 4.0 mg/day 4.0 mg/day 6 mg/day 4 mg/day 5 mg/day 6 mg/day	· Widely distributed in foods, but not in highly refined foods · Meat · Liver, kidney · Egg yolks · Whole grain	· Irritability, restlessness, fatigue, apathy, sleep disturbance.	· No reports of adverse effects of oral pantothenic acid in either humans or animals.
Biotin (vitamin B-7) · Cofactor for carboxylase enzymes in mitochondria and cytosol.	**Adequate Intake (AI)** **Children** 1–3 yrs 4–8 yrs **Boys** 9–13 yrs 14–18 yrs **Girls** 9–13 yrs 14–18 yrs **Adults (19+ yrs)** Men Women **Pregnancy (19+ yrs)** **Lactation (19+ yrs)**	8 µg/day 12 µg/day 20 µg/day 30 µg/day 20 µg/day 25 µg/day 30 µg/day 25 µg/day 30 µg/day 35 µg/day	· Liver · Meats · Cereals	· Dermatitis, conjunctivitis, alopecia and central nervous system abnormalities. · Biotin deficiency is seen in people who consume raw egg white over long periods. Avidin, a protein found in raw egg white, binds biotin in the gut and prevents its absorption.	· No evidence of adverse effects in humans and animals.

Functions	Nutrient Reference Values*	Food sources	Deficiency	Toxicity

Choline
• Precursor for the neurotransmitter acetyl choline and membrane constituents phospholipid and sphingomyelin, platelet activating factor and betaine.
• May improve cognitive function and memory.
	Adequate Intake (AI)
	Children
	1–3 yrs 200 mg/day
	4–8 yrs 250 mg/day
	Boys
	9–13 yrs 375 mg/day
	14–18 yrs 550 mg/day
	Girls
	9–13 yrs 375 mg/day
	14–18 yrs 400 mg/day
	Adults (19+ yrs)
	Men 550 mg/day
	Women 425 mg/day
	Pregnancy (19+ yrs)
	            440 mg/day
	Lactation (19+ yrs)
	            550 mg/day
		• Milk
		• Liver
		• Eggs
		• Peanuts
		• Wheat germ and soybeans (for vegetarians)
				• Hypotension, cholinergic responses and fishy body odour have been reported after large doses of choline therapy.

Vitamin C (ascorbic acid)	*Recommended Dietary Intake (RDI)*
	Children
	1–3 yrs 35 mg/day
	4–8 yrs 35 mg/day
	Boys and girls
	9–13 yrs 40 mg/day
	14–18 yrs 40 mg/day
	Adults (19+ yrs)
	Men 45 mg/day
	Women 45 mg/day
	Pregnancy (19+ yrs)
	             60 mg/day
	Lactation (19+ yrs)
	             85 mg/day
		• Fruits
		• Vegetables
		• Vitamin C can rapidly be lost from food during preparation
			• Scurvy
			• Delay in wound healing
			• Susceptibility to infections.
				• Gastrointestinal disturbances are the most common adverse effects associated with high doses of vitamin C given over a short period of time.
				• Risks of **megadose** therapy include rebound scurvy after discontinuation of megadoses of vitamin C, metabolic acidosis, changes in prothrombin activity and vitamin B-12 deficiency.

Note: * Usual intake at or above Adequate Intake (AI) or Recommended Dietary Intake (RDI) level has a low probability of inadequacy

Sources: Briggs & Wahlqvist (1988); NHMRC (2006)

vitamin B-2 in foods is in the forms of riboflavin phosphate and flavin adenine dinucleotide (FAD). These are hydrolysed to yield free riboflavin in the intestinal lumen and then absorbed in the upper small intestine. Relatively large amounts of free riboflavin can be found in milk and eggs. Much of the absorbed free riboflavin is converted by the addition of phosphate, and enters the bloodstream as riboflavin phosphate.

The active forms of riboflavin are FAD and flavin mononucleotide. Bound to enzymes and functioning as coenzymes, riboflavin and its derivatives act as electron carriers in a wide variety of oxidation and reduction reactions central to all metabolic processes, including the mitochondrial electron transport chain. They are important for the body's handling of some other nutrients, including conversion of vitamin B-6 to pyridoxal phosphate, conversion of tryptophan to niacin and conversion of methylene tetrahydrofolate to methyl tetrahydrofolate. Riboflavin is a constituent of all metabolising cells but, as with thiamin, there is limited storage in the body. Riboflavin deficiency is often associated with hypochromic anaemia, which may result from problems in the body's handling of iron. In addition, marginal riboflavin status may be a factor in hyperhomocysteinaemia, which is associated with increased CVD risk. There is some evidence that riboflavin supplements may be beneficial in lowering plasma homocysteine. Excess riboflavin is excreted by the kidneys in the urine, a possible explanation for its low toxicity.

Niacin

Niacin or vitamin B-3 has been identified in two forms: niacin (nicotinic acid) and niacinamide (nicotinamide). The best dietary sources of niacin are foods rich in protein, such as organ and muscle meats, poultry, legumes and peanuts (Table 16.5). Niacin can also be synthesised in the body from an amino acid, tryptophan. It is estimated that approximately 60 mg of the precursor tryptophan is needed to produce 1 mg of niacin in the body. This relationship between niacin and tryptophan has been taken into account in the development of the unit known as the niacin equivalent (NE). The NE value of a diet is calculated as follows:

$$\text{Niacin equivalent (mg)} = \text{dietary niacin (mg)} + (0.16 \times \text{dietary protein in grams})$$

The roles of niacin and riboflavin in cell metabolism are closely related, and clinical evidence of both deficiencies is often seen in the same individual. The niacin-deficiency disease pellagra produces the symptoms of diarrhoea, dermatitis, dementia and, eventually, death.

Vitamin B-6

Vitamin B-6 occurs naturally in food in three forms—pyridoxine, pyridoxal and pyridoxamine—and it is widely distributed in a variety of animal and plant food sources. Legumes, nuts, potatoes and bananas are among the best sources of pyridoxine; pork, fish and organ meats are the richest sources of pyridoxal and pyridoxamine. The bioavailability of vitamin B-6 varies with the type of food and losses can occur during storage and preparation. Consumption of a high-protein diet increases the need for vitamin B-6 because it acts as a coenzyme in the metabolism of amino acids. Generally, protein intake is taken into consideration in setting requirements for vitamin B-6. The amount of vitamin B-6 required is small and deficiency is rare. Vitamin B-6 is required for the conversion of tryptophan to niacin, as well as for folate metabolism; therefore, symptoms of vitamin B-6 deficiency resemble those of pellagra and can lead to niacin deficiency.

Unlike other water-soluble vitamins, vitamin B-6 is stored in muscle tissue. It is not safe to consume large amounts of this vitamin. The recommended upper limit in Australia should probably not exceed 10 mg daily on a regular basis (Table 16.5). A 'sensory neuropathy' (damage to nerve fibres conducting sensation) has been described with intakes of 200 mg daily, contained in some supplements. There is limited evidence that premenstrual tension may be ameliorated by vitamin B-6 supplements. In this situation, the individual must be careful not to take excessive amounts (Wyatt et al. 1999).

Vitamin B-12

Three predominant forms of vitamin B-12 in food are methylcobalamin, adenosylcobalamin and hydroxocobalamin. Vitamin B-12 is supplied almost entirely by animal foods, with organ meats, eggs, seafood, dairy products and fermented foods being excellent sources. The occurrence of vitamin B-12 in nature is the result of microbial synthesis, but the amount available from the intestinal bacteria of humans is not known. Intestinal absorption of vitamin B-12 requires the presence of a molecule called intrinsic factor, which is secreted by the stomach and facilitates the transfer of vitamin B-12 into the cells lining the ileum. Calcium is also thought to be necessary for this transfer. The human body has a good storage capacity for vitamin B-12, as well as

a very efficient method of recycling the vitamin, so the amount required for normal metabolism appears to be small. The onset of deficiency symptoms due to depletion may be delayed by up to ten years, and is rarely seen within two years.

Folate

Folate is the generic name for many compounds that exhibit the biological activity of folic acid or pteroyl glutamic acid. Folate occurs widely in a variety of foods, including leafy vegetables, liver, citrus fruit and nuts, which are particularly good sources. Folate is present usually in the form of tetrahydrofolate and conjugated with the amino acid glutamic acid. Different forms of folates vary widely in their biological activity, stability and availability to the

FOLATE AND CANCER

Folate intake in Australia and New Zealand has dramatically increased over the past decade, owing partly to mandatory folic acid fortification and partly to the consumption of supplemental folic acid. A large body of epidemiological evidence suggests that folate deficiency could increase the risk of several major cancers, including those of the colorectum, pancreas, prostate and breast. However, several randomised clinical trials of folic acid supplementation have reported either an increase in or null effect on cancer incidence and/or mortality.

Folic acid, which is a synthetic form of folate, is inactive until it is metabolised into the natural reduced forms, including 5-methyltetrahydrofolate (5m-THF), the prevailing circulating folate species. Because unmetabolised folic acid enters the folate metabolic cycles differently to 5m-THF, and has a distinct metabolism, it may have biological effects that differ from those of the naturally occurring folates. High circulating concentrations of unmetabolised folic acid have been reported in the post-fortification period, likely due to a high folic acid intake from both supplementation and fortification.

While there has been sufficient evidence to conclude that folic acid supplements provide no benefit for cancer risk reduction among people with adequate background folate status, there are still a number of questions about the benefits (and/or risks) of folic acid supplementation and food fortification. These questions include whether or not high circulating unmetabolised folic acid poses a health risk, including the tumour-promoting effect; whether or not 5m-THF is a safer and effective alternative to folic acid in providing supplemental concentrations of folate; and, ultimately, whether folic acid and naturally occurring folates have different biochemical and carcinogenic effects. These considerations may also apply to folic acid intervention to reduce neural tube defects, which is not uniformly successful, perhaps because of related nutrient deficiencies (Li et al. 2016).

body. In animal foods, such as liver, most of the folate is present as 5-methyl tetrahydrofolate or 'free form', which is readily absorbed unaltered in the duodenum and jejunum of the small intestine. In plant foods, most of the folate is present as polyglutamates. This 'conjugated form' has to be hydrolysed, probably in the lumen of the gut by intestinal bacteria, prior to absorption. The larger the number of glutamate residues in the polyglutamate chain, the less well the compound is absorbed. Bioavailability of folates in food is about 50–60 per cent, whereas that of the folic acid used to fortify foods or as a supplement is about 85 per cent. To accommodate the varying degrees of bioavailability, the term 'dietary folate equivalent' (DFE) has been used in the assessment of folate requirements. 1 μg dietary folate equivalent (DFE):

= 1 μg food folate

= 0.5 μg folic acid on an empty stomach

= 0.6 μg folic acid with meals or as fortified foods.

Folate deficiency can be caused by diets that do not include enough fruits and vegetables, diseases in which folic acid is not well absorbed in the digestive system (such as Crohn's disease or coeliac disease), some genetic disorders that affect levels of folate, and certain medicines, such as phenytoin or sulfasalazine. Folate deficiency impairs cell division and protein synthesis. Without folate, DNA synthesis slows and cells lose their ability to divide. In folate deficiency, the replacement of red blood cells and gastrointestinal tract cells falters—therefore, two of the first symptoms of folate deficiency are anaemia, characterised by large, immature blood cells (macrocytic anaemia), and gastrointestinal tract deterioration. Results from epidemiological and randomised controlled studies indicate that folate can be useful in the prevention of diseases such as neural tube defects in newborn babies. Folate fortification of wheat flour used in breadmaking has been mandatory since 2008 (FSANZ 2016) (see also Chapter 20).

FOLATE CONTENT OF FOODS AND IN YOUR DIET

The complex nature of folate, along with its different forms and stability, makes it difficult to measure folate in food. Analytical methods using different principles have been developed; these include microbiological assays for total folate content, and high-performance liquid chromatography (HPLC) methods for different forms of the vitamin. The Australian Food Composition Database (previously called NUTTAB) contains a wide range of foods and folate content data using improved methods of analysis. Some of the values of free and total folates reported in 2010 were determined using the triple enzyme (conjugase, protease and amylase) microbiological method, while values reported in previous versions of NUTTAB were determined using a single enzyme (conjugase) microbiological assay.

Following the release of NUTTAB 2010, FSANZ conducted a small analytical program in 2014–2015 to improve the quality and robustness of the food composition data. It was found that the levels of total folates in certain fruits, vegetables and dairy products were substantially different from the previous data. The explanations for this could include natural variation, advances in analytical techniques over the past decade leading to greater extraction of folates from foods, or changes in transport, processing and/or storage that affect post-harvest folate losses.

Explore the Australian Food Composition Database to develop a list of foods with high folate content. Look at this across a range of culturally diverse foods. Check your own diet and reflect on the amount of folate you are consuming. What foods do you need to increase?

Source: Nutrient tables for use in Australia (Australian Food Composition Database) (FSANZ 2012)

The RDI for folate in Australia is 400 μg DFE for both men and women. Women capable of or planning pregnancies are encouraged to consume 400 μg/day of folic acid as a supplement or in the form of fortified foods for at least one month before and the first three months of pregnancy, in addition to increasing their daily intake of folate-rich foods (Table 16.5). Indicators of folate requirement include erythrocyte, serum or urinary folate, plasma homocysteine and haematological status measures. Of these, erythrocyte folate is generally regarded as the primary indicator, as it reflects tissue folate storage.

As vitamin B-12 is required for the activation of folate, its deficiency manifests as the anaemia of folate deficiency. Before receiving folate treatment, patients with megaloblastic anaemia need to be tested for vitamin B-12 deficiency by measuring methyl malonic acid levels. If the patient has vitamin B-12 deficiency, taking folate supplement can remove the anaemia symptoms, but it can also worsen neurologic problems. By doing so, folate masks vitamin B-12 deficiency. Therefore, the folate fortification in cereal products may cause a problem in those at risk of vitamin B-12 deficiency, such as the elderly.

Folate deficiency, along with vitamin B-6 and B-12 deficiencies, may—even when marginal by the usual criteria of its blood concentration— lead to an increase in homocysteine in the blood. Homocysteine can be toxic to blood vessels and increase the risk of thrombosis. Its mildly raised concentration is a risk factor for CVD, including stroke and ischaemic heart disease. Doses of folate from 500 μg/day to 5 mg/day have been shown to reduce homocysteine by about 25 per cent depending on pre-treatment blood homocysteine and folate concentrations. Since folate contributes to DNA synthesis and repair, it has been suggested that folate may have a role in reducing the risk of cancer by preventing the occurrence and reducing the progression of certain cancers, notably cervical cancer in women, although not all studies agree. A systematic review in 2017 found no relationship between taking folate supplements and cancer risk (Schwingshackl et al. 2017).

Ascorbic acid (Vitamin C)

Vitamin C exists in two forms: L-ascorbic acid (predominant form) and its oxidised form, L-dehydroascorbic acid. The best sources of vitamin C include readily available fruits and vegetables. Vitamin C is easily destroyed by high temperatures and exposure to air, drying, alkalis and prolonged storage. It is very soluble in water, and losses during the preparation and cooking of fruit and vegetables can be considerable. Large amounts of vitamin C are also added to the food supply in the preservation of food and in the process of nutrient restoration.

Ascorbic acid performs numerous physiological functions in the human body. These functions include the synthesis of collagen, carnitine and neurotransmitters; the synthesis and catabolism of tyrosine; and the metabolism of microsome. The biological role of ascorbate is to act as a reducing agent, donating electrons to various enzymatic and a few non-enzymatic reactions. The one- and two-electron oxidised forms of vitamin C (semi-dehydroascorbic acid and dehydroascorbic acid, respectively) can be reduced in the body by glutathione and NADPH-dependent enzymatic mechanisms. The presence of glutathione in cells and extracellular fluids helps maintain ascorbate in a reduced state. In humans, vitamin C is essential to a healthy diet as well as being a highly effective antioxidant, acting to lessen oxidative stress, and an enzyme cofactor for the biosynthesis of many important chemicals in the body. Ascorbic acid can be broken down by the L-ascorbate oxidase enzyme. Ascorbate that is not directly excreted in the urine as a result of body saturation or destroyed in other body metabolism is oxidised by this enzyme and removed.

Deficiency of vitamin C can lead to scurvy. Without this vitamin, collagen made by the body is too unstable to perform its function. Scurvy leads to the formation of brown spots on the skin, spongy gums, and bleeding from all mucous membranes. In advanced scurvy there are open, suppurating wounds, loss of teeth and, eventually, death. The human body can store only a certain amount of vitamin C, and so the body stores are depleted if fresh supplies are not consumed. The timeframe for onset of symptoms of scurvy in unstressed adults on a completely vitamin C-free diet, however, may range from one month to more than six months, depending on previous loading of vitamin C.

The RDI of vitamin C is 45 mg/day for adult men and women, and intakes of no more than 1000 mg/day for adults would be prudent (NHMRC 2006). A varied diet without supplementation usually contains enough vitamin C to prevent scurvy in an average healthy adult, while those who smoke tobacco or are under stress require slightly more. Clinical scurvy is a rare disease in Australia and most other industrialised countries, where the population generally consume far more than sufficient vitamin C. Subclinical deficiency represents a state of 'nutritional risk', but whether it impairs overall health is uncertain. Many of the original claims of beneficial effects of large doses of vitamin C, up to one gram or more per day, have not been substantiated. Routine vitamin C supplementation does not reduce the incidence or severity of the common cold in the general population, though it may reduce the duration of illness.

There has been substantial growth in interest in the role of antioxidants, such as vitamins A, C and E, in health and disease prevention. The antioxidant functions of vitamin C include scavenging oxygen free radicals, which can cause cellular damage, and in regenerating vitamin E from the tocopheroxyl radical. High intakes of vitamin C have been linked to a reduction in risk of certain cancers (especially gastric cancers) and cataracts. However, many systemic reviews and meta-analyses have failed to find support for the prevention of lung, prostate, colorectal and breast cancer with vitamin C supplementation. Similarly, there is no evidence that vitamin C supplementation reduces the risk of myocardial infarction, stroke, CVD mortality or all-cause mortality. While a favourable effect of vitamin C on endothelial function was observed when taken at doses greater than 500 mg/day, it was noted that the effect of vitamin C supplementation appeared to be dependent on health status, with stronger effects in those at higher CVD risk (Ashor et al. 2014).

High intake of vitamin C is implicated in the development of diarrhoea and other gastrointestinal disturbances, kidney stones, withdrawal scurvy, dental erosion and increased toxicity of certain metals such as iron. Vitamin C in the excessive amounts, such as above 500 mg/day, may actually be pro-oxidant and damage DNA. Due to these adverse effects, recommendations to the general public to increase intake of vitamin C to gram amounts are unjustified on the basis of the available evidence (Table 16.5).

Pantothenic acid

The name 'pantothenic acid' derives from the Greek 'pantothen', meaning 'from everywhere', and small quantities of pantothenic acid or vitamin B-5 are found in nearly every food, with high amounts in liver, kidney, egg yolks and dried mushrooms. Dietary deficiency of pantothenic acid is, therefore, exceptionally rare and has not been thoroughly studied. In the few cases where deficiency was seen—in victims of starvation or those fed synthetic diets—nearly all symptoms can be reversed with the return of pantothenic acid.

Pantothenic acid (or pantothenate) is essential in the synthesis of coenzyme A (CoA), which, in the form of acetyl CoA and succinyl CoA, plays an important role in the synthesis of fatty acids, membrane phospholipids, and also of amino acids, steroid hormones, porphyrin and neurotransmitters. Pantothenic acid in the form of CoA is also required for acylation and acetylation, which are involved, for example, in signal transduction and enzyme activation and deactivation respectively. Since pantothenic acid participates in a wide array of key biological roles, it is essential to all forms of life. As such, deficiencies in pantothenic acid may have numerous effects.

Symptoms of pantothenic acid deficiency are similar to other vitamin B deficiencies. There is impaired energy production, due to low CoA levels, which could cause symptoms of irritability, fatigue and apathy. Acetylcholine synthesis is also impaired; therefore, neurological symptoms including numbness, burning or prickling sensation and muscle cramps can also appear in the deficiency. Lack of pantothenic acid can also cause hypoglycaemia, or an increased sensitivity to insulin. Additional symptoms could include restlessness, malaise, sleep disturbances, nausea, vomiting and abdominal cramps. In a few rare circumstances, more serious (but reversible) conditions have been seen, such as adrenal insufficiency and hepatic encephalopathy.

Biotin

Biotin or vitamin B-7 is a cofactor in carboxylation reactions, and is important in fatty acid synthesis, branched-chain amino acid catabolism and gluconeogenesis. It is found in free and protein-bound form in food, but little is known about its bioavailability. It is present in a variety of foods; good sources include egg yolks, brewer's yeast, soybeans and liver, while smaller amounts occur in meat, fruit and vegetables. Significant amounts of biotin are produced by intestinal bacteria, which makes the dietary requirement uncertain.

Biotin is necessary for cell growth, assisting in various metabolic reactions involving the transfer of carbon dioxide, and may also be helpful in maintaining a steady blood glucose concentration. Biotin is often recommended as a dietary supplement for strengthening hair and nails, though scientific data supporting this outcome are weak.

An average varied diet is likely to provide 50–300 mg/day of biotin, and this appears to be sufficient for most healthy adults (Table 16.5). Biotin deficiency, although rare, has been seen in people who consume raw egg white over long periods. The protein avidin in egg white binds biotin, rendering it unavailable. There is increasing evidence that sub-optimal biotin status may be relatively common. Symptoms of biotin deficiency, hair loss, dermatitis, conjunctivitis and central nervous system abnormalities have been observed in patients receiving **total parenteral nutrition** for prolonged periods.

Choline

Choline is a quaternary amine containing four methyl groups and can act as a methyl donor for many important metabolic pathways. Choline also serves as a precursor for neurotransmitter acetylcholine, and the membrane constituents phospholipid and sphingomyelin. Choline can be synthesised in the body from phosphatidylethanolamine, but the ability of the body to produce enough choline depends on the methyl-exchange relationships between choline and folate, vitamin B-12 and amino acid methionine. Endogenous biosynthesis of choline does not meet physiological requirements, so the body would need choline from food or supplements. Choline is widely distributed in foods, being part of the phospholipid lecithin. Milk, eggs, liver, soybeans and peanuts are good sources of choline.

Choline is often grouped with the vitamin B family because the two are closely related; however, some researchers do not truly consider choline a vitamin because they cannot agree on any common definitions of its deficiency symptoms (Zeisel 2000). Choline deficiencies have not been reported in the general population, but they can be seen in experimental situations and in total parenteral nutrition. Vegetarians consuming significant quantities of refined products have a risk of becoming choline deficient. Chronic deficiency of choline can lead to liver dysfunction. Fatty liver develops with choline deficiency, a reflection of its importance as a part of the phospholipid lecithin in lipoprotein (membrane and plasma) structure and in the turnover of the molecule carnitine, involved in free fatty acid transport in cells.

There is evidence that excessive intake of choline might increase the likelihood of atherosclerotic macrovascular disease and cardiac dysfunction. This is because trimethylamine (TMA) can be formed by gut microbiota from choline, and then in the liver converted to trimethylamine-N-oxide (TMAO), which damages the arterial wall (Tang et al. 2013). However, the likelihood of this may depend on the dietary choline source, gut microbiome or duration of exposure, since when as much as two eggs per day are consumed, plasma TMAO production is not measurably altered (Missimer et al. 2018).

SUMMARY

- Vitamins are organic compounds essential for normal growth and metabolic processes.
- Most vitamins cannot be synthesised by humans in adequate amounts, and therefore must be obtained from food.
- Vitamins A, D, E and K are fat-soluble and are present in animal and plant fats and oils. They can be stored in body tissues and, if excessive amounts are consumed, toxicity can occur.
- The water-soluble B vitamins and vitamin C are normally excreted in the urine if excessive amounts are consumed.
- A single vitamin deficiency seldom occurs in isolation; more often a multi-vitamin deficiency occurs.
- The major vitamin deficiency disorders affecting the socioeconomically and geographically disadvantaged have organ, system and mental effects, such as vitamin A deficiency affecting vision; vitamin D deficiency affecting bone and the immune and endocrine systems; and folate and vitamin B-12 deficiencies affecting haemapoietic tissue and the nervous system.

KEY TERMS

Coenzyme: a small molecule that combines with a particular protein molecule to make an enzyme; an enzyme is a protein molecule that acts as a catalyst to facilitate chemical reactions.

Endogenous: originating from inside the body and not from the diet.

Exogenous: originating from outside the body and needing to be provided by the diet.

Megadose: A dose of a substance such as a vitamin or a drug that far exceeds the normal or recommended amount, and is usually given intentionally.

Micronutrients: nutrients that are needed in small amounts, but which play crucial roles in human development and wellbeing.

Provitamins: vitamin precursors with chemical structures closely related to the vitamins. In the body, the inactive provitamin is converted to the active form of the vitamin.

Total parenteral nutrition: a way of supplying all the nutritional needs of the body by bypassing the digestive system and dripping nutrient solution directly into a vein.

REFERENCES

Ashor, A.W., Lara, J., Mathers, J.C. & Siervo, M., 2014, 'Effect of vitamin C on endothelial function in health and disease: A systematic review and meta-analysis of randomised controlled trials', *Atherosclerosis, 235*(1): 9–20, doi:10.1016/j.atherosclerosis.2014.04.004

Beulens, J.W., Bots, M.L., Atsma, F., Bartelink, M.-L.E., Prokop, M. et al., 2009, 'High dietary menaquinone intake is associated with reduced coronary calcification', *Atherosclerosis, 203*(2): 489–93, doi:10.1016/j.atherosclerosis.2008.07.010

Briggs, D.R. & Wahlqvist, M.L., 1988, *Food Facts: The complete no-fads-plain-facts guide to healthy eating*, Melbourne: Penguin Books

de Pee, S., West, C.E., Hautvast, J.G.A.J., Muhilal, Karyadi, D. & West, C.E., 1995, 'Lack of improvement in vitamin A status with increased consumption of dark-green leafy vegetables', *Lancet, 346*(8967): 75–81, doi:10.1016/S0140-6736(95)92111-7

Ferland, G., 2012, 'Vitamin K', in J.W.J. Erdman, I.A. Macdonald & S.H. Zeisel (eds), *Present Knowledge in Nutrition*, Oxford: John Wiley & Sons, pp. 230–47

Fisker, A.B. & Greiner, T., 2017, 'High dose vitamin A capsules–Rusty bullets?', *World Nutrition, 8*(1): 52–61, doi:10.26596/wn.20178152-61

FSANZ, 2012, *NUTTAB 2010*, <www.foodstandards.gov.au/science/monitoringnutrients/nutrientables/nuttab/Pages/default.aspx>, accessed 5 April 2018

—— 2016, *Folate Fortification*, <www.foodstandards.gov.au/consumer/nutrition/folicmandatory/Pages/default.aspx>, accessed 23 November 2018

Gast, G.-C.M., de Roos, N.M., Sluijs, I., Bots, M.L., Beulens, J.W. et al., 2009, 'A high menaquinone intake reduces the incidence of coronary heart disease', *Nutrition, Metabolism and Cardiovascular Diseases, 19*(7): 504–10, doi:10.1016/j.numecd.2008.10.004

GISSI-Prevenzione Investigators, 1999, 'Dietary supplementation with n-3 polyunsaturated fatty acids and vitamin E after myocardial infarction: Results of the GISSI-Prevenzione trial', *Lancet, 354*(9177): 447–55, doi:10.1016/S0140-6736(99)07072-5

Huang, T., Chen, Y., Yang, B., Yang, J., Wahlqvist, M.L. & Li, D., 2012, 'Meta-analysis of B vitamin supplementation on plasma homocysteine, cardiovascular and all-cause mortality', *Clinical Nutrition, 31*(4): 448–54, doi:10.1016/j.clnu.2011.01.003

Huang, Z.-B., Wan, S.-L., Lu, Y.-J., Ning, L., Liu, C. & Fan, S.-W., 2015, 'Does vitamin K2 play a role in the prevention and treatment of osteoporosis for postmenopausal women: A meta-analysis of randomized controlled trials', *Osteoporosis International, 26*(3): 1175–86, doi:10.1007/s00198-014-2989-6

Knapen, M.H., Braam, L.A., Drummen, N.E., Bekers, O., Hoeks, A.P. & Vermeer, C., 2015, 'Menaquinone-7 supplementation improves arterial stiffness in healthy postmenopausal women', *Thrombosis and Haemostasis, 114*(05): 1135–44, doi:10.1160/TH14-08-0675

Li, K., Wahlqvist, M. & Li, D., 2016, 'Nutrition, one-carbon metabolism and neural tube defects: A review', *Nutrients, 8*(11): 741, doi:10.3390/nu8110741

Lonn, E., Bosch, J., Yusuf, S., Sheridan, P., Pogue, J. et al., 2005, 'Effects of long-term vitamin E supplementation on cardiovascular events and cancer: A randomized controlled trial', *JAMA, 293*(11): 1338–47, doi:10.1001/jama.293.11.1338

Mason, J., Benn, C., Sachdev, H., West, K.P., Palmer, A.C. & Sommer, A., 2018, 'Should universal distribution of high dose vitamin A to children cease?', *BMJ, 360*: k927, doi:10.1136/bmj.k927

Miller, E.R., Pastor-Barriuso, R., Dalal, D., Riemersma, R.A., Appel, L.J. & Guallar, E., 2005, 'Meta-analysis: high-dosage vitamin E supplementation may increase all-cause mortality', *Annals of Internal Medicine, 142*(1): 37–46, doi:10.7326/0003-4819-142-1-200501040-00110

Missimer, A., Fernandez, M.L., DiMarco, D.M., Norris, G.H., Blesso, C.N. et al., 2018, 'Compared to an oatmeal breakfast, two eggs/day increased plasma carotenoids and choline without increasing trimethyl amine n-oxide concentrations', *Journal of the American College of Nutrition, 37*(2): 140–8, doi:10.1080/07315724.2017.1365026

NHMRC, 2006, *Nutrient Reference Values for Australia and New Zealand. Version 1.2. Updated September 2017*, <www.nrv.gov.au>, accessed 28 November 2018

Norman, A.W. & Bouillon, R., 2010, 'Vitamin D nutritional policy needs a vision for the future', *Experimental Biology and Medicine, 235*(9): 1034–45, doi:10.1258/ebm.2010.010014

Rimm, E.B., Stampfer, M.J., Ascherio, A., Giovannucci, E., Colditz, G.A. & Willett, W.C., 1993, 'Vitamin E consumption and the risk of coronary heart disease in men', *New England Journal of Medicine, 328*(20): 1450–6, doi:10.1056/NEJM199305203282004

Schweiggert, R.M. & Carle, R., 2017, 'Carotenoid deposition in plant and animal foods and its impact on bioavailability', *Critical Reviews in Food Science and Nutrition, 57*(9): 1807–30, doi:10.1080/10408398.2015.1012756

Schwingshackl, L., Schwedhelm, C., Hoffmann, G., Knüppel, S., Iqbal, K. et al., 2017, 'Food groups and risk of hypertension: A systematic review and dose-response meta-analysis of prospective studies', *Advances in Nutrition, 8*(6): 793–803, doi:10.3945/an.117.017178

Shea, M.K., O'Donnell, C.J., Hoffmann, U., Dallal, G.E., Dawson-Hughes, B. et al., 2009, 'Vitamin K supplementation and progression of coronary artery calcium in older men and women', *American Journal of Clinical Nutrition, 89*(6): 1799–807, doi:10.3945/ajcn.2008.27338

Solomons, N.W., 2012, 'Vitamin A', in J.W.J. Erdman, I.A. Macdonald & S.H. Zeisel (eds), *Present Knowledge in Nutrition*, Oxford: John Wiley & Sons, pp. 149–84

Stampfer, M.J., Hennekens, C.H., Manson, J.E., Colditz, G.A., Rosner, B. & Willett, W.C., 1993, 'Vitamin E consumption and the risk of coronary disease in women', *New England Journal of Medicine, 328*(20): 1444–9, doi:10.1056/NEJM199305203282003

Tang, W.W., Wang, Z., Levison, B.S., Koeth, R.A., Britt, E.B. et al., 2013, 'Intestinal microbial metabolism of phosphatidylcholine and cardiovascular risk', *New England Journal of Medicine, 368*(17): 1575–84, doi:10.1056/NEJMoa1109400

Turner, P.L. & Mainster, M.A., 2008, 'Circadian photoreception: Aging and the eye's important role in systemic health', *British Journal of Ophthalmology, 92*: 1439–44, doi:10.1136/bjo.2008.141747

Wahlqvist, M.L. & Lee, M.S., 2007, 'Regional food culture and development', *Asia Pacific Journal of Clinical Nutrition 16*(S1): 2–7, doi:10.6133/apjcn.2007.16.s1.02

Walsh, J.S., Bowles, S. & Evans, A.L., 2017, 'Vitamin D in obesity', *Current Opinion in Endocrinology & Diabetes and Obesity, 24*(6): 389–94, doi:10.1097/MED.0000000000000371

WHO/FAO, 2004, *Vitamin and Mineral Requirements in Human Nutrition*, <www.who.int/nutrition/publications/micronutrients/9241546123/en/>, accessed 24 November 2018

Wyatt, K.M., Dimmock, P.W., Jones, P.W. & O'Brien, P.S., 1999, 'Efficacy of vitamin B-6 in the treatment of premenstrual syndrome: Systematic review', *BMJ, 318*(7195): 1375–81, doi:10.1136/bmj.318.7195.1375

Yusuf, S., Dagenais, G., Pogue, J., Bosch, J. & Sleight, P., 2000, 'Vitamin E supplementation and cardiovascular events in high-risk patients', *New England Journal of Medicine, 342*(3): 154–60, doi:10.1056/NEJM200001203420302

Zeisel, S.H., 2000, 'Choline: An essential nutrient for humans', *Nutrition, 16*(7–8): 669–71, doi:10.1016/S0899-9007(00)00349-X

{CHAPTER 17}
MICRONUTRIENTS: MINERALS

Mark L. Wahlqvist and Naiyana Wattanapenpaiboon

OBJECTIVES

- Outline the biological roles fulfilled by minerals and understand the reasons for their daily requirements.
- Describe the symptoms of deficiencies and toxicities of these minerals, and identify the circumstances under which deficiency occurs and the vulnerable population groups.
- Identify food sources of these minerals.
- Recognise that interactions between some minerals can have biological consequences.

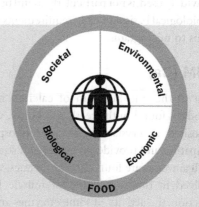

INTRODUCTION

Minerals are widely distributed in food, and the physiological need is usually quite small. It might therefore be expected that mineral intakes would be far in excess of requirements, but deficiencies are much more common than are toxic overloads. This is because there are a number of factors controlling the supply to tissues of specific minerals in forms that can be used for functional purposes. These include alterations to absorptive processes by food components that enhance or diminish mineral uptake, as well as physiological influences on the efficiency of mineral utilisation; for example, by homeostatic regulation. The fraction of a dietary mineral that is absorbed and biologically utilised is a measure of its 'bioavailability' (ranging from almost 100 per cent for sodium and chloride down to 5–10 per cent for iron, copper and manganese).

THE BIOLOGICAL ROLES OF MINERALS

The biological roles of minerals are diverse, as is their relationship to diet and health, and some are still poorly understood. Only the more important ones are dealt with here; more comprehensive information can be found elsewhere (see, for example, O'Dell & Sunde 1997). The *Nutrient Reference Values for Australia and New Zealand* (NHMRC 2006) includes a Recommended Dietary Intake (RDI) for eight minerals (calcium, magnesium, iodine, iron, zinc, phosphorus, molybdenum and selenium) and an Adequate Intake (AI) for a further six (sodium, potassium, copper, fluoride, chromium and manganese). An Upper Limit (UL) for some minerals is also included.

There are about 22 minerals needed for specific metabolic functions or whose absence results in physiological impairment. These minerals, also called essential 'elements' or essential 'mineral elements' (Table 17.1), make up a small but significant component of the adult body, and they must be obtained by absorption in the gut from the available food supply.

Minerals required in large amounts, such as sodium, potassium and calcium, are often called 'major minerals', while those required in very small amounts (such as copper and iodine) are called 'microminerals', 'trace elements' or 'micro-elements'. This distinction, although widely used, is not particularly useful because it has no biological basis, and daily requirements range from grams to micrograms.

CALCIUM (Ca)

Nearly all of the one kilogram of calcium in the human body is found in the teeth and bones, where it is deposited as crystals of calcium phosphates (hydroxyapatite) and provides structure and strength. Only small amounts are found in other tissues, where it is involved in the contraction of muscle fibres, nerve function, the activity of some enzymes and the cascade of reactions that cause blood clotting.

Table 17.1: List of essential mineral elements

Minerals required in >10 mg amounts	Minerals required in <10 mg amounts
Calcium (Ca)*	Arsenic (As)
Chloride (Cl)	Boron (B)
Magnesium (Mg)*	Chromium (Cr)*
Phosphorus (P)*	Copper (Cu)*
Potassium (K)*	Fluoride (F)*
Sodium (Na)*	Iodine (I)*
	Iron (Fe)*
	Lead (Pb)
	Lithium (Li)
	Manganese (Mn)*
	Molybdenum (Mb)*
	Nickel (Ni)
	Selenium (Se)*
	Silicon (Si)
	Vanadium (V)
	Zinc (Zn)*

Note: * Mineral elements that are included in *Nutrient Reference Values for Australia and New Zealand* (NHMRC 2006)

Source: O'Dell & Sunde (1997)

Calcium in foods occurs as inorganic calcium salts (carbonates, phosphates, silicates), complexes with oxalates and phytates, and complexes with proteins (for example, milk caseins). Only dissolved calcium can move across the intestinal epithelium. One aspect of calcium bioavailability, then, is the extent to which it can be solubilised during digestion. This will vary with the type of food consumed and whether there has been prior processing (for example, yeast breaks down phytate in wheat flour during fermentation of bread dough before baking). Calcium in the inorganic salts is poorly absorbed because they have very limited solubility under physiological conditions. Similarly, calcium complexes formed with phytic acid (a strong acid found in cereals and legumes) or oxalic acid (found in spinach, beetroot, rhubarb and tea) have low solubility at physiological pH. During the passage down the gastrointestinal tract, much of the inorganic calcium in food dissolves in stomach acid, but further on in the small intestine the pH of digesta increases, making the calcium salts less soluble, which results in the precipitation of calcium. On the other hand, calcium complexed with protein in milk and cheese is soluble and more easily taken up from the gut. Lactose (milk sugar) promotes the absorption of calcium, as do other dietary sugars.

The absorption of calcium is an adaptive physiological response to diet, because people on low intakes can absorb a larger proportion of calcium than those on high intakes. The net effect for consumers of Australian diets is that only about 30–40 per cent of intake is absorbed and 60–70 per cent is excreted in the faeces. If the diet is adequate, then adults can absorb enough calcium to balance losses until they reach 40–50 years of age. Pregnant women, infants and children, however, must eat more calcium-rich foods and maintain positive calcium balance (so that utilisation exceeds losses) to support the synthesis of new tissue. All these factors are taken into account when making estimates of the dietary calcium intakes needed to maintain health throughout life.

It is well-documented that sodium, in the form of sodium chloride, induces **calciuria**, and this evokes compensatory responses that may lead to increased bone remodelling and bone loss. Calciuria

Table 17.2: Nutrient Reference Values and food sources for selected minerals

Minerals	Nutrient Reference Values*	Food sources
CALCIUM (Ca)	**Recommended Dietary Intake (RDI)**	

Needed for normal development and maintenance of bones and teeth. Serves as the most common signal transmitter for neuromuscular and cardiac function. Essential for normal clotting of blood, and regulation of enzymes and muscle function.	**Children**
	1–3 yrs 500 mg/day
	4–8 yrs 700 mg/day
	Boys and girls
	9–11 yrs 1000 mg/day
	12–13 yrs 1300 mg/day
	14–18 yrs 1300 mg/day
	
	Men
	19–30 yrs 1000 mg/day
	31–50 yrs 1000 mg/day
	51–70 yrs 1000 mg/day
	>70 yrs 1300 mg/day
	Women
	19–30 yrs 1000 mg/day
	31–50 yrs 1000 mg/day
	51–70 yrs 1300 mg/day
	>70 yrs 1300 mg/day
	Pregnancy (19+ yrs)
	  1000 mg/day
	Lactation (19+ yrs)
	  1000 mg/day
		• Milk and milk products
		• Cheese
		• Sardines (canned)
		• Nuts, especially almonds, brazil nuts and pistachio nuts
		• Sesame seeds

CHROMIUM (Cr)	**Adequate Intake (AI)**	

Possibly potentiates the effects of insulin.	**Children**
	1–3 yrs 11 µg/day
	4–8 yrs 15 µg/day
	Boys
	9–13 yrs 25 µg/day
	14–18 yrs 35 µg/day
	Girls
	9–13 yrs 21 µg/day
	14–18 yrs 25 µg/day
	
	Adults (19+ years)
	Men 35 µg/day
	Women 25 µg/day
	Pregnancy (19+ yrs)
	  30 µg/day
	Lactation (19+ yrs)
	  45 µg/day
		• Crustacean seafoods (prawns, crab, lobster)
		• Organ meats (liver and kidney)
		• Wheat bran
		• Bread
		• Yeast
		• Nuts

COPPER (Cu)	**Adequate Intake (AI)**	

Serves as an essential catalytic cofactor for several copper-dependent enzymes. These enzymes are involved in fundamental processes in energy production, iron utilisation, activation of neuropeptides and neurotransmitter synthesis.	**Children**
	1–3 yrs 0.7 mg/day
	4–8 yrs 1.0 mg/day
	Boys
	9–13 yrs 1.3 mg/day
	14–18 yrs 1.5 mg/day
	Girls
	9–13 yrs 1.1 mg/day
	14–18 yrs 1.1 mg/day
	
	Adults (19+ yrs)
	Men 1.7 mg/day
	Women 1.2 mg/day
	Pregnancy (19+ yrs)
	  1.3 mg/day
	Lactation (19+ yrs)
	  1.5 mg/day
		• Crustacean seafoods (oysters, crab, lobster)
		• Liver
		• Wheat bran
		• Yeast
		• Nuts, particularly brazil nuts

Minerals	Nutrient Reference Values*		Food sources

FLUORINE (F)

Protects calcified tissues, such as tooth enamel, against demineralisation.

Adequate Intake (AI) of fluoride

Children		Adults (19+ yrs)	
1–3 yrs	0.6 mg/day	Men	4 mg/day
4–8 yrs	1.1 mg/day	Women	3 mg/day
Boys and girls		**Pregnancy (19+ yrs)**	
9–13 yrs	2 mg/day		3 mg/day
14–18 yrs	3 mg/day	**Lactation (19+ yrs)**	
			3 mg/day

Food sources:
- Crude sea salt
- Fish and seafoods
- Fluoridated water

IODINE (I)

Essential component of thyroid hormone, thyroxine T4 and triiodothyronine T3. Thyroid hormone regulates a variety of physiological processes including growth and development, and reproductive function.

Recommended Dietary Intake (RDI)

Children		Adults (19+ yrs)	
1–3 yrs	90 µg/day	Men	150 µg/day
4–8 yrs	90 µg/day	Women	150 µg/day
Boys and girls		**Pregnancy (19+ yrs)**	
9–13 yrs	120 µg/day		220 µg/day
14–18 yrs	150 µg/day	**Lactation (19+ yrs)**	
			270 µg/day

Food sources:
- Iodised salt
- Fish and seafoods
- Vegetables
- Meat
- Eggs

IRON (Fe)

- Component of ferroproteins, such as haemoglobin in red blood cells, and myoglobin in muscle.
- Iron-containing haeme enzymes are involved with electron transfer and oxidase activities.
- Serves as a cofactor of amino acid hydroxylase enzymes.

Recommended Dietary Intake (RDI)

Children		Men (19+ yrs)	8 mg/day
1–3 yrs	9 mg/day	**Women**	
4–8 yrs	10 mg/day	19–30 yrs	18 mg/day
Boys		31–50 yrs	18 mg/day
9–13 yrs	8 mg/day	>50 yrs	8 mg/day
14–18 yrs	11 mg/day	**Pregnancy (19+ yrs)**	
Girls			27 mg/day
9–13 yrs	8 mg/day	**Lactation (19+ yrs)**	
14–18 yrs	15 mg/day		9 mg/day

Food sources:
- Meat, especially organ meats, and meat products
- Nuts
- Cereals and cereal products
- Eggs
- Condiments such as curry powder, ground ginger, pepper, mustard powder

Not all of the iron consumed is available to our bodies.

Minerals	Nutrient Reference Values*		Food sources

MAGNESIUM (Mg)

- Needed for metabolic reactions including glycolysis and oxidative phosphorylation.
- Required for the active transport of potassium.
- Serves as 'nature's physiological calcium channel blocker' – counteracting the effects of calcium on skeletal and smooth muscle contraction.

Recommended Dietary Intake (RDI)

Children		Men	
1–3 yrs	80 mg/day	19–30 yrs	400 mg/day
4–8 yrs	130 mg/day	>30 yrs	420 mg/day
Boys		**Women**	
9–13 yrs	240 mg/day	19–30 yrs	310 mg/day
14–18 yrs	410 mg/day	>30 yrs	320 mg/day
Girls		**Pregnancy (19+ yrs)**	
9–13 yrs	240 mg/day	19–30 yrs	350 mg/day
14–18 yrs	360 mg/day	31–50 yrs	360 mg/day
		Lactation (19+ yrs)	
		19–30 yrs	310 mg/day
		31–50 yrs	320 mg/day

Food sources: Magnesium occurs widely in foods.
- Nuts
- Cereals and cereal products
- Vegetables
- Milk and cheese

MANGANESE (Mn)

Part of several metallo-enzymes, such as manganese superoxide dismutase enzyme. This enzyme is an important antioxidant defence in nearly all living cells exposed to oxygen, which can cause cell damage.

Adequate Intake (AI)

Children		Adults (19+ yrs)	
1–3 yrs	2.0 mg/day	Men	5.5 mg/day
4–8 yrs	2.5 mg/day	Women	5.0 mg/day
Boys		**Pregnancy (19+ yrs)**	
9–13 yrs	3.0 mg/day		5.0 mg/day
14–18 yrs	3.5 mg/day	**Lactation (19+ yrs)**	
Girls			5.0 mg/day
9–13 yrs	2.5 mg/day		
14–18 yrs	3.0 mg/day		

Food sources:
- Nuts
- Cereals and cereal products
- Vegetables
- Fruits
- Meat

MOLYBDENUM (Mb)

- Serves as a cofactor for a number of enzymes, particularly sulphite oxidase enzyme. The lack of this sulphite oxidase can cause death in early childhood.
- Part of enzymes that are involved in the production of waste products prior to excretion.

Recommended Dietary Intake (RDI)

Children		Adults (19+ yrs)	
1–3 yrs	17 µg/day	Men	45 µg/day
4–8 yrs	22 µg/day	Women	45 µg/day
Boys and girls		**Pregnancy (19+ yrs)**	
9–13 yrs	34 µg/day		50 µg/day
14–18 yrs	43 µg/day	**Lactation (19+ yrs)**	
			50 µg/day

Food sources: Plant foods, especially potatoes, cabbage, carrots, legumes and grains

Minerals	Nutrient Reference Values*	Food sources

PHOSPHORUS (P)

- In combination with calcium, it is needed for the formation of bones and teeth.
- Involved in cell membrane structure as phospholipids, in energy metabolism as ATP and GTP, in information coding as DNA and RNA, and in enzymatic activation by phosphorylation of catalytic proteins.

Recommended Dietary Intake (RDI)

Children
1–3 yrs   460 mg/day
4–8 yrs   500 mg/day
Boys and girls
9–13 yrs   1250 mg/day
14–18 yrs   1250 mg/day

Adults (19+ yrs)
Men   1000 mg/day
Women   1000 mg/day
Pregnancy (19+ yrs)
   1000 mg/day
Lactation (19+ yrs)
   1000 mg/day

Food sources:
- Seafoods
- Meat and meat products
- Eggs
- Dairy products (milk and cheese)
- Nuts such as brazil nuts, walnuts, pistachio nuts, almonds and cashews
- Sesame seeds

POTASSIUM (K)

- As the predominant cation in intracellular fluids, potassium ions interact with sodium and chloride ions in controlling water balance.
- Involved in the electrical stimulation of muscles and nerves.

Adequate Intake (AI)

Children
1–3 yrs   2000 mg/day
4–8 yrs   2300 mg/day
Boys
9–13 yrs   3000 mg/day
14–18 yrs   3600 mg/day
Girls
9–13 yrs   2500 mg/day
14–18 yrs   2600 mg/day

Children
1–3 yrs   50 mmol/day
4–8 yrs   60 mmol/day
Boys
9–13 yrs   76 mmol/day
14–18 yrs   92 mmol/day
Girls
9–13 yrs   64 mmol/day
14–18 yrs   66 mmol/day

Adults (19+ yrs)
Men   3800 mg/day
Women   2800 mg/day
Pregnancy (19+ yrs)
   2800 mg/day
Lactation (19+ yrs)
   3200 mg/day

Adults (19+ yrs)
Men   100 mmol/day
Women   72 mmol/day
Pregnancy (19+ yrs)
   72 mmol/day
Lactation (19+ yrs)
   82 mmol/day

Food sources:
- Potassium is present in a wide range of foods, including:
  - Fruits
  - Vegetables
  - Nuts
  - Meat and meat products
  - Eggs
  - Fish and seafoods

Use of potassium salts as substitutes for common salt (sodium chloride) is potentially harmful, and overuse can be fatal.

SELENIUM (Se)

- Selenium-containing enzymes play an important role in the body's antioxidant defence system. The important selenoenzymes include glutathione peroxidase enzymes (cellular antioxidant systems) and selenoprotein P.
- Another selenoenzyme, iodothyronine 5'-deiodinase enzymes (for thyroxine activation), remove excess thyroid hormones from circulation.

Recommended Dietary Intake (RDI)

Children
1–3 yrs   25 µg/day
4–8 yrs   30 µg/day
Boys
9–13 yrs   50 µg/day
14–18 yrs   70 µg/day
Girls
9–13 yrs   50 µg/day
14–18 yrs   60 µg/day

Adults (19+ yrs)
Men   70 µg/day
Women   60 µg/day
Pregnancy (19+ yrs)
   65 µg/day
Lactation (19+ yrs)
   75 µg/day

Food sources:
- Seafood
- Organ meats, muscle meats
- Cereals

The content of selenium in plant foods depends on the soil concentration, and therefore varies with geographic sources of the food.

Minerals	Nutrient Reference Values*		Food sources

SODIUM (Na)

- Sodium ions work with chloride ions in maintaining the volume and osmotic balance of extracellular fluids.
- Plays an essential role in the electrical activity of muscles and nerves.

Adequate Intake (AI)

Children		Adults (19+ yrs)	
1–3 yrs	200–400 mg/day	Men	460–920 mg/day
4–8 yrs	300–600 mg/day	Women	460–920 mg/day
Boys and girls		**Pregnancy (19+ yrs)**	
9–13 yrs	400–800 mg/day		460–920 mg/day
14–18 yrs	460–920 mg/day	**Lactation (19+ yrs)**	
			460–920 mg/day
Children		**Adults (19+ yrs)**	
1–3 yrs	9–17 mmol/day	Men	20–40 mmol/day
4–8 yrs	13–26 mmol/day	Women	20–40 mmol/day
Boys and girls		**Pregnancy (19+ yrs)**	
9–13 yrs	17–34 mmol/day		20–40 mmol/day
14–18 yrs	20–40 mmol/day	**Lactation (19+ yrs)**	
			20–40 mmol/day

Food sources:
- Table salt, soy sauce
- Processed meats (bacon, ham, salami)
- Cheese
- Cereals and cereal products, including bread

ZINC (Zn)

- Needed for many different functions including protein and carbohydrate metabolism, wound healing, growth and vision.
- Important component of over 50 catalytic metallo-enzymes.
- Serves to stabilise the structure of proteins including those involved in DNA replication and transcription.
- Maintains cell membrane structure and function.

Recommended Dietary Intake (RDI)

Children		Adults (19+ yrs)	
1–3 yrs	3 mg/day	Men	14 mg/day
4–8 yrs	4 mg/day	Women	8 mg/day
Boys		**Pregnancy (19+ yrs)**	
9–13 yrs	6 mg/day		11 mg/day
14–18 yrs	13 mg/day	**Lactation (19+ yrs)**	
Girls			12 mg/day
9–13 yrs	6 mg/day		
14–18 yrs	7 mg/day		

Food sources:
- Dried yeast
- Wheat bran
- Meat and meat products
- Brazil nuts, peanuts, walnuts, almonds

Note: * Usual intake at or above Adequate Intake (AI) or Recommended Dietary Intake (RDI) level has a low probability of inadequacy

Sources: Briggs & Wahlqvist (1988); NHMRC (2006)

occurs due partly to salt–induced volume expansion and partly to the competition between sodium and calcium ions in the renal tubule. With calcium intakes at or above recommended levels, there appear to be no detrimental effects of prevailing salt intakes on bone or the calcium economy, mainly because adaptive increases in calcium absorption offset the increased urinary loss (Heaney 2006). However,

IS CALCIUM SUPPLEMENTATION NECESSARY?

For men and women aged 70 years and over, the average dietary intake of calcium is 700–800 mg/day (ABS 2015), while the recommended intake is 1300 mg of calcium daily for bone health and fracture prevention (NHMRC 2006). This means most older people may need to take calcium supplements to meet these recommendations.

Calcium supplementation at doses of 1000 mg/day, however, could have adverse effects, including cardiovascular events, kidney stones and hospital admissions for acute gastrointestinal symptoms. Consequently, older people are encouraged to improve bone health by increasing their calcium intake through food rather than by taking supplements. This advice assumes that increasing dietary calcium intake to the recommended level of 1300 mg/day can prevent fractures without causing the adverse effects of calcium supplements.

A prospective longitudinal cohort study involving over 61,000 women and a 19-year follow-up has reported higher rates of death from all causes and higher rates of CVD and ischaemic heart disease (but not of stroke) among those with high intakes of calcium (sum of dietary and supplemental), i.e. above 1400 mg/day (Michaëlsson et al. 2013). However, these results are not supported by the Cancer Prevention Study II Nutrition Cohort, which involved more than 130,000 men and women followed up for 17.5 years (Yang et al. 2016). Despite these inconsistent results, emphasis should be placed on people with a low intake of calcium rather than increasing the intake of those already consuming satisfactory amounts.

- Determine how much food an older person would need to consume in order to meet the daily recommended intake of calcium. Is this feasible?
- Review a range of studies looking at the risks of calcium supplementation. What is your recommendation?

Here are some references to get you started.
- Harvey, N.C. et al., 2018, 'Calcium and vitamin D supplementation are not associated with risk of incident ischaemic cardiac events or death: Findings from the UK biobank cohort', *Journal of Bone and Mineral Research*, 33(5): 803–11
- Michaëlsson, K. et al., 2013, 'Long-term calcium intake and rates of all cause and cardiovascular mortality: Community-based prospective longitudinal cohort study', *BMJ*, 346: F228
- Tankeu, A.T., Ndip Agbor, V. & Noubiap, J.J., 2017, 'Calcium supplementation and cardiovascular risk: A rising concern', *Journal of Clinical Hypertension*, 19(6): 640–6
- Yang, B. et al., 2016, 'Calcium intake and mortality from all causes, cancer, and cardiovascular disease: The Cancer Prevention Study II Nutrition Cohort', *American Journal of Clinical Nutrition*, 103(3): 886–94.

such compensation is likely to be incomplete at low calcium intakes. Potassium intakes in the recommended range can reduce or prevent sodium chloride-induced calciuria. The optimal strategy to protect the skeleton is to ensure adequate calcium and potassium intakes. Excessive protein intake has a similar effect to sodium on urinary calcium, and this is particularly important in the older population (see also Chapter 32). When diets are high in protein, a reduction in sodium intake can reduce the physiological need for calcium and so improve calcium nutrition.

Milk and dairy foods are by far the richest dietary sources of calcium. Although lower in calcium, bread makes a significant contribution to overall intakes because it is such a regular component of diets. Intakes of dietary calcium seem to vary over a much wider range than do other nutrients. Over half of the Australian population aged two years and over has inadequate usual intakes of calcium; the 2011–2012 Australian Health Survey revealed that 54 per cent of adult males and 79 per cent of adult females, particularly those aged 70 years or older, had usual calcium intake from foods lower than the Estimated Average Requirement (EAR) (ABS 2015).

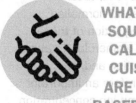

WHAT ARE SOURCES OF CALCIUM IN CUISINES THAT ARE NOT DAIRY-BASED?

Not all cuisines of the world are based on dairy. For those cuisines—for example, the cuisines of East and Southeast Asia—what are the primary sources of calcium in the diet? List these and compare the calcium content with high sources of calcium in Australia and New Zealand.

MAGNESIUM (Mg)

An adult body contains about 25 g of magnesium, with 60 per cent in the skeleton, 39 per cent intracellular (20 per cent in skeletal muscle) and 1 per cent extracellular. Magnesium plays a variety of important metabolic roles in many of the biochemical reactions that take place in the cell, and particularly in processes involving the formation and utilisation of ATP and those that use other nucleotides to synthesise DNA and RNA.

Magnesium is an element that occurs ubiquitously in nature. Legumes, cereals, nuts and green leafy vegetables are rich sources of magnesium. Moreover, there is evidence that magnesium intake's contribution to survival is dependent on the background diet being biodiverse (Huang et al. 2015). Absorption of magnesium occurs in the small intestine by both **active transport** and **passive diffusion** mechanisms. The proportion absorbed varies with diet and is usually in the range of 20–30 per cent, depending on the amount of magnesium in the diet and on calcium intake.

The most frequent causes of hypomagnesaemia, or low plasma magnesium, in children are reduced intake, impaired intestinal absorption, renal loss and genetic diseases. Hypomagnesaemia is reflected clinically in the nervous system, and there are neurophysiological and metabolic changes. Magnesium probably plays an important role in vitamin D metabolism. Some patients with hypocalcaemia and magnesium deficiency are resistant to pharmacological doses of vitamin D or may have a form of magnesium-dependent vitamin D-resistant rickets.

Hypomagnesaemia is common. The primary cause of deficiency is low dietary intake; about 40 per cent of Australians do not meet the EAR (ABS 2015). Additional causes are other illnesses, such as alcoholism, diabetes, malabsorption, starvation or kidney disease. Most magnesium deficiencies are asymptomatic, but symptoms such as neuromuscular, cardiovascular and metabolic dysfunction may occur. Magnesium toxicity is also rare and is secondary to other pathologies where magnesium-containing drugs have been used. However, sub-optimal magnesium status is likely to be an important factor that increases the risk of osteoporosis, hypertension, insulin resistance and heart disease.

PHOSPHORUS (P)

Phosphorus in the body occurs in several different forms. A total of 600 g out of the 700 g found in an adult human is located in bone, where inorganic phosphate is an integral part of the hydroxyapatite crystals of bone matrix. Inorganic phosphate also plays important roles as a component of genetic material (DNA and RNA), and phosphorus, in the form of pyrophosphate $(P_2O_7^{4-})$ is central to the biochemistry of energy production. In the form of organic phosphates (RPO_4^{2-}), it forms part of the structural components of tissue phosphoproteins, phospholipids and phosphosugars. It is absorbed all along the gastrointestinal tract, but most is taken up in the small intestine by both active transport and passive diffusion. Absorption is enhanced by 1,25-OH vitamin D and is inhibited by formation of insoluble complexes with calcium. Also, high levels of calcium in the gut lumen diminish serum 1,25-OH vitamin D concentrations, thereby suppressing vitamin-enhanced absorption of phosphorus. There has been much discussion of what constitutes ideal proportions of calcium and phosphorus in diets in order to minimise the formation of insoluble complexes and maximise absorption of both minerals, particularly in population groups vulnerable to calcium deficiency. The relatively large amounts of phosphate present in cow's milk reduce calcium absorption, and some infants fed on whole cow's milk can develop muscular spasms (tetany) if blood calcium falls too low. On the other hand, human milk has a higher calcium:phosphorus ratio, and its calcium is better absorbed. In general, about 65 per cent of phosphorus is absorbed from a mixed diet.

Many factors control phosphate balance (that is, intake and excretion), and regulation is effected mainly by the kidneys, where typically 600–800 mg is excreted in the urine each day. Because phosphorus is ubiquitously distributed in foods,

HOMEOSTASIS OF CALCIUM, PHOSPHORUS AND MAGNESIUM

Calcium, phosphorus and magnesium are multivalent cations that are important for many biological and cellular functions. In the gut, calcium and magnesium may compete for the active transport carrier in intestinal absorption. If there is a small amount of calcium but an abundance of magnesium in the contents of the intestine, magnesium gets more actively absorbed. However, a high intake of calcium can reduce the absorption of both calcium and magnesium. The amount of calcium or magnesium absorbed depends on the dietary ratio of calcium to magnesium.

The kidneys play a central role in homeostasis of calcium, magnesium and phosphorus. Gastrointestinal absorption is balanced by renal excretion. When body stores of these ions decline significantly, gastrointestinal absorption, bone resorption, and renal tubular reabsorption increase to normalise their levels. Renal regulation of these ions occurs through glomerular filtration and tubular reabsorption and/or secretion and is therefore an important determinant of plasma ion concentration. Phosphate depletion has been observed to be accompanied by an increase in urinary magnesium and calcium. Under physiological conditions, the whole-body balance of calcium, phosphate and magnesium is maintained by fine adjustments of urinary excretion to equal the net intake.

Source: Blaine et al. (2015)

dietary deficiencies are almost unknown, except in starvation. Most Australians' diets exceed the RDI, the main foods supplying phosphorus being cereal products, milk products and meat.

SODIUM (AND CHLORIDE)

Sodium (Na) and chloride (Cl) are the principal electrolytes (as Na^+ and Cl^-) in extracellular body fluids such as blood plasma. They are involved in maintaining the volume and osmotic balance of extracellular fluids by controlling water movements within and between tissues (see Chapter 14). They also play an essential role in the electrical activity of muscles and nerves. About 20 per cent of total body sodium is found in bone, but this exchanges only slowly with the extracellular pool. There appears to be no control of the gastrointestinal absorption of sodium or chloride, and they are extensively and readily taken up from food and drink. Physiological control of whole-body sodium levels is regulated by excretion via the kidneys, and sodium excretion is passively accompanied by chloride ions to maintain electrolyte balance. The amount of sodium lost in sweat is usually minimal (2–4 **mmol**/day) in comparison with urine excretion, but these may be increased (up to 350 mmol/day) during prolonged and unaccustomed heavy exercise.

Sodium is largely consumed as sodium chloride, or 'salt'. Sodium may also be found in food additives such as sodium phosphate, sodium bicarbonate and sodium benzoate; however, these contribute much less to total sodium intakes than dietary salt. Approximately 90 per cent of the total sodium intake is excreted in the urine, so studies utilise the 24-hour urinary sodium measure as indication of sodium intake.

Sodium levels are low in raw ingredients and in unprocessed foods, but are often increased by the addition of salt during cooking or at the table. Discretionary salt intake is usually much lower than that obtained from manufactured and processed or takeaway food products. The 2011–2012 Australian Health Survey reported average sodium daily intakes for adults (19 years or over) of 2400 mg or about 100 mmol (ABS 2015). A reduction in systolic blood pressure of 2 mm Hg (when corrected to the Australia and New Zealand population) is shown in a meta-analysis when mean sodium excretion was lowered from about 3500 mg/day to 2100 mg/day (NHMRC 2006). This has led to the recommendation of the **Suggested Dietary Target** (SDT) of 2000 mg/day for adults. This value is consistent with international recommendations, including the 2012 WHO Guideline for sodium intake (WHO 2012), which strongly recommends a reduction to less than 2 g/day (equivalent to 5 g/day of salt) for adults, and the recommended maximum intake level of sodium in adults should be adjusted downward based on the energy requirements of children relative to those of adults.

The kidneys normally act to guard the body's stores of sodium; however, abnormal losses causing low blood sodium (hyponatraemia) may arise from excessive sweating, severe or chronic diarrhoea, use of diuretics or osmotic diuresis. An increased intake of salt does not necessarily increase the amount of sodium in the body, because the kidneys normally excrete the extra sodium and keep the volume of extracellular fluids constant. However, the kidneys can malfunction and retain too much sodium; and this, if not corrected, can lead to excessive extracellular fluid, which consequently impairs normal organ function.

POTASSIUM (K)

Potassium is the predominant cation (K^+) found in intracellular cell fluids; this is in contrast to sodium, which is mainly located in extracellular fluids. As well as controlling water balance by its interaction with sodium ions (Na^+) and chloride ions (Cl^-), potassium is involved in the electrical stimulation of nerves and muscles. Uptake of potassium in the gut from foods is close to 100 per cent, occurring primarily in the small intestine as a consequence of bulk fluid absorption. Its excretion is controlled largely by the kidney, which ensures close control of blood plasma levels (3.5–5.0 mmol/L) at a much lower concentration than is found inside most cells of the body (150 mmol/L).

The wide distribution of potassium in food supply means that dietary deficiency is rare. Low blood potassium (hypokalaemia) are associated with other factors such as use of diuretics or laxatives, diarrhoea, hyperinsulinaemia and protein energy malnutrition, especially if accompanied by diarrhoea. Excessive potassium intake (more than about 200 mmol/day or 8 g/day), resulting in high blood levels (hyperkalaemia), is also rare.

COPPER (Cu)

The amount of copper in the human body is small, about 80 mg in total, and it is widely distributed among the various tissues. Its main biological role is as a key component in a variety of **metallo-enzymes** involved in processes such as energy production, collagen synthesis and the manufacture of neurotransmitters (such as noradrenalin). Most of these enzymes are oxidases. In blood, for example, most of the copper is found in red blood cells as part of the enzyme ceruloplasmin involved in the oxidation of ferrous iron ($Fe2^+$) to ferric iron ($Fe3^+$).

Good food sources of copper are shellfish, legumes, wholegrain cereals, nuts and liver. In foods, it occurs in organic complexes and the acid environment of the stomach dissociates this bound copper. Some is absorbed by passive diffusion across the stomach wall. Most copper, however, is absorbed from the duodenum, but the rising pH limits its solubility and, in order to remain soluble and therefore absorbable, free copper must form a complex with amino acids or organic acids that may be present in the lumen. Many factors limit copper uptake, including zinc, which competes for proteins that would normally transport copper out of the mucosal cells lining the gut. Less than 50 per cent of ingested copper is absorbed; the remainder is lost to the faeces. Absorption decreases as intake increases. Significant amounts of copper are found in the skeleton, muscle and liver. Body organs are supplied with copper by ceruloplasmin and other copper-containing proteins in the blood. Control of body levels is obtained by altering secretion in bile, although the mechanisms for this are not clear.

Copper deficiency is rare in humans. The diverse roles played by copper in metabolism means that severe deficiency results in malfunction of many systems, including the blood (hypochromic anaemia and neutropenia) and connective tissue (abnormal bone formation and vascular abnormalities). These symptoms are usually associated with some other underlying illness. A marginal deficiency due to inadequate diet in otherwise healthy people has not been clearly identified in human populations. Infants receiving breastmilk appear to obtain sufficient copper to meet their requirements, but clinical deficiency resulting in growth retardation has been shown in infants fed with formulas, particularly in some soy-based formulas.

Excess intakes of copper salts can be acutely toxic but rarely fatal because the mineral is an irritant and causes vomiting. Copper intoxication is very rare, although there are instances of mortality in Indian infants fed buffalo milk previously stored in copper vessels.

FLUORIDE

Fluoride is an inorganic anion of fluorine (F) with the chemical formula F^-. The body content of about 2.5 g of fluoride is mainly (>98 per cent) found in bone and teeth, with negligible amounts in blood and other tissues. Its biological functions are not clearly established, but its incorporation into tissues increases the degree of crystallinity of mineral structures. This is particularly noticeable in teeth, where its incorporation into dental enamel causes hardening and increased resistance to dissolution by acids produced by cariogenic bacteria resident in the oral cavity. Fluoride can also stimulate new bone formation. The absorption of fluoride from drinking water or from tablets is almost 100 per cent, whereas dietary components like calcium can form insoluble complexes with fluoride that reduce absorption from food to 50–80 per cent of intake. Absorption occurs from the stomach and the small intestine by passive diffusion, and it is excreted mainly in the urine with smaller amounts lost to sweat. It is not clear whether the balance between intake, excretion and blood levels is under homeostatic control or whether the observed changes are merely incidental responses imposed by other factors.

With the exception of seafood and tea, most foods are low in fluoride (less than 30 µg/100 g) and drinking water levels can also be low in some regions. As a result, the Water Resources Council of Australia and the NHMRC have recommended that the reticulated water supply should be fortified with added fluoride to the level of 1 mg/L, a level that has been associated with marked reductions in the incidence of childhood dental caries (NHMRC 2006). Research consistently shows that children growing up in areas with optimal levels of ingested fluoride can have up to 70 per cent fewer caries than those not exposed to fluoride (Kaminsky et al. 1990).

However, the range of intakes compatible with health is extremely narrow and, as the fluoride content of drinking water exceeds 1 mg/L, a variety of clinical symptoms of toxicity (fluorosis) can develop. The earliest sign is a mottling of tooth enamel, and it is estimated that 12.5 per cent of exposed people will develop fluorosis to an extent that they will find aesthetically concerning even when fluoride is added to water at only 1 mg/L.

IODINE (I)

About 70–80 per cent of iodine in the body is concentrated in the thyroid gland, where it is employed in the manufacture of iodine-containing hormones thyroxine (T4) and triiodothyronine (T3). These important hormones influence growth, maturation, thermogenesis and the metabolism of all tissues by stimulating the synthesis of many different enzymes involved in these processes. Neural tissues are extremely sensitive to T3 and T4, especially when they are growing during early fetal life. Therefore, these hormones have a direct effect on fetal brain development.

In contrast to many other essential minerals, iodine in the form of iodide salts is almost completely absorbed and organic forms in animal products have a lesser bioavailability. Most iodine is excreted via the urine and sweat and this normally balances uptake.

Iodine occurs in the soil, and the iodine content of plant and animal foods reflects the iodine content of the soil, which is typically deficient in parts of the world where iodine has been leached from the soil by high rainfall or glaciation. Foods grown in the soil of mountainous areas or high rainfall areas are low in iodine content, and they are the cause of iodine-deficiency disorders (IDDs). Iodine deficiency is a major cause of preventable mental retardation (Hetzel 2012). At intakes below about 25 µg/day, a spectrum of IDD develops that can affect all age groups, but the most damaging occurs during pregnancy and in early childhood. These include abortion, stillbirths, infant mortality, congenital abnormalities, **cretinism**, goitre, impaired mental function and hypothyroidism.

There are a number of substances in foods, collectively called goitrogens, that interfere with the uptake of iodine by the thyroid gland and thereby impair the production of T3 and T4. Brassica vegetables, such as cabbage, cauliflower, broccoli and brussels sprouts, contain inactive glucosinolates which, upon breakdown by myrosinase enzyme, release biologically active isothiocyanates and other hydrolytic products (see Chapter 18). These compounds are absorbed from the gut and metabolised to thiocyanates, which interferes with iodine uptake by the thyroid gland. Overconsumption of these vegetables uncooked can lead to enlargement of the thyroid (goitre). However, the myrosinase enzyme can be destroyed by heat from cooking, and therefore less goitrogenic thiocyanate amount is produced.

The cyanogenic glycosides found in cassava, corn, bamboo shoots, sweet potatoes, lima beans and millet produce cyanide and glycoside, which is then metabolised into goitrogenic thiocyanates. These glycosides do not cause a major problem because they are located in the inedible parts of the plant (except in cassava) or occur in very small amounts. The food of major concern is cassava, a root vegetable that is a staple for large populations in Africa. Although some glycosides are removed by traditional processing, a portion remains. When this occurs in geographical regions where iodine intakes are already low (for example, the Democratic Republic of the Congo), serious clinical disorders can result, such as an

IODINE FORTIFICATION IN AUSTRALIA AND NEW ZEALAND: DOES IT WORK?

In Australia and New Zealand, iodine deficiency has re-emerged as an important public health problem. In some states of Australia, up to half of all school-age children may have mild iodine deficiency. A mild deficiency is enough to cause measurable reductions in mental function. The reasons for the re-emergence of iodine deficiency are not fully understood, but may relate to a decline in the use of iodine-based cleaning products in the dairy industry and reduced consumption of iodised salt added to cooking and at the table.

Mandatory iodine fortification implemented in Australia and New Zealand by FSANZ in 2009 requires non-iodised salt be replaced with iodised salt in bread at 25–65 mg of iodine/kg of salt. In 2014, it was reported that the proportion of all New Zealand children with inadequate iodine intakes had declined from 95 per cent pre-fortification to 21 per cent post-fortification. Similar results were reported in 2016; the mean daily intake of dietary iodine for all Australians increased from 107 µg/day pre-fortification to 168 µg/day post-fortification, and the proportion of Australian children (2–16 years) with dietary iodine intake below EAR was less than 1 per cent (FSANZ 2018). The expected positive health outcome from the increase in dietary iodine intake is a reduction in the incidence of iodine deficiency-related health problems, including impaired neurological function in children.

However, while the national iodine fortification program addressed the needs of most Australians, it did not meet the increased iodine requirements of pregnant and breastfeeding women, especially among those residing in the most iodine-deficient areas (Rahman et al. 2011). This put the most vulnerable group (the unborn, babies and infants) at risk of irreversible neurological underdevelopment and its adverse effects on mental capability throughout life. The NHMRC recognised the inadequacy of the mandatory iodine fortification program for pregnant and breastfeeding women and, in January 2010, released a statement recommending that all women who are pregnant, intending to become pregnant, or breastfeeding take an iodine supplement of 150 µg each day (NHMRC 2010) (see also Chapter 20).

Find out whether the combination of fortification and supplementation has been effective in reducing the risk of iodine deficiency. If it has not, what might be the long-term repercussions? Here are some additional articles to get you started:

- Condo, D., et al., 2017, 'Iodine status of pregnant women in South Australia after mandatory iodine fortification of bread and the recommendation for iodine supplementation', *Maternal & Child Nutrition*, 13(4): e12410
- Hine, T., et al., 2018, 'Iodine-containing supplement use by pregnant women attending antenatal clinics in Western Australia', *Australian and New Zealand Journal of Obstetrics and Gynaecology*, 58(6): 636–42
- Mitchell, E.K.L., et al., 2018, 'Maternal Iodine dietary supplements and neonatal thyroid stimulating hormone in Gippsland, Australia', *Asia Pacific Journal of Clinical Nutrition*, 27(4): 848–52.

increased prevalence of cretinism, goitre and other iodine-deficiency disorders.

Some goitrogenic foods include:

- cruciferous vegetables: cabbage (all types), broccoli, cauliflower, brussels sprouts, kale, kohlrabi
- mustard greens, spinach, Chinese greens, bamboo shoots
- corn
- sweet potato, swede, turnip
- cassava (tapioca)
- garlic, onion, millet
- soy (flour, milk and tofu)—only a problem if also iodine-deficient but best to limit intake if on thyroxine
- lima beans
- linseed oil and linseeds
- mustard oil
- stone fruit
- peanuts, pine nuts, almonds, brazil nuts.

Soy isoflavones may directly inhibit the function of the thyroid gland, although this inhibition may only be significant in people who are deficient in iodine. Therefore, it is probably prudent for people with impaired thyroid function to avoid consuming large amounts of soy products, especially if those products are iodine-deficient. While some clinicians recommend that people with hypothyroidism avoid these goitrogen-containing foods, none has been proven to cause hypothyroidism in humans, except for cassava (Hetzel 2000).

There are well-documented cases of over-consumption of iodine in Japan through eating too much iodine-rich seaweed and in Tasmania through iodine supplementation of individuals suffering from goitre. Excessive iodine intake can result in hyperthyroidism (overactive thyroid), thyrotoxicosis (thyroid malfunction) and may cause sensitivity reactions and thyroid cancer. An early effect of iodine excess is an elevated level of thyroid-stimulating hormone (TSH). Although exposure to high levels of iodine from food or supplements can increase TSH for about 24 hours, most healthy individuals compensate by reducing the uptake of iodine into the thyroid gland and excreting the excess iodine in urine. However, in some parts of China and Japan where iodine-rich seaweeds are consumed in large quantities, the sustained high intake of iodine (>1100 µg/day) may inhibit the iodine uptake into the thyroid gland, resulting in reduced synthesis of T4 and elevated secretion of TSH, which stimulates the thyroid follicles to enlarge and multiply, producing a goitre (Mu et al. 1987; Suzuki et al. 1965).

IRON (Fe)

Most of the iron in the human body is found in the form of two metallo-proteins, haemoglobin in red blood cells and myoglobin in muscle cells. These molecules contain non-protein structures called haem, each containing a single iron atom at their centre. Haemoglobin contains four haem groups, each one anchored to a discrete polypeptide in a globular protein, whereas myoglobin has one. The iron in these haem molecules has the important property of reversibly binding to oxygen. Haemoglobin in red blood cells is responsible for taking up oxygen in the lungs and transporting it to peripheral tissues, where the oxygen readily leaves haemoglobin to be used by cells for oxidative metabolism. Myoglobin, on the other hand, is found only in muscle cells, where it acts as an oxygen reserve in periods of peak metabolic activity during exercise. The remainder of the body's iron is found in a range of other metallo-proteins, such as ferritin (an iron-storage protein), transferrin (an iron-transport protein), cytochromes (proteins involved in oxidation–reduction reactions where the iron atom plays a crucial role) and non-haem iron-containing enzymes.

The iron content in the body is maintained within a fairly narrow range to provide sufficient iron for its bodily functions in oxygen transport and catalysis, and yet avoid the toxic effects of excess. Hepcidin, a peptide hormone from the liver, plays a crucial role, through the actions of **ferroportin**, in regulating dietary iron absorption and body iron distribution or iron homeostasis in response to body iron stores, demand for iron in red blood cell production, infection, inflammation and **hypoxia**.

Unlike other mineral elements, there is no physiological mechanism for the excretion of iron. Although it is very effectively recycled within the body, losses occur continuously when epithelial cells are sloughed from the skin and from the gut, and periodically when blood is shed during menstruation or injury. Therefore, body stores are effectively controlled by the amounts absorbed from the diet. The absorption of iron from the gut is affected by two factors: the form in which it occurs in foods and the presence of food components that inhibit absorption.

In acidic conditions in the stomach, inorganic iron from cereals and vegetables is converted to its reduced state, ferrous iron (Fe^{2+}), and in this form it is then liberated from food complexes that would otherwise prevent its subsequent absorption. The conversion to ferrous iron is enhanced by vitamin C and other reducing substances in food. Further down the gastrointestinal tract, in alkaline conditions in the duodenum, ferrous iron (Fe^{2+}) is oxidised to ferric iron (Fe^{3+}), and in this form the free iron is extensively absorbed by mucosal cells. In meats, iron occurs as haem compounds; the haem molecules can be directly absorbed into the mucosa and the central iron atom is released within the cells. Overall, dietary iron from meat is much more readily absorbed (bioavailable) than is inorganic iron from cereals and vegetables. Food components such as oxalates in spinach, phytates in cereals or polyphenols in tea can form complexes with inorganic iron, making it unabsorbable. However, cooking improves availability and the consumption of vitamin C-rich foods (fruits and some vegetables) in the same meal can further improve absorption, by up to 50 per cent. Nonetheless, no more than about 20 per cent of total dietary intake is absorbed from the gut in a typical mixed diet, and the figure is nearer 10 per cent for vegetarian diets. Results of the Australian Health Survey in 2011–2012 show that the main sources of iron in Australian diets are cereals and cereal products (47 per cent), meat (17 per cent) and vegetables (10 per cent) (ABS 2015).

Iron is very active chemically, binds non-specifically to many proteins and can catalyse undesirable oxidations. Therefore, in the body it is usually transported and stored bound to specific proteins and only small amounts exist as free iron. Following absorption from the gut, the absorbed iron is transported by the serum protein transferrin to other tissues for storage, mainly in the liver, or for uses in metabolism (for example, to the bone marrow for haemoglobin synthesis). Iron is stored in a protein called ferritin, which is a very efficient iron store—one single molecule can hold up to 3000 iron atoms. In humans, ferritin acts as a buffer against iron deficiency and iron overload. It is found in most tissues as a cytosolic protein, but small amounts are secreted into the serum where it functions as an iron carrier. Significant amounts of ferritin are stored in gut mucosa and the constant sloughing of cells causes some of the absorbed iron to be returned to the gut lumen and lost in the faeces. When ferritin stores are full, iron forms a complex with phosphate called haemosiderin, found only within cells as opposed to circulating in blood. The iron within deposits of hemosiderin is very poorly available to supply iron when needed.

Iron is constantly being turned over in various tissue compartments, but it is very effectively recycled, with the result that only small additional amounts (approximately 1 mg/day) are normally required from the diet to 'top up' the body's stores. However, the low bioavailability of iron (15–20 per cent) means that considerably larger quantities than this must be consumed to ensure that this requirement is met. In individuals with low iron stores, however, the absorption of iron from foods is increased to more than 40 per cent. Presumably this is an adaptive physiological response. The amount of dietary iron needed each day varies with the stages of life. During gestation, the fetus stores about 250 mg of iron, and these stores are sufficient for the first four months after birth; breastfed babies will get what they need from their mother's milk during the first six months of life (Oski 1993). After this time iron must be consumed in amounts adequate to meet the needs of maintenance and growth (Fomon 1993) (see also Chapter 20).

Women who are pregnant or breastfeeding are at high risk of iron deficiency because of the increased demand to meet the needs of the growing fetus or for milk. When supplies of iron are not enough to meet daily losses, this can lead to a reduction in body iron stores (ferritin). Ultimately, ferritin stores become exhausted and the synthesis of haemoglobin in the bone marrow becomes compromised. Low haemoglobin in red blood cells is therefore an indicator of a late stage in iron deficiency. Chronic deficiency of iron results in low haemoglobin, low serum ferritin, elevated transferrin and reductions of tissue iron (myoglobin and iron-containing enzymes). Iron deficiency, if not treated, can contribute to reduced fitness and productivity, cognitive impairment, morbidity from infectious disease, child mortality, perinatal mortality and maternal mortality (Stoltzfus 2003).

Some possible clinical consequences of prolonged iron deficiency include:

- anaemia
- decreased memory, impaired learning ability and concentration
- fatigue and decreased capacity for physical activity
- decreased work productivity
- impaired immune function and increased risk of infections
- adverse pregnancy outcomes:
  - increased risk of low birthweight
  - increased risk of prematurity
  - increased risk of maternal morbidity
  - developmental delays in infants and young children. (Horton & Ross 2003; Zimmermann & Hurrell 2007)

Low haemoglobin can lead to anaemia, a condition in which the number or the oxygen-carrying capacity of red blood cells is insufficient to meet physiological needs. The most common cause of anaemia globally is iron deficiency; other causes include folate, vitamin B-12 and vitamin A deficiencies, chronic inflammation, parasitic infections, and inherited disorders. In its severe form, it is associated with fatigue, weakness, dizziness and drowsiness. Pregnant women and children are particularly vulnerable (see also Chapter 29). In Australia, it is estimated that in 2016 about 20 per cent of pregnant women and 14 per cent of children under five years were anaemic (Institute for Health Metrics and Evaluation 2018).

Approximately one in 300 Australians suffers from haemochromatosis, the inherited iron-overload disorder characterised by increased iron absorption relative to stores. Deficiency of the hormone hepcidin is the cause of hereditary hemochromatosis. Excess iron stored as haemosiderin is deposited in the liver and heart, causing an increased risk of these organs malfunctioning. Avoidance of dietary iron altogether (and other medical treatment) is required in this situation (Dietitians Association of Australia (DAA) 2018).

ZINC (Zn)

Zinc is present in all tissues of the body, with about 60 per cent of the 2 g total body content occurring in muscle, 30 per cent in bone, and smaller but significant amounts in the skin, liver and brain. Its major function is as a constituent of hundreds of different metalloenzymes involved in a wide range of key metabolic processes, including carbohydrate metabolism, DNA synthesis, protein synthesis, protein digestion, bone metabolism, and the synthesis of brain receptors and neurotransmitters. There is no body store of zinc as such, but during periods of low dietary intake the activity of zinc-containing enzymes and plasma zinc concentrations are maintained within normal limits for several months. This is probably achieved by transport of zinc from tissues—for example, from muscle and bone undergoing **catabolism** during normal turnover.

The acid environment of the stomach solubilises zinc salts in food, and this is absorbed from the small intestine. At the same time, zinc is lost from the body in digestive juices, sloughed cells, urine, hair and sweat. Since very little is lost in urine, the amount retained in the body appears to be controlled by adjustment to the rate of absorption. As the levels of zinc in tissues increase, absorption decreases and vice versa.

As with iron, there are a number of intrinsic and extrinsic factors that affect zinc's bioavailability in diets. Consequently, bioavailability from food covers a wide range, and on average only 25–40 per cent of intake is absorbed. Foods that contain most zinc (2–8 mg/100 g fresh weight) and that have the highest bioavailability are the muscles of animals. Cereals and vegetables have a lower content (0.2–2.0 mg/100 g), and this is also less well absorbed because some zinc may be bound to phytate, fibre or undigested plant protein. Results of the Australian Health Survey in 2011–2012 show that the main sources of zinc in Australian diets are cereals and cereal products (32 per cent), meat (32 per cent), and milk and milk products (11 per cent) (ABS 2015).

The principal clinical features of severe deficiency are growth retardation, delay in skeletal and sexual maturation, skin lesions, diarrhoea and behavioural changes. Zinc deficiency is rare in Australia and is usually secondary to some other diseases, but mild deficiency is common in many economically poor countries and in individuals who have a limited intake of muscle meat. It is characterised by impaired growth, increased susceptibility to infections and impaired neurophysiological function. This improves rapidly when additional zinc is supplied. It might be expected that vegetarians would be at risk of deficiency but among adult vegetarians dietary zinc intakes appear to be adequate because they have a low requirement. Children, however, have a much greater requirement because they are still growing and thus are vulnerable to zinc deficiency when eating a vegetarian diet. Zinc deficiency often accompanies iron deficiency and affects many young women, pregnant women and lactating mothers.

Excess or accidental consumption of zinc causes

MULTIFACTORIAL MICRONUTRIENT DEFICIENCY AND ANAEMIA

Nutritional anaemia is generally multifactorial, although most commonly attributable to iron deficiency, which is where the cells are pale (hypochromic) and small (microcytic) respectively. It is divided into morphological types by the size (microcytic (smaller), normocytic (normal/average) or macrocytic (larger)), appearance including colour (hypochromic or normochromic) and shape (sickle cell, spherocytic and others) of red blood cells. However, these colours, types and shapes are not precise when deductions are made about the contributing micronutrient deficiencies. For example, hypochromic microcytic anaemia may not be nutritional but due to thalassaemia, which is a genetic disorder of haemoglobin structure. The enlargement of red blood cells, called macrocytosis, may be seen with both folic acid and vitamin B-12 deficiencies. If iron and folic acid deficiencies co-exist, the net effect on red blood cell appearance may be that it is normochromic. Other nutrient deficiencies may contribute to anaemia of no specific type, but be clinically important; these include vitamin C, copper, essential fatty acids, and general malnutrition associated with chronic inflammatory disease. The storage iron ferritin is actually an inflammatory marker and makes the assessment of iron storage difficult.

The gender difference in haemoglobin concentrations—women have lower haemoglobin than men—may have considerable physiological and health significance. It is thought that the regular loss of iron by way of menstruation in women may protect them against the oxidative damage of iron, a benefit that men do not have unless they lose blood through injury or intestinal bleeding. On the other hand, if women have heavy menstrual periods, they can develop anaemia, which will be associated with at least iron if not other nutrient deficiencies on account of blood loss.

nausea and vomiting, and this helps prevent toxicity. However, amounts in excess of 50 mg/day, while not acutely toxic, interfere with the absorption of copper, and larger amounts (400–600 mg/day) can result in copper deficiency-induced anaemia.

SELENIUM (Se)

The essential biological function of selenium is its role at the active site of enzymes that make up part of antioxidant defence and other systems in the body. Selenium is usually incorporated into proteins as part of the amino acid selenocysteine, and the selenoenzymes containing this amino acid include glutathione peroxidases and thyroid hormone de-iodinating enzymes. The former are responsible for removing active oxygen species produced in cells during metabolism that might otherwise cause damage; the latter are responsible for removing excess thyroid hormones from circulation.

Absorption of selenium from the diet is not under homeostatic control, and its uptake in the gut as selenoproteins from foods or as inorganic selenium in mineral supplements is greater than 90 per cent. It is absorbed from both the small and large intestine and excretion occurs mainly via the urine and the faeces, the latter comprising selenium from diet as well as from biliary and pancreatic secretions. Levels of selenium in foods reflect the amounts in the soil and its accumulation in the food chain. Analyses of

foods in Australian state capitals showed that the most concentrated sources of selenium were fish and liver but, according to the 2011–2012 Australian Health Survey, the food groups that contributed most to intakes were cereals and meat (ABS 2015). Results of the Australian Health Survey in 2011–2012 show that the main sources of selenium in Australian diets are cereals and cereal products (31 per cent), meat (26 per cent) and fish and seafood (12 per cent) (ABS 2015).

Dietary deficiency of selenium has not been unequivocally demonstrated in humans, although animals on a deficient diet develop a number of symptoms, including retarded growth, muscular dystrophy and necrosis of the heart, kidney and liver. In regions of the world where soil selenium levels are low and intakes are correspondingly low (11 µg/day), such as the Keshan region of China, there is a significant occurrence of cardiomyopathy associated with low plasma selenium (Keshan disease). The prevalence of Keshan disease slowly diminishes when selenium supplementation is introduced. However, the disease is not common in other countries that also experience low selenium soils and low dietary intakes (for example, New Zealand and Finland).

OTHER MINERALS

There are a range of other minerals with important biological functions; these are summarised in Table 17.3.

Table 17.3: Other minerals with important biological functions

Mineral	Biological functions	Food sources
Cadmium (Cd)	Possibly involved in the function of certain proteins.	Wheat, fruits, vegetables and nuts
Cobalt (Co)	Part of vitamin B-12.	Green leafy vegetables, organ and muscle meats
Nickel (Ni)	Plays several possible roles in maintenance and production of body cells.	Green leafy and tuberous vegetables, fruits and grains
Silicon (Si)	Shown in animals to be essential for bone mineralisation and formation of connective tissues. Whether this applies to humans is not known.	Wholegrain cereals and citrus fruits
Tin (Sn)	Appears to be important for normal growth in rats, but whether this applies to human growth is not known.	Cereals, fresh meat and fresh vegetables
Vanadium (V)	Might affect glucose metabolism by mimicking action of insulin.	Vegetables, wheat, seafoods

Source: Briggs & Wahlqvist (1988)

SUMMARY

- Minerals are vital components of organic tissues. They fulfil a diversity of functions as structural components of bone, as central atoms in oxygen-carrying proteins, as constituents of numerous enzymes and as electrolytes responsible for the movement of water through tissues.
- If minerals are not provided in the diet, normal metabolic processes can be disturbed and deficiency symptoms arise. In some cases, toxicity occurs due to an oversupply.
- Mineral requirements vary from a few micrograms to hundreds of milligrams per day, and the proportion absorbed from food in the intestine ranges from ten to 100 per cent. The balance between the absorption of minerals from food and their rate of excretion determines body levels, which must be maintained within limits for optimal health.
- The amount of a mineral absorbed from the diet and available for metabolic use is a measure of its bioavailability.
- Minerals are widely but unevenly distributed in foods, and the consumption of a diet comprising many foods should protect against the possibility of deficiency or excess.
- The major mineral deficiency disorders affecting the socioeconomically and geographically disadvantaged have organ, system and mental effects, such as iodine deficiency affecting mental health and iron deficiency affecting haemopoietic, muscular and central nervous systems.

KEY TERMS

Active transport: the movement of ions or molecules across a membrane against their concentration gradient (i.e. from an area of lower concentration to an area of higher concentration). Active transport mechanisms require energy, usually in the form of adenosine triphosphate (ATP).

Calciuria: the presence of calcium in the urine. Sometimes it is used to describe increased urinary calcium excretion or hypercalciuria.

Catabolism: the set of metabolic pathways that breaks down molecules into smaller units.

Cretinism: the condition of severely stunted physical and mental growth due to untreated congenital deficiency of thyroid hormone (congenital hypothyroidism).

Ferroportin: a membrane protein that allows iron to move from the inside of a cell to the outside of a cell. It helps dietary iron, after being absorbed, to be transported out of the cells of the small intestine into the circulation. Ferroportin is a critical iron transporter in terms of acquisition and distribution between tissues.

Hypoxia: a state in which the body or part of the body is deprived of a sufficient oxygen supply, as opposed to anoxia, which is the condition where oxygen is entirely absent.

Metallo-enzymes: enzymes that, in the active form, contain one or more metal ions, such as copper, iron and zinc, which are essential for the enzyme's biological function.

mmol: the concentration of sodium and potassium in body fluids is usually expressed in moles rather than grams (e.g. Na 23 mg = 1 mmol; K 39 mg = 1 mmol) because their interactions with other ions in biological systems are more easily understood when expressed in this way.

> **Passive diffusion:** the movement of ions or molecules across a membrane along their concentration gradient (i.e. from an area of higher concentration to an area of lower concentration). Passive transport requires no energy input and its rate depends on the permeability of the membrane. For example, water passes through semi-permeable membranes by passive diffusion, equalising the concentration on either side of the membrane.
>
> **Suggested Dietary Target (SDT):** a daily average intake from food and beverages for certain nutrients that may help in prevention of chronic disease risk at a population level; in the case of sodium, for example, the relationship between sodium intake and high blood pressure is addressed.

ACKNOWLEDGEMENT

This chapter has been modified and updated from the 'Minerals' chapter written by Gwynn P. Jones and Jonathan M. Hodgson which appeared in the third edition of *Food and Nutrition*.

REFERENCES

ABS, 2015, *Australian Health Survey: Usual Nutrient Intakes, 2011–12,* <www.abs.gov.au/ausstats/abs@.nsf/Lookup/by%20Subject/4364.0.55.008~2011-12~Main%20Features~Key%20findings~100>, accessed 22 November 2018

Blaine, J., Chonchol, M. & Levi, M., 2015, 'Renal control of calcium, phosphate, and magnesium homeostasis', *Clinical Journal of the American Society of Nephrology, 10*(7): 1257–72, doi:10.2215/CJN.09750913

Briggs, D.R. & Wahlqvist, M.L., 1988, *Food Facts. The complete no-fads-plain-facts guide to healthy eating,* Melbourne: Penguin Books

Condo, D., Huyhn, D., Anderson, A.J., Skeaff, S., Ryan, P. et al., 2017, 'Iodine status of pregnant women in South Australia after mandatory iodine fortification of bread and the recommendation for iodine supplementation', *Maternal & Child Nutrition, 13*(4): e12410, doi:10.1111/mcn.12410

Dietitians Association of Australia (DAA), 2018, *Things to Consider with Haemochromatosis,* <https://daa.asn.au/smart-eating-for-you/smart-eating-fast-facts/medical/things-to-consider-with-haemochromatosis/>, accessed 28 November 2018

Fomon, S.J., 1993, *Nutrition of Normal Infants,* St Louis: Mosby

FSANZ, 2018, *Iodine Fortification,* <www.foodstandards.gov.au/consumer/nutrition/iodinefort/Pages/default.aspx>, accessed 23 March 2018

Harvey, N.C., D'Angelo, S., Paccou, J., Curtis, E.M., Edwards, M. et al., 2018, 'Calcium and vitamin D supplementation are not associated with risk of incident ischaemic cardiac events or death: Findings from the UK biobank cohort', *Journal of Bone and Mineral Research, 33*(5): 803–11, doi:10.1002/jbmr.3375

Heaney, R.P., 2006, 'Role of dietary sodium in osteoporosis', *Journal of the American College of Nutrition, 25*(suppl. 3): 271S–276S, doi:10.1080/07315724.2006.10719577

Hetzel, B.S., 2000, 'Iodine-deficiency disorders', in J.S. Garrow, W.P.T. James & A. Ralph (eds), *Human Nutrition and Dietetics,* Edinburgh: Churchill Livingstone, pp. 621–4

—— 2012, 'The development of a global program for the elimination of brain damage due to iodine deficiency', *Asia Pacific Journal of Clinical Nutrition, 21*(2): 164–70, doi:10.6133/apjcn.2012.21.2.01

Hine, T., Zhao, Y., Begley, A., Skeaff, S. & Sherriff, J., 2018, 'Iodine-containing supplement use by pregnant women attending antenatal clinics in Western Australia', *Australian and New Zealand Journal of Obstetrics and Gynaecology, 58*(6): 636–42, doi:10.1111/ajo.12785

Horton, S. & Ross, J., 2003, 'The economics of iron deficiency', *Food Policy, 28*(1): 51–75, doi:10.1016/S0306-9192(02)00070-2

Huang, Y.-C., Wahlqvist, M.L., Kao, M.-D., Wang, J.-L. & Lee, M.-S., 2015, 'Optimal dietary and plasma magnesium statuses depend on dietary quality for a reduction in the risk of all-cause mortality in older adults', *Nutrients,* 7(7): 5664–83, doi:10.3390/nu7075244

Institute for Health Metrics and Evaluation, 2018, *Global Burden of Disease Study 2016 (GBD 2016) Data Resources,* <http://ghdx.healthdata.org/gbd-2016>, accessed 10 August 2018

Kaminsky, L.S., Mahoney, M.C., Leach, J., Melius, J. & Miller, M.J., 1990, 'Fluoride: Benefits and risks of exposure', *Critical Reviews in Oral Biology & Medicine, 1*(4): 261–81, doi:10.1177/10454411900010040501

Michaëlsson, K., Melhus, H., Lemming, E.W., Wolk, A. & Byberg, L., 2013, 'Long-term calcium intake and rates of all cause and cardiovascular mortality: Community-based prospective longitudinal cohort study', *BMJ, 346,* p. F228, doi:10.1136/bmj.f228

Mitchell, E.K.L., Martin, J.C., D'Amore, A., Francis, I. & Savige, G.S., 2018, 'Maternal iodine dietary supplements and neonatal thyroid stimulating hormone in Gippsland, Australia', *Asia Pacific Journal of Clinical Nutrition, 27*(4): 848–52, doi:10.6133/apjcn.022018.02

Mu, L., Chengyi, Q., Qidong, Q., Qingzhen, J., Eastman, C. et al., 1987, 'Endemic goitre in central China caused by excessive iodine intake', *Lancet, 330*(8553): 257–9, doi:10.1016/S0140-6736(87)90838-5

NHMRC, 2006, *Nutrient Reference Values for Australia and New Zealand,* <www.nrv.gov.au>, accessed 28 November 2018

—— 2010, *Public Statement: Iodine supplementation for pregnant and breastfeeding women,* <www.nhmrc.gov.au/about-us/publications/iodine-supplementation-pregnant-and-breastfeeding-women>, accessed 1 April 2018

O'Dell, B.L. & Sunde, R.A. (eds), 1997, *Handbook of Nutritionally Essential Mineral Elements,* New York, NY: Marcel Dekker

Oski, F.A., 1993, 'Iron deficiency in infancy and childhood', *New England Journal of Medicine, 329*(3): 190–3, doi:10.1056/NEJM199307153290308

Rahman, A., Savige, G.S., Deacon, N.J., Chesters, J.E. & Panther, B.C., 2011, 'Urinary iodine deficiency in Gippsland pregnant women: The failure of bread fortification', *Medical Journal of Australia, 194*(5): 240–3, <www.mja.com.au/system/files/issues/194_05_070311/rah10861_fm.pdf>, accessed 18 January 2019

Stoltzfus, R.J., 2003, 'Iron deficiency: Global prevalence and consequences', *Food and Nutrition Bulletin, 24*(4_suppl. 2): S99–S103, doi:10.1177/15648265030244S106

Suzuki, H., Higuchi, T., Sawa, K., Ohtaki, S. & Horiuchi, Y., 1965, 'Endemic coast goitre in Hokkaido, Japan', *Acta Endocrinologica, 50*(2): 161–76, doi:10.1530/acta.0.0500161

Tankeu, A.T., Ndip Agbor, V. & Noubiap, J.J., 2017, 'Calcium supplementation and cardiovascular risk: A rising concern', *Journal of Clinical Hypertension, 19*(6): 640–6, doi:10.1111/jch.13010

WHO, 2012, *Guideline: Sodium intake for adults and children,* <www.who.int/nutrition/publications/guidelines/sodium_intake_printversion.pdf>, accessed 22 November 2018

Yang, B., Campbell, T., Gapstur, S.M., Jacobs, E.J., Bostick, R.M. et al., 2016, 'Calcium intake and mortality from all causes, cancer, and cardiovascular disease: The Cancer Prevention Study II Nutrition Cohort', *American Journal of Clinical Nutrition, 103*(3): 886–94, doi:10.3945/ajcn.115.117994

Zimmermann, M.B. & Hurrell, R.F., 2007, 'Nutritional iron deficiency', *Lancet, 370*(9586): 511–20, doi:10.1016/S0140-6736(07)61235-5

{CHAPTER 18}
PHYTONUTRIENTS AS BIOACTIVE FOOD COMPONENTS

Mark L. Wahlqvist and Naiyana Wattanapenpaiboon

OBJECTIVES

- Identify a range of phytonutrients and other healthful bioactive food components recognised as essential for health.
- Describe the possible biological roles fulfilled by certain phytonutrients and their contribution to the health effects of plant-based foods.
- Explain the role for and limitations of nutrient supplementation.

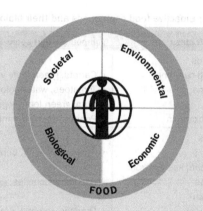

INTRODUCTION

Foods contain many compounds in addition to traditional nutrients. Many of these compounds have an ability to alter chemical and enzymatic reactions, and therefore may affect human health positively, adversely or both. These biologically active compounds in food, especially plant food, have become known by names such as phytochemicals, phytonutrients and non-traditional nutrients. Although the term 'phytochemicals' may include all plant chemicals, it is applied to chemically minor components and those that have not already been classified as nutrients for humans. These compounds usually exist in plants as secondary metabolites used by the plant for defence and survival. They may also appear in animal tissue eaten by humans.

However, the term 'phytonutrients' (plant-based nutrients) may be preferable, as it implies favourable nutritional properties rather than those which are health-neutral, adverse or even naturally occurring plant toxicants. However, as with all bioactive factors affecting human biology, phytonutrients themselves have a functional and safety range.

Classifications of phytonutrients can be made in accordance with plant source, chemistry or functions. No one classification is satisfactory, because plants are sources of various chemical and functional classes of compounds; the chemistry is complex and the compounds myriad. What has become clear is that one class of phytonutrients may have several functions, i.e. there are multifunctional compounds. On the other hand, a particular function may be provided by more than one class of phytonutrients (Table 18.1). The interaction between the compounds is also likely to be considerable and complex, causing both masking of effects and synergy.

THE POSSIBLE BIOLOGICAL ROLES OF PHYTONUTRIENTS

A problem in considering the place of phytonutrients in human health is that they are numerous, alongside a few known essential nutrients, and therefore, their net interactive effect ultimately requires a study of food itself and food patterns. The health–promoting use of plants has been known in food cultural folklore for many centuries, but identification of active chemical compound(s), clear understanding of mechanisms of action and reproducibility of proposed therapeutic benefits have not been easy to demonstrate. Advances in analytical technology and in molecular biology have identified phytonutrient components of popular foods used in health promotion, which may explain traditional beliefs and help quantify possible health benefits.

Results from intervention trials of the health

Table 18.1: Bioactive food compounds and their biological properties

Compound class	Compounds and some important food sources	Biological properties
Carotenoids • α- and β-carotene • Lycopene • Lutein • β-cryptoxanthin	• Carrots, green leafy vegetables • Tomatoes, watermelon, pink grapefruit • Corn, green leafy vegetables • Pepper, pumpkin, winter squash	Antioxidant Antimutagen Anticarcinogen

Flavonoids
• Flavonols
  (quercetin, kaempferol)
• Flavones
  (apigenin)
• Flavanones
  (naringenin, hesperidin)
• Anthocyanins
  (cyanidin)
	• Apples, currants, berries
	
	• Parsley, artichokes, green pepper
	
	• Oranges, lemons, grapefruit
	
	• Currants, berries
		Antioxidant

Catechins	Tea	Antioxidant Anticariogen
Isoflavonoids • isoflavones (genistein, daidzein)	Soy, red clover	Oestrogen-like Immuno-modulating Antioxidant
Isothiocyanates & indoles	Cruciferous vegetables, such as broccoli, cabbage, kale	Anticarcinogen Antimicrobial
Lignans	Linseed (or flaxseed), chickpea	Oestrogen-like
Organic sulphur compounds	Garlic, onions, leeks	Anticarcinogen Antibacterial
Phytosterols	Pumpkin seeds	Reduce symptoms of prostate enlargement
Curcumin	Turmeric	Antioxidant Anti-inflammatory
Salicylates	Grapes, dates, cherries, pineapples	Protective against macrovascular disease
L-dopa	Broad beans	Parkinson's disease

Sources: Cerella et al. (2011); Hewlings & Kalman (2017); International Agency for Research on Cancer et al. (2004); Kozlowska & Szostak-Wegierek (2014); Miadoková (2009); Wahlqvist, Wattanapenpaiboon et al. (1998)

benefits of phytonutrients do not always support—and sometimes even contradict—the epidemiological research findings. This can in part be explained by the notion that there is an inter-individual variation in the way the human body handles the bioactive compounds, as well as the heterogeneity in the biological response to them (Manach et al. 2017), as illustrated in Figure 18.1. While this is the case, it is advisable to encourage the consumption of a varied diet.

Phytonutrients may almost be regarded as pharmaceuticals rather than dietary nutrients when they are used to manage clinical conditions. This is not surprising, as many important drugs were, at least initially, derived from plants. An alternative viewpoint is that conditions for which they are used as treatment may have occurred because of inadequate intakes from foods (Wahlqvist, Kouris-Blazos et al. 1998). The emergence of new familial

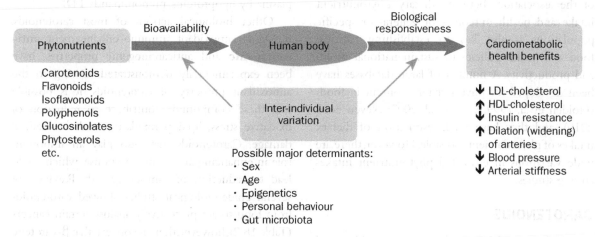

Figure 18.1: Potential factors responsible for inter-individual variation in bioavailability and biological responsiveness to phytonutrient intake in relation to cardiometabolic health

Source: Adapted from (Manach et al. 2017). Reprinted with permission. Creative Commons BY-NC-ND 4.0

POSSIBLE ROLE OF CERTAIN PHYTONUTRIENTS IN CANCER PREVENTION

Since the 1980s, research has shown that several phytonutrients exert their anticancer effects by modulating the enzymatic systems responsible for counteracting **carcinogens**, either by reducing their carcinogenic potential or by increasing their excretion. Some phytonutrients, such as curcumin from turmeric and resveratrol from grapes, inhibit tumour growth by directly inducing cancer cell death by apoptosis. Several phytonutrients modify the tumour's microenvironment and create physiological conditions that are hostile to tumour growth. For example, catechins, an abundant phytonutrient found in tea, inhibit the formation of new blood vessel networks that provide oxygen and nutrients to tumour cells and sustain the development of cancer. This anti-angiogenic activity is an important factor of the chemopreventive properties of these phytonutrients.

Sources: Linnewiel-Hermoni et al. (2015); Weng & Yen (2012)

diseases may reflect a change in food culture, exposing genetic predispositions. The growing array of phytonutrients opens up opportunities for more healthful food choices, and for the development of functional foods to serve particular physiological or pathological needs.

Considerable effort has been made to determine phytonutrient content in various food sources, and to establish optimal human dietary consumption levels for each category of phytonutrients. Examination of the associations between dietary phytonutrient intake and health outcomes of general or specific populations is also key to establishing national food and health policies to sustain national health and productivity. A number of large databases have been developed for phytonutrient content in foods (Holden et al. 1999; Lako et al. 2007; Neveu et al. 2010), and they have made estimation of dietary intakes of phytonutrients possible. However, there are wide variations in estimated phytonutrient intakes among studies.

CAROTENOIDS

Carotenoids are the most abundant and widespread pigments, responsible for many of the brilliant red, orange and yellow colours of edible fruit, vegetables and flowers, as well as the colours of certain animals, such as lobsters and trout. They are a class of hydro-carbons (carotenes) and their oxygenated derivatives (xanthophylls), consisting of eight isoprenoid units. The symmetrical structure of the molecule found in β-carotene and many carotenes is a precursor of vitamin A in both humans and animals.

Humans are not capable of carotenoid synthesis and are dependent on those found in the diet. Major circulating carotenoids in blood are α-carotene, β-carotene, lycopene, β-cryptoxanthin, lutein and zeaxanthin. Carotenoids of fruit, vegetables and animal products are usually fat-soluble and are associated with lipid fractions. During digestion, carotenoids are released from complex proteins and then incorporated into micelles and transported to the mucosal cells (see also Chapter 16). Absorption efficiency of carotenoids is affected by the presence or absence of other components in the diet, such as dietary fat and protein, and by bile salts. Therefore, carotenoids in foods are usually less well absorbed from the intestine than preformed vitamin A. After absorption, provitamin A carotenoids are cleaved in the intestinal mucosal cells to form retinal, which is then reduced to retinol (vitamin A). Some unconverted carotenoids are directly absorbed and pass into the blood where their composition reflects the diet. These carotenoids are transported in human plasma by lipoproteins, predominantly LDL.

Other biological actions of most carotenoids, including antioxidant, immuno-enhancement, **antimutagenic** and anticarcinogenic properties, have been experimentally demonstrated. Owing to the antioxidant property of carotenoids, it is possible that these compounds contribute to reduction of oxidative stress, lipid peroxidation and free radical damage. Carotenoids may also play an important role in enhancing an immune response, which could lead to reduction of tumour growth. Reviews of several epidemiological studies showed carotenoids from food to act protectively against certain cancers (Table 18.2); however, there is concern that β-carotene supplements may increase the risk of certain cancers (Albanes et al. 1995; MacLennan et al. 1999).

The physiological functions of carotenoids may be highly specialised—as indicated, for instance, by the presence of zeaxanthin and lutein in the macular area of the retina in the virtual absence of β-carotene. The macular pigment density could be raised by increasing dietary intake of lutein and zeaxanthin from spinach and corn. These carotenoids accumulated in the retina, and other antioxidant vitamins may help retard some of the destructive processes in the retina and the retinal pigment epithelium that lead to age-related degeneration of the macula.

FLAVONOIDS

Flavonoids are the most common and widely distributed large group of polyphenolic compounds to occur naturally in vegetables and fruit, as well as in beverages such as tea and wine. Over 4000

Table 18.2: Summary of systemic reviews and meta-analyses on carotenoids from dietary sources and cancer

Type of cancer	Results
Lung cancer (Vieira et al. 2015)	Intakes of fruits and vegetables up to 400 g/day ➔ reduced risk (8–18%)
Colorectal cancer (Panic et al. 2017)	No association between the consumption of carotenoids and colorectal cancer
Head and neck cancer (Leoncini et al. 2015)	• β-carotene intake ➔ reduced risk for cancer of oral cavity and laryngeal cancer • Lycopene and β-cryptoxanthin ➔ reduced laryngeal cancer • Lycopene, α-carotene, β-cryptoxanthin ➔ reduced oral and pharyngeal cancer
Breast cancer (Chajès & Romieu 2014)	β-carotene intake ➔ reduced risk Blood concentrations of total carotenoids, β-carotene, α-carotene and lutein ➔ reduced risk

individual flavonoids occur in nature. The range and structural complexity of flavonoids have led to their subclassification as flavonols, flavones, flavanones, flavan-3-ols (and their oligomers, proanthocyanidins), isoflavones, and anthocyanins. Flavonoids have been studied in relation to their improvement of vascular fragility, their ability to increase cellular permeability and their vitamin C–sparing activities. Some flavonoids, such as quercetin, kaempferol and myricetin, have antimutagenic and anticarcinogenic effects *in vitro* and *in vivo*.

Based on 24-hour dietary recalls of the European Prospective Investigation into Cancer and Nutrition (EPIC) study of 36,000 adults aged 35–74 years, the average intake of total phenols in Europe was estimated to be 1187 mg/day, which included flavonoids (526 mg/day) and phenolic acids (605 mg/day). Its main sources were apple and pear, tea, coffee and wine (Zamora-Ros et al. 2016). There appears to be a large heterogeneity in the intakes of various polyphenolic compounds across ten European countries, particularly between Mediterranean and non-Mediterranean countries.

A protective effect of the consumption of vegetables and fruit on various forms of cancer has been reported in a large number of epidemiological studies investigating relations between diet and cancer. This protective effect is generally believed to be attributed to the vitamin C and carotenoids present in these foods. However, the significance of other potentially protective compounds, such as flavonoids, present in vegetables and fruit has become

an important issue. It appears that a number of the biological effects of flavonoids may be explained by their antioxidative activity and ability to scavenge free radicals. Other mechanisms for their reported anticarcinogenic potential include their capacity to inhibit the promotion phase of carcinogens and to modulate the balance between activation and inactivation processes of specific enzymes in the liver.

ISOFLAVONOIDS

Isoflavonoids are another group of plant polyphenolic compounds having important antimicrobial activities. They occur principally, although not exclusively, in legumes such as soy, lentils and chickpeas. They are at particularly high levels in certain legumes regularly consumed by humans and animals. A small number of isoflavones, such as genistein and daidzein, display oestrogenic activity (Wilcox et al. 1990). This hormonal effect is attributed to the similar spatial arrangement of functional groups on both isoflavones and oestrogens, allowing those isoflavones to bind to the oestrogen receptors. Furthermore, genistein is also found to inhibit endothelial cell proliferation and *in vitro* angiogenesis.

ISOTHIOCYANATES AND INDOLES

Isothiocyanates in vegetable foods are responsible for the pungent and acrid flavour and odour of mustard, radish, and watercress, and the familiar biting taste that develops when some cruciferous vegetables, such as broccoli and brussels sprouts, are eaten. These plants are members of the Brassicales order, which is characterised by the production of glucosinolates, and of the enzyme myrosinase, which acts on glucosinolates to release isothiocyanates. This group of compounds has a variety of pharmacological and toxic activities, which include goitrogenic, antibacterial, antifungal and antiprotozoal actions (see also 'Iodine' in Chapter 16). Several substances in this group could block the toxic and neoplastic effects of a wide variety of chemical carcinogens.

PLANT STEROLS

Plant foods do not contain cholesterol. However, some plants, such as sesame, linseed, corn, soy and peanuts, contain phytosterols (plant sterols) which have a similar chemical structure to cholesterol. Plant sterols can help to lower circulating cholesterol by inhibiting the incorporation of cholesterol into micelles in the gastrointestinal tract and decreasing cholesterol absorption. Despite the potential positive impact on cardiovascular risk due to cholesterol lowering, concerns have been raised that plant sterols may also exert adverse cardiovascular effects. However, in a systemic review and meta-analysis of seventeen studies involving 11,182 participants, no evidence of an association, either favourable or unfavourable, between serum concentrations of plant sterols and cardiovascular risk was observed (Genser et al. 2012). This situation is a reminder that a consideration of effects of an intervention like phytosterol fortification of foods on serum cholesterol status is not necessarily

HOW EFFECTIVE ARE PHYTOSTEROLS?

Many food products in Australia, such as margarine, milk, yoghurt and breakfast cereals, are fortified with plant sterols. It is proposed that adults with high absolute risk (i.e. those who are likely to have a cardiovascular event within a five-year period), could benefit from the cholesterol-lowering effect of consuming naturally occurring phytosterols in plant foods and phytosterol-enriched foods. The Heart Foundation of Australia (2018) recommends consumption of 2–3 g of phytosterols per day from fortified food products. Apparently, eating more than 3 g/day does not further reduce LDL cholesterol.

Using the information on the product label shown, and additional peer-reviewed literature, discuss the following.

- How much (in grams and in teaspoons) of this product do you have to eat to obtain 3 g plant sterols?
- How much energy would this amount of product provide?
- Is there any evidence that fortification of foods with phytosterols increases life expectancy or reduces cardiovascular events?
- To what extent could a diet rich in legumes provide phytosterols without the need for their isolation and reutilisation in other foods?
- To what extent are health authorities unnecessarily encouraging the population at large to purchase more expensive edible fats with questionable health value and uncertain risk?

NUTRITION INFORMATION			
SERVINGS PER PACK: 75	SERVING SIZE: 10g		
	Qty^ per Serving	% Daily Intake* per Serving	Qty^ per 100g
Energy	239kJ	3%	2390kJ
Protein	<1.0g	<0.1%	<1.0g
Fat, total	6.4g	9%	64.3g
saturated	1.4g	6%	13.5g
trans	0.05g		0.5g
polyunsaturated	2.8g		27.5g
monounsaturated	2.3g		22.8g
Plant sterols	0.8g		8.0g
Carbohydrate	<1.0g	<0.1%	<1.0g
sugars	<1.0g	<0.1%	<1.0g
Sodium	36mg	2%	360mg
Potassium	3mg		27mg

^ Average values unless otherwise stated. *Percentage Daily Intakes are based on an average adult diet of 8700kJ. Your daily intakes may be higher or lower depending on your energy needs.

No artificial colours or flavours

Made in Australia from at least 46% Australian ingredients

INGREDIENTS Vegetable oils, water, phytosterol esters (8% plant sterols), salt, milk solids, emulsifiers (soy lecithin, 471), preservative (202), food acid (lactic acid), natural flavours, vitamins (A, D), natural colour (β-carotene). Contains milk and soy

indicative of health outcomes in general, or even CVDs alone.

OTHER PHYTONUTRIENTS

Allicin is an organosulphur compound found in garlic, onions and leeks. When fresh garlic is chopped or crushed, allicin—which is responsible for the aroma of fresh garlic—is produced. The allicin is unstable and rapidly changes into a series of other sulphur compounds, such as diallyl disulphide. Several studies reveal that diallyl disulphide is a major component responsible for protection against colorectal cancer and CVDs.

Avenanthramides, phenolic alkaloids found in oats but not in other cereal grains, are reported to have antioxidant and anti-inflammation properties (Sang & Chu 2017). Their ability to reduce oxidative stress and inflammatory responses may partly explain how oats could protect against atherosclerosis, in addition to their ability to improve the function of blood vessel endothelial cells, which help regulate blood pressure and blood flow. In addition, the antiproliferative effects of avenanthramides on several cancerous cell lines could be one of the possible mechanisms for the protective effect of oats against colon cancer (Meydani 2009).

Curcumin is the main bioactive compound in turmeric, which is an Indian herb used in curry powder. Owing to its antioxidant and anti-inflammatory effects, curcumin has been extensively studied for its potential role in the prevention and treatment of various medical conditions, including atherosclerosis, cystic fibrosis, arthritis and certain cancers. In addition, a growing body of evidence indicates that curcumin has a potential role in the prevention and treatment of dementia and Alzheimer's disease (Lee et al. 2014; Small et al. 2018) (see also Chapter 34). The beneficial effects of curcumin on cognitive function may be attributable to its anti-inflammatory properties and/or its ability to reduce β-amyloid plaques and delay degradation of neurons (Mishra & Palanivelu 2008).

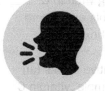 **'SUPERFOODS'—ARE THEY REALLY MAGIC BULLETS?**

Superfoods are so called due to their high nutrient-density and most are plant foods. Information on superfoods is common in the popular literature and some of these reports have some basis in the evidence. However, the effects are often overstated and it is unclear as to whether distilling or extracting the active ingredient(s) into a pill has the same effect as consuming the food. Superfoods also have trends; in recent years, kale, acai and turmeric have been trending with combinations such as kale shakes and turmeric lattes.

Choose a superfood from the list below and use the literature to find out why it is considered a superfood, what the active ingredient(s) are, what the evidence-based benefits are and, finally, what quantities need to be consumed to have an effect. Write a blog for the general public to communicate your message.

- blueberries
- turmeric
- acai
- goji berries
- avocados
- oats
- kale

Extension question: plants are currently being genetically modified to increase their bioactive components. What is your opinion on this development?

NUTRIENT SUPPLEMENTS

As far as possible, dietary diversity should be the basis of adequate intakes of nutrients, especially micronutrients and phytonutrients. This is generally achievable if enough food is eaten, avoiding energy intake excess through being physically active. The food system may, however, fail to deliver some healthful components in areas where the soil and water supply are deficient as in iodine or selenium. Food trade into such areas sometimes offsets this risk, but certainty is provided by supplementation or food fortification. Supplementation is also needed where the food system fails—for example, where there is restricted access to arable land and land reform is required. Another is where beliefs or taboos limit use of nutritious foods. For example, tropical fruits like papaya are good sources of provitamin A carotenoids, but in some areas of southern India girls and young women are reluctant to eat them because they are

ANTIOXIDANT RELEVANCE TO HUMAN HEALTH: TO USE OR NOT TO USE?

The oxidation process is essential in the body's defence against infection or in response to tissue damage. Reactive oxygen species (ROS) are used by the immune system as a way to attack and kill pathogens. Free radicals and ROS can also play roles as cellular secondary messengers, which are one of the initiating components of intracellular signal transduction cascades, or signalling molecules. However, free radicals, peroxides and other reactive species cause chain reactions, and excessive free radicals and chain reactions can result in cell damage or even cell death. For the homeostasis of oxidant status, antioxidant capacity is required both intra- and extracellularly. The body's antioxidant system is acquired from food intake and generated in the body. Many plant-derived foods have a range of antioxidant compounds, including vitamin C, vitamin E, polyphenols, carotenoids and ubiquinols. With some being water-soluble and others fat-soluble, these compounds appear to complement each other for effective antioxidant functions in biological systems.

However, some antioxidant compounds can be pro-oxidants and induce oxidative stress (an imbalance between oxidants and antioxidants in favour of the oxidants). For example, vitamin C has antioxidant activity when it reduces oxidising substances such as hydrogen peroxide, and it can reduce metal ions leading to the generation of free radicals. The metal ion in this reaction can be reduced, oxidised, and then re-reduced, in a process that generates ROS.

When there is oxidative stress, damage can potentially occur to all components of the cell, including proteins, lipids and DNA (Sies 1985). Oxidative stress can also cause disruptions in normal mechanisms of cellular signalling. In humans, oxidative stress is thought to be involved in the development of chronic diseases, particularly CVD and cancer. The use of antioxidants as supplements to prevent some diseases is controversial. A 2007 meta-analysis revealed that some popular antioxidant supplements, such as vitamin A, β-carotene and vitamin E, may increase mortality risk (Bjelakovic et al. 2007).

While there is a lack of evidence that the antioxidant level present in a food translates into a related antioxidant effect in the body, food plays a major role in determining and setting the body's intrinsic antioxidant capacity, and food matrices and patterns, especially with diversity, can contribute to the safety of antioxidant consumption (Wahlqvist 2013).

considered abortifacients; this places them at risk of xerophthalmia. In such cases, it would be better to have the foods which are much more nutritionally replete than an isolated nutrient.

However, supplements may be considered for women in their reproductive years if they would be deficient coming into and during pregnancy. With iron and zinc deficiencies the problem is commonly one not of intake but of excessive loss on account of intestinal parasitosis, such as hookworm or ascariasis. Clinically, it may be recognised that a disease process or its treatment may increase micronutrient requirements. Thus, the case for supplementation is justifiable principally where there is a definable public health need, or where there is clinical deficiency, but not for healthy populations. In the latter case, there is evidence that micronutrient supplements may actually increase mortality (Mursu et al. 2011).

Where supplements are found necessary for any reason, it is best that they are used for the shortest period possible and at doses near to the physiological requirements (unless catch-up is needed), and only while the underlying problem is addressed. Rarely, vitamins may be used therapeutically for reasons different to those based on their known physiology. Niacin (nicotinic acid or vitamin B-3), for example, is used in mega-dosage for treatment of some forms of hyperlipidaemia, which is not a feature of its nutritional physiology.

SUMMARY

- Foods contain many compounds in addition to traditional nutrients. Many of these compounds are biologically active, and therefore may affect human health positively, adversely or both. Bioactive food components with beneficial health properties are referred to as phytonutrients because they usually exist in plants.
- Nutrient supplementation is not necessary for individuals who consume a wide variety of foods, and who are physically active enough to consume, commensurately, enough energy.
- Where nutrient supplements are found necessary for any reason, it is best that they are used for the shortest period possible and at doses near to the physiological requirements, unless catch-up is needed, and while the underlying problem is addressed.

KEY TERMS

Anticarcinogen: A substance that counteracts the effects of a carcinogen (a substance or agent that causes cancer) or prevents the development of cancer by deactivating carcinogens and/or blocking the action of carcinogens such as damage to DNA.

Antimutagen: A substance that can counteract the effects of a mutagen, which is a substance or agent that causes genetic mutation. Antimutagens can counteract mutagenic effects by preventing the transformation of a mutagenic compound into a mutagen, inactivating mutagen, or preventing the mutagen-DNA reaction.

REFERENCES

Albanes, D., Heinonen, O.P., Huttunen, J.K., Taylor:R., Virtamo, J. et al., 1995, 'Effects of alpha-tocopherol and beta-carotene supplements on cancer incidence in the Alpha-Tocopherol Beta-Carotene Cancer Prevention Study', *American Journal of Clinical Nutrition, 62*(6): 1427S–30S, doi:10.1093/ajcn/62.6.1427S

Bjelakovic, G., Nikolova, D., Gluud, L.L., Simonetti, R.G. & Gluud, C., 2007, 'Mortality in randomized trials of antioxidant supplements for primary and secondary prevention: systematic review and meta-analysis', *JAMA, 297*(8): 842–57, doi:10.1001/jama.297.8.842

Cerella, C., Dicato, M., Jacob, C. & Diederich, M., 2011, 'Chemical properties and mechanisms determining the anti-cancer action of garlic-derived organic sulfur compounds', *Anti-Cancer Agents in Medicinal Chemistry, 11*(3): 267–71, doi:10.2174/187152011795347522

Chajès, V. & Romieu, I., 2014, 'Nutrition and breast cancer', *Maturitas, 77*(1): 7–11, doi:10.1016/j.maturitas.2013. 10.004

Genser, B., Silbernagel, G., De Backer, G., Bruckert, E., Carmena, R. et al., 2012, 'Plant sterols and cardiovascular disease: A systematic review and meta-analysis', *European Heart Journal, 33*(4): 444–51, doi:10.1093/eurheartj/ehr441

Heart Foundation of Australia, 2018, 'Plant Sterols', <www.heartfoundation.org.au/healthy-eating/food-and-nutrition/fats-and-cholesterol/plant-sterols>, accessed 13 May 2018

Hewlings, S.J. & Kalman, D.S., 2017, 'Curcumin: A review of its effects on human health', *Foods, 6*(10): 92, doi:10.3390/foods6100092

Holden, J.M., Eldridge, A.L., Beecher, G.R., Marilyn Buzzard, I., Bhagwat, S. et al., 1999, 'Carotenoid content of U.S. foods: An update of the database', *Journal of Food Composition and Analysis, 12*(3): 169–96, doi:10.1006/jfca.1999.0827

International Agency for Research on Cancer, IARC Working Group on the Evaluation of Cancer-Preventive Strategies & World Health Organization, 2004, *Cruciferous Vegetables, Isothiocyanates and Indoles*, Lyon: IARC

Kozlowska, A. & Szostak-Wegierek, D., 2014, 'Flavonoids-food sources and health benefits', *Roczniki Państwowego Zakładu Higieny, 65*(2): 79–85, <http://wydawnictwa.pzh.gov.pl/roczniki_pzh/download-article?id=1017>, accessed 1 June 2019

Lako, J., Trenerry, V.C., Wahlqvist, M., Wattanapenpaiboon, N., Sotheeswaran, S. & Premier, R., 2007, 'Phytochemical flavonols, carotenoids and the antioxidant properties of a wide selection of Fijian fruit, vegetables and other readily available foods', *Food Chemistry, 101*(4): 1727–41, doi:10.1016/j.foodchem.2006.01.031

Lee, M.-S., Wahlqvist, M.L., Chou, Y.-C., Fang, W.-H., Lee, J.-T. et al., 2014, 'Turmeric improves post-prandial working memory in pre-diabetes independent of insulin', *Asia Pacific Journal of Clinical Nutrition, 23*(4): 581–91, doi:10.6133/apjcn.2014.23.4.24

Leoncini, E., Nedovic, D., Panic, N., Pastorino, R., Edefonti, V. & Boccia, S., 2015, 'Carotenoid intake from natural sources and head and neck cancer: A systematic review and meta-analysis of epidemiological studies', *Cancer Epidemiology and Prevention Biomarkers, 24*(7): 1003–11, doi:10.1158/1055-9965.EPI-15-0053

Linnewiel-Hermoni, K., Khanin, M., Danilenko, M., Zango, G., Amosi, Y. et al., 2015, 'The anti-cancer effects of carotenoids and other phytonutrients resides in their combined activity', *Archives of Biochemistry and Biophysics, 572*: 28–35, doi:10.1016/j.abb.2015.02.018

MacLennan, R., Macrae, F., Bain, C., Newland, R.C., Russell, A. et al., 1999, 'Effect of fat, fibre, and beta carotene intake on colorectal adenomas: Further analysis of a randomized controlled dietary intervention trial after colonoscopic polypectomy', *Asia Pacific Journal of Clinical Nutrition, 8*(Suppl): S54–S58, <http://apjcn.nhri. org.tw/server/MarkWpapers/Papers/Papers%201999/P267.pdf>, accessed 18 January 2019

Manach, C., Milenkovic, D., Van de Wiele, T., Rodriguez-Mateos, A., De Roos, B. et al., 2017, 'Addressing the inter-individual variation in response to consumption of plant food bioactives: Towards a better understanding of their role in healthy aging and cardiometabolic risk reduction', *Molecular Nutrition & Food Research, 61*(6): 1600557, doi:10.1002/mnfr.201600557

Meydani, M., 2009, 'Potential health benefits of avenanthramides of oats', *Nutrition Reviews, 67*(12): 731–5, doi:10.1111/j.1753-4887.2009.00256.x

Miadoková, E., 2009, 'Isoflavonoids—an overview of their biological activities and potential health benefits', *Interdisciplinary Toxicology, 2*(4): 211–18, doi:10.2478/v10102-009-0021-3

Mishra, S. & Palanivelu, K., 2008, 'The effect of curcumin (turmeric) on Alzheimer's disease: An overview', *Annals of Indian Academy of Neurology, 11*(1): 13, doi:10.4103/0972-2327.40220

Mursu, J., Robien, K., Harnack, L.J., Park, K. & Jacobs, D.R., 2011, 'Dietary supplements and mortality rate in older women: The Iowa Women's Health Study', *Archives of Internal Medicine, 171*(18): 1625–33, doi:10.1001/archinternmed.2011.445

Neveu, V., Perez-Jiménez, J., Vos, F., Crespy, V., du Chaffaut, L. et al., 2010, 'Phenol-Explorer: An online comprehensive database on polyphenol contents in foods', *Database, 2010*: bap024, doi:10.1093/database/bap024

Panic, N., Nedovic, D., Pastorino, R., Boccia, S. & Leoncini, E., 2017, 'Carotenoid intake from natural sources and colorectal cancer: A systematic review and meta-analysis of epidemiological studies', *European Journal of Cancer Prevention, 26*(1): 27–37, doi:10.1097/CEJ.0000000000000251

Sang, S. & Chu, Y., 2017, 'Whole grain oats, more than just a fiber: Role of unique phytochemicals', *Molecular Nutrition & Food Research, 61*(7): 1600715, doi:10.1002/mnfr.201600715

Sies, H., 1985, *Oxidative Stress,* London: Academic Press

Small, G.W., Siddarth:, Li, Z., Miller, K.J., Ercoli, L. et al., 2018, 'Memory and brain amyloid and tau effects of a bioavailable form of curcumin in non-demented adults: A double-blind, placebo-controlled 18-month trial', *American Journal of Geriatric Psychiatry, 26*(3): 266–77, doi:10.1016/j.jagp.2017.10.010

Vieira, A.R., Abar, L., Vingeliene, S., Chan, D., Aune, D. et al., 2015, 'Fruits, vegetables and lung cancer risk: A systematic review and meta-analysis', *Annals of Oncology, 27*(1): 81–96, doi:10.1093/annonc/mdv381

Wahlqvist, M.L., 2013, 'Antioxidant relevance to human health', *Asia Pacific Journal of Clinical Nutrition, 22*(2): 171–6, doi:10.6133/apjcn.2013.22.2.21

Wahlqvist, M.L., Kouris-Blazos, A., Dalais, F., Kannar, D. & Wattanapenpaiboon, N., 1998, 'Phytochemical deficiency disorders: Inadequate intake of protective foods', *Current Therapeutics, 39*(7): 53–6, 58–60, <http://apjcn.nhri.org.tw/server/MarkWpapers/Papers/Papers%201998/P250.pdf>, accessed 24 May 2019

Wahlqvist, M.L., Wattanpenpaiboon, N., Kouris-Blazos, A., Mohandoss: & Savige, G.S., 1998, 'Dietary reference values for phytochemicals?', *Proceedings of the Nutrition Society of Australia, 22*: 34–40, <http://apjcn.nhri.org.tw/server/MarkWpapers/Papers/Papers%201998/P261.pdf>, accessed 24 May 2019

Weng, C.-J. & Yen, G.-C., 2012, 'Chemopreventive effects of dietary phytochemicals against cancer invasion and metastasis: Phenolic acids, monophenol, polyphenol, and their derivatives', *Cancer Treatment Reviews, 38*(1): 76–87, doi:10.1016/j.ctrv.2011.03.001

Wilcox, G., Wahlqvist, M.L., Burger, H.G. & Medley, G., 1990, 'Oestrogenic effects of plant foods in postmenopausal women', *BMJ, 301*(6757): 905, <www.ncbi.nlm.nih.gov/pmc/articles/PMC1664107/>, accessed 18 January 2019

Zamora-Ros, R., Knaze, V., Rothwell, J.A., Hémon, B., Moskal, A. et al., 2016, 'Dietary polyphenol intake in Europe: The European Prospective Investigation into Cancer and Nutrition (EPIC) study', *European Journal of Nutrition, 55*(4): 1359–75, doi:10.1007/s00394-015-0950-x

{CHAPTER 19}
FOOD-BASED GUIDANCE SYSTEMS

Danielle Gallegos

OBJECTIVES

- Describe the elements of a food-based guidance system.
- Understand how elements of food-based guidance systems are developed.
- Evaluate a range of different food-based guidance systems in different cultural contexts.

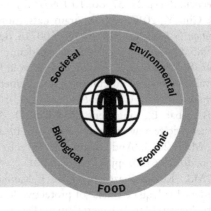

INTRODUCTION

A national food and nutrition policy may be defined as a statement of intent about governmental action to achieve nutrient or dietary goals, explicitly taking into account the relationship between diet and health. Food and nutrition guidance systems are a series of tools that are used by countries to inform these policies and assist in guiding populations to develop eating patterns that are conducive for health. With the triple burden of disease (wasting/stunting (see Chapter 25); micronutrient deficiencies; obesity and chronic conditions) becoming more commonplace, these guidance systems are increasingly focused on achieving sustenance as well as reducing the risk of chronic conditions.

Food-based guidance systems highlight the importance of a dietary pattern approach to the maintenance of health and a reduction in risk for nutritionally related diseases and conditions. Food and nutrition guidance systems recognise that no single food (with the exception of breastmilk for infants in the first six months of life) can provide all the nutrients needed for health. It also recognises that a whole-of-diet approach with a focus on dietary patterns is more effective in building health and minimising disease risk. This chapter builds on your understanding of food groups and nutrients to look at how the messages for healthy eating are developed and transmitted.

ELEMENTS OF FOOD AND NUTRITION GUIDANCE SYSTEMS

Food and nutrition guidance systems form the cornerstone of international efforts to improve action on nutrition as outlined at the Second International Conference on Nutrition (ICN2) in 2014. Specifically the framework calls for the development of international guidelines on healthy eating, and the implementation of nutrition interventions based on dietary guidelines and coherent policies (FAO & WHO 2014). There are five elements to food guidance systems, each informing the other, culminating in visual representations known as food-based dietary guidelines (FBDGs). These elements are outlined in Table 19.1.

Table 19.1: Elements of food and nutrition guidance systems

Element	Description
Food composition data	Sound food composition data within country are essential for informing dietary guidelines and FBDGs. Values for certain food categories, and accurate food composition data, will inform the inherent messages for populations. Food composition data that include accurate data for indigenous foods for countries such as Australia and New Zealand, and include a range of foods consumed by ethnically diverse populations, should also inform the development of FBDGs (Greenfield & Southgate 2003; Leclercq et al. 2001).
Food consumption data	Food supply and systems are constantly evolving and impact on the types and amounts of foods consumed by the population. Dietary guidelines are aspirational but need to reflect the consumption patterns of the population they are targeting. This requires up-to-date, accurate food consumption data, as derived, for example, from national nutrition surveys. Monitoring of trends in nutrient intakes is linked to the accuracy of food consumption data; some changes may well be occurring but apparent trends may relate to the accuracy of or definitions used within food composition data (Leclercq et al. 2009). In Australia, this is most recently represented by the Australian Health Survey 2011–2012, and in New Zealand by the Nutrition Survey 2008–2009. Chapter 24 provides a more in-depth discussion of national nutrition surveys.
Nutrient Reference Values (NRVs)	NRVs are a composite of a number of reference values, including the Estimated Average Requirement (EAR); Recommended Dietary Intake (RDI); Adequate Intake (AI); and Upper Limit (UL) (NHMRC 2018). These are based on extensive review of the evidence to provide the physiological basis for dietary guidelines and are mainly used by professionals. They are discussed in more depth later in this chapter. See the *Nutrient Reference Values for Australia and New Zealand* (NHMRC 2018).
Food-based dietary guidelines	Dietary guidelines translate nutrient recommendations (NRVs) into food and dietary patterns for the community. For example, the recommendation for a diet to consist of 45–65% carbohydrate would be expressed in a dietary guideline as: eat more bread and cereals (preferably wholegrain), vegetables and fruits. Guidelines do not have to be quantified, but do need to be based on a national dietary vision. The guidelines may incorporate other elements of the vision such as food safety, sustainability or **commensality**.
Visual representations of dietary guidelines	Dietary guidelines can be complemented by food guides and visual representations, such as pyramids, plates or other diagrams, that provide information on the types and quantities of different food groups that are recommended to make up a diet. Food-based dietary guidelines are 'tailored to the specific nutritional, geographical, economic and cultural conditions within which they operate' (Fischer & Garnett 2016).

Nutrient Reference Values

The Nutrient Reference Values (NRVs) were developed for Australia and New Zealand in 2006 after an extensive review of the current evidence. The NRVs replaced the previous Recommended Dietary Intakes (RDI), which were designed for use for populations but were misused through their application to individuals. The NRVs consist of seven reference values that attempt to describe the recommendations to prevent deficiencies but also chronic conditions. The definitions and scope for use of these individual reference values are outlined in Table 19.2. The NRVs for individual nutrients are included with each macro- and micronutrient in chapters 10–17. This section provides an overview of the NRVs and their application as it informs the development of dietary guidelines.

In the Australian context, the NRVs are used as the basis for dietary guidelines via a food modelling system which translates the NRVs into food consumption patterns that:

- deliver the nutrient requirements for people of varying age/gender, activity levels and life-stages
- are culturally acceptable, socially equitable and environmentally sustainable

Table 19.2: Nutrient Reference Values definitions and scope for use

Reference Value	Definition	Scope for use	
		Individual	Groups
REFERENCE VALUES FOR GENERAL HEALTH AND WELLBEING			
EAR (Estimated Average Requirement)	The level estimated to meet the requirements of half of the healthy individuals in a particular life stage and gender group.	Used to examine the probability that usual intake is inadequate.	Used to estimate the prevalence of inadequate intakes within a group.
RDI (Recommended Dietary Intake)	The average daily dietary intake level that is sufficient to meet the nutrient requirements of nearly all (97–98%) healthy individuals in a particular life stage and gender group. RDIs are greater than the average physiological requirement for each group and include generous allowances to allow for differences in the absorption and metabolism of nutrients between individuals of the same age, sex and physiological state. If the data are normally distributed and sufficiently robust to calculate an EAR, then a Recommended Dietary Intake is defined as the EAR plus two standard deviations—that is, most EAR values are 20 per cent less than the RDIs.	RDIs are used to plan diets or assess if an individual's dietary intake is likely to be adequate.	Do not use to assess intakes of groups.
AI (Adequate Intake)	The median intake of a given nutrient in apparently healthy people as obtained from the National Nutrition Surveys of Australia and New Zealand (available at the time) that are assumed to be adequate.	Usual intake at or above this level has a low probability of inadequacy.	Mean usual intake at or above this level implies a low prevalence of inadequate intakes.
UL (Upper Level of intake)	The highest average daily nutrient intake likely to pose no adverse health effects to almost all individuals in the general population. As intake increases above the UL, the potential risk of adverse effects increases.	Usual intake above this level may place an individual at risk of adverse effects from excessive nutrient intake.	Use to estimate the percentage of the population at potential risk of adverse effects from excessive nutrient intake.
REFERENCE VALUES FOR THE PREVENTION OF CHRONIC CONDITIONS			
AMDR (Acceptable Macronutrient Distribution Range)	An estimate of the range of intake for each macronutrient for individuals expressed in terms of total energy consumed that would allow adequate intake of all the other nutrients. Only apply to adults and children over the age of 14.	If an individual exceeds the AMDR there is the potential for increasing chronic disease risk.	By determining the proportion of a group that falls below, within and above the AMDR, a population's adherence to recommendations can be assessed.
SDT (Suggested Dietary Target)	A daily average intake from food and beverages for certain nutrients that may help in prevention of chronic disease. Only apply to adults and children over the age of 14.	Not applicable.	Used to inform guidelines at the population level.

Source: AIHW (2012); NHMRC (2018)

- reflect the current Australian food supply and food consumption patterns
- provide some flexibility in food choice
- promote health and wellbeing, consider chronic disease.

The dietary models are called the **Foundation Diets** and **Total Diets** and highlight that nutritional requirements are met through the whole diet and not via single foods, making the combination of foods critical. The key nutrients used to drive the modelling and those assessed as outputs from the modelling, as well as those not considered, are outlined in Table 19.3. Foundation diets included omnivore, ovo-lacto vegetarian, pasta-based and rice-based models, accounting for some cultural and social variations. Environmental sustainability was another consideration and influenced, for example, serves of meat and fish. Sustainable diets including the influence of dietary guidelines are discussed in more detail in Chapter 26.

The food selection guides are used by individuals, so RDI was the basis for planning in the Foundation Diet but was cross-checked with 100 seven-day simulations against the EAR, with individual food choices aimed at exceeding the EAR. Total Diets were all checked against the UL, AMDR and SDT for those above 14 years of age. The diets are presented as serves per week rather than per day to convey the message that daily meal patterns can vary, but that the average weekly intake should be consistent with the recommended pattern.

FOOD-BASED DIETARY GUIDELINES

Nutrition advice continually evolves as new evidence comes to light and contexts, including social, cultural and food supply, change. FBDGs are therefore dynamic documents that require periodical review and updating. As the documents that communicate a national dietary vision for a population, they are the mandated and approved guidelines that provide the basis for public food and nutrition, health and agricultural policies and nutrition education programs (FAO 2018). The guidelines, however, will only impact on people's lives if they are incorporated and enacted in a range of policies, education, legislation and strategies. They provide the vision, but not necessarily the action; consequently, the first recommendation of the ICN2 was for 'political commitment and social participation for improving nutrition at the country level' (FAO & WHO 2014).

Food-based dietary guidelines use modelling and evidence to translate the technical nutrition science

Table 19.3: Nutrients used and not used in the dietary modelling

Key nutrients driving modelling	Nutrients with AI only assessed as outputs from modelling	Not included as drivers due to inadequate food composition data
Energy	Linoleic acid	Selenium
Protein	α-linolenic acid	Vitamin B-6
Thiamin	Long-chain n-3 fatty acids	Vitamin B-12
Vitamin A as retinol equivalents	Dietary fibre	**Not included as drivers due to abundance in Australian diet**
Vitamin C	Vitamin D	Riboflavin
Folate as dietary folate equivalents	Vitamin E	Niacin
Calcium	Potassium	Phosphorus
Iodine	Sodium	
Iron		
Magnesium		
Zinc		

inherent in the NRVs into simple information that the public can easily understand and that focuses on foods commonly consumed, portion sizes and behaviours. They go beyond addressing 'foods' simply as 'food groups', and avoid reference to nutrients at the point of guidance. At the same time, they take account of the best nutrition (including nutrients) science available.

Increasingly, there are calls for FBDGs to also incorporate learnings from environmental and social sciences recognising that food is a commodity that requires inputs and creates outputs with environmental impact, and that eating is a social act. Internationally, 92 countries (out of a possible 195) have

dietary guidelines; of these, the majority are high- or high–middle-income countries, with only four (8 per cent) low-income countries (Afghanistan, Benin, Nepal and Sierra Leone) having guidelines as of 2019 (FAO 2019). In some countries the guidelines are difficult to find, indicating that their use to provide clear direction to the public and as a vision informing policies is perhaps limited. In developing and implementing national dietary guidelines and their accompanying visual representations, a number of key tenets are recommended; these are outlined in Table 19.4.

To describe the process of developing FBDGs as solely scientific is naive; the development of FBDGs

Table 19.4: Key tenets for the development and implementation of dietary guidelines

Evidence-based. Dietary guidelines should be premised on the best available evidence and incorporate up-to-date information on food and nutrition science. They should consider all of the evidence, including trials of macronutrient manipulation, cohort and ecological studies (Mann et al 2016).
Actionable and applicable. FBDGs should reflect the nutrition situation of the country and refer to foods that are commonly available, affordable, culturally relevant and socially acceptable. They should be developed in a cultural context, recognising the social, economic and environmental aspects of foods and eating patterns. They should be practical and take into consideration factors such as available resources, including time.
Food. FBDGs need to reflect food patterns and cuisines rather than numeric goals. These food patterns can vary significantly but still be consistent with good health. Consuming a variety of foods to make up a composite diet should be a primary goal. They incorporate food that is: produced (agriculture, horticulture); processed (food industry); developed (novel/ functional foods); prepared and traditional (cuisine).
Targeted. Sub-populations have differing nutritional requirements at critical points in the lifecourse. FBDGs need to ensure that all sub-populations are catered for.
Inclusive. The process of developing dietary guidelines needs to include a broad range of stakeholders, bringing together diverse academic expertise and undergo a consultation process with civil society and industry.
Transparent. FBDGs are political documents and as such are subject to influence from vested interests (the food industry and primary producers would be two examples). Any process should minimise the impact of these interests and be transparent in how decisions were reached.
Aspirational. While the FBDGs need to be based on current consumption patterns and be realistic, they also need to promote a clear change in dietary patterns that can be achievable through a series of stepped changes. Public health issues should determine their relevance.
Championed. FBDGs need to be owned by the government and be clearly championed by one government agency but involve multiple agencies in their deployment.
Pleasure. FBDGs need to communicate and encourage the enjoyment of food. They should promote pleasure and taste.
Ecological. FBDGs have impacts that go beyond the individual. They have the potential to influence the symbiosis between humans, animals, plants and the environment, where human and environmental health are outcomes of interest.
Translatable. FBDGs at the national level need to be translated into action at the local level in communities, schools and households. FBDGs should foster difference in approaches with an agreed underpinning of broad-based science.
Food literacy. The translation of FBDGs will purportedly allow greater scope and choice from the foods available as well as control over the food supply. However, this presupposes a level of food literacy that needs to be developed and integrated throughout other systems and needs to occur concurrently with the implementation of FBDGs (see the Japan example later in this chapter).

Source: FAO (2018); Fischer & Garnett (2016); Keller & Lang (2008); Wahlqvist (2009)

is a political process and is subject to a range of influences from other agendas. The development of FBDGs in many countries utilises a collaborative approach combining the expertise of predominantly nutrition experts to arrive at a consensus. The evidence for the dietary guidelines has been gradually strengthening, as have the processes around the declaration of conflict of interests for those involved. However, each member of the committee has their own set of opinions and agendas and reaching consensus is often an 'interplay of give–and–take, bullying, boredom, and (eventually) compromise' (Nestle 2013, p. 71). The arrival at a consensus can often be at the expense of clarity.

There is a lot at stake in determining guidelines that will influence the dietary intake of a population. They have the potential to drive agricultural practice as well as business across the food chain, from product development to processing to retail. Therefore, it is not unreasonable for the food industry and primary producers to want to participate in the process. That the food industry is influential with government and with the development of policy around nutrition has been noted by Nestle (2013). In Australia, the close relationship between individuals within the food industry and those with the power to make decisions has been described in an analysis of nutrition policy (Cullerton et al. 2017). The vested interests of the scientists, food industry and primary producers have all influenced the FBDGs in different ways. In the USA, the influence of the food industry has been described in relation to softening 'eat less' messages (Nestle 2013). While FBDGs emphasise foods over nutrients, most guidelines exhort populations to eat less fat, especially saturated fat, and to moderate sugar intake, albeit without appropriate messaging on what foods to avoid in order to achieve this. The US government's commitment to promoting US agricultural products (meat, sugar, oil) has hampered the development of key messages that embrace the

THE ROLE OF THE FOOD INDUSTRY

The food industry plays an important role in the food system—ensuring that foods are grown and processed to meet the needs of consumers. However, there are some tactics of the food industry that directly undermine food-based dietary guidelines and need to be questioned. These tactics have led to food companies being described as 'BIG food', which aligns with the strategies used previously by 'BIG tobacco'.

Your task is to review the peer-reviewed scientific literature and see where you stand ethically on some of these issues:
- industry-sponsored scientific research or reviews promoting a certain food item
- sponsorship of sport, particularly children's sport, by multinational fast-food companies
- undermining the implementation of sugar taxes
- sponsorship or support of dietetic and nutrition associations
- the use of toys, playgrounds and online games to attract children
- marketing of energy-dense/nutrient-poor foods to children
- using free trade agreements to flood markets in low-income countries with energy-dense/nutrient-poor foods
- preventing restaurants making free water available to customers.

Thinking broadly, what strategies do you think could be put in place to reduce the consumption of energy-dense/nutrient-poor foods? Be as creative and outrageous as you like.

best available evidence (Hite 2011). Recently, the role of the sugar industry in commissioning and influencing research and researchers in producing 'evidence' in its favour has been equated to the practices of the tobacco industry (Kearns et al. 2016).

Criticisms of FBDGs have emerged, especially in high-income countries, with critics describing the guidelines' exhortations to eat less fat with no caveats on carbohydrate intake as the primary reason for the obesity epidemic. However, these arguments focus on nutrients and not on whole foods. The evidence is clear and robust for diets that are predominantly plant-based and minimally processed (eat more fruit, vegetables, grain foods) and low in saturated fat and sugars. The guidelines are designed for predominantly healthy populations. They are not intended to be used for dietary issues such as weight loss, diabetes management and sports performance; these issues require targeted dietary advice.

Part of the issue is that FBDGs provide a vision but are not necessarily detailed enough as actionable policy documents (Keller & Lang 2008). The development of FBDGs has occurred largely in isolation from policies that develop the food and nutrition literacy of the population and integrate these guidelines into different settings (workplaces, schools, communities, households).

The average number of recommendations in FBDGs is ten, with the range between six (Nigeria) and sixteen (Greece). The recommendations can be as non-specific as 'consume a variety of foods' or as specific as 'eat two tablespoons of beans per tortilla' (Guatemala) or 'eat at least one dark green and one orange vegetable per day' (Canada).

Many countries exhort their populations to 'enjoy' a varied diet or particular foods, but only a few extend this to explicitly link the pleasure of eating, commensality and social aspects to quality diets and improved eating. For example, in Mexico one of the guidelines advises people, 'Take your time to eat and enjoy your meals by sharing them with family and friends whenever possible'; similarly, in Uruguay there is a guideline that says, 'Enjoy your food: eat slowly and, when possible, eat in company' and a second that highlights the importance of

traditional foods and cooking: 'Cooking traditional foods is good for you: discover the joy of cooking and make it a shared activity' (FAO 2016). The notion of pleasure and satisfaction is crucial in encouraging people to change their eating habits (Oliveira & Silva-Amparo 2017).

Four FBDG case studies are explored in more depth below to illustrate different approaches:
- Australia: the Dietary Guidelines and the Australian Guide to Healthy Eating, visually represented as a plate.
- Japan: the Dietary Guidelines and its representation as a spinning top as an exemplar of promoting dietary variety and having an accompanying national **food literacy** policy, 'Shokuiku'.
- Brazil: the Dietary Guidelines and their pictorial representation, as an exemplar of the inclusion of sustainability, commensality and food preparation.
- The Mediterranean diet—as an example of an international portrayal of a regional diet.

Australia

Dietary guidelines for Australians were first developed in 1981 and revised in 1992 (NHMRC 1992), 2003 (NHMRC 2003) and 2013 (NHMRC 2013b). These guidelines are represented in Table 19.5. Dietary guidelines for children and adolescents were released for the first time in 1995 (NHMRC 1995) and for older Australians in 1999 (NHMRC 1999), but have since been rescinded. Infant Feeding Guidelines for Health-workers were first published in 1996 (NHMRC 1996) and updated in 2012 (NHMRC 2013c). The guidelines are accompanied by the Australian Guide to Healthy Eating, which was first released in 1998 and updated again in 2010 and 2013 (NHMRC 2013a).

The Dietary Guidelines and the Australian Guide to Healthy Eating are premised on an extension of the five food groups. The five food groups were developed by the Australian Commonwealth Department of Health in the 1940s and were Australia's food selection guide from the 1940s until the early 1990s. They were the mainstay of dietary advice before the articulation of dietary guidelines in the 1980s. They generally grew out of concerns to ensure that during wartime, as well as in periods of economic difficulty and famine, the population was adequately and nutritionally fed. They were principally concerned with the adequacy of the diet and its relationship to deficiency states (such as vitamin A deficiency and anaemia), not with excesses (such as fat) or deficits (such as carbohydrate, fibre) and their relationship to chronic diseases (such as heart disease, obesity or colon cancer). They used an adequacy or minimal requirement approach rather than a total diet concept. This type of food selection guide is no longer favoured, as it does not address the problems of macronutrient excesses (fat, protein, energy, refined carbohydrates, alcohol) and macronutrient inadequacies (unrefined carbohydrates, fibre).

In the early 1980s, Nutrition Australia's Healthy Eating Pyramid also came into use and has been continually evolving, with formal updates in 2004 and 2015 (Figure 19.1, see colour section). The Healthy Eating Pyramid is essentially a qualitative food guide that addresses the issue of dietary balance of the total diet through the use of descriptive terms such as 'eat more', 'eat moderately' and 'eat less' in relation to various food groups and the Dietary Guidelines. The updated version depicts whole foods and minimally processed foods (identified as food groups) plus healthy fats as the foundation of a varied diet. It also encourages drinking water, enjoying herbs and spices (in recognition of their important role in a varied diet and adding pleasure and taste), and limiting salt and added sugar. It was designed as a simple conceptual model for people to use as a first step to adequate nutrition and is used in conjunction with the Australian Guide to Healthy Eating in many settings.

Australian Guide to Healthy Eating

The Australian Guide to Healthy Eating is based on the core food groups and has not been designed to replace other food guides; rather, it is intended to clarify and build upon the tools already available to the public. It is in the shape of a plate or pie, with 'slices' for fruit, vegetables (and legumes), cereals, animal-derived foods such as meat, fish and eggs (and legumes/nuts

as meat alternatives), and milk and dairy products. This guide addresses the 'total diet' by providing recommendations about 'extras' or 'indulgences' and fats. It does have a number of limitations.

- There are no recommendations for varying energy needs and physical activity levels; it does not provide a guide to serves to assist with portion sizes (this is provided as ancillary material but is not incorporated into the primary guide).
- Food sustainability, security and commensality are not addressed.
- The growing importance of legumes, nuts and seeds, herbs and spices in promoting and maintaining health has not been addressed.
- The re-emergence of nutrient deficiency-related disease, especially in at-risk groups—lower income households, house/office-bound people, the elderly, obese people, pregnant women, children, those with excess alcohol consumption, vegetarians, excessive fast-food consumers, people with gastric banding, people on certain medications (e.g. diuretics, proton pump inhibitors)—is not addressed. Nutrients that need particular attention include vitamin D, iodine, iron and possibly zinc, selenium and magnesium.
- Beverages with possible positive benefits and with high levels of consumption, including tea and coffee, are not included.

The guide does attempt to provide a guide to those consuming a vegetarian diet and is inclusive of some limited culturally diverse foods. However, its applicability to the eating patterns of Australia's diverse population must be questioned. An Aboriginal and Torres Strait Islander version of the plate is available (Figure 19.2, see colour section). However, despite the fact that 11 per cent of Australians do not speak English at home and there is significant variety in dietary patterns, there does not appear to be a Commonwealth commitment to providing tailored guides to healthy eating. The NSW government has provided a repository of translated versions of the guide. The box 'Local development of food-based guidelines' provides an example of a guide to healthy

Table 19.5: Australian dietary guidelines, main messaging 1981, 1992, 2003, 2013

	1981	1992	2003	2013
Explicitly recommends diet variety	Choose a nutritious diet from a variety of foods.	Enjoy a wide variety of nutritious foods.	Enjoy a wide variety of nutritious foods.	Enjoy a wide variety of nutritious foods from these five food groups every day.
Recommends increased fruit and vegetable consumption	Eat more breads and cereals (preferably wholegrain) and vegetables and fruits.	Eat plenty of breads and cereals (preferably wholegrain), vegetables (including legumes) and fruits.	Eat plenty of vegetables, legumes and fruits.	Plenty of vegetables, including different types and colours, legumes/beans and fruit.
Recommends reducing fat and changing fat type	Avoid eating too much fat.	Eat a diet low in fat and, in particular, low in saturated fat.	Limit saturated fat and moderate total fat intake.	Limit intake of foods high in saturated fat such as many biscuits, cakes, pastries, pies, processed meats, commercial burgers, pizza, fried foods, potato chips, crisps and other savoury snacks. Replace high-fat foods which contain predominantly saturated fats, such as butter, cream, cooking margarine, coconut and palm oil, with foods which contain predominantly polyunsaturated and monounsaturated fats, such as oils, spreads, nut butters/pastes and avocado. Low fat diets are not suitable for children under the age of 2 years.
Recommends reducing salt	No reference	Choose low-salt foods and use salt sparingly.	Choose foods low in salt.	Limit intake of foods and drinks containing added salt. Read labels to choose lower sodium options among similar foods. Do not add salt to foods in cooking or at the table.
Recommends reducing sugar	Avoid eating too much sugar.	Eat only a moderate amount of sugars and foods containing sugars.	Consume only moderate amounts of sugars and foods containing added sugars.	Limit intake of foods and drinks containing added sugars such as confectionery, sugar-sweetened soft drinks and cordials, fruit drinks, vitamin waters, energy and sports drinks.
Recommends moderating meat intake	No reference	Eat foods containing iron. This applies particularly to girls, women, vegetarians and athletes.	Include lean meat, fish, poultry and/or alternatives.	[Include] lean meats and poultry, fish, eggs, tofu, nuts and seeds, and legumes/beans.
Recommends dairy intake	No reference	Eat foods containing calcium. This is particularly important for girls and women.	Include milks, yoghurts, cheeses and/or alternatives. Reduced-fat varieties should be chosen, where possible.	[Include] milk, yoghurt, cheese and/or their alternatives, mostly reduced-fat (reduced-fat milks are not suitable for children under the age of 2 years).

	1981	1992	2003	2013
Recommends bread, cereals, grain foods	Eat more breads and cereals (preferably wholegrain) and vegetables and fruits.	Eat plenty of breads and cereals (preferably wholegrain), vegetables (including legumes) and fruits.	Eat plenty of cereals (including breads, rice, pasta and noodles), preferably wholegrain.	Grain (cereal) foods, mostly wholegrain and/or high-cereal fibre varieties, such as breads, cereals, rice, pasta, noodles, polenta, couscous, oats, quinoa and barley.
Recommends limiting alcohol consumption	Limit alcohol consumption.	If you drink alcohol, limit your intake.	Limit your alcohol intake if you choose to drink.	If you choose to drink alcohol, limit intake. For women who are pregnant, planning a pregnancy or breastfeeding, not drinking alcohol is the safest option.
Recommends controlling weight		Control your weight.	Maintain a healthy body weight by balancing physical activity and food intake.	Prevent weight gain: be physically active and eat according to your energy needs. / To achieve and maintain a healthy weight, be physically active and choose amounts of nutritious food and drinks to meet your energy needs. Children and adolescents should eat sufficient nutritious foods to grow and develop normally. They should be physically active every day and their growth should be checked regularly. Older people should eat nutritious foods and keep physically active to help maintain muscle strength and a healthy weight.
Addresses food safety and hygiene	No reference	No reference	No reference	Care for your food: prepare and store it safely. / Care for your food; prepare and store it safely.
Water consumption actively encouraged	No reference	No reference	No reference	Drink plenty of water. / ... and drink plenty of water.
Breastfeeding actively encouraged	No reference	No reference	Encourage and support breastfeeding.	Encourage, support and promote breastfeeding.

LOCAL DEVELOPMENT OF FOOD-BASED GUIDELINES

There is a significant **diaspora** of Pacific peoples in New Zealand and Australia. The largest communities outside the Pacific islands live in New Zealand and the second largest in Queensland, Australia. The Pasifika diaspora in both New Zealand and Australia have high levels of chronic disease, lower life expectancy and poorer overall health. Pasifika communities tend to consume larger portion sizes and increased serves of energy-dense/nutrient-poor foods (Perkins et al. 2016). Food and feasting is an important cultural element within Pasifika culture and larger stature remains associated with beauty, social standing, health and wealth (Hawley & McGarvey 2015). In Queensland, the Good Start program has been funded by Queensland Health to develop and implement a range of strategies aimed at Pacific Islander and Māori children. These strategies are designed for the school setting and aim to improve nutrition and increase physical activity using culturally appropriate methods.

With this in mind the Good Start staff members, including multicultural health workers from the targeted communities and in conjunction with community members, redesigned the Australian Guide to Healthy Eating to provide a pictorial representation (Figure 19.3, see colour section) that had more meaning for the community. The key features of the new version included:

* use of the taro leaf shape—this is a commonly eaten vegetable by the community and has a distinctive shape that is immediately recognised
* inclusion in each food group of both traditional foods and foods that have been adopted from Australian culture
* adaptation of 'sometimes' foods to include commonly consumed items such as coconut and canned corned beef/camp pie
* careful design and use of colours to represent the seven largest Māori and Pasifika communities in Queensland—for example, the fala (the weaving in the background) has significant cultural value for these communities.

This is a case study of how food-based guidelines can be adapted for local contexts in order to retain their applicability within culturally diverse groups. For more information on the Good Start program, visit <www.childrens.health.qld.gov.au/chq/our-services/community-health-services/good-start-program/> (CHQ 2018).

eating that has been developed with a community in order to provide cultural context.

Japan

Japan has one of the healthiest diets in the world, and this is underpinned by a strong food culture. However, this healthy diet and food culture is being threatened by increases in food imports and an increased reliance on readily available processed foods. One of the criticisms of FBDGs is that they occur in isolation from policy that develops food and nutrition literacy. Japan is an example of where dietary guidelines and their communication visually are underpinned by the Shokuiku—a law enforcing food education. This section looks at the features of the Japanese dietary guidelines, their representation as a spinning top (Figure 19.4, see colour section) and the role of the Shokuiku.

The typical Japanese diet is low in meat and saturated fats and includes moderate intakes of alcohol along with high intakes of legumes and n-3 plant/marine fats and fish, which contribute to longevity. The traditional Japanese diet is, however, high in salt and salty foods, which contribute to higher rates of stomach cancer and stroke. Adherence to the Japanese Food Guide Spinning Top is associated with a 15 per cent reduction in total mortality rate, mainly attributable to a reduction in deaths from stroke (Kurotani et al. 2016). The Japanese Dietary Guidelines are presented in Table 19.6. In previous versions of the dietary guidelines mention was made of dietary variety—namely, consuming at least 30 different types of food per day. However, this was removed in 2000 in response to concerns about the potential for eating too much and the lack of evidence around the target of 30 types (Katanoda & Matsumura 2005). Of note in these guidelines is the reference to the timing and the components of meals (rhythms), as well as weight, and to eating locally.

The Basic Law of Shokuiku was enacted in 2005 and is defined as the 'acquisition of knowledge about food and nutrition, as well as the ability to make appropriate food choices through various experiences related to food'. The law is enforced in schools, workplaces and in the community and focuses on production to plate, food safety, food preparation and eating together (Ishikawa et al. 2015).

The spinning top is an example of food guides referencing cultural artefacts (in this case a top, but in other countries a plate or, in China, a pagoda). The key feature of the spinning top that is different to most other countries is that it refers to dishes rather than foods. The aim is to make it readily understandable by those who rarely cook; a dish is classified according to the main ingredients (Yoshiike et al. 2007).

Brazil

The FBDGs for Brazil were first developed in 2006 and reviewed in 2014. With the incorporation of environmental, cultural and social sustainability they are described internationally as the gold standard for FBDGs (Fischer & Garnett 2016). The messages are made up of five principles which provide the underpinning framework (these echo the principles of FBDGs established by the FAO and WHO) and are summarised in the '10 steps to a healthy eating plan' (Table 19.7). The main difference of the Brazilian guidelines is that they have forgone the commonly used food group model (which is typically nutrient-based) with a model that critiques the industrial

Table 19.6: Japanese Dietary Guidelines

- Enjoy your meals.
- Establish a healthy rhythm by keeping regular hours for meals.
- Eat well-balanced meals with staple food, as well as main and side dishes.
- Eat enough grains, such as rice and other cereals.
- Combine vegetables, fruits, milk products, beans and fish in your diet.
- Avoid too much salt and fat.
- Maintain a healthy body weight and balance the calories you eat with physical activity.
- Take advantage of your dietary culture and local food products, while incorporating new and different dishes.
- Reduce leftovers and waste through proper cooking and storage methods.
- Track your daily food intake to monitor your diet.

Source: FAO (2010)

Table 19.7: Brazilian recommendations for choices of foods and meals

- Make natural or minimally processed foods the basis of your diet.
- Use oils, fats, salt and sugar in small amounts for seasoning and cooking foods and to create culinary preparations.
- Limit consumption of processed foods.
- Avoid consumption of ultra-processed foods.
- Eat regularly and carefully in appropriate environments and, whenever possible, in company.
- Shop in places that offer a variety of natural or minimally processed foods.
- Develop, exercise and share cooking skills.
- Plan your time to make food and eating important in your life.
- Out of home, prefer places that serve freshly made meals.
- Be wary of food advertising and marketing.

Source: FAO (2014)

DIETARY VARIETY

Dietary variety is a key tenet of food-based dietary guidelines (see also Chapter 8). Nutrition advocacy has tended to focus on staples, which has more to do with increasing energy and protein to ensure adequate intake rather than looking at optimal health. The focus on staples also does not encourage biodiversity, which in itself is increasingly crucial for healthy environments (see Chapter 26). The more explicit nutritional significance of achieving biological variety in one's diet is that it helps ensure an adequate intake of essential nutrients and other components; it dilutes potential adverse food factors; and it recognises the factors in food that are important for health, namely, phytochemicals or phytonutrients. Some protective foods may be low in nutrients, but are nearly always high in phytonutrients—for example, tea, spices and herbs (see Chapter 18).

To increase food variety, it is recommended to choose foods that already provide variety, such as eating multigrain breads and natural mueslis. Rather than having a meal comprising a few different ingredients in large portions (e.g. steak, potato and peas), it is more desirable to have meals with many ingredients in smaller portions. Stir-fries, casseroles, soups and salads are an easy way to increase 'vegetable' variety by adding lots of different ingredients, especially onions, garlic, parsley, herbs and spices. Adapting traditional recipes by adding extra vegetables and legumes is another simple way to increase variety. Varying breakfast cereals, breads and sandwich fillings daily and finding ways to sneak in little extras (such as adding handfuls of herbs to salads or nuts in stir-fry) or serving accompaniments such as salads, dips/sauces (pesto, caviar dip), chutney, jams and nut spreads will also help increase food variety.

The FAO has a Household Dietary Diversity Score, used more often in low-income countries; alternatively, have a look at the Nutrition Australia Food Variety Checklist <www.nutritionaustralia.org/sites/default/files/Food%20Variety%20Checklist_0.pdf> (Nutrition Australia n.d.) or take the online Healthy Eating Quiz developed by the University of Newcastle <http://healthyeatingquiz.com.au/>.

Report on your diet variety, relate whether this is a usual occurrence, reason why this might be the case, and identify the changes you will make to improve the situation.

diet and highlights the risk of industrialisation for traditional diets. The **NOVA** model classifies foods according to the extent and purpose of the industrial processes used to preserve, extract, modify or create them (Table 19.8) (Monteiro et al. 2016). This type of classification is being increasingly used globally to determine the contribution of ultra-processed foods to total diets (Monteiro, Cannon, et al. 2017; Monteiro, Moubarac, et al. 2017; Pulker et al. 2017).

While these guidelines are a welcome development and herald a new approach that not only looks at human health but embraces social and environmental sustainability, there are two areas that need to be explored and debated so that this approach can be retained. The first is that health is still not the central focus of food provisioning; profit remains the primary motivator. Governments have a mandate to build the overall economic position of the state, and to do this they actively need to maximise consumption and profits. Profits can be increased by adding fat, sugar, salt and other additives to whole foods to make them cheap. Governments, therefore, have a

Table 19.8: NOVA classification of foods

Category	Definition
GROUP 1 Natural or minimally processed	Unprocessed/natural foods include all edible parts of plants, animals, fungi, algae and water. Minimally processed foods are those altered by processes that remove inedible or unwanted parts or extend shelf life without the addition of other substances such as sugar, salt, fat or vinegar. Processes include grinding, crushing, pasteurisation, freezing and non-alcoholic fermentation.
GROUP 2 Processed cooking ingredients	These are substances obtained directly from Group 1 foods or from nature by processes such as pressing, refining, grinding and milling. The purpose of processing in this group is to prepare, season and cook Group 1 foods to make them varied and enjoyable. They are not meant to be consumed by themselves.
GROUP 3 Processed foods	These are relatively simple products made by adding sugar, oil, salt or other Group 2 substances to Group 1 foods. Most processed foods have one to three ingredients and are recognised as modified Group 1 foods. The main purpose of processing in this group is to increase the longevity/durability of the items or to enhance their sensory qualities.
GROUP 4 Ultra-processed foods	These are industrial formulations with five or more ingredients. These ingredients can include those used in processed foods as well as substances not commonly used in culinary preparations whose addition is designed to imitate qualities or Group 1 foods or to disguise undesirable qualities of the final product. These substances can be: directly extracted from foods such as whey and gluten; derived from the further processing of food constituents (for example, hydrogenated oils, hydrolysed proteins, maltodextrin); or are completely processed, such as dyes, stabilisers, non-sugar sweeteners, firming, bulking, anti-caking agents. Industrial processes with no equivalent in the domestic kitchen, such as extrusion and moulding, can also be used. The main purpose of ultra-processing is to create products that are ready to eat or drink and are likely to replace unprocessed or minimally processed foods. Common attributes of ultra-processed foods include: hyper-palatability, attractive packaging, aggressive marketing and ownership by transnational companies.

Source: Monteiro et al. (2016); Monteiro, Cannon et al. (2017)

conflict of interest in trying to reduce consumption and maximise health. Secondly, the drive for healthy eating and use of minimally processed foods has not considered who will be undertaking the labour involved. While there is advocacy for the building of cooking skills in both men and women, women still undertake the majority of foodwork in a household. Cooking at home is increasingly associated with better diet quality (Tiwari et al. 2017), but the question remains: who will do the cooking?

The Mediterranean diet

The Mediterranean diet, which is currently promoted as a model for 'good health', came from the Greek island of Crete and southern Italy around the 1960s, when a prospective longitudinal study (30-year mortality follow-up)—known as the Seven Countries Study—began. In 2010, the Mediterranean diet was placed on the UNESCO representative list of the Intangible Cultural Heritage of Humanity. The essential characteristics of the Mediterranean diet are outlined in Table 19.9. The importance of the Mediterranean diet is that its benefits derive from the diet as a whole rather than individual dietary elements. The Mediterranean diet is not homogeneous but, rather, varies across the region based on differences in crops and dietary patterns, traditions, religious practices, and historical, geographical and ecological environments. The Mediterranean diet represents a dietary pattern that has been widely reported as a model of healthy eating, contributing not only to longevity in seniors (Kouris-Blazos et al. 1999) but also to favourable health status (Sofi et al. 2013), including prevention and slowing the progression of **metabolic syndrome** (Esposito et al. 2013), diabetes (Koloverou et al. 2014), cancer (Schwingshackl & Hoffmann 2014), heart disease (Tong et al. 2016), dementia and declining cognitive function (Petersson & Philippou 2016), rheumatoid arthritis (Tedeschi & Costenbader

Table 19.9: Characteristics of the Mediterranean diet

Nutritional features	Food features
A balanced ratio of n-6 and n-3 fatty acids due to low intake of polyunsaturates and higher intake of n-3 fatty acids.	Lower meat intake, higher fish intake.
A higher intake of n-3 linolenic acids.	Higher intakes of nuts (especially walnuts), green leafy vegetables and legumes.
A lower intake of saturated fats.	Lower intakes of meat and butter. Meat is also higher in n-3 fatty acids due to grazing on wild plants and herbs rather than on grains, which increases n-6 fatty acid content.
A higher intake of monounsaturated fats.	Higher intakes of olive oil. Olive oil is also implicated in increased absorption of some vitamins (e.g. tocopherols) and phytonutrients (e.g. carotenoids, certain polyphenols).
Lower energy density.	Higher intake of vegetables, especially dark green leafy vegetables and legumes. Vegetables are an integral part of meals, not served 'on the side'.
Higher fibre, antioxidants, flavonoids and phytonutrient intake.	Higher intake of legumes, nuts, vegetables, fruits and olive oil.
Higher intake of short-chain fatty acids.	Intakes of fermented dairy products and cheese.
Moderate intake of alcohol.	Moderate intake of alcohol and mainly consumed with meals.
Conviviality: cooking, sitting around a table and sharing food in the company of family and friends.	

Source: Sofi et al. (2013)

2016) and obesity/weight loss (Mancini et al. 2016). The social aspects of the Mediterranean diet should not be underestimated and are thought to contribute to its success in reducing chronic conditions and promoting longevity. Importantly, the characteristics of the Mediterranean diet can be found or embedded in other food cultures, with comparable benefits (Kouris–Blazos et al. 1999).

The Mediterranean diet has been captured as a food pyramid (https://oldwayspt.org/traditional-diets/mediterranean–diet) conveying both the types and quantities of foods to be consumed (Figure 19.5, see colour section).

The fundamental features of the pyramid are designed to decrease meat intake and to increase fish and vegetable consumption. Another distinguishing feature of this pyramid is the separation of legumes from vegetables and fruits, with their consumption encouraged on a daily basis. Legume (dried beans, peas, lentils, soy products) consumption is common in many Mediterranean countries (as well as many Asian countries), and legumes are traditionally

consumed in place of meat at least twice a week in soups and salads or roasted and eaten as a snack (for example, roasted chickpeas). Legume intake of Australian-born persons is low (<15 g/day) compared with Mediterranean and Asian ethnic groups (>30 g/day). Legumes are considered to be meat alternatives because they are nutrient-dense, being a good source of protein, iron, zinc, calcium, folate and soluble fibre. Legumes (and olive oil) are also a good source of phytoestrogens, such as lignans (enterolactone, enterodiol) and isoflavones (genistein, daidzein). Critics of the Mediterranean food guide have expressed concerns, however, that it may be inadequate in calcium (restricted in cheese and yoghurt) and iron (red meat restricted to a few times a month)—two problem nutrients for many people, especially women.

The Mediterranean diet varies markedly and there appears to be a large variation in the constituents of the diet when it is studied. For example, intakes of olive oil vary from 16 to 80 mL per day and legumes from 5 to 61 g, which could have implications for

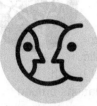

TAKE THE MEDITERRANEAN DIET CHALLENGE

Find a partner and complete the Mediterranean Diet Score (see below) and identify where in your partner's diet changes could be made to make the diet more Mediterranean.

		Criteria for one point
1.	Do you use olive oil as the main culinary fat?	Yes
2.	How much olive oil do you consume in a given day (including oil used for frying, salads, out-of-house meals etc.)?	≥4 tbsp
3.	How many vegetable servings do you consume per day (1 serving = 200 g)?	≥2 (≥1 if raw or salad)
4.	How many fruit serves (including natural fruit juice) do you consume per day?	≥3
5.	How many servings of red meat, mince, or meat products (ham, sausage etc.) do you consume per day (1 serving = 100–150 g)?	<1
6.	How may servings of butter, margarine or cream do you consume per day (1 serving = 1 tbsp)?	<1
7.	How many sweet or carbonated beverages do you drink per day?	<1
8.	How much wine do you drink per week? (glasses, a glass = 200 mL)	≥7
9.	How many legume servings do you consume per week (1 serving = 150 g)?	≥3
10.	How many fish/shellfish servings do you consume per week (1 serving = 100–150 g fish or 4–5 units or 200 g shellfish)?	≥3
11.	How many times a week do you consume commercial sweets or pastries (not homemade) such as cakes, biscuits or custards?	<3
12.	How many servings of nuts (including peanuts) do you consume per week (1 serving = 30 g)?	≥3
13.	Do you preferentially consume chicken, turkey or rabbit meat instead of veal, pork, mince or sausage?	Yes
14.	How many times a week do you consume vegetables, pasta, rice or other dishes seasoned with sofrito (sauce made with tomato and onion, leek, or garlic and simmered with olive oil)?	≥2

Source: Martínez-González et al. (2012)

Translate this information into three key specific food-based changes to be made, or three key specific food-based activities to continue. Discuss how easy or difficult this will be.

specific and all-cause mortality risk (Davis et al. 2015). Due to the cultural variability there does seem to be some value in defining the diet by the nutrients it provides, rather than by the foods. This means that the active constituents of the Mediterranean diet can be applied to range of dietary patterns, allowing for preservation of unique foods and dishes (Davis et al. 2015).

The imperative for dietary guidelines across the globe to take account of and mitigate climate change is being recognised internationally and nationally, with a much stronger focus on plant-based diets and ecologically sensitive food production (Fischer & Garnett 2016; Lucas & Horton 2019; Willett et al. 2019). See Chapter 26 for further discussion of this issue.

SUMMARY

- Food-based dietary guidelines (FBDGs) are complex policy documents that take into consideration a wide range of scientific research and principles to provide the public with simple messaging around foods arranged into dietary patterns to consume for health.
- FBDGs are important for translating nutrient information into practical recommendations around the types of foods to consume.
- The development of FBDGs is about operationalisation as well as the integrative science of food and food systems, which takes into consideration a number of viewpoints and positions.
- Visual representation of guidelines needs to resonate with the communities in which they are used. It is important that the messages are clear and able to be actioned regardless of the audience's level of education, income or region.
- The development of guidelines without political and economic support to implement them across a wide variety of contexts means that FBDGs, in and of themselves, have potentially limited value.
- The emphasis of FBDGs is shifting towards the sustainability of food systems with climate change.

KEY TERMS

Commensality: eating and drinking at the same table as a fundamental social act which creates and consolidates relationships.

Diaspora: the dispersal or spread of a people from their original homeland.

Food literacy: the 'scaffolding that empowers individuals, households, communities or nations to protect diet quality through change and strengthen dietary resilience over time. It is composed of a collection of interrelated knowledge, skills and behaviours required to plan, manage, select, prepare and eat food to meet needs and determine intake' (Vidgen & Gallegos 2014).

Foundation Diet: provides overall numbers of serves of each of the major food groups using composite foods to cover RDI for ten key nutrients within the least energy required for age/gender groups. No discretionary or extra foods added.

Metabolic syndrome: a health condition characterised by abdominal obesity, dyslipidaemia, elevated blood pressure and impaired glucose tolerance.

NOVA: a food system that classes foods according to the degree and purpose of food processing rather than the food's inherent qualities in terms of nutrition. The NOVA model (NOVA is a name, not an acronym), which was developed at the University of Sao Paulo in Brazil, uses four categories: unprocessed or minimally processed foods, processed culinary ingredients, processed foods, and ultra-processed food and drink products.

Total Diet: a variety of approaches to total diets building on a foundation for each age/gender to reach various energy levels. Discretionary or extra foods added.

REFERENCES

AIHW, 2012, *Australia's Food and Nutrition*, <www.aihw.gov.au/reports/food-nutrition/australias-food-nutrition-2012/contents/table-of-contents>, accessed 17 January 2019

CHQ, 2018, *Good Start Program*, <www.childrens.health.qld.gov.au/chq/our-services/community-health-services/good-start-program/>, accessed 19 June 2018

Cullerton, K., Donnet, T., Lee, A. & Gallegos, D., 2017, 'Joining the dots: The role of brokers in nutrition policy in Australia', *BMC Public Health, 17*: 307, doi:10.1186/s12889-017-4217-8

Davis, C., Bryan, J., Hodgson, J. & Murphy, K., 2015, 'Definition of the Mediterranean diet; a literature review', *Nutrients, 7*(11): 9139–53, doi:10.3390/nu7115459

Esposito, K., Kastorini, C.-M., Panagiotakos, D.B. & Giugliano, D., 2013, 'Mediterranean diet and metabolic syndrome: An updated systematic review', *Reviews in Endocrine and Metabolic Disorders, 14*(3): 255–63, doi:10.1007/s11154-013-9253-9

FAO, 2010, *Food-based Dietary Guidelines—Japan*, <www.fao.org/nutrition/education/food-based-dietary-guidelines/regions/countries/japan/en/>, accessed 19 June 2018

—— 2014, *Food-based Dietary Guidelines—Brazil*, <www.fao.org/nutrition/education/food-dietary-guidelines/regions/countries/brazil/en/>, accessed 19 June 2018

—— 2016, *Food-based dietary guidelines—Uruguay*, <www.fao.org/nutrition/education/food-based-dietary-guidelines/regions/countries/uruguay/en/>, accessed 19 June 2018

—— 2018, *Food and Nutrition Education*, <www.fao.org/nutrition/education/en/>, accessed 19 June 2018

—— 2019, *Food-based Dietary Guidelines*, <www.fao.org/nutrition/nutrition-education/food-dietary-guidelines/en/>, accessed 15 May 2019

FAO & WHO, 2014, *Conference Outcome Document: Framework for action*, <www.fao.org/3/a-mm215e.pdf>, accessed 17 January 2019

Fischer, C.G. & Garnett, T., 2016, *Plates, Pyramids and Planets: Developments in national healthy and sustainable dietary guidelines—A state of play assessment*, <www.fao.org/3/a-i5640e.pdf>, accessed 19 January 2019

Greenfield, H. & Southgate, D.A.T., 2003, *Food Composition Data: Production, management and use* (2nd edn), Rome: Food and Agriculture Organization, <www.fao.org/docrep/pdf/008/y4705e/y4705e.pdf>, accessed 1 June 2019

Hawley, N.L. & McGarvey, S.T., 2015, 'Obesity and diabetes in Pacific Islanders: The current burden and the need for urgent action', *Current Diabetes Reports, 15*(5): 29, doi:10.1007/s11892-015-0594-5

Hite, A.H., 2011, 'Is the science behind the 2010 Dietary Guidelines for Americans unquestioned?', *Nutrition, 27*(4): 385–6, doi:10.1016/j.nut.2011.02.005

Ishikawa, M., Kusama, K. & Shikanai, S., 2015, 'Food and nutritional improvement action of communities in Japan: lessons for the world', *Journal of Nutritional Science and Vitaminology, 61*: S55–7, doi:10.3177/jnsv.61.S55

Katanoda, K. & Matsumura, Y., 2005, 'Letter to the editor: Dietary diversity in the Japanese national dietary guidelines', *Nutrition Reviews, 63*(1): 37, doi:10.1111/j.1753-4887.2005.tb00109.x

Kearns, C.E., Schmidt, L.A. & Glantz, S.A., 2016, 'Sugar industry and coronary heart disease research: A historical analysis of internal industry documents', *JAMA Internal Medicine, 176*(11): 1680–5, doi:10.1001/jamainternmed.2016.5394

Keller, I. & Lang, T., 2008, 'Food-based dietary guidelines and implementation: Lessons from four countries—Chile, Germany, New Zealand and South Africa', *Public Health Nutrition, 11*(8): 867–74, doi:10.1017/S1368980007001115

Koloverou, E., Esposito, K., Giugliano, D. & Panagiotakos, D., 2014, 'The effect of Mediterranean diet on the development of type 2 diabetes mellitus: A meta-analysis of 10 prospective studies and 136,846 participants', *Metabolism, 63*(7): 903–11, doi:10.1016/j.metabol.2014.04.010

Kouris-Blazos, A., Gnardellis, C., Wahlqvist, M.L., Trichopoulos, D., Lukito, W. & Trichopoulou, A., 1999, 'Are the advantages of the Mediterranean diet transferable to other populations? A cohort study in Melbourne, Australia', *British Journal of Nutrition, 82*(1): 57–61, doi:10.1017/S0007114599001129

Kurotani, K., Akter, S., Kashino, I., Goto, A., Mizoue, T. et al., 2016, 'Quality of diet and mortality among Japanese men and women: Japan Public Health Center based prospective study', *BMJ, 352*: i1209, doi:10.1136/bmj. i1209

Leclercq, C., Arcella, D., Piccinelli, R., Sette, S., Le Donne, C. & Turrini, A., 2009, 'The Italian National Food Consumption Survey INRAN-SCAI 2005-06: Main results in terms of food consumption', *Public Health Nutrition, 12*(12), p.2504–32, doi:10.1017/s1368980009005035

Leclercq, C., Valsta, L.M. & Turrini, A., 2001, 'Food composition issues—Implications for the development of food-based dietary guidelines', *Public Health Nutrition, 4*(2B): 677–82, doi:10.1079/PHN2001153

Lucas, T. & Horton, R., 2019, 'The 21st-century great food transformation', *Lancet, 393*(10170): 386–7, doi:10.1016/S0140-6736(18)33179-9

Mancini, J.G., Filion, K.B., Atallah, R. & Eisenberg, M.J., 2016, 'Systematic review of the Mediterranean diet for long-term weight loss', *American Journal of Medicine, 129*(4): 407–15.e404, doi:10.1016/j.amjmed.2015.11.028

Mann, J., Morenga, L.T., McLean, R., Swinburn, B., Mhurchu, C.N. et al., 2016, 'Dietary guidelines on trial: The charges are not evidence based', *Lancet, 388*(10047): 851–3, doi:10.1016/S0140-6736(16)31278-8

Martínez-González, M.A., García-Arellano, A., Toledo, E., Salas-Salvado, J., Buil-Cosiales, P. et al., 2012, 'A 14-item Mediterranean diet assessment tool and obesity indexes among high-risk subjects: The PREDIMED trial', *PloS One, 7*(8): e43134, doi:10.1371/journal.pone.0043134

Monteiro, C.A., Cannon, G., Levy, R., Moubarac, J.-C., Jaime, P. et al., 2016, 'NOVA: The star shines bright', *World Nutrition, 7*(1–3): 28–38, <https://worldnutritionjournal.org/index.php/wn/article/view/5>, accessed 18 January 2019

Monteiro, C.A., Cannon, G., Moubarac, J.-C., Levy, R.B., Louzada, M.L.C. & Jaime, C., 2017, 'The UN Decade of Nutrition, the NOVA food classification and the trouble with ultra-processing', *Public Health Nutrition, 21*(1): 5–17, doi:10.1017/S1368980017000234

Monteiro, C.A., Moubarac, J.-C., Levy, R.B., Canella, D.S., Louzada, M.L.d.C. & Cannon, G., 2017, 'Household availability of ultra-processed foods and obesity in nineteen European countries', *Public Health Nutrition, 21*(1): 18–26, doi:10.1017/S1368980017001379

Nestle, M., 2013, *Food Politics: How the food industry influences nutrition and health* (10th anniversary edn), Oakland CA: University of California Press

NHMRC, 1992, *Dietary Guidelines for Australians* (N4), <www.nhmrc.gov.au/guidelines-publications/n4>, accessed 22 November 2018

—— 1995, *Dietary Guidelines for Children and Adolescents* (N1), <www.nhmrc.gov.au/guidelines-publications/n1>, accessed 22 November 2018

—— 1996, *Infant Feeding Guidelines for Health Workers* (N20), <www.nhmrc.gov.au/guidelines-publications/n20>, accessed 22 November 2018

—— 1999, *Dietary Guidelines for Older Australians* (N23), <www.nhmrc.gov.au/guidelines-publications/n23>, accessed 22 November 2018

—— 2003, *Dietary Guidelines for All Australians* (N29–34), <www.nhmrc.gov.au/guidelines-publications/n29-n30-n31-n32-n33-n34>, accessed 22 November 2018

—— 2013a, *Australian Guide to Healthy Eating* <www.eatforhealth.gov.au/sites/default/files/content/The%20 Guidelines/n55i_australian_guide_to_healthy_eating.pdf>, accessed 1 April 2018

—— 2013b, *Eat for Health: Australian dietary guidelines*, <www.eatforhealth.gov.au/>, accessed 22 November 2018

—— 2013c, *Infant Feeding Guidelines: Information for Health Workers (2012)* (N56), <www.nhmrc.gov.au/guidelines-publications/n56>, accessed 22 November 2018

—— 2018, *Nutrient Reference Values for Australia and New Zealand* (Vol. 2006), <www.nhmrc.gov.au/sites/default/files/images/nutrient-refererence-dietary-intakes.pdf>, accessed 22 November 2019

Nutrition Australia, n.d., *Food Variety Checklist* <www.nutritionaustralia.org/sites/default/files/Food%20Variety%20 Checklist_0.pdf>, accessed 19 January 2019

Oliveira, M.S.d.S. & Silva-Amparo, L., 2017, 'Food-based dietary guidelines: A comparative analysis between the dietary guidelines for the Brazilian population 2006 and 2014', *Public Health Nutrition, 21*(1): 210–17, doi:10.1017/S1368980017000428

Perkins, K.C., Ware, R., Tautalasoo, L.F., Stanley, R., Scanlan-Savelio, L. & Schubert, L., 2016, 'Dietary habits of Samoan adults in an urban Australian setting: A cross-sectional study', *Public Health Nutrition, 19*(5): 788–95, doi:10.1017/S1368980015001998

Petersson, S.D. & Philippou, E., 2016, 'Mediterranean diet, cognitive function, and dementia: A systematic review of the evidence', *Advances in Nutrition: An International Review Journal, 7*(5): 889–904, doi:10.3945/an.116.012138

Pulker, C.E., Scott, J.A. & Pollard, C.M., 2017, 'Ultra-processed family foods in Australia: Nutrition claims, health claims and marketing techniques', *Public Health Nutrition, 21*(1): 38–48, doi:10.1017/S1368980017001148

Schwingshackl, L. & Hoffmann, G., 2014, 'Adherence to Mediterranean diet and risk of cancer: A systematic review and meta-analysis of observational studies', *International Journal of Cancer, 135*(8): 1884–97, doi:10.1002/ijc.28824

Sofi, F., Macchi, C., Abbate, R., Gensini, G.F. & Casini, A., 2013, 'Mediterranean diet and health status: An updated meta-analysis and a proposal for a literature-based adherence score', *Public Health Nutrition, 17*(12): 2769–82, doi:10.1017/S1368980013003169

Tedeschi, S.K. & Costenbader, K.H., 2016, 'Is there a role for diet in the therapy of rheumatoid arthritis?', *Current Rheumatology Reports, 18*(5): 23, doi:10.1007/s11926-016-0575-y

Tiwari, A., Aggarwal, A., Tang, W. & Drewnowski, A., 2017, 'Cooking at home: A strategy to comply with U.S. dietary guidelines at no extra cost', *American Journal of Preventive Medicine, 52*(5): 616–24, doi:10.1016/j.amepre.2017.01.017

Tong, T.Y.N., Wareham, N.J., Khaw, K.-T., Imamura, F. & Forouhi, N.G., 2016, 'Prospective association of the Mediterranean diet with cardiovascular disease incidence and mortality and its population impact in a non-Mediterranean population: The EPIC-Norfolk study', *BMC Medicine, 14*(1): 135, doi:10.1186/s12916-016-0677-4

Vidgen, H.A. & Gallegos, D., 2014, 'Defining food literacy and its components', *Appetite, 76*: 50–59, doi:10.1016/j.appet.2014.01.010

Wahlqvist, M.L., 2009, 'Connected Community and Household Food Based Strategy (CCH–FBS): Its importance for health, food safety, sustainability and security in diverse localities', *Ecology of Food and Nutrition 48*(6): 457–81, doi:10.1080/03670240903308596

Willett, W.C., Rockstrom, J., Loken, B., Lang, T., Vermeulen, S. et al., 2019, 'Food in the Anthropocene: The EAT–Lancet Commission on healthy diets from sustainable food systems', *Lancet, 393*(10170): 447–92, doi:10.1016/S0140-6736(18)31788-4

Yoshiike, N., Hayashi, F., Takemi, Y., Mizoguchi, K. & Seino, F., 2007, 'A new food guide in Japan: The Japanese Food Guide spinning top', *Nutrition Reviews, 65*(4): 149–54, doi:10.1111/j.1753-4887.2007.tb00294.x

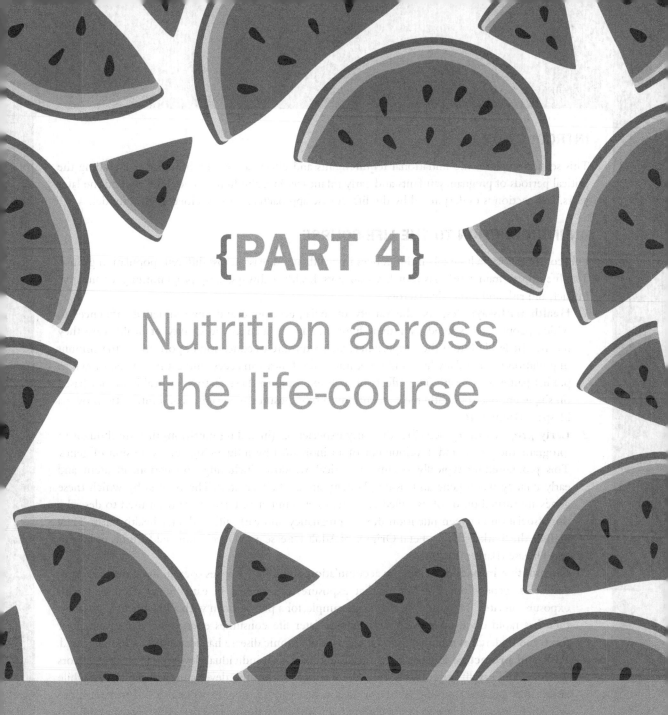

{PART 4}

Nutrition across the life-course

INTRODUCTION

This section explores the nutritional requirements and effects across the life-course, including the critical periods of pregnancy, infants and early infant feeding, children and adolescents, and the later years. This section is underpinned by the life-course approach and the socioecological model.

AN INTRODUCTION TO THE LIFE-COURSE

Life-course theory helps explain differences in health and disease across different population groups. The life-course framework has four key concepts: health pathways, early programming, cumulative impact, and risk and protective factors.

1. **Health pathways** describe the variety of social, economic and environmental influences to which people are exposed over their lifespan. Factors such as the quality of health care they receive, the level of stress they experience, their exposure to education opportunities, the amount of pollution in their daily lives and the kinds of food they can access and eat have been shown to predict patterns of health. The effects of such exposure to these factors on health are not based on single episodes but, rather, on a continuum of exposures, experiences and interactions over a lifespan (Baum 2016).

2. **Early programming** describes the early experiences (including nutrition) that are thought to 'program' the health and development of an individual by influencing the expression of genes. This programming typically occurs at critical windows including conception, in-utero and early infancy when gene and tissue plasticity are at their greatest. The process by which these genes are turned on or off is called epigenetics. A number of terms have been used to describe this association between nutrition during pregnancy and early life and later health status. They include the 'Barker' theory, Fetal Origins of Adult Disease and Developmental Origins of Health and Disease (Barker 2012).

3. **Cumulative impact** describes the accumulation of multiple stresses over an individual's lifespan and across generations. This means that exposure to a stressor in early life is combined with exposures in later life to increase risk. For example, for a person born with a low birthweight who then has rapid catch-up growth, and then in later life consumes energy-dense/nutrient-poor foods and undertakes minimal exercise, the risk of chronic disease has accumulated and increased.

4. **Risk and protective factors** dynamically interact as an individual develops. Protective factors (such as eating well) improve health and contribute to healthy developmental outcomes, while risk factors (such as smoking and poor diet) will negatively impact on health and make it more difficult to realise full developmental potential. This interaction means that pathways of health can be influenced at any point in the life-course.

Figure 4.A highlights the relationship between risk of chronic or non-communicable diseases, age and accumulated risk.

The life-course approach can be useful when looking at nutrition across the lifespan, but the perspective has also been criticised. First, it has been argued that it is too deterministic; in other words, the approach encourages an attitude that once an individual has been exposed to adverse events (such as poor nutrition *in utero*) the pathway has been set and there is no possibility of

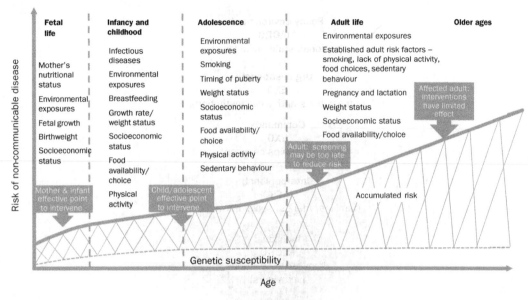

Notes: Interventions are cumulative; maximum benefit in one age group can be derived from interventions in earlier age groups; interventions need to be multi-faceted and focused at various points in the life-cycle to ensure sustainability, especially for the most vulnerable groups; interventions in one generation will bring benefits to successive generations

Figure 4.A: The life-course approach to diet, nutrition and the prevention of chronic disease
Source: Adapted from Darnton-Hill et al. (2004); Uauy & Solomons (2005); Hanson & Gluckman (2014)

achieving better outcomes. The alternative view is that the risk can be managed at all life-stages and that with optimal eating and physical activity, for example, risk can be reduced. Secondly, it has been criticised for leading to the front-loading of interventions for maternal and child health outcomes as the primary critical window for influence. However, if a whole-of-life approach is taken then the life-course framework can provide opportunities for intervening and for influencing both risk and protective factors to maximise positive health outcomes.

AN INTRODUCTION TO THE SOCIOECOLOGICAL MODEL

In addition to the life-course approach, another useful model to guide our understanding of the range of personal, environmental and system factors that determine behaviour is the socioecological model.

The socioecological model has been adapted for use in other contexts, as shown in Figure 4.B. The model was developed by Bronfenbrenner using an ecological systems theoretical approach to describe the multifaceted, interconnecting influences on child development (Bronfenbrenner & Ceci 1994). The model is now used in a range of contexts and describes macro (broad societal), exo (institutional), meso (interpersonal) and micro (individual) influences on health. The model acknowledges that behaviour affects and is affected by multiple levels of influence (CDC 2018). These are described in Table 4.A. The ecological model treats the interaction between factors at

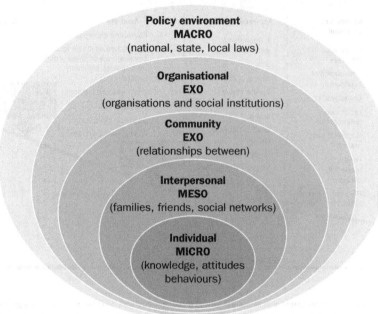

Notes: EXO = institutional; MACRO = broad societal; MESO = interpersonal; MICRO = individual

Figure 4.B: The socioecological model

Source: Adapted from CDC (2018)

Table 4.A: Description of the levels of influences in the socioecological model

Level of influence	Description
Intrapersonal	Individual characteristics that influence behaviour: knowledge, attitudes, gender, religious identity, sexual orientation, values, goals, literacy, skills, self-efficacy.
Interpersonal	Family, friends, peers; formal and informal networks and social support systems that influence individual behaviours.
Community	Relationships among organisations, institutions, and informational networks within defined boundaries, including the built environment, businesses, transportation.
Organisational	Organisations and social institutions with rules and regulations. Churches, schools, work places, stores; rules, regulations, policies, structures constraining or promoting behaviours.
Public policy	Local, state, federal and international policies and laws that regulate or support healthy practices and actions and influence the allocation of resources.

the different levels with equal importance to the influence of factors within a single level. There is consistent evidence that implementing multiple changes in a range of different settings across the levels of the socioecological model are effective in improving eating and physical activity behaviours.

Reference will be made to both the life–course and socioecological frameworks throughout the next chapters.

REFERENCES

Barker, D.J.P., 2012, 'Developmental origins of chronic disease', *Public Health Nutrition, 126*(3): 185–9, doi:10.1016/j.puhe.2011.11.014

Baum, F.E., 2016, *The New Public Health* (4th edn), Melbourne: Oxford University Press

Bronfenbrenner, U. & Ceci, S.J., 1994, 'Nature-nurture reconceptualized in developmental perspective: A bioecological model', *Psychological Review, 101*(4): 568–86, doi:10.1037/0033-295X.101.4.568

CDC, 2018, *The Social-Ecological Model: A framework for prevention,* <www.cdc.gov/violenceprevention/overview/social-ecologicalmodel.html>, accessed 21 June 2018

Darnton-Hill, I., Nishida, C., James, W.P.T., 2004, 'A life-course approach to diet, nutrition and the prevention of chronic disease', *Public Health Nutrition,* 7(1A): 101–21, doi:10.1079/PHN2003584

Hanson, M.A. & Gluckman, P.D., 2014, 'Early developmental conditioning of later health and disease: Physiology or pathophysiology?', *Physiological Reviews, 94*(4): 1027–76, doi:10.1152/physrev.00029.2013

Uauy, R. & Solomons, N., 2005, 'Diet, nutrition and the life-course approach to cancer prevention', *Journal of Nutrition, 135*(12): 2934S–2945S, doi:10.1093/jn/135.12.2934S

{CHAPTER 20}
PREGNANCY AND LACTATION

Danielle Gallegos

OBJECTIVES

- Summarise the significance of nutrition during periconception, pregnancy and lactation and its implications across the life-course.
- Describe key nutritional requirements during pregnancy based on physiological and metabolic changes.
- Discuss food-based recommendations to address common concerns and issues during pregnancy and lactation.

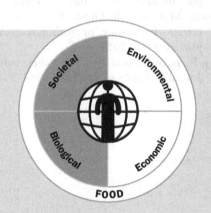

INTRODUCTION

The life-course approach underpins our understanding of the critical nature of the period around conception, pregnancy and lactation for a child's development. Nutritional status prior to, during and after pregnancy influences maternal and infant health outcomes in the short term and the development of chronic disease later in life. The importance of this time has led to a strong focus on the first 1000 days, which covers the time from conception to a child's second birthday. We will look at the physiological and metabolic changes that occur during pregnancy and lactation, weight gain and critical periods in fetal growth, and the nutritional requirements of and dietary recommendations for the mother.

NUTRITION DURING PERICONCEPTION

The prefix 'peri' refers to something being 'around' or 'near'; periconception therefore refers to the time period near or around conception and can include up to ten weeks gestation (Steegers-Theunissen et al. 2013). It includes oocyte (cell in an ovary) formation, fertilisation, implantation and development. The influence of the maternal nutritional environment on the growing fetus and the subsequent programming that takes place in the development of disease is well-accepted (Barker 2004). However, there is growing evidence that exposure of the ova and sperm to environmental challenges, including nutrition, has an impact on the growth and development of not only the fetus but also subsequent generations (Lane et al. 2015).

NUTRITIONAL INFLUENCES ON FERTILITY

Nutrition influences the fertility of both men and women. Fertility issues in men include three primary disorders: low sperm counts, absence of sperm motility and low sperm motility. In women, fertility problems relate to ovulation and tubal problems, endometriosis (a condition where tissue similar to the lining of the womb grows outside in other parts of the body) or, in about a third of cases, are unexplained (Fontana & Torre 2016; Giahi et al. 2015). The influences of weight and nutrition on fertility are summarised in Table 20.1.

Figure 20.1 summarises the key role diet plays in improving sperm parameters, by improving sperm motility, concentration or structure. Long-chain polyunsaturated fatty acids (PUFAs), especially docosahexaenoic acid (DHA) (see Chapter 11), are in higher concentration in sperm and the testes and are integral to the structure of the spermatozoa cell membrane. The increased consumption of PUFAs could therefore improve the integrity of the membrane. However, consuming PUFAs in isolation may not be enough. Consuming seafood high in PUFAs also provides high levels of fat-soluble vitamins that may also play a crucial role (Giahi et al. 2016). A dietary pattern high in fruits and vegetables is also rich in antioxidants. Antioxidants have the ability to protect spermatozoa against oxidative damage, improving their motility and their concentration. Environmental contaminants now appearing in the food and water supply, such as endocrine disruptors, may also be contributing to

Table 20.1: Weight and fertility in men and women

Weight status	Men	Women
Underweight (BMI <19 kg/m²)	Having a BMI <20 kg/m² is associated with a reduction in sperm concentration and count.	Underweight women require an average of 29 months to conceive as compared to 6.8 months in women within the healthy weight range.
Overweight and obese (BMI >25 kg/m²)	With increasing BMI, sperm concentration and motility decrease, testosterone decreases, impacting on spermatogenesis, and there are increased levels of DNA damage.	The chance of spontaneous conception decreases by 5% for each unit increase in BMI greater than 29 kg/m².

Source: Fontana & Torre (2016); Giahi et al. (2015); Jensen et al. (2004)

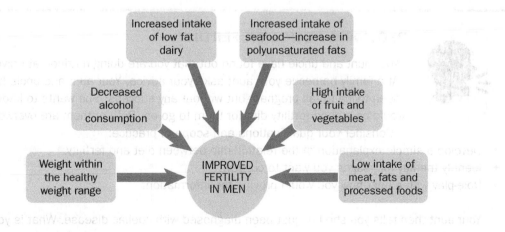

Figure 20.1: Dietary factors associated with fertility in men
Source: Developed from Giahi et al. (2016); Sermondade et al. (2012)

declining male fertility (Maffini et al. 2006; Reddy et al. 2018; Sikka & Wang 2008). Taste preference and bitter tastants consumed by men can also alter spermatogenesis (Lu et al. 2017; Xu et al. 2012) (see Chapter 30). These food pattern associations with spermatogenesis and fertility are also of relevance to epigenetic, life-course and intergenerational health outcomes.

For women, replacing trans fatty acids with monounsaturated fatty acids is associated with a lower risk of impaired ovarian function, but it is still unclear as to whether changes in protein, carbo-

hydrate and/or other micronutrients are also involved. Women who receive a folic acid supplement have better, more mature oocytes compared to women who do not receive folic acid.

CHANGES IN MATERNAL METABOLISM DURING PREGNANCY

Many metabolic adjustments occur during pregnancy that have a profound effect on nutritional requirements. In general, these changes are the result of the action of hormones secreted by the placenta.

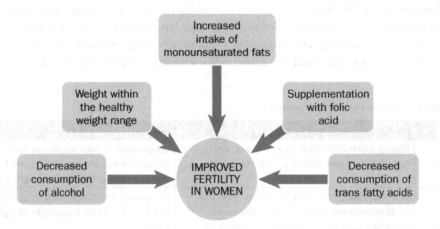

Figure 20.2: Dietary influences associated with improved fertility in women
Source: Developed from Gaskins et al. (2015); Lane et al. (2015)

PROVIDING ADVICE ON FERTILITY

Your aunt and uncle have found out that you are doing nutrition at university. At a family barbecue your aunt asks your advice. Your aunt and uncle have been trying to fall pregnant but without any success. She wants to know what would be a good fertility diet for them to go on. Both of them are overweight.
Consider your qualifications and scope of practice:
- Develop a simple explanation of the relationship between diet and fertility.
- Identify the key messages you want to convey.
- Role-play with a peer how you would provide the information.

Your aunt then tells you she has just been diagnosed with coeliac disease. What is your response?

The role of these hormones and the placenta is to create the most favourable environment for the development of the fetus.

The two principal hormones secreted by the placenta are progesterone and oestrogen. Progesterone has the effect of relaxing smooth muscle tissue, which helps with expansion of the uterus. It also reduces activity in the gastrointestinal tract and, as a result, allows more time for nutrient absorption. Progesterone also favours maternal fat deposition. Oestrogen, on the other hand, leads to increased fluid retention and plays an important regulatory role in both thyroid hormone production and adjustments to basal metabolism. Other hormones are responsible for raising blood glucose, promoting nitrogen retention and increasing calcium absorption during pregnancy.

Blood volume increases in order to supply the placenta, which, as well as being the main source of the hormones regulating maternal metabolism, also provides the means by which nutrients and oxygen are transferred to the fetus and waste products are excreted. Since the increase in blood volume is approximately 35–40 per cent of the blood volume before pregnancy, it is not surprising that the concentration of some constituents (such as haemoglobin, total plasma protein and many vitamins and minerals) falls as the volume increases (Picciano 2003). This does not mean that the reduced concentration is a sign of deficiency, as the total amount of these constituents is not reduced. In fact, the total amounts circulating are frequently the same or higher.

PHYSIOLOGY OF LACTATION

Regardless of whether or not a woman breastfeeds, her breasts (mammary glands) are prepared for lactation by hormones secreted during pregnancy by the ovary and the placenta. The breasts are mainly composed of glandular and adipose tissues. The glandular component comprises between fifteen and twenty sections called lobes, which consist of alveoli, as seen in Figure 20.3.

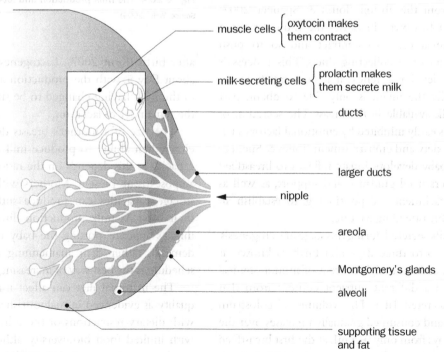

muscle cells { oxytocin makes them contract

milk-secreting cells { prolactin makes them secrete milk

ducts

larger ducts

nipple

areola

Montgomery's glands

alveoli

supporting tissue and fat

Figure 20.3: Anatomy of the breast
Source: WHO (2009)

During pregnancy, the alveoli increase in number and undergo other changes in preparation for milk production. This is known as mammogenesis. Three stages of lactogenesis occur as part of the lactation development process. Lactogenesis I, where the glands develop the ability to secrete milk components, occurs in the second trimester of pregnancy. Following birth, Lactogenesis II, or the onset of copious milk production, is triggered by changes in hormone levels such as drops in progesterone levels and an increase in prolactin levels (Jones & Spencer 2007). Putting the baby to the breast further stimulates prolactin secretion and increases milk production. This stage of lactogenesis usually occurs about 60 hours after the birth but can range from 24 to 102 hours, and is often called the 'coming in' of the milk supply (Kent 2007). If the baby is not breastfed, the prolactin level falls and milk secretion stops.

Suckling or expressing milk from the breast is also necessary to stimulate the production of the hormone oxytocin by the posterior part of the pituitary gland, which then allows the milk to be released from the alveoli (Jones & Spencer 2007) (Figure 20.4). Oxytocin causes the muscular tissue (myoepithelial cells) to contract and so to push the milk into the collecting ducts. This process is called the 'let-down' reflex; if it does not function satisfactorily, the infant is only able to obtain part of the milk available in the breast. The secretion of oxytocin is easily inhibited by emotional factors such as pain, anxiety and embarrassment (Jones & Spencer 2007). A baby develops innate reflexes to breastfeed but mothers need guidance and support, as well as correct attachment and positioning, to establish an exclusive breastfeeding routine.

The milk secreted during this stage of lactogenesis, the first two to three days after birth, is known as colostrum and has a high content of immunological factors and a different nutrient content from that of milk secreted later. The volume of colostrum produced and consumed gradually increases over the first few days from only 0–5 mL at the first breastfeed within 60 minutes of birth, to a total of 395–868 mL (over 5–10 breastfeeding sessions) at two to six days

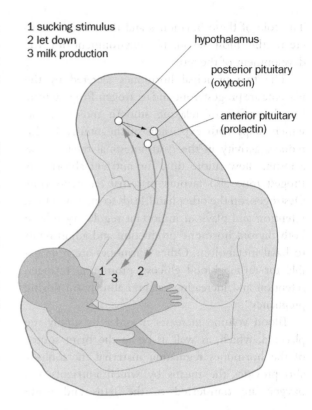

1 sucking stimulus
2 let down
3 milk production

hypothalamus

posterior pituitary (oxytocin)

anterior pituitary (prolactin)

Figure 20.4: The milk production and let-down reflex
Source: WHO (2009)

after birth (Kent 2007). Lactogenesis III begins by about Day 5, with the production and composition of the milk having changed to be similar to that for the remainder of lactation.

The size of a mother's breasts does not indicate either their ability to produce milk or their storage capacity, as this depends on the ratio of glandular to adipose tissue present. Mothers with large or small storage capacities can produce sufficient milk for their baby. As milk production directly reflects the infant's appetite, putting the baby to the breast on demand, rather than maintaining a rigid feeding schedule, is the best way of increasing the milk supply.

The maternal diet can affect milk quantity and quality, as evidenced in malnourished women, those with dietary restrictions or those living in locations with limited food biodiversity, although breastmilk can be remarkably nutrient-sufficient until around the sixth month of lactation (Dal Pont et al. 2016;

Jelliffe & Jelliffe 1978). Some traditional feeding practices may enhance lactation without loss of quality; for example, in Simalungun, North Sumatra, postpartum women consume a torbangun vegetable soup to increase milk supply (Damanik et al. 2006; Mortel & Mehta 2013).

WEIGHT GAIN DURING PREGNANCY

The mother's pre-pregnancy weight, rate of weight gain and total weight gained during pregnancy are key indicators of fetal development and likely pregnancy outcomes (Institute of Medicine 2009). Pregnancy weight gains within recommended ranges are associated with the most favourable outcomes for both mother and infant for women of different pre-pregnancy weights (Institute of Medicine 2009). An infant birthweight of 3–4 kg is associated with fewer problems and more favourable outcomes (Institute of Medicine 2009).

Being overweight or obese prior to pregnancy is associated with **pre-eclampsia**, **gestational diabetes** and caesarean delivery (Institute of Medicine 2009). International and Australian studies show maternal obesity is increasing in prevalence and is also associated with obstetric difficulties and increased costs and with negative neonatal outcomes such as macrosomia (an infant significantly larger than average), birth defects, prematurity, stillbirth and perinatal deaths (Aune et al. 2014; Godfrey et al. 2017; Santangeli et al. 2015). Large-size infants increase the risk of delivery complications, birth trauma and caesarean section, thus increasing the risk of complications and death of both mother and infant (Institute of Medicine 2009).

A BMI below the recommended range may lead to pre-term delivery and small-for-gestational-age babies (Institute of Medicine 2009; Lynch et al. 2014). Intra-uterine growth restriction has been associated with low maternal BMI but the amount of weight gained during the pregnancy and the effect of maternal micronutrient deficiencies also need to be considered (Grivell et al. 2009). Smaller size at birth has been associated with increased fetal and infant mortality, cerebral palsy, hypoglycaemia, hypocalcaemia and persistent deficits in both size and neurocognitive performance (Institute of Medicine 2009). There are also long-term outcomes for infants born to women with inadequate or excessive weight gains during pregnancy, including lifelong risk of obesity, metabolic dysregulation, increased insulin resistance, hypertension and dyslipidaemia (Herring et al. 2012). There are some indications that extremely inadequate weight gain during pregnancy is linked to the development of schizophrenia (Mackay et al. 2017).

Recommended amounts or ranges for weight gain over the term of the pregnancy vary depending on the initial weight of the mother prior to the pregnancy, with higher gains recommended for underweight women and lower gains (but at least 6.8 kg) for heavier women. The US Institute of Medicine guidelines (2009) are given in Table 20.2, with variation among individuals acknowledged by the use of ranges rather than specific weights. There is growing evidence that Asian cut-offs for overweight and obesity, that is, $23.0–24.9$ kg/m^2 for overweight and 25 kg/m^2 for obese, should be used to assess weight gain in these populations (Morisaki et al. 2017).

Table 20.2: Recommendations for total and rate of weight gain during pregnancy, by pre-pregnancy BMI

Pre-pregnancy BMI	BMI (kg/m²)	Total weight gain (kg)	Rates of weight gain* 2nd and 3rd trimester kg/week [range]
Underweight	<18.5	12.5–18	0.51 [0.44–0.58]
Normal weight	18.5–24.9	11.5–16	0.42 [0.35–0.50]
Overweight	25.0–29.9	7–11.5	0.28 [0.23–0.33]
Obese (all classes)	30.0	5–9	0.22 [0.17–0.27]

Source: Institute of Medicine (2009)

PREGNANCY WEIGHT GAIN

Mavis is a 22-year-old woman who had a pre-pregnancy BMI of 23 kg/m². She has just found out she is pregnant and is very conscious she does not want to gain too much weight. As a result, she begins to restrict her energy intake, limiting foods such as bread, pasta, dairy products and meat.

MAVIS'S WEIGHT:

Pre-pregnancy:	62 kg
Week 8:	63 kg
Week 12:	63.5 kg
Week 14:	64 kg
Week 18:	64.5 kg
Week 26:	66.5 kg

QUESTIONS

- Using the weight gain charts, is Mavis's weight gain adequate?
- How much weight should she have gained by Week 26?
- In terms of both weight gain and nutrients, what are the risks of restricting dietary intake in the short and long term?

The pattern of weight gain is most commonly described as sigmoidal, with body weight increasing very slowly at first—with gains of only 1–2 kg in the first trimester (three months)—and much more rapidly later (Hytten 1991); again, this can vary between individuals (Institute of Medicine 2009). Components of maternal weight gain include the products of conception (fetus, placenta, amniotic fluid), maternal tissues (uterus, breasts, blood), extravascular fluid and maternal fat stores, as shown in Figure 20.5.

In recognition of this variation, pregnancy weight gain charts have been developed and are increasingly used in clinical practice (Figure 20.6, see colour section). Given the importance of gestational weight gain for short- and long-term health outcomes, the value of regular weight-gain monitoring and follow-up as part of standard antenatal care is now recognised. There are charts for women with BMIs <25 kg/m² and ≥25 kg/m², and for women carrying twins.

FOOD AND NUTRIENT NEEDS

Based on data from doubly labelled water studies (see Chapter 13), the gold standard for body composition, the size of maternal pre-pregnancy energy stores appears to be a major determinant of the overall metabolic response to pregnancy and lactation. Thin or marginally nourished women appear to have the ability to conserve energy during pregnancy, while better-nourished women appear not to do so (Prentice & Goldberg 2000). Although the adaptation appears to be of benefit and allows the survival of the fetus despite low energy intakes by the mother, the long-term risks associated with developing in these sub-optimal nutritional and physiologic conditions are of concern, especially with the increasing evidence supporting the importance of fetal programming and critical periods (Prentice & Goldberg 2000).

The current Australian recommendation for pregnant women is for an additional dietary energy intake of 1.4 MJ and 1.9 MJ per day during the second and third trimesters respectively (NHMRC 2006). It is not possible to predict the energy requirements of individual women reliably and there is significant variation between women; therefore, it is unrealistic to establish a single value for the additional energy requirements of pregnancy (Institute of Medicine 2009; NHMRC 2006). Adequate weight gain should be used as an indicator of adequate energy intake, with requirements varying depending on pre-pregnancy weight. Later in pregnancy, appetite and energy intake will be influenced both by maternal energy stores and by the level of activity that is maintained. Unless weight gain is excessive, appetite

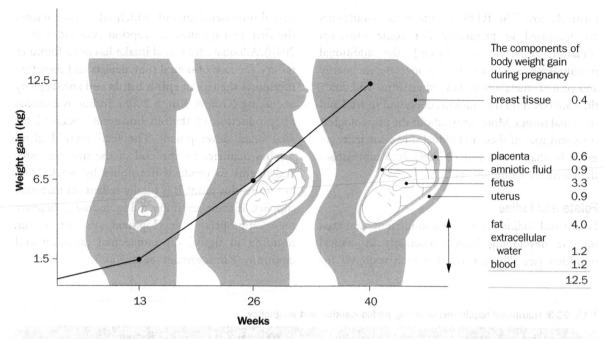

The components of
body weight gain
during pregnancy

breast tissue	0.4
placenta	0.6
amniotic fluid	0.9
fetus	3.3
uterus	0.9
fat	4.0
extracellular water	1.2
blood	1.2
	12.5

Weight gain (kg)

12.5

6.5

1.5

13   26   40

Weeks

Figure 20.5: Weight gain in pregnancy

is the best guide to an adequate level of energy intake. A varied diet is more likely to ensure that nutrient needs are met.

Current estimates for energy requirement in lactation are for an additional 2.0–2.1 MJ per day assuming full breastfeeding to six months and partial feeding thereafter (NHMRC 2006). This is an average figure, as individual energy needs for lactation vary considerably depending on individual metabolism, stage of lactation and extent of weaning, weight loss occurring and physical activity level (Butte & King 2005). This figure assumes milk production of 0.78 L/day, an energy content of milk of 2.8 kJ/g, 80 per cent efficiency and an assumed weight loss equivalent to 720 kJ per day in the mother in the first few months of lactation, with no change in physical activity level and milk production of an average 0.60 L/day in the second six months (NHMRC 2006). Weight loss during lactation is usually in the first three to six months, and is greater in those who are exclusively breastfeeding (Butte and King 2005). Excessive energy restriction during lactation in order to lose weight gained during pregnancy is not recommended, although overweight or obese

women are advised to consume a healthy intake that is nutrient-dense and not to increase their energy intake to compensate for the milk production.

During the period of fetal growth, considerable amounts of nutrients are needed, both to grow fetal tissues and to provide stores of energy and iron for the immediate postnatal period. In a normal pregnancy, these nutrients are obtained both from the mother's diet and from her own stores. The metabolic adjustments that occur during pregnancy tend to increase both absorption and storage of a number of nutrients from early in pregnancy in readiness to meet later fetal demands. In this way, the contribution of the maternal diet to the nutrients required for pregnancy is effectively spread throughout the whole of the pregnancy and not concentrated in the last trimester, when fetal demands for a number of nutrients are high.

Many nutrients, such as amino acids, water-soluble vitamins (but not fat-soluble vitamins) and minerals (see chapters 10, 16 and 17), are found at higher levels in the fetal circulation. The ability to concentrate these nutrients enables the fetus to obtain the nutrients even when maternal levels are relatively low. The RDIs for many micronutrients are increased in pregnancy. For some nutrients (thiamin, riboflavin and niacin), the additional requirements are linked to the increase in energy and protein metabolism. For others (iron and zinc), they are based on the amounts deposited in fetal and maternal tissues. More details about the physiological basis and role of these individual micronutrients are given in chapters 16 and 17. Table 20.3 summarises the increased requirements.

Folate and iodine

Folate and iodine are two micronutrients essential for the developing fetus, particularly at critical windows (see Chapter 16). Folate is required for neural tube development, which takes place within the first 28 days after conception (van Gool et al. 2018). Adequate folic acid intake has been found to reduce the risk of neural tube defects and therefore minimises the risk of **spina bifida** and anencephaly occurring (Goh & Koren 2008). Iodine is essential for production of thyroid hormones, essential for fetal brain development. The fetal thyroid gland reaches maturity by the end of the first trimester and begins to produce hormones by week 16—but up to this point it is totally reliant on maternal supplies. If these are impacted by iodine deficiency then appropriate development cannot occur, resulting in significant intellectual disability and cretinism (Zimmermann et al. 2008).

Table 20.3: Nutritional requirements during periconception and pregnancy

Periconception Trimester 1	Trimester 2	Trimester 3	Lactation
Energy requirements unchanged	Additional 1.4 MJ	Additional 1.9 MJ	Additional 2.0–2.1 MJ
Protein 0.8 g/kg/day or about 60 g	An additional 0.2 g/kg/day but really no change as most women in Australia consume more than 0.8 g/kg/day.		0.88–1.1 g/kg/day No change as most women in Australia consume more than 0.8 g/kg/day.
DHA requirements unchanged	DHA consumption increased to promote fetal nervous system and brain development. Consider fish safety.		DHA requirements increase again during lactation.
Folate requirements increased; consume supplement with a minimum of 400 mg of folate plus folic acid rich and folate fortified foods.			Folate requirements slightly increased; increase should be achievable through dietary changes.
Calcium requirements unchanged	Calcium requirements unchanged as absorption increased. However, women with low calcium intakes should consider increasing as there may be skeletal benefits in the newborn. Calcium supplementation for pre-eclampsia.		Calcium requirements unchanged as absorption increased.
Iron requirements unchanged	Iron requirements increased. Iron deficiency anaemia during pregnancy associated with pre-term delivery, low birthweight, delays in the development of the central nervous system. Requirements may not be met by diet and supplements may be needed.		Iron requirements decreased as assumed menstruation does not recommence until six months after exclusive breastfeeding is discontinued.
Iodine requirements increased; consume supplement of at least 150 mg daily.			Iodine requirements increase again during breastfeeding; consume supplement of at least 150 mg daily.

Strategies to improve the folate and iodine intake of females of childbearing age have included education and promotion programs, supplementation and fortification. As many pregnancies are unplanned, and the neural tube and other central nervous system elements develop before many women know they are pregnant, fortification and promotion programs to encourage an increased intake by the population have been determined to be the strategy most likely to be effective. Supplementation in Australia is an individual responsibility and there have been limited education campaigns calling for increased consumption or supplementation. As a result, the population is almost entirely reliant on fortification programs (see chapters 16 and 17).

In Australia, there is mandatory fortification of folic acid and iodine. Folic acid is added to bread-making flour, while iodine is added to salt used in breadmaking. Results from the Australian Health Survey indicate that less than 1 per cent of women aged 16–44 in 2011–12 had a red cell folate concentration less than 906 nmol/L, indicative of increased risk of neural tube defects (ABS 2013). For iodine, however, one in five women aged 16–44 had a urinary iodine concentration less than 50 mg/L, indicative of moderate deficiency (ABS 2013).

During lactation, iodine requirements increase again to replace the iodine lost through breastmilk and to ensure adequate iodine is consumed by the breastfeeding infant. For women with lower intakes of iodine, it appears that the iodine is preferentially funnelled into breastmilk, ensuring that the infant receives a steady supply (Dold et al. 2017). The RDI for folate during lactation (500 mg) is less than during pregnancy (600 mg) but more than when not lactating (400 mg).

Iron

Iron-absorption rates during pregnancy are thought to be dependent on the maternal iron status (for more general information on iron, see Chapter 17). As iron stores are depleted during pregnancy, serum ferritin levels fall and iron absorption rates increase (Fisher & Nemeth 2017). The regulation of iron availability in pregnancy is dependent, in part, on maternal **hepcidin** concentrations. Hepcidin is a hormone that affects iron absorption. When iron is abundant, hepcidin is produced, switching off dietary absorption in the duodenum as well as the release of recycled iron from **macrophages** and of stored iron from the liver. When iron is deficient, little or no hepcidin is produced (Ganz & Nemeth 2012). Hepcidin levels are decreased during the second and third trimesters allowing increased circulation of iron and transfer to the fetus (Fisher & Nemeth 2017). Barrett et al. (1994) found iron absorption increased from an average of 7 per cent at twelve weeks to 36 per cent at 24 weeks and 66 per cent at 36 weeks of gestation in subjects with normal iron status at the outset of pregnancy.

Of concern, however, is that many women do not have normal iron status at the outset of pregnancy; this can compromise neonatal iron stores and early development of the brain (Radlowski & Johnson 2013). Iron supplementation at variable levels has become routine practice in many countries to minimise the risk of deficiency and its consequences and has been effective in reducing maternal iron deficiency anaemia (Peña-Rosas et al. 2012). It should

WHICH WOMEN ARE MOST AT RISK OF FOLATE AND IODINE DEFICIENCY?

Folate and iodine intakes are determined by a range of factors including the types of foods consumed due to cultural background, foods avoided due to medical conditions, trends in food consumption and where you live (in the case of iodine). Exploring what you know about the fortification program and investigating trends in food consumption, provide a description of which groups in Australia and New Zealand are at highest risk of folate and iodine deficiency.

be noted that the RDI for iron during lactation falls to nine milligrams, the same as for post-menopausal women or girls prior to puberty, since menstruation usually ceases during lactation and hence no increased iron requirements exist (NHMRC 2006).

Other nutrients

Low maternal vitamin D in pregnancy may be associated with increased risk of pre-eclampsia, gestational diabetes, preterm birth and small-for-gestational-age babies (Wei et al. 2013). Women most at risk of vitamin D deficiency are those who are dark-skinned and who remain covered or indoors for cultural reasons (Munns et al. 2006).

DIETARY INTAKES AND RECOMMENDATIONS IN PREGNANCY AND LACTATION

If a healthy, well-nourished woman is consuming an adequate and varied diet before pregnancy, little adjustment is required during pregnancy. The poorer the mother's nutritional status prior to pregnancy, the greater the importance of the diet during pregnancy. Despite the significance of dietary intake on maternal and infant outcomes, concern exists as to the quality of diets of many women in Australia during and prior to pregnancy, with many appearing not to meet the current recommendations (Malek et al. 2016). Current food recommendations during

pregnancy and lactation, according to the Australian Guide to Healthy Eating, are presented in Table 20.4.

Breastfeeding mothers are advised to eat whatever nutritious foods they choose. Some infants seem to become uncomfortable and may be sensitive to certain foods, such as onions or garlic. If a particular food appears to be causing discomfort to the infant, the mother is advised to remove that food from her diet for a few days and see whether symptoms go away. Care should be taken, however, that the mother's diet does not become unnecessarily restricted.

COMMON CONCERNS IN PREGNANCY AND LACTATION

Pregnant and breastfeeding women are usually concerned about the foods and beverages they consume and how they can safely minimise the effects of pregnancy. Some of the most frequently asked questions relate to alcohol consumption, morning sickness, indigestion, constipation, dieting, tea and coffee consumption, artificial sweeteners, food safety and vegetarianism.

Alcohol intake

I am going to a wedding next week and I am 16 weeks pregnant, one glass of wine won't hurt, will it?
Drinking alcohol is not recommended during pregnancy, as noted in the background material prepared for the development of the 2009 Australian Guidelines

Table 20.4: Current food recommendations for pregnancy and lactation in Australia

	Vegetables[1] (serves)	Fruit[2] (serves)	Grains[3] (serves)	Meat/Alternative[4] (serves)	Dairy[5] (serves)
Pregnant up to age 18	5	2	8	3.5	3.5
Pregnant over age 18	5	2	9	2.5	2.5
Lactating up to age 18	5.5	2	8.5	3.5	2.5
Lactating over age 18	7/5	2	9	2.5	4

Notes: A serve is equivalent to:
1. ½ cup cooked vegetables; 1 cup raw leafy green vegetables; ½ cup legumes or beans; ½ medium potato
2. 1 medium piece of fruit; ½ cup 100% fruit juice
3. 1 slice bread; ½ bread roll; ½ cup cooked pasta/rice; 3 crispbreads; ¼ cup of flour
4. 65 g cooked lean meat; 80 g cooked poultry; 100 g fish; 2 large eggs; 1 cup lentils, legumes; 175 g tofu
5. 1 cup milk; 1 200-g carton of yoghurt; 40 g cheese.

Source: Australian Department of Health and Ageing (2013)

to Reduce Health Risk from Drinking Alcohol (NHMRC 2009) (see Chapter 15). Exposure of the fetus to alcohol may result in a broad spectrum of effects grouped together as Fetal Alcohol Spectrum Disorder.

Limited research exists to support definitive advice on recommended intakes of alcohol while breastfeeding, but the consumption of two standard drinks or more per day during lactation has been associated with:

- decreased lactation performance (in terms of the milk ejection reflex, milk production by the mother and milk consumption by the baby)
- earlier cessation of breastfeeding
- deficits in infant psychomotor development
- disrupted infant sleep–wake behavioural patterns
- deficits in infant and child cognitive function (Gibson & Porter 2018; Giglia & Binns 2006).

I drank a glass of wine every night and then I found out that I was pregnant. Have I harmed my baby?

Small amounts of alcohol consumed before pregnancy is known to represent a small risk. Once pregnancy is known, however, the safest option is to stop drinking alcohol completely.

Morning sickness

I have just found out I am pregnant and I am nauseous all day and I vomit some of my meals. I am worried that I am not eating enough for the baby.

During the first trimester, probably the major influence on diet will be the extent to which 'morning sickness' occurs. It is thought to be caused by changes in hormones during pregnancy (Wylde et al. 2016) and may make eating difficult. Although it is called 'morning sickness', nausea (with or without vomiting) can happen at any time of the day and may last all day in some pregnant women. Generally, 'morning sickness' goes away after about twelve to thirteen weeks gestation, but it may continue for longer and even up until birth in some women.

To manage the symptoms of 'morning sickness', small and frequent meals, which consist chiefly of easily digested foods such as carbohydrates, are usually suggested. Other common suggestions include:

- Eat smaller meals more often. Missing meals can make nausea worse.
- Avoid large drinks. Have frequent small drinks between meals.
- Separate liquid and solid foods.
- Limit fatty, spicy and fried foods.
- Food has a stronger odour or smell when it is heated, which may make nausea worse. If possible, have other people help with cooking, or prepare your food at times of the day when you feel better.
- Try eating a dry biscuit before getting out of bed in the morning.
- Eat a healthy snack before going to bed at night. This might include fruit (fresh, canned, dried), crackers with hard cheese or yoghurt.
- Avoid foods if their taste, smell or appearance makes you feel sick.
- If vomiting, it is important to drink enough fluids. It may be easier to have lots of small drinks than to try to drink a large amount in one go. Try a variety of fluids such as water, fruit juice, lemonade and clear soups. Sometimes it can be helpful to try crushed ice, slushies, ice blocks, or even suck on frozen fruit such as grapes or orange segments. Note that the stomach acids in vomiting can soften teeth enamel. It is best not to use a toothbrush to clean the teeth straight after vomiting as this may damage them. (Brown 2008)

Some evidence supports the use of ginger and vitamin B-6 as a safe and effective treatment option for nausea and vomiting during pregnancy, with its use being recommended by midwives as a non-medication treatment (Sharifzadeh et al. 2018).

Severe vomiting, if prolonged, can result in electrolyte imbalance, dehydration and malnutrition, a condition called hyperemesis gravidarum. This requires close monitoring and ongoing care.

Indigestion and constipation

I am in my last three months of pregnancy and I am not eating very well. I seem to have either indigestion or constipation and this is reducing my appetite.

The later stages of pregnancy are often accompanied by indigestion and a tendency to constipation due to relaxation of gastrointestinal muscles and also to the pressure of the growing baby on the mother's internal organs (Brown 2008). Indigestion is best dealt with by:

- avoiding foods that trigger it
- maintaining a pattern of small, frequent meals and snacks
- separating drinking from eating
- limiting high-fat foods and highly spiced foods.

The tendency to constipation, which is often accentuated by consumption of iron supplements, can be assisted by a diet that contains plenty of fluid and fibre-rich foods (fruit, vegetables and wholegrain cereals). Laxatives are not recommended during pregnancy, but other suggestions to increase fibre and fluid are similar to those for the rest of the population.

Dieting

I don't want to gain too much weight while I am pregnant so I think I might go on a diet.

Dieting during pregnancy should be avoided. As noted earlier, appropriate weight gain for optimal pregnancy outcomes is dependent on pre-pregnancy weight. Obese or overweight women should preferably achieve a healthy weight prior to pregnancy to minimise risk of excess weight gain in pregnancy and future obesity. If this is not possible, excessive weight gain during the pregnancy should be avoided and weight loss strategies postponed until after the baby's birth.

Caffeine intake

I enjoy my cup of espresso every morning; do I need to give this up now I am pregnant?

Consumption of caffeine has been linked to delayed conception, spontaneous miscarriages, fetal growth restriction and low birthweight, but not birth defects (Temple et al. 2017). Approximately three cups of coffee a day (>350 mg caffeine) was associated with a 60 per cent increase in low birthweight (Chen et al. 2014).

Energy drinks are not recommended during pregnancy as they may contain high levels of caffeine and other ingredients not recommended for pregnant women. As with alcohol, avoidance of caffeine during pregnancy clearly minimises any possible risk from this source (see Table 20.5 for current levels of caffeine).

Intake of teas

I enjoy herbal teas before I go to bed but will any of these pose a risk to my baby?

Conflicting evidence exists as to the risks or benefits associated with the consumption of various teas during pregnancy. As with caffeine, minimal intake appears to be the most prudent advice until more research is able to establish safety and efficacy of the range of teas, such as raspberry leaf, currently available (Holst et al. 2009). There is some evidence to indicate that raspberry leaf tea should only be consumed in the last trimester due to its effects on the uterus (Holst et al. 2009).

Artificial sweeteners

I have been trying to reduce my consumption of sugar, so I now use artificial sweeteners and eat foods and drinks containing these—do I need to stop doing this now I am pregnant?

There is increased controversy regarding the use of artificial sweeteners and their efficacy in reducing weight gain and improving glycaemic control. There is limited but emerging evidence that the use of non-nutritive sweeteners (particularly aspartame) during pregnancy may contribute to obesity and chronic

Table 20.5: Caffeine content of some foods

Food	Caffeine content
Espresso	145 mg/50 mL cup
Formulated caffeinated beverages or 'energy' drinks	80 mg/250 mL can
Instant coffee (1 teaspoon/cup)	80 mg/250 mL cup
Black tea	50 mg/250 mL cup
Cola	50 mg/375 mL can
Milk chocolate	10 mg/50 g bar

Source: FSANZ (2018a)

conditions in children later in life (Reid et al. 2016). This is thought to be due to changes in the gut microbiota, increases in intestinal glucose absorption and appetite dysregulation (Araújo et al. 2014). Women during pregnancy should be encouraged to limit their consumption of artificial sweeteners. Women with **phenylketonuria** should avoid sweeteners containing aspartame; and those with high sorbitol content can cause diarrhoea if consumed in large amounts.

Food safety

Are there any foods that are unsafe for me to consume while I am pregnant?

Contaminated foods causing food poisoning in pregnant women can be debilitating and dangerous, mostly due to the dehydration that results. Taking special care to follow correct hygiene practices and avoid foods at risk of being contaminated is strongly recommended. One particular foodborne bacterium of special concern during pregnancy is *Listeria monocytogenes*. Pregnant women are about eighteen times more likely than other healthy adults to get listeriosis and account for 35 per cent of all cases of listeriosis (Madjunkov et al. 2017). The consequences of listeriosis for the mother are relatively mild, with mostly only flu-like or general non-specific symptoms, making diagnosis difficult (Madjunkov et al. 2017). For infants, listeriosis in the first trimester is more likely to result in miscarriage (65 per cent risk); in the second and third trimesters there is a 26 per cent risk of stillbirth, miscarriage or fetal death and a 10–15 per cent chance of premature labour (Madjunkov et al. 2017).

To prevent listeriosis, care with particular foods is recommended, together with standard food safety precautions such as personal hygiene, and appropriate food handling and storage practices, to minimise the risk of food contamination (Buchanan et al. 2017). As certain foods pose particular risk of contamination, and as *L. monocytogenes* can continue to multiply in food at refrigerator temperatures and survive freezing, guidelines have been developed by FSANZ as provided in Table 20.6 (FSANZ 2018b). The advice for women who are pregnant and eating out is to only buy ready-to-eat food that is steaming hot, and to only order hot meals that are cooked to order and served hot.

Another dietary contaminant of particular concern during pregnancy is mercury. This heavy metal contaminant can cross the placenta and have severe negative effects on the developing brain and nervous system. Mercury content of larger fish, if consumed in large quantities, can be of concern. As fish consumption is often recommended due to its n-3 fatty acid content, women who may become pregnant, pregnant or lactating women, and children up to the age of twelve are advised by FSANZ (2011) to consume the following:

- two to three serves* per week of any fish and seafood not specified in the following serve options, or
- one serve per week of orange roughy (deep sea perch) or catfish and no other fish that week, or
- one serve per fortnight of shark (flake) or billfish (swordfish/broadbill and marlin) and no other fish that fortnight.

* A serve for an adult woman and a child over the age of six years is 150 g and for a child up to six years it is 75 g.

Can I keep eating a vegetarian diet while I am pregnant?

Vegetarian diets can be adequate for pregnancy requirements if care is taken with food selection and consumption. Certain nutrients have been identified as being at risk of inadequate intake, such as vitamins B-12 and D, calcium, zinc, n-3 fatty acids and riboflavin. Vegan mothers will need vitamin B-12 supplementation throughout pregnancy in sufficient amounts to ensure adequate supplies for themselves and their child (NHMRC 2006). If breastfeeding, women following vegan or vegetarian diets need to take care with their food selection to ensure adequate nutrient intakes.

Table 20.6: Higher risk vs safer food options in relation to *Listeria* contamination

Food type	Examples	Safer alternatives
Cold meats	Cold meats from delicatessen counters and sandwich bars, and packaged, sliced ready-to-eat meats.	Home-cooked, stored in the fridge and used within a day of cooking. If it is going to be longer than 24 hours, freeze until ready to use.
Cold, cooked chicken	Cold cooked ready-to-eat chicken (whole, portions, or diced).	Home-cooked. Ensure chicken is cooked thoroughly, use immediately. Store leftovers in the fridge and use within a day; if it is going to be longer, freeze. Hot takeaway cooked chicken. Eat immediately, store any leftovers in fridge and eat within a day of purchase. Reheat until steaming hot.
Paté	Refrigerated paté or meat spreads.	Paté from non-meat sources such as mushrooms.
Salads (fruit and vegetables)	Pre-prepared or pre-packaged fruit or vegetables as well as salads, including those from supermarkets, buffets and salad bars.	Freshly prepared homemade salads. Wash all vegetables and fruits thoroughly. Store any leftover prepared vegetables and fruits in the fridge, use within a day of preparation.
Chilled seafood	Chilled seafood such as raw oysters, sashimi and sushi, smoked ready-to-eat seafood and cooked ready-to-eat prawns.	All freshly cooked seafood. Use immediately, store leftovers in fridge and use within a day of cooking.
Cheese	Soft, semi-soft and surface-ripened cheeses such as brie, camembert, ricotta, blue and feta.	Hard cheese (e.g. cheddar, gouda, edam); processed cheese, cheese spreads, plain cream cheese, plain cottage cheese. Store in fridge. Purchase cheeses packaged by the manufacturer and within their use-by dates.
Ice cream	Soft serve.	Packaged frozen ice cream, that has been maintained as frozen (that is, has not melted or previously melted).
Other dairy products	Unpasteurised dairy products (e.g. raw milk).	Pasteurised dairy products (e.g. pasteurised milk, yoghurt, custard, dairy dessert).

Source: FSANZ (2018b)

SUMMARY

- Just prior to pregnancy and during pregnancy is a critical window for the future health and functioning of women and children.
- The life-course framework identifies this period as instrumental in 'programming' genetic material impacting on health and disease in later life. Social, environmental and nutritional factors combine to influence health across the lifespan.
- Pregnancy and lactation are normal physiological processes and a successful outcome is the rule rather than the exception, provided that maternal health and nutritional status are good at the outset of pregnancy.
- Weight status prior to pregnancy, rate of weight gain during pregnancy and total amount gained during pregnancy (including inadequate and excessive weight gains) are key indicators of fetal development and pregnancy outcomes.

- Nutritional status and dietary intake of the mother prior to and during pregnancy can affect critical development stages of the infant, which can have both short- and long-term health consequences.
- Increased nutritional requirements during pregnancy and lactation can often be met without major changes in food intake.
- As the nutritional status and dietary intakes of women of reproductive age do not appear to be optimal prior to or during pregnancy, mandatory fortification of foods with folate and iodine has been undertaken as a public health strategy. In some cases, supplementation with other nutrients may be required.
- Provision of appropriate advice and support to help pregnant and lactating women manage common challenges and areas of concern is essential to optimise dietary intake and nutritional status.

KEY TERMS

Gestational diabetes: the diabetes that occurs during pregnancy. Having gestational diabetes is a risk factor for developing type 2 diabetes later in life. About 12–14 per cent of women will develop diabetes during pregnancy and all women should be tested at 24–28 weeks of pregnancy. Pregnancy hormones increase insulin resistance; in other words, the hormones block the action of insulin and so about two to three times more insulin is required. Some women are not able to cope with the additional requirements for insulin, resulting in an increase in blood glucose concentrations.

Hepcidin: identified as the key iron regulation hormone, hepcidin regulates intestinal iron absorption, plasma iron concentrations, and tissue iron distribution by inducing degradation of its receptor, the cellular iron exporter ferroportin.

Macrophage: a type of white blood cell which is a part of the immune system that ingests foreign material.

Phenylketonuria (PKU): an inborn error of metabolism that leads to decreased metabolism of the amino acid phenylalanine. Untreated PKU can lead to intellectual disability, seizures and mental health issues. Treatment is a diet low in phenylalanine and supplements. All newborns are screened for PKU through the blood spot test.

Pre-eclampsia: occurs in the second half of pregnancy or just after birth. The signs of pre-eclampsia are high blood pressure (hypertension), protein in the urine and swelling of the face, hands and feet. Pre-eclampsia affects one in ten pregnancies and can cause circulation issues, limiting the supply of oxygen and nutrients to the baby.

Spina bifida: refers to a range of birth defects (called neural tube defects) that affect the spinal cord. Spina bifida is Latin for 'split spine' and is an abnormality in the growing embryo which means that the vertebral column does not form properly. As a result, the nerves and spinal cord are exposed and can be easily damaged. This means that the nerves supplying the lower half of the body do not function properly, resulting in motor and sensory issues including bowel and bladder control.

ACKNOWLEDGEMENT

This chapter has been modified and updated from previous versions in earlier editions of *Food and Nutrition*. Thank you to Ingrid H.E. Rutishauser, Kelly Stewart, Jan Payne and Sue Ash for their contributions.

REFERENCES

ABS, 2013, *Australian Health Survey: Biomedical Results for Chronic Diseases, 2011–12,* <www.abs.gov.au/AUSSTATS/abs@.nsf/0/D31F2F311CA9936ACA257BBB00121DB8?Opendocument>, accessed 20 June 2018

Araújo, J.R., Martel, F. & Keating, E., 2014, 'Exposure to non-nutritive sweeteners during pregnancy and lactation: Impact in programming of metabolic diseases in the progeny later in life', *Reproductive Toxicology, 49*: 196–201, doi:10.1016/j.reprotox.2014.09.007

Aune, D., Saugstad, O.D., Henriksen, T. & Tonstad, S., 2014, 'Maternal body mass index and the risk of fetal death, stillbirth, and infant death: A systematic review and meta-analysis', *JAMA, 311*(15): 1536–46, doi:10.1001/jama.2014.2269

Australian Department of Health and Ageing, 2013, *Australian Guide to Healthy Eating,* <www.eatforhealth.gov.au/guidelines/australian-guide-healthy-eating>, accessed 28 November 2018

Barker, D.J.P., 2004, 'The developmental origins of chronic adult disease', *Acta Pædiatrica, 93*: 26–33, doi:10.1111/j.1651-2227.2004.tb00236.x

Barrett, J.F., Whittaker, P.G., Williams, J.G. & Lind, T., 1994, 'Absorption of non-haem iron from food during normal pregnancy', *BMJ, 309*(6947): 79–82, doi:10.1136/bmj.309.6947.79

Brown, J.E., 2008, *Nutrition Through the Life Cycle,* Belmont, CA: Thomas Wadsworth

Buchanan, R.L., Gorris, L.G.M., Hayman, M.M., Jackson, T.C. & Whiting, R.C., 2017, 'A review of *Listeria monocytogenes*: An update on outbreaks, virulence, dose-response, ecology, and risk assessments', *Food Control, 75*: 1–13, doi:10.1016/j.foodcont.2016.12.016

Butte, N.F. & King, J.C., 2005, 'Energy requirements during pregnancy and lactation', *Public Health Nutrition, 8*(7a): 1010–27, doi:10.1079/PHN2005793

Chen, L., Bell, E.M., Browne, M.L., Druschel, C.M. & Romitti, P.A., 2014, 'Exploring maternal patterns of dietary caffeine consumption before conception and during pregnancy', *Maternal and Child Health Journal, 18*(10): 2446–55, doi:10.1007/s10995-014-1483-2

Dal Pont, A., Ferraroni, M., Bravi, F., Decarli, A., Agostoni, C. & Wiens, F., 2016, 'Impact of maternal nutrition on breast-milk composition: A systematic review', *American Journal of Clinical Nutrition, 104*(3): 646–62, doi:10.3945/ajcn.115.120881

Damanik, R., Wahlqvist, M.L. & Wattanapenpaiboon, N., 2006, 'Lactagogue effects of Torbangun, a Bataknese traditional cuisine', *Asia Pacific Journal of Clinical Nutrition, 15*(2): 267–73, <http://211.76.170.15/server/MarkWpapers/Papers/Papers 2006/Rizal.pdf>, accessed 17 July 2019

Dold, S., Zimmermann, M.B., Aboussad, A., Cherkaoui, M., Jia, Q. et al., 2017, 'Breast milk iodine concentration is a more accurate biomarker of iodine status than urinary iodine concentration in exclusively breastfeeding women', *Journal of Nutrition, 147*(4): 528–37, doi:10.3945/jn.116.242560

Fisher, A.L. & Nemeth, E., 2017, 'Iron homeostasis during pregnancy', *American Journal of Clinical Nutrition, 106*(Suppl. 6): 1567S–74S, doi:10.3945/ajcn.117.155812

Fontana, R. & Torre, S.D., 2016, 'The deep correlation between energy metabolism and reproduction: A view on the effects of nutrition for women fertility', *Nutrients, 8*(2): 87, doi:10.3390/nu8020087

FSANZ, 2011, *FSANZ Advice on Fish Consumption,* <www.foodstandards.gov.au/consumer/chemicals/mercury/documents/mif%20brochure.pdf>, accessed 29 November 2018

—— 2018a, *Caffeine,* <www.foodstandards.gov.au/consumer/generalissues/Pages/Caffeine.aspx>, accessed 29 November 2018

—— 2018b, *Listeria,* <www.foodstandards.gov.au/consumer/safety/listeria/Pages/default.aspx>, accessed 29 November 2018

Ganz, T. & Nemeth, E., 2012, 'Hepcidin and iron homeostasis', *Biochimica et Biophysica Acta (BBA)—Molecular Cell Research, 1823*(9): 1434–43, doi:10.1016/j.bbamcr.2012.01.014

Gaskins, A.J., Toth, T.L. & Chavarro, J.E., 2015, 'Prepregnancy nutrition and early pregnancy outcomes', *Current Nutrition Reports, 4*(3): 265–72, doi:10.1007/s13668-015-0127-5

Giahi, L., Mohammadmoradi, S., Javidan, A. & Sadeghi, M.R., 2015, 'Nutritional modifications in male infertility: A systematic review covering 2 decades', *Nutrition Reviews, 74*(2): 118–30, doi:10.1093/nutrit/nuv059

—— 2016, 'Nutritional modifications in male infertility: A systematic review covering 2 decades', *Nutrition Reviews, 74*(2): 118–30, doi:10.1093/nutrit/nuv059

Gibson, L. & Porter, M., 2018, 'Drinking or smoking while breastfeeding and later cognition in children', *Pediatrics, 142*(2): e20174266, doi:10.1542/peds.2017-4266

Giglia, R. & Binns, C., 2006, 'Alcohol and lactation: A systematic review', *Nutrition & Dietetics, 63*(2): 103–16, doi:10.1111/j.1747-0080.2006.00056.x

Godfrey, K.M., Reynolds, R.M., Prescott, S.L., Nyirenda, M., Jaddoe, V.W. et al., 2017, 'Influence of maternal obesity on the long-term health of offspring', *The Lancet Diabetes & Endocrinology, 5*(1): 53–64, doi:10.1016/S2213-8587(16)30107-3

Goh, Y. & Koren, G., 2008, 'Folic acid in pregnancy and fetal outcomes', *Journal of Obstetrics and Gynaecology, 28*(1): 3–13, doi:10.1080/01443610701814195

Grivell, R., Dodd, J. & Robinson, J., 2009, 'The prevention and treatment of intrauterine growth restriction', *Best Practice & Research Clinical Obstetrics & Gynaecology, 23*(6): 795–807, doi:10.1016/j.bpobgyn.2009.06.004

Herring, S.J., Rose, M.Z., Skouteris, H. & Oken, E., 2012, 'Optimizing weight gain in pregnancy to prevent obesity in women and children', *Diabetes, Obesity and Metabolism, 14*(3): 195–203, doi:10.1111/j.1463-1326.2011.01489.x

Holst, L., Haavik, S. & Nordeng, H., 2009, 'Raspberry leaf—should it be recommended to pregnant women?', *Complementary Therapies in Clinical Practice, 15*(4): 204–8, doi:10.1016/j.ctcp.2009.05.003

Hytten, F.E., 1991, 'Weight gain in pregnancy', in F.E. Hytten & G. Chamberlain (eds), *Clinical Physiology in Obstetrics,* London: Blackwell Scientific, pp. 173–203

Institute of Medicine, 2009, *Nutrition During Pregnancy—Part I, Weight Gain,* <www.ncbi.nlm.nih.gov/books/NBK32813/pdf/Bookshelf_NBK32813.pdf>, accessed 22 November 2018

Jelliffe, D.B. & Jelliffe, E.P., 1978, 'The volume and composition of human milk in poorly nourished communities: A review', *American Journal of Clinical Nutrition, 31*(3): 492–515, doi:10.1093/ajcn/31.3.492

Jensen, T.K., Andersson, A.-M., Jørgensen, N., Andersen, A.-G., Carlsen, E. et al., 2004, 'Body mass index in relation to semen quality and reproductive hormones among 1,558 Danish men', *Fertility and Sterility, 82*(4): 863–70, doi:10.1016/j.fertnstert.2004.03.056

Jones, E. & Spencer, S., 2007, 'The physiology of lactation', *Paediatrics and Child Health, 17*(6): 244–8, doi:10.1016/j.paed.2007.03.001

Kent, J.C., 2007, 'How breastfeeding works', *Journal of Midwifery & Women's Health, 52*(6): 564–70, doi:10.1016/j.jmwh.2007.04.007

Lane, M., Zander-Fox, D.L., Robker, R.L. & McPherson, N.O., 2015, 'Peri-conception parental obesity, reproductive health, and transgenerational impacts', *Trends in Endocrinology & Metabolism, 26*(2): 84–90, doi:10.1016/j.tem.2014.11.005

Lu, P., Zhang, C.-H., Lifshitz, L.M. & ZhuGe, R., 2017, 'Extraoral bitter taste receptors in health and disease', *Journal of General Physiology, 149*(2): 181–97, doi:10.1085/jgp.201611637

Lynch, A.M., Hart, J.E., Agwu, O.C., Fisher, B.M., West, N.A. & Gibbs, R.S., 2014, 'Association of extremes of pre-pregnancy BMI with the clinical presentations of preterm birth', *American Journal of Obstetrics and Gynecology, 210*(5): 428. e421–9, doi:10.1016/j.ajog.2013.12.011

Mackay, E., Dalman, C., Karlsson, H. & Gardner, R.M., 2017, 'Association of gestational weight gain and maternal body mass index in early pregnancy with risk for nonaffective psychosis in offspring', *JAMA Psychiatry, 74*(4): 339–49, doi:10.1001/jamapsychiatry.2016.4257

Madjunkov, M., Chaudhry, S. & Ito, S., 2017, 'Listeriosis during pregnancy', *Archives of Gynecology and Obstetrics, 296*(2): 143–52, doi:10.1007/s00404-017-4401-1

Maffini, M.V., Rubin, B.S., Sonnenschein, C. & Soto, A.M., 2006, 'Endocrine disruptors and reproductive health: The case of bisphenol-A', *Molecular and Cellular Endocrinology, 254–255*: 179–86, doi:10.1016/j.mce.2006.04.033

Malek, L., Umberger, W., Makrides, M. & Zhou, S.J., 2016, 'Adherence to the Australian Dietary Guidelines during pregnancy: Evidence from a national study', *Public Health Nutrition*, *19*(7): 1155–63, doi:10.1017/S1368980015002232

Morisaki, N., Nagata, C., Jwa, S.C., Sago, H., Saito, S. et al., 2017, 'Pre-pregnancy BMI-specific optimal gestational weight gain for women in Japan', *Journal of Epidemiology*, *27*(10): 492–8, doi:10.1016/j.je.2016.09.013

Mortel, M. & Mehta, S.D., 2013, 'Systematic review of the efficacy of herbal galactogogues', *Journal of Human Lactation*, *29*(2): 154–62, doi:10.1177/0890334413477243

Munns, C., Zacharin, M.R., Rodda, C.P., Batch, J.A., Morley, R. et al., 2006, 'Prevention and treatment of infant and childhood vitamin D deficiency in Australia and New Zealand: A consensus statement', *Medical Journal of Australia*, *185*(5): 268–72, doi:10.5694/j.1326-5377.2006.tb00558.x

NHMRC, 2006, *Nutrient Reference Values for Australia and New Zealand* <www.nrv.gov.au/home>, accessed 14 February 2019

—— 2009, *Australian Guidelines to Reduce Health Risks From Drinking Alcohol* <www.nhmrc.gov.au/health-topics/alcohol-guidelines>, accessed 14 February 2019

Peña-Rosas, J.P., De-Regil, L.M., Dowswell, T. & Viteri, F.E., 2012, 'Daily oral iron supplementation during pregnancy', *The Cochrane Database of Systematic Reviews*, *12*: CD004736, doi:10.1002/14651858.CD004736.pub4

Picciano, M.F., 2003, 'Pregnancy and lactation: Physiological adjustments, nutritional requirements and the role of dietary supplements', *Journal of Nutrition*, *133*(6): 1997S–2002S, doi:10.1093/jn/133.6.1997S

Prentice, A.M. & Goldberg, G.R., 2000, 'Energy adaptations in human pregnancy: Limits and long-term consequences', *American Journal of Clinical Nutrition*, *71*(5): 1226S–32S, doi:10.1093/ajcn/71.5.1226s

Radlowski, E. & Johnson, R., 2013, 'Perinatal iron deficiency and neurocognitive development', *Frontiers in Human Neuroscience*, *7*: 585, doi:10.3389/fnhum.2013.00585

Reddy, A., Parikh, M.J., Gabrielson, A.T. & Sikka, S.C., 2018, 'Environmental health policy regarding men's reproductive and sexual health,' in S.C. Sikka & W.J.G. Hellstrom (eds), *Bioenvironmental Issues Affecting Men's Reproductive and Sexual Health*, Boston, MA: Academic Press, pp. 515–29

Reid, A.E., Chauhan, B.F., Rabbani, R., Lys, J., Copstein, L. et al., 2016, 'Early exposure to nonnutritive sweeteners and long-term metabolic health: A systematic review', *Pediatrics*, *137*(3): e20153603, doi:10.1542/peds.2015-3603

Santangeli, L., Sattar, N. & Huda, S.S., 2015, 'Impact of maternal obesity on perinatal and childhood outcomes', *Best Practice & Research Clinical Obstetrics & Gynaecology*, *29*(3): 438–48, doi:10.1016/j.bpobgyn.2014.10.009

Sermondade, N., Faure, C., Fezeu, L., Shayeb, A.G., Bonde, J.P. et al., 2012, 'BMI in relation to sperm count: An updated systematic review and collaborative meta-analysis', *Human Reproduction Update*, *19*(3): 221–31, doi:10.1093/humupd/dms050

Sharifzadeh, F., Kashanian, M., Koohpayehzadeh, J., Rezaian, F., Sheikhansari, N. & Eshraghi, N., 2018, 'A comparison between the effects of ginger, pyridoxine (vitamin B6) and placebo for the treatment of the first trimester nausea and vomiting of pregnancy (NVP)', *Journal of Maternal-Fetal & Neonatal Medicine*, *31*(19): 2509–14, doi:10.1080/14767058.2017.1344965

Sikka, S.C. & Wang, R., 2008, 'Endocrine disruptors and estrogenic effects on male reproductive axis', *Asian Journal of Andrology*, *10*(1): 134–45, doi:10.1111/j.1745-7262.2008.00370.x

Steegers-Theunissen, R.P.M., Twigt, J., Pestinger, V. & Sinclair, K.D., 2013, 'The periconceptional period, reproduction and long-term health of offspring: The importance of one-carbon metabolism', *Human Reproduction Update*, *19*(6): 640–55, doi:10.1093/humupd/dmt041

Temple, J.L., Bernard, C., Lipshultz, S.E., Czachor, J.D., Westphal, J.A. & Mestre, M.A., 2017, 'The safety of ingested caffeine: A comprehensive review', *Frontiers in Psychiatry*, *8*: 80, doi:10.3389/fpsyt.2017.00080

van Gool, J.D., Hirche, H., Lax, H. & De Schaepdrijver, L., 2018, 'Folic acid and primary prevention of neural tube defects: A review', *Reproductive Toxicology*, *80*: 73–84, doi:10.1016/j.reprotox.2018.05.004

Wei, S.-Q., Qi, H.-P., Luo, Z.-C. & Fraser, W.D., 2013, 'Maternal vitamin D status and adverse pregnancy outcomes: A systematic review and meta-analysis', *The Journal of Maternal-Fetal & Neonatal Medicine*, *26*(9): 889–99, doi:10.3109/14767058.2013.765849

WHO, 2009, *Infant and Young Child Feeding: Model Chapter for Textbooks for Medical Students and Allied Health Professionals,* <http://apps.who.int/iris/bitstream/handle/10665/44117/9789241597494_eng.pdf;jsessionid= 172FFE84A7E00C4176292406D8E6655E?sequence=1>, accessed 12 January 2019

Wylde, S., Nwose, E. & Bwititi, P., 2016, 'Morning sickness in pregnancy: Mini review of possible causes with proposal for monitoring by diagnostic methods', *International Journal of Reproduction, Contraception, Obstetrics and Gynecology, 5*(2): 261–7, doi:10.18203/2320-1770.ijrcog20160356

Xu, J., Cao, J., Iguchi, N., Huang, L. & Riethmacher, D., 2012, 'Functional characterization of bitter-taste receptors expressed in mammalian testis', *MHR: Basic Science of Reproductive Medicine, 19*(1): 17–28, doi:10.1093/molehr/gas040

Zimmermann, M.B., Jooste, P.L. & Pandav, C.S., 2008, 'Iodine-deficiency disorders', *Lancet, 372*(9645): 1251–62, doi:10.1016/S0140-6736(08)61005-3

{CHAPTER 21}
INFANCY, CHILDHOOD AND ADOLESCENCE

Gayle S. Savige and Danielle Gallegos

OBJECTIVES

- Describe the normal pattern of growth during infancy, childhood and adolescence.
- Explain the basis for energy and nutrient requirements during infancy and childhood.
- Identify and discuss the issues that commonly influence nutrition in infancy, childhood and adolescence.

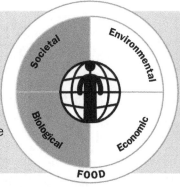

INTRODUCTION

Early childhood and adolescence is recognised as a critical period in child development, which encompasses physical, cognitive, social and emotional health. Nutrition is integral to this development. In infancy and early childhood, parents and caregivers are primarily responsible for nutrition but as children get older they have increasing autonomy or control over their food preferences and food choices. Parents, caregivers, children and adolescents need to navigate an increasingly complex food system in order to maintain optimal health. While it is recognised that nutrition is a key factor, other elements are also important in what has been described as nurturing care (WHO, UNICEF & World Bank Group 2016) (Figure 21.1). For optimal growth and development that will impact on the choices available and

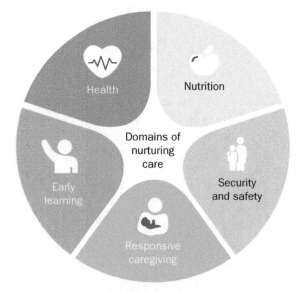

Figure 21.1: The domains of nurturing
Source: Bundy et al. (2017) License: Creative Commons Attribution CC BY 3.0 IGO

trajectory for health in adulthood, care of infants, children and adolescents needs to incorporate:

- optimal nutrition and health
- opportunities for early learning and ongoing education
- responsive caregiving
- security and safety.

Chapter 20 focuses on nutrition prior to conception, during pregnancy and lactation. This chapter focuses on the life-stages of infancy, childhood and adolescence. Infancy, childhood and adolescence are life-stages that are not necessarily biologically determined but rather are socially and culturally constructed. They are usually given age brackets for ease but there is large variation in the physiological changes that mark each stage.

GROWTH IN CHILDHOOD AND ADOLESCENCE

Optimal nutrition is fundamental to achieving normal growth and development in children. Chapter 22 provides details on how growth is measured and monitored.

Weight and height

During infancy there is a rapid rate of physical growth and development. Birthweight more than doubles by six months and trebles by the end of the first year, while length increases by about 50 per cent. After birth, most infants lose weight with about half of infants regaining their birthweight up to ten days after birth (Paul et al. 2016). Typical weight gains for infants are 150–200 g/week during the

DEFINING INFANCY, CHILDHOOD AND ADOLESCENCE

INFANCY

Infancy generally describes the first year of life. During this phase there is rapid growth and development. Infants move from a predominantly liquid diet (breastmilk or formula) to eating family foods.

CHILDHOOD

Childhood typically describes the time period between infancy and adolescence. It is defined by the *Convention on the Rights of the Child* as a person younger than 18 years, unless the legal definition of 'adult' is younger in a particular country. In this context, however, a physiological definition of child would be from the age of one to approximately ten when there is the onset of puberty. However, taking a settings approach typically schooling defines the age brackets with children attending pre-school and primary school (that is, up to 12–13 years of age).

ADOLESCENCE

The World Health Organization (WHO) defines adolescence as the period between ten and nineteen years. It is characterised by the onset of puberty and rapid growth in early adolescence (10–14 years) with slower growth in late adolescence. The term 'teenager' is taken to be between the ages of thirteen and eighteen years. In countries such as Australia and New Zealand adulthood is defined as being from eighteen years when individuals are legally responsible and have, for example, the right to vote. Taking a settings approach secondary school is the age bracket that most commonly defines adolescence from 12–13 years to 17 years.

first three months, 100–150 g/week from three to six months and 70–90 g/week from six to twelve months (NHMRC 2013b). Ideally, the pattern of growth by the infant should be monitored over time using growth charts to compare to population standards (see Chapter 23).

During childhood, the rate of growth (height and weight) is relatively steady and linear until adolescence. At this time, there is at sudden increase in growth velocity known as the **pubertal** growth spurt (Figure 21.2).

On average, the growth spurt begins at ten to eleven years in girls and at twelve to thirteen years in boys, and usually lasts for two to two-and-a-half years (Tanner et al. 1975); see figures 21.3 (weight) and 21.4 (height). More than 80 per cent of growth in attained height occurs in early adolescence (10–15 years) and then slows in the postpubertal stage (WHO 2006a). The timing of the growth spurt varies widely between males and females and among individuals but its duration is fairly uniform. The peak velocity for weight gain tends to occur

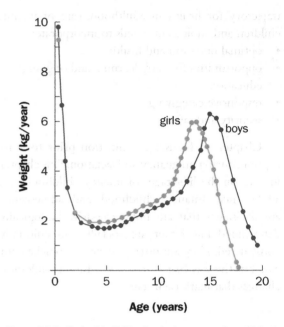

Figure 21.3: Typical individual velocity curves for weight in boys and girls

Source: Gracey et al. (1989)

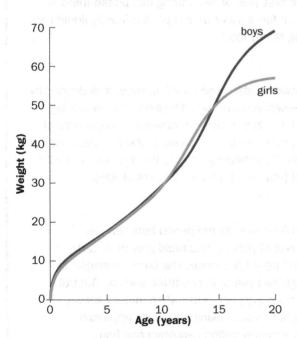

Figure 21.2: Typical individual weight-attained curves in boys and girls

Source: WHO (2007)

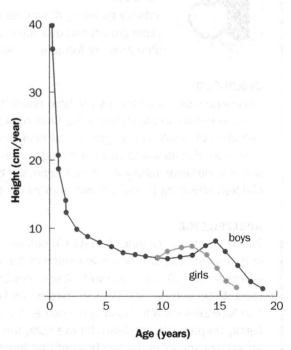

Figure 21.4: Typical individual velocity curves for height in boys and girls

Source: Gracey et al. (1989)

about three months later than that for height. In girls, menarche (or the onset of menstruation) generally occurs after the peak in height velocity, while in boys the development of secondary sexual characteristics (development of pubic and facial hair, Adam's apple) is much less closely related to the adolescent growth spurt. Hormonal changes associated with the growth spurt interact and are modulated by nutritional status. For instance, malnutrition is associated with a later onset of menstruation and overnutrition (obesity) usually results in early maturity.

It is important to assess and monitor growth over time to ensure optimal health and wellbeing. Assessing growth is also useful in diagnosing disease and monitoring treatment. In 2006, the World Health Organization developed a set of growth standards for infants and young children. These standards, developed from a multicentre study, found that all children up to the age of five years, regardless of ethnicity and socioeconomic status, follow a similar growth pattern when their health and nutritional needs are met (WHO 2006b). In older children, assessing growth relies on growth charts that use cross-sectional reference data from an existing population to generate percentile values. These percentile lines allow an individual's growth to be compared with that of his or her peers. These charts and their development are discussed in more depth in Chapter 23.

Internationally, wasting (low weight-for-height) and stunting (low height-for-age) (between −3 and −2 z-scores) of children are used as indicators of extreme hunger, and both are strong predictors of mortality in children under five years. To be attributed to nutritional factors, what the parents and child eats, and episodes of infection with growth retardation need to be documented. Shortness can be adaptive in many areas and can be healthy if growth faltering is not in evidence.

Organ and tissue growth

The organs and tissues of the body do not all grow at the same rate. Skeletal muscle growth reflects overall body growth, unlike the brain, lymphoid, adrenal and reproductive tissue (Figure 21.5). Almost all of

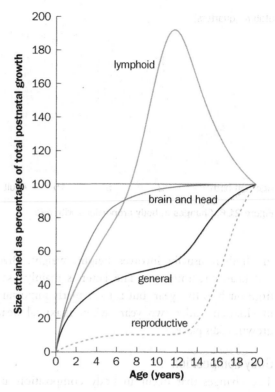

Figure 21.5: Growth curves of different parts and tissues of the body
Source: Tanner (1962)

the postnatal growth in the brain occurs in the first five years of life, whereas there is virtually no growth in the reproductive organs until adolescence. The early rapid growth of the brain and head is one of the reasons why adequate nutrition in early childhood is particularly important. Malnutrition during sensitive periods of cognitive development, such as those associated with language development, may have lasting negative consequences (Benton & ILSI Europe 2008). The reproductive system grows slowly until puberty, whereas the lymph tissue grows rapidly before reducing in size.

The differences in growth rate of the various parts of the body are also evident in the changes in body proportions that occur with age. Figure 21.6 shows the marked decrease in the size of the head relative to the whole body, and the increase in length of the lower limbs with age that occurs during the process of growth and development. Assessment of growth

Stature (quarters)

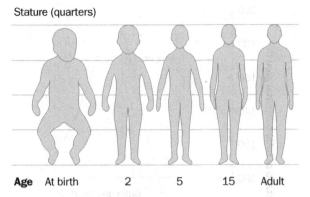

| Age | At birth | 2 | 5 | 15 | Adult |

Figure 21.6: Changes in body proportions with age

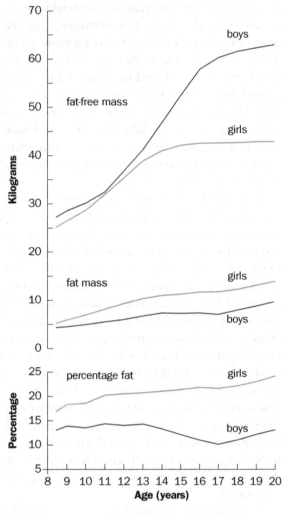

Figure 21.7: Growth curves for fat-free mass, fat mass and percentage fat

Source: Malina et al. (1988). Republished with permission of *Annual Reviews*, conveyed through Copyright Clearance Center, Inc.

in children usually involves height, weight, BMI and head circumference. The latter is mainly used from birth to five years but is particularly important in children under two years when maximal head growth takes place.

Body composition

The changes that occur in body composition are less obvious. At birth, the lean tissues contain more water and less protein than later on in life, while the body as a whole contains less fat. In the full-term infant, body fat content is around 15 per cent and differs more with **gestational age** than with gender. During childhood, girls tend to have slightly more fat than boys, but the marked differences in body composition with gender that are seen in adults do not emerge until adolescence. Adolescence is also accompanied by major differences in the rate and amount of lean tissue gained (Figure 21.7).

Boys show a rapid and sustained spurt in lean weight and only a modest increase in body fat, while girls experience a smaller gain in lean weight and a larger gain in body fat. During the second decade of life, boys double their **fat-free mass** (FFM) while in girls FFM increases by only about 50 per cent. That is, boys gain FFM at a greater rate and for a longer time, so young adult values of FFM are reached in females at 15–16 years of age compared with 19–20 years in males (Rogol et al. 2002). FFM in females, therefore, is only about 70 per cent of that of a mature male. This difference in body composition is physiological

and provides mature females with an energy reserve for the demands of pregnancy and lactation.

ENERGY AND NUTRITION REQUIREMENTS

Adequate intake of energy and nutrients essential for normal growth in children can be estimated by observing the food intake of healthy infants and children, and by basing requirements on the amounts of nutrients accumulated in the body during growth.

In most instances, the Recommended Dietary Intake (RDI) relies on both kinds of information. The energy requirement for basal metabolism and activity increases proportionately with body size, while the energy requirement for growth is relatively small after the first year of life (see Chapter 13). Small body size influences infant nutrition by limiting the amount of food that can be consumed at any one time, and is one of the reasons why newborn infants need to be fed frequently. It also means that the infant has a larger surface area and a higher resting metabolic rate relative to body weight, resulting in higher maintenance requirements for water, energy and nutrients.

Activity is a major component of the energy requirement and varies considerably among individuals. Substantial differences in energy intake can be found among healthy children of similar age and body size due largely to differences in the energy expended in physical activity. The dietary recommendation for energy intake therefore represents an estimate of the average needs of a specific age group and does not apply to all individuals of that age group. Energy requirements per kilogram of body weight fall between 300–400 kJ/kg in the first year to around 200 kJ/kg in late adolescence. Nutrient requirements increase with age and body size during childhood and adolescence, but decrease when expressed relative to body weight. These are reflected in the recommended serves for children of different ages, summarised in Table 21.1. The amount of food required will vary depending on activity levels, presence of a disability and other factors.

Nutrient requirements of infants

The nutrient requirements of infants are outlined in Table 21.2. For full-term healthy infants, these requirements can be met through breastmilk or formula.

Table 21.1: Recommended average daily number of serves of each of the five food groups

		Recommended average daily number of serves* from each of the five food groups					Additional serves* for more active/taller or older children/ adolescents
	Age	Vegetable/ legumes/ beans	Fruit	Grain (cereal) foods	Lean meat/ poultry/fish/ eggs/tofu/nuts/ seeds/legumes	Milk/yoghurt/ Cheese and/ or alternatives mainly low fat	Additional number of serves from other groups, unsaturated oils or discretionary choices
Boys	2–3	2.5	1	4	1	1.5	0–1
	4–8	4.5	1.5	4	1.5	2	0–2.5
	9–11	5	2	5	2.5	2.5	0–3
	12–13	5.5	2	6	2.5	2.5	0–3
	14–18	5.5	2	7	2.5	2.5	0–3
Girls	2–3	2.5	1	4	1	1.5	0–1
	4–8	4.5	1.5	4	1.5	1.5	0–1
	9–11	5	2	4	2.5	3	0–3
	12–13	5	2	5	2.5	3.5	0–2.5
	14–18	5	2	7	2.5	3.5	0–2.5

*A serve is equivalent to:
½ cup cooked vegetables; 1 cup raw leafy green vegetables; ½ cup legumes or beans; ½ medium potato
1 medium piece of fruit; ½ cup 100% fruit juice
1 slice bread; ½ bread roll; ½ cup cooked pasta/rice; 3 crispbreads; ¼ cup of flour
65 g cooked lean meat; 80 g cooked poultry; 100 g fish; 2 large eggs; 1 cup lentils, legumes; 175 g tofu
1 cup milk; 1 200-g carton of yoghurt; 40 g cheese.

Table 21.2: Nutrient requirements of infants

Water	Healthy breastfed infants, if fed on demand, can meet all their water needs from breastmilk, even in hot climates. Breastmilk itself is 88% water, and is enough to satisfy a baby's thirst and water requirements. Formula-fed infants may need additional plain boiled water between feeds in very hot weather. It is important that the water does not replace a formula feed.
Energy	For the first six months of life, the infant's energy requirements are met primarily from fat and lactose, either from human milk or from a commercial artificial formula, usually based on cow's milk. After this time, a gradually increasing proportion of the energy comes from foods other than milk, and from macronutrients other than fat and lactose. Breastmilk can supply all energy requirements up to about six months. From six months, a combination of breastmilk and solid food is required to meet energy requirements.
Protein	In infants under the age of six months, the amount of protein received in breastmilk allows for adequate growth even though it constitutes only 6–7% of the total energy. Infants fed human milk receive approximately 2–2.4 g/kg/day of protein during the first six months and about 1.5 g/kg/day after six months (Rutishauser 2002).
Carbohydrate	The main carbohydrate in both human and cow's milk is lactose. Mature human milk and infant formulae contain around 7% and cow's milk 4–5% (Mann & Truswell 2007; NHMRC 2009). Infants fed human milk obtain about a third of their total energy intake from lactose. Lactose facilitates the absorption of minerals such as calcium and magnesium.
Fat	Fat is the principal source of energy for the newborn infant, supplying 40–55% of the total energy intake (Andreas et al. 2015). It is an important component of infant diets for several reasons, in that it is a: • concentrated source of energy when capacity for food intake is limited • vehicle for the fat-soluble vitamins A, D, E and K • source of essential fatty acids • source of energy which does not increase the renal solute load or lead to loss of water in the small intestine. Intakes of DHA (see Chapter 11) have also been associated with better infant neurodevelopment and/or visual acuity, with the content of breastmilk depending on the maternal diet and varying widely (Jensen & Lapillonne 2009). While the long-chain polyunsaturated n-6 and n-3 acids form only a small proportion of the total lipids (<2 per cent), they have important roles in promoting growth, neural development and vascular function. Low-fat diets in infancy are not advised.
Vitamins and minerals	The basis for vitamin and mineral allowances in the first six months of life is the amounts estimated to be provided, on average, by human milk from a well-nourished mother. Since not all babies are breastfed, other considerations also apply in making nutrient recommendations for this age group. Some nutrients— for example, thiamin, vitamin B-6 and vitamin C—are destroyed by heat and may be destroyed during the process of preparing infant formulas. In order to allow for these losses, the amounts recommended are greater than those received, on average, by infants who are breastfed. In the case of the minerals—calcium, iron and zinc—for which the percentage absorption from human milk is generally much greater than from cow's milk-based infant formulas, a range of values is given in order to allow for differences in absorption between breastfed and formula-fed babies.

Breastmilk is a living fluid and, as such, can change in composition from the beginning to the end of a feed and as the infant matures.

• Concentrations of proteins such as protective immunoglobulins in the colostrum (the thick, initial secretion at the beginning of lactation) change to an increased concentration of lactose, casein and fat in the more watery–appearing breastmilk that follows.

• Composition can change within a feed, with the degree of fullness of the breast an indicator for the fat or cream content of the milk. The milk taken from a full breast will have a lower fat content than that taken at the end of a feed when the breast is drained and the volume minimal.

• The range of antibodies, cells and other non-specific components varies. Antibodies in human milk are produced by the mother in response to bacteria and viruses to which she is exposed via the intestine and respiratory tract, and thus provide protection against those pathogens that the infant is most likely to encounter.

- There is minimal variation between population groups as to volume produced, with mothers in low-income countries able to produce the same as those in high income countries, regardless of mothers' diets.
- The reflection of the mother's diet in breastmilk concentrations of certain vitamins and minerals may vary (NHMRC 2013b).

WHY IS BREASTMILK CALLED A LIVING FLUID?

Read the following reviews and other peer-reviewed literature on human milk and write two pages summarising:
- the unique composition of breastmilk
- the specific changes to breastmilk composition within a feed and over time.

Write a 'nutrition label' for breastmilk and compare this to an artificial infant formula.

Andreas, N.J., Kampmann, B. & Le-Doare, K.M., 2015, 'Human breast milk: A review on its composition and bioactivity', *Early Human Development*, 91(11): 629–35.

Eriksen, K.G. et al., 2018, 'Human milk composition and infant growth', *Current Opinion in Clinical Nutrition and Metabolic Care*, 21(3): 200–6.

WHAT ARE AUSTRALIAN INFANTS EATING?

Breastmilk

Breastfeeding is the physiological norm for infants and there is overwhelming evidence to support breastfeeding over artificial feeding in most instances. Internationally, exclusive breastfeeding is recommended until infants are around six months of age, with appropriate introduction of complementary (solids or first) foods and ongoing breastfeeding until two years (WHO & UNICEF 2003). In Australia, the same recommendations apply but with continued breastfeeding to twelve months or for as long as the mother and infant desire (NHMRC 2013b). Internationally, there are agreed definitions for initiation, exclusive and predominant breastfeeding as well as complementary feeding. These are outlined in Table 21.3.

Extensive research has shown immunological, health, nutritional, physiological, psychological, practical and economic benefits and advantages associated with breastmilk and breastfeeding (Horta et al. 2013a; 2013b). Breastmilk is protective against disease both in the short and long term. Exclusive breastfeeding

Table 21.3: Population indicators used for breastfeeding

Breastfeeding initiation	Infant put to the breast within an hour of birth.
Exclusive breastfeeding	Breastmilk (including milk expressed from the breast or provided by a wet nurse). Allows the infant to receive oral rehydration solution, drops, syrups (vitamins, minerals, medicines). Allows no other foods or fluids.
Predominant breastfeeding	Breastmilk (including milk expressed from the breast or provided by a wet nurse). Allows the infant to receive water and water-based drinks, fruit juices, ritual fluids, oral rehydration solution, drops, syrups (vitamins, minerals, medicines). Does not allow non-human milk or food-based fluids.
Complementary feeding	Breastmilk (including milk expressed from the breast or provided by a wet nurse) and solid or semi-solid foods.

Source: WHO (2008)

for six months reduces the risk of gastrointestinal infection more than exclusive breastfeeding for three to four months without any adverse effects on growth (Kramer & Kakuma 2012). There is growing evidence of the influence of breastmilk on the gut microbiota, with breastmilk providing a pathway for the transfer of maternal microbes as well as providing selective prebiotics (Munyaka et al. 2014) (see Chapter 30 for more information on the microbiome). Human breastmilk contains exosomes or microvesicles with a complex composition including RNA. This provides breastmilk with a mechanism to regulate immune and gut function and for person-to-person transfer of genetic material other than by reproduction. This knowledge represents a paradigm shift in our understanding of lactation and nutrition, and what can and cannot be imitated by breastmilk substitutes at present (Admyre et al. 2007; de la Torre Gomez et al. 2018; Lässer et al. 2011).

Conflicting advice is emerging regarding the duration of exclusive breastfeeding and the development of food allergies and intolerances, with some suggesting that introducing foods at four months reduces the risk of allergy. However, the evidence is weak and the benefits outweighed by those of exclusive breastfeeding to six months. A compromise suggested by the Australasian Society of Clinical Immunology and Allergy is to recommend food be introduced 'at around six months but not before four months' (ASCIA 2016); this window is not strict, but introduction of a diversity of complementary foods should not be delayed beyond twelve months. In addition, evidence indicates that egg and peanuts should be introduced in the first year of life regardless of allergy risk factors, and hydrolysed formula (partially or extensively) is not recommended for the prevention of allergic disease (Joshi et al. 2019).

While breastfeeding is the physiological norm, few women exclusively breastfeed their infants at six months. In Australia, 96 per cent of women initiate breastfeeding—that is, put the infant to breast within one hour of birth. Over two-thirds of infants were receiving some breastmilk up to four months of age. Exclusive breastfeeding dropped to 39 per cent at three months with 15 per cent exclusively

BREASTMILK AS PERSONALISED MEDICINE

The benefits of breastmilk may be mediated directly or indirectly by the infant microbiome. The microbiome may have a role in immune regulation, metabolic responses and regulation as well as cognitive development. How babies are born (vaginally or by caesarean section) initially establishes the preliminary gut microbiota and this is followed by feeding mode.

Read the panel on breastmilk as personalised medicine in Victora, C.G. et al., 2016, 'Breastfeeding in the 21st century: Epidemiology, mechanisms, and lifelong effect', *Lancet*, 387(10017): 475–90.

Search the academic databases for breastmilk AND microbiome—restrict the search to the last two years.

Read another two articles that talk about the infant microbiome and breastmilk and discuss what factors impact on the development of the microbiome. What are the likely consequences?

breastfeeding at six months of age (AIHW 2011). In New Zealand these rates were (as of 2010), 42 per cent exclusively breastfeeding at three months dropping to 16 per cent at six months (Royal New Zealand Plunket Society 2017).

Possible contraindications to breastfeeding

Almost all mothers can breastfeed successfully, but for a small minority this is not possible or there are medical reasons why breastfeeding should not occur, either temporarily or permanently (NHMRC 2013b; WHO & UNICEF 2009). Breastfeeding can usually continue with the following conditions if they are being medically managed: breast abscess, mastitis, hepatitis B, hepatitis C and tuberculosis. For mothers living with HIV the recommendation is for breastfeeding for at least twelve months and possibly up to 24 months while being fully supported by antiretroviral therapy (WHO 2016b). Situations in which breastfeeding is not recommended include:

- illness in the mother that is very severe (e.g. **sepsis**) or transmissible (e.g. herpes) or requires treatment with drugs that have adverse side effects in the infant in the amounts likely to be excreted in human milk (e.g. chemotherapy drugs)
- breastfeeding is also contraindicated when the infant has some inherited metabolic disorders such as **galactosaemia** (NHMRC 2013b)
- very low birthweight or preterm infants may have higher requirements than can be provided by breastmilk and so may require fortified breastmilk delivered via alternative routes (NHMRC 2013b).

Factors that influence the success of breastfeeding

Breastfeeding is a learned behaviour and affected by a range of cultural, social and individual factors. Figure 21.8 and Table 21.4 outline these factors at the individual, group and society levels. Strategies to improve breastfeeding have included:

- education and social marketing
- individual support, including peer (such as the Australian Breastfeeding Association and La Leche League) and professional support
- health service policy and practices, including the 'ten steps to a baby-friendly hospital', implementation of the international agreement on marketing of infant formula and training of health professionals
- legislation such as maternity leave provisions, workplace policies and creating supportive environments in public places.

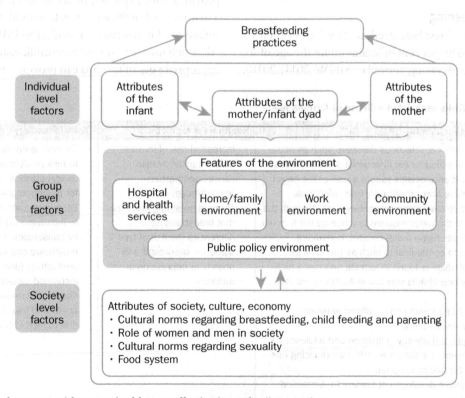

Figure 21.8: A conceptual framework of factors affecting breastfeeding practices

Source: Hector et al. (2005)

Table 21.4: Individual factors influencing breastfeeding

Factors	Rationale
Intention	Intention to breastfeed—when women make a decision to breastfeed before or during pregnancy they are more likely to breastfeed. This intention is affected by knowledge, attitudes, family support and previous experience.
Self-efficacy or confidence	Believing you can breastfeed and can solve issues associated with breastfeeding is strongly linked to breastfeeding commencement and duration. Self-efficacy is supported by role models (peers or family) and support from partners, peers and professionals.
Physical factors	Many women stop breastfeeding due to nipple pain or they believe they are not producing enough milk. Most of these issues can be overcome with support and encouragement.
Social factors	Returning to work or study is one of the primary reasons for ceasing to breastfeed. Feeling embarrassed about feeding in public is another reason given for cessation of breastfeeding. It is now illegal to discriminate against a breastfeeding woman: a woman cannot be asked to leave a cafe for breastfeeding her baby; a woman cannot be refused employment because she is breastfeeding.

Breastmilk is the biological norm and formula is unable to match breastmilk's biological superiority and environmental sustainability. Table 21.5 highlights the risks associated with the use of formula feeds.

Formula feeding

Based on the latest breastfeeding statistics, between 75 per cent and 85 per cent of infants under the age of six months are receiving formula (AIHW 2011; 2018).

In addition to known indicators for not breastfeeding, described earlier, there will be situations where the mother, despite efforts to continue breastfeeding, will not be able to fully meet the infant's nutritional requirements. If an infant is not to be breastfed, or provided with expressed or donor human breastmilk, a commercial artificial formula should be used for infants aged under twelve months (NHMRC 2013b). Although unable to mimic breastmilk exactly, safe and appropriate use of formula can provide a nutritionally

Table 21.5: Risks associated with use of formula feeds

Health risks for infants	Health risks for mothers	Risks for society
• Increased risk of infectious diseases such as acute otitis media (middle ear infections), gastroenteritis, necrotising enterocolitis (where a part of the bowel dies), severe lower respiratory tract infections. • Exposure to environmental contaminants through the formula or the water required to make up the formula (for example, heavy metal content, melamine). • Exposure to contaminants such as *Cronobacter sakazakii* which is found in formula and has a high mortality rate (risk is very low in Australia and New Zealand). • Sudden infant death and childhood leukaemia. • Poor jaw development. • Overweight and obesity in children and adolescents (the evidence is weak for an effect on reducing risk of other chronic conditions). • Poor cognitive development leading to decreased intelligence.	• Increased risk of invasive breast cancer, ovarian cancer, postpartum haemorrhage. • There is no strong evidence that breastfeeding decreases the risk of type 2 diabetes, overweight and obesity or depression in mothers.	• Environmental costs related to milk production, water usage, plastics production for paraphernalia. • Economic costs related to increased expenditure by households, increased healthcare costs, lost productivity (due to increased maternal and child deaths, decreased cognitive ability and lost days of work due to morbidity).

Source: Rollins et al. (2016); Stuebe (2009); Victora et al. (2016)

GLOBALISATION OF INFANT FORMULA

The growth of the globalisation of infant formula is strongly linked to the globalisation of milk production. The largest global dairy exporter is the New Zealand-based Fonterra, which promotes industrial-style milk production in Brazil, Chile, Uruguay, the US Midwest, Hawaii and, increasingly, China.

This dairy industry provides the milk powder for most infant formula. In 2013, US$41 billion was spent on infant formula, with rapid market growth in Latin America and the Asia-Pacific. Formula companies are starting to build factories in low-income countries to meet the demands of an emerging middle class and to lower production costs (Kent 2015). The cost of not breastfeeding is, however, far greater with the WHO estimating the total cost of not breastfeeding in China to be US$66 billion per year (UNICEF et al. 2017).

DISCUSSION QUESTIONS:
- Who benefits from growing the formula market? Who is disadvantaged?
- Is the increase in the formula market sustainable?
- What are some alternatives to formula for women unable to breastfeed but who wish their infant to receive breastmilk?

adequate intake and should be used in preference to cow's, goat's or any other milks. All infant formulas in Australia and New Zealand are regulated by the *Australia New Zealand Food Standards Code* and in particular Standard 2.9.1.

In Australia and New Zealand, the array of infant formulas available from supermarkets and pharmacies potentially makes selection a difficult task. There is a variety of formulations, including different brands of starter, follow-on, standard, 'Gold', 'HA', soy-based, lactose-free or anti-reflux formula. Formulas also vary with respect to casein-to-whey ratios and the addition of nucleotides, *Lactobacillus bifidus* bacterium, inulin or DHA. A brief summary of some of the main types of formula and their key differences is provided in Table 21.6, but mothers should seek individual advice as to the most appropriate product for their infant if formula is required.

Marketing of breastmilk substitutes

Aggressive marketing of formula continues to undermine the promotion of exclusive breastfeeding for the recommended periods of time. In 1981, the World Health Organization released an International Code for the Marketing of Breastmilk Substitutes. The code is a public health strategy to ensure that mothers are not unduly influenced by formula companies to substitute artificial feeding for breast-feeding. The code stipulates that there should be no marketing of formula, bottles or teats to the public, that health facilities and health professionals should not have a role in promoting formula and that free samples should not be given to pregnant women or new parents. The code is not anti-formula and recognises that breastmilk substitutes have a role to play; what it aims to do is protect the community against irresponsible and biased marketing of formula that seriously undermines the role of breastfeeding.

As of March 2016, 135 countries had at least some form of legal measure in place covering some provisions of the Code. Thirty-nine countries have legislation or legal measures that cover all or most provisions of the code; 31 countries have some legal provision for many provisions of the code; 65 countries have legal measures for a few provisions; while 49 countries have non-legal or no measures (WHO, UNICEF & IBFAN 2016).

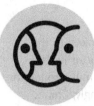

WET NURSING AND MILK BANKS

Breastmilk has been informally shared through wet nursing and donations for millennia. Wet nursing is when a woman other than the mother breastfeeds the infant. This was a very common practice prior to the 20th century when alternatives to breastmilk were not available and there were high rates of maternal death during childbirth.

Milk banks are formalised bodies that collect, store, process and dispense donated human milk. Milk banks were common up to the AIDS epidemic in the 1980s, when there were concerns about the transmission of the virus. As of 2017 there were five milk banks operating in Australia (Perth, Sydney, Melbourne, Brisbane and the Gold Coast) and two informal networks of milk sharing (Human Milk 4 Human Babies and Eats on Feets) in Australia and Mother's Milk in New Zealand. Many of the milk banks are associated with hospitals to assist in the care of premature babies. There are issues when money is paid for milk, with dilution of breastmilk a potential issue.

When a mother's own milk is not available, donated human milk is the next best option. With the sexualisation of the breast and the perception of breastmilk as a bodily fluid, however, there are mixed feelings regarding the use of donated milk or the use of wet nurses.

Think about your own attitudes and beliefs regarding the use of wet nursing and donated human milk. Is it something that you can rationalise or do you find it difficult to accept? What might be some of the concerns around wet nursing or donated breastmilk? After identifying these concerns, use your skills in searching the literature to find the evidence to discuss these concerns.

Table 21.6: Types of infant formula

Type of formula	Key features and indications for use
Cow's milk-based	Several forms available. Varying casein–whey ratios with whey-dominant (that is, those that more closely match human milk) causing less metabolic stress and preferred for low birthweight babies. Carbohydrate usually lactose.
Soy-based	May be suitable for vegans and some medical conditions; usually have sucrose or corn syrup solids as carbohydrate; not recommended for allergy and could contribute to allergy development.
Anti-regurgitation/ anti-reflux (AR)	Formulas containing thickening agent such as rice starch, potato starch or carob-bean gum to try to reduce regurgitation.
Partially hydrolysed or hypoallergenic (HA)	Suggested for infants not being breastfed. Was once used for treatment of eczema, food allergy, asthma or allergic rhinitis (runny nose) but is no longer recommended for allergic disease.
Specialised: Extensively hydrolysed (EH), amino acid (AA)	Available on prescription only. Protein is broken down. Used for cow's milk protein allergy. Amino acid formula may be indicated in infants with complex multiple allergies, gastrointestinal symptoms that are severe and cannot be resolved.
Goat's milk formula	Becoming popular. No indications for use preferentially over cow's milk.
Bone broth formula	Not indicated for infants under any circumstances. The paleo diet trend has created an increase in homemade bone broths for infants. These are dangerous and should not be used.

Source: ASCIA (2016); Gray (2017); Joshi et al. (2019); Meyer et al. (2018); NHMRC (2013b)

Australia, New Zealand and the United States have no legal measures.

In Australia, the WHO code manifests as the Marketing in Australia of Infant Formula (MAIF) agreement. The MAIF is a self-regulatory code of conduct overseen by the Commonwealth Department of Health. The MAIF is much more limited than the code and does not cover bottles, teats, retailers or pharmacists and only covers infant formula for babies under twelve months of age. The MAIF only applies to those manufacturers who are signatories to the agreement.

Examples of breaches include:

- the Autumn 2015 edition of *Australian Family Magazine* contained an advertisement for a toddler milk product featuring an image of a pre-toddler baby (The Ethics Centre 2018)
- a two-page lift-out promoting infant formula appeared in the October 2014 issue of *Practical Parenting* magazine, published by the Amcal pharmacy chain. It was argued that promotion of infant formula by retailers is not within scope of the MAIF Agreement. In this case a breach was upheld, as the manufacturers contributed financially to the publication and provided content (The Ethics Centre 2016).

Toddler milks

'Follow-on formulas' recommended by manufacturers for use from six months usually have a slightly higher protein content and many are casein-dominant, with increased levels of some **electrolytes** and iron. As there are no significant nutritional differences between these and starter formulas, changing at six months is not absolutely necessary (NHMRC 2013b). The so-called 'follow-on milks' or 'toddler formulas' for infants aged over twelve months are not necessary as children can receive adequate nutrients from a mixed diet (Romo-Palafox & Harris 2017).

Introducing first foods

Complementary feeding or the introduction of first foods or 'solids' plays an important role in preventing nutritional deficiencies in infancy and early childhood, and for longer-term development (Udall 2007; WHO & UNICEF 2003). In general, full-term healthy infants who are breastfed or who are fed an infant formula do not require any other food for about the first six months of life. After six months, exclusively breastfed full-term infants may be at risk of deficiencies of vitamin D (if the infant or mother have had very little sun exposure), iron and zinc, and vitamins A, B-12 and riboflavin (Foote & Marriott 2003; Krebs & Hambidge 2007). The timing and sequence of the introduction of foods is logically based on the:

- nutritional needs of the infant
- advantages and disadvantages of introducing specific foods
- physiological readiness to utilise foods other than milk
- physical capacity to handle semi-solid and solid foods.

The message to introduce foods at around six months is a public health message. Many healthy full-term infants may be ready to consume complementary foods earlier, but recommendations are not before four months (ASCIA 2016). In Australia, 28 per cent of infants aged four months had been introduced to first foods, increasing to 56.2 per cent at five months and 91.6 per cent at six months (AIHW 2011). The median age for the introduction of first foods was 4.7 months (AIHW 2011). Physiologically, eating requires the development of oral sensory, motor and swallowing skills, adequate pulmonary and gastrointestinal function, central nervous system integration and adequate musculoskeletal tone in order to effectively coordinate the timing of simultaneous breathing, sucking and swallowing to progressively manage the transition of feeding that occurs over the first twelve months from birth (Udall 2007). Infant developmental skills that are thought to occur by about six months, and that indicate readiness for complementary foods, include:

- upright sitting with minimal support
- midline head position maintained for several minutes without support
- hand-to-mouth motor skills

- dissociation of lip and tongue motions
- anatomic changes resulting in more space for the tongue in the oral cavity, allowing vertical motion of the tongue in addition to the previously restricted movements of 'in and out' suckling (extrusion reflex—when a food placed on the tongue is pushed out the front of the mouth). (Udall 2007)

Traditionally in Australia, the first food given to babies has been an infant cereal preparation usually

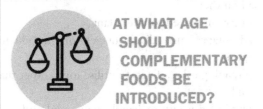

AT WHAT AGE SHOULD COMPLEMENTARY FOODS BE INTRODUCED?

Child feeding is a very culture-specific practice, and the age at introduction and types of foods introduced vary. There is strong evidence supporting exclusive breastfeeding to six months but it should be remembered that this is a public health message—that is, a general message that will elicit the most appropriate behaviour to maximise health in a majority of the population. Individual infants may be developmentally ready for complementary foods before or after this six-month milestone. There is some debate regarding introducing foods at around four months to reduce the risk of food allergy.

Manufacturers of infant foods routinely market food products to infants aged four months.

Visit supermarkets and go to the websites of food manufacturers, and review the types of foods marketed to infants under the age of six months. Do these match the guidelines for infants in terms of timing, texture and type? Develop an opinion on whether the food manufacturers are engaging in ethical behaviour.

based on rice fortified with iron. In other countries, gruels based on the staple cereals of that country are commonly used. There is no set requirement for the types of foods (as long as they are high in iron) to introduce or the speed at which they should be introduced. From six months, infants mainly tolerate purees and mashed foods, followed by minced/chopped foods; by eight months these are 'finger foods' leading to family foods at twelve months of age (NHMRC 2013b).

In addition to being concerned about what infants are eating, attention is also turning to how infants are being fed. Non-responsive feeding practices—such as pressuring a child to eat and using food as a reward to encourage eating—may interfere with a child's ability to recognise and respond to internal hunger and satiety (feeling full) cues (Byrne et al. 2017; Finnane et al. 2017). Responsive feeding practices—which can be summarised as 'parent provide, child decide'—have been associated with less food fussiness and a decreased risk of obesity (Magarey et al. 2016).

WHAT ARE AUSTRALIAN CHILDREN EATING?

In 2014–2015, just over two-thirds (68.1 per cent) of children aged 2–18 years ate enough fruit to meet the Australian Dietary Guidelines, which was in stark contrast to the very small proportion (5.4 per cent) meeting the guidelines for serves of vegetables (ABS 2015). In the 2011–2012 Australian Health Survey, the proportion of energy from **discretionary foods** was lowest among the two- to three-year-olds (30 per cent) and highest among the fourteen- to eighteen-year-olds (41 per cent). Biscuits were the largest discretionary food contributor to the energy intake of two- to three-year-olds (4.8 per cent) and among 14- to 18-year-olds it was confectionery and cereal/nut/fruit/seed bars (3.7 per cent) and soft drinks/flavoured mineral waters (3.6 per cent) (ABS 2014).

Tables 21.7 and 21.8 summarise children's food group and nutrient intakes relative to recommendations.

Table 21.7: Food and nutrient intakes for boys aged 2–18 years

Years	2–3	4–8	9–13	14–18
Five food groups: mean intake against recommended serves				
Vegetables	X	X	X	X
Fruits	✓	✓	X	X
Grains	X	✓	✓ (9–11) X (12–13)	X
Meat	X	X	X	X
Dairy	✓	X	X	X
Discretionary food: % of energy (broad recommendation is to limit intake)				
	29	39	39	41
Added sugars: % of energy (broad recommendation is to limit intake)				
	8.4	11	11	13
Trans and saturated fat: % energy (recommendation is less than 10% for those 14 years and over)				
	14	14	14	13
Sodium: mean intake (mg) versus adequate intake (mg)				
	1517 (200–400)	2236 (300–600)	2657 (400–800)	3117 (460–920)
Calcium: proportion of population (%) with intakes less than the estimated requirement				
	0.7	11	46 (9–11) 67 (12–13)	71
Iron: proportion of population (%) with intakes less than the estimated requirement				
	8.5	5.9	3.3	8.3
Dietary folate equivalents: proportion of population (%) with intakes less than the estimated requirement				
	–	–	0.4	1.2
Iodine: proportion of population (%) with intakes less than the estimated requirement				
	0.1	0.1	0.3	0.8
Fibre: mean intake (g/day) as a proportion (%) of the adequate intake level				
	121	112	95	80

Source: AIHW (2018)

Table 21.8: Food and nutrient intakes for girls aged 2–18 years

Years	2–3	4–8	9–13	14–18
Five food groups—mean intake against recommended serves				
Vegetables	X	X	X	X
Fruits	✓	✓	X	X
Grains	X	X	✓ (9–11) X (12–13)	X
Meat	X	X	X	X
Dairy	✓	X	X	X
Discretionary food: % of energy (broad recommendation is to limit intake)				
	32	36	40	41
Added sugars: % of energy (broad recommendation is to limit intake)				
	8.1	11	12	13
Trans and saturated fat: % energy (recommendation is less than 10% for those 14 years and over)				
	14	13	14	13
Sodium: mean intake (mg) versus adequate intake (mg)				
	1448 (200–400)	1868 (300–600)	2263 (400–800)	2399 (460–920)
Calcium: proportion of population (%) with intakes less than the estimated requirement				
	2.4	2.1	54 (9–11) 84 (12–13)	90
Iron: proportion of population (%) with intakes less than the estimated requirement				
	15	11	11	40
Dietary folate equivalents: proportion of population (%) with intakes less than the estimated requirement				
	–	–	1.2	7.9
Iodine: proportion of population (%) with intakes less than the estimated requirement				
	0.5	0.3	0.5	6.4
Fibre: mean intake (g/day) as a proportion (%) of the adequate intake level				
	109	96	96	88

Source: AIHW (2018)

A SETTINGS APPROACH TO NUTRITION FOR INFANTS, CHILDREN AND ADOLESCENTS

Most children and adolescents in Australia and New Zealand spend a large proportion of their time outside of the home environment in educational settings. These can be early education and care settings (long day care, family day care, kindergarten), primary schools and high schools. Sporting clubs and venues have been identified as other sites influential with respect to access and availability of healthy food choices. The availability of and access to healthy

---

EXAMPLES OF NUTRITION INTERVENTIONS BASED ON A SETTINGS APPROACH

EARLY EDUCATION AND CARE

There are two types of food provisioning in early education and care; food is either cooked on site or parents are required to provide all food. The Department of Health has developed the *Healthy Eating and Physical Activity Guidelines for Early Childhood* to assist these settings in establishing supportive environments for health (www.health.gov.au/internet/main/publishing.nsf/content/phd-early-childhood-nutrition-resources). Examples of programs that have been developed include:

- Munch and Move (NSW Government & Heart Foundation 2018) <www.healthykids.nsw.gov.au/campaigns-programs/about-munch-move.aspx>
- Learning Eating Active Play Sleep (LEAPS) (Nutrition Australia QLD 2018) <https://training.naqnutrition.org/courses/#/filter/early-years/leaps>

PRIMARY AND HIGH SCHOOL SETTINGS

National and state guidelines have been developed to govern the provisioning of food on school grounds and, in particular, by school canteens and tuckshops. These guidelines stipulate the types of foods and beverages that should be sold in the canteen and, in some cases, appropriate foods for fundraising activities. Examples include:

- The National Guidelines for Healthy Food and Drinks Supplied in School Canteens (Australian Government 2014) <www.health.gov.au/internet/main/publishing.nsf/content/5FFB6A30ECEE9321CA257BF0001DAB17/$File/Canteen%20guidelines.pdf>
- SMART choices based in Queensland (Queensland Government 2016) <https://education.qld.gov.au/student/Documents/smart-choices-strategy.pdf>
- Western Australian School Canteen Association StarCAP accreditation program (WASCA 2018) <www.waschoolcanteens.org.au/star-cap/>
- In New Zealand, the Heart Foundation has developed Fuelled4life (Heart Foundation 2018) <www.fuelled4life.org.nz/>.

SPORTING VENUES

Participation in sport is strongly encouraged for children and adolescents and sporting clubs and venues are another site where healthy food provisioning can be modelled. The national Good Sports program provides resources for clubs to provide healthier food choices, promote mental health and minimise the consumption of alcohol <http://goodsports.com.au/this-is-good-sports/>.

food and beverage choices is therefore an important consideration. In many other countries (such as the USA and UK) children are provided with lunch, and in some cases breakfast, but this is not the case in Australia. The 'Examples of nutrition interventions' box gives examples of programs, initiatives or guidelines that attempt to govern food provisioning in these settings through the development of supportive environments.

NUTRITION-RELATED CONCERNS DURING CHILDHOOD AND ADOLESCENCE

Restricted diets—vegetarian, vegan, low fat

Strict vegan, macrobiotic and fruitarian diets are not suitable for babies, due to the numerous nutrient deficiencies that could result in cognitive impairment. Due to the high energy and nutrient requirements in infancy, it is difficult to provide sufficient energy and nutrients for an infant on a vegan diet that does not include milk, eggs and milk products, and these diets are therefore not recommended. Mothers following a vegan diet and breastfeeding should also ensure adequate energy and nutrient intakes to decrease the risk of severe cognitive impairment of the infant due to vitamin B-12 deficiency (Agostoni et al. 2008; Truswell 2007). Low-fat diets are also not appropriate for infants, with low-fat milk not encouraged for those under the age of two (NHMRC 2013b).

Food refusal

During the early preschool years, the rate of growth is relatively slow compared with that during infancy. The toddler also learns new skills and becomes more interested in activities other than eating. It is not uncommon for many children in this age group to accept only one or two foods for short periods of time, or to reject new foods (food **neophobia**). This behaviour does not usually pose a nutritional problem and is usually self-limiting. Other children of the same age may continuously demand food. It is important to remember that children will eat when they are hungry unless there is a relevant medical

VEGETARIAN CASE STUDY

Emma is a 16-year-old teenager who has been an ovo-lacto vegetarian for the past two years. Recently, she has been finding it difficult to concentrate and sometimes falls asleep in class. A visit to the GP and subsequent blood tests identify iron deficiency. A diet history reveals the following about Emma's usual food habits.

Meal	Typical example
Breakfast	2 slices of toast 1 glass apple juice
Morning snack	1 muffin or doughnut
Lunch	1 cheese sandwich (white bread) 1 apple 1 can of diet coke or fruit box
Afternoon snack	1 slice of cake 1 mug of hot chocolate
Dinner	1 bowl of pasta with mushroom or tomato sauce with salad 2 scoops of ice cream with chocolate topping 1 cup of tea
Supper	2 sweet biscuits
Other snacks	Chocolate bars, potato crisps, muesli bars
Eats takeaway (2–3/week)	Favourites include Mexican (tacos) or Chinese (fried rice and spring rolls)

ACTIVITY:
- Compare Emma's intake against the Australian Guide to Healthy Eating.
- Using the Australian Food Composition Database or a dietary intake computer program, estimate the amount of dietary iron in her diet.
- What dietary changes would you recommend and why?
- What are the most common causes of iron deficiency?

condition. Alternative foods do not need to be offered if they do not eat the main meal and energy-dense foods and drinks are not required.

Anaemia

Iron deficiency anaemia is the most common nutritional deficiency in both low- and high-income countries. The consequences are particularly important in children because anaemia can impair learning and concentration and weaken immune function. During infancy, anaemia can also cause a delay in both physical and mental development. It also has a serious negative impact on growth and development during adolescence. The Australian Health Survey (2011–2012) found 2.8 per cent of children aged 12–17 years were at risk of anaemia (ABS 2013). The onset of menstruation places adolescent girls at greater risk of iron deficiency, especially in girls with heavy menstrual loss. Adolescent boys also have increased iron requirements due to the considerable growth that goes on during this time (NHMRC 2013b).

In Australia, dietary causes of iron deficiency anaemia are most likely to occur when there is an inadequate intake of foods that are good sources of iron. Children who are particularly susceptible include young children given large quantities of cow's milk (in the absence of foods that are good sources of iron) and children on a vegetarian diet, which is bulky, high in fibre and from which iron is not readily absorbed.

Allergies or intolerances

The prevalence of **food allergies** and intolerances has been increasing, in Australia and globally (Tang & Mullins 2017). The Australasian Society of Clinical Immunology and Allergy has released infant feeding advice to parents aiming to minimise the risk of allergy in their infant (ASCIA 2016). Their advice includes:

- At around six months but not before four months, start to introduce a variety of solid foods, starting with iron-rich foods, while continuing breastfeeding.
- All infants should be given allergenic solid foods including peanut butter, cooked egg, dairy and wheat products in the first year of life. This includes infants at high risk of allergy.
- Exclusion of any particular foods from the maternal diet during pregnancy or breastfeeding is not recommended as this has not been shown to prevent allergies.

Dental caries

Dental caries (tooth decay) affects children from all socioeconomic backgrounds and is largely preventable. A report published by the WHO in 2015 recommended reducing the intake of free sugars to less than 10 per cent of total energy intake to protect against dental caries (WHO 2015). In Australia, the majority of free sugars (81 per cent) are consumed as discretionary foods. In 2011–2012, sugary drink consumption (the main source of added sugars) peaked among 14- to 18-year-olds, with 51 per cent of males and 38 per cent of females in this age group consuming soft drink on the day prior to interview (ABS 2014). The cariogenicity (ability to cause dental decay) of a food is not simply a function of the sugar content or the amount consumed but also depends on frequency of use, effects on saliva production, plaque formation, time of retention on the tooth and its ability to dissolve enamel. These factors can be mitigated with good dental hygiene, fluoride toothpaste and water fluoridation. Tooth decay in children under the age of two is typically due to the consumption of high-sugar fluids and foods. Typically, dental caries occur in children who have access to bottles with milk and other fluids; the teeth are constantly exposed to the sugars in these fluids, leading to decay.

Weight

Worldwide, obesity (an excessive deposition of adipose tissue) is a significant contributor to the burden of chronic disease and disability. Its prevalence is increasing due to overconsumption of energy, a decline in physical activity and an increase in sedentary behaviour. Obesity can develop at any time during childhood and, once established, is difficult to treat. Regular growth monitoring during childhood enables the early detection of excess weight gain relative to height gain, but such monitoring is unfortunately neither routinely practised nor reported in Australia. The prevalence of overweight and obesity in children and adolescents in Australia varies between 18 and 33 per cent (refer to Table 21.9).

In treating obesity in childhood and adolescence, two factors need to be considered. First, very low-energy diets are not suitable as it is difficult to ensure an adequate intake of essential nutrients when energy intake is low; instead, limiting foods that contribute to excess energy, such as discretionary foods (energy-dense/nutrient-poor foods) and beverages (sugar-sweetened) is recommended. Second, obese children and adolescents are often **sedentary** and so more physical activity should be encouraged. Family participation in both dietary and activity strategies is important to ensure children maintain their current weight while growing taller, and to enable their BMI to reach a healthy level.

The WHO Commission on Ending Childhood Obesity has identified a range of actions that should take place in order to address growing global incidence and prevalence of overweight and obesity (WHO 2016a). These strategies for preventing childhood obesity include:

- Implement comprehensive programs that promote the intake of healthy foods and reduce the intake of unhealthy foods and sugar-sweetened beverages. For example: tax on sugar-sweetened beverages.
- Implement comprehensive programs that promote physical activity and reduce sedentary behaviours. For example: ensure that adequate facilities are available on school premises and in public spaces for physical activity.
- Integrate and strengthen guidance for non-communicable disease prevention with current guidance for preconception and antenatal care to reduce risk of childhood obesity. For example: diagnose and manage gestational diabetes.
- Provide guidance on and support for healthy diet, sleep and physical activity in early childhood to ensure children grow appropriately and develop healthy habits. For example: support mothers to breastfeed.
- Implement comprehensive programs that promote healthy school environments, health and nutrition literacy and physical activity. For example: require inclusion of nutrition and health education within the core curriculum of schools.
- Provide family-based, multicomponent, personal behaviour weight management services for children and young people who are obese. (WHO 2016a)

The role of sleep in childhood obesity

Sleep duration and quality in children appear to influence weight gain in children. There are a variety of mechanisms that have been suggested to explain this, including an increase in insulin resistance, changes in the appetite hormones ghrelin and leptin or as-yet unexplained pathways (Felső et al. 2017; Okely et al. 2018).

Adolescent eating patterns

The hallmark of adolescence is change. This includes change in physical characteristics, in psychological development, and in social roles and responsibilities.

Table 21.9: Rates of overweight and obesity and compliance with physical activity recommendations in children aged 2–18

Years	2–3	4–8	9–13	14–18
BOYS				
Overweight/obesity: proportion (%) of population overweight and obese				
	25	20	32	33
Physical activity: proportion (%) of population meeting physical activity recommendations				
	73	46	19	17
GIRLS				
Overweight/obesity: proportion (%) of population overweight and obese				
	18	25	26	28
Physical activity: proportion (%) of population meeting physical activity recommendations				
	78	40	15	15

Source: AIHW (2018)

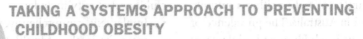

TAKING A SYSTEMS APPROACH TO PREVENTING CHILDHOOD OBESITY

The prevention of obesity in children and adolescents crosses a number of systems: health, business, marketing and so on. Look at the following website, reports and articles. What are the key take-home messages? Discuss possible government and industry solutions. What role can families play in tackling childhood obesity?

Lobstein, T. et al., 2015, 'Child and adolescent obesity: Part of a bigger picture', *Lancet*, 385(9986): 2510–20

Swinburn, B. et al., 2015, 'Strengthening of accountability systems to create healthy food environments and reduce global obesity', *Lancet*, 385(9986): 2534–45

WHO, 2016, *Report of the Commission on Ending Childhood Obesity*, <http://apps.who.int/iris/bitstream/handle/10665/204176/9789241510066_eng.pdf?sequence=1>

World Cancer Research Fund, 2018, *Nourishing: Our policy framework to promote healthy diets and prevent obesity*, <www.wcrf.org/int/policy/nourishing/our-policy-framework-promote-healthy-diets-reduce-obesity>.

One important consequence of these changes is adolescents' increasing control over their own eating patterns. The foods eaten will now depend not solely on family food patterns, but also on many other factors including self-image, peers, the media, cultural and social expectations in relation to body shape and size, access to money for food and the proximity of food outlets. Consumption of snacks both between and instead of meals is a common feature of adolescent diets. The fact that adolescents have higher total energy requirements than young adults is often overlooked. On average, adolescent energy requirements are about 1000 kJ higher per day than those of adults, and consequently there is room for the consumption of some foods with a higher energy density. Although many snacks (chocolate bars, potato chips, crisps, cakes, pies, biscuits and soft drinks) may be high in energy (fat and/or sugar) and relatively low in nutrient content, others can be more nutrient-dense. Fruit, raw vegetables, nuts, cheese, bread, breakfast cereals, eggs, meat and fish can all be eaten in the form of snacks that have a high nutrient concentration.

Other issues for adolescents include dieting behaviour and alcohol consumption. The fear of becoming overweight is particularly strong in adolescent girls, so dieting and other forms of weight-control behaviour are common in this age group. Controlling weight by means of extreme diets (sometimes combined with excessive physical exercise) tends to result in the loss of more water and lean tissue from the body than fat. Moreover, behaviours that adversely affect growth and development during adolescence may also lead to poorer health in later life. When such behaviours continue for any length of time, they constitute an eating disorder. Adolescence can also be a time for experimenting with alcohol and other drugs. Alcohol consumption in this age group is discussed in Chapter 15.

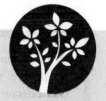

SUMMARY

- Growth occurs throughout childhood but increases markedly at adolescence before ceasing altogether.
- Since different parts of the body develop at different rates, changes occur not only in body size but also in body proportions, body composition and in the stage of maturity of different body systems.
- Recommendations for energy and nutrient intake during infancy, childhood and adolescence are based mainly on the observed intakes of healthy children and on data about the amounts of nutrients accumulated in the body during the period of growth.
- Energy requirements of children and adolescents are higher than those of adults when expressed per kilogram of body weight; however, with the possible exception of calcium, children and adolescents do not require a diet that has a higher nutrient density than that of adults.
- Breastfeeding exclusively for the first six months of life is internationally recommended for optimal growth and wellbeing. Thereafter there should be the appropriate introduction of complementary foods, including those high in iron.
- Breastfeeding is a learned skill and requires a range of policy, community and individual factors to ensure that it is a cultural norm.
- Australian children are not consuming the required numbers of vegetable serves, are obtaining more than one-third of their energy from discretionary foods, are receiving inadequate calcium (especially in older age groups) and are consuming over three times the acceptable limit of sodium.
- The most commonly encountered nutrition-related concerns during childhood and adolescence include food refusal, anaemia, dental caries, allergies and intolerances, and obesity.
- Ensuring optimal nutrition across the lifespan and the prevention of childhood overweight and obesity requires a systems approach with engagement of a wide range of stakeholders in a range of settings.

KEY TERMS

Discretionary foods: foods and drinks that are not necessary to provide the nutrients the body needs, but that may add variety. Many of these are high in saturated fats, sugars, salt and/or alcohol, and are therefore described as energy dense. They can be included sometimes in small amounts by those who are physically active, but are not a necessary part of the diet (NHMRC 2013a).

Electrolytes: substances that produce electrically conducting solution when dissolved in solvents such as water. They help move nutrients into and waste products out of the body's cells. The five electrolytes are calcium, chlorine, magnesium, potassium and sodium.

Fat-free mass (FFM): lean body mass plus the mass of the skeleton.

Food allergy: where a food causes an immunology reaction involving immunoglobulin E (IgE), causing a range of symptoms that can be severe and life-threatening. Onset is usually immediate. Food intolerance does not involve IgE but the chemicals in foods can cause symptoms. Food intolerances can occur immediately but typically take 12–24 hours before onset; they are dependent on how much of the food is consumed.

Galactosaemia: an inborn error of metabolism. Those born with this error cannot break down galactose, which makes up half of lactose. Other inborn errors of metabolism include maple sugar urine disease and phenylketonuria.

Gestational age: the developmental age of the newborn from the point of conception.

Neophobia: dislike of the new; in food terms, refers to an innate distrust of new foods. Neophobia was thought to have developed as an evolutionary trait protecting humans from consuming foods that were potentially life threatening. Food neophobia manifests as picky or fussy eating in children. A child needs to try a new food between ten and fifteen times before it will be accepted.

Puberty: the onset of physical changes that occur in a child's body as it matures towards sexual reproduction.

Sedentary: refers to the time spent sitting or lying down. This can be in relation to watching TV, screen time or desk time. There is evidence that the amount of sedentary time, independent of physical activity, is related to increased risk of non-communicable disease.

Sepsis: overwhelming and life-threatening response to infection that can lead to tissue damage, organ failure and death.

ACKNOWLEDGEMENT

This chapter has been modified and updated from chapters written by Jan Payne (Infant Nutrition), which appeared in the third edition of *Food and Nutrition*, and by Ingrid H.E. Rutishuaser and Kelly L. Stewart (Childhood and Adolescence), which appeared in the second and third editions of *Food and Nutrition* respectively.

REFERENCES

ABS, 2013, *Australian Health Survey: Biomedical results for chronic diseases 2011–12'*, <www.abs.gov.au/AUSSTATS/abs@.nsf/0/D31F2F311CA9936ACA257BBB00121DB8?Opendocument>, accessed 20 June 2018

—— 2014, *Australian Health Survey: Nutrition First Results—Food and nutrients, 2011–12*, <www.abs.gov.au/ausstats/abs@.nsf/Lookup/by%20Subject/4364.0.55.007~2011-12~Main%20Features~Key%20Findings~1>, accessed 20 June 2018

—— 2015, *National Health Survey: First results, 2014–15*, <www.abs.gov.au/ausstats/abs@.nsf/Lookup/by%20Subject/4364.0.55.001~2014-15~Main%20Features~Children's%20risk%20factors~31>, accessed 20 June 2018

Admyre, C., Johansson, S.M., Qazi, K.R., Filén, J.-J., Lahesmaa, R. et al., 2007, 'Exosomes with immune modulatory features are present in human breast milk', *Journal of Immunology, 179*(3): 1969, doi:10.4049/jimmunol.179.3.1969

Agostoni, C., Decsi, T., Fewtrell, M., Goulet, O., Kolacek, S. et al., 2008, 'Complementary feeding: A commentary by the ESPGHAN Committee on Nutrition', *Journal of Pediatric Gastroenterology and Nutrition, 46*(1): 99–110, doi:10.1097/01.mpg.0000304464.60788.bd

AIHW, 2011, *2010 Australian National Infant Feeding Survey: Indicator results* <www.aihw.gov.au/getmedia/af2fe025-637e-4c09-ba03-33e69f49aba7/13632.pdf.aspx?inline=true>, accessed 30 November 2018

—— 2018, *Nutrition Across the Life Stages* <www.aihw.gov.au/getmedia/fc5ad42e-08f5-4f9a-9ca4-723cacaa510d/aihw-phe-227.pdf.aspx?inline=true>, accessed 30 November 2018

Andreas, N.J., Kampmann, B. & Mehring Le-Doare, K., 2015, 'Human breast milk: A review on its composition and bioactivity', *Early Human Development, 91*(11): 629–35, doi:10.1016/j.earlhumdev.2015.08.013

ASCIA, 2016, *ASCIA Guidelines: Infant feeding and allergy prevention*, <www.allergy.org.au/patients/allergy-prevention/ascia-guidelines-for-infant-feeding-and-allergy-prevention>, accessed 30 November 2018

Australian Government, 2014, *National Healthy School Canteens: Guidelines for healthy foods and drinks supplied in school canteens*, <www.health.gov.au/internet/main/publishing.nsf/content/5FFB6A30ECEE9321CA257BF0001DAB17/$File/Canteen%20guidelines.pdf>, accessed 14 February 2019

Benton, D. & ILSI Europe, 2008, 'The influence of children's diet on their cognition and behavior', *European Journal of Nutrition, 47*(3): 25–37, doi:10.1007/s00394-008-3003-x

Bundy, D.A.P., de Silva, N., Horton, S., Jamison, D.T. & Patton, G.C. (eds), 2017, *Child and Adolescent Health and Development: Disease control priorities* (3rd edn), Washington, DC: World Bank.

Byrne, R., Jansen, E. & Daniels, L., 2017, 'Perceived fussy eating in Australian children at 14 months of age and subsequent use of maternal feeding practices at 2 years', *International Journal of Behavioral Nutrition and Physical Activity, 14*(1): 123, doi:10.1186/s12966-017-0582-z

de la Torre Gomez, C., Goreham, R.V., Bech Serra, J.J., Nann, T. & Kussmann, M., 2018, '"Exosomics"—a review of biophysics, biology and biochemistry of exosomes with a focus on human breast milk', *Frontiers in Genetics, 9*(92), doi:10.3389/fgene.2018.00092

Eriksen, K.G., Christensen, S.H., Lind, M.V. & Michaelsen, K.F., 2018, 'Human milk composition and infant growth', *Current Opinion in Clinical Nutrition and Metabolic Care, 21*(3): 200–6, doi:10.1097/MCO.0000000000000466

The Ethics Centre, 2016, *Annual Report: Marketing in Australia of Infant Formula 2014–2015*, <www.health.gov.au/internet/main/publishing.nsf/Content/phd-brfeed-apmaif_14>, accessed 14 February 2019

—— 2018, *Annual Report: Marketing in Australia of Infant Formula 2016–2017* <http://health.gov.au/internet/main/publishing.nsf/Content/E7680032A4A919CCCA2582940013C096/$File/MAIF-Tribunal-Annual-Report-2016-17-300118.pdf>, accessed 14 February 2019

Felső, R., Lohner, S., Hollódy, K., Erhardt, É. & Molnár, D., 2017, 'Relationship between sleep duration and childhood obesity: Systematic review including the potential underlying mechanisms', *Nutrition, Metabolism and Cardiovascular Diseases, 27*(9): 751–61, doi:10.1016/j.numecd.2017.07.008

Finnane, J.M., Jansen, E., Mallan, K.M. & Daniels, L.A., 2017, 'Mealtime structure and responsive feeding practices are associated with less food fussiness and more food enjoyment in children', *Journal of Nutrition Education and Behavior, 49*(1): 11–18.e11, doi:10.1016/j.jneb.2016.08.007

Foote, K.D. & Marriott, L.D., 2003, 'Weaning of infants', *Archives of Disease in Childhood, 88*(6): 488–92, doi:10.1136/adc.88.6.488

Gracey, M., Hetzel, B., Smallwood, R., Strauss, B. & Tasman-Jones, C., 1989, *Responsibility for Nutrition Diagnosis: A report by the Nutrition Working Party of the Social Issues Committee of the Royal Australasian College of Physicians*, London: Smith-Gordon

Gray, S., 2017, 'Education extra: Breastfeeding and the role of infant formula', *Australian Pharmacist, 36*(9): 34–37, <https://search.informit.com.au/documentSummary;dn=638022959858747;res=IELHEA>, accessed 14 February 2019

Heart Foundation, 2018, *Fuelled 4 Life*, <www.fuelled4life.org.nz/>, accessed 20 June 2018

Hector, D., King, L., Webb, K. & Heywood, P., 2005, 'Factors affecting breastfeeding practices: Applying a conceptual framework', *New South Wales Public Health Bulletin, 16*(4): 52–5, doi:10.1071/NB05013

Horta, B., Victora, C. & WHO, 2013a, *Long-Term Effects of Breastfeeding: A systematic review*, <http://apps.who.int/iris/handle/10665/79198>, accessed 14 February 2019

—— 2013b, *Short-Term Effects of Breastfeeding: A systematic review on the benefits of breastfeeding on diarrhoea and pneumonia mortality*, <http://apps.who.int/iris/handle/10665/95585>, accessed 14 February 2019

Jensen, C.L. & Lapillonne, A., 2009, 'Docosahexaenoic acid and lactation', *Prostaglandins Leukotrienes and Essential Fatty Acids, 81*(2–3): 175–8, doi:10.1016/j.plefa.2009.05.006

Joshi, P.A., Smith, J., Vale, S. & Campbell, D.E., 2019, 'The Australasian Society of Clinical Immunology and Allergy infant feeding for allergy prevention guidelines', *Medical Journal of Australia, 210*: 89–93, doi:10.5694/mja2.12102

Kent, G., 2015, 'Global infant formula: Monitoring and regulating the impacts to protect human health', *International Breastfeeding Journal, 10*: 6, doi:10.1186/s13006-014-0020-7

Kramer, M.S. & Kakuma, R., 2012, 'Optimal duration of exclusive breastfeeding', *Cochrane Database of Systematic Reviews, 8*: Cd003517, doi:10.1002/14651858.CD003517.pub2

Krebs, N.F. & Hambidge, K.M., 2007, 'Complementary feeding: Clinically relevant factors affecting timing and composition', *American Journal of Clinical Nutrition, 85*(2): 639S–45S, doi:10.1093/ajcn/85.2.639S

Lässer, C., Seyed Alikhani, V., Ekström, K., Eldh, M., Torregrosa Paredes, P. et al., 2011, 'Human saliva, plasma and breast milk exosomes contain RNA: Uptake by macrophages', *Journal of Translational Medicine, 9*(1): 9, doi:10.1186/1479-5876-9-9

Lobstein, T., Jackson-Leach, R., Moodie, M.L., Hall, K.D., Gortmaker, S.L. et al., 2015, 'Child and adolescent obesity: Part of a bigger picture', *Lancet, 385*(9986): 2510–20, doi:10.1016/S0140-6736(14)61746-3

Magarey, A., Mauch, C., Mallan, K., Perry, R., Elovaris, R. et al., 2016, 'Child dietary and eating behavior outcomes up to 3.5 years after an early feeding intervention: The NOURISH RCT', *Obesity, 24*(7): 1537–45, doi:10.1002/oby.21498

Malina, R.M., Bouchard, C. & Beunen, G., 1988, 'Human growth: Selected aspects of current research on well-nourished children', *Annual Review of Anthropology, 17*(1): 187–219, doi:10.1146/annurev.an.17.100188.001155

Mann, J. & Truswell, S., 2007, *Essentials of Human Nutrition* (3rd edn), Oxford: Oxford University Press

Meyer, R., Groetch, M. & Venter, C., 2018, 'When should infants with cow's milk protein allergy use an amino acid formula? A practical guide', *Journal of Allergy and Clinical Immunology: In practice, 6*(2): 383–99, doi:10.1016/j.jaip.2017.09.003

Munyaka, P.M., Khafipour, E. & Ghia, J.-E., 2014, 'External influence of early childhood establishment of gut microbiota and subsequent health implications', *Frontiers in Pediatrics, 2*: 109, doi:10.3389/fped.2014.00109

NHMRC, 2009, *Nutrient Reference Values for Australia and New Zealand (2006)*, <www.nrv.gov.au/home>, accessed 20 June 2018

—— 2013a, *Australian Dietary Guidelines*, <www.nhmrc.gov.au/about-us/publications/australian-dietary-guidelines>, accessed 17 July 2019

—— 2013b, *Infant Feeding Guidelines: Information for Health Workers (2012)* (N56), <www.nhmrc.gov.au/guidelines-publications/n56>, accessed 14 February 2019

NSW Government & Heart Foundation, 2018, *Healthy Kids: About Munch & Move*, <www.healthykids.nsw.gov.au/campaigns-programs/about-munch-move.aspx>, accessed 20 June 2018

Nutrition Australia QLD, 2018, *LEAPS*, <https://naqld.org/category/leaps/>, accessed 20 June 2018

Okely, A.D., Tremblay, M.S., Reilly, J.J., Draper, C.E. & Bull, F., 2018, 'Physical activity, sedentary behaviour, and sleep: Movement behaviours in early life', *Lancet Child & Adolescent Health, 2*(4): 233–5, doi:10.1016/S2352-4642(18)30070-1

Paul, I.M., Schaefer, E.W., Miller, J.R., Kuzniewicz, M.W., Li, S.X. et al., 2016, 'Weight change nomograms for the first month after birth', *Pediatrics, 138*(6): e20162625, doi:10.1542/peds.2016-2625

Queensland Government, 2016, *Smart Choices: Healthy food and drink supply strategy for Queensland schools*, <http://education.qld.gov.au/schools/healthy/food-drink-strategy.html>, accessed 14 February 2019

Rogol, A.D., Roemmich, J.N. & Clark, P.A., 2002, 'Growth at puberty', *Journal of Adolescent Health, 31*(6, Suppl.): 192–200, doi:10.1016/S1054-139X(02)00485-8

Rollins, N.C., Bhandari, N., Hajeebhoy, N., Horton, S., Lutter, C.K. et al., 2016, 'Why invest, and what it will take to improve breastfeeding practices?', *Lancet, 387*(10017): 491–504, doi:10.1016/S0140-6736(15)01044-2

Romo-Palafox, M.J. & Harris, J.L., 2017, 'Toddler formulas: Nutritional value and marketing claims', *FASEB Journal, 31*(1 Suppl.): 169.165, doi:10.1096/fasebj.31.1_supplement.169.5

Royal New Zealand Plunket Society, 2017, *Breastfeeding Data: Analysis of 2010–2015 data, New Zealand'*, <www.plunket.org.nz/assets/PDFs/Breast-feeding-Data-2010-2015.pdf>, accessed 17 February 2019

Rutishauser, I., 2002, 'Infant nutrition', in M. Wahlqvist (ed.), *Food and Nutrition: Australia and New Zealand* (2nd edn), Sydney: Allen & Unwin, pp. 302–11

Stuebe, A., 2009, 'The risks of not breastfeeding for mothers and infants', *Reviews in Obstetrics and Gynecology, 2*(4): 222, doi:10.3909/riog0093

Swinburn, B., Kraak, V., Rutter, H., Vandevijvere, S., Lobstein, T. et al., 2015, 'Strengthening of accountability systems to create healthy food environments and reduce global obesity', *Lancet, 385*(9986): 2534–45, doi:10.1016/S0140-6736(14)61747-5

Tang, M.L. & Mullins, R.J., 2017, 'Food allergy: Is prevalence increasing?', *Internal Medicine Journal, 47*(3): 256–61, doi:10.1111/imj.13362

Tanner, J.M., 1962, *Growth at Adolescence* (2nd edn), Oxford: Blackwell Scientific Publications

Tanner, J.M., Whitehouse, R.H., Marshall, W.A. & Carter, B.S., 1975, 'Prediction of adult height from height, bone age, and occurrence of menarche, at ages 4 to 16 with allowance for midparent height', *Archives of Disease in Childhood, 41*(1): 14–26, doi:10.1136/adc.50.1.14

Truswell, A.S., 2007, 'Vitamin B12', *Nutrition & Dietetics, 64*(suppl 4): S120–25, doi:10.1111/j.1747-0080.2007.00198.x

Udall, J.N., 2007, 'Infant feeding: Initiation, problems, approaches', *Current Problems in Pediatric and Adolescent Health Care, 37*(10): 374–99, doi:10.1016/j.cppeds.2007.09.001

UNICEF, WHO, 1000 Days, & Alive & Thrive, 2017, *Nurturing the Health and Wealth of Nations: The investment case for breastfeeding,* <www.who.int/nutrition/publications/infantfeeding/global-bf-collective-investmentcase/en/>, accessed 14 February 2019

Victora, C.G., Bahl, R., Barros, A.J.D., França, G.V.A., Horton, S. et al., 2016, 'Breastfeeding in the 21st century: Epidemiology, mechanisms, and lifelong effect', *Lancet, 387*(10017): 475–90, doi:10.1016/S0140-6736(15)01024-7

WASCA, 2018, *Western Australia School Canteen Association Inc.*, <www.waschoolcanteens.org.au/star-cap/>, accessed 20 June 2018

WHO, 2006a, *Adolescent Nutrition: A review of the situation in selected South-East Asian countries* (SEA-NUT-163), <http://apps.who.int/iris/handle/10665/204764>, accessed 14 February 2019

—— 2006b, *WHO Child Growth Standards: Length/height for age, weight-for-age, weight-for-length, weight-for-height and body mass index-for-age, methods and development,* <www.who.int/childgrowth/standards/Technical_report.pdf>, accessed 14 February 2019

—— 2007, *Growth Reference Data for 5–19y,* <www.who.int/growthref/en/>, accessed 21 June 2018

—— 2008, *Indicators for Assessing Infant and Young Child Feeding Practices, Part 1: Definitions* (1), <www.who.int/maternal_child_adolescent/documents/9789241596664/en/>, accessed 14 February 2019

—— 2015, *Guideline: Sugars intake for adults and children* (WHO/NMH/NHD/15.2), <www.who.int/nutrition/publications/guidelines/sugars_intake/en/>, accessed 14 February 2019

—— 2016a, *Report of the Commission on Ending Childhood Obesity,* <http://apps.who.int/iris/bitstream/handle/10665/204176/9789241510066_eng.pdf>, accessed 30 November 2018

—— 2016b, *Updates on HIV and Infant Feeding,* <www.who.int/maternal_child_adolescent/documents/hiv-infant-feeding-2016/en/>, accessed 14 February 2019

WHO & UNICEF, 2003, *Global Strategy for Infant and Young Child Feeding,* <www.who.int/nutrition/publications/infantfeeding/9241562218/en/>, accessed 14 February 2019

—— 2009, *Acceptable Medical Reasons for Use of Breast-Milk Substitutes,* <www.who.int/nutrition/publications/infantfeeding/WHO_NMH_NHD_09.01/en/>, accessed 14 February 2019

WHO, UNICEF & IBFAN, 2016, *Marketing of Breast-Milk Substitutes: National implementation of the international code* (Status report 2016), <www.who.int/nutrition/publications/infantfeeding/code_report2018/en/>, accessed 14 February 2019

WHO, UNICEF & World Bank Group, 2016, *Advancing Early Childhood Development: From science to scale* (The Lancet Series), <www.who.int/maternal_child_adolescent/documents/early-child-development-lancet-series/en/>, accessed 14 February 2019

World Cancer Research Fund, 2018, *Nourishing: Our policy framework to promote healthy diets and prevent obesity,* <www.wcrf.org/int/policy/nourishing/our-policy-framework-promote-healthy-diets-reduce-obesity>, accessed 14 February 2019

{CHAPTER 22}
ADULTS AND THE LATER YEARS

Danielle Gallegos

OBJECTIVES

- Describe the impact of ageing on nutritional status and the role of nutrition in ageing.
- Explain the risk factors for altered nutrition in ageing.
- Formulate food-based recommendations for healthy ageing.

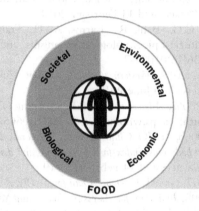

INTRODUCTION

Life is a journey and adulthood, and the later years of life that follow it, represent no less of a changing experience than the childhood and adolescence that precede them. The life-course approach identifies the early years and pregnancy as key points where adult risk can be minimised. However, this approach also recognises that each life-stage, including adulthood and old age, have unique nutritional requirements and opportunities to maximise health. Adulthood is recognised as a period of independence and self-sufficiency, with responsibilities attributed according to expectations of society, family, community, workplace or various organisations, which may range from high to low, or even zero. However, an adult's nutritional wellbeing may often be precarious, depending on the socioecological frameworks supporting that individual.

An adult's nutritional security is affected by a range of considerations.

- Is there a functional extended family in the form of a spouse or partner, siblings, children,
a network consisting of friends or workmates or organisational associates?
- How accessible and responsive might these human resources be?
- What are the individual's physical resource development and management skills like?
- Does or could food play a social role in this person's life?
- Do stressful events or periods evoke food or eating as a possible risk or solution?

Our ability to live longer is partly attributable to better nutrition (from the intra-uterine environment right through to old age) but also to a range of other factors such as:

- reducing substance abuse (alcohol, drugs)
- greater recreational opportunities
- improved health care (for example, reduced infant and maternal mortality, earlier diagnosis and management of cancers and heart disease)
- better educational and economic opportunities
- improved housing (especially less crowding)
- more supportive social systems.

Keeping an elderly population well is of great importance for the individuals themselves, for the wellbeing of society in general (the transfer of knowledge and skills to younger people and a reduced burden on others), and for reasons related to managing available resources to care for the aged. As you will see later in this chapter, the accumulating effects of years of poor eating habits can increase the risk of many health conditions as one grows older. Yet it is never too late to change.

This chapter will focus on the later years, when an individual is an adult and then enters into old age. It will explore the specific food and nutrition elements that affect people as they get older.

WHAT IS OLD AGE?

Age as described for children and adolescents is a biological as well as a sociocultural construct. Adulthood is culturally considered to be eighteen years and over in Australia and New Zealand. Ageing may be defined as **chronological age** or **biological age**.

Recent studies have indicated that people are less biologically old than they used to be at the same chronological age and that this difference may be as much as ten years of biological age (Rowe & Kahn 2015). In Australia, 65 years and over is often referred to as elderly, as this is the age adults become eligible for the age pension. In other cultures, 'old age' begins at 50.

The global average life expectancy at birth in 2015 was 71.4 years. In African nations, average life expectancy ranges from 50.1 years (in Sierra Leone) to 66.7 years (Senegal) (WHO 2017). In other countries the average life expectancy has exceeded 80 years: the Japanese population live the longest, at 83.7 years; Australia has an average life expectancy of 82.8 years and New Zealand 81.6 years. Women tend to live longer than men and in Australia and New Zealand average life expectancy for women is 84.8 and 83.3 years respectively, compared to 80.0 years for men in both countries. Life expectancy takes into consideration all-cause mortality, including conflict and natural disasters.

HOW LONG-LIVED IS YOUR FAMILY?

Think about your own ancestors (great-grandparents, great-aunts, great-uncles). What were their main causes of death? How old were they when they died? Were they rich or poor? How much education did they have? What factors may have contributed to their deaths? Think about where they grew up, the level of health care they had access to and any other factors that may have contributed to either a longer or shorter lifespan.

Think about your relatives over the age of 65.

- Are they still living independently?
- What do you think contributes to them being able to live independently?
- If they are reliant on care, why is this the case?
- What sort of support do they rely on from others and from your own family?

IS THE POPULATION AGEING?

It is predicted that between 2015 and 2030 the number of older people (aged over 60 years) in the world will grow by 56 per cent to more than 1.4 billion; and that by 2030 the number of older people will outnumber those aged 0–9 years. Worldwide, 60 per cent of women and 52 per cent of men born in 2000–2005 will survive to their 80th birthday (except in Africa), compared to 40 per cent of men and women born in 1950–1955 (UN 2015). By 2052, it is predicted that six million people (25 per cent of the population) will be 65 and over (US Census Bureau 2018). Like other nations, Australia is ageing (Figure 22.1). Centenarians have increased by 8.5 per cent per year over the past 25 years. The 85+ age group represented 0.12 per cent of the Australian population aged 65 years and over in 2006 (3000 individuals); by 2020, this number is expected to increase to 12,000 (Richmond 2008) (see Figure 22.2 for changes over time). However, individuals do not appear to exceed a maximal lifespan of about 120 years. This may change as biotechnology, ways of living, and health care develop in favour of greater longevity.

THE PHYSIOLOGICAL, BEHAVIOURAL AND SOCIAL CONTRIBUTORS TO AGEING

Genes have a strong influence on biological age; it is now believed that factors such as healthy eating, physical activity, the management of stress, decreased substance abuse (including tobacco and alcohol) and

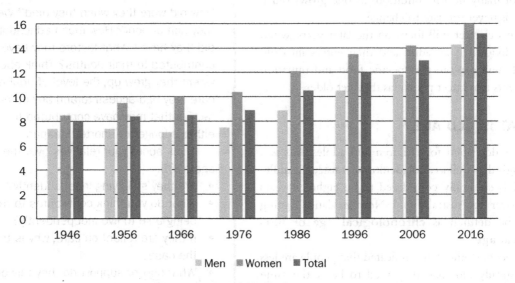

Figure 22.1: Proportion (%) of the population aged 65+ (1946–2016)
Source: ABS (2014b), (2017a)

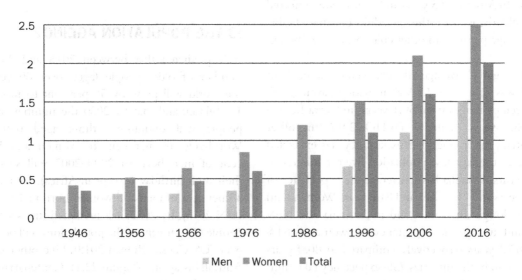

Figure 22.2: Proportion (%) of the population aged 85+ (1946–2016)
Source: ABS (2014b), (2017a)

quality of life also have a strong influence. You may be able to remain biologically younger as you age, if you look after yourself in your younger adult years. The question remains: what aspects of ageing are biologically inevitable—having to do, for example, with the programmed death of cells (apoptosis)—and how much is related to accumulation of risk over time?

Successful ageing from a life-course perspective is not a static snapshot of function at a point in time. Rather, ageing is considered lifelong with late-life health outcomes meaning there are opportunities for growth and adaptation as well as intervention across the lifespan (Stowe & Cooney 2014). The three key factors for successful ageing have been identified as:
1. low risk of disease and disease-related disability
2. maintenance of high mental and physical function
3. continued engagement with life, which includes relations with others and productive activity, either paid or volunteered (Rowe & Kahn 2015).

Poor eating habits accumulated over the life-course can increase the risk of health conditions and disease. Food habits, however, are amenable to modification. The prevention of chronic diseases should commence early in life, but significant reductions in **morbidity** and **mortality** in those aged over 70 are also possible by more optimal healthy eating and physical activity — in other words, it is never too late to start. In fact, it is possible to compress morbidity into the last years of life—not necessarily to increase lifespan but to increase **health–span**.

Several of the health problems and bodily changes experienced by older adults, which previously have been attributed to the 'normal ageing process', are increasingly being recognised as being linked to personal behaviour or environmental factors. For example, declines in lean body mass and increases in body fat which tend to occur as people grow older cannot entirely be due to the ageing process. Social and physical activity and adequate nutrient and phytonutrient intakes are now thought to be instrumental in the ability to compress morbidity towards the end of life. That is, you only become unwell or unable to function for a very short period prior to death. This compression of morbidity is one of the cornerstones of successful ageing (Seals et al. 2016).

Sometimes the assumption is made that, after the age of 65 or 70, changes made to the way you live will no longer have significant benefits. However, several recent studies reveal that improvements in nutrition and regular physical activity can benefit health even in advanced old age (Marengoni et al. 2018; Martinez-Gomez et al. 2017). For example, older muscles are just as responsive to strength training exercises as young muscles. Nonagenarians have shown impressive increases in muscle mass, muscle strength and walking speed with weight training programs (Cadore et al. 2014). Chronological age is, therefore, not a justification for deciding whether it is worthwhile to pursue change. Behavioural risk factors (such as not eating regularly, lack of regular physical activity, overweight and smoking) have been shown to remain predictors of seventeen-year mortality even in people aged over 70 (Horwath et al. 1999).

What happens at the cellular level in ageing?

Bodily processes do age and there is recognition that there is progressive deterioration of cellular processes in all cells. The accumulation of cellular damage limits the capacity of tissues to regenerate and this damage may explain why it is difficult to maintain control over biological **homeostasis**. These changes at the cellular level are summarised in Figure 22.3.

The process of cellular ageing eventually alters physiological functioning. However, many bodily functions remain relatively unaffected to about 75 years of age when, on average, they start to decrease more noticeably. Nutritionally related health problems are often compounded in later life by the reduced physiological function of many organs. For example, reduced cardiac reserve means that an added salt load may tip someone into heart failure when otherwise it would not.

Social changes in adulthood and later life

In addition to the physiological and functional changes that occur as bodies get older, there are a number of social changes as individuals move

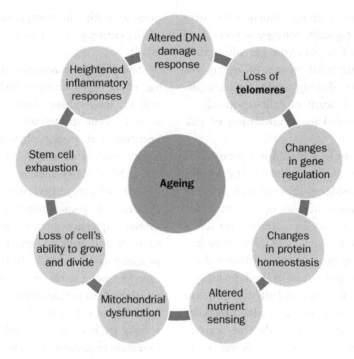

Figure 22.3: Cellular changes that occur with ageing

Source: Developed from López-Otín et al. (2013)

through adulthood. One of the first is moving away from the parental home and creating a new family unit. Food purchases and preparation, as well as eating patterns, are likely to change. There are many opportunities for preventive nutrition and health in families, through growing food, shopping, cooking, eating and minimising food waste together. The family unit can begin, therefore, to secure food-related

EXPLORING THE FOOD OF YOUR GRANDPARENTS OR GREAT-GRANDPARENTS

We all have an individual food culture that is developed over time from our early childhood experiences, shaped by our economic and environmental circumstances and by beliefs. All of us have family food practices that transcend time. Some of these may be based on certain cultural or religious patterns; others may be family-generated.

Find a member of your extended family and talk to them about the foods of their youth and what their parents prepared for everyday meals or for celebrations. What were the major influences on the types of foods they consumed? What was their favourite dish/meal? Are there any foods/dishes that they still prepare that were handed down through the generations?

If you have the opportunity, take the time to get the family member to teach you how to make the food/dish. Note the recipe and share with others. What are the similarities/differences in these dishes?

advantages for later years. In individualistic societies, such as Australia and New Zealand, the elderly are often left to fend for themselves. However, this is potentially a missed opportunity for intergenerational transfer of experience, knowledge and skills.

Employment

Not every adult person easily finds a job, and this can mean limited food-purchasing power and a need to choose foods carefully in order to maintain an adequate nutrient intake. Employment brings with it new eating routines, changed economic circumstances and new peer group pressures, each with possible effects on nutritional status and physical activity. The transition out of full-time paid employment also

impacts on food choices and eating patterns. There are changes in economic circumstances (positive and negative, which can increase and decrease food consumption respectively) as well as changes in routines and influential others.

Household and housing conditions

In Australia in 2011, 56 per cent of older people lived in a private dwelling with their partner, although this was the case for only 23 per cent of those aged 85 years or more. One-quarter of older people lived alone, and 64 per cent lived with at least one relative (spouse, sibling or children). Two per cent of those aged 65–74, 6 per cent of 75- to 84-year-olds and 26 per cent of those 85 years

---

AGED CARE SYSTEMS IN AUSTRALIA

Unlike many other countries, care for older people in Australia is not necessarily left solely to families. As women have increasingly entered the paid workforce, the traditional role of caring for the elderly has been outsourced. In Australia, there are a number of options that are primarily focused on keeping older people in their homes for as long as possible. To be eligible for government-funded services, all older people need to undergo an Aged Care Assessment to determine their eligibility for different levels of care.

CARE IN THE HOME

There are four levels of care in the home available:

- basic care needs, such as help with shopping and cooking, social support and activities of daily living
- low-level care adds the loan of equipment and some nursing assistance
- intermediate care needs add on medication management, assistance with memory and allied health support
- high care needs are for complex cases who would be eligible to enter into an aged care facility.

RESIDENTIAL AGED CARE

For older people unable to stay in their own home due to significant disability and who require ongoing 24-hour support, residential aged care may be an option. Residential aged care is subsidised by the Commonwealth government and is regulated under the *Aged Care Act 1997*. Providers of residential care are regularly assessed and accredited by the Aged Care Quality Agency to ensure quality standards are met. The reports are available publicly (Australian Government 2017).

and over lived in accommodation where they were cared for. In the older age group, this is a decrease from 1991, when 39 per cent of older adults were living in aged care accommodation; this reflects policies related to 'ageing in place' strategies (ABS 2013b).

A household is where there is commensality or food-sharing, which enables it to be the basic food system unit in a community. Housing of the adult and family can influence food intake patterns in several ways—for example according to:

- whether there is a designated eating place in the home
- the availability of cooking facilities and what kind, food storage and what type (shelf, refrigeration, freezer, access of pests) and food preparation hygiene and safety
- the extent to which home production of fruits, vegetables, and herbs is possible
- proximity of neighbourhood shops, shopping centre or food market (for fruit, vegetables, fish and meat)
- locality—whether the household is located in a rural town, a provincial city or a major metropolitan centre.

Maintaining a separate independent household is often a goal for older people. However, housing can be expensive, and cognitive and physical declines can interrupt the ability to source and prepare foods. Services such as Meals on Wheels, transportation to shopping centres and in-home assistance can help to maintain independence and food security. However, a small number of older people are unable to continue to manage in their own homes; in these cases, aged care facilities may provide the assistance required.

Physical activity

Sporting and recreational patterns are likely to change in adulthood, usually in the direction of reduced physical activity, with the risks of positive energy balance and overweight. Finding sporting and recreational activities that give enjoyment and fit in with time, economic and social constraints is

important to ensure lifelong physical activity. The type of physical activity can play an important role in the health of older people. In addition to **aerobic activity**, older people are encouraged to undertake activities to enhance their balance on three or more days a week and resistance (or strength) training to prevent declines in muscle mass on two or more days a week (Bauman et al. 2016).

FOOD AND NUTRIENT REQUIREMENTS IN THE LATER YEARS

Several landmark studies by the International Union of Nutritional Sciences, known as 'Food Habits in Later Life' (FHILL) and the SENECA studies, have shown that in long-lived cultures in Australia, Europe and Asia, a biodiverse dietary pattern, rather than any nutrient or food alone in later life, was most able to predict survival (Kouris-Blazos et al. 2007; Lee et al. 2011; Trichopoulou et al. 1995). Foods that have disproportionate advantage appear to be legumes (Chang et al. 2011; Darmadi-Blackberry et al. 2004; Foyer et al. 2016) and fish (Li et al. 2019; Wahlqvist et al. 1989). The findings in Greece, which were assessed in relation to the traditional diet in Crete, have provided the basis of what has come to be known as the Mediterranean diet, which provides a simplification of the generalisability of biodiversity as a dietary principle for optimal health (Knoops et al. 2004; Kouris-Blazos et al. 1995) (see Chapter 19).

As people age, nutrient requirements may be altered. The major challenge for older adults is ensuring a nutrient-dense diet that has, among other characteristics, adequate protein to maintain muscle mass and micronutrients/phytonutrients for health and wellbeing.

Some of these at-risk nutrients in older adults and the potential reasons for changes in requirements are summarised below. Table 22.1 summarises the changes to macronutrient and fluid requirements in older adults. Tables 22.2 and 22.3 summarise changes to micronutrient requirements for vitamins and minerals respectively.

Table 22.1: Changes to macronutrient and fluid requirements in older adults

Nutrient	Changes to requirements	Causes
Energy	Energy requirements in the elderly are reduced. Basal metabolic rate (BMR) (see Chapter 13) progressively declines by 1–2% per decade. Adjusted for changes in fat-free mass, BMR is 5% lower in older adults than in younger adults (Baum et al. 2016).	Loss of appetite (related to taste acuity, decreased activity, medications, mood), changes in social circumstances—limiting the ability to procure or prepare food or chronic conditions including changes in cognitive function.
Protein	Protein requirements in the elderly increase. It is more difficult for older people to maintain positive nitrogen balance (see Chapter 10), as there is age-related **anabolic resistance** to dietary protein. Optimal intake is thought to be 1.0–1.3 g/kg body weight (Nowson & O'Connell 2015). Protein balance tends to decline due to a loss of fat-free mass and gain of less metabolically active fat; increased sedentary behaviour and reduced physical activity; and insulin resistance (Haran et al. 2012).	Decreased appetite, changes in social circumstances and the presence of chronic conditions. Poor dentition and dysphagia (the inability to swallow) (see Table 22.7 for more detail) can also contribute by making consumption of some protein sources (for example, meat) difficult to chew and swallow.
Fluid	Fluid consumption decreases with age (Scherer et al. 2016). The amount of fluid required on a daily basis fluctuates based on environmental conditions and health. The NRVs recommend between 2.8 and 3.4 L/day for women and men respectively (NHMRC 2006). Fluid balance in older adults is much more difficult to maintain; mild dehydration or overload can cause significant shifts in electrolytes. Acute illness that causes diarrhoea or vomiting or heat stress can easily tip older people into dangerous dehydration.	Water homeostasis is challenging in the elderly for a number of reasons including: physiological changes to body composition (decreased plasma volume), kidneys (decreased **glomerular filtration rates**) and the brain (decreased thirst perception, increased **arginine vasopressin** (Cowen et al. 2013); social/ physical and psychological effects including dementia (forgetting to drink), dysphagia, limited mobility reducing free access to fluids, and beliefs that reducing intake will minimise incontinence.

Table 22.2: Changes to selected micronutrients—vitamins in older adults

Nutrient	Changes to requirements	Causes
Folate	Folate requirements stay consistent with age. Folate deficiency is higher in older people, with folate concentrations in serum and **cerebrospinal fluid** falling and plasma homocysteine (see Chapter 16) rising with age (Reynolds 2002).	Poor appetite; atrophic gastritis and hypochlorhydria (see 'What is atrophic gastritis?' box); poor utilisation of folate due to **genetic polymorphisms**. Those with T polymorphism (TT genotype) in the enzyme methylenetetrahydrofolate reductase have impaired folate metabolism, lower serum and red cell folate and higher plasma homocysteine concentrations (Hughes et al. 2013); folate may also be produced by bacteria in the gut, and so the gut microbiome may influence folate status (Jeffery & O'Toole 2013).

Nutrient	Changes to requirements	Causes
Vitamin B-12	The requirement for vitamin B-12 stays consistent with age but those with decreased absorption may require more. B-12 deficiency increases with age predominantly due to decreased absorption. In adults aged over 50 living in Sydney, 22.9% had low serum B-12. According to the Australian Health Survey, serum B-12 falls by 7% between the ages of 55 and 75+ (ABS 2013a). B-12 deficiency also contributes to sensory disturbances in the extremities (tingling and numbness) and loss of sense of joint position, which can lead to changes in gait and increased falls; impaired cognition and depression; impaired vision, impotency, impaired bladder and bowel control (Dangour et al. 2015; NHMRC 2006).	An autoimmune disease that destroys the gastric mucosa resulting in loss of intrinsic factor; atrophic gastritis; increased prevalence of *Helicobacter pylori* resulting in vitamin B-12 malabsorption; and antagonistic medications such as metformin for diabetes management.
Vitamin D	Vitamin D requirements increase for the over-50s to 10 µg/day and then to 15 µg/day for those over the age of 70. The increased requirement accounts for the prevalence of vitamin D deficiency (blood levels <50 nmol/L) which has become a public health concern in Australia, with nearly one-third of adults being deficient. In those aged over 75, 28% of men and 57% of women were Vitamin D deficient (Daly et al. 2012).	Limited sun exposure (in particular for housebound, institutionalised, darker skinned and for those who cover their skin for cultural reasons); reduced efficiency of the skin to produce; compromised or impaired liver and/or kidney function (Lips 2001); decreased intake—fatty fish are a good source but can be expensive, in Australia the primary food source is margarine; those aged over 70 years consume less than two teaspoons of margarine per day (ABS 2016).

Table 22.3: Changes to selected micronutrients—minerals in older adults

Nutrient	Changes to requirements	Causes
Zinc	Requirements for zinc remain the same in the elderly as for other adults. There are no recent studies on the prevalence of zinc deficiency in the elderly. However, in high-income countries it is estimated that nearly 30% of the elderly are zinc-deficient (Prasad 2014).	Poor appetite, and psychosocial factors limiting purchase and preparation of foods rich in zinc; altered intestinal absorption; inadequate chewing; and drug interactions.
Iron	Although physiological iron requirements do not vary between adult and elderly men and postmenopausal and elderly women, iron deficiency anaemia increases with age. Serum ferritin levels also decrease with age with the National Health Survey indicating a 13.5% decrease in ferritin levels between the 55–64 and the 75+ years age groups (ABS 2013a). There is no evidence to suggest that a decrease in iron stores is an inevitable effect of ageing; it is instead more likely due to poor intakes and absorption (Fairweather-Tait et al. 2014).	Loss of appetite; changes in social circumstances (as above); poor dentition and dysphagia which may make consumption of high-quality iron sources difficult; chronic low-grade inflammation increases circulating hepcidin levels, leading to a suppression of circulating iron that is available for **erythropoiesis** (Lane et al. 2016); low circulating levels of ascorbate, decreasing iron absorption (Lane et al. 2016); atrophic gastritis and hypochlorhydria; some medical conditions such as hypothyroid, coeliac disease; medication use (antacids, proton-pump inhibitors, aspirin and non-steroidal anti-inflammatory drugs (NSAIDs)) can cause gastrointestinal bleeding; and blood loss that is not immediately apparent or visible (this could be from gastrointestinal bleeding, bleeding gums or teeth).

Nutrient	Changes to requirements	Causes
Calcium	Calcium requirements increase by 300 mg from 1000 to 1300 mg in women after menopause and for men over the age of 70. In susceptible individuals, incidence of osteoporosis increases and there is also an increased rate of hip and vertebral fractures. Low serum 25-hydroxyvitamin D [25(OH)D] concentrations (see Vitamin D above) and dietary calcium intake have also been associated with impaired insulin sensitivity in people at high risk of type 2 diabetes (Gagnon et al. 2014). Adequate calcium, magnesium and vitamin D intake plus weight-bearing exercise can attenuate bone loss as people age. There is no evidence to support the use of calcium supplements (Reid 2014) but other meta-analyses argue that calcium and vitamin D supplementation can reduce total and hip fractures (Tang et al. 2007; Weaver et al. 2016). The benefit of supplementation is greater for those living in institutions, with low bodyweight, poor dietary calcium intake and with a higher baseline risk for osteoporotic fractures.	Increased bone mass loss from about 40 years of age, of approximately 0.5–1% loss per year; in postmenopausal women there is an accelerated loss of 1–2% per year for up to ten years; increased urinary calcium excretion; decreased intestinal absorption; decreased intake of foods containing bioavailable calcium sources.
Magnesium	Screening for chronic magnesium deficiency is difficult because a normal serum level may still be associated with moderate to severe deficiency (Reddy & Edwards 2017). Magnesium intake in older adults in Australia is generally below recommended levels.	Decreased capacity of the skeleton to store and release magnesium with age; increased renal excretion; lower intake of magnesium-rich foods (a majority of these are unprocessed foods such as whole grains, vegetables, nuts and fruits) as well as diminished bioavailability.

CASE STUDIES ON NUTRITION AND AGEING

CASE STUDY 1: MENOPAUSAL MUM

Your mum is going through menopause. She is relatively active and a healthy weight. She is worried about her bone density and getting osteoporosis after your grandmother recently had a fall and broke her wrist. She is asking you if you think she should start taking calcium supplements.

1. Go through the steps to determine if your mother is consuming sufficient calcium.
2. If she is consuming sufficient calcium, what would be your recommendation?
3. If she is not consuming sufficient calcium, what would be your 'food-first' approach?
4. Under what circumstances would you recommend calcium supplementation to your mother?

CASE STUDY 2: GRUMPY GRANDPA

Your Grandpa has recently become much more irritable and he also appears to be losing weight. Knowing what you do about nutrition:

1. What sorts of nutrients may be at risk?
2. What questions might you ask Grandpa about his social circumstances and psychological state?
3. What may be some food recommendations you would make?

WHAT IS ATROPHIC GASTRITIS?

Atrophic gastritis is a chronic inflammation of the stomach leading to atrophy of the mucosa, which in turn results in reduced gastric acid secretion (hypochlorhydria). This results in a reduced ability to release components from food and subsequently absorb them. This atrophy of the stomach mucosa becomes more common with ageing and appears to affect about one-third of those aged over 60 years. This can reduce the availability for absorption of vitamin B-12 (gastric acid is needed to liberate food-bound B-12), calcium, iron and folate, and results in elevated homocysteine levels.

FOOD AND NUTRIENT INTAKES OF ADULTS AND OLDER ADULTS

Recent analysis of the dietary intake of Australian adults up to the age of 50 revealed that very few are eating the recommended serves of any of the food groups. They are also exceeding the recommendations for sodium, added sugars and saturated/trans fat intake. Two in five and seven in ten women have inadequate iron and calcium intakes respectively; while two in five men have inadequate calcium intakes. Aboriginal and Torres Strait Islander adults are consuming less fruit, vegetables and dairy products than non-Indigenous adults (AIHW 2018) (Table 22.4).

A survey of older adults in the USA indicated that adults over the age of 60 ate a greater variety of foods and had a greater variety of micronutrient-dense foods than their younger counterparts (Roberts et al. 2005). However, in Australia the dietary patterns of older adults have generally been found to be similar to or only slightly healthier than those of their

Table 22.4: Food and nutrient intakes for adults aged 19–50

Years	19–30	31–50	19–30	31–50
	Males		**Females**	
Five food groups: mean intake against recommended serves				
Vegetables	X	X	X	X
Fruits	X	X	X	X
Grains	X	X	X	X
Meat	X	X	X	X
Dairy	X	X	X	X
Discretionary food: % of energy (broad recommendation is to limit intake)				
	36	37	35	33
Added sugars: % of energy (broad recommendation is to limit intake)				
	11	9.4	11	8.9
Trans and saturated fat: % energy (recommendation is less than 10% for those 14 years and over)				
	12	12	13	12
Sodium: mean intake (mg) versus adequate intake (mg)				
	3120 (460–920)	2303 (460–920)	2915 (460–920)	2154 (460–920)
Calcium: proportion of population (%) with intakes less than the estimated requirement				
	44	43	71	67
Iron: proportion of population (%) with intakes less than the estimated requirement				
	2.2	2.2	38	38
Dietary folate equivalents: proportion of population (%) with intakes less than the estimated requirement				
	2.8	2.3	11	11
Iodine: proportion of population (%) with intakes less than the estimated requirement				
	1.5	1.6	12	9
Fibre: mean intake (g/day) as a proportion of the adequate intake level				
	81	83	81	83

Source: AIHW (2018)

younger counterparts. Older people are eating more energy-dense food as they age (see Table 22.5) but have reduced their consumption of added sugars. Nevertheless, intakes of fruit, vegetables and grains

Table 22.5: Food and nutrient intakes for adults aged 51–71+ (excluding those who are institutionalised)

Years	51–70	71+	51–70	71+
	Males		Females	
Five food groups: mean intake against recommended serves				
Vegetables	X	X	X	X
Fruits	X	X	X	X
Grains	X	X	X	✓
Meat	X	X	X	X
Dairy	X	X	X	X
Discretionary food: % of energy (broad recommendation is to limit intake)				
	35	36	31	32
Added sugars: % of energy (broad recommendation is to limit intake)				
	7.8	8.5	7.7	8.0
Trans and saturated fat: % energy (recommendation is less than 10% for those 14 years and over)				
	12	12	12	12
Sodium: mean intake (mg) versus adequate intake (mg)				
	2510 (460–920)	1972 (460–920)	2217 (460–920)	1773 (460–920)
Calcium: proportion of population (%) with intakes less than the estimated requirement				
	63	90	91	94
Iron: proportion of population (%) with intakes less than the estimated requirement				
	2.8	3.1	5.0	6.7
Dietary folate equivalents: proportion of population (%) with intakes less than the estimated requirement				
	2.5	1.6	7.6	6.1
Iodine: proportion of population (%) with intakes less than the estimated requirement				
	3.5	4.2	11	9.2
Fibre: mean intake (g/day) as a proportion of the adequate intake level				
	83	84	89	84

Source: AIHW (2018)

remain below the recommended intakes. Dietary intakes due to greater disability, disease and cognitive decline tend to be lower in the institutionalised elderly.

Energy intakes tend to fall from 11,000 kJ to 8000 kJ for men and from 8000 kJ to 6500 kJ for women (ABS 2014a). Protein intakes fall by 30 per cent from the 19–30 age group to the 71 and over age group, with Australians in this age group consuming 83 g per day (ABS 2014a). The recent nutrition survey in Australia also identified that a proportion of men and women over the age of 70 are not consuming adequate nutrients for health; these are summarised in Table 22.6.

What factors increase risk of nutritional vulnerability in older adults?

Some subgroups of older people are more likely to consume inadequate diets, including:

* the institutionalised elderly (living in aged care or mental health facilities)
* the physically and socially inactive
* those with physical disabilities, impaired motor performance and/or mobility
* those exhibiting the presence of chronic conditions
* those taking prescribed multiple medications (polypharmacy).

Older adults are nutritionally vulnerable due to a range of physiological, psychological and social factors, which are outlined in Table 22.7.

Table 22.6: Nutrient intakes of older Australians

Nutrient	% of 71+ not meeting EAR	
	Men	Women
Calcium	89.5	94.3
Magnesium	63.9	48.5
Vitamin B-6	56.7	72.1
Riboflavin	20.3	20.3
Zinc	66.3	12.1
Thiamin	9.7	18.5
Iodine	4.2	9.2
Iron	3.1	6.7
Folate equivalents	1.6	6.1
Vitamin B-12	0.8	5.8

Source: ABS (2014a)

Table 22.7: Contributors to altered dietary intakes in older adults

Social factors	
Social isolation	With 25% of older adults living alone, social isolation is a strong likelihood. Social isolation is a risk factor for meal-skipping. Older men living alone are particularly vulnerable.
Poverty	Almost 70% of older Australians rely in full or part on the age pension (AIHW 2017). One in four older Australians live in poverty and 7% of the homeless population are aged 65 years or over (Australian Human Rights Commission 2015). The poverty rate in the 55–64 year age group is 15.5% and increases to 29.2% in those aged 75 years and over. Home ownership protects older households from poverty by allowing their incomes—largely from the pension—to cover non-housing costs. Increases in utility (gas, electricity, telephone) costs will seriously impact on the amount of income remaining for other expenses. While food prices have remained relatively stable, affording nutrient-dense foods continues to be an issue.
Psychological factors	
Mental health	Poor dietary intake both contributes to and is an outcome of sub-optimal mental health. Mental health issues can range from depression and/or anxiety to dementia. Mental health in older people may be affected by bereavement, losing the ability to live independently, a drop in income, or a major health impairment that impacts on the activities of daily living (AIHW 2015). The highest age-specific suicide death rate in 2016 was among males aged 85 and over (34 per 100,000) (ABS 2017b).
Food beliefs, food faddism, avoidance	Older people are not immune to the effects of food beliefs in their later years. Factors contributing to disordered eating behaviour include prolongation of an eating disorder from earlier life (Mangweth-Matzek et al. 2014), preoccupation with the major morbidities and mortalities associated with later life (e.g. fluid restriction due to incontinence, avoidance of certain foods due to misguided beliefs about their impact on their medical condition) and continuation and extension of food restrictions associated with long-term chronic conditions (e.g. restriction of carbohydrates or fats).
Physical factors	
Poor appetite or anorexia	Ageing is associated with a decrease in the opioid (dynorphin) feeding drive and an increase in the satiety effect of cholecystokinin, which is a peptide hormone produced in the gut with eating (Landi et al. 2016). There is also delayed gastric emptying, meaning that older people feel full for longer, and loss of gastric compliance due to decreased secretion of nitric oxide. Chronic gastritis and some drugs (e.g. proton-pump inhibitors) may cause hypochlorhydria, which further delays gastric emptying (Landi et al. 2016). Appetite is also affected by medication, taste changes, mental health and other factors. Poor appetite has comparable predictability to loss of weight as a determinant of survival in later life (Huang et al. 2014).
Polypharmacy	The many medications that seniors are often prescribed can affect nutrient absorption/utilisation and appetite. Polypharmacy is associated with a higher incidence of frailty, with the more medications prescribed leading to higher rates of frailty (Veronese et al. 2017). Polypharmacy is a known risk factor for malnutrition in the elderly. One of the key strategies for older people is to have a regular medication review by a pharmacist to minimise medications and reduce potential adverse interactions.
Poor dentition and chewing difficulty	Poor dentition is often cited as a contributor to poor intake. Older people may have higher tooth loss due to lower exposure to fluoride and dental care. Although dentition and chewing ability only explains part of the variance in food and nutrition intake, it is still important to consider (Mudge et al. 2011). Nevertheless, chewing disability is a predictor of survival, especially in association with dietary quality and cardiometabolic dysfunction (Lee et al. 2010).
Loss of taste	Taste sensation in the elderly can be compromised. This can be due to smoking, medications or loss of cognitive function. Older people retain their ability to taste sweet but salty and bitter taste sensation is diminished (Ogawa et al. 2017). This could explain increases in consumption of salt and caffeine. Other sensory losses (smell and eyesight) can also contribute to poor intake.
Decreases in cognitive ability	Losses in cognitive function can create confusion and memory loss. Depending on its severity this can result in forgetting how to prepare foods, forgetting to shop or forgetting to eat. As it progresses, loss of cognitive function can also interfere with feeding, chewing and swallowing.

Physical factors	
Dysphagia	Dysphagia can be caused by a range of conditions such as stroke, Parkinson's disease and other neurological conditions. In addition, sarcopenia can cause dysphagia due to loss of muscle mass associated with the swallowing muscles (Nishioka et al. 2017). Difficulty in swallowing contributes to both malnutrition and dehydration. The risk of being malnourished is almost double in those showing signs of dysphagia (Namasivayam-MacDonald et al. 2017). Treatment is usually thickening of fluids, and this can reduce the availability of water for hydration.
Disability	Disability in older people is a result of multiple factors, some associated with chronic conditions. Loss of hearing and sight as well as musculoskeletal impairments associated with back pain, osteoporosis and arthritis are relatively common (AIHW 2017). These issues impact on the ability to procure, prepare and consume food.

NUTRITION AND THE MANAGEMENT OF CONDITIONS ASSOCIATED WITH AGEING

There is growing awareness that the major health problems, and even mortality, in the aged do have nutritional contributors and can (in part) be prevented with food intake of sufficient quality (variety) and quantity. These health problems do not necessarily need to occur with ageing, and death can be delayed. As the number of chronic conditions increases with age, these contribute to disability and frailty, which in turn reduces a person's level of independence, sometimes resulting in institutionalisation. This next section goes through some of the common issues with underlying nutritional determinants in older people, their **aetiology** and how they can be managed.

Protein energy dysnutrition and sarcopenia

As described above, the most common nutritional scenario in the aged is a decrease in lean mass (comprising water and protein–dominant tissues such as muscle and organs such as the liver, and also bone) and an increase in abdominal fat. This disorder can be described as protein energy **dysnutrition** (PED). Illness or inadequate food intake may result in PED, a condition more common among elderly adults, especially in institutional care. It is associated with impaired immune responses, infections, poor wound healing, anaemia, osteoporosis/hip fracture, reduced cognitive function, delayed recovery from surgery, decreased muscle strength (frailty) (risk factor for falls

WORKING WITH OLDER PEOPLE

If an older person's food intake is lower due to poor appetite or other issues, then the foods that are consumed need to be more nutrient-dense. In a group or with a partner:

- Brainstorm ways to increase the energy, protein and nutrient density of commonly consumed foods.
- Identify what foods/beverages to recommend in order to improve nutrient density.
- Identify what foods/beverages to discourage and why.
- Discuss the economic consequences of and cooking skills required by the suggestions you have made. How would you adjust your suggestions if the person was on a tight budget or had limited cooking skills?
- Identify factors you would need to consider when communicating with an older person.

in the elderly) and, ultimately, increased morbidity and mortality. Intervention studies have shown that an increase in protein can help increase muscle mass in seniors when combined with high-intensity

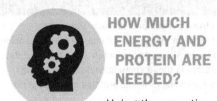

HOW MUCH ENERGY AND PROTEIN ARE NEEDED?

Using the equations to calculate energy requirements from Chapter 13, calculate the energy requirements for a 65-year-old man (height 180 cm, weight 80 kg, moderately active, good appetite) and an 85-year-old man (height 178 cm, weight 70 kg, mainly sedentary, poor appetite).

Using a suitable diet and nutrient analysis package, work out a suitable meal plan to meet protein and energy requirements for each man.

resistance exercise training (Artaza–Artabe et al. 2016; Deutz et al. 2014).

Sarcopenia is defined as the loss of skeletal muscle mass and body weight accompanied by a reduction in strength and mobility. It has the potential to reduce quality of life and increase disability. Sarcopenia can result in:

- functional impairments (slow walking speed, poor balance)
- physical disability (difficulty in performing activities of daily living; increased risk of falls)
- increased risk of cardiovascular disease, type 2 diabetes and obesity
- increased risk of all–cause mortality. (Witard et al. 2016)

Sarcopenia can be caused by poor nutrition, inactivity, disease and the ageing process. Ageing is associated with a rise in **catabolic inflammatory cytokines**, which can result in sarcopenia due to their effect on muscle mass (Farshidfar et al. 2015). Figure 22.4 describes the contributors to sarcopenia.

Frailty

Frailty is now considered to be a distinct health dimension and is a precursor to disability (Santos-Eggimann & Sirven 2016). Protein–energy dys-nutrition and sarcopenia can develop into frailty. In addition, magnesium deficits facilitate oxygen-derived free radical formation and low–grade inflam-

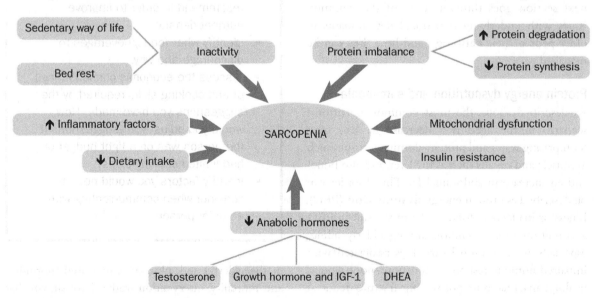

Figure 22.4: Contributors to sarcopenia

Source: Farshidfar, F. et al. (2015). Reprinted with permission from IOS Press

mation and may lead to frailty, to which sarcopenia may contribute (Huang et al. 2015). Frailty is described as a multisystem reduction in reserve capacity of physiological systems where there are at least three of the following five characteristics:

- poor appetite accompanied by weight loss
- exhaustion
- muscle weakness
- slow walking speed and unsteady gait
- low physical activity. (Clegg et al. 2013)

As a result of these factors, the frail person is at increased risk of disability (increased risk of falling, impaired cognition and mental health), osteopenia (low bone-density and fracture susceptibility) and death (Campbell & Buchner 1997). It has been estimated that 6–25 per cent of people aged 65 years or more could be considered to be frail, rising to 25–40 per cent of those aged over 80 years (Strandberg & Pitkala 2007). See 'The FRAIL scale' box.

Obesity

The health implications of being overweight in old age are controversial. Loss of muscle is a greater health hazard than being overweight. The healthy range of BMI for older people is higher (27–30 kg/m^2) than in younger adults (20–25 kg/m^2) with respect to survival rates (Winter et al. 2017). However, greater body fatness, especially if centrally distributed, still increases the risk of insulin resistance, hypertension and hypercholesterolaemia in the aged. However, it is not evidence-based to advise even a mildly obese older person to lose weight. To advise an elderly person to restrict intake to prolong life could result in loss of lean body mass and frailty, potentially shortening lifespan and health-span.

Obesity in the elderly does continue to contribute to loss of quality of life and increased healthcare usage. The aim for obese adults, therefore, would be to replace energy-dense/nutrient-poor foods with nutrient- and phytonutrient-dense foods. Intervention studies are indicating successful weight loss in older obese people (under the age of 80) using a combination of nutrient-dense foods or supplements and resistance training in order to preserve lean muscle mass (Porter Starr & Bales 2015; Verreijen et al. 2015). Weight maintenance is still recommended for older obese people over the age of 80. These findings must be viewed cautiously, since elderly people who are overweight by the criteria for younger adults have longer life expectancies than those with lower BMIs. Mortality is highest for those with BMIs less than 20 kg/m^2 and greater than 28.0–28.9 kg/m^2 (Winter et al. 2017).

Immune dysfunction

The decline observed in immune function with ageing may be prevented with nutrient intakes greater than that currently recommended for 'normal' health. Nutrients found to be important in immune function include protein, zinc, iron, vitamin C, vitamin B-6, tocopherols and vitamin D (see chapters 17, 18 and 19). Other components of food not considered to be essential for health may become so with age. For example, glutamine, a dispensable amino acid stored primarily in skeletal muscle, is utilised by intestinal cells, lymphocytes and macrophages and is required for the synthesis of DNA and RNA. The rate of glutamine formation and availability may be compromised in older people as a consequence of the reduced contribution of skeletal muscle to whole-body protein metabolism. This in turn may adversely affect immune function, resulting in a less favourable response to infection or trauma. Glutamine can be synthesised from glutamic acid. Glutamic acid is found in wheat, soybeans, lean meat and eggs. Glutathione, together with phytonutrients such as flavonoids and carotenoids, also appears to play a role in immune function.

Macular degeneration

Age-related macular degeneration is a progressive, chronic disease of the central retina and is the leading cause of blindness and low vision among older adults. It is the main cause of vision impairment in 9 per cent of the population and of bilateral blindness in 71 per cent (Foreman et al. 2017). Studies are indicating that diets high in lutein and zeaxanthin (the two predominant carotenoids of the macular pigment found in the yellow spot of the retina) are

THE FRAIL SCALE

The FRAIL scale (Fatigue, Resistance, Ambulation, Illnesses and Loss of Weight) (Morley et al. 2012) is a simple five-question tool that can be used in primary care to screen for frailty.

	Question	Scoring	Result
F	FATIGUE *How much of the time during the past 4 weeks did you feel tired?*	1 = All of the time 2 = Most of the time 3 = Some of the time 4 = A little of the time 5 = None of the time Responses of 1 or 2 = 1 All others = 0	
R	RESISTANCE *By yourself and not using aids, do you have any difficulty walking up ten steps without resting?*	1 = Yes 0 = No	
A	AMBULATION *By yourself and not using aids, do you have any difficulty walking several hundred metres?*	1 = Yes 0 = No	
I	ILLNESS Has a doctor ever told you that you have: • hypertension • diabetes • cancer (other than a minor skin cancer) • chronic lung disease • heart attack • congestive heart failure • angina • asthma • arthritis • stroke • kidney disease?	Responses of 0 to 4 (total illnesses) = 0 Responses of 5–11 = 1	
L	LOSS OF WEIGHT *How much do you weigh with your clothes on but without shoes?* [current weight] *One year ago in [MONTH, YEAR], how much did you weigh without your shoes and with your clothes on?* [weight 1 year ago]	A 5% loss of weight is scored as 1 and < 5% as 0	
Total score:			
Scoring: 0 = robust; 1–2 = pre-frail; 3 or more = frail			

protective against eye disease. These carotenoids are found in yellow and orange foods such as rockmelon, carrots, orange/yellow capsicums, salmon and egg yolks (Abdel-Aal et al. 2013). In addition to these carotenoids, vitamins C and E, zinc and n-3 fatty acids all contribute to eye health. This would require consumption of a variety of fruits (kiwi, grapes, berries, citrus), vegetables (green leafy vegetables, broccoli, corn, orange/yellow capsicum), nuts and seeds (sunflower seeds, almonds, walnuts, hazelnuts) and seafood (oysters, salmon, sardines) (McCusker et al. 2016).

A large study—the Age-related Eye Diseases Study—has identified that the use of these nutrients as supplements can slow the progression of existing macular degeneration. However, little is known about the adverse effect of using such high-dose antioxidants for long periods. Consequently, improving the quality of the diet by eating whole foods is recommended (Age-Related Eye Disease Study Research Group 2001).

Chronic conditions: Diabetes, cardiovascular disease, cancer

With ageing, the accumulation of risk over the life-course increases the prevalence of chronic conditions such as diabetes, cardiovascular disease and cancer. Many older people have been managing a chronic condition for significant periods of time. Nutritional prevention and management of chronic conditions are covered in Part 7. For older people, management of chronic conditions needs to be balanced with minimising protein energy dysnutrition, sarcopenia, frailty and maintaining quality of life. Diagnosis and prognosis potentially changes the treatment options. Late diagnosis of cancer, for example, where the prognosis is poor may, with family consultation, result in palliative care rather than aggressive medical and nutrition treatment.

The higher homocysteine levels caused by inadequate folate and vitamins B-6 and B-12 are associated with an elevated risk of CVD, stroke (as a result of increased inflammatory plaque formation) and lower bone mineral density (Hughes et al. 2013) as well as macular degeneration in over-75-year-olds

(Rochtchina et al. 2007). Zinc deficiency has been implicated in chronic inflammation and increased oxidative stress contributing to atherosclerosis and diabetes.

Issues associated with joints

Older people are more likely to experience issues with joints and bones. This is most commonly osteoarthritis, but elderly people also sometimes have rheumatoid arthritis or gout (deposition of uric acid crystals in joints). Degenerative osteoarthritis is commonly seen in weight-bearing joints like hips and knees and in the high-usage small joints of the hands. Obesity is generally regarded as a risk factor for osteoarthritis in weight-bearing joints. In rheumatoid arthritis, the immune system mistakenly attacks the bone coverings as if they were made of foreign tissue. Rheumatoid arthritis has a possible link to diet through the immune system—that is, a poor diet may worsen this type of arthritis. Marine long-chain n-3 fatty acids may help reduce the inflammation in the joints that makes arthritis so painful. In the older age groups, vitamin D deficiency is associated with decreased muscle strength increasing the risk of falls; in combination with osteoporosis, an increase in the risk of fractures; colorectal cancer, prostate cancer, multiple sclerosis, diabetes, cardiovascular diseases, and tuberculosis (Hughes et al. 2004; Hypponen et al. 2001; Luscombe et al. 2001; van der Mei et al. 2003; van der Mei et al. 2007; Zittermann 2003). Additionally, as the receptors for vitamin D are in the brain it is highly likely to play a role in cognition (and in particular memory) and depression (Miller et al. 2015).

Cognitive impairment, Alzheimer's disease and depression

Dementia covers a range of neurological conditions characterised by memory loss and cognitive impairment. Alzheimer's disease is the most common of these, accounting for 50–70 per cent of dementia cases (Dementia Australia 2018). Some deterioration can be attributed to atherosclerotic disease, and thus interventions such as aspirin or particular dietary patterns that reduce cardiovascular risk may also prevent dementia. High educational status early in life and continued mental stimulation may also be protective. It is generally accepted that dementias and depression have a strong genetic background. However, the genetic susceptibility to a certain disease is strongly influenced by environmental factors. Thus, nutrients may have a disease-accelerating or protective effect. Risk factors for Alzheimer's disease include heavy alcohol consumption, high saturated fat intake, elevated homocysteine and deficiencies in vitamins B-6, B-12 and folate as well as iron (Durga et al. 2007; Fairweather-Tait et al. 2014). For more information on mental health disorders see Chapter 34.

Inadequate fluid intake can lead to dehydration, which, in turn, can contribute to cognitive impairment, confusion, constipation and increased risk of falls. For healthy individuals, it is advisable to consume at least four large cups of water or other fluids like tea (which has the added benefit of containing antioxidant phytonutrients), irrespective of thirst. Consuming food with high water content, such as fruit, will also help hydration status. For those with loss of appetite and other factors limiting intake, care needs to be taken to ensure that non-caloric fluids do not displace more nutrient-dense fluids.

Depression in the elderly is a very common symptom. There is a growing body of evidence to suggest n-3 polyunsaturated fatty acids may play an important role in the aetiology and treatment of depression (Grosso et al. 2014). Caffeine ingested as either tea or coffee has been shown to improve mood and reduce anxiety.

Skin integrity and wrinkling

Collagen and elastin give skin its firmness and elasticity, but with age these gradually decline and the skin becomes looser, weaker, less elastic and drier. Disappearance of fat pads under the skin, and for women decreasing oestrogen after menopause, accelerate the formation of wrinkles and the skin begins to sag. This in turn can make elderly skin more prone to sun damage, skin cancer and skin lesions.

Loss of skin integrity is affected by:
- genetic programming

- cumulative sun damage (photoageing)
- direct chemical effects from cigarette smoking and/or abrasive chemicals
- diet.

Several nutrients have been found to improve skin texture by strengthening collagen and elastin, reducing the risk of sunburn and promoting wound healing. These include:
- lycopene, β-carotene, lutein, zeaxanthin, bioflavonoids (Greul et al. 2002; Heinrich et al. 2003; Heinrich et al. 2006)
- isoflavones (Irrera et al. 2017; Izumi et al. 2007)
- green tea (Chiu et al. 2005)
- vitamin C (Pullar et al. 2017)
- selenium (Zhu et al. 2015).

A high intake of fat, especially monounsaturated fat, olive oil, olives, vegetables (especially leafy greens, spinach, eggplant, asparagus, celery, onions/leeks and garlic), legumes, fruit (especially prunes, cherries and apples), eggs, reduced-fat dairy products, tea and water is linked to less wrinkling. In contrast, a high intake of saturated fat, meat/processed meat, full-fat dairy products, ice cream, cakes/pastries/sweets, potatoes, butter and margarine were linked to more wrinkling (Purba et al. 2001).

NUTRITIONAL AND GENERAL STRATEGIES FOR HEALTHY AGEING

The nutritional and dietary requirements which might prevent or manage the development of key conditions associated with ageing have been discussed. However, a range of strategies can contribute to healthy ageing. These revolve around nutritional health, physical activity and social and emotional wellbeing. Messages for healthy longevity might be:
- Maintain a sense of community and companionship as a security network.
- Be active lifelong.
- Eat a variety of nutrient- and phytonutrient-dense foods and reduce energy-dense/nutrient-poor food intakes
- Stay hydrated.
- Eat regularly and share meals.

- Maintain a healthy weight: beware unintended weight loss.
- Avoid stressful situations.
- Cultivate and maintain a sense of purpose.
- Develop and maintain restful sleep habits.
- Exercise your mind and practice meditation.
- Develop an active social network.
- Default to healthy habits.

While a younger person will be able to consume an inadequate diet with no immediately foreseeable consequences, an elderly person is more likely to experience problems because of diminished physiological function and capacity to adjust to adverse events. There are three key nutritional and one physical activity recommendations for the elderly. These recommendations have been incorporated into an assessment tool, the Healthy Ageing Nutrition Index (HANI), that predicts survival based on eating alone, cooking and food choice and may represent early markers for the development of risk providing impetus for early intervention (Huang et al. 2018).

Recommendation 1–Consume a biodiverse, nutrient-dense diet

Older individuals who live longer have, in general, more biodiverse diets. Compared with younger adults, older adults have lower energy requirements but increased requirements for protein, riboflavin, vitamin B-6, calcium and vitamin D, and some seniors may require extra vitamin B-12. Essential amino acids (EAA) are potent stimulators of maximal protein synthesis and this occurs with the consumption of 15 g of EAA, translating to 35 g of high-quality protein at each meal (Baum et al. 2016). The average 50-year-old needs to eat around 25 per cent less than they ate at age eighteen. An alternative would be to increase the amount of movement during the day by 25 per cent. Given the tendency for activity levels to decline and total food intakes to fall with advancing years, there is less room for energy-dense foods (such as cakes, biscuits, pastries, crisps) that supply few of the essential nutrients bodies continue to need. Therefore, older adults need be selective about what they eat to avoid excessive

fat gain and select foods that are nutrient dense and high in protein, such as nuts, lean red meat, low-fat dairy products, legumes and seeds.

Recommendation 2–Eat regularly and with others

It is recommended that elderly people consume meals regularly and not skip meals (Fulkerson et al. 2014). There is also evidence that spreading protein throughout the day has maximum benefits for muscle mass and strength (Nowson & O'Connell 2015). Eating regular meals also seems to contribute to higher cognitive function (Kim et al. 2017; Kuczmarski et al. 2014). There is, however, no evidence on what 'regular' meals actually means and whether there are benefits conferred by eating meals and snacks (that is, six meals a day), whether three meals is adequate or, indeed, if two meals would suffice (as occurs in some cultural groups). Common sense, however, would indicate that if appetite is poor and satiety high, as occurs in many older adults, then the likelihood of consuming a nutrient-rich diet in a smaller number of meals a day is unlikely. Regular mealtimes also assist in setting a rhythm to the day that may coincide with fluid consumption, thereby alleviating the risk of dehydration. Mealtimes also provide an opportunity for social interaction.

Social activity and relationships are now thought to be one of the most important determinants of longevity. A meta-analysis indicated that individuals with adequate social relationships had a 50 per cent greater likelihood of survival; this is comparable to quitting smoking (Holt-Lunstad et al. 2010). The impact of social activity on longevity could be through its impact on psychological wellbeing and through nutrition. For example, elderly people who are socially isolated, lonely, institutionalised, recently bereaved or socially inactive have been found to have inadequate food intakes (Horwath 1989). Eating alone increases the likelihood of skipping meals, and of consuming lower intakes of energy after controlling for age, gastrointestinal problems, poor appetite, income and not eating snacks (Fulkerson et al. 2014). Commensal meal patterns in late adulthood are associated with better nutritional health (Fulkerson et al. 2014) and, especially for men, greater survival (Huang et al. 2017). Enhancing mealtime experiences for the elderly living in institutionalised care also improves intake (Mahadevan et al. 2014).

Recommendation 3—Maintain a healthy weight and avoid unintentional weight loss

A healthy weight for an older person is slightly higher that recommended for younger adults. Over the age of 65 years, individuals should be aiming for a BMI of about 27 kg/m². Lower weights increase the risk of osteoporosis, falls and frailty, while higher weights can impact on mobility, chronic disease management and quality of life. Again, the focus should be on eating nutrient-dense foods, minimising consumption of foods that contribute energy and little else. Dieting through the restriction of energy is not recommended as it can contribute to sarcopenia. Instead, older people should be encouraged to watch their weight but enjoy their food and eat with others. If weight starts to fall (without the presence of a causative diagnosis)

strategies should be implemented early to seek medical advice, determine body compositional basis, and increase the intake of energy- and nutrient-dense foods.

Recommendation 4—Undertake regular activity and resistance training

Physical activity in older adults has multiple benefits, including aerobic fitness, maintenance of muscle mass, maximisation of functionality, improved mental health and wellbeing, reduced risk of falls, and reduced risk and/or better management of chronic conditions. The recommendation is to be active every day, doing a range of activity that incorporates fitness, strength, balance and flexibility. This can be achieved through incidental activities, such as housework or walking to the bus-stop; leisure, such as dancing or golf; structured activities, such as yoga, tai chi or strength training; or supervised physical activity for those with health problems. Older people should accumulate 30 minutes of moderate intensity physical activity every day.

SUMMARY

- The global population is ageing, with those over the age of 85 one of the fastest-growing demographics.
- Taking a life-course approach, it is known that risk of chronic conditions accumulates over time. Healthy ageing requires compression of morbidity towards the end of life. This will partly be achieved by delaying the loss of organ function (or physiological reserve) and the onset of frailty, and by improving nutritional reserves. It is never too late to make changes to diet (achieving food variety with nutrient- and phytonutrient-dense food), physical activity (including endurance and strength exercises), avoiding substance abuse and strengthening social engagement to improve outcomes.
- Australian adults and older adults are not eating the recommended serves of any of the food groups. In addition, discretionary foods contribute one-third of energy intake, while very few older adults meet their calcium requirements.
- Compared with their younger counterparts, older adults do not require as much energy but do need more protein to ensure that muscle mass is retained. Requirements for micronutrients (apart from vitamin D and calcium) tend to remain the same throughout adulthood but deficiency can occur due to poor consumption, absorption and increased excretion.

- Mild vitamin, mineral and phytonutrient deficiencies are common in older adults and have been associated with several 'diseases of ageing' (e.g. cognitive impairment, arthritis, poor wound healing and skin wrinkling) and medications.
- Nutritionally vulnerable 'at-risk' groups within older populations who are more likely to consume inadequate diets (especially protein, calcium, zinc, magnesium, vitamins B-6, B-12 and folate) include older men living alone, the socially isolated or the lonely, those with low socioeconomic status and the recently bereaved.
- The primary nutritionally related health problems affecting the elderly are protein energy dysnutrition (PED), frailty, sarcopenia, obesity, joint issues (including osteoporosis), chronic conditions, immune dysfunction, cancer and cognitive impairment.
- The healthy range of BMI for older people is higher than in younger adults with respect to survival rates. However, greater body fatness, especially if centrally distributed, still increases the risk of insulin resistance, hypertension and hypercholesterolaemia in the aged. It is not evidence-based to advise even a mildly obese older person to lose weight. Sarcopenic obesity—where there is a combination of excess weight and reduced muscle mass and/or strength—significantly increases the risk of disability, osteoporosis, insulin resistance and mortality.

KEY TERMS

Aerobic activity: any physical activity that makes you sweat, causes you to breathe harder, and gets your heart beating faster than at rest.

Aetiology: the cause, set of causes, or manner of causation of a disease or condition.

Anabolic resistance: the phenomenon in which muscle does not respond to stimulus with normal muscle protein synthesis, but produces a reduced response.

Arginine vasopressin: a hormone, also known as the antidiuretic hormone, produced by the hypothalamus.

Biological age: the decline in function that occurs in every human being, given sufficient time.

Catabolic inflammatory cytokines: a type of signalling molecules that are produced by the body in response to an injury or infection. Examples include interferon and tumour necrosis factor. They can have positive and negative effects. Some of the negative effects are their contribution to the inflammation associated with a number of chronic diseases.

Cerebrospinal fluid: the fluid that surrounds the brain and spinal cord, providing a mechanical and immunological buffer.

Chronological age: a person's age in years since birth.

Dysnutrition: a term commonly used and associated with the aged. It refers to under, over and disordered nutrition, and can be used interchangeably with malnutrition. The triple burden of disease, i.e. the coexistence of underweight, overweight and micronutrient deficiencies, is an example of dysnutrition.

Erythropoiesis: a complex physiological process that maintains oxygen in the blood through the production of red blood cells. Low oxygen is detected in the kidneys which control red blood cell production by the bone marrow via the hormone erythropoietin.

Genetic polymorphism: where the same gene in different people may produce a different effect or outcome. Single nucleotide polymorphisms or SNPs are the most common type of genetic variation in humans.

Glomerular filtration rate: how well the kidneys are filtering waste products from the blood.

Health-span: the length of time you are healthy and thriving, as opposed to the lifespan, the length of time you are alive.

Homeostasis: the tendency to maintain stable, relatively constant bodily functions.

Morbidity: the lack of physical or psychological wellbeing resulting from disease, illness or injury, especially when the individual is aware of their condition. For example, morbidity could refer to the state of a person who is living with diabetes, has had amputations and reduced sight due to diabetes-related complications.

Mortality: relating to death. All-cause mortality refers to deaths attributed to all causes.

Telomeres: DNA-protein complexes at the end of chromosomes that protect against loss of sequences (genetic modifications) during DNA replication. Shorter telomeres have been associated with poor health behaviours, age-related diseases, and early mortality. Telomere length is regulated by the enzyme telomerase, and is linked to exposure to pro-inflammatory cytokines and oxidative stress. Nutrition, and in particular lower n-6:n-3 PUFA ratios can lower the impact of cell ageing and inflammation and potentially reduce disease (Kiecolt-Glaser et al. 2013).

ACKNOWLEDGEMENT

This chapter is based on the chapters 'Nutrition in Adulthood' written by Mark L. Wahlqvist and 'Nutrition in Maturity and Ageing' written by Mark L. Wahlqvist and Antigone Kouris-Blazos, which appeared in the third edition of *Food and Nutrition*.

REFERENCES

Abdel-Aal, E.-S.M., Akhtar, H., Zaheer, K. & Ali, R., 2013, 'Dietary sources of lutein and zeaxanthin carotenoids and their role in eye health', *Nutrients*, 5(4): 1169, doi:10.3390/nu5041169

ABS, 2013a, *Australian Health Survey: Biomedical results for nutrients, 2011–12*, <www.abs.gov.au/AUSSTATS/abs@.nsf/DetailsPage/4364.0.55.0062011-12?OpenDocument>, accessed 27 June 2018

—— 2013b, *Reflecting a Nation: Stories from the 2011 Census, 2012–13*, <www.abs.gov.au/ausstats/abs@.nsf/Lookup/2071.0main+features602012-2013>, accessed 18 December 2017

—— 2014a, *Australian Health Survey: Nutrition First Results—Food and nutrients, 2011–12*, <www.abs.gov.au/ausstats/abs@.nsf/Lookup/by%20Subject/4364.0.55.007~2011-12~Main%20Features~Key%20Findings~1>, accessed 20 June 2018

—— 2014b, *Australian Historical Population Statistics, 2014*, <www.abs.gov.au/AUSSTATS/abs@.nsf/DetailsPage/3105.0.65.0012014?OpenDocument>, accessed 21 June 2018

—— 2016, *Australian Health Survey: Consumption of food groups from the Australian Dietary Guidelines, 2011–12*, <www.abs.gov.au/ausstats/abs@.nsf/0/CBBD84445CA4BA4ACA2581F400773E44?Opendocument>, accessed 20 June 2018

—— 2017a, *Australian Demographic Statistics, December 2016*, <www.abs.gov.au/AUSSTATS/abs@.nsf/DetailsPage/3101.0Dec%202016?OpenDocument>, accessed 1 December 2018

—— 2017b, *Causes of Death, Australia, 2016*, <www.abs.gov.au/ausstats/abs@.nsf/Lookup/by%20Subject/3303.0~2016~Main%20Features~Intentional%20self-harm:%20key%20characteristics~7>, accessed 26 June 2018

Age-Related Eye Disease Study Research Group, 2001, 'A randomized, placebo-controlled, clinical trial of high-dose supplementation with vitamins C and E and beta carotene for age-related cataract and vision loss: AREDS Report No. 9', *Archives of Ophthalmology, 119*(10): 1439–52, doi:10.1001/archopht.119.10.1439

AIHW, 2015, *Australia's Welfare 2015* (Series no. 12), <www.aihw.gov.au/reports/australias-welfare/australias-welfare-2015/contents/table-of-contents>, accessed 14 February 2019

—— 2017, *Older Australia at a Glance* (21 April 2017), <www.aihw.gov.au/reports/older-people/older-australia-at-a-glance/contents/social-and-economic-engagement/employment-and-economic-participation>, accessed 14 February 2019

—— 2018, *Nutrition Across the Life Stages*, <www.aihw.gov.au/getmedia/fc5ad42e-08f5-4f9a-9ca4-723cacaa510d/aihw-phe-227.pdf.aspx?inline=true>, accessed 30 November 2018

Artaza-Artabe, I., Sáez-López, P., Sánchez-Hernández, N., Fernández-Gutierrez, N. & Malafarina, V., 2016, 'The relationship between nutrition and frailty: Effects of protein intake, nutritional supplementation, vitamin D and exercise on muscle metabolism in the elderly. A systematic review', *Maturitas, 93*: 89–99, doi:10.1016/j.maturitas.2016.04.009

Australian Government, 2017, *Ageing and Aged Care: About residential care*, <https://agedcare.health.gov.au/programs-services/residential-care/about-residential-care>, accessed 26 June 2018

Australian Human Rights Commission, 2015, *Face the Facts: Older Australians*, <www.humanrights.gov.au/face-facts-older-australians>, accessed 26 June 2018

Baum, J.I., Kim, I.-Y. & Wolfe, R.R., 2016, 'Protein consumption and the elderly: What is the optimal level of intake?', *Nutrients, 8*(6): 359, doi:10.3390/nu8060359

Bauman, A., Merom, D., Bull, F.C., Buchner, D.M. & Fiatarone Singh, M.A., 2016, 'Updating the evidence for physical activity: Summative reviews of the epidemiological evidence, prevalence, and interventions to promote "active aging"', *Gerontologist, 56*(Suppl. 2): S268–280, doi:10.1093/geront/gnw031

Cadore, E.L., Casas-Herrero, A., Zambom-Ferraresi, F., Idoate, F., Millor, N. et al., 2014, 'Multicomponent exercises including muscle power training enhance muscle mass, power output, and functional outcomes in institutionalized frail nonagenarians', *Age, 36*(2): 773–85, doi:10.1007/s11357-013-9586-z

Campbell, A.J. & Buchner, D.M., 1997, 'Unstable disability and the fluctuations of frailty', *Age and Ageing, 26*(4): 315–18, <https://pdfs.semanticscholar.org/c294/ef1e66f97ba1dd88ecaf6df8f96438836191.pdf>, accessed 31 May 2019

Chang, W.-C., Wahlqvist, M.L., Chang, H.-Y., Hsu, C.-C., Lee, M.-S. et al., 2011, 'A bean-free diet increases the risk of all-cause mortality among Taiwanese women: The role of the metabolic syndrome', *Public Health Nutrition, 15*(4): 663–72, doi:10.1017/S1368980011002151

Chiu, A.E., Chan, J.L., Kern, D.G., Kohler, S., Rehmus, W.E. & Kimball, A.B., 2005, 'Double-blinded, placebo-controlled trial of green tea extracts in the clinical and histologic appearance of photoaging skin', *Dermatologic Surgery, 31*(Suppl. 1): 855–60, doi:10.1111/j.1524-4725.2005.31731

Clegg, A., Young, J., Iliffe, S., Rikkert, M.O. & Rockwood, K., 2013, 'Frailty in elderly people', *Lancet, 381*(9868): 752–62, doi:10.1016/S0140-6736(12)62167-9

Cowen, L.E., Hodak, S.P. & Verbalis, J.G., 2013, 'Age-associated abnormalities of water homeostasis', *Endocrinology and Metabolism Clinics of North America, 42*(2): 349–70, doi:10.1016/j.ecl.2013.02.005

Daly, R.M., Gagnon, C., Lu, Z.X., Magliano, D.J., Dunstan, D.W. et al., 2012, 'Prevalence of vitamin D deficiency and its determinants in Australian adults aged 25 years and older: A national, population-based study', *Clinical Endocrinology, 77*(1): 26–35, doi:10.1111/j.1365-2265.2011.04320.x

Dangour, A.D., Allen, E., Clarke, R., Elbourne, D., Fletcher, A.E. et al., 2015, 'Effects of vitamin B-12 supplementation on neurologic and cognitive function in older people: A randomized controlled trial', *American Journal of Clinical Nutrition, 102*(3): 639–47, doi:10.3945/ajcn.115.110775

Darmadi-Blackberry, I., Wahlqvist, M.L., Kouris-Blazos, A., Steen, B., Lukito, W. et al., 2004, 'Legumes: The most important dietary predictor of survival in older people of different ethnicities', *Asia Pacific Journal of Clinical Nutrition, 13*(2): 217–20, <http://apjcn.nhri.org.tw/SERVER/MarkWpapers/Papers/Papers%202004/P330.pdf>, accessed 16 February 2019

Dementia Australia, 2018, *Types of Dementia*, <www.dementia.org.au/about-dementia/types-of-dementia/alzheimers-disease>, accessed 2 December 2018

Deutz, N.E.P., Bauer, J.M., Barazzoni, R., Biolo, G., Boirie, Y. et al., 2014, 'Protein intake and exercise for optimal muscle function with aging: Recommendations from the ESPEN Expert Group', *Clinical Nutrition, 33*(6): 929–36, doi:10.1016/j.clnu.2014.04.007

Durga, J., van Boxtel, M.P., Schouten, E.G., Kok, F.J., Jolles, J. et al., 2007, 'Effect of 3-year folic acid supplementation on cognitive function in older adults in the FACIT trial: A randomised, double blind, controlled trial', *Lancet, 369*(9557): 208–16, doi:10.1016/s0140-6736(07)60109-3

Fairweather-Tait, S.J., Wawer, A.A., Gillings, R., Jennings, A. & Myint, P.K., 2014, 'Iron status in the elderly', *Mechanisms of Ageing and Development, 136–137*: 22–8, doi:10.1016/j.mad.2013.11.005

Farshidfar, F., Shulgina, V. & Myrie, S.B., 2015, 'Nutritional supplementations and administration considerations for sarcopenia in older adults', *Nutrition and Aging, 3*(2–4): 147–70, doi:10.3233/NUA-150057

Foreman, J., Xie, J., Keel, S., van Wijngaarden, P., Sandhu, S.S. et al., 2017, 'The prevalence and causes of vision loss in indigenous and non-indigenous Australians: The National Eye Health Survey', *Ophthalmology, 124*(12): 1743–52, doi:10.1016/j.ophtha.2017.06.001

Foyer, C.H., Lam, H.-M., Nguyen, H.T., Siddique, K.H., Varshney, R.K. et al., 2016, 'Neglecting legumes has compromised human health and sustainable food production', *Nature Plants, 2*(8): 16112, doi:10.1038/nplants.2016.112

Fulkerson, J.A., Larson, N., Horning, M. & Neumark-Sztainer, D., 2014, 'A review of associations between family or shared meal frequency and dietary and weight status outcomes across the lifespan', *Journal of Nutrition Education and Behavior, 46*(1): 2–19, doi:10.1016/j.jneb.2013.07.012

Gagnon, C., Daly, R.M., Carpentier, A., Lu, Z.X., Shore-Lorenti, C. et al., 2014, 'Effects of combined calcium and vitamin D supplementation on insulin secretion, insulin sensitivity and beta-cell function in multi-ethnic vitamin D-deficient adults at risk for type 2 diabetes: A pilot randomized, placebo-controlled trial', *PLoS One, 9*(10): e109607, doi:10.1371/journal.pone.0109607

Greul, A.K., Grundmann, J.U., Heinrich, F., Pfitzner, I., Bernhardt, J. et al., 2002, 'Photoprotection of UV-irradiated human skin: An antioxidative combination of vitamins E and C, carotenoids, selenium and proanthocyanidins', *Skin Pharmacology and Applied Skin Physiology, 15*(5): 307–15, doi:10.1159/000064534

Grosso, G., Pajak, A., Marventano, S., Castellano, S., Galvano, F. et al., 2014, 'Role of omega-3 fatty acids in the treatment of depressive disorders: A comprehensive meta-analysis of randomized clinical trials', *PLoS One, 9*(5): e96905, doi:10.1371/journal.pone.0096905

Haran, P.H., Rivas, D.A. & Fielding, R.A., 2012, 'Role and potential mechanisms of anabolic resistance in sarcopenia', *Journal of Cachexia, Sarcopenia and Muscle, 3*(3): 157–62, doi:10.1007/s13539-012-0068-4

Heinrich, U., Gartner, C., Wiebusch, M., Eichler, O., Sies, H. et al., 2003, 'Supplementation with beta-carotene or a similar amount of mixed carotenoids protects humans from UV-induced erythema', *Journal of Nutrition, 133*(1): 98–101, doi:10.1093/jn/133.1.98

Heinrich, U., Tronnier, H., Stahl, W., Bejot, M. & Maurette, J.M., 2006, 'Antioxidant supplements improve parameters related to skin structure in humans', *Skin Pharmacology and Applied Skin Physiology, 19*(4): 224–31, doi:10.1159/000093118

Holt-Lunstad, J., Smith, T.B. & Layton, J.B., 2010, 'Social relationships and mortality risk: A meta-analytic review', *PLoS Medicine 7*(7): e1000316, doi:10.1371/journal.pmed.1000316

Horwath, C., Kouris-Blazos, A., Savige, G.S. & Wahlqvist, M.L., 1999, 'Eating your way to a successful old age, with special reference to older women', *Asia Pacific Journal of Clinical Nutrition, 8*(3): 216–25, doi:10.1046/j.1440-6047.1999.00116.x

Horwath, C.C., 1989, 'Dietary intake studies in elderly people', *World Review of Nutrition and Dietetics, 59*: 1–70, doi:10.1159/000417073

Huang, Y.-C., Cheng, H.-L., Wahlqvist, M.L., Lo, Y.-T.C. & Lee, M.-S., 2017, 'Gender differences in longevity in free-living older adults who eat-with-others: A prospective study in Taiwan', *BMJ Open, 7*(9): e016575, doi:10.1136/bmjopen-2017-016575

Huang, Y.-C., Wahlqvist, M.L., Kao, M.-D., Wang, J.-L. & Lee, M.-S., 2015, 'Optimal dietary and plasma magnesium statuses depend on dietary quality for a reduction in the risk of all-cause mortality in older adults', *Nutrients, 7*(7): 5664–83, doi:10.3390/nu7075244

Huang,Y.-C.,Wahlqvist,M.L.& Lee,M.-S.,2014,'Appetite predicts mortality in free-living older adults in association with dietary diversity: A NAHSIT cohort study', *Appetite, 83*: 89–96, doi:10.1016/j.appet.2014.08.017

Huang,Y.C.,Wahlqvist, M.L., Lo,Y.C., Lin, C., Chang, H.Y. & Lee, M.S., 2018,'A non-invasive modifiable Healthy Ageing Nutrition Index (HANI) predicts longevity in free-living older Taiwanese', *Scientific Reports, 8*(1): 7113, doi:10.1038/s41598-018-24625-3

Hughes,A.M.,Armstrong,B.K.,Vajdic, C.M.,Turner,J., Grulich,A.E. et al., 2004,'Sun exposure may protect against non-Hodgkin lymphoma: A case-control study', *International Journal of Cancer, 112*(5): 865–71, doi:10.1002/ijc.20470

Hughes, C.F., Ward, M., Hoey, L. & McNulty, H., 2013, 'Vitamin B12 and ageing: Current issues and interaction with folate', *Annals of Clinical Biochemistry, 50*(4): 315–29, doi:10.1177/0004563212473279

Hypponen, E., Laara, E., Reunanen, A., Jarvelin, M.R. & Virtanen, S.M., 2001, 'Intake of vitamin D and risk of type 1 diabetes: A birth-cohort study', *Lancet, 358*(9292): 1500–3, doi:10.1016/s0140-6736(01)06580-1

Irrera, N., Pizzino, G., D'Anna, R.,Vaccaro, M., Arcoraci,V. et al., 2017, 'Dietary management of skin health: The role of genistein', *Nutrients, 9*(6): 622, doi:10.3390/nu9060622

Izumi, T., Saito, M., Obata, A., Arii, M.,Yamaguchi, H. & Matsuyama, A., 2007, 'Oral intake of soy isoflavone aglycone improves the aged skin of adult women', *Journal of Nutritional Science and Vitaminology, 53*(1): 57–62, doi:10.3177/jnsv.53.57

Jeffery, I.B. & O'Toole, P.W., 2013,'Diet-microbiota interactions and their implications for healthy living', *Nutrients, 5*(1): 234–52, doi:10.3390/nu5010234

Kiecolt-Glaser, J.K., Epel, E.S., Belury, M.A., Andridge, R., Lin, J. et al., 2013, 'Omega-3 fatty acids, oxidative stress, and leukocyte telomere length: A randomized controlled trial', *Brain Behavior and Immunity, 28*: 16–24, doi:10.1016/j.bbi.2012.09.004

Kim, C.J., Park,J., Kang, S.W. & Schlenk, E.A., 2017,'Factors affecting aging cognitive function among community-dwelling older adults', *International Journal of Nursing Practice, 23*(4): e12567, doi:10.1111/ijn.12567

Knoops, K.T.B., de Groot, L.C.P.G.M., Kromhout, D., Perrin,A.-E., Moreiras-Varela, O. et al., 2004,'Mediterranean diet, lifestyle factors, and 10-year mortality in elderly European men and women:The HALE project', *JAMA, 292*(12): 1433–9, doi:10.1001/jama.292.12.1433

Kouris-Blazos, A., Gnardellis, C., Wahlqvist, M.L., Trichopoulos, D., Lukito, W. & Trichopoulou, A., 2007, 'Are the advantages of the Mediterranean diet transferable to other populations? A cohort study in Melbourne, Australia', *British Journal of Nutrition, 82*(1): 57–61, doi:10.1017/S0007114599001129

Kouris-Blazos, A., Trichopoulou, A., Gnardellis, C., Trichopoulos, D., Polychronopoulos, E. et al., 1995, 'Diet and survival of elderly Greeks: A link to the past', *American Journal of Clinical Nutrition, 61*(6): 1346S–50S, doi:10.1093/ajcn/61.6.1346S

Kuczmarski, M.F.,Allegro, D. & Stave, E., 2014,'The association of healthful diets and cognitive function:A review', *Journal of Nutrition in Gerontology and Geriatrics, 33*(2): 69–90, doi:10.1080/21551197.2014.907101

Landi, F., Calvani, R., Tosato, M., Martone, A.M., Ortolani, E. et al., 2016, 'Anorexia of aging: Risk factors, consequences, and potential treatments', *Nutrients, 8*(2): 69, doi:10.3390/nu8020069

Lane, D.J., Jansson, P.J. & Richardson, D.R., 2016, 'Bonnie and Clyde:Vitamin C and iron are partners in crime in iron deficiency anaemia and its potential role in the elderly', *Aging, 8*(5): 1150–2, doi:10.18632/aging.100966

Lee, M.-S., Huang, Y.-C., Su, H.-H., Lee, M.-Z. & Wahlqvist, M.L., 2011, 'A simple food quality index predicts mortality in elderly Taiwanese', *Journal of Nutrition, Health & Aging, 15*(10): 815–21, doi:10.1007/s12603-011-0081-x

Lee, M.S., Huang,Y.C. & Wahlqvist, M.L., 2010,'Chewing ability in conjunction with food intake and energy status in later life affects survival in Taiwanese with the metabolic syndrome', *Journal of the American Geriatrics Society, 58*(6): 1072–80, doi:10.1111/j.1532-5415.2010.02870.x

Li, D., Wahlqvist, M.L. & Sinclair, A.J., 2019, 'Advances in n-3 polyunsaturated fatty acid nutrition', *Asia Pacific Journal of Clinical Nutrition, 28*(1): 1–5, doi:10.6133/apjcn.201903_28(1).0001

Lips, P., 2001,'Vitamin D deficiency and secondary hyperparathyroidism in the elderly: Consequences for bone loss and fractures and therapeutic implications', *Endocrine Reviews, 22*(4): 477–501, doi:10.1210/edrv.22.4.0437

López-Otín, C., Blasco, M.A., Partridge, L., Serrano, M. & Kroemer, G., 2013,'The hallmarks of aging', *Cell, 153*(6): 1194–217, doi:10.1016/j.cell.2013.05.039

Luscombe, C.J., Fryer, A.A., French, M.E., Liu, S., Saxby, M.F. et al., 2001, 'Exposure to ultraviolet radiation: Association with susceptibility and age at presentation with prostate cancer', *Lancet, 358*(9282): 641–2, doi:10.1016/s0140-6736(01)05788-9

McCusker, M.M., Durrani, K., Payette, M.J. & Suchecki, J., 2016, 'An eye on nutrition: The role of vitamins, essential fatty acids, and antioxidants in age-related macular degeneration, dry eye syndrome, and cataract', *Clinics in Dermatology, 34*(2): 276–85, doi:10.1016/j.clindermatol.2015.11.009

Mahadevan, M., Hartwell, H.J., Feldman, C.H., Ruzsilla, J.A. & Raines, E.R., 2014, 'Assisted-living elderly and the mealtime experience', *Journal of Human Nutrition and Dietetics, 27*(2): 152–61, doi:10.1111/jhn.12095

Mangweth-Matzek, B., Hoek, H.W., Rupp, C.I., Lackner-Seifert, K., Frey, N. et al., 2014, 'Prevalence of eating disorders in middle-aged women', *International Journal of Eating Disorders, 47*(3): 320–4, doi:10.1002/eat.22232

Marengoni, A., Rizzuto, D., Fratiglioni, L., Antikainen, R., Laatikainen, T. et al., 2018, 'The effect of a 2-year intervention consisting of diet, physical exercise, cognitive training, and monitoring of vascular risk on chronic morbidity—the FINGER randomized controlled trial', *Journal of the American Medical Directors Association, 19*(4): 355–60.e1, doi:10.1016/j.jamda.2017.09.020

Martinez-Gomez, D., Bandinelli, S., Del-Panta, V., Patel, K.V., Guralnik, J.M. & Ferrucci, L., 2017, 'Three-year changes in physical activity and decline in physical performance over 9 years of follow-up in older adults: The Invecchiare in Chianti study', *Journal of the American Geriatrics Society, 65*(6): 1176–82, doi:10.1111/jgs.14788

Miller, J.W., Harvey, D.J., Beckett, L.A., Green, R., Farias, S.T. et al., 2015, 'Vitamin D status and rates of cognitive decline in a multiethnic cohort of older adults', *JAMA Neurology, 72*(11): 1295–303, doi:10.1001/jamaneurol.2015.2115

Morley, J.E., Malmstrom, T.K. & Miller, D.K., 2012, 'A simple frailty questionnaire (FRAIL) predicts outcomes in middle aged African Americans', *Journal of Nutrition Health & Aging, 16*(7): 601–8, doi:10.1007/s12603-012-0084-2

Mudge, A.M., Ross, L.J., Young, A.M., Isenring, E.A. & Banks, M.D., 2011, 'Helping understand nutritional gaps in the elderly (HUNGER): A prospective study of patient factors associated with inadequate nutritional intake in older medical inpatients', *Clinical Nutrition, 30*(3): 320–5, doi:10.1016/j.clnu.2010.12.007

Namasivayam-MacDonald, A.M., Morrison, J.M., Steele, C.M. & Keller, H., 2017, 'How swallow pressures and dysphagia affect malnutrition and mealtime outcomes in long-term care', *Dysphagia, 32*(6): 785–96, doi:10.1007/s00455-017-9825-z

NHMRC, 2006, *Nutrient Reference Values for Australia and New Zealand (2006)*, <www.nrv.gov.au>, accessed 14 February 2019

Nishioka, S., Okamoto, T., Takayama, M., Urushihara, M., Watanabe, M. et al., 2017, 'Malnutrition risk predicts recovery of full oral intake among older adult stroke patients undergoing enteral nutrition: Secondary analysis of a multicentre survey (the APPLE study)', *Clinical Nutrition, 36*(4): 1089–96, doi:10.1016/j.clnu.2016.06.028

Nowson, C. & O'Connell, S., 2015, 'Protein requirements and recommendations for older people: A review', *Nutrients, 7*(8): 6874–99, doi:10.3390/nu7085311

Ogawa, T., Uota, M., Ikebe, K., Arai, Y., Kamide, K. et al., 2017, 'Longitudinal study of factors affecting taste sense decline in old-old individuals', *Journal of Oral Rehabilitation, 44*(1): 22–9, doi:10.1111/joor.12454

Porter Starr, K.N. & Bales, C.W., 2015, 'Excessive body weight in older adults', *Clinics in Geriatric Medicine, 31*(3): 311–26, doi:10.1016/j.cger.2015.04.001

Prasad, A.S., 2014, 'Impact of the discovery of human zinc deficiency on health', *Journal of Trace Elements in Medicine and Biology, 28*(4): 357–63, doi:10.1016/j.jtemb.2014.09.002

Pullar, J.M., Carr, A.C. & Vissers, M.C.M., 2017, 'The roles of vitamin C in skin health', *Nutrients, 9*(8): 866, doi:10.3390/nu9080866

Purba, M.B., Kouris-Blazos, A., Wattanapenpaiboon, N., Lukito, W., Rothenberg, E.M. et al., 2001, 'Skin wrinkling: Can food make a difference?', *Journal of the American College of Nutrition, 20*(1): 71–80, doi:10.1080/07315724.2001.10719017

Reddy, P. & Edwards, L.R., 2017, 'Magnesium supplementation in vitamin D deficiency', *American Journal of Therapeutics, 26*(1): e124–32, doi:10.1097/mjt.0000000000000538

Reid, I.R., 2014, 'Should we prescribe calcium supplements for osteoporosis prevention?', *Journal of Bone Metabolism*, *21*(1): 21–8, doi:10.11005/jbm.2014.21.1.21

Reynolds, E.H., 2002, 'Folic acid, ageing, depression, and dementia', *BMJ*, *324*(7352): 1512–5, doi:10.1136/bmj.324.7352.1512

Richmond, R.L., 2008, 'The changing face of the Australian population: Growth in centenarians', *Medical Journal of Australia*, *188*(12): 720–3, doi:10.1086/589867

Roberts, S.B., Hajduk, C.L., Howarth, N.C., Russell, R. & McCrory, M.A., 2005, 'Dietary variety predicts low body mass index and inadequate macronutrient and micronutrient intakes in community-dwelling older adults', *Journals of Gerontology: Series A, Biological Sciences and Medical Sciences*, *60*(5): 613–21, doi:10.1093/gerona/60.5.613

Rochtchina, E., Wang, J.J., Flood, V.M. & Mitchell, P., 2007, 'Elevated serum homocysteine, low serum vitamin B12, folate, and age-related macular degeneration: The Blue Mountains Eye Study', *American Journal of Ophthalmology*, *143*(2): 344–6, doi:10.1016/j.ajo.2006.08.032

Rowe, J.W. & Kahn, R.L., 2015, 'Successful aging 2.0: Conceptual expansions for the 21st century', *Journals of Gerontology: Series B*, *70*(4): 593–6, doi:10.1093/geronb/gbv025

Santos-Eggimann, B. & Sirven, N., 2016, 'Screening for frailty: Older populations and older individuals', *Public Health Reviews*, *37*: 7, doi:10.1186/s40985-016-0021-8

Scherer, R., Maroto-Sanchez, B., Palacios, G. & Gonzalez-Gross, M., 2016, 'Fluid intake and recommendations in older adults: More data are needed', *Nutrition Bulletin*, *41*: 167–74, doi:10.1111/nbu.12206

Seals, D.R., Justice, J.N. & LaRocca, T.J., 2016, 'Physiological geroscience: Targeting function to increase healthspan and achieve optimal longevity', *Journal of Physiology*, *594*(8): 2001–24, doi:10.1113/jphysiol.2014.282665

Stowe, J.D. & Cooney, T.M., 2014, 'Examining Rowe and Kahn's concept of successful aging: Importance of taking a life course perspective', *Gerontologist*, *55*(1): 43–50, doi:10.1093/geront/gnu055

Strandberg, T.E. & Pitkala, K.H., 2007, 'Frailty in elderly people', *Lancet*, *369*(9570): 1328–9, doi:10.1016/s0140-6736(07)60613-8

Tang, B.M., Eslick, G.D., Nowson, C., Smith, C. & Bensoussan, A., 2007, 'Use of calcium or calcium in combination with vitamin D supplementation to prevent fractures and bone loss in people aged 50 years and older: A meta-analysis', *Lancet*, *370*(9588): 657–66, doi:10.1016/s0140-6736(07)61342-7

Trichopoulou, A., Kouris-Blazos, A., Wahlqvist, M.L., Gnardellis, C., Lagiou, P. et al., 1995, 'Diet and overall survival in elderly people', *BMJ*, *311*(7018): 1457–60, doi:10.1136/bmj.311.7018.1457

UN, 2015, *World Population Ageing 2015* (ST/ESA/SER.A/368), <www.un.org/en/development/desa/population/publications/pdf/ageing/WPA2015_Highlights.pdf>, accessed 14 February 2019

US Census Bureau, 2018, *U.S. and World Population Clock*, <www.census.gov/popclock/world>, accessed 21 June 2018

van der Mei, I.A., Ponsonby, A.L., Dwyer, T., Blizzard, L., Simmons, R. et al., 2003, 'Past exposure to sun, skin phenotype, and risk of multiple sclerosis: Case-control study', *BMJ*, *327*(7410): 316, doi:10.1136/bmj.327.7410.316

van der Mei, I.A., Ponsonby, A.L., Dwyer, T., Blizzard, L., Taylor, B.V. et al., 2007, 'Vitamin D levels in people with multiple sclerosis and community controls in Tasmania, Australia', *Journal of Neurology*, *254*(5): 581–90, doi:10.1007/s00415-006-0315-8

Veronese, N., Stubbs, B., Noale, M., Solmi, M., Pilotto, A. et al., 2017, 'Polypharmacy is associated with higher frailty risk in older people: An 8-year longitudinal cohort study', *Journal of the American Medical Directors Association*, *18*(7): 624–8, doi:10.1016/j.jamda.2017.02.009

Verreijen, A.M., Verlaan, S., Engberink, M.F., Swinkels, S., de Vogel-van den Bosch, J. & Weijs, P.J., 2015, 'A high whey protein-, leucine- and vitamin D-enriched supplement preserves muscle mass during intentional weight loss in obese older adults: A double-blind randomized controlled trial', *American Journal of Clinical Nutrition*, *101*(2): 279–86, doi:10.3945/ajcn.114.090290

Wahlqvist, M., Lo, C. & Myers, K., 1989, 'Fish intake and arterial wall characteristics in healthy people and diabetic patients', *Lancet*, *334*(8669): 944–6, doi:10.1016/S0140-6736(89)90954-9

Weaver, C.M., Alexander, D.D., Boushey, C.J., Dawson-Hughes, B., Lappe, J.M. et al., 2016, 'Calcium plus vitamin D supplementation and risk of fractures: An updated meta-analysis from the National Osteoporosis Foundation', *Osteoporosis International*, 27(1): 367–76, doi:10.1007/s00198-015-3386-5

WHO, 2017, *Life Expectancy at Birth (Years), 2000–2016*, <http://gamapserver.who.int/gho/interactive_charts/mbd/life_expectancy/atlas.html>, accessed 18 December 2017

Winter, J.E., MacInnis, R.J. & Nowson, C.A., 2017, 'The influence of age on the BMI and all-cause mortality association: A meta-analysis', *Journal of Nutrition, Health & Aging*, 21(10): 1254–8, doi:10.1007/s12603-016-0837-4

Witard, O.C., McGlory, C., Hamilton, D.L. & Phillips, S.M., 2016, 'Growing older with health and vitality: A nexus of physical activity, exercise and nutrition', *Biogerontology*, 17(3): 529–46, doi:10.1007/s10522-016-9637-9

Zhu, X., Jiang, M., Song, E., Jiang, X. & Song, Y., 2015, 'Selenium deficiency sensitizes the skin for UVB-induced oxidative damage and inflammation which involved the activation of p38 MAPK signaling', *Food and Chemical Toxicology*, 75: 139–45, doi:10.1016/j.fct.2014.11.017

Zittermann, A., 2003, 'Vitamin D in preventive medicine: Are we ignoring the evidence?', *British Journal of Nutrition*, 89(5): 552–72, doi:10.1079/bjn2003837

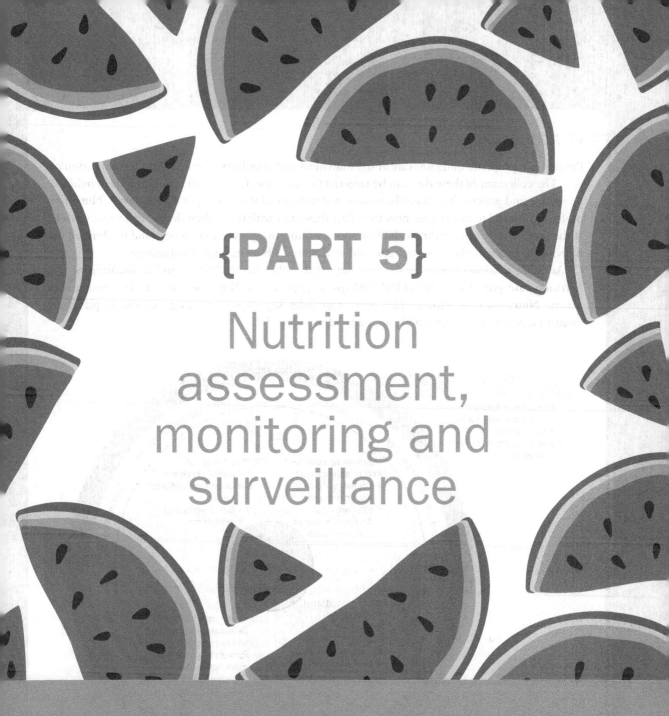

{PART 5}

Nutrition assessment, monitoring and surveillance

INTRODUCTION

Providing appropriate nutrition care at the individual and population level requires the collection of data. The collection of these data can be targeted (for example, for a specific condition or individual) or routine and general (for example, to monitor nutritional status at a population level). Nutrition professionals need to understand how to collect these data with the highest degree of accuracy, while at the same time balancing this with the resources (time, manpower and money) and the burden on individuals. Every method has strengths and weaknesses, advantages and disadvantages.

Assessing nutritional status is the first step in the planning, evaluating and monitoring of the nutrition care provided to individuals, groups or populations. Nutrition care can be summarised via the Nutrition Care Process. This process includes key steps—screening, assessment, planning, evaluation and monitoring—and is summarised in Figure 5.A.

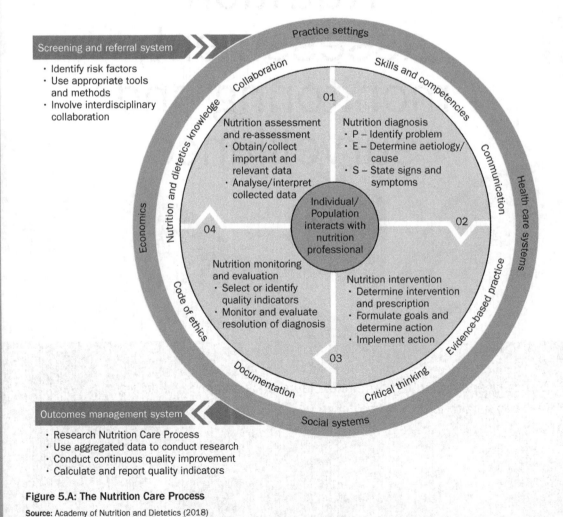

Figure 5.A: The Nutrition Care Process

Source: Academy of Nutrition and Dietetics (2018)

This process can be applied to individual care, as when a practitioner, for example, prescribes a nutritional approach for a particular condition; or at the population level, as when a state or country assesses the risk of a particular condition, implements an intervention and evaluates for effectiveness (see Table 5.A).

Table 5.A: Examples of using the Nutrition Care Process at the individual and population level

	Individual	Population
Scenario	Gestational diabetes	High blood pressure
Screening	Pregnant women screened for gestational diabetes.	Elevated blood pressure identified as issue through national health surveys.
Assessment	Blood glucose levels, weight status (pre-pregnancy and gestational weight gain), micronutrient status, dietary intake.	Review of epidemiological studies, national health surveys for at-risk populations, national nutrition surveys for foods consumed.
Diagnosis	Based on individual parameters.	Elevated blood pressure due to excessive sodium in food supply.
Intervention	Individualised, tailored dietary advice plus/minus insulin or oral medication.	Legislated reduction of sodium in processed foods; public health campaign to reduce salt usage.
Evaluation and monitoring	Regular blood glucose monitoring, diet diary, weight monitoring.	Nationally representative surveys reviewing blood pressure and dietary intake.

Nutrition monitoring and surveillance refers to the assessment of nutritional status and health in large population groups. For example, it could involve collection of data of a representative sample of people to draw conclusions about citizens of a country. It could also involve data collection in specific regions of a country, or in specific high-risk population subgroups.

Chapter 23 covers assessing and evaluating nutritional status, diets and physical activity across the life-course. Chapter 24 reviews the monitoring and surveillance of the nutritional status of populations and its importance in contributing to the nutritional status of a population.

REFERENCE

Academy of Nutrition and Dietetics, 2018, *Electronic Nutrition Care Process Terminology*, <www.ncpro.org/nutrition-care-process>, accessed 18 February 2019

{CHAPTER 23}
ASSESSING AND EVALUATING NUTRITIONAL STATUS, DIETS AND PHYSICAL ACTIVITY

Danielle Gallegos

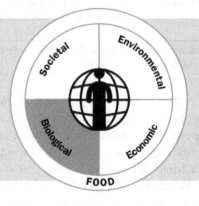

OBJECTIVES

- Identify and apply methods for assessing nutritional status, dietary intakes and physical activity for individuals at different stages of the life-course.
- Evaluate the strengths and weaknesses of each method of assessment.

INTRODUCTION

Nutritional status is measured using a variety of methods that can be summarised using the acronym ABCDE. The components of ABCDE assessment are used to gain an overall picture of the individual. These are outlined in Table 23.1 and will be discussed in relation to children, adults and the elderly.

ANTHROPOMETRY

Anthropometry is the study of the physical dimensions of the body and has been used as a simple, non-invasive, quick and reliable form of obtaining objective information about an individual's nutritional status. Body composition is complex and it is important to have a critical understanding of the

strengths and weaknesses of each physical assessment method.

In this section the use of height, weight, BMI, the circumference measurements of waist, hips, mid-arm, calf, head and skinfold thicknesses for children, adults and older adults is reviewed.

Height

Height is routinely assessed in children and adults to ascertain nutritional status. It is commonly used in conjunction with weight. In adults, the level of energy stores rather than the rate of growth is the indicator most commonly used to assess nutritional status. While in theory the mass of the body (body weight) provides an absolute measure of the body's store of energy, differences in height mean that it is

Table 23.1: Summary of nutrition assessment

A	Anthropometry	Measurement of body weight, and lengths, circumferences and thicknesses of parts of the body. This assesses changes in tissue stores and relevant anatomical changes.
B	Biochemistry	Measurement of biochemical functions related to a nutrient's function. This assesses changes to tissue stores, body fluids and metabolism.
C	Clinical assessment	Examination of medical history, general appearance, physical signs, medications that may be associated with nutritional health. This assesses changes in clinical status.
D	Dietary assessment	Estimation of dietary intake taking into consideration diet patterns, cuisine, cultural factors, food variety and nutritional intake.
E	Environment and social assessment	Details of cultural and social background, living conditions, education level, income and other factors that impact the ability to plan, prepare and transport food. Physical activity levels can also be included.

not possible to compare the weights of individuals of various heights. Consequently, BMI is used. Height as a measure of growth in children is assessed against charts that take their age into consideration.

Accurate measurement of height requires a standardised procedure and the use of appropriate, calibrated measuring equipment. For children under the age of two years, height is measured in the recumbent (lying down) position; children over the age of two can have their standing height measured. The difference between recumbent and standing height is about 0.7 cm, which has been taken into consideration in the growth charts (WHO 2008). This means that if a child under the age of two will not lie down to have their height measured, 0.7 cm needs to be added to the measurement; and if a child older than two cannot stand then 0.7 cm needs to be subtracted from the measurement. A length board is typically used for children under the age of two and a **stadiometer** for children over the age of two, adolescents and adults.

Measuring recumbent height needs two people: one to hold the head of the child, to ensure the shoulders are touching the board, and a second person to apply minimal pressure to straighten the knees and move the foot-board to measure the height. For standing height, shoes should be removed and the measured person should be standing upright with arms loosely at their side, back straight, heels against a vertical measure and the head in the Frankfort plane (Figure 23.1). The person taking the measurement may need to adjust the head to the right position.

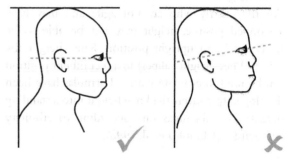

Figure 23.1: The Frankfort plane

Height is measured after a deep in-breath (WHO 2008).

Standing height can vary by as much as six millimetres across the day (Coles et al. 1994) and longitudinal studies suggest that height reduces by approximately one millimetre per year after the age of 40 years (Dey et al. 1999). Minor issues to consider when measuring height include hairstyles (braiding, ponytails and ornaments); more significant issues include abnormal spine curvatures.

Three alternative measures for height can be used if standing is not an option: self-report, arm span and knee height.

Self-report

When height cannot be measured an approximation can be obtained from self-reported values or from estimations made by an observer. Self-report of height tends to overestimate when compared to measured height, with mean differences ranging from 1.3 cm in young Australian adults (Pursey et al.

2014) up to 18.5 cm in adults over 65 years of age, where height losses can occur (Gorber et al. 2007).

Arm span

Arm span is another substitute for height and happens to be the same as maximal height achieved. A formula is used to convert arm span to height. There is, however, significant ethnic variation, with arm span being approximately equivalent to height in some subjects but much greater than height in others (Quanjer et al. 2014).

Knee height

For the elderly who are not agile and may have a stooped posture, height may not be able to be measured in an upright position. Knee height (by using a knee-height caliper) in a recumbent position can be used to estimate stature. Formulas have been developed to convert the knee height into a standing height; these formulas vary according to ethnicity and gender (Chumlea et al. 1998).

Weight

Weight loss is the single best factor for predicting persons at risk of protein-energy dysnutrition. Body weight represents the sum of protein, fat, water and bone mineral mass—that is, fat-free and fat mass—but does not distinguish between these. Hence, changes in body weight may reflect a change in one or more of these compartments. A standardised technique should be used. For infants, measuring of weight requires the removal of all clothes and nappies; and for children over two years and adults, weighing is undertaken in light clothing only. No allowances are made for clothing or for variations that may occur across a day which can be as much as two kilograms as a result of food/fluid intake or bowel/bladder evacuation.

When using weight in the clinical setting, consideration needs to be given to shifts in fluid that can occur; for example, in renal disease with dialysis, in liver disease with the presence of **ascites**, and in cases where **oedema** is present. Shifts in this fluid balance could mask weight changes attributed to loss of muscle and fat mass. Adjustments to body

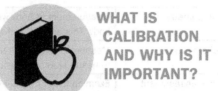

WHAT IS CALIBRATION AND WHY IS IT IMPORTANT?

The accuracy of measurement tools degrades over time due to use. The time to degradation can vary according to frequency of use and how often the measurement tool is moved. Calibration should take place according to the manufacturer's recommendations if there has been a shock to the equipment and periodically (for example, annually). Calibration is a process of comparing the measurement values delivered under test with those of a standard of known accuracy.

weight also need to be undertaken in the presence of amputations.

Weight is measured using a number of devices in different clinical settings. For infants under the age of two years there are two methods. The first is using a reclining baby scale. The second is using a tared standing scale. This involves having an adult stand on the scales and taring the scale to zero, then handing the undressed infant to the adult and recording the weight. Children over the age of two who are able to stand still can be weighed using a standing scale. Standing scales should be electronic, able to measure up to 150 kg and measure to a precision of 0.1 kg (WHO 2008).

For adults, weight can be measured on standing scales which are on a hard, firm surface and calibrated daily. Alternatively, sitting, bed or wheelchair balance-beam scales can be used. Scales should be calibrated for maximum weights. In the event that a weight cannot be measured it can be self-reported; however, there is a tendency to underestimate actual weight.

Ambulatory adults are weighed on an upright balance-beam scale or digital scale. A movable wheelchair balance-beam scale can also be used for adults who can only sit. A bed scale should be available in hospitals for measuring the weight of bed-bound patients.

Assessment of height and weight in children

Chronic under- or overnutrition is reflected in growth rates, and thus the monitoring of growth is an integral part of nutritional assessment. When interpreting the pattern of growth, clinicians use growth charts to 'plot' a child's growth (both weight and length) and to observe any changes in the trajectory of growth (usually done by comparing the individual trajectory against '**percentile** lines' on a growth chart). The fiftieth centile represents the median weight (or height)—that is, the mid-range value below which the weights or heights of 50 per cent of healthy children are expected to fall. Information about a child's growth and the interpretation and response to growth measurements, should always be considered alongside other clinical information. Growth charts may suggest that an infant or child who is above the 95th centile or below the fifth centile is unusually large or small; however, the growth of a well-nourished individual will typically follow a growth curve.

A greater cause for concern is when a child crosses centiles, particularly if this happens over a short period, suggesting inappropriate weight gain or acute growth failure or retardation, such as wasting or stunting. This could be due to chronic undernutrition or an underlying disease condition. Wasting is detectable on weight-for-age growth charts and by reduced skinfold measures, while stunting is seen as impairment of linear growth as detected by length or height-for-age growth charts. There are large variations between individuals in rates and patterns of growth, and these variations must be taken into consideration when determining whether a child's growth is abnormal.

Which growth charts to use?

There are two primary sets of growth charts in circulation internationally, the WHO 2006 growth standards for infants and children aged 0–2 years (WHO 2006) and the US Centers for Disease Control (CDC) growth charts for children aged 2–18 years (Centers for Disease Control and Prevention 2000). In 2012, all Australian and New Zealand jurisdictions agreed to adopt the WHO 2006 growth charts for Australian and New Zealand children aged 0–2 years. The WHO has found that the infant breastfed exclusively for the first six months of life provides the best and most internationally consistent reference point for healthy growth and development. Growth charts have been developed using these criteria based on internationally pooled data. The WHO charts are based on children from a range of ethnic groups and are considered relevant for all Australian children regardless of their cultural background.

Different growth charts are needed to assess the growth of older children to allow for differences in the timing of the adolescent growth spurt. Australia and New Zealand have adopted the CDC charts for two- to 18-year-olds. Table 23.2 shows the charts recommended for use in Australia and New Zealand and Table 23.3 compares and contrasts the WHO and CDC charts.

Body mass index

Body mass index (BMI) has been used widely to estimate total body fatness. BMI can be obtained by using the formula:

$$BMI = weight\ (kg)/height\ (m)^2$$

In theory, the mass of the body (body weight) provides an absolute measure of the body's store of

INFANT GROWTH

A mother is concerned about the growth of her baby. Her baby is following the third percentile for growth without deviating. Work with a partner and role-play your response.

Table 23.2: Recommended charts for Australia and New Zealand

		Girls and boys	Percentiles
0–24 months	WHO (2006)	Head circumference	3rd—97th
		Weight for age	3rd—97th
		Length for age	3rd—97th
2–18 years	CDC (2000)	Weight for age	3rd—97th
		Height for age	3rd—97th
		BMI for age	3rd—97th

Table 23.3: Comparison of CDC and WHO growth charts

	CDC 2000 Charts <www.cdc.gov/growthcharts/clinical_charts.htm>	WHO Child Growth Standards (2006) <www.who.int/childgrowth/standards/en/>
Data collection	Cross-sectional (one measurement point)	Longitudinal (0–24 months) (21 measurement points) Cross-sectional 18 months–5 years
Sample size	4697 (<100 per age group)	For 0–24 months: 18,973 observations for 882 distinct children For 18 months–5 years: 6669 observations
Exclusion criteria	Very low birth weight (<1500 g)	Low socioeconomic status Birth at altitude >1500 m Birth at <37 weeks or ≥42 weeks Multiple births Perinatal morbidities Child health conditions known to affect growth Maternal smoking during pregnancy or lactation Any breastfeeding for <12 months Introduction of complementary foods before age 4 months or after age 6 months Weight-for-length measurements >3SD above or below study median for sex
Feeding method	Mixture of breastfed and formula-fed, reflective of breastfeeding rates in the USA at the time: 50% ever breastfed 33% breastfed at 3 months	100% ever breastfed 100% predominantly breastfed at 4 months 100% still breastfed at 12 months Mean age of introduction of solids was 5.4 months

Source: de Onis et al. (2007)

energy; differences in height, however, mean that it is not possible to compare the weights of individuals of various heights. For this reason, BMI, which corrects body mass for differences in height, is now widely used for this purpose.

Interpreting BMI z-scores for children

For children, the preference has been to use weight–height. However, many countries have now developed BMI-for-age charts for children and BMI cut-offs for children aged two to eighteen years have been developed by pooling data from six large nationally representative cross-sectional growth studies to provide an international standard for the definition of overweight and obesity in childhood (Cole & Lobstein 2012). While these cut-offs are linked to the widely accepted adult cut-off points for overweight and obesity (BMI 25.0 and 30.0 respectively), they are not based on data on the health risks associated with overweight and obesity, as is the case for adults.

The long-term health consequences for children defined as overweight or obese by these cut-offs are not known. Interpretation of BMI **z-scores** is outlined in Table 23.4.

BMI for adults

BMI can be calculated to help classify whether the subject is in the reference range. A BMI below 20.0 kg/m² suggests inadequate nutrition and a BMI below 18.5 kg/m² is indicative of malnutrition in adults. Values in the healthy range for BMI are consistent with low mortality and morbidity. There is evidence that higher BMIs are associated with increased risk of mortality and morbidity from obesity, diabetes, cardiovascular disease and some cancers. Alternatively, a low or decreasing BMI is also associated with an increased risk of mortality, infection, slower recovery rates from surgery and longer hospital stays.

Table 23.4: Interpretation of BMI z-scores

z-score	BMI for age
Above +3	Obese
Above +2	Overweight
Above +1	Possible risk of overweight
0 (median)	Healthy
Below –1	Healthy
Below –2	Wasted
Below –3	Severely wasted

Source: WHO (2018b)

There is evidence of different ranges of BMI in different ethnic groups that are indicative of risk. Asian populations, in particular, appear to suffer much higher levels of illness such as diabetes or hypertension at a BMI well below 25 kg/m² and countries such as China define obesity at a BMI of 28 kg/m² or greater (Zhou et al. 2002). A WHO expert consultation concluded that there was insufficient evidence to recommend BMI cut-points for different ethnic groups; however, it did propose a range of public health 'action points' to guide the development of local interventions (WHO Expert Consultation 2004). See Table 23.5 for classification of adult weight according to BMI.

As BMI is derived from body weight, it does not distinguish between muscle and fat mass and so cannot differentiate between individuals with higher values due to greater muscle and those with higher fat mass. BMI also does not take into consideration where the fat is located. Abdominal distribution of fat is a known risk factor for chronic diseases. This is why other measures such as waist circumference are often used in conjunction with BMI.

Absolute weight loss

While BMI and the other tools are useful, absolute weight loss is another tool to use, especially in clinical settings. It is associated with an increased risk of morbidity, infection and mortality. Low body weight and/or unintended weight loss are significant risk factors, especially among ageing adults (see Chapter 22).

Table 23.5: Adult classifications of BMI

Classification	BMI (kg/m²)		Risk of chronic disease
	Caucasian	Asian	
Underweight	<18.5	<18.5	Low (but confers other risks)
Healthy range	18.5–24.9	18.5–23.9	Average
Overweight	25.0–29.9	24.0–26.0	Increased
Obese Class I	30.0–34.9	27.0–39.0	Moderate
Obese Class II	35.0–39.9		Severe
Obese Class III	>40		Very severe

Source: IDF (2006)

INTERPRETING BMI

Using the following scenarios calculate and interpret BMI.

- Mr Jones is a 67-year-old man. His height is 179 cm and he weighs 83 kg. How would you describe his BMI in terms of risk for his age?
- Mrs Smith is a 32-year-old woman. Her height is 168 cm and her weight is 54 kg. How would you describe her BMI in terms of risk for her age?
- Mr Nguyen is a 40-year-old man of Vietnamese origin. His height is 170 cm and his weight is 72 kg. How would you describe his BMI in terms of risk for his age and ethnic origins?
- Miss Phillips is a 19-year-old woman. Her height is 175 cm and her weight is 94 kg. How would you describe her BMI in terms of risk for her age?

INTERPRETING WEIGHT LOSS

Calculate the percentage loss of weight for the following individuals and decide if there is cause for concern or action.

- Fred is an 81-year-old man who has developed pneumonia. At the beginning of the week he was 85 kg and he had lost one kilogram by the end of the week. What was his percentage weight loss and is it cause for concern? After another month he had lost an additional four kilograms. Is there now cause for concern?
- Joan is a 40-year-old woman and has been trying to lose weight. She was 105 kg and lost thirteen kilograms in the last six months. Are you concerned?
- Phillip is a 36-year-old who was 79 kg. He went to his doctor complaining of nausea and had lost three kilograms over the last month. Are you concerned?

When considering weight loss, general guidelines requiring action would be:

- 2 per cent decrease of body weight in one week
- 5 per cent decrease of body weight in one month
- 7 per cent decrease of body weight in three months
- 10 per cent decrease of body weight in six months.

Interpretation of the weight losses and gains in clinical settings and older people should be done with caution. Increases in body weight may indicate overweight/obesity or oedema. On the other hand, decreases in body weight can signify the correction of oedema, development of dehydration or emergence of nutritional disorders. Weight loss is the single best factor for predicting persons at risk of protein–energy dysnutrition.

Circumferences

Head circumference (infants and children)

Head circumference is a routine measure at birth and in the first few months of life. It is indicative of the level of malnutrition *in utero* and in the first few months. Chronic malnutrition at these stages can decrease the number of brain cells and result in abnormally low head circumferences. It can also be used as an indicator of chronic protein–energy malnutrition in the first two years.

Waist circumference

Although obesity is generally considered a health hazard, results from several prospective and metabolic studies have shown that it is not the absolute excess of adipose tissue that is associated with an increased prevalence of diabetes, hypertension, hyperlipidaemia and cardiovascular disease, but rather the regional distribution of body fat. Abdominal fatness, irrespective of body size, will predispose an individual to these conditions (Després & Lemieux 2006).

Accurate measurement of waist circumference requires a standardised procedure. The measurement should be taken with a non-stretch tape. The person being measured should remove any bulky outer or tight garments and shoes with heels, empty their bladder, then stand upright with arms loosely to the side. The tape is passed round the body and positioned midway between the iliac crest (the prominent bone of the hip) and costal margin of the lower rib, ensuring it is horizontal and untwisted. The tape should be parallel to the floor at the time the measurement is taken. The tape itself should be snug but not pulled so tight that it is constricting. The subject should be looking ahead and breathe out with the measurement taken at the end of expiration and the procedure repeated (WHO 2011). A number of studies have shown that abdominal measurements alone can be used to safely decide whether weight loss is necessary to reduce the risk from diseases such as heart disease and diabetes. The International Diabetes Federation (IDF) has identified waist circumference cut-offs according to gender and ethnicity; these are outlined in Table 23.6. In ethnic

groups where the average build is slight, such as in many Asian countries, a lesser degree of abdominal fatness may still put the person at risk of developing chronic diseases, especially if BMI is over 23 kg/m^2.

Waist–hip ratio

The simplest measure that reflects body type is waist-to-hip ratio (WHR), which is calculated by dividing the abdominal/waist circumference (midway between the lowest rib margin and iliac crest or hip bone) by the hip circumference (greatest gluteal protuberance). A WHR greater than 0.9 in men and 0.8 in women indicates central or **android fat** distribution and is comparable to BMI and waist circumference alone as a predictor of health risk.

Waist–height ratio

The waist–height ratio is increasingly recognised as a good predictor of metabolic risk and superior to BMI or waist circumference in men and women. A cut-off of less than 0.5 is recommended in order to reduce risk of diabetes, hypertension, dyslipidaemia, metabolic syndrome and other cardiovascular outcomes. There is one cut-off for adults, children, men, women and various ethnic groups. The public health message is also simple—to keep waist circumference less than half height (Ashwell et al. 1996; Ashwell et al. 2012).

Table 23.6: Waist circumference cut-offs indicative of higher metabolic risk

Country/Ethnic group		Waist circumference
Europeans	Male	≥ 94 cm
	Female	≥ 80 cm
South Asians	Male	≥ 90 cm
	Female	≥ 80 cm
Chinese	Male	≥ 90 cm
	Female	≥ 80 cm
Japanese	Male	≥ 85 cm
	Female	≥ 90 cm
Ethnic South and Central Americans	Use South Asian recommendations until more specific data are available	
Sub-Saharan Africans	Use European data until more specific data are available	
Eastern Mediterranean and Middle East populations	Use European data until more specific data are available	

Source: IDF (2006).

Mid-arm muscle circumference (MAMC)

MAMC or mid-upper arm circumference (MUAC) is taken at the mid-point between **acromion** and olecranon and can be used to identify chronic energy deficiency. Population studies indicate that a lower MAMC in adults is associated with a higher mortality risk (Wu et al. 2017). MAMC is routinely used in the field as a quick and non-invasive measure of nutrition status, particularly among children.

The WHO has percentile charts for arm circumference-for-age (WHO 2018a). There is also a range of disposable MAMC measuring tapes that are colour-coded to allow for quick identification of malnutrition (UNICEF n.d.).

The MAMC can also be used in conjunction with triceps skinfold to calculate mid-arm muscle area (MAMA), which is an index of total body protein mass. The use of MAMA is preferable to MAMC as it reflects the true change in muscle mass. However, the complexities of collecting two measurements in the field and a complex calculation means the disadvantages outweigh the increased sensitivity. Corrected MAMA equations account for the non-circular nature of muscles and the inclusion of non-skeletal muscle tissue. The equation to estimate MAMA is (all measurements in centimetres):

$$cAMA = \frac{(MUAC - (\pi \times TSF))^2 - k}{4\pi}$$

MUAC = Mid-upper arm circumference
TSF = Triceps skinfold
k = 6.5 for women and 10.0 for men (Gibson 2005).

Calf circumference

Calf circumference (taken at the largest circumference by using non-stretchable flexible measuring tape), in the absence of lower limb oedema, can be used to calculate weight. It can be measured in either leg, seated or lying down and can therefore be used for those who are bed-bound. Calf circumference is being increasingly used as a predictor for care needs in older adults. Lower calf circumferences indicate decreased muscle mass of the lower extremities and therefore potentially poorer functional performance (Hsu et al. 2016).

Skinfolds

Skinfold thickness measurements are a simple field method for estimating body fat. However, as intra-abdominal adipose tissue cannot be assessed the technique is more useful in lean individuals with smaller fat stores than in overweight individuals (Madden & Smith 2016). Measurement of skinfold thicknesses is particularly relevant in situations where it is desirable to differentiate large muscle mass from fat (for example, in bodybuilders) or if there is a changing proportion of muscle mass to fat mass (for example, if exercising). In these situations, BMI, which relies on weight and height alone, will not adequately assess body fat, since the weight component may be fat or muscle. The method relies on the use of portable skinfold calipers but does require standardised techniques, training and monitoring to ensure reliability of measurements.

The skinfolds are used to calculate body fat, because about 50 per cent of body fat is normally located in the subcutaneous (under the skin) region. The calculations are based on a number of studies in which skinfold thicknesses have been measured in addition to measurements of body fat by the generally more accurate laboratory methods described later. This has enabled the preparation of equations and tables relating measured body fat to the thicknesses of folds of skin measured at specific positions on the body. One or several skinfolds may be used. The most used sites are:

- triceps skinfold, at the mid-point of the back of the upper arm
- biceps skinfold, at the same mark as the triceps skinfold rotated to the front of the arm
- suprailiac, just above the crest of the hip bone at the side of the body
- subscapular, just below the lower corner of the scapula (shoulder blade) on the back.

All skinfolds to be measured are picked up between the thumb and forefinger; the skin is gently pinched and pulled away from the underlying muscle; calipers are applied one centimetre in from the edge of the fold and the reading taken three seconds after application of the calipers to standardise the effect of compression of the tissue. The value recorded is the average of three readings. There are a variety of equations used to infer body weight from skinfolds. The best ones to use are based on data from populations.

Other measures of body composition
Total body fat
Body composition can be measured or estimated in a number of ways. These are usually grouped into laboratory methods, which require specialised and expensive equipment, and field methods (described above), which are relatively simple but inevitably less accurate. There are six laboratory methods that are widely used:

- underwater weighing
- air displacement plethysmography
- measurement of body water
- measurement of body potassium
- dual energy x-ray absorptiometry (DEXA)
- body impedance analysis.

The first four are direct and have similar accuracy. The latter two are indirect and rely on complex equations and are, therefore, subject to a greater degree of uncertainty.

Underwater weighing
The person is weighed in air and weighed again while fully submerged in water, which allows for determination of the specific gravity (or relative density) of the body. The method requires the person to be fully submersed in water and they are required to perform repeated maximal voluntary exhalations. A correction must be calculated to allow for the small amount of air remaining in the lungs. Since the specific gravity of fat (0.900) and lean tissues (1.100) are known with a fair degree of accuracy, it is possible to calculate the amounts of fat and lean tissues. This method requires specialised equipment that is expensive to install and to maintain.

Air displacement plethysmography
Air displacement plethysmography is a method designed to measure body volume and therefore fat mass. It uses the same principles as underwater weighing but is less invasive. In this method, the volume of an object is measured indirectly by determining the volume of air that is displaced inside an enclosed chamber. During the measurement, the chamber produces a very small volume change inside the chamber and measures the pressure responses to these small volume changes. Firstly, the volume of the empty chamber is determined; then the volume is determined when the subject is seated inside. Chambers, known commercially as the BODPOD and the PEABOD, have been developed for infants, children and adults.

Measurement of body water
The person consumes a drink containing a measured amount of water labelled with deuterium (^{2}H heavy hydrogen). Over the following three hours or so, the water becomes evenly distributed throughout the body, except for the areas occupied by fat, which cannot be mixed with water. A saliva, urine or blood sample can then be taken and the dilution of the labelled water measured. This permits calculation of the 'water space' of the body and thus the mass of lean tissue and fat.

Measurement of body potassium
A small proportion of the potassium in the body is of the radioactive form, ^{41}K. A person can be placed inside a large whole-body radioactivity counter and the natural radioactivity measured. Since potassium is contained in the cells of the lean tissue, and fat contains no potassium, the amount of lean tissue and fat can be calculated. The methods described above are reasonably accurate, but are primarily research methods rather than methods that can be applied to everyday measurements.

Dual energy x-ray absorptiometry (DEXA)
Twin x-ray beams are used to scan across the body and the x-ray absorption is measured at intervals down the body. The use of beams of different energies allows the differential measurement of fat, lean tissue and bone, and these values are integrated to give a map of body composition.

Body impedance analysis

In body impedance analysis, electrodes are attached to one hand and one foot. A small alternating current is passed through the body and impedance (resistance to alternating current) is measured. The method relies on the greater conductivity of lean tissue as compared to fat, and a pre-established equation that includes body weight is used to determine a value for fat.

Body impedance analysis is so simple and easy to apply that it is becoming widely used in places such as gymnasiums; however, it should be noted that measured body fat levels have an acceptable level of accuracy when determined for groups of people but may be relatively inaccurate when determined for one individual.

BIOCHEMISTRY

Biochemical, haematological and immunological assessments are useful to confirm nutritional disorders and to identify specific complications that accompany them. Laboratory tests are useful in several ways in that they can be used to:

- provide the earliest indications of some nutrient deficiencies and excesses
- confirm a nutrition diagnosis based on clinical signs and symptoms
- assess the effect of nutritional therapy.

Table 23.7 lists some of the more commonly used laboratory tests to identify nutrition problems. A range of factors influence the interpretation of laboratory tests and these need to be taken into

Table 23.7: Commonly used laboratory blood tests to assess nutritional status

Laboratory test	Nutritional problem	What the test measures
Red cell indices	Anaemia	The number and size of red cells. For example, as iron deficiency anaemia progresses blood cells become smaller and paler.
Haematocrit	Anaemia	Proportion of cells to plasma in blood.
Serum iron	Reduced iron transport	The amount of iron bound to iron transport protein in the blood. Transferrin, the protein that binds iron, may also be measured in iron deficiency anaemia—this will be increased.
Serum ferritin	Lack of iron stores	The total body store of iron.
Red cell folate	Anaemia due to folate deficiency	Amount of folate in cells.
Serum cholesterol	Risk factor for cardiovascular disease	Measure of total circulating (both high and low density) cholesterol.
Serum triglyceride	Risk factor for cardiovascular disease and diabetes mellitus	Measure of blood lipid in fasting state.
Blood glucose	Risk factor for diabetes mellitus	Usually taken in a fasting state. Can be measured as a single measure or as an oral fasting blood glucose tolerance test.
HbA1c Glycated haemoglobin	Risk factor for poorly controlled diabetes mellitus	Provides an indication of prevailing blood glucose concentration over the last 2–3 months.
Vitamin K	Vitamin K deficiency	Prothrombin time. Determines the clotting tendency of the blood.
Serum albumin/ pre-albumin/ C-reactive protein	Risk factor for poor nutritional status	Protein status. Albumin is not a sensitive measure of nutritional status, with a half-life of 14–20 days, and is affected by inflammation. Pre-albumin has a much shorter half-life (2–3 days) but is still affected by inflammation. CRP has a half-life of 19 hours and is constant under all medical conditions.
Potassium/ creatinine/urea	Kidney function	These measures are all elevated when kidney function is disrupted.

consideration and indicate why holistic assessment of the individual is required.

Blood and urine tests are the most commonly performed biochemical tests, mainly because they are readily obtained and there is a system in place for collection and analysis. Blood tests vary little due to homeostatic control. Urine testing varies between nutrients and is influenced by a variety of factors, including volume. Multiple samples are usually required. Hair and nails may be used to test for information on trace elements; other tests, such as gut biopsies, used for the diagnosis of gluten intolerance, are more invasive.

CLINICAL ASSESSMENT

A clinical assessment encompasses sociodemographics, medical history, signs and **symptoms** and medications. This information provides clues as to the likely nature of the nutritional problem and why it is occurring. **Signs** and symptoms should not be used in isolation as they often manifest late in the development of a nutrition problem and can be quite non-specific and occur for non-nutritional reasons. Tissues with faster turnover rates (hair, skin and tongue) are the most likely to show signs of nutritional deficiencies. Some of these signs and symptoms are outlined in Table 23.8.

One of the tools now routinely used for the assessment of malnutrition in clinical settings is the Subjective Global Assessment (SGA) or the Patient-Generated Subjective Global Assessment (PG-SGA). The SGA takes into consideration weight loss, dietary intake, gastrointestinal symptoms (nausea, vomiting, diarrhoea, lack of appetite), and functional capacity. It also involves a physical assessment looking at subcutaneous fat losses, muscle wasting, oedema and ascites (Detsky et al. 1984). The PG-SGA includes four patient-generated elements related to weight, food intake, symptoms and function/activities (Bauer et al. 2002). It is then followed by a professional assessment of the disease and its stages, components of metabolic stress (for example, infection, fever, use of corticosteroids) and a physical examination as for the SGA. Both the SGA and the PG-SGA classify individuals as: A—well nourished; B—mildly malnourished; or C—severely malnourished. The SGA and PG-SGA are subjective assessments and, as such, require training and practice to ensure consistent results.

Table 23.8: Signs and symptoms of nutritional deficiencies

Signs and symptoms	Nutrients to consider
GENERAL	
Poor growth	Protein, energy, essential fatty acids (EFA); iron, zinc, calcium, vitamin D, vitamin A
Poor immunity	Iron, zinc, selenium, vitamin D, vitamin A, vitamin C
Fatigue/irritability	Protein, iron, zinc, chromium, pyridoxine, B-12, folate, vitamin C
Moody/depressed/impaired memory	Protein, energy, iron, zinc, iodine, magnesium, thiamin, niacin, pyridoxine, B-12, vitamin C, vitamin D
Sleep disturbance	Magnesium, calcium, pyridoxine, niacin, vitamin C, vitamin D
HAIR	
Hair loss/dry/brittle/slow growth	Protein, EFA, zinc, iron, iodine, riboflavin, biotin, vitamin A (deficiency and excess)
EYES	
Dark circles under eyes	Iron
Pale conjunctiva	Iron
Impaired night vision	Zinc, vitamin A
Twitching eye lid/facial spasms	Magnesium, calcium

Signs and symptoms	Nutrients to consider
NOSE/TASTE/TONGUE/MOUTH	
Poor smell/impaired taste	Zinc, vitamin A
Pale tongue	Iron
Magenta/blue tongue	Riboflavin, biotin
Smooth bright red tongue	Riboflavin, pyridoxine, B-12, folate, biotin
Large, pale, swollen tongue	Iodine
Raw, painful, dark red tongue	Niacin, B-12, folate
Cherry-tip tongue	Niacin, pyridoxine
Angular stomatitis (inflammation at the corners of the mouth)	Iron, thiamin, riboflavin, niacin, pyridoxine, folate, B-12
Bleeding gums	Vitamin C, riboflavin, vitamin K
NAILS	
Vertical ridges (pronounced)	Protein, riboflavin, zinc
Pronounced central ridge	Protein, iron, folate
Horizontal grooves	Past severe illness; protein, zinc, selenium, calcium
White spots (leukonychia)	Zinc
Pale half-moon at base of nails	Pyridoxine
Dry, thin, brittle nails	Protein, EFA, iron, calcium
Peeling/splitting nails	Protein, calcium
Yellow nails	Vitamin E
Eggshell nails	Vitamin A
MUSCLES	
Muscle pains/aches	Calcium, magnesium, selenium, potassium, thiamin, vitamin C, vitamin E, vitamin D, coenzyme Q
Cramps	Calcium, magnesium, iron, potassium, vitamin D, vitamin C, water (dehydration)
Twitching/spasms	Calcium, magnesium, potassium, pyridoxine, vitamin D
SKIN	
Excessive ageing of skin/wrinkling	EFA, vitamin E, iodine
Perifollicular hyperkeratosis (toad skin)	Zinc, vitamin A, B-vitamins, vitamin C, EFA
Oily scaly seborrheic dermatitis (nasolabial folds, eyebrows, forehead)	EFA, riboflavin, niacin, pyridoxine, biotin, copper
Dry, scaly/coarse/itchy dermatitis	EFA, zinc, iodine, niacin, biotin, vitamin A, vitamin E, vitamin C
Dry 'fish scale' 'flaky paint' especially on legs	Vitamin A, zinc
Hyperpigmented scaly dermal patches on face/limbs (pellagra)	EFA, thiamin, niacin, biotin, zinc
NERVES	
Impaired coordination/balance disorientation/ataxic gait	Thiamin, B-12, niacin, vitamin E
Neuropathy (weakness, ataxia, pins and needles, paraesthesia, foot/wrist drop, reduced tendon reflexes, numbness)	Thiamin, riboflavin, pyridoxine, B-12, carnitine, folate, magnesium, calcium, potassium, EFA, chromium, iron, vitamin E

MYTH BUSTING

There are often many myths that circulate regarding signs and symptoms from eating too much or too little of specific nutrients. Using your skills in searching the peer-reviewed literature, gather evidence to write a page to refute or support the following claims.

- Muscle cramps are caused by a lack of salt.
- Acne is caused by eating too much fat and sugar.
- Pre-menstrual tension is caused by a lack of magnesium.
- Mouth ulcers are a result of a deficiency in the B vitamins.

DIETARY INTAKE

Dietary intake data provide information on the kinds and amounts of foods consumed by an individual. These data can be difficult to obtain as the food supply is extremely varied, individuals eat widely varying amounts and combinations of food from day to day, and there are variations in recipes and nutrient contents of the same food. Depending on the information obtained, it is possible to estimate the amount of nutrients consumed (by referring to tables of food composition), dietary variety or quality, and diet patterns. They are also used at the population level and the application of these tools for populations is discussed in Chapter 24. Each method has advantages and disadvantages.

Retrospective dietary data collection methods rely on remembering what has been consumed over a set period of time. Prospective data collection requires documentation of dietary intake as it is occurring. Advantages and disadvantages of these methods are outlined in Table 23.9.

Retrospective methods
Diet history
The diet history has been used for over 75 years (Burke 1947). In a clinical situation, the most relevant information is that which describes an individual's usual pattern of intake and not just their intake on a particular day. There are typically three components to a diet history. Firstly, an interview about actual intake (usually over the last 24 hours). Secondly, information is collected on usual intake, covering overall dietary patterns at mealtimes and between meals. A trained nutritionist probes for types and amounts of food and drink items. Thirdly, there is a cross-check with a list of key foods to determine the number of times a day, week or month specific foods

Table 23.9: Advantages and disadvantages of dietary intake assessment measures

Method	Examples	Advantages	Disadvantages
Retrospective	· Diet history · 24-hour recall · Food frequency questionnaires	· Quick and inexpensive. · Low burden for the participant. · Lower literacy and numeracy skills required. · Good cooperation. · Can be undertaken using a variety of methods.	· Reliant on memory. · Conceptualisation skills necessary to describe frequency of consumption and portion sizes. · Observer bias possible. · Reported diet may be different to usual diet. · May not measure day-to-day variation. · Requires regular eating habits. · Dependent on food composition tables.
Prospective	· Food diaries · Weighed food records	· Measures current diet. · Direct observation. · Daily variation described. · Length of recording can be varied.	· Labour-intensive. · Requires literacy and numeracy skills. · Under-reporting likely. · Changes to usual intake can occur. · Expensive.

DETERMINING PORTION SIZES

Every dietary assessment method relies on recalling portion sizes. How much of a particular food is consumed is important in determining diet and nutrient intake qualitatively and quantitatively. Determining this is important in ensuring the accuracy of the information collected. In some situations, examples or pictures of common household utensils can be used. Using three-dimensional food models, common household measures and common objects have been routinely used. However, these are not always available in settings outside the clinical or research environment. Dietitians and nutritionists need to become familiar with other means to estimate portion sizes. Using hand, fist or finger/thumb sizes can vary if you rely on those dimensions in others, but if you know the portion size of your own hands this can be a useful tool.

Using ordinary household utensils measure out a serve of:

- pasta
- cooked vegetables
- salad vegetables
- cheese
- rice.

Is this more or less than you expected? How could you describe this to potential clients?

are consumed. A dietary history interview may take an hour or longer to complete.

24-hour recall method

The 24-hour recall is an in-depth interview conducted by a trained interviewer, usually with the aid of pictures or examples of commonly used tools (cups, spoons, bowls) to allow more accurate estimation of serve sizes. Detailed information is gathered on all foods and drinks from midnight to midnight on the previous day or in the previous 24 hours. The interview often requires probing for food preparation methods, recipe ingredients, and brand names of commercial products.

A major source of error for the recall is that it relies on memory, and the ability to remember accurately is dependent on age, intelligence, mood, attention and the consistency of eating patterns. The principal advantage of the 24-hour recall is that it minimises the demands made on individuals and is widely acceptable. The main limitation of the 24-hour recall is that it provides information for each individual for only one day. For most individuals, one day is unlikely to be characteristic of their food consumption patterns in the longer term. For this reason, it is not possible to use the data from single 24-hour recall data to classify individuals in terms of the nutrient adequacy of their diet or to relate the 24-hour recall data from an individual to his or her health status. This can be minimised with the use of multi-pass recalls, which take into account multiple days over a week (typically non-adjacent days that include a weekday or weekend day).

A 24-hour recall has validity when taken over the phone, although some detail may be lost as examples of serve sizes cannot be used. Increasingly, 24-hour recalls are taken interactively using computer software in order to improve accuracy through standardisation. These systems are typically used at the population level rather than at the individual level and include the US National Health and Nutrition Examination Survey (NHANES) Automated Multiple Pass Method and the menu-driven standardised program (EPIC-soft) used in the European Prospective Investigation into Cancer and Nutrition. Work is being undertaken to validate self-administered web-based 24-hour recalls in adults and children (Conrad et al. 2018; Kirkpatrick et al. 2017). Typically, the 24-hour recall is not useful for individual dietary intake data collection except as the first step in a diet history.

Food frequency questionnaires

The fact that 24-hour recall data cannot provide reliable information about an individual's habitual longer-term food intake has led to the development of methods of dietary assessment that are designed to obtain information on habitual intake. Food frequency questionnaires (FFQs) largely overcome the first of these problems. The FFQ is a list of foods for each of which the respondent is asked to indicate how frequently they usually consumed the food over the last year or other nominated time period. Sometimes the individual is also asked to estimate the amount of each food that is usually consumed, either in relation to a reference serve size given in the questionnaire or in relation to one or more illustrations of commonly consumed amounts.

The length of the food list varies with the specific purpose of the questionnaire, but if the objective is to obtain an estimate of the total diet then the list usually contains between 100 and 150 foods. The main problem with the food frequency approach is that it is, at best, only semi-quantitative and cannot provide the level of descriptive or quantitative detail provided by 24-hour recall data and by records of food intake. The results obtained are also dependent on the ability of individuals to provide reliable data on their long-term average food intake amounts and on the reference serve sizes and nutrient values assigned to the food categories in the questionnaire. Shorter FFQs can be developed that assist in the measurement of individual nutrients—for example, calcium or fibre. One of the disadvantages is that the foods listed need to reflect the cultural variations within a population. For example, foods listed on an FFQ for a person who follows a more Mediterranean dietary pattern may be different from those listed by someone who follows an Asian eating pattern.

Versions of FFQs are increasingly being used as online indicators of healthy eating. This is allowing individuals to assess their own diet against pre-determined indicators. In these cases, FFQs are often adapted to form short questions that ask about the type, amount and frequency of different foods consumed. An example is the CSIRO Healthy Diet Score, which is available freely online and asks 38 questions (Hendrie et al. 2017).

Prospective methods

Estimated food records

For an estimated food record, the individual is asked to list all the food (type, amount) consumed at the time of consumption over a certain period of time. A food diary such as this can provide useful data, but people can change what they eat due to the process of recording. A food diary may be used clinically to ascertain the relationship between food consumption and other symptoms, such as consistency and frequency of bowel motions, or symptoms related to intolerances or allergies. A range of technologies is increasingly being developed to enhance the use of food records. These include mobile phone applications which provide an opportunity to record all food eaten and are linked to food composition tables. The use of mobile phone technologies to collect food record data has been shown to be more acceptable to some groups and is just as accurate as using pen and paper (Hutchesson et al. 2015). Features of applications that improve the process include integrated food composition databases, search ability for foods, suggested food lists, saved

USING AN APP TO RECORD YOUR FOOD INTAKE

1. Search for a free diet-recording application—for example, Easy Diet Diary, My Diet Tracker.
2. Assess the app according to the criteria in Chapter 3.
3. Record your dietary intake for seven days.
   - What was easy or difficult?
   - Did you change your intake?
   - What days were more accurate than others? Why?

favourite foods and recipes, barcode scanners, and push notifications or text message to remind users to record intake (Allman-Farinelli & Gemming 2017).

Image-assisted food records

Photographic food records are an extension of estimated food records and rely on active image capture using a mobile phone or digital camera or passive capture using wearable devices. Analysis of the images may be automated or semi-automated and rely on computer vision techniques that quantify the food in the images. Manual analysis requires input from a trained analyst who can identify and quantify the foods and beverages in the images. Photographic record approaches have been found to be easier than weighed records and passive recording has shown to reduce mis- and under-reporting of foods (Rollo et al. 2016). Other advantages include increased objectivity (in comparison to self-report) and the ability to re-review images if inconsistencies are found (Allman-Farinelli & Gemming 2017). Table 23.10 provides examples of some of these approaches that have been used on their own or in conjunction with other methods.

Weighed records of food intake

Weighed food records are the most precise method for estimating usual food and nutrient intakes for individuals. The number of days can vary, with seven days considered the optimum; however, due to the significant burden placed on the respondent weighed records are generally limited to three to four days. The method requires the individual to weigh and record all foods and beverages before and after consumption. Consideration needs to be given to the days selected and their representativeness of usual intake, and to the difficulties posed by weighing food if the respondent is not eating at home.

Until recently, weighed food records have been regarded as the 'gold standard', mainly because they do not rely on memory for either what is eaten or the estimation of portion size. It is now recognised that, while the method can provide an accurate estimate of what is actually eaten during the period of recording, this may not represent habitual food intake. The tendency is for individuals to either eat less than usual or to simplify their diet in other ways. As a consequence, when energy intakes measured by this method have been compared with measurements of energy expenditure obtained by the doubly labelled water method, or with the amount of food required to maintain body weight, it has been found that on average the method frequently underestimates usual food intake by as much as 20 per cent.

For the respondent, this method of measuring food intake is undoubtedly the most demanding,

Table 23.10: Examples of image-assisted food records

Name	Principles	Reference
ACTIVE		
DietCam	DietCam utilises the position of a credit card next to the food to give a reference size—three photographs around the dish every 120° or a video is taken before eating and after eating.	Kong et al. 2015; Kong & Tan 2012
NutriCam	NutriCam is an active image-assisted food record that requires the individual to capture a photograph of a food item and store a voice recording of the photograph.	Rollo et al. 2015
PASSIVE		
eButton	eButton is a wearable technology, worn on the chest, and is a continuous sensor and camera. For diet assessment applications the eButton, without the awareness of the wearer, takes pictures of food on the plate at a rate of one picture every two seconds.	Gemming et al. 2014; Jia et al. 2013; Sun et al. 2014
SenseCam	SenseCam is a small lightweight camera worn around the neck. Sensors detect movement, heat and light to trigger images every 20 seconds.	Gemming et al. 2014; O'Loughlin et al. 2013

WHAT ARE THE ADVANTAGES AND DISADVANTAGES OF EACH DIETARY ASSESSMENT METHOD?

Develop a table that outlines the advantages and disadvantages of each dietary assessment method.

Consider the individuals below and identify and justify an appropriate dietary assessment method.

- Jane has chronic kidney disease and the dietitian needs to know her consumption of high-sodium foods in the last three months.
- June is the community nutritionist who is collecting dietary intake data from a school prior to implementing an intervention.
- John is about to have surgery and the staff need to know what he ate yesterday.
- Jim is undertaking a dietary randomised controlled trial where 50 per cent of his saturated fat will be replaced with monounsaturated fat.
- Josephine is trying to lose weight. She is seeing a dietitian every month.

---

particularly if all food is weighed and not simply recorded in terms of standard household measures.

Assessing food intake

Food intake using these methods can be assessed qualitatively and quantitatively.

Qualitative assessment

Qualitative assessment is achieved by comparing the number of food servings consumed from each food group against the recommended servings according to the local food–based dietary guidelines (in Australia this would be the *Australian Guide to Healthy Eating*). If the food consumed (for a healthy individual) matches the recommended serves, it can be assumed that the person's diet is adequate. If the recommended serves are not reached for a particular food group, or a food group is missing from an individual's diet, then counselling on particular nutrients may be given. For example, if the recommended number of serves of dairy are not being consumed and there are no other sources of calcium, then calcium may be an at–risk nutrient. Some of these consumption patterns are outlined in Table 23.11.

Quantitative assessment

Quantitative assessment can be undertaken in one of two ways. The first relies on entering the data into a nutrient analysis computer program. These programs are based on the best available food composition data in which some (but not all) foods have been periodically updated (some fruit and vegetable composition data are 30 years old) and in which some nutrients may be missing. In Australia there are a number of programs, including FoodWorks (Xyris Software).

In the clinical setting, ready reckoners are often used to estimate nutrient intakes. Ready reckoners are a summary tool to provide average energy, protein and nutrient intakes for grouped menu items. This method does allow for the accumulation of error and so may not provide an accurate estimation of intake (Paciepnik & Porter 2017). Ready reckoners have been developed for specific nutrients relevant for particular disease states—for example, a renal ready reckoner would provide information on energy, protein, fat, carbohydrate, sodium, potassium and phosphorus for commonly eaten foods.

Environment

Dietary intake and nutrition status is as much a product of environment as it is about the individual. It is essential when doing a full assessment to take into consideration social and environmental factors, as these will impact on the type of strategies that are developed. Table 23.12 provides an example of

Table 23.11: Examples of food habits or circumstances that place individuals at risk of nutrient deficiency

Food pattern	At-risk nutrients
At-risk individuals based on clinical assessment, especially those following diets less than 6300 kJ/day for several months, elderly, polypharmacy, bowel/stomach disorders.	Multiple nutrients: calcium, magnesium, iron, zinc, B vitamins, fibre
High intakes of refined carbohydrate, processed foods, pre-cooked meals, takeaway.	Multiple nutrients: magnesium, chromium, zinc, fibre
Excess alcohol.	Multiple nutrients: calcium, magnesium, potassium, iron, zinc, selenium, folate, thiamine, vitamins C, D, E
Eating out more than twice a week for the main meal, especially at fast-food restaurants.	Multiple nutrients, fibre
Fatty fish consumed less than three times a week.	n-3 fatty acids, EPA/DHA
Low intake of animal foods (with no nut consumption).	Iron, zinc, selenium, vitamins B-12, B-6
Total avoidance of animal foods and fish (vegan diet).	Iodine, iron, zinc, calcium, omega-3 fatty acids, vitamins A, B-12, D
Low intake of dairy or calcium-fortified soy foods. In cultural groups where dairy is not commonly consumed, also look for low consumption of fish with bones/shells, green leafy vegetables.	Calcium, vitamin B-2
Low intake of dairy, eggs, carrots, sweet potato, green leafy vegetables, and avoidance of organ meats such as liver.	Vitamin A
Focus on low-carbohydrate diets and where there is little intake of whole grains.	Thiamin, magnesium, zinc, chromium, fibre
Low intake of dark green leafy vegetables.	Magnesium, zinc, folate, fibre
Low intake of fruit and vegetables.	Vitamin C, folate, β-carotene, magnesium, fibre

some of the information that could be collected. It is important to remember that many of these questions can be sensitive in nature and therefore need to be asked or determined tactfully. It is important not to make assumptions based on social information.

PHYSICAL ACTIVITY ASSESSMENT

Being physically active is an important component of building and maintaining wellbeing (refer to Chapter 30 for definitions and the guidelines). Physical activity contributes to not only physical but also mental health. There are a number of elements of **physical activity** that need to be measured to enable an assessment of its contribution. These elements include type, frequency, duration and intensity.

Intensity of activity is divided into three categories (Norton et al. 2010):

- low-intensity physical activity requires little effort, does not cause the individual to sweat

under moderate conditions and lets you carry on a normal conversation—for example, slow walking, doing the dishes.
- Moderate-intensity physical activity requires some effort but still allows you to hold a conversation easily—for example, brisk walking, recreational swimming, dancing, social tennis, riding a bike, gardening.
- Vigorous-intensity physical activity requires more effort and makes you breathe harder or 'huff and puff'—for example, running, fast cycling, digging.

Methods for measuring physical activity

As for the measurement of dietary intake, there are a number of measures of physical activity, each with their own advantages and disadvantages. The type of measurement used will depend on the context and how the data will be used. These measures are outlined in Table 23.13.

Table 23.12: Social, cultural and environmental factors in undertaking a nutrition assessment

Social	
Employment	What do they do for a living? Are they working, on benefits or retired?
	What is their income? How is this income achieved?
	Income will determine how much money a person has to spend on food. Whether that income comes from employment or benefits may provide insight into economic capacity.
	How much sunlight exposure do they receive?
Housing	What type of housing do they have?
	This can often go hand-in-hand with living arrangements. They may have stable housing or this may not be the case—they may be 'couch surfing' or moving around a lot, or they could be in a share house arrangement or hostel. Are they living in an apartment or in a house?
Living arrangements	Who do they live with?
	Are they married?
	Do they have children living with them?
	Are they a carer?
	How much sunlight exposure do they receive?
	Food intake will vary depending on whether you live alone or with somebody else and whether you have dependants.
Literacy	Can they read and write?
	Can they read and write in English or are they more comfortable doing this in another language?
Food literacy	How well are they able to plan and prepare meals?
	How often are meals prepared?
	Do they eat with others?
Family history	Is there a family history of any particular diseases or illnesses?
Alcohol, smoking, illicit drug use	Alcohol consumption, smoking and illicit drug use will impact on nutritional status, income available for food and ability to prepare foods.
Cultural	
Identity	Do they identify with any particular ethnicity?
	Do they identify as Indigenous?
Religion	Do they have any religious practices that may influence what they eat? Do they have any religious practices that may influence how much of their body is covered? (for exposure to sunlight see Chapter 16)
	How strictly do they follow these religious practices?
	Individuals will identify as practising a particular religion but there will be varying degrees of orthodoxy.
Language	Do they speak or read a language other than English?
	If they speak English how proficient are they?
	Do they have a preference for another language?
Environmental	
Location	This is assessing where a person lives—is it in the inner city, suburbs of a major city, in a regional or rural area, do they live remotely? This may determine their ability to access foods in the long term and exposure to sunlight (which impacts on mental health and vitamin D status).
Transport	Do they have access to transport?
	This may determine if they are able to access shops or markets for food. If they do not have a car, the use of public transport may limit what types and quantities of food can be purchased at any one time.
Cooking equipment	Do they have access to storage and cooking facilities?
	The types of equipment available may determine what meals they are able to prepare.

Table 23.13: Methods for measuring physical activity (PA)

Measure	Unit of measurement	Advantages	Disadvantages	Examples
SUBJECTIVE				
Physical activity diaries	Bouts of PA	Quantitative and qualitative information. Detailed data on type, duration, frequency, intensity for all activities. Minimal recall bias. Information is able to determine estimated energy expenditure. Logs can be low-tech, using pen and paper, or more high-tech, relying on mobile phone or web applications.	Time-consuming. High participant burden. Multiple day records are required and they will not necessarily reflect seasonal variations. May alter participants' PA patterns. Require literacy and numeracy skills.	Bouchard Physical Activity Record. 3-day Physical Activity Recall (3DPAR) (adolescents) (Sallis & Saelens 2000).
Physical activity self-report questionnaires	Bouts of PA	Quantitative and qualitative information. Inexpensive, low participant burden and can be administered quickly. Information is able to determine estimated energy expenditure. Tend to look at compliance against PA guidelines.	Reliability and validity issues associated with recall bias. Potential content validity issues associated with misinterpretation of physical activity in different populations.	Active Australia Survey (AIHW 2003). International Physical Activity Questionnaire (Craig et al. 2003).
OBJECTIVE				
Accelerometers	Movement counts	Objective indicator of movement. Useful in laboratory and field settings. Provides indicator of intensity, frequency, duration, and energy expenditure. Non-invasive. Provides for minute-to-minute information.	Expensive. Inaccurate assessment of a range of activities, including those involving upper-body movements and in the water. Reliable data are dependent on placement of monitor.	There are a range of commercially available devices. Devices are getting increasingly sophisticated, with accelerometers being inserted into watches and shirts linked to mobile phone technology. (Trost et al. 2005)
Pedometers	Step counts	Inexpensive, non-invasive. Potential for use in a variety of settings. Easy to set up and administer. Objective measure of a common activity (walking).	Accuracy limited when measuring jogging or running. Unable to measure other activities involving the upper body, cycling, water sports. Possibility of participant tampering. Can change behaviour (which is an advantage if that is a goal, but a disadvantage if there is an attempt to obtain an objective measure of PA).	Like the accelerometer there are a range of commercially available devices. Devices are getting increasingly sophisticated and linked to mobile phone technology. Original pedometers were worn at the hip, newer models are worn on the wrist. (Bravata et al. 2007)

SUMMARY

- Assessment of nutritional status is informed by the Nutrition Care Process, which provides a standardised process to provide tailored care at individual and population levels.
- Assessment of nutritional status includes anthropometry, biochemistry, clinical signs and symptoms, dietary intake and environmental conditions, which include social and cultural considerations.
- Anthropometric measurements include analysis of height, weight and growth for children. BMI—that is, weight which takes height into consideration—is used as a guide to ascertaining risk for chronic diseases. Waist circumference, which is used as an indicator of abdominal fat, is used in combination with hip and height to provide ratios that are also indicators of chronic risk.
- In addition to height, weight and waist measurements, a range of circumferences (head, arm and calf) are used to indicate nutritional status. Skinfold thicknesses in various locations are also used as a measure of subcutaneous fat.
- Biochemical markers in blood and urine are used to provide a guide to nutritional status. These include markers for protein status, blood lipids and micronutrients.
- Dietary intakes are measured using a variety of retrospective and prospective methods. These include diet histories, food frequency questionnaires, 24-hour food recalls, food diaries and weighed food records. Increasingly, technology is being used to increase the accuracy of these tools.
- Nutritional assessment cannot be complete without an examination of environmental, social, economic and cultural factors.
- Physical activity is the other side of the energy equation that impacts on overall nutritional status. Physical activity can be measured via recall methods, by observation or through the use of wearable technologies such as accelerometers and pedometers, which provide a more objective indication.

KEY TERMS

Acromion: the bony process at the top of the shoulder. The olecranon is the prominent bony projection of the ulna bone that can be felt at the elbow.

Android fat: fat that is deposited in areas such as the abdomen, chest, shoulders and nape of the neck. This pattern may lead to an 'apple shape'.

Ascites: the abnormal accumulation of fluid in the abdomen.

Oedema: the presence of abnormally large amounts of fluid in the intercellular tissue spaces of the body, usually applied to demonstrable accumulation of excessive fluid in the subcutaneous tissues.

Percentiles:
- 97th percentile—three in approximately 100 children are above this line
- 3rd percentile—three in approximately 100 children are below this line
- 50th percentile—half the children at any age are above this line and half are below.

Physical activity: elements measured include duration, frequency, intensity and type:
- *Duration* is the time of the activity bout (minutes or hours) during a specified timeframe.
- *Frequency* is the number of sessions over a specified time period. Frequency can often be further defined as the number of bouts ≥ 10 minutes.
- *Intensity* is an indicator of metabolic demand of an activity that can be objectively measured (e.g. oxygen consumption, heart rate) and subjectively assessed (e.g. perceived exertion, walk-and-talk test) or quantified by body movement (e.g. stepping rate). Intensity is often described in terms of METs—metabolic equivalents.
- *Type* is the specific activity performed, e.g. walking, gardening. Can be defined in the context of physiological or biomechanical types such as aerobic/anaerobic; resistance training; stability training.

Signs: observations made by a suitably qualified professional.

Stadiometer: a ruler calibrated in metres, centimetres or millimetres, which is fixed to the wall and has a movable head-plate.

Symptoms: manifestations reported by the individual.

z-score: the reference lines on the growth charts are called z-score lines because they are based on standard deviation scores. These scores are used to describe how far a measurement is away from the median. The z-scores are calculated differently for height, which is normally distributed, and weight, which is not. The WHO has a software package (WHO Anthro, www.who.int/childgrowth/software/en/) that is used for the calculation of z-scores, particularly in research.

ACKNOWLEDGEMENT

This chapter is based on the chapters 'Nutrition Assessment and Monitoring' and 'Nutritional Standards of Reference' written by Mark L. Wahlqvist and Antigone Kouris-Blazos, which appeared in the third edition of *Food and Nutrition*.

REFERENCES

AIHW, 2003, *The Active Australia Survey: A guide and manual for implementation, analysis and reporting* Canberra, <www.aihw.gov.au/reports/physical-activity/active-australia-survey>, accessed 23 May 2018

Allman-Farinelli, M. & Gemming, L., 2017, 'Technology interventions to manage food intake: Where are we now?', *Current Diabetes Reports, 17*(11): 103, doi:10.1007/s11892-017-0937-5

Ashwell, M., Cole, T.J. & Dixon, A.K., 1996, 'Ratio of waist circumference to height is strong predictor of intra-abdominal fat', *BMJ, 313*(7056): 559, doi:10.1136/bmj.313.7056.559d

Ashwell, M., Gunn, P. & Gibson, S., 2012, 'Waist-to-height ratio is a better screening tool than waist circumference and BMI for adult cardiometabolic risk factors: Systematic review and meta-analysis', *Obesity Reviews, 13*(3): 275–86, doi:10.1111/j.1467-789X.2011.00952.x

Bauer, J., Capra, S. & Ferguson, M., 2002, 'Use of the scored Patient-Generated Subjective Global Assessment (PG-SGA) as a nutrition assessment tool in patients with cancer', *European Journal of Clinical Nutrition, 56*: 779–85, doi:10.1038/sj.ejcn.1601412

Bravata, D.M., Smith-Spangler, C., Sundaram, V., Gienger, A.L., Lin, N. et al., 2007, 'Using pedometers to increase physical activity and improve health: A systematic review', *JAMA, 298*(19): 2296–304, doi:10.1001/jama.298.19.2296

Burke, B.S., 1947, 'The dietary history as a tool in research', *Journal of the American Dietetic Association, 23*: 1041–6

Centers for Disease Control and Prevention, 2000, *CDC Growth Charts*, <www.cdc.gov/growthcharts/cdc_charts.htm>, accessed 25 February 2019

Chumlea, W.C., Guo, S.S., Wholihan, K., Cockram, D., Kuczmarski, R.J. & Johnson, C.L., 1998, 'Stature prediction equations for elderly non-Hispanic white, non-Hispanic black, and Mexican-American persons developed from NHANES III data', *Journal of the American Dietetic Association, 98*: 137–42, doi:10.1016/S0002-8223(98)00036-4

Cole, T.J. & Lobstein, T., 2012, 'Extended international (IOTF) body mass index cut-offs for thinness, overweight and obesity', *Pediatric Obesity, 7*(4): 284–94, doi:10.1111/j.2047-6310.2012.00064.x

Coles, R.J., Clements, D.G. & Evans, W.D., 1994, 'Measurement of height: Practical considerations for the study of osteoporosis', *Osteoporosis International, 4*: 353–6, doi:10.1007/BF01622197

Conrad, J., Koch, S.A.J. & Nöthlings, U., 2018, 'New approaches in assessing food intake in epidemiology', *Current Opinion in Clinical Nutrition & Metabolic Care, 21*(5): 343–51, doi:10.1097/mco.0000000000000497

Craig, C.L., Marshall, A.L., Sjöström, M., Bauman, A.E., Booth, M.L. et al., 2003, 'International physical activity questionnaire: 12-country reliability and validity', *Medicine & Science in Sports & Exercise, 35*(8): 1381–95, doi:10.1249/01.MSS.0000078924.61453.FB

de Onis, M., Garza, C., Onyango, A.W. & Borghi, E., 2007, 'Comparison of the WHO Child Growth Standards and the CDC 2000 Growth Charts', *Journal of Nutrition, 137*(1): 144–8, doi:10.1093/jn/137.1.144

Després, J.-P. & Lemieux, I., 2006, 'Abdominal obesity and metabolic syndrome', *Nature, 444*: 881–7, doi:10.1038/nature05488

Detsky, A.S., Baker, J.P., Mendelson, R.A., Wolman, S.L., Wesson, D.E. & Jeejeebhoy, K.N., 1984, 'Evaluating the accuracy of nutritional assessment techniques applied to hospitalized patients: Methodology and comparisons', *Journal of Parenteral and Enteral Nutrition, 8*(2): 153–9, doi:10.1177/0148607184008002153

Dey, D.K., Rothenberg, E., Sundh, V., Bosaeus, I. & Steen, B., 1999, 'Height and body weight in the elderly: A 25-year longitudinal study of a population aged 70 to 95 years', *European Journal of Clinical Nutrition, 53*: 905–14, doi:10.1093/gerona/56.12.M780

Gemming, L., Rush, E., Maddison, R., Doherty, A., Gant, N. et al., 2014, 'Wearable cameras can reduce dietary under-reporting: Doubly labelled water validation of a camera-assisted 24 h recall', *British Journal of Nutrition, 113*(2): 284–91, doi:10.1017/S0007114514003602

Gibson, R.S., 2005, *Principles of Nutritional Assessment*, Oxford: Oxford University Press

Gorber, S.C., Tremblay, M., Moher, D. & Gorber, B., 2007, 'A comparison of direct vs. self-report measures for assessing height, weight and body mass index: A systematic review', *Obesity Reviews, 8*(4): 307–26, doi:10.1111/j.1467-789X.2007.00347.x

Hendrie, G., Baird, D., Golley, R. & Noakes, M., 2017, 'The CSIRO healthy diet score: An online survey to estimate compliance with the Australian Dietary Guidelines', *Nutrients, 9*(1): 47, doi:10.3390/nu9010047

Hsu, W.-C., Tsai, A.C. & Wang, J.-Y., 2016, 'Calf circumference is more effective than body mass index in predicting emerging care-need of older adults—results of a national cohort study', *Clinical Nutrition, 35*(3): 735–40, doi:10.1016/j.clnu.2015.05.017

Hutchesson, M.J., Rollo, M.E., Callister, R. & Collins, C.E., 2015, 'Self-monitoring of dietary intake by young women: Online food records completed on computer or smartphone are as accurate as paper-based food records but more acceptable', *Journal of the Academy of Nutrition and Dietetics, 115*(1): 87–94, doi:10.1016/j.jand.2014.07.036

IDF, 2006, *The IDF Consensus Worldwide Definition of Metabolic Syndrome*, <www.idf.org/e-library/consensus-statements/60-idfconsensus-worldwide-definitionof-the-metabolic-syndrome>, accessed 24 February 2019

Jia, W., Chen, H.-C., Yue, Y., Li, Z., Fernstrom, J. et al., 2013, 'Accuracy of food portion size estimation from digital pictures acquired by a chest-worn camera', *Public Health Nutrition, 17*(8): 1671–81, doi:10.1017/S1368980013003236

Kirkpatrick, S., Raffoul, A., Sacco, J., Lee, K., Chen, E. et al., 2017, 'Evaluation of the Automated Self-Administered 24-hour Dietary Assessment Tool (ASA24) for use with children: An observational feeding study', *The FASEB Journal, 31*(suppl. 1): 149–7, doi:10.1096/fasebj.31.1_supplement.149.7

Kong, F., He, H., Raynor, H.A. & Tan, J., 2015, 'DietCam: Multi-view regular shape food recognition with a camera phone', *Pervasive and Mobile Computing, 19*(Suppl. C): 108–21, doi:10.1016/j.pmcj.2014.05.012

Kong, F. & Tan, J., 2012, 'DietCam: Automatic dietary assessment with mobile camera phones', *Pervasive and Mobile Computing*, 8(1): 147–63, doi:10.1016/j.pmcj.2011.07.003

Madden, A.M. & Smith, S., 2016, 'Body composition and morphological assessment of nutritional status in adults: A review of anthropometric variables', *Journal of Human Nutrition and Dietetics*, 29(1): 7–25, doi:10.1111/jhn.12278

Norton, K., Norton, L. & Sadgrove, D., 2010, 'Position statement on physical activity and exercise intensity terminology', *Journal of Science and Medicine in Sport*, 13(5): 496–502, doi:10.1016/j.jsams.2009.09.008

O'Loughlin, G., Cullen, S.J., McGoldrick, A., O'Connor, S., Blain, R. et al., 2013, 'Using a wearable camera to increase the accuracy of dietary analysis', *American Journal of Preventive Medicine*, 44(3): 297–301, doi:10.1016/j.amepre.2012.11.007

Paciepnik, J. & Porter, J., 2017, 'Comparing computerised dietary analysis with a ready reckoner in a real world setting: Is technology an improvement?', *Nutrients*, 9(2): 99, doi:10.3390/nu9020099

Pursey, K., Burrows, T.L., Stanwell, P. & Collins, C.E., 2014, 'How accurate is web-based self-reported height, weight, and body mass index in young adults?', *Journal of Medical Internet Research*, 16(1): e4, doi:10.2196/jmir.2909

Quanjer, P.H., Capderou, A., Mazicioglu, M.M., Aggarwal, A.N., Banik, S.D. et al., 2014, 'All–age relationship between arm span and height in different ethnic groups', *European Respiratory Journal*, 44(4): 905–12, doi:10.1183/09031936.00054014

Rollo, M., Ash, S., Lyons-Wall, P. & Russell, A., 2015, 'Evaluation of a mobile phone image-based dietary assessment method in adults with type 2 diabetes', *Nutrients*, 7(6): 4897–910, doi:10.3390/nu7064897

Rollo, M.E., Williams, R.L., Burrows, T., Kirkpatrick, S.I., Bucher, T. & Collins, C.E., 2016, 'What are they really eating? A review on new approaches to dietary intake assessment and validation', *Current Nutrition Reports*, 5(4): 307–14, doi:10.1007/s13668-016-0182-6

Sallis, J.F. & Saelens, B.E., 2000, 'Assessment of physical activity by self-report: Status, limitations, and future directions', *Research Quarterly for Exercise and Sport*, 71(Suppl. 2): 1–12, doi:10.1080/02701367.2000.11082780

Sun, M., Burke, L.E., Mao, Z.-H., Chen, Y., Chen, H.-C. et al., 2014, 'eButton: A wearable computer for health monitoring and personal assistance', *Proceedings of the Design Automation Conference, 2014*, 1–6, doi:10.1145/2593069.2596678

Trost, S.G., McIver, K.L. & Pate, R.R., 2005, 'Conducting accelerometer-based activity assessments in field-based research', *Medicine and Science in Sports and Exercise*, 37(11 Suppl.): S531–43, doi:10.1249/01.mss.0000185657.86065.98

UNICEF, n.d., *Measuring MUAC*, <www.unicef.org/nutrition/training/3.1.3/1.html>, accessed 6 December 2018

WHO, 2006, *WHO Child Growth Standards: Methods and development*, <www.who.int/childgrowth/standards/technical_report/en/>, accessed 18 February 2019

—— 2008, *Training Course on Child Growth Assessment*, <www.who.int/childgrowth/training/module_b_measuring_growth.pdf>, accessed 18 February 2019

—— 2011, *Waist Circumference and Waist-Hip Ratio: Report of a WHO Expert Consultation, Geneva, 8–11 December 2008*, <http://apps.who.int/iris/bitstream/10665/44583/1/9789241501491_eng.pdf>, accessed 18 February 2019

—— 2018a, *Arm Circumference for Age*, <www.who.int/childgrowth/standards/ac_for_age/en/>, accessed 6 December 2018

—— 2018b, *Global Database on Child Growth and Malnutrition*, <www.who.int/nutgrowthdb/about/introduction/en/index5.html>, accessed 6 December 2018

WHO Expert Consultation, 2004, 'Appropriate body-mass index for Asian populations and its implications for policy and intervention strategies', *Lancet*, 363(9403): 157–63, doi:10.1016/S0140-6736(03)15268-3

Wu, L.-W., Yuan-Yung, L., Tung-Wei, K., Chien-Ming, L., Fang-Yih, L. et al., 2017, 'Mid-arm muscle circumference as a significant predictor of all-cause mortality in male individuals', *PLoS One*, 12(2): e0171707, doi:10.1371/journal.pone.0171707

Zhou, B., Wu, Y., Yang, J., Li, Y., Zhang, H. & Zhao, L., 2002, 'Overweight is an independent risk factor for cardiovascular disease in Chinese populations', *Obesity Reviews*, 3(3): 147–56, doi:10.1046/j.1467-789X.2002.00068.x

{CHAPTER 24}
NUTRITION MONITORING AND SURVEILLANCE

Jolieke C. van der Pols

OBJECTIVES

- Describe nutrition monitoring and surveillance and its importance in contributing to the nutritional status of a population.
- Report on the types of nutrition monitoring and surveillance taking place in Australia and New Zealand.
- Discuss the advantages and disadvantages of different types of nutrition monitoring and surveillance.

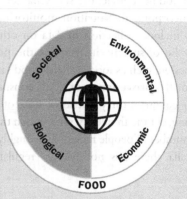

WHAT IS NUTRITION MONITORING AND SURVEILLANCE?

Nutrition monitoring and surveillance refers to the assessment of nutritional status and health in large population groups. For example, it could involve collection of data of a representative sample of people to draw conclusions about citizens of a country. It could also involve data collection in specific regions of a country, or in specific high-risk population subgroups.

Nutrition monitoring is important for the regular reviewing of the health status of people in a nation, or within high-risk groups within a country. Governments need to be able to draw on high-quality and up-to-date data to make decisions about food and nutrition issues in a country. Nutrition monitoring data can be used for the detection of emerging health problems that need to be acted upon, or for an assessment of how common certain known health problems are, and whether these have changed over

time. For example, nutrition monitoring activities can aim to estimate the proportion of pregnant women that have iodine deficiency; whether this proportion has gone up or down compared to previous years; and the effectiveness of public health strategies in alleviating deficiency.

Nutrition monitoring and surveillance typically involves data collection on large groups of people. In that respect it is different from smaller research studies, which are specifically designed to assess certain nutritional indicators in a group of people to address a particular research question. However, research aims are often integrated into the design of large nutrition monitoring surveys.

As discussed in more detail below, nutrition monitoring activities can draw on different types of data, such as data collections on individual persons, or by using routinely collected data such as mortality data, or hospital data. Nutrition surveys which collect data from individual persons usually include an assessment of the person's dietary intake, anthropometry (e.g. height, weight, waist circumference), general demographic information (e.g. socioeconomic indicators; characteristics of the person's living environment, such as whether they live with other people and in an urban or rural area) and assessments of biomarkers in biological samples, such as blood or urine (see also Chapter 23). Clinical measurements (e.g. detection of symptoms of micronutrient deficiency, such as palpation of the neck to detect goitre in iodine deficiency; see Chapter 17) may also be incorporated. Nutrition monitoring surveys may also include collection of data on other topics that may be of specific interest for the population being assessed, such as food security, food safety, food literacy, or the **provenance** of foods consumed.

Many countries carry out some type of nutrition monitoring, but the frequency with which this is done and the number of people included are highly variable. In Australia, there has not been a regular, routine program of nutritional monitoring and surveillance; however, national surveys of adults were undertaken in 1983, of children in 1985, of adults and children in 1995, and of children again in 2007. Most recently, in 2011–2013, the Australian Bureau of Statistics carried out an expanded version of the National Health Survey (a regular general health survey), which included the National Nutrition and Physical Activity Survey, a collection of detailed data on dietary intake, physical activity, food avoidance and food security in a subgroup of more than 12,000 National Health Survey participants (Figure 24.1); an additional, smaller group of people also provided a blood and urine sample for biomarker assessments and underwent other assessments of health risk factors. A separate survey in a representative sample of Aboriginal and Torres Strait Islander people was also carried out.

Internationally, large nutrition surveys take place in many countries, particularly high-income countries in Europe, North America and Asia. In the

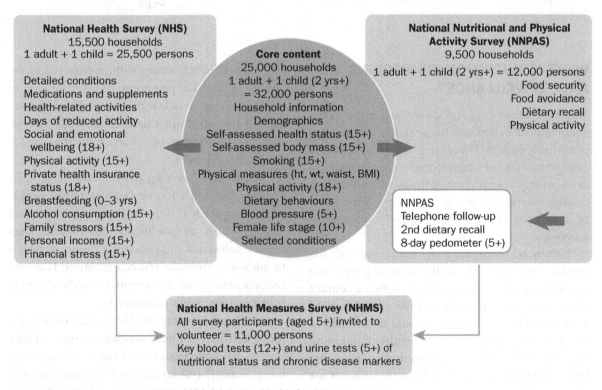

Figure 24.1: Structure of the 2011–2013 Australian Health Survey
Source: ABS (2013) © Creative Commons BY 4.0 Licence

USA, for example, the National Health and Nutrition Examination Survey (NHANES) is a program of national surveys that started in the 1960s. In 1999, the NHANES program became a continuing, yearly round of surveys of around 5000 persons each year. These surveys have provided a wealth of information to support health policy development and research worldwide—for example, by building evidence that it is acceptable to use self-reported weight and height data (rather than measured weight and height) to study health and the health consequences of being overweight or obese (Stommel & Schoenborn 2009). In the UK, national surveys have been carried out under the National Diet and Nutrition Survey (NDNS) program, which started in 1992 with a round of surveys in limited age groups (children, adults, older adults), after which it became a rolling program of surveys in a national sample of people aged 1.5 years and over (Public Health England 2014b), similar to the NHANES surveys in the USA.

Many European and Nordic countries carry out nutrition monitoring and surveillance at a national level (European Food Safety Authority 2017; Fagt et al. 2012). Due to the use of different methodologies, it can be difficult to compare results between different countries. The European Food Safety Authority is therefore working to collate all European food consumption data, and is aiming to improve standardisation of future national surveys so that comparisons between different countries can be made more reliably. Many countries in other parts of the world have carried out large national nutrition surveys; however, very few countries have done this on a regular basis (De Keyzer et al. 2015).

For low-income countries, nutrition monitoring and surveillance is more often organised as a response to acute crisis situations—for example, when severe drought or crop failure affects large parts of a country or region. In such situations, the data collection and nutrition monitoring activities may particularly focus on the region affected, or on the population subgroups at highest risk of malnutrition. In a low-income country context, nutrition monitoring is also often designed to investigate particular nutritionally related health problems that are known to exist—

such as to assess the prevalence of wasting and stunting, or to show the prevalence of micronutrient deficiencies. For example, a large survey of vitamin A deficiency in Uganda showed that in eastern parts of the country, 31 per cent of women of childbearing age were vitamin A deficient, compared to 14 per cent of women in the capital city, Kampala, and 19 per cent on average nationally (FANTA 2010). Results of such nutrition monitoring surveys can thus identify important health disparities within a country, and provide information for the planning of health interventions and for development of health policies.

When a nutrition monitoring activity is particularly aiming to assess severe malnutrition, it is also common for data to be collected from sources other than sampling of the general population. Observations from community-based sites can be used; for example, measurements taken on people visiting health clinics in a region, or data on the proportion of children who presented with symptoms of vitamin A deficiency at a particular clinic or hospital. For such alternative data sources, it is always important to evaluate whether the persons attending the clinics can be considered representative of the population at large (for example, severely ill persons may not be able to travel to a clinic).

WHY NUTRITION MONITORING?

There are several reasons why governments, health organisations and policy-makers want to use information from nutrition monitoring surveys. Information such as the usual dietary intake of people in a country or region, understanding of what foods and combination of foods are commonly eaten, and measures of how common nutritionally related health problems are, are used when dietary recommendations are being developed for a country, and when it needs to be decided which recommendations for dietary change need to be prioritised. Monitoring of dietary intake can also be used to evaluate compliance with dietary guidelines, and it can support decision-making on food regulation (for example, whether certain ingredients, such as trans fats or added sugar, need to be restricted in processed foods). Monitoring of nutritional status can be used to evaluate the success of nutrition interventions, such as new mandatory food fortification or taxation laws, or healthy eating campaigns. In the Republic of Korea, a long-term national health and nutrition monitoring program (the Korea National Health and Nutrition Examination Survey), has helped to develop growth charts and dietary reference values for that country (Kweon et al. 2014).

In the international context, nutrition monitoring is needed worldwide to evaluate progress towards ending hunger and malnutrition, and for the safeguarding of safe, nutritious and sufficient food for all. In 2015, the United Nations General Assembly decided on a list of seventeen Sustainable Development Goals (SDGs) that it hopes will be achieved by the year 2030 (see also Chapter 29). The second of these development goals is to 'end hunger, achieve food security and improved nutrition, and promote sustainable agriculture' (United Nations 2018). All other development goals have direct or indirect relevance to nutrition as well. Nutrition monitoring will be needed to evaluate the success of these goals—for example, the indicators that will be used to evaluate progress towards the second development goal include the prevalence of undernourishment, measurements of food insecurity, and prevalence of stunting and malnutrition in children (United Nations 2018). In addition to committing to the SDGs, in 2016 the UN General Assembly declared a 'United Nations Decade of Action on Nutrition', with the aim of ending hunger and eradicating all forms of malnutrition by 2025 (WHO 2016). Nutrition monitoring data will be required to evaluate these high-stakes international goals for years to come.

NUTRITION MONITORING IN POPULATION SUBGROUPS

Sometimes there is particular concern about nutritional health in a subgroup of people in a country—for example, children, women of childbearing age, or the elderly. Nutrition surveys of a general sample of people may include some persons that fall into these high-risk groups, but it is likely that their numbers will not be sufficiently large enough to be able to draw reliable conclusions about them. In such circumstances, it is better and more efficient to conduct a nutrition survey that is specifically designed to collect data on the high-risk group of interest. Such surveys are sometimes particularly focused on a certain diet- or nutrition-related issue. For example, in Australia a special survey was organised in 2010 to review breastfeeding practices, so data were collected from only new mothers (AIHW 2011). Large surveys are therefore sometimes specifically designed to support policy development and decision-making on important priority topics.

When a general population survey is sufficiently large and designed to sample enough participants from subgroups that are of interest, the data can be 'disaggregated' (analysed in subgroups) to evaluate and compare these subgroups (for example, males

USING NATIONAL DATA TO GET AN INTERNATIONAL PICTURE

An example of how national data are being used to review the nutrition situation globally can be seen at the Global Burden of Disease and Institute for Health Metrics and Evaluation website. Visit <www.healthdata.org> and, using any of the tools or research publications, explore how data from national surveys have been used to investigate a range of health issues within and between countries and regions.

- What does the information say about sub-optimal dietary risks in 195 countries?
- What is the global, regional and national burden of stroke?

vs females, or different age groups or regions). For instance, the Department of Health in Queensland, Australia, carries out regular surveys of the Queensland population, and these surveys involve a sample of people from regions of varying remoteness within the state. These data have helped to identify relevant differences between regions, such as discrepancies in the prevalence of overweight and obesity in adults (Table 24.1)—see the 'Remoteness' box for how regions are categorised.

Table 24.1: Self-reported BMI in adults by region, Queensland, Australia

Remoteness	Adult, self-reported BMI % (95% CI)			
	Healthy weight	Overweight	Obese	Overweight/obese
Major cities	40.5 (38.5–42.5)	35.0 (33.2–37.0)	22.0 (20.4–23.8)	57.1 (55.1–59.1)
Inner regional	35.8 (33.4–38.4)	33.6 (31.4–36.0)	28.4 (26.3–30.7)	62.1 (59.5–64.5)
Outer regional	36.5 (33.6–39.5)	33.9 (31.3–36.7)	26.8 (24.4–29.4)	60.8 (57.8–63.7)
Remote/very remote	29.9 (26.3–33.8)	36.2 (32.1–40.5)	30.0 (26.4–33.9)	66.2 (61.7–70.5)

Source: Queensland Government (2016)

REMOTENESS

Remoteness in Australia has been categorised by the Australian Bureau of Statistics into five categories based on relative access to services. This is a geographic classification and does not include any other social or economic indicators. The index is called the Accessibility and Remoteness Index of Australia, or ARIA (ABS 2018). It recognises areas as:

- major cities
- inner regional
- outer regional
- remote
- very remote.

New Zealand divides areas into urban and rural. Urban areas are divided into three categories and rural areas into four categories (Table 24.2).

Table 24.2: New Zealand regional categories and subcategories

Urban	Rural
· Main urban areas	· Rural areas with high urban influence
· Satellite urban areas	· Rural areas with moderate urban influence
· Independent urban areas	· Rural areas with low urban influence
	· Highly rural/remote areas

Source: Statistics New Zealand (2018)

People who live in rural areas or in remote or very remote areas are known to have disparities in disease prevalence. This could be due to a range of issues, lack of access to services, poor food access, poor physical activity opportunities or low incomes.

DIFFERENT DATA SOURCES FOR NUTRITION MONITORING AND SURVEILLANCE

In an ideal world, diet and nutrition data are collected on a large number of individuals, using the best possible methods and without restrictions on funds and other resources. Unfortunately, this ideal situation very rarely occurs. The design of large nutrition surveys of individuals always needs to be tailored carefully to fit with the resources and budget available. Other sources of data can also be used to draw conclusions about the nutritional status and health of populations.

Nutrition surveys

In nutrition surveys, data are usually collected on individual persons or households selected based on a pre-decided strategy, usually a statistical sampling method that considers the probability of a unit (person or household) being selected. For the purpose of nutrition monitoring and surveillance, such surveys typically involve data collection on a large sample, often at least a couple of thousand people; sometimes tens of thousands of people are included in such surveys. The large scales of these surveys means that costs for data collection and data processing can quickly become very high. Thus, careful planning is needed from the outset to assess what topics and variables are considered a priority, what methods for data collection and analysis will provide results that are valid yet affordable, and how many people need to be included to obtain reliable results. If the design of such surveys involves multiple stakeholders, this can help to make sure that the data collected provide good value for money (Zezza et al. 2017).

Selection of participants and methods

Nutrition surveys usually select participants by first deciding what the specific population groups of interest are—for example, whether information is needed about adults of any age, elderly people aged 65 years and over, or children aged 6–36 months. As a next step it becomes important what the subgroups

of interest are—for example, is a comparison between urban and rural areas desirable, or between men and women. Such decisions about subgroup comparisons become relevant for decisions about the number of participants required in each of these subgroups, and about how these will be selected and invited for participation. For example, if it is expected that in a general sample of the population few rural households would be included, but urban versus rural comparisons are a priority, then oversampling of rural households, or **stratified sampling**, to make sure that there is equal representation of these groups, may be warranted. The details of approaches to sample size calculations for large surveys are available elsewhere (Swinburn et al. 2015) and typically involve decisions about the allowable level of uncertainty in the data collected (in other words, how certain do you want to be that the data collected provide a true representation of the population at large?). It also involves assumptions about the extent to which the indicator of interest varies within the population that is being studied.

The number of people who actually participate in nutrition surveys is always smaller than the number of persons selected and invited for participation. Also, the level of participation is often lower than average in certain groups—for example, in younger adults who have busy jobs, or in people who have little interest in diet and health (who are also more likely to have unhealthy personal behaviours, including smoking and poor diets). In some circumstances, statistical techniques can be used to correct for the lower levels of participation in some groups (e.g. weighting or **imputation**) in order to make the data more representative of the population that was targeted for investigation.

The choice of methods used for estimating dietary intake requires careful consideration of the exact aims of such data (e.g. assessing current intake vs usual intake, estimation of total diet and total energy intake vs. collecting data on specific food groups only), and an evaluation of the specific advantages and disadvantages of the dietary intake methods available (see Chapter 23 for more details on methods to assess dietary intake). Challenges include the continuing debate about which methods provide the best and most valid data in different circumstances, the increasing share of foods consumed away from home in total dietary intake in many countries (Zezza et al. 2017), and the constant developments of new technologies that can be used to collect data on dietary intake and other indicators. In this decision-making process, a set of questions could be asked to help choose the preferred methods:

- Does the method result in data that provide the information that is required (e.g. assessment of short-term intake vs long-term status)?
- Does the method result in valid data (what is the probability of bias, misreporting or lack of reporting, for example; has the method been validated in other studies)?
- Is the method acceptable and feasible for the survey participants (what level of literacy is required, how much time and effort are involved for the participants)?
- Is the method affordable (what are the costs for data collection and analysis, including laboratory costs, staff time)?
- Does the method facilitate comparisons with other surveys (with what other surveys should the results be compared, and what methods did they use)?

Similar issues apply to the choice of laboratory methods for assessment of biomarkers and genetic markers, for which new technologies and platforms constantly become available, and new methods supersede older ones very quickly.

Repeated nutrition surveys in the same population

Surveys of diet and nutritional status (with measurements on individual persons) are often repeated over time to establish how the health of that population changes—this is usually a situation when nutrition monitoring is used for 'surveillance'. Evidence of changes over time can give important information about factors that cause increases or decreases in nutritionally related health and wellbeing—for example, as a result of national programs to reduce

food insecurity. Repeated cross-sectional surveys can help identify population subgroups in which average nutritional status, food security or other indicators are worsening, and thus help to identify priorities for interventions. Repeated cross-sectional surveys involve a new sample of people in each survey—in contrast, repeated measurement on the same person is common in longitudinal research studies, but is not often done in nutrition monitoring surveys (due to the extra effort involved in keeping track of people's whereabouts, and the high probability of people dropping out of the study at later time points).

One example of how repeated nutritional surveys can be used is the monitoring of salt intake in the population of the UK. In the early years of the 21st century, the UK government began to work with the food industry to try to reduce the salt content of processed foods, after survey data had indicated that the average intake of salt in the

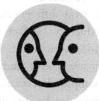

SALT CONSUMPTION

Report on your own or a member of your family's salt consumption.
- What foods do you eat that are high in salt?
- Do you add salt at the table?
- Do you like salty foods?

Using this experience, what are the possible explanations for the decreases in salt intake in the UK? What processed foods are highest in sodium?

The gold standard method for estimating a person's salt intake is measurement of sodium excreted in a 24-hour urine sample.
- Why is it difficult to assess people's salt intake reliably through dietary questionnaires?

UK population was higher than the recommended five grams per day for women and seven grams per day for men. There is compelling evidence that lowering a population's average salt intake helps to decrease the health burden of cardiovascular diseases. By using data from nutrition surveys that collected information on urinary sodium excretion every three years between 2005 and 2014, it became possible to monitor changes in average estimated salt intake over time. The 2015 data indicated that average salt intake was still too high (seven grams per day for women and nine grams per day for men), but that the mean estimated salt intake had reduced by around 11 per cent over this observation period (Public Health England 2014a).

A key point in the design of repeated surveys is that the methods used for data collection should ideally be the same, or at least similar enough to facilitate reliable comparisons. When two separate surveys use different methodologies, it will often remain unclear whether differences between observations in the two surveys are true differences, or whether these differences are due to the fact that different data collection methods were used. This applies to comparisons between any type of study or survey in different population samples. For example, when estimating people's dietary intake, use of a 24-hour recall method would give different estimates than when a food frequency questionnaire is used.

When vitamin D status is assessed in a population, the difference between two surveys may be due to seasonal effects if the surveys were not carried out around the same time of the year.

General population surveys

Some health conditions, such as obesity or cardiovascular diseases, have a strong national presence and are caused by a range of individual, social and environmental factors. Assessment of the prevalence of such conditions is often included in large general health surveys and can therefore be used to give indirect evidence about dietary intake (and physical activity) in a population. In New Zealand, for example, a national health survey of 13,000 adults and 4000 children is conducted annually (MOH 2018b). The survey collects data on a range of health topics, including height, weight, and waist circumference measurements. The 2016–2017 data indicated that around 12 per cent of children aged 2–14 years were obese (Figure 24.2). The survey also indicated that children who lived in lower socioeconomic neighbourhoods were 2.5 times as likely to be obese as children in the wealthiest neighbourhoods, independent of their age, sex or ethnicity (MOH 2018b). This is an example of how such large-scale nutrition and health surveys can provide information that can be used to set public health priorities and identify subgroups most affected.

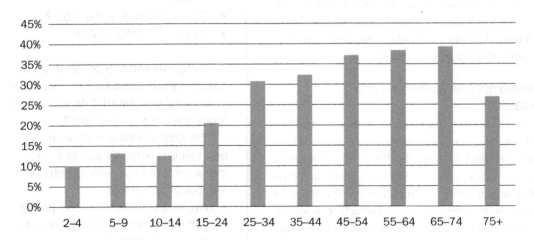

Figure 24.2: Percentage of children and adults who are obese in New Zealand, 2016–2017

Source: MOH (2018b). Creative Commons BY 4.0 Licence

Mortality and morbidity data, burden of disease data

Most (but not all) countries in the world have a central system for recording deaths, including the causes of deaths. Data on the most common causes of death in a population can give some clues about the relative importance of health risk factors in that population, such as infectious diseases (e.g. deaths due to HIV), smoking (lung cancer, chronic obstructive pulmonary disease), alcohol use (certain cancer types, accidents) and nutrition (deaths due to cardiovascular diseases, diabetes, certain cancer types). Besides death registry data, data on the occurrence of cancer types can also often be obtained from cancer registries, if notification of diagnosis of certain cancer types is mandatory and cancer registries exist (not all countries have these).

The factors that cause death and chronic diseases are complex, and multiple risk factors usually play a role. Thus, without data collected on individual persons (e.g. estimation of dietary intake), it is difficult to tease out the exact contribution of nutritional factors by using these general population-level death and morbidity data. This applies, for example, to the interpretation of data on the declining rate of ischaemic heart disease in Māori and non-Māori

New Zealanders (Figure 24.3). This decline could be due to improvements in risk factor profiles (including diet), but may also be due to improvements in early diagnosis and treatment of ischaemic heart disease, or to other unknown factors, or (most likely) a combination of different factors.

One major international initiative that summarises the relative contribution of risk factors for diseases, including nutritionally related risk factors, is the Global Burden of Disease project (www.healthdata.org/gbd) (Institute for Health Metrics and Evaluation 2018). There are also specific country-level burden of disease studies organised by local governments and research organisations. The strength of the burden of disease approach lies in the fact that it does not simply count the number of deaths and number of people affected by a disease. The burden of disease method also allows for the fact that some diseases cause people to die at a young age compared to older age. A substantially larger part of a person's potential life is lost when they die young; thus, the impact on life and the burden to society from that disease is much larger. Similarly, this approach considers the time that a person's life is affected by disability due to a particular disease or health condition, which is also incorporated when estimating the impact of

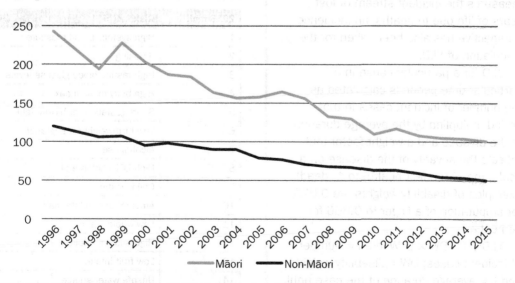

Figure 24.3: Mortality rates due to ischaemic heart disease (per 100,000 persons) for Māori and non-Māori men and women in New Zealand, 1996–2015

Source: Ministry of Health (2018a). Creative Commons BY 4.0 Licence

that disease to a population. A key indicator used is the disability-adjusted life years (DALYs) lost. This is defined in the box below.

DISABILITY-ADJUSTED LIFE YEARS (DALYs)

DALYs for a disease or health condition are calculated as the sum of the Years of Life Lost (YLL) due to premature mortality in the population and the Years Lost due to Disability (YLD) for people living with the health condition or its consequences. It is calculated as DALY = YLL + YLD (WHO 2018).

YLL corresponds to the number of deaths multiplied by the standard life expectancy at the age at which death occurs. The basic formula for YLL for a given cause, age and sex is YLL = N × L, where N = number of deaths due to condition and L = standard life expectancy at age of death. As YLL measures the incident stream of lost years of life due to deaths, an incidence perspective has also been taken for the calculation of YLD.

YLD for a particular cause in a particular time period is calculated as the number of incident cases in that period multiplied by the average duration of the disease and a weight factor that reflects the severity of the disease on a scale from 0 (perfect health) to 1 (dead). Examples of disability weights are 0.023 for amputation of a finger to 0.666 for dementia.

YLD = I × DW × L. Where I = number of incident cases; DW = disability weight; and L = average duration of the case until remission or death (years) (WHO 2018).

In the 2011 Australian Burden of Disease study, a detailed estimate was made of the relative importance of risk factors that cause disease and death (expressed as DALYs), including behavioural, metabolic, environmental and dietary risk factors. The data used for such estimates include data from nutrition monitoring surveys, which would have provided information on how common low fruit intake or high saturated fat intake was in the Australian population. These estimations also use knowledge of the extent to which dietary and other risk factors are an actual cause (or preventive factor) in the disease or health conditions being studied. Note, however, that there is a level of overlap between the different risk factors considered, and that risk factors considered separately—such as obesity, high blood pressure, and high fasting glucose—have a strong dietary component as underlying risk factor (Table 24.3).

Globally, when considering all major risk factors for disease, the ten factors that are estimated to cause the largest burden of disease include dietary risks (the number one risk factor), child and maternal malnutrition, high systolic blood pressure, high fasting glucose levels, high body mass index, and

Table 24.3: Leading risk factors for DALYs globally

2016 rank	Risk factor
1	High systolic blood pressure
2	Smoking
3	High fasting blood glucose levels
4	High body mass index
5	Short gestation for birthweight
6	Low birthweight for gestation
7	Alcohol use
8	High LDL cholesterol
9	Child wasting
10	Ambient particulate matter
11	Low whole grains
12	High sodium intake
13	Low fruit intake
14	Unsafe water source
15	Impaired kidney function

Source: Gakidou et al. (2017)

high cholesterol levels—thus, six of the ten largest causes of death and disability around the world are related to nutrition (with alcohol use also in the top ten risk factors for men, but not for women) (Global Burden of Disease Study 2016). Globally, dietary risks were the leading risk factor for death in 2016, and the second-leading risk factor for DALYs (Gakidou et al. 2017).

Food security data

The costs of paying for sufficient nutritious food can be a major factor influencing dietary intake and health. Food insecurity exists when the food that a person eats is insufficient in quantity or quality to meet their needs for a healthy and active life (see also Chapter 25). It also exists when a person is worried about their access to food; additionally, beside the costs of food there can be other barriers, such as the availability of healthy foods or clean water

with which to prepare food. Affordability of food has been a focus in nutrition monitoring for many years—for example, in surveys that assess how much money households spend on food and other costs of living (see Chapter 27). The Household Expenditure Survey of Australia, for example, established that in 2015–2016, on average 17 per cent of the expenditure of households was spent on foods and non-alcoholic beverages, which is similar to 2009–2010, but less (as a proportion of expenditure) than in 1984 (when the relative costs of housing were lower than in recent years) (ABS 2017).

Food security is very complex and no one tool measures all elements. Table 24.4 provides examples of food security measurement tools that have been used in different contexts for different purposes.

In 2011–2012, 4 per cent of participants in the Australian Health Survey reported that in the past twelve months their household had run out of food

Table 24.4: Food insecurity measures

National indicators of food insecurity	
Prevalence of undernourishment	Based on the availability and adequacy of the dietary energy supply relative to dietary energy requirement of the average individual in the population.
Global Hunger Index	Calculated using four different indicators: proportion of undernourished people (in this context defined as people not able to acquire enough food to meet the daily minimum dietary energy requirements); proportion of wasted children under five years old; proportion of stunted children under five years old; and mortality rates of children under the age of five.
The Global Food Security Index	A national-level 28-indicator index that assesses three dimensions qualitatively and quantitatively: 'affordability' (cost and capacity to pay for food), 'availability' (food supply and food availability), and 'quality and safety' (quality of diets and food safety).
Household food access	
Household Consumption and Expenditure Surveys	Used to estimate food consumption patterns at the household level, assess poverty and household economic status, and calculate consumer price indices.
Dietary intake	Dietary intake methods directly assess food and energy intake as well as individual dietary quality. Dietary intake methods can provide dietary information on intra-household distribution of food intakes as well as dietary patterns at the national and local levels.
Dietary diversity measures	Can be useful as indicators or proxies of food insecurity; capture food access by identifying the number of foods or food groups consumed over a specified time-period.
Measures based on participatory adaptation	This includes the Coping Strategies Index and experience-based food insecurity scales, which include the United States Food Security Survey Module (the most commonly used tool internationally), the Household Food Insecurity Access Scale, Household Hunger Scale, Latin American and Caribbean Household Food Security Scale and the Food Insecurity Experience Scale.

Source: Adapted from Pérez-Escamilla et al. (2017)

MEASURING FOOD INSECURITY

Read the following article:

• Perez-Escamilla, R. et al., 2017, 'Food security measurement and governance: Assessment of the usefulness of diverse food insecurity indicators for policy-makers', *Global Food Security*, 14: 96–104.

Based on this article, draw up a table that identifies the advantages and disadvantages of each measure of food insecurity.

and could not afford to buy more (ABS 2014). The sensitivity of this question is low, failing to identify additional households that are or may be at risk of food insecurity (McKechnie et al. 2018). Work has commenced on developing an Australian Household Food and Nutrition Security Survey (Archer et al. 2017; Kleve et al. 2018). Such national average data give some indication of the extent of food insecurity, but regional differences exist, and of course lower socioeconomic households would be at higher risk of food insecurity—thus, monitoring of food insecurity relies on data collection across a range of different regions and socioeconomic subgroups in order to provide valuable information. In the USA, food security is assessed in large annual surveys that include a representative sample of around 45,000 households as part of the Current Population Survey, and the data are then analysed by the US Department of Agriculture. In 2016, around 12 per cent of all households were estimated to be food insecure (USDA 2018). More recently, the FAO has undertaken an international survey using an eight-item tool, finding that food insecurity in high-income countries is between 9 and 11 per cent (FAO 2016).

Food supply data

Country-level food production data have been used for many years to assess food availability for citizens and to estimate dietary intake of people in a country. Such data are sometimes called food disappearance data, or apparent consumption data. For many years, the FAO has collated such data in 'food balance sheets' for different countries (FAO 2017). The food balance sheets consider on one hand the food *supply*, including food produced in the agricultural and livestock production systems as well as food available from food imports and food produced by industry. On the other hand, they consider food *utilisation*, which includes food that is used for animal feed, seeding, food lost during food processing, food that is wasted, exported, and other uses of food.

Interpretation of the food supply data can be difficult because they lack the detailed understanding that is gained from data collected from individuals on their actual food intake. However, food balance sheets have been used for higher-level policy development and decision-making. For example, these data can provide insights into the extent to which a country is reliant on food imports to feed the people in that country, which can then be used to set priorities for supporting agriculture and livestock industries. Governments also use these data to make projections about the food requirement in future years, when the population of a country may grow, again helping to set priorities that help safeguard sufficient and nutritious food for all people within a country.

Birth weight, infant mortality and child growth data

Poor nutritional status is a main risk factor for low birthweight. Monitoring of birthweight data has therefore traditionally been an important method for identifying at-risk populations and for evaluation of nutrition intervention programs. An underweight infant is at increased risk of disease and death, so birth weight is a major indicator used to review the health of populations (see Chapter 21). Large international organisations such as UNICEF collate birth weight data from countries around the world.

The World Health Assembly has set a target of reducing the number of children born with low birthweight by 30 per cent before the year 2025 (UNICEF 2013). Country-level data show that low birthweight is particularly high in Southeast Asia (including India), where on average 28 per cent of babies are born with a birthweight below 2500 grams (the cut-off used to define low birthweight), compared to 12 per cent in Sub-Saharan Africa and 6 per cent in East Asia and the Pacific (UNICEF 2013).

Growth indicators of children are also used to assess the nutritional health of populations. Wasting is an indicator of acute forms of undernutrition, and stunting an indicator of chronic undernutrition during critical periods of growth and development in a child's life (see chapters 21 and 23 for more detail on how wasting and stunting are defined). Nutrition monitoring and surveillance programs will often incorporate a review of these measures where possible.

Wasting and stunting of children is still relatively common, but there is an increasing number of countries where childhood overweight and obesity are also rapidly increasing. This is referred to as the 'double burden of malnutrition' (WHO 2016), and it particularly affects countries that go through a 'nutrition transition', moving from a predominance of traditional food patterns and subsistence farming to food patterns rich in energy-dense/nutrient-poor foods combined with sedentary behaviours. China is an example of a country that is undergoing such a nutrition transition. By combining the data from a number of different large surveys carried out over several years in China, it becomes clear that wasting and stunting have become less common (but still exist), while childhood overweight and obesity are increasing rapidly (Zong & Li 2014).

OTHER DATA SOURCES FOR NUTRITION MONITORING AND SURVEILLANCE

There are other sources of data that can be used to review indicators of diet and nutrition in large population groups. Routine laboratory observations can sometimes be used to draw conclusions about the nutritional status of populations. For example, a review of all samples analysed in a large diagnostic pathology laboratory in Australia was helpful in assessing that there was a 77 per cent reduction in the prevalence of low serum and red blood cell folate concentrations in the year following the introduction of mandatory fortification of bread flour in 2009 (Brown et al. 2011). Of course, the samples analysed in a hospital laboratory are not fully representative of all Australians, but such data do give some reassurance about the impact of the mandatory food fortification program designed to prevent neural tube defects in newborn infants. Another way in which this mandatory folic acid

LARGE DIET AND NUTRITION SURVEYS

Large diet and nutrition surveys for the purpose of nutrition monitoring and surveillance programs are usually organised by governmental departments or not-for-profit organisations. They commonly involve collaboration between several different institutions and involve the expertise of professionals from different disciplines.

- What do you think are the core areas of knowledge and key skills that a nutrition professional would bring to the planning and execution of such large diet and nutrition surveys?
- What do you think are some of the other professions and skills required for the successful completion of such large diet and nutrition surveys?
- What considerations need to be given when collecting data from a culturally diverse population?

fortification program was evaluated was by using data from the Register of Developmental Anomalies in Western Australia. The data showed that, compared to the period before the introduction of mandatory fortification of bread flour, the rate of neural tube defects in Aboriginal infants in Western Australia had reduced by 68 per cent in the following year (Bower et al. 2016). Thus, alternative data sources can become useful, depending on the particular topic or health issue being assessed.

SUMMARY

- Nutrition monitoring and surveillance refers to the collection of data from populations in order to ascertain information on food and nutrient intake and health impacts. These data are essential to inform policy changes across systems, including in agriculture (what should we grow?), trade (what food do we need to import?) and health (what do we need to encourage or discourage with regard to consumption?) laws and regulations.
- Internationally, large national surveys take place regularly and routinely. This is not the case in Australia, where there is no regular schedule for collecting data related to food consumption and nutritional status.
- A range of data sources are used to collect information regarding nutrition intake and the impact of nutrition on health. These include nutrition surveys, mortality and morbidity data, and data on food security and the food supply and infant birthweight and mortality.
- When undertaking nutrition surveys, it is important to make a decision on the best method used according to population to be sampled, time available and cost. Participant selection needs to take into consideration what will be measured, how many people will actually participate and how the data will be analysed.
- If surveys are to be undertaken on a regular basis, consideration needs to be given to ensuring that the questions asked can be compared across years to determine trends.

KEY TERMS

Imputation: the assignment of a value by inference so that there is reduced missing data.
Provenance: the source of foods.
Stratified sampling: the process of dividing members of the population into homogeneous subgroups before sampling. For example, you could stratify the sample according to economic status and make sure you select participants from each sample. If the numbers are very different in each strata, you could select different numbers from each to minimise bias.

REFERENCES

ABS, 2013, *Australian Health Survey: User's guide 2011–2013,* <www.abs.gov.au/ausstats/abs@.nsf/Lookup/4363.0.
55.001Chapter1102011-13>, accessed 9 December 2018
—— 2014, *Australian Health Survey: Nutrition First Results—Food and nutrients, 2011–12,* <www.abs.gov.au/ausstats/
abs@.nsf/Lookup/by%20Subject/4364.0.55.007~2011-12~Main%20Features~Key%20Findings~1>,
accessed 20 June 2018

—— 2017, *Household Expenditure Survey, Australia: Summary of results, 2015–16*, <www.abs.gov.au/ausstats/abs@.nsf/Latestproducts/6530.0Main%20Features32015-16?opendocument&tabname=Summary&prodno=6530.0&issue=2015-16&num=&view=>, accessed 18 February 2019

—— 2018, *The Australian Statistical Geography Standard (ASGS) Remoteness Structure*, <www.abs.gov.au/websitedbs/D3310114.nsf/home/remoteness+structure>, accessed 9 December 2018

AIHW, 2011, *2010 Australian National Infant Feeding Survey: Indicator results*, <www.aihw.gov.au/getmedia/af2fe025-637e-4c09-ba03-33e69f49aba7/13632.pdf.aspx?inline=true>, accessed 30 November 2018

Archer, C., Gallegos, D. & McKechnie, R., 2017, 'Developing measures of food and nutrition security within an Australian context', *Public Health Nutrition, 20*(14): 2513–22, doi:10.1017/S1368980017001288

Bower, C., Maxwell, S., Hickling, S., D'Antoine, H. & O'Leary, P., 2016, 'Folate status in Aboriginal people before and after mandatory fortification of flour for bread-making in Australia', *Australian and New Zealand Journal of Obstetrics and Gynaecology, 56*(3): 233–7, doi:10.1111/ajo.12425

Brown, R.D., Langshaw, M.R., Uhr, E.J., Gibson, J.N. & Joshua, D.E., 2011, 'The impact of mandatory fortification of flour with folic acid on the blood folate levels of an Australian population', *Medical Journal of Australia, 194*(2): 65–7, doi:10.5694/j.1326–5377.2011.tb04169.x

De Keyzer, W., Bracke, T., McNaughton, S.A., Parnell, W., Moshfegh, A.J. et al., 2015, 'Cross-continental comparison of national food consumption survey methods—a narrative review', *Nutrients, 7*(5): 3587, doi:10.3390/nu7053587

European Food Safety Authority, 2017, *EU Food Consumption Data*, <www.efsa.europa.eu/en/data/food-consumption-data>, accessed 18 February 2019

Fagt, S., Gunnarsdottir, I., Hallas-Møller, T., Helldán, A., Halldorsson, T.I. et al., 2012, *Nordic Dietary Surveys. Study Designs, Methods, Results and Use in Foodbased Risk Assessments*, <http://orbit.dtu.dk/files/12310307/TN2012529%20web%20(1).pdf>, accessed 25 February 2019

FANTA, 2010, *The Analysis of the Nutrition Situation in Uganda*, <www.fantaproject.org/sites/default/files/resources/Uganda_NSA_May2010.pdf>, accessed 24 May 2018

FAO, 2016, *Voices of the Hungry: Methods for estimating comparable rates of food insecurity experienced by adults throughout the world*, <www.fao.org/3/a-i4830e.pdf>, accessed 14 February 2019

—— 2017, *The State of Food Security and Nutrition Around the World, 2017*, <www.fao.org/3/a-I7695e.pdf>, accessed 18 February 2019

Gakidou, E., Afshin, A., Abajobir, A.A., Abate, K.H., Abbafati, C. et al., 2017, 'Global, regional, and national comparative risk assessment of 84 behavioural, environmental and occupational, and metabolic risks or clusters of risks, 1990–2016: A systematic analysis for the Global Burden of Disease Study 2016', *Lancet, 390*(10100): 1345–422, doi:10.1016/S0140-6736(17)32366-8

Global Burden of Disease Study, 2016, 'Global, regional, and national comparative risk assessment of 79 behavioural, environmental and occupational, and metabolic risks or clusters of risks, 1990–2015: A systematic analysis for the Global Burden of Disease Study 2015', *Lancet, 388*(10053): 1659–724, doi:10.1016/S0140-6736(16)31679-8

Institute for Health Metrics and Evaluation, 2018, *Global Burden of Disease*, <www.healthdata.org/gbd>, accessed 9 December 2018

Kleve, S., Gallegos, D., Ashby, S., Palermo, C. & McKechnie, R., 2018, 'Preliminary validation and piloting of a comprehensive measure of household food security in Australia', *Public Health Nutrition, 21*(3): 526–34, doi:10.1017/S1368980017003007

Kweon, S., Kim, Y., Jang, M.-j., Kim, Y., Kim, K. et al., 2014, 'Data resource profile: The Korea National Health and Nutrition Examination Survey (KNHANES)', *International Journal of Epidemiology, 43*(1): 69–77, doi:10.1093/ije/dyt228

McKechnie, R., Turrell, G., Giskes, K. & Gallegos, D., 2018, 'Single-item measure of food insecurity used in the National Health Survey may underestimate prevalence in Australia', *Australian and New Zealand Journal of Public Health, 42*(4): 389–95, doi:10.1111/1753-6405.12812

MOH, 2018a, *Mortality: Historical summary 1948–2015*, <www.health.govt.nz/publication/mortality-historical-summary-1948-2015>, accessed 9 December 2018

—— 2018b, *New Zealand Health Survey*, <www.health.govt.nz/nz-health-statistics/national-collections-and-surveys/surveys/new-zealand-health-survey?mega=Health%20statistics&title=NZ%20Health%20Survey>, accessed 9 December 2018

Pérez-Escamilla, R., Gubert, M.B., Rogers, B. & Hromi-Fiedler, A., 2017, 'Food security measurement and governance: Assessment of the usefulness of diverse food insecurity indicators for policy makers', *Global Food Security, 14*: 96–104, doi:10.1016/j.gfs.2017.06.003

Public Health England, 2014a, 'National Diet and Nutrition Survey: Assessment of dietary sodium—Adults (19 to 64 years) in England', <https://assets.publishing.service.gov.uk/government/uploads/system/uploads/attachment_data/file/773836/Sodium_study_2014_England_Text_final.pdf>, accessed 21 May 2019

—— 2014b, *National Diet and Nutrition Survey. Headline results from Years 1, 2 and 3 (combined) of the Rolling Programme (2008/2009–2010/11)*, <https://assets.publishing.service.gov.uk/government/uploads/system/uploads/attachment_data/file/207708/NDNS-Y3-report_All-TEXT-docs-combined.pdf>, accessed 20 May 2019

Queensland Government, 2016, *2016 Chief Health Officer's Report*, <www.health.qld.gov.au/research-reports/reports/public-health/cho-report/current/full>, accessed 18 February 2019

Statistics New Zealand, 2018, *Defining Urban and Rural New Zealand*, <http://archive.stats.govt.nz/browse_for_stats/Maps_and_geography/Geographic-areas/urban-rural-profile/defining-urban-rural-nz.aspx>, accessed 9 December 2018

Stommel, M. & Schoenborn, C.A., 2009, 'Accuracy and usefulness of BMI measures based on self-reported weight and height: Findings from the NHANES & NHIS 2001–2006', *BMC Public Health, 9*(1): 421, doi:10.1186/1471-2458-9-421

Swinburn, B., Kraak, V., Rutter, H., Vandevijvere, S., Lobstein, T. et al., 2015, 'Strengthening of accountability systems to create healthy food environments and reduce global obesity', *Lancet, 385*(9986): 2534–45, doi:10.1016/S0140-6736(14)61747-5

UNICEF, 2013, *Improving Child Nutrition: The achievable imperative for global progress*, <https://data.unicef.org/wp-content/uploads/2015/12/NutritionReport_April2013_Final_29.pdf>, accessed 18 February 2019

United Nations, 2018, *Sustainable Development Goal 2*, <https://sustainabledevelopment.un.org/sdg2>, accessed 18 February 2019

USDA, 2018, *Food Security Status of U.S. Households*, <www.ers.usda.gov/topics/food-nutrition-assistance/food-security-in-the-us/measurement/>, accessed 18 February 2019

WHO, 2016, *The Double Burden of Nutrition: Policy brief*, <www.who.int/nutrition/publications/doubleburden malnutrition-policybrief/en/>, accessed 18 February 2019

—— 2018, *Metrics: Disability-adjusted life year (DALY)*, <www.who.int/healthinfo/global_burden_disease/metrics_daly/en/>, accessed 9 December 2018

Zezza, A., Carletto, C., Fiedler, J.L., Gennari, P. & Jolliffe, D., 2017, 'Food counts: Measuring food consumption and expenditures in household consumption and expenditure surveys (HCES)—Introduction to the special issue', *Food Policy, 72*: 1–6, doi:10.1016/j.foodpol.2017.08.007

Zong, X.-N. & Li, H., 2014, 'Physical growth of children and adolescents in China over the past 35 years', *Bulletin of the World Health Organization, 92*: 555–64, doi:10.2471/BLT.13.126243

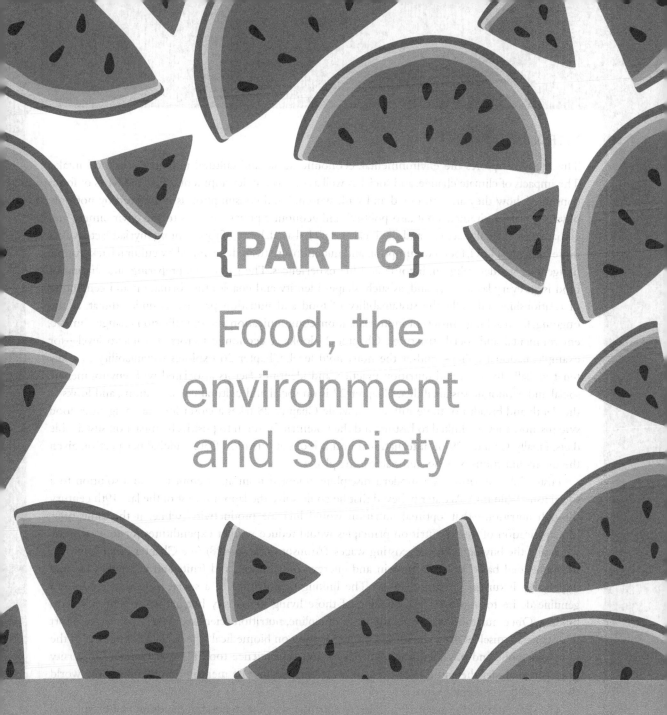

INTRODUCTION

This section explores the environmental, economic, social and cultural influences on food intake. The impacts of climate change, and social as well as economic development, affect the types of foods consumed, how they are consumed and with whom. Food consumption is influenced by not only physiological requirements but also political and economic policy, changes to the environment and climate, agricultural practices, and the local and global availability of food among myriad factors. At a more individual level, food consumption and nutritional status is determined by cultural background, indigeneity, gender, religion, income and life experiences. The gathering, preparing and sharing of food is an everyday activity and, as such, shapes identity and enables the formation and cementing of relationships. Globally, the sustainability of food and nutrition practice is under threat, as the ongoing, far-reaching impacts of industrialisation, communication and globalisation change climatic, environmental and social structures. Chapter 25 looks at economic factors at a macro level—for example, national policy—and at the household level. Chapter 26 explores sustainability as a key tenet globally for food and nutrition practice, and identifies factors associated with environmental, social and economic sustainability. Chapter 27 is on social and cultural considerations, and looks at the depth and breadth of these influences, while Chapter 28 takes a closer look at Indigenous food systems, how they are linked to history and the potential for them to positively impact on sustainable diets. Finally, Chapter 29 on international health looks at nutrition from a global perspective, given the interconnections of ecosystems across the planet.

Historically, nutrition as a modern discipline emerged from an attempt to find a solution to a social issue. Wilbur O. Atwater believed that he could solve the labour unrest of the late 19th century through nutrition—that 'optimal nutrition would increase productivity' while, at the same time, 'the application of sound nutrition principles would reduce worker expenditures for food, thereby increasing the buying power of existing wages' (Aronson 1982, p. 428) (see Chapter 25). Diets were recommended based on their protein and energy contribution, and fruits and vegetables became dispensable luxuries (Carpenter 2003). The linking of nutrition to a social issue was not from a genuine desire to improve the wellbeing of those living in poverty but, rather, to gain access to funding. Once nutrition was established as a discipline, nutrition scientists made a concerted effort to distance themselves from the social aspects, focusing on biomedical aspects. The beginnings of the more metabolic and physiological approach to nutrition science took place at Giessen University in Germany under the auspices of Justus von Liebig and those he mentored from around the world (Brock 2002) (see also Chapter 1).

The same approach is occurring today, as nutrition scientists trained in the dominant biomedical approaches turn to linking social conditions with nutritional deficits with a view to providing 'evidence' for who and what should be targeted via interventions. This reductionist approach has given rise to a call for more socially engaged nutrition practice that gives equal weight to the exploration of the complex social and cultural narratives that underpin food consumption and dietary intake (Schubert et al. 2012). Such an approach also acknowledges that while food consumption performs a utilitarian task of keeping bodies alive and healthy, it also expresses the complexity of our social, cultural, political, environmental and economic relationships. The Public Interest Civil Society Organizations acknowledge this broad role of food, stating:

It is our common understanding that food is the expression of values, cultures, social relations and people's self-determination, and that the act of feeding oneself and others embodies our sovereignty, ownership and empowerment. When nourishing oneself and eating with one's family, friends, and community, we reaffirm our cultural identities, our ownership over our life course and our human dignity. Nutrition is foundational for personal development and essential for overall wellbeing. (cited in FAO 2014, p. 2)

In this section, a range of factors that contribute to the social and cultural context of food and nutrition intake are explored. Figure 6.A depicts some social and cultural factors that influence food choice and, therefore, nutritional status. This follows the socioecological model of health (see Part 4) that identifies factors at the policy, organisational, community, interpersonal and individual level. The model is used extensively by international organisations to frame health interventions for prevention and management.

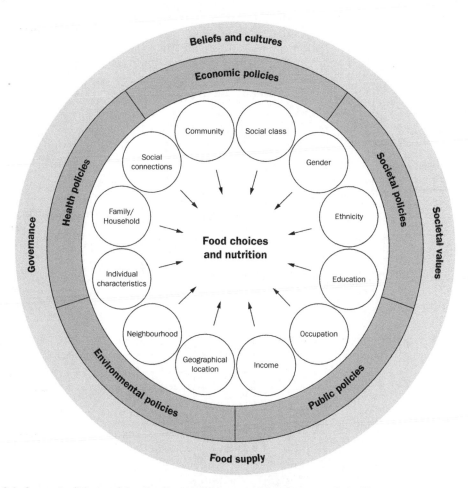

Figure 6.A: Conceptualising social and cultural influences on food choices and nutrition

REFERENCES

Aronson, N., 1982, 'Nutrition as a social problem: A case study of the entrepreneurial strategy in science', *Social Problems, 29*(5): 474–87, doi:10.2307/800397

Brock, W.H., 2002, *Justus von Liebig: The chemical gatekeeper*, Cambridge: Cambridge University Press

Carpenter, K.J., 2003, 'A short history of nutritional science: Part 2 (1885–1912)', *Journal of Nutrition, 133*(4): 975–84, doi:10.1093/jn/133.4.975

FAO, 2014, *Public Interest Civil Society Organizations' and Social Movements' Forum Declaration to the Second International Conference on Nutrition (ICN2)*, <www.fao.org/3/a-at641e.pdf>, accessed 16 December 2018

Schubert, L., Gallegos, D., Foley, W. & Harrison, C., 2012, 'Re-imagining the "social" in the nutrition sciences', *Public Health Nutrition, 15*(2): 352–9, doi:10.1017/S1368980011001297

CHAPTER 25

NUTRITIONAL ECONOMICS

Mark L. Wahlqvist

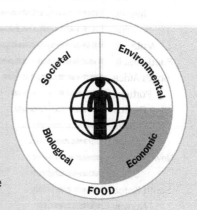

OBJECTIVES

- Recognise nutritional economics as a dimension of nutritional science.
- Describe how economic factors affect food and health systems.
- Relate how food choices and nutritional status contribute to livelihoods.
- Explain how household and community economics are interdependent with sustainable food systems.

FOOD

ECONOMICS AS A DIMENSION OF NUTRITION SCIENCE

'Nutritional economics' is a concept that deals with the connections between economic systems, nutritional status and food security, and how changes in the former affect the latter. Nutritional economics is not a new concept; it must be acknowledged that the present imperatives to think and plan in terms of nutritional economics were pioneered throughout human agrarian history by women managing household budgets and food security. As a discipline, nutrition (via Wilbur Atwater) had its origins in developing appropriate regimens to fuel workers for increased productivity (Aronson 1982) and through the development of home economics, which emerged as a way to teach women to manage households more effectively.

National comparison by the US Department of Agriculture of the proportion of household expenditure on food consumed at home (Figure 25.1) demonstrates that richer countries spend a smaller fraction of their income on food.

According to Amartya Sen, nutrition insufficiency is one of the major sources of '**unfreedom**' and limits human development (Sen 2001) (see Chapter 27 for further discussion of Sen's notion). The direction of this relationship is not one-way. Economic factors are also determinants of nutritional status and both influence human wellbeing, directly and indirectly.

Economists see nutrition as an important input to economic growth and development. The Copenhagen Consensus (a panel of economists) in 2012 ranked 'bundled micronutrient interventions on the basis of cost effectiveness and desirability as the top ranking investment to improve human welfare' (Copenhagen Consensus 2012). At this macro-level nutrition is fundamental for human development, but in circumstances of ongoing resource scarcity nutrition policies must compete with other public

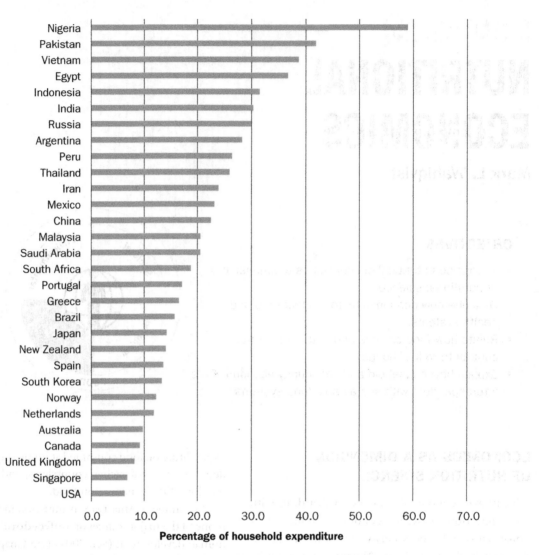

Figure 25.1: How much countries spend on food at home, 2016

Source: Developed from data located at USDA ERS (2016)

health and education programs. This is an ongoing challenge for nutrition scientists, who need to contextualise the policy implications as the interaction between nutrition and economics becomes stronger than ever. Food as a commodity is traded globally and, as such, is an integral part of the macroeconomics that contributes to a country's overall **gross domestic product** (GDP). Global supply and demand and trade agreements set food prices, which in turn affect the food purchasing at the household and individual level. The agricultural and

food industries are among the largest employers as food travels from production to consumption.

The volatility of global food prices in the early 21st century threatens public health and is also jeopardising the health of the most disadvantaged. The factors which most commonly contribute to this crisis include the costs of food production, processing and marketing, linked to sharply higher oil prices; the use of food crops for biofuel production in the USA and Europe; speculative trade in food commodities and associated derivatives and debt; growing meat consumption that stimulates increased demand for animal feed; poor harvests in certain major agriculture regions; and consistent underinvestment in agriculture over past decades, resulting in agricultural production that lags behind population growth or broader economic growth (see chapters 4 and 26 for more information). The impact of increasing food prices focuses the attention of international agencies and national governments. The 2018 Organisation for Economic Co-operation and Development (OECD) report on food policy predicts that spikes and volatility in food prices and associated food security will increasingly reflect climate change (OECD 2018). To this will be added natural disasters (exacerbated by climate change), conflict (including over food and water), mass migration and displacement, politically driven food trade-wars, and further financial crises. The OECD, in conjunction with other international agencies, is encouraging local resilience in food systems as an unfolding priority in food security.

Economic factors play a crucial role within households (the place of commensality or where food is shared) and for individuals and affects personal nutrition status and health. Economics impacts on nutritional status and diet quality across a number of dimensions: (a) consumer behaviour, or how food pricing affects food choice and health; (b) provider behaviour, the influences of material cost and trade on food safety and availability; and (c) how diet costs relate to dietary quality.

In taking all of these factors into consideration, the sustainable livelihoods framework provides a useful way of thinking about what is required in order to build a sustainable means of living.

The sustainable livelihoods framework

Livelihoods refers to the capabilities (skills, education, ability to work), assets (cash, material resources) and activities required to secure the necessities of life. A livelihood is sustainable when it can cope with stresses and shocks, where capabilities and assets are maintained and the opportunities can be forwarded to the next generation. Figure 25.2 summarises the model.

As noted in Chapter 4, more opportunities and better livelihoods mean more people have sufficient, better-quality and more varied food; and food growers, harvesters or producers have more certain and enduring roles. A livelihoods approach does not

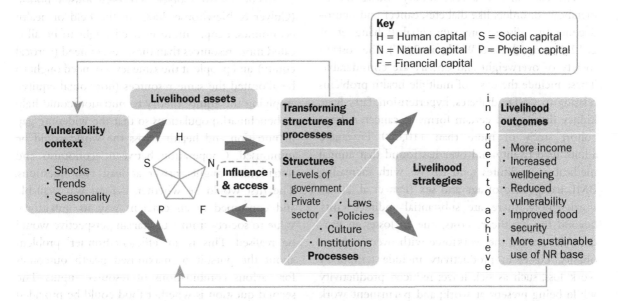

Figure 25.2: The sustainable livelihoods framework

Source: Ashley & Carney (1999). Used with permission of Department for International Development

necessarily assume employment. With an ageing population and the rise of automation and technology, employment as it is currently conceptualised will be contested. As Wahlqvist (2016) notes, 'Technology and ageing demographics encroach on employment as we have known it and create social ills which need not eventuate if we each had defined livelihoods. These need to be contractual within our evolving communities and with rural to urban shifts' (p. 76).

FOOD PRICES AND HEALTH

Rising food prices can have severe impacts on population health and nutritional status (Lee et al. 2013). Food prices surged in 2007–2009, raising serious concerns about food security around the world. The link between socioeconomic status and the purchase of more nutritious foods, as judged by diet diversity and overall health, is significant. From a public health perspective, poor-quality diet has been linked to significant increases in medical costs as well as costs to the economy through lost productivity (Turner et al. 2018). Those who consume more plant-based foods appear to have lower health service usage and medical costs (Lo et al. 2016).

The costs of overfatness, obesity and associated metabolic disorders like diabetes, cancer and neuro-degenerative disease are substantial (Chang et al. 2012; Kouris-Blazos & Wahlqvist 2007). The costs to society of overweight and obesity are considerable. These include the costs of multiple health problems relating to CVDs, diabetes, hypertension, fatty liver, kidney disease, and certain forms of cancer. A large cohort study of more than 110,000 Taiwanese adults aged twenty and over has found that annual medical expenditures tend to rise with increasing BMI, irrespective of age and sex (Pan et al. 2012). Furthermore, there are substantial indirect costs, beyond the healthcare costs, due to losses in productivity among the workforce with overweight or obesity. Losses in productivity include temporary work loss, such as sick leave; reduced productivity while being present at work; and permanent work loss (Goettler et al. 2017). Achieved nutritional status, insofar as muscle mass and avoidance of sarcopenia

are concerned, is also associated with less medical expenditure (Lo et al. 2013). However, among older people a higher BMI, rather than underweight, is associated with greater survival (see Chapter 22). Some of this advantage may depend on the availability of healthcare resources (Pan et al. 2012). This is an example of how nutritional economics needs a contextual interpretation.

Policy decision models such as cost–effectiveness, cost–benefit analysis and cost–utility analysis are used to determine which interventions require investment. Due to resource scarcity, policy-makers must make choices between alternative nutritional intervention programs. This scarcity is being exacerbated by climate change, with loss of arable land, compromised fisheries and diminished water supplies as major rivers and ground water disappear. Comparable criteria and standards for alternative health interventions allow varying degrees and types of resource input improvement for various health outcomes to be evaluated. Thus, novel nutrition programs or interventions can be prioritised and ranked by health outcome, related costs, equitable distribution and ethical considerations (Friel & Baker 2009).

According to Culyer and Newhouse's notion (Culyer & Newhouse 2000) in the field of health economics, people more in need ought to be allocated more resources than those less in need (vertical equity), and people at the same level of need ought to be allocated the same resources (horizontal equity). Applying the equity theory to nutrition could help to benchmark populations so that the widening gap in nutrition and health across the world could be minimised. Cooperation between economists and nutritionists might answer at least two questions. The first would be whether, if food was available and consumed in an efficient way, its nutritional value to society from a utilitarian perspective would be realised. This is an 'efficient-frontier' problem about the pursuit of maximised health outcomes for various combinations of resource inputs. The second question is whether food could be provided and consumed in a way that equalises nutritional status; this would achieve egalitarian goals. The various interventions used to date, or planned, should be amenable to structural analysis of this kind to improve cost–benefit–risk performance (Cobiac et al. 2013; Horton 2017); however, they tend to be limited to single-factor interventions addressing, for example, micronutrient supplementation or salt reduction; or particular outcomes, such as stature in the SUN (Scaling Up Nutrition) program (WHO 2014). More effort is required for interventions to be food- and food system-based, as with urban gardens or women's food and nutritional literacy.

Trade agreements

The adequacy and quality of the food supply depends first on the combination of local production and trade, with more or less of one or the other. Economic globalisation has a significant role to play in the sustainability of agriculture, diets and nutrition. Global trade liberalisation can have many positive outcomes, including stimulating economic growth, reducing poverty, improving investments in health care, sanitation and education, and increasing access to life-saving and environmental technologies (Schram et al. 2015). Promotion of trade is viewed as a mechanism to improve food system sustainability by reducing inefficiencies that can result in environmental degradation, and as an economic adaptation to climate change. In other words, countries likely to see their agricultural production decrease will still be able to access food from other parts of the world without having to resort to measures that would deplete their natural resources further (Clapp 2016; Gordon et al. 2017). Increasingly, however, trade liberalisation has been identified as a significant risk to sustainable diets and the ensuing nutrition of nations. Table 25.1 defines some of the terms commonly used.

Trade agreements can have a range of impacts, but freeing up market access (that is, the flow of imports and exports) changes the availability and affordability of health-harmful commodities (tobacco, alcohol, ultra-processed foods) (Friel et al. 2013b; Schram et al. 2018). Figure 25.3 provides a framework for identifying the impact of trade agreements on the development of chronic

Table 25.1: Glossary of trade terms

Term	Definition
HHC	Health-harmful commodities.
Non-tariff barriers to trade	Government measures other than tariffs that restrict trade flows (e.g. import licensing, quantitative restrictions on goods or services).
Quota	A quantitative restriction that limits the number or volume of foreign products that can enter a domestic market.
Subsidy	A direct or indirect incentive or benefit granted by government for the production or distribution (through export) of a product.
Tariff	A custom duty or tax applied on imported goods at the border.
Trade agreement	A negotiated agreement between two or more countries to limit or alter their policies with respect to trade. Trade agreements can be bilateral (between two countries), regional (within a regional area) or multilateral (between multiple countries).
Trade liberalisation	The reduction or removal of barriers in order to create a 'free' market in goods, services or finance. A political philosophy that supports reduced government involvement in the economy.

Source: Adapted from Thow (2010)

conditions (Schram et al. 2018). Trade liberalisation is presented as a mechanism through which there could be a more equitable global distribution of food. However, in effect it offers a mechanism through which high-income countries, who can subsidise their agriculture, dump surplus products on lower-income countries, displacing local producers. These processes marginalise poor farm households, which lack appropriate transport routes and market access mechanisms and are unable to compete with multinationals (Sonnino et al. 2014).

Examples of some of these macroeconomic impacts include:

- Samoa: market competition where cheaper processed and hydrogenated oils replaced locally produced coconut oils (Thow et al. 2011)
- Fiji: reduction of import tariffs increased import of ultra-processed foods (Thow et al. 2011)

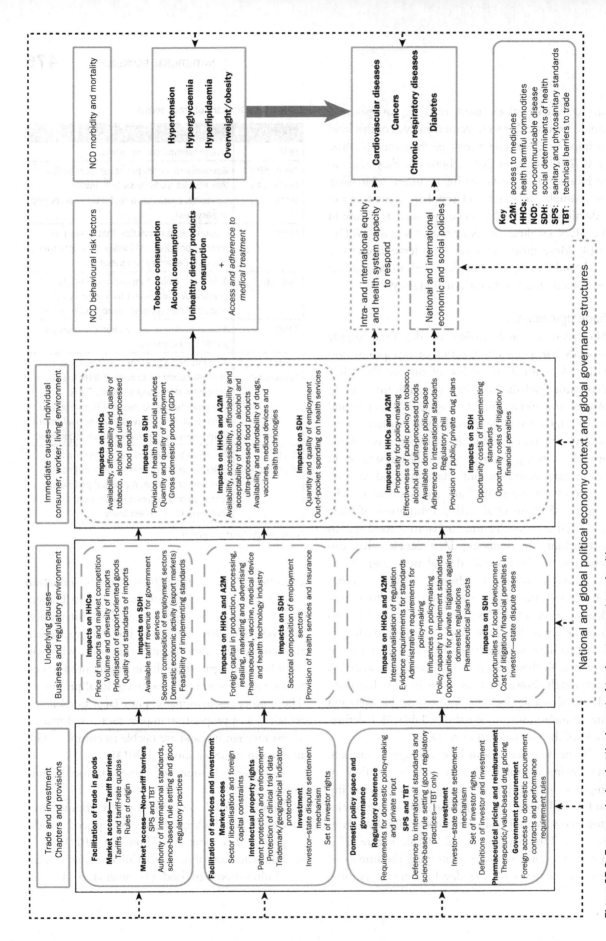

Figure 25.3: Framework showing the impact of trade agreements on health

Source: Schram et al. (2018)

- Central America: free trade agreement with the United States increasing imports of chocolate, confectionery, biscuits, crisps (Thow & Hawkes 2009)
- Thailand: 2006 proposal for the introduction of front-of-label traffic light labelling on snack-food products; the USA and other countries claimed this contravened the Agreement on Technical Barriers to Trade and the traffic light system was abandoned (Friel et al. 2013a)
- Low- and middle-income countries: lower tariffs increase imports of sugar-sweetened beverages, leading to greater sales (Mendez Lopez et al. 2017).

The arrival of these foods is often accompanied by increased entry of transnational companies and direct foreign investment, as well as intensive global marketing and advertising that shift consumer expectations (Friel et al. 2015). This was demonstrated in Vietnam, where trade liberalisation increased the exposure of markets to transnational food and beverage corporations, resulting in aggressive marketing strategies, strategic partnerships with retail distributors and major consumer food-service chains. In the year after Vietnam opened its markets to foreign companies there was a significant increase in the sales of sugar-sweetened carbonated beverages, with the main beneficiaries being foreign beverage companies while domestic companies lost market share (Schram et al. 2015). Combined with aggressive marketing (an example of which is shown in Figure 25.4), consumption of these items has increased markedly.

CONSUMER BEHAVIOUR: PRICE AND INCOME EFFECTS ON FOOD CHOICE

The determinants of food choice are complex and multifactorial, and are not well understood. Studies have focused on structural factors, such as access to grocery stores, transportation, and neighbourhood safety, as well as inequities in access to healthy foods. There is also an increasing awareness that healthier foods are associated with monetary factors

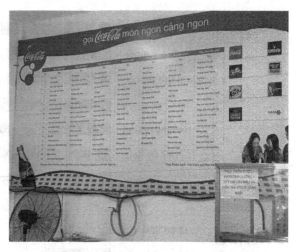

Figure 25.4: Menu board at a Vietnamese hospital showing commercial product logos
Source: Danielle Gallegos

(Figure 25.5). Food prices are identified as the highest-ranking contributor to food choices.

Individual food choices interact with environmental and individual factors. Environmental factors that influence eating behaviour include a changing food supply, increased eating out, food advertising, healthy eating promotion, education and food pricing. For individuals, taste, perceived value (such as price and portion size) and perceived nutrition value are the three main dimensions related to food choice. Presumably, confidence in a food's safety is a key determinant as well. Thus, food prices can operate as both environmental and individual factors, which can affect people's food choices.

Microeconomic policy tools within public and welfare economics include regulation, licensing, taxation and subsidisation. These may be employed by governments to influence access to and choice of food. Consumers and providers may adjust their behaviours to a changed policy environment—or bargain for it to reflect their interests. Nutritional economic analysis can discover how the behavioural aspects of policies affect the food system, from producers to consumers. For example, such analysis may better encourage an equality in which diets and health reach different populations in various food systems (Friel & Baker 2009; Wahlqvist et al. 2009).

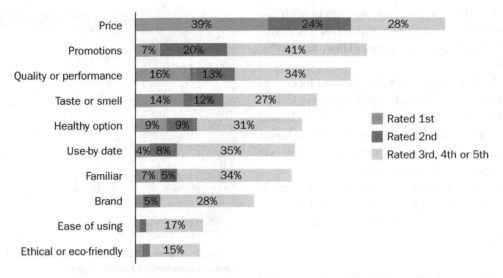

Figure 25.5: Factors influencing consumer product choice

Source: UK Department for Environment, Food & Rural Affairs (2014, p. 23). Reprinted under Open Government Licence. Department for Environment, Food and Rural Affairs UK, © Crown 2014

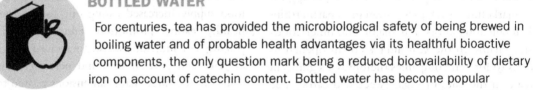

BOTTLED WATER

For centuries, tea has provided the microbiological safety of being brewed in boiling water and of probable health advantages via its healthful bioactive components, the only question mark being a reduced bioavailability of dietary iron on account of catechin content. Bottled water has become popular and profitable, even where it can be safely consumed from reticulated water facilities at no cost to the consumer. Where bottles for water, sugary drink or tea (or cups for coffee), are made of plastic, the WHO has raised concerns about increased exposure to micro- and even nano-plastic, which is likely to add to the environmental risk posed by endocrine disruptors (see also Chapter 29). Governments are tackling this unnecessary use of plastic by promoting sustainable alternative containers and increasing recyclability or returnability by paid deposit. Beverage manufacturers are seeking alternative markets to ensure market share, as with iced tea, but not necessarily with non-plastic containers. An unintended consequence of a sugar-sweetened beverage tax may be an increased consumption of alcoholic beverages (Quirmbach et al. 2018).

In a departure from its traditional sugar-sweetened beverage business, Coca-Cola launched three lemon-flavoured fizzy alcoholic drinks in Japan in 2018. The drinks are described as 'chu-hi'—canned, flavoured drinks typically made with sparkling water and shochu, a Japanese spirit distilled from grains (Detrick 2018).

If you are interested in the tactics of beverage companies, read Marion Nestle's *Soda Politics: Taking on Big Soda (and winning)* (2015).

Regulatory approaches are being considered more often as a suitable approach to change people's food consumption. This includes carefully manipulating the price of foods to either encourage or discourage consumption (Lee et al. 2013). As food prices have a strong effect on food choices, price reduction intervention strategies could increase healthful food purchases (Afshin et al. 2017). The success of tobacco tax regulation indicates the potential power of price changes in changing purchasing behaviours.

Price reduction strategies to increase fruit and vegetable purchasing from supermarkets have been successful. A Melbourne study showed that a 20 per cent reduction in fruit and vegetable prices resulted in a 35 per cent and 15 per cent increase in fruit and vegetable purchases respectively (Ball et al. 2015). Another example is the sugar tax. There continues to be strong advocacy for a 'sugar tax' on sugar-sweetened beverages to reduce the risk of obesity and associated health problems. The tax has been introduced in the UK and in some localities in the USA. Evidence from countries like Mexico (Colchero et al. 2016), where it has been introduced, is that the use of sugar-sweetened beverages (SSBs) may have been reduced by such a tax, but the long-term health consequences are yet to be determined. For example, an unintended consequence might be a shift from such beverages to alcoholic beverages. However, there is growing evidence that a sugar tax would decrease SSB consumption and improve the health of those most disadvantaged, especially if the tax revenue was used to fund initiatives benefiting those living with the most disadvantage (Lal et al. 2017). Price reduction strategies are increasingly being explored in Aboriginal and Torres Strait Islander communities to encourage healthier food choices (Ferguson et al. 2017; Magnus et al. 2018).

Price elasticity

When looking at these price changes, economists refer to the price elasticity (PE) of demand. This concept refers to the percentage change in purchased quantity or demand with a 1 per cent change in price (Andreyeva et al. 2010). There is own-PE, which is the change in demand for a food due to changes in

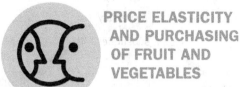

PRICE ELASTICITY AND PURCHASING OF FRUIT AND VEGETABLES

Think about your own purchasing of fruit and vegetables and the contributors to price elasticity of demand.

- When are fruit and vegetables too expensive to buy?
- What determines 'too expensive'?
- What do you substitute if they are too expensive?
- How would this impact somebody on a low income?

its own price, and cross-PE, which is the change in demand for a food due to changes in the price of another food. The concern with taxes or subsidies on food is that while, for example, a decrease in the price of fruit and vegetables should increase demand (own-PE), it may in fact increase purchasing of less desirable nutrient-poor foods because of cross-PE effects or increased disposable income. Research has shown that these effects are minimal and that low-income households have a greater sensitivity to price (Mhurchu et al. 2013). Price elasticity of demand is affected by a range of factors, illustrated in Figure 25.6.

Diet cost and dietary quality

Consumer behaviour in food choice appears to be greatly influenced by food price and household income. When certain foods are price sensitive, people are likely to make food choices related to their current economic status, and, with time and advocacy, this could lead to changes in provider or market price structures. This is most evident when food prices are rising and elastic and when demand is determined by health considerations as well as basic energy needs.

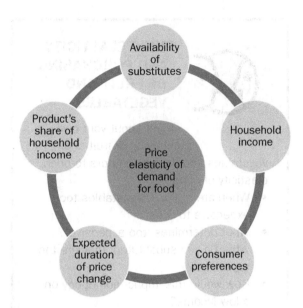

Figure 25.6: Factors affecting price elasticity of demand for food

Source: Developed from Andreyeva et al. (2010)

Healthy diets cost more if healthy food costs more. Thus, higher food prices will have a greater impact on the most vulnerable groups (Cade et al. 1999; Darmon & Drewnowski 2008). Low-income families are more sensitive to price than those with higher incomes and are more likely to choose less healthy foods (Brimblecombe & O'Dea 2009; Drewnowski & Specter 2004). Food diversity, reported as an index of dietary quality, health outcome and food security, might be relevant to diet costs (Lo et al. 2012). Households respond to increasing food prices by eating more monotonous diets of lower nutritional quality. Characteristically, less foods rich in essential micronutrients, such as fresh produce, fish, lean meat, fruits and vegetables are eaten, as the cheapest sources of food energy are sought (Drewnowski & Specter 2004). People who change their dietary patterns due to financial considerations may develop complex nutritionally related disorders, which may be referred to (albeit simplistically) as overnutrition (especially of energy) and undernutrition (especially of biologically active protective food components). This phenomenon tends to increase in precarious transitional economies

and is seen within communities, households and even individuals. Other critical household expenditures, such as education and health care, are also affected. To maintain income sources through expenditure on work-related travel, food and health expenditures may suffer in competition (see Chapter 27).

From an economic perspective, personal or household income and food prices are important determinants of food choice. Low-income households spend a higher proportion of their income on food than do higher income households (Ward et al. 2013). Wealthier households, however, spend more of their food budgets on away-from-home food than other households. Food costs are a barrier for low-income families to healthier food choices (Darmon & Drewnowski 2015). Lower income groups are less likely to make food purchasing choices consistent with dietary guideline recommendations. This is called the economics of food choice, where dietary decisions are made to maximise the energy value for money (kJ/$) (Drewnowski & Specter 2004). For example, Brimblecombe and O'Dea (2009) found that in a remote Aboriginal and Torres Strait Islander community, foods with higher energy density were associated with lower costs. Thus, food consumption behaviours are complex in an economic system. People eat food to acquire biological, psychological or social wellbeing, and they value the food-relevant wellbeing by a comparison with other uses of their manageable resources as opportunity costs that are reflected in a monetary unit. Economic factors such as income and food price shape consumers' food choice behaviours, and eventually influence nutritional status.

National monitoring of food prices is not undertaken in Australia and there is some debate regarding which tools to use (Lewis & Lee 2016). There are calls for an international approach that would allow comparison within and between countries (Lee et al. 2013; 2018). Queensland is the only state that has undertaken regular monitoring of a healthy food basket over time (Harrison et al. 2007; 2010). Surveys have been undertaken in 2000, 2001, 2004, 2006, 2010 and 2014 (Queensland Department of Health 2015). The 2014 survey indicated that food prices are higher in regional and remote areas, further disadvantaging those living in these areas (Queensland Department of Health 2015). However, comparisons need to be made between unhealthy foods—which in Australia is the habitual diet—and healthier food choices (Lee et al. 2013).

INFLUENCES OF MATERIAL COSTS AND TRADE ON FOOD SAFETY AND AVAILABILITY

The prices of food products available in the retail market can be affected by costs of food production and processing. Retail food cost is composed of the price of raw food product (farm-gate price) and the costs of marketing and advertising, along with transportation, processing, packaging and preparation. In general, farm-gate value on animal products contributes a greater share of retail price than those for crop-based foods, and foods that require more manufacturing processes yield a lower return to the farm gate level. Moreover, the distribution of food cost between production and marketing components varies with time. Together with marketing costs, increased payouts for labour and energy as a result of economic growth keep retail food prices at a higher level than would otherwise be the case. Higher oil prices make it more expensive to operate food production machinery and transport agricultural products. At the same time, high oil prices encourage the energy industry to produce biofuels instead of petrol, which diverts maize and other feed and food crops to biofuel production and, eventually, forces up crop prices.

The demand side also plays a role in the costs of food production. There have been major shifts in the sources and types of agricultural products destined for different foods. Much of this is made possible by innovative food technology, with extrusion techniques and taste profiling able to support sophisticated food product simulation. With rising incomes, millions of people in low-income countries have experienced significant changes in food patterns, moving from grains and staple crops to animal products—sometimes with higher nutrient densities, like meat, dairy, and fish and plant foods like fruits, vegetables and nuts. Rising incomes also have allowed a proliferation of processed foods of lesser nutritional value using inexpensive ingredients like refined carbohydrates, fat, salt and sugar. Foodstuffs that are more nutritious generally have higher production costs than those that are less nutritious. Moreover, processed foods are increasingly dominant in the food market. On the one hand, food companies are more likely to develop and promote pre-packaged foods that allow for added 'value' (i.e. profit and commercial advantage) through processing. Examples include breakfast cereals, fruit juices, canned fruits or frozen vegetables. The societal value of such processing has more to do with reduced post-harvest loss, increased storage times without hazardous preservatives (like salt and curing) and availability at a distance from source. On the other hand, there is a trend for consumers to devote less time to food preparation and to seek more processed and pre-packaged foods for convenience. More food processing requires more labour and capital inputs. Thus, increased food costs are driven directly by the supply side and indirectly from the demand side.

Costs are also related to food safety, which requires investment and maintenance expenditure. Efficiencies with better outcomes can be achieved through new methodologies and regulatory regimes, such as those offered by HACCP (see Chapter 5). However, problems arise when food companies pursue financial benefits by reducing costs through cheaper, but less safe, methods or materials. There is growing circumstantial evidence that food price hikes affect food safety. For example, melamine was used as an adulterant in dairy products in China to simulate protein nitrogen. The demand for milk at cheaper prices was met by unscrupulous suppliers through dilution of milk with water and addition of a tailor-made non-protein nitrogen source—plastics industry waste—to meet the required standard (Wen et al. 2016). Similarly, recycled cooking oils may be overused and over-acidic, which is a compromise to save costs in industry, by small vendors and even in households.

WASTE MANAGEMENT TO IMPROVE FOOD SAFETY AND SECURITY: A CASE STUDY FROM TAIWAN

The price of food waste is often neglected in nutritional economics (FAO 2011; Parfitt et al. 2010; White et al. 2011). It may amount to 30–40 per cent of food harvest and production costs, along with associated packaging, transport and storage inefficiencies. Methods are available to estimate and remedy these problems (Huang 2010). In Taipei, the separate and almost daily collection of biodegradable household waste—which is recycled into fertiliser and animal feed—has dramatically reduced net waste by more than 80 per cent, although it still contributes about a third of municipal solid waste, along with its contribution to plastic and paper waste from packaging (Figure 25.7) (Lin et al. 2009). Food spending is more circumspect when the consequences of over-purchase are apparent with upstream benefits on both the food and health systems. This approach can be captured in national dietary guidelines.

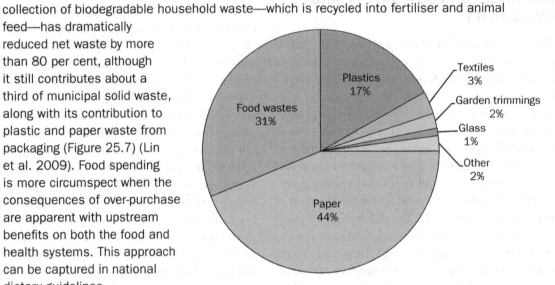

Figure 25.7: Composition of municipal solid waste in Taiwan

Source: Reproduced with permission from Lin et al. (2009)

PLASTIC MATTERS

Plastic is ubiquitous in our lives. Most food containers are made with plastics that use phthalates or bisphenol A (BPA) in the manufacturing process; both of these compounds have endocrine disruptor properties— that is, if they enter the body, they could interfere with the endocrine system. Another problem with plastic is that, instead of biodegrading, it breaks down into very tiny particles called microplastics (or nanoplastics, if even smaller). The physiology, metabolism, growth and reproduction of marine life that eats or draws in microplastics can be impacted. Microplastics from sewage-based fertilisers and plastic field coverings can also infiltrate the soil. There is increasing scientific and public concern over the impact of microplastics on the natural environment and eventually in our food systems on human health. Consumers and industry are encouraged to reduce plastic consumption, re-use when possible, and use proper disposal (see also the 'Bottled water' box in this chapter).

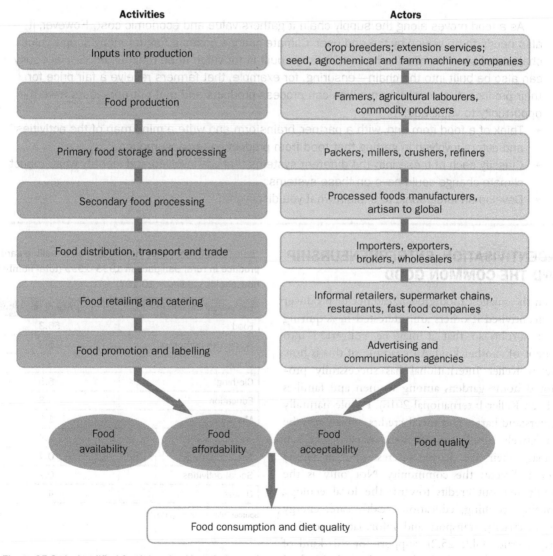

FOOD SUPPLY VALUE CHAIN ANALYSIS

Food supply value chain analysis refers to the value added to a product as it moves through the supply chain. The two components are 'value' and 'chain'. For a single food product, the chain comprises the processes and actors that take the food from its production on a farm to the consumer and on to its disposal as waste. Supply chains can be highly complex or very simple. A simplified representation is depicted in Figure 25.8. What you will notice is that it involves the integration of several different systems, all with different desired outcomes.

Activities

- Inputs into production
- Food production
- Primary food storage and processing
- Secondary food processing
- Food distribution, transport and trade
- Food retailing and catering
- Food promotion and labelling

Actors

- Crop breeders; extension services; seed, agrochemical and farm machinery companies
- Farmers, agricultural labourers, commodity producers
- Packers, millers, crushers, refiners
- Processed foods manufacturers, artisan to global
- Importers, exporters, brokers, wholesalers
- Informal retailers, supermarket chains, restaurants, fast food companies
- Advertising and communications agencies

- Food availability
- Food affordability
- Food acceptability
- Food quality

Food consumption and diet quality

Figure 25.8: A simplified food supply value chain

Source: Reproduced from Hawkes & Ruel (2012). Reproduced with permission from the International Food Policy Research Institute (www.ifpri.org)

Value refers to the value added to the product by activities undertaken at each step. Across the chain the value can be upgraded by:
- process upgrading—improving the efficiency of processing, decreasing waste
- product upgrading—introducing new products or improving old products, complying with standards
- volume upgrading—producing more of the product
- functional upgrading—changing the mix of activities occurring at various points in the chain (for example, farmers engaged in processing as well as growing)
- improving value-chain coordination (Hawkes & Ruel 2012).

As a food moves along the supply chain it gathers value and economic cost. However, it also needs to be valued by the end user. Climate change poses a risk for many supply value chains and so many need to have adaptation built in for value to be maintained. Social equity can also be built into the chain—ensuring, for example, that farmers receive a fair price for their produce, that local communities can process products and that entrepreneurs have the opportunity to value-add.
- Think of a food item and, with a partner, brainstorm and write a mind map of the activities and actors involved in getting that food from production to consumption.
- Classify each of these into the different systems that are involved and identify what impact climate change could have on these systems.
- Develop an infographic to explain what you discovered.

INCENTIVISATION, ENTREPRENEURSHIP AND THE COMMON GOOD

Even the smallest food grower, catcher or producer is incentivised if others are interested in acquiring their surplus so that it may be converted into benefit of another kind. An example of this is how Helen Keller International has successfully promoted home gardens among women and families (Helen Keller International 2018). People naturally understand barter and social credits, which may be a relatively simple way. Women, in particular, can manage their lives in the interest of their family and, indirectly, the community. Not only is the family fed, but credits towards the local ecology, housing, clothing, education, health care, energy for electricity, transport and information services may accrue (Table 25.2). Support for this kind of entrepreneurship, which favours household food security, can come from **microcredit** financing or some other form of societal exchange within, between or beyond communities. Nowadays, this may be facilitated by smart phones or other forms of digital technology.

Table 25.2: Main use of income earned by selling garden produce in rural Bangladesh 1998–1999 (total number of households studied = 10,107)

Household commodities	Percentage of households
Food	56.3
Productive purposes	15.3
Saved	9.7
Clothing	5.5
Education	4.8
Medicine	1.6
Housing	1.4
Amusement	0.4
Social activities	0.2
Others	4.8

Source: Talukder et al. (2001)

There is growing concern about inequality and inequity and what that signifies for present and future food security (Friel & Baker 2009). A relatively small number of individuals now control most of the world's wealth measured in monetary terms (Oxfam International 2017) and, implicitly, much of the global food systems. In the USA at least, with its focus on individualism, and perhaps more widely, some inequality is tolerated if it is 'fair' (Norton & Ariely 2011). What is unlikely to be regarded as 'fair inequality' is the presence of poverty associated with hunger, a situation deemed unacceptable by the United Nations as evidenced in its Sustainable Development Goals (see chapters 26 and 29). Unless they are better understood and effectively addressed, it can be expected that inequity and food insecurity will lead to increasing social unrest and conflict as they have done in the past.

SUMMARY

- Nutritional economics has its origins in the development of nutrition and home economics as discipline areas. It can help to understand how socioeconomic status interacts with human nutritional status and health.
- The sustainable livelihoods framework describes the capabilities (skills, education, ability to work), assets (cash, material resources) and activities required to secure the necessities of life. It provides a useful way to conceptualise the importance of economics in maintaining health and wellbeing. It focuses on livelihood and the efficient, sustainable, affordable, equitable and ethical distribution of food to support optimal health for as many as possible.
- Food prices reflect both environmental and individual factors that affect people's food choices. Higher food prices are a barrier to healthier food choices for low-income families. Rapid increases in food prices, along with financial crises, have contributed to global food insecurity and threatened population-level nutrition and health. Malnutrition—either as undernutrition or overnutrition—has significant impacts on economies through increased healthcare costs and lost productivity. Interventions are assessed based on their cost-effectiveness.
- Food availability and prices can be affected by global trade agreements. Trade agreements have resulted in the increased availability of ultra-processed foods and other health-harmful commodities in low- to middle-income countries.
- As consumers are very sensitive to price, governments can manipulate food prices by introducing subsidies to increase consumption of healthy foods and taxes to discourage unhealthy choices.
- Economists refer to the price elasticity of food, which is important to consider when changing food prices to ensure there are no unintended consequences.
- Households respond to increasing food prices by eating more monotonous diets of lower nutritional quality. People on lower incomes may choose foods that are energy-dense rather than nutrient-dense to minimise the risk of hunger.
- Food prices are a greater issue for low-income families as they account for a higher percentage of income. Healthy food tends to be more expensive than unhealthier food options and foods in general are more expensive in regional and remote areas.
- The prices of food products available in the retail market can be affected by costs of food production and processing. Retail food cost is composed of the price of raw food product (farm-gate price) and the costs of marketing and advertising, transportation, processing,

packaging and preparation. The food supply value chain is a way to conceptualise all the value embedded in the food system, from production to plate to waste.

* When biodegradable food waste must be disposed of by consumers for known utilisation as fertiliser or animal feed, the awareness and incentive to purchase food in amounts closer to need is greater. Any excess purchase becomes burdensome.

KEY TERMS

Gross domestic product: GDP is one of the primary indicators used to measure the health of a country's economy. It represents the total dollar value of all goods and services produced over a specific time period.

Microcredit: the lending of small amounts of money to low-income earners, effectively increasing their assets to either enable the further accumulation of assets or to enhance capabilities as part of the sustainable livelihoods framework. Critics argue that it is the privatisation of welfare and can lead to accumulation of debt rather than assets.

Unfreedom: another term for lack of freedom. Amartya Sen argues that people have a right to a set of freedoms: political, opportunity, access to credit, and protection from poverty. For Sen, development is a part of obtaining freedom, and this is enhanced by democracy and protection of human rights (Sen 2001).

ACKNOWLEDGEMENT

This chapter drew on the following journal publication and shared authorship with this book through Professor Mark L. Wahlqvist and with the copyright approval of HEC Press: Lo, Y.T., Chang, Y.H., Lee, M.S. & Wahlqvist, M.L., 2009, 'Health and nutrition economics: Diet costs are associated with diet quality', *Asia Pacific Journal of Clinical Nutrition, 18*(4): 598–604.

REFERENCES

Afshin, A., Peñalvo, J.L., Del Gobbo, L., Silva, J., Michaelson, M. et al., 2017, 'The prospective impact of food pricing on improving dietary consumption: A systematic review and meta-analysis', *PloS One, 12*(3): e0172277, doi:10.1371/journal.pone.0172277

Andreyeva, T., Long, M.W. & Brownell, K.D., 2010, 'The impact of food prices on consumption: A systematic review of research on the price elasticity of demand for food', *American Journal of Public Health, 100*(2): 216–22, doi:10.2105/ajph.2008.151415

Aronson, N., 1982, 'Nutrition as a social problem: A case study of the entrepreneurial strategy in science', *Social Problems, 29*(5): 474–87, doi:10.2307/800397

Ashley, C. & Carney, D., 1999, *Sustainable Livelihoods: Lessons from early experience*, London: Department for International Development

Ball, K., McNaughton, S.A., Le, H.N., Gold, L., Ni Mhurchu, C. et al., 2015, 'Influence of price discounts and skill-building strategies on purchase and consumption of healthy food and beverages: Outcomes of the Supermarket Healthy Eating for Life randomized controlled trial', *American Journal of Clinical Nutrition, 101*(5): 1055–64, doi:10.3945/ajcn.114.096735

Brimblecombe, J.K. & O'Dea, K., 2009, 'The role of energy cost in food choices for an Aboriginal population in northern Australia', *Medical Journal of Australia, 190*(10): 549–51, doi:10.5694/j.1326-5377.2009.tb02560.x

Cade, J., Upmeier, H., Calvert, C. & Greenwood, D., 1999, 'Costs of a healthy diet: analysis from the UK Women's Cohort Study', *Public Health Nutrition, 2*(4): 505–12, doi:10.1017/S1368980099000683

Chang, Y.-H., Chen, R.C.-Y., Lee, M.-S. & Wahlqvist, M.L., 2012, 'Increased medical costs in elders with the metabolic syndrome are most evident with hospitalization of men', *Gender Medicine, 9*(5): 348–60, doi:10.1016/j.genm.2012.08.005

Clapp, J., 2016, *Trade and the sustainability challenge for global food governance*, Paper presented at the Global Governance/Politics, Climate Justice & Agrarian/Social Justice Linkages and Challenges: An International Colloquium, The Hague, The Netherlands, <www.iss.nl/sites/corporate/files/1-ICAS_CP_Clapp.pdf>, accessed 29 May 2019

Cobiac, L.J., Veerman, L. & Vos, T., 2013, 'The role of cost-effectiveness analysis in developing nutrition policy', *Annual Review of Nutrition, 33*: 373–93, doi:10.1146/annurev-nutr-071812-161133

Colchero, M.A., Popkin, B.M., Rivera, J.A. & Ng, S.W., 2016, 'Beverage purchases from stores in Mexico under the excise tax on sugar sweetened beverages: Observational study', *BMJ, 352*: h6704, doi:10.1136/bmj.h6704

Copenhagen Consensus, 2012, *Outcome: The Expert Panel findings,* <www.copenhagenconsensus.com/copenhagen-consensus-iii/outcome>, accessed 9 December 2018

Culyer, A.J. & Newhouse, J.P., 2000, *Handbook of Health Economics*, Oxford: Elsevier

Darmon, N. & Drewnowski, A., 2008, 'Does social class predict diet quality?', *American Journal of Clinical Nutrition, 87*(5): 1107–17, doi:10.1093/ajcn/87.5.1107

—— 2015, 'Contribution of food prices and diet cost to socioeconomic disparities in diet quality and health: A systematic review and analysis', *Nutrition Reviews, 73*(10): 643–60, doi:10.1093/nutrit/nuv027

Detrick, H., 2018, 'Coca-Cola just started selling its first alcoholic drink ever', *Fortune*, 28 May, <http://fortune.com/2018/05/28/coca-cola-first-alcoholic-drink-japan/>, accessed 9 December 2018

Drewnowski, A. & Specter, S.E., 2004, 'Poverty and obesity: The role of energy density and energy costs', *American Journal of Clinical Nutrition, 79*(1): 6–16, doi:10.1093/ajcn/79.1.6

FAO, 2011, *Global Food Losses and Food Waste: Extent, causes, and prevention,* <www.fao.org/docrep/014/mb060e/mb060e.pdf>, accessed 23 February 2018

Ferguson, M., O'Dea, K., Holden, S., Miles, E. & Brimblecombe, J., 2017, 'Food and beverage price discounts to improve health in remote Aboriginal communities: Mixed method evaluation of a natural experiment', *Australian and New Zealand Journal of Public Health, 41*(1): 32–7, doi:10.1111/1753-6405.12616

Friel, S. & Baker, P.I., 2009, 'Equity, food security and health equity in the Asia Pacific region', *Asia Pacific Journal of Clinical Nutrition, 18*(4): 620–32, doi:10.6133/apjcn.2009.18.4.23

Friel, S., Gleeson, D., Thow, A.-M., Labonte, R., Stuckler, D. et al., 2013a, 'A new generation of trade policy: Potential risks to diet-related health from the Trans-Pacific Partnership Agreement', *Globalization and Health, 9*(1): 46, doi:10.1186/1744-8603-9-46

Friel, S., Hattersley, L., Snowdon, W., Thow, A.M., Lobstein, T. et al., 2013b, 'Monitoring the impacts of trade agreements on food environments', *Obesity Reviews, 14*(Suppl. 1): 120–34, doi:10.1111/obr.12081

Friel, S., Hattersley, L. & Townsend, R., 2015, 'Trade policy and public health', *Annual Review of Public Health, 36*(1): 325–44, doi:10.1146/annurev-publhealth-031914-122739

Goettler, A., Grosse, A. & Sonntag, D., 2017, 'Productivity loss due to overweight and obesity: A systematic review of indirect costs', *BMJ Open, 7*(10): e014632, doi:10.1136/bmjopen-2016-014632

Gordon, L.J., Bignet, V., Crona, B., Henriksson, P.J., Van Holt, T. et al., 2017, 'Rewiring food systems to enhance human health and biosphere stewardship', *Environmental Research Letters, 12*(10): 100201, doi:10.1088/1748-9326/aa81dc

Harrison, M., Lee, A., Findlay, M., Nicholls, R., Leonard, D. & Martin, C., 2010, 'The increasing cost of healthy food', *Australian and New Zealand Journal of Public Health, 34*(2): 179–86, doi:10.1111/j.1753-6405.2010.00504.x

Harrison, M.S., Coyne, T., Lee, A.J., Leonard, D., Lowson, S. et al., 2007, 'The increasing cost of the basic foods required to promote health in Queensland', *Medical Journal of Australia, 186*(1): 9–14, doi:10.5694/j.1326-5377.2007.tb00778.x

Hawkes, C. & Ruel, M.T., 2012, 'Value chains for nutrition', in S. Fan & R. Pandya-Lorch (eds), *Reshaping Agriculture for Nutrition and Health,* Washington, DC: International Food Policy Research Institute, pp. 73–82

Helen Keller International, 2018, *Nourishing Families,* <www.hki.org/our-work/nourishing-families>, accessed 12 December 2018

Horton, S., 2017, 'Economics of nutritional interventions', in S. de Pee, D. Taren & M.W. Bloem (eds), *Nutrition and Health in a Developing World,* Cham: Springer International Publishing, pp. 33–45

Huang, S.T.-Y., 2010, 'A recycling index for food and health security: Urban Taipei', *Asia Pacific Journal of Clinical Nutrition, 19*(3): 402–11, doi:10.6133/apjcn.2010.19.3.15

Kouris-Blazos, A. & Wahlqvist, M.L., 2007, 'Health economics of weight management: Evidence and cost', *Asia Pacific Journal of Clinical Nutrition, 16*(Suppl. 1): 329–38, doi:10.6133/apjcn.2007.16.s1.63

Lal, A., Mantilla-Herrera, A.M., Veerman, L., Backholer, K., Sacks, G. et al., 2017, 'Modelled health benefits of a sugar-sweetened beverage tax across different socioeconomic groups in Australia: A cost-effectiveness and equity analysis', *PLoS Medicine, 14*(6): e1002326, doi:10.1371/journal.pmed.1002326

Lee, A., Mhurchu, C.N., Sacks, G., Swinburn, B., Snowdon, W. et al., 2013, 'Monitoring the price and affordability of foods and diets globally', *Obesity Reviews, 14*(Suppl. 1): 82–95, doi: 10.1111/obr.12078

Lee, A.J., Kane, S., Lewis, M., Good, E., Pollard, C.M. et al., 2018, 'Healthy diets ASAP—Australian Standardised Affordability and Pricing methods protocol', *Nutrition Journal, 17*(1): 88, doi:10.1186/s12937-018-0396-0

Lewis, M. & Lee, A., 2016, 'Costing "healthy" food baskets in Australia: A systematic review of food price and affordability monitoring tools, protocols and methods', *Public Health Nutrition, 19*(16): 2872–86, doi:10.1017/S1368980016002160

Lin, A.Y.-C., Huang, S.T.-Y. & Wahlqvist, M.L., 2009, 'Waste management to improve food safety and security for health advancement', *Asia Pacific Journal of Clinical Nutrition, 18*(4): 538–45, doi:10.6133/apjcn.2009.18.4.12

Lo, Y.-T., Chang, Y.-H., Lee, M.-S. & Wahlqvist, M.L., 2012, 'Dietary diversity and food expenditure as indicators of food security in older Taiwanese', *Appetite, 58*(1): 180–7, doi:10.1016/j.appet.2011.09.023

Lo, Y.-T., Wahlqvist, M.L., Chang, Y.-H., Kao, S. & Lee, M.-S., 2013, 'Dietary diversity predicts type of medical expenditure in elders', *American Journal of Managed Care, 19*(12): e415–23, <www.ajmc.com/journals/issue/2013/2013-1-vol19-n12/dietary-diversity-predicts-type-of-medical-expenditure-in-elders>, accessed 29 May 2019

Lo, Y.-T.C., Wahlqvist, M.L., Huang, Y.-C. & Lee, M.-S., 2016, 'Elderly Taiwanese who spend more on fruits and vegetables and less on animal-derived foods use less medical services and incur lower medical costs', *British Journal of Nutrition, 115*(5): 823–33, doi:10.1017/S0007114515005140

Magnus, A., Cobiac, L., Brimblecombe, J., Chatfield, M., Gunther, A. et al., 2018, 'The cost-effectiveness of a 20% price discount on fruit, vegetables, diet drinks and water, trialled in remote Australia to improve Indigenous health', *PloS One, 13*(9): e0204005, doi:10.1371/journal.pone.0204005

Mendez Lopez, A., Loopstra, R., McKee, M. & Stuckler, D., 2017, 'Is trade liberalisation a vector for the spread of sugar-sweetened beverages? A cross-national longitudinal analysis of 44 low- and middle-income countries', *Social Science & Medicine, 172*: 21-7, doi:10.1016/j.socscimed.2016.11.001

Mhurchu, C.N., Eyles, H., Schilling, C., Yang, Q., Kaye–Blake, W. et al., 2013, 'Food prices and consumer demand: Differences across income levels and ethnic groups', *PLoS One, 8*(10): e75934, doi:10.1371/journal.pone.0075934

Nestle, M., 2015, *Soda Politics: Taking on Big Soda (and winning)*, New York, NY: Oxford University Press

Norton, M.I. & Ariely, D., 2011, 'Building a better America—one wealth quintile at a time', *Perspectives on Psychological Science, 6*(1): 9–12, doi:10.1177/1745691610393524

OECD, 2018, *Towards Better Food Policies,* <www.oecd.org/tad/policynotes/oecd-agriculture-brochure.pdf>, accessed 22 February 2019

Oxfam International, 2017, *An Economy for the 99%,* <www.oxfam.org/en/research/economy-99>, accessed 3 April 2018

Pan, W.-H., Yeh, W.-T., Chen, H.-J., Chuang, S.-Y., Chang, H.-Y. et al., 2012, 'The U-shaped relationship between BMI and all-cause mortality contrasts with a progressive increase in medical expenditure: A prospective cohort study', *Asia Pacific Journal of Clinical Nutrition, 21*(4): 577–87, doi:10.6133/apjcn.2012.21.4.13

Parfitt, J., Barthel, M. & Macnaughton, S., 2010, 'Food waste within food supply chains: Quantification and potential for change to 2050', *Philosophical Transactions of the Royal Society B: Biological Sciences, 365*(1554): 3065–81, doi:10.1098/rstb.2010.0126

Queensland Department of Health, 2015, *Healthy Food Basket Access Survey 2014*, <www.health.qld.gov.au/research-reports/reports/public-health/food-nutrition/access/overview>, accessed 12 December 2018

Quirmbach, D., Cornelsen, L., Jebb, S.A., Marteau, T. & Smith, R., 2018, 'Effect of increasing the price of sugar-sweetened beverages on alcoholic beverage purchases: An economic analysis of sales data', *Journal of Epidemiology & Community Health*, 72(4): jech-2017–209791, doi:10.1136/jech-2017-209791

Schram, A., Labonte, R., Baker, P., Friel, S., Reeves, A. & Stuckler, D., 2015, 'The role of trade and investment liberalization in the sugar-sweetened carbonated beverages market: A natural experiment contrasting Vietnam and the Philippines', *Globalization and Health*, 11(1): 41, doi:10.1186/s12992-015-0127-7

Schram, A., Ruckert, A., VanDuzer, J.A., Friel, S., Gleeson, D. et al., 2018, 'A conceptual framework for investigating the impacts of international trade and investment agreements on noncommunicable disease risk factors', *Health Policy and Planning*, 33(1): 123–36, doi:10.1093/heapol/czx133

Sen, A.K., 2001, *Development as Freedom*, Oxford: Oxford University Press

Sonnino, R., Moragues Faus, A. & Maggio, A., 2014, 'Sustainable food security: An emerging research and policy agenda', *International Journal of Sociology of Agriculture and Food*, 21(1): 173–88, <http://orca.cf.ac.uk/id/eprint/58308>, accessed 29 May 2019

Talukder, A., de Pee, S., Taher, A., Hall, A., Moench-Pfanner, R. & Bloem, M.W., 2001, 'Improving food and nutrition security through homestead gardening in rural, urban and peri-urban areas in Bangladesh', *UA-Magazine*, 5: 45–6, <www.ruaf.org/improving-food-and-nutrition-security-homestead-gardening-bangladesh>, accessed 12 December 2018

Thow, A., 2010, 'Glossary of trade terms', in C. Hawkes, C. Blouin, S. Henson, N. Drager & L. Dube (eds), *Trade, Food, Diet, and Health: Perspectives and policy options*, West Sussex: John Wiley & Sons Ltd, pp. 299–300

Thow, A.M. & Hawkes, C., 2009, 'The implications of trade liberalization for diet and health: A case study from Central America', *Globalization and Health*, 5(1): 5, doi:10.1186/1744-8603-5-5

Thow, A.M., Heywood, P., Schultz, J., Quested, C., Jan, S. & Colagiuri, S., 2011, 'Trade and the nutrition transition: Strengthening policy for health in the Pacific', *Ecology of Food and Nutrition*, 50(1): 18–42, doi:10.1080/03670244.2010.524104

Turner, G.M., Larsen, K.A., Candy, S., Ogilvy, S., Ananthapavan, J. et al., 2018, 'Squandering Australia's food security—the environmental and economic costs of our unhealthy diet and the policy path we're on', *Journal of Cleaner Production*, 195: 1581–99, doi:10.1016/j.jclepro.2017.07.072

UK Department for Environment, Food & Rural Affairs, 2014, *Food Statistics Pocketbook 2013—In Year Update*, <https://assets.publishing.service.gov.uk/government/uploads/system/uploads/attachment_data/file/315418/foodpocketbook-2013update-29may14.pdf>, accessed 22 February 2019

USDA ERS (Economic Research Service), 2016, *Data on Expenditures on Food and Alcoholic Beverages in Selected Countries*, <www.ers.usda.gov/topics/international-markets-us-trade/international-consumer-and-food-industry-trends/#outputs>, accessed 26 February 2019

Wahlqvist, M.L., 2016, 'Ecosystem dependence of healthy localities, food and people: IUNS News', *Annals of Nutrition and Metabolism*, 69: 75–8, doi:10.1159/000449143

Wahlqvist, M.L., Keatinge, J.D.H., Butler, C.D., Friel, S., McKay, J. et al., 2009, 'A Food in Health Security (FIHS) platform in the Asia-Pacific Region: The way forward', *Asia Pacific Journal of Clinical Nutrition*, 18(4): 688–702, doi:10.6133/apjcn.2009.18.4.34

Ward, P.R., Verity, F., Carter, P., Tsourtos, G., Coveney, J. & Wong, K.C., 2013, 'Food stress in Adelaide: The relationship between low income and the affordability of healthy food', *Journal of Environmental and Public Health*, article ID 968078, doi:10.1155/2013/968078

Wen, J.-G., Liu, X.-J., Wang, Z.-M., Li, T.-F. & Wahlqvist, M.L., 2016, 'Melamine-contaminated milk formula and its impact on children', *Asia Pacific Journal of Clinical Nutrition*, 25(4): 697–705, doi:10.6133/apjcn.072016.01

White, A., Gallegos, D. & Hundloe, T., 2011, 'The impact of fresh produce specifications on the Australian food and nutrition system: A case study of the north Queensland banana industry', *Public Health Nutrition*, 14(8): 1489–95, doi:10.1017/S1368980010003046

WHO, 2014, *Global Nutrition Targets 2025: Stunting policy brief*, <http://apps.who.int/iris/bitstream/10665/149019/1/WHO_NMH_NHD_14.3_eng.pdf>, accessed 7 April 2018

{CHAPTER 26}
SUSTAINABLE FOOD AND NUTRITION PRACTICE

Danielle Gallegos

OBJECTIVES

- Define and describe sustainability within a food and nutrition context.
- Describe the impact of climate change on human health.
- Identify sustainable food and nutrition practices at the population, community and individual levels.
- Apply the principles of sustainable food and nutrition practices at the individual level.

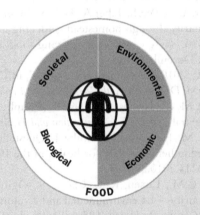

INTRODUCTION

There is growing recognition that the human race lives in a symbiotic relationship with the environment, with its very survival dependent on connectedness to animate and inanimate elements (Wahlqvist 2014). People eat foods that are assembled as diets—that is, selections of foods chosen by an individual from those made available by the food system (Meybeck & Gitz 2017). Consequently, diets are both outcomes and drivers of the food system (see Chapter 4). The food system, at each stage from production to consumption, has the potential to be affected by and to contribute to environmental degradation (Friel & Ford 2015). The food system is recognised as one of the primary contributors to greenhouse gas emissions, water scarcity, loss of biodiversity and

land misuse contributing to climate change. In turn, climate change—with average global increases of ambient temperature and extreme weather (drought, intense rain events)—will decrease the availability and affordability of food (that is, food security; see chapters 4 and 26). Yet sustainability is not just about the environment but incorporates economic, cultural and social practices as well.

This chapter defines and describes sustainability and its impact on food and nutrition. It will describe the impact of climate change on human health generally and then for food and nutrition more specifically. The chapter then outlines strategies that have been identified to improve the sustainability of the food system and how you, as a nutrition professional, can integrate this into nutrition advice. These strategies will be explored at the population, community and individual levels. Finally, the chapter will assist you to apply sustainable food and nutrition practices to your own diet.

WHAT IS SUSTAINABILITY?

Sustainability as a concept first emerged in 1987 from the Brundtland Report, which defined sustainable development as development that 'meets the needs of the present without compromising the ability of future generations to meet their own needs' (United Nations 1987). Sustainability is conceptualised as having three pillars, environmental, economic and social (see the 'Definitions of sustainability' box). The key features of sustainability are, therefore, the intergenerational component—that is, that it is not about just the present but also about the future— and the integration of alleviating poverty, tackling climate change and fighting inequalities.

These tenets now underpin the United Nations Sustainable Development Goals (see Chapter 29), which provide a global framework for strategies to 'end poverty, protect the planet and ensure prosperity for all' for the next 15 years (United Nations 2015). All of these goals underpin health either directly or indirectly through the promotion of education or equity, and all are linked to environmental, economic and social sustainability. Remember, though, that without the environment, social and economic goals are not attainable.

Sustainability within a food and nutrition context

Sustainability within the food and nutrition context encompasses the entire food system, from production to consumption and post-consumption to waste. Within the context of an ecological framework, sustainability for food and nutrition includes

DEFINITIONS OF SUSTAINABILITY

Environmental sustainability means living responsibly to avoid depletion or degradation of our natural resources, so that future generations are not disadvantaged. This means consuming materials such as energy, land and water at sustainable rates. Some resources are less abundant than others, and scarcity and damage to the environment from extraction of these materials needs to be taken into consideration. The environment underpins both society and the economy. This includes, for example, reducing carbon dioxide emissions, stopping rainforest destruction, finding alternatives to fossil fuels (coal, petrol), and consuming fish only from sources that are renewable.

Social sustainability occurs when formal and informal processes, systems, structures (including the built environment) and relationships actively support the creation of healthy and liveable communities. These communities are equitable, diverse, connected, harmonious and democratic and provide a good quality of life (Sen 2000). The overlap between the social and the environment is how we choose to live—it is about how homes and cities are created and how resources are used.

Economic sustainability requires the use and distribution of resources efficiently, equitably and responsibly so that economic growth, in balance with social factors and the environment, produces an operational profit. The overlap between the social and the economic is about equitable solutions; the overlap between the economic and the environment is about viable solutions.

economic, environmental and social elements to encompass health, quality and governance (Lang 2016). Importantly, sustainability needs to ensure that both the health of humans and the health of the environment are maintained, and one is not possible without the other. This has been described as an ecological approach to nutrition—the idea that nutrition, human and agricultural productivity and environmental sustainability are interlinked (see Chapter 1). This concept is further strengthened when it is noted that areas in which biodiversity has diminished correlate to areas with the highest levels of hunger and where there is a need for improved agricultural systems (Declerck et al. 2011).

Sustainability is integral to the conceptualisation of food security (see chapters 4 and 27). The environment, climate and the ability to harness natural resources are required to ensure the availability of food as well as preserving biodiversity. Economic and social sustainability are necessary for the accessibility of food (be that around food affordability or infrastructure to transport food from where it is grown to where it is consumed). Finally, the utilisation component of food security also requires economic and social sustainability (Berry et al. 2015).

The importance of sustainability with respect to food and nutrition has led to the concept of sustainable diets. The term 'sustainable diet' was first introduced by nutritionist Joan Dye Gussow in 1986 (Gussow & Clancy 1986). Gussow and Clancy argued that food sustainability and environmental and ecological harmony were essential to build and maintain human health. In 2010, the FAO and Biodiversity International formulated the definition of sustainable diets as:

> those diets with low environmental impacts which contribute to food and nutrition security and to healthy life for present and future generations. Sustainable diets are protective and respectful of biodiversity and ecosystems, culturally acceptable, accessible, economically fair and affordable; nutritionally adequate, safe and healthy; while optimizing natural and human resources. (Burlingame et al. 2010)

Sustainable diets therefore include a range of economic, environmental, social, quality, governance and health standards, as outlined in Table 26.1. They are protective and respectful of biodiversity and ecosystems, are culturally acceptable, economically fair and affordable and able to deliver diets of a quantity and quality to build and maintain health. The outcomes of sustainable diets will be multidimensional and include: reduced health-related chronic conditions and nutrient deficiencies; mitigation of climate change and natural resource depletion; sustainable employment and trade opportunities; reduced impact of the social determinants on health; enhanced health and wellbeing; cultural and social diversity; and animal welfare (Johnston et al. 2014).

Table 26.1: Dimensions of sustainable diets

Quality	Social values
• Taste • Seasonality • Cosmetic • Fresh (where appropriate) • Authenticity	• Pleasure • Identity • Religion • Animal welfare • Equality and justice • Cultural appropriateness • Skills (food citizenship)
Environment	**Health**
• Climate change • Energy use • Water • Land use • Soil • Biodiversity • Waste reduction and circularity	• Safety • Nutrition • Equal access • Availability • Social determinants of health, e.g. affordability • Information and education • Protection from marketing
Economy	**Governance**
• Food security and resilience • Affordability (price) • Efficiency • True competition • Fair return to primary producers • Jobs and decent working conditions • Fully internalised costs • Circular economy (full recycling)	• Science and technology evidence base • Transparency • Democratic accountability • Ethical values (fairness) • International aid and development • Trust

Source: Mason & Lang (2017)

Figure 26.1 demonstrates the elements of sustainable diets, underpinned by sustainable food systems.

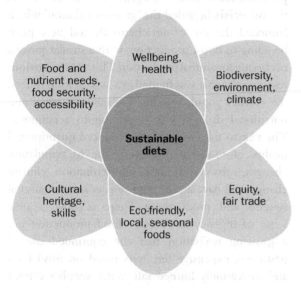

Figure 26.1: Elements of a sustainable diet

Source: Lairon (2012). Reproduced with permission

THREATS TO SUSTAINABLE FOOD SYSTEMS

Climate change

One of the biggest environmental threats to the ongoing supply of food and to dietary quality and diversity is climate change (FAO 2018; Rockström et al. 2018). Climate change refers to the increases in ambient temperatures, changes to sea levels, changes to rainfall patterns and acidification of oceans as a result of elevated and ongoing greenhouse gas emissions. There are predictions that if global warming is limited to 1.5°C vulnerability to reductions in food production will be less than if it increases to 2°C (Betts et al. 2018). There are, however, still serious ramifications if temperatures increase by the predicted 1.5°C (IPCC 2018).

In Australia, climate change has resulted in:

- increases in mean surface air and sea surface temperatures by around 1°C since 1910; globally, 2015 was the warmest year since recording began in 1880
- extreme heat events and extreme fire weather increasing in duration, frequency and intensity
- increased rainfall across northern Australia

GREENHOUSE GASES

Greenhouse gases are compounds that trap longwave radiation at the earth's surface, causing an increase in temperatures. Greenhouse gases enter our atmosphere in two ways. The first is through natural processes such as animal and plant respiration. The second is via human sources, including fossil fuel usage, intensive livestock farming, use of synthetic fertilisers and industrial processes.

Greenhouse gases include:

- carbon dioxide, the main sources of which are the burning of coal, oil and gas; deforestation contributes to increased concentrations due to a reduced uptake of carbon dioxide by plants
- nitrous oxide, with agriculture (animal manure, use of fertilisers) and burning of fossil fuels the primary sources
- methane, produced by fossil fuel extraction and burning, livestock farming, landfill and waste, rice production, biomass burning (i.e. of crops) and use of biofuels (in particular, animal dung, wood or agricultural waste)
- fluorinated gases, with the main sources being refrigeration, foams and aerosols.

- an 11 per cent decrease in rainfall during the April–October peak south-east growing season since the mid-1990s
- an increase in mean sea level—increasing the effects of high tides and storm surges—directly influenced by the melting of the Greenland and Antarctic ice sheets and glaciers
- an increase of about 25 per cent in ocean acidity levels, with the potential to impact the marine biosphere. (Australian Government et al. 2016)

Climate change is linked to health in a number of ways. These are described in Figure 26.2 (see colour section). In summary, climate change will:

- contribute to undernutrition by reducing agricultural productivity and increasing the incidence of diarrhoea through flood-borne disease
- increase mortality and morbidity (particularly in older people) due to heatwaves
- decrease the ability to work due to hot conditions—this will affect farmers and further contribute to decreased food production
- cause heat stress, exacerbating pre-existing heart and renal disease
- increase the incidence of **vector-borne diseases** such as dengue fever
- lead to poor air quality, directly contributing to increased incidence of cardiovascular disease, stroke, lung disease and acute and chronic lung infections (Fanzo et al. 2018; Watts et al. 2017).

Climate change, agriculture and the food system

In 1798, Thomas Malthus predicted that as the world's population was increasing exponentially (1, 2, 4, 8, 16, 32, 64 …) and agricultural productivity was increasing arithmetically (1, 2, 3, 4, 5, 6 …), at some point in time demand would outstrip supply. Critics of the Malthusian equation argue that this approach does not take into consideration birth control, fertilisers and technology, which have slowed population growth and increased production. There are indications that the fertility rate has decreased; however, population growth continues, with estimates indicating that the world population of 7.7 billion (June 2019) will increase to 9.7 billion in 2050 (United Nations 2019).

After World War 2, when countries became anxious about supply interruptions and food shortages, industrialised countries (the USA, the UK, Australia) made a conscious decision that more and cheaper food was needed. This began the **productionist** phase of agriculture. In the 1970s, the **oil crisis** heralded the 'green revolution' which launched the use of agrichemicals and new plant breeding to boost production, with a similar process occurring for animal production. This was the obvious response to what was framed as a lack of food to feed the world's population, but the environmental and nutritional damage was beginning to accumulate. The risk to the food system—reduced quantity and quality of food—is not over. Due to population changes, urbanisation and industrialisation, climate change will have a profound impact on agricultural systems and productivity. There is now a new sense of urgency to increase food production but a growing realisation that the continued use of pesticides, expensive fertilisers based on fossil fuels and increasingly limited safe water supplies cannot continue. In Australia, predictions are that climate change could decrease agricultural production by up to 10 per cent by 2030, and 19 per cent by 2050 (Gunasekera et al. 2007).

Agricultural practices

There is a range of agricultural practices that currently threaten the sustainability of the food system. The consequences of these practices include degradation and loss of agricultural land, the loss of biodiversity, pressure on water resources, pollution, and resource depletion (Sonnino et al. 2014).

Degradation and loss of agricultural land

Approximately 40 per cent of the earth's land surface is being used for agriculture with an estimated 16–40 per cent of this land already lightly to severely degraded. Degradation of agricultural land is caused by intensive farming practices and climate change. These losses have been attributed to suboptimal practices, including inadequate use of soil conservation techniques such as slope coverage, lying fallow, and reincorporation and recycling of

PLANT MICROBIOTA

The impact of climate change could also affect other ecological systems essential for plant health. The plant microbiota is being increasingly recognised as influential in productivity and health.

Read the following article and summarise the key points on the impact of climate change on agricultural productivity via plant microbiota.

- Müller, D.B., Vogel, C. Bai, Y., Vorholt, J.A., 2016, 'The plant microbiota: Systems-level insights and perspectives', *Annual Review of Genetics*, 50: 211–34, doi:10.1146/annurev-genet-120215-034952.

THE STORY OF BEES

Bee populations worldwide are in decline. Bees are an important component of the agricultural and food system as essential pollinators of both wild and cultivated plants. Of the 100 crop species that provide 90 per cent of the world's food, over 70 are pollinated by bees. Bees are facing multiple threats, including:

- destruction by insecticides and pesticides used in agriculture that interfere with the bee's brain metabolism and gut microbiota
- air pollution interfering with the bee's ability to find flowering plants, masking the scent
- electromagnetic fields that may interfere with bees' ability to navigate back to their hives
- the spread globally of parasites and fungi that invade hives and destroy bees; in Australia, likely points of entry for such pests are shipping ports via coal, sugar and grain ships
- competition from 'alien' species such as the Africanised bee in the United States; in Australia, the major threat to native bee species is from the European honey bee
- climate change-induced changes in the flowering of plants, affecting the production of nectar and potentially reducing the bee's food supply.

(Kluser & United Nations Environment Programme 2010; Motta et al. 2018; Sandilyan 2017)

manure; underuse of green manure; deforestation; and overgrazing (Sonnino et al. 2014). Degradation occurs in the form of erosion, soil salinity and soil acidity. In Australia, dryland soil salinity is expected to affect seventeen million hectares by 2050. Soil acidity, predominantly caused by the use of high-ammonia fertilisers, is predicted to affect over 50 per cent of Australia's current agricultural land (Commonwealth of Australia 2017). Acidity reduces nutrient availability and microbial activity, restricting root access to water and nutrients, thereby reducing productivity.

Loss of biodiversity

There are two aspects to the loss of biodiversity. The first is that human activities—through population growth, increased mobility, deforestation and over-exploitation of species—have reduced biodiversity. Deforestation and the destruction of native vegetation that acts as **biodiversity sinks** is accompanied by increasing opportunities for the introduction of invasive species which can change native ecosystems by destroying the balance between predation and competition. In addition, overfishing and overhunting have led to the loss of species, destabilising ecosystems (Chappell & LaValle 2011).

The other contributor to loss of biodiversity is the agricultural practice of monocropping—that is, large-scale specialisation of a single crop, which is designed to increase productivity and efficiency. Monocropping is often accompanied by the use of genetically uniform, high-yielding crop varieties that are often less resistant to pathogens and pests and more susceptible to new or adapted pests (Chappell & LaValle 2011). Other agricultural practices that impact on biodiversity are frequent, short or bare **fallows**, which disrupt the communities of soil organisms—as does the increased mechanisation of tillage (Chappell & LaValle 2011). Intact ecosystems of indigenous plants and animals appear to protect or buffer against the effects of invasive plants and animals, pathogens and toxins (Burlingame et al. 2010).

There is still some debate about the relative value of large corporate farms that focus on a single crop versus smaller farms that are more diverse. The resource requirements, including land tenure, for food production may be financially burdensome, even prohibitive, discouraging small and family producers and favouring agribusiness. However, smaller-scale food production may be mixed, more environmentally sensitive, a whole-of-family or community investment, and more directed towards local livelihoods These smaller family-operated farms are less reliant on the price of a single commodity for income, make more efficient use of irrigation, have higher quality labour (that is, family) who have a stake in the success of operations, and have lower costs associated with the use of agrochemicals (Chappell & LaValle 2011). Family farms have greater potential for biodiversity and sustainable food systems than does agribusiness (Quintana 2014). There is a trade-off, however: large corporate agricultural businesses can keep food prices lower. People want their food to be inexpensive, but farmers need a good price for the food they produce so that they can pay for

---

HOW CAN A DECREASE IN DIET DIVERSITY THREATEN FOOD SECURITY AND HEALTH?

Khoury and colleagues (2014), based on the FAO national per capita food supply data, reported a convergence in crop commodities towards a universal diet in more than 150 countries from 1961 to 2009. There has been a global rise in the consumption of foods including wheat, rice, soybeans and sunflower, while crops of regional importance, including sorghum, millet, rye and root crops such as sweet potato, cassava and yam, have lost ground. Globally, national food supplies have become increasingly similar in composition. The importance of crop commodities in our food supplies—particularly their contribution to protein and fat, but also other nutrients—may shift in response to health, natural resources and climate pressures. The narrowing of the diversity of crop species, both in production systems and in the overall food supply, has the potential to compromise food security and health outcomes (Khoury et al. 2014; Lee et al. 2011).

Read the following articles or search for additional material and explore whether this interpretation of food supply trends and their health relevance is valid:

- Khoury, C.K. et al., 2014, 'Increasing homogeneity in global food supplies and the implications for food security', *Proceedings of the National Academy of Sciences, 111*(11): 4001–06
- Lee, M.S. et al., 2011, 'A simple food quality index predicts mortality in elderly Taiwanese', *Journal of Nutrition, Health and Aging, 15*: 815–21.

WHAT IS THE EVIDENCE FOR THE BENEFITS OF ORGANIC FARMING?

'Organic' agriculture is defined as 'a production system that sustains the health of soils, ecosystems and people. It relies on ecological processes, biodiversity and cycles adapted to local conditions, rather than the use of inputs with adverse effects. Organic agriculture combines tradition, innovation and science to benefit the shared environment and promote fair relationships and a good quality of life for all involved' (International Federation of Organic Agriculture Movements 2014, p. 31).

Growers wanting to label their foods 'organic' or 'biodynamic' must voluntarily adhere to standards. Internationally, the term 'organic' is covered by provisions in the *Codex Alimentarius* and in Australia by Standards Australia (ASD6000-2015). Certification is provided by private companies after an assessment process. However, the producer of any foods that are claimed to be organic must be able to substantiate that claim. The standards cover all aspects of production including use of genetically modified items, land care, plant production, livestock handling, preparation and transport.

Consumers tend to choose organic food for a variety of reasons, including health, taste, animal welfare, environmental impact or because they do not trust the conventional food production systems (Hansen et al. 2018). The Australian Organic Market Report (Australian Organic Ltd 2017) identified the key perceived benefit of organic food as being food free from:

- chemicals
- additives
- hormones and antibiotics
- genetic modification
- cruelty.

The main barriers to consuming organic foods are price, limited availability and perceived quality.

Are organic foods healthier? There are indications that, in some parts of the world, organic foods lower an individual's exposure to pesticide residues, are more environmentally friendly and may be better for animal welfare. It does, however, largely depend on local practices. Some studies indicate that organically grown items are superior nutritionally; for example, containing higher levels of vitamins and minerals in fruits and vegetables, higher levels of beneficial fatty acids in milk and meat and lower levels of heavy metals in cereals. The differences, however, are quite small and may have little impact on the health of well-nourished populations, especially given the price premium paid (Brantsaeter et al. 2017).

Questions to think about and explore further include:

- Can people trust organic labelling and what does this actually mean?
- What motivates people to consume organic food?
- Do the benefits of organic food outweigh the costs?
- Are we creating a bigger division between the rich and poor given that organic food costs more?

Read the evidence on organic food and develop the key points you would argue in a radio interview on the benefits of consuming organic food.

better seed, machinery, fertiliser, and other inputs with which to produce more and better food. Technological answers may depend on general economic development. More opportunities and better livelihoods mean more people have sufficient, better quality and more varied food; and food growers, harvesters or producers have more certain and enduring roles.

Resource depletion

Agricultural practices are contributing to the depletion of global resources and, conversely, production is being limited by these resources. One of the key points made by The EAT–*Lancet* Commission on Healthy Diets from Sustainable Food systems is the need for radical improvements in the efficiency of fertiliser and water use, recycling phosphorus and mitigating climate change (Willett et al. 2019). There are a range of resources affected, but the depletion of two particular resources is currently critical: phosphorus and water. Phosphorus is a non-renewable resource, while water is renewable.

Phosphorus

Phosphorus is an essential element within ecological systems. As part of phosphate, it makes up important physiological structures essential for genetic material, bone structure, and energy release. The phosphorus cycle in the environment begins with the removal of phosphorus from the weathering of sedimentary rock; it is then distributed through soils and water. Plants take up the phosphate ions from soils and the element passes into animals through the consumption of these plants. The phosphates absorbed by animal tissue return to the soil through excretion of urine and faeces and as part of the final decomposition of animals and plants.

Phosphorus is essential for food production and its availability in soils limits crop yields globally. On the other hand, excess phosphorus is polluting waterways due to fertiliser run-off. Phosphorus availability has been severely limited by the actions of humans. Geological phosphate reserves have been mined to produce fertilisers, creating a large one-way flow from rocks to farms to lakes and oceans (Elser &

Bennett 2011). Phosphorus supply and demand is a good example of the intersection of social, economic and biological influences within the ecosystem (Cordell et al. 2009).

Eighty-five per cent of phosphorus reserves are controlled by five countries: Morocco, China, Algeria, Syria and South Africa. The United States used to be the world's largest exporter but now has approximately 20 years of reserves left. China has imposed a 135 per cent export tariff to secure domestic fertiliser supply, effectively halting exports (Weber et al. 2014). Morocco controls the bulk of phosphate rock in the Western Sahara, claiming the land and resources. However, this occupation of the Western Sahara is condemned as unlawful by the United Nations and is not recognised internationally. The occupation of this area has resulted in the displacement of the local Saharawi people and there are calls to divest from supporting the industry in this region (Kingsbury 2015). The concentration of power for control of phosphate reserves is much greater than that for oil and could lead to political turmoil as prices for fertiliser increase and affordability decreases.

Due to the low reserves of phosphate, other ways of recycling and reducing the use of phosphate are being explored. Approximately eight million tonnes of phosphorus is lost from farms through soil leaching and erosion. Practices such as optimising the timing and placement of fertiliser and **no-till cultivation** can significantly reduce those losses (Elser & Bennett 2011). Extracting phosphorus from excrement is also under development. It has been estimated that extraction of phosphorus from human urine and faeces could meet 22 per cent of the global demand for phosphorus (Mihelcic et al. 2011). For example, in less industrialised areas where sanitation remains an issue, single-use biodegradable bags have been developed in which human faeces can be safely composted for agricultural use (Vinnerås et al. 2009).

Water

Water scarcity—that is, the lack of water availability to meet demand—is expected to intensify with the combined effects of increased urbanisation, pollution and climate change. The agricultural sector currently accounts for 70 per cent of global freshwater use (FAO 2014); consequently, there can be no food security without water security. Globally, there have been a number of suggestions to improve the availability of water for agriculture, including:

- increasing rainwater availability via rainwater harvesting and soil and water conservation practices
- minimising evaporative losses by improved water and crop management; for example, by layering a protective cover over the top of the soil (mulching)
- improving the efficiency of irrigation
- use of crop variants that are tolerant to drought
- promotion of safe and productive use of low-quality water. (Steduto et al. 2018)

In Australia, water security is critical for ongoing agricultural production. For irrigated agriculture there is a complex system of entitlements to and allocation of surface and groundwater, creating a water market. The level of water security will depend on what is being grown and will vary depending on the levels and flows of rivers, demand relative to supply and the complexity of the environmental and social values being protected. At its simplest, the rules would limit extraction of water in dry years and the water would be shared according to the water access entitlements (Horne 2018). For rain-fed agriculture in Australia (the two largest users being beef and cereal crop production), climate change with decreasing rainfall will have a large impact. The cereal industry has responded by improving agricultural practices such as improved cropping systems, no-till cultivation, effective use of herbicides, and better seeds that allowed the crops to use moisture more effectively (Richards et al. 2014).

Water usage is increasingly recognised as another critical element along with greenhouse gas emissions in determining the environmental sustainability of the food system. Recent research indicates that healthier diets use less water. A diet consistent with dietary guidelines uses less water, with reductions in the water footprint thought to be 11–35 per cent for a healthy diet with meat, 33–55 per cent with fish and 35–55 per cent for a vegetarian diet (Vanham et al. 2018).

Accessing water from natural waterways is a key element of water security. Low availability of safe water from these sources affects the livelihoods of all of those relying on the waterway as a source of income, transport, irrigation or food. The Mekong River is an international example, flowing through six countries (Cambodia, China, Laos, Myanmar, Thailand and Vietnam) and providing direct employment, food, energy and transportation for an estimated 70 million people. Political cooperation is essential to ensure the viability of the waterway, but indications are that controlling the waterway means controlling the economy of most of Southeast Asia.

An Australian example is the Murray–Darling Basin. This river system is one of Australia's most important water systems, flowing through three states (New South Wales, Victoria and South Australia). Extraction or mismanagement of the water upstream will have significant impacts on those relying on the water source downstream. In 2017 there were allegations of theft by New South Wales from the system that impacted negatively on South Australia.

Agroecology

Agroecology is both a science and a political movement. It is fundamentally about sustainable farming practices with a strong emphasis on diversity, efficient use of resources, recycling, the co-creation and sharing of knowledge and the link between human values and sustainable livelihoods. It also explicitly includes social and ethical issues (Béné et al. 2019). It privileges peasant and Indigenous agricultural practices.

Post-production practices

While agricultural production accounts for a good proportion of greenhouse gas emissions, post-production activities—including transportation, refrigeration, waste disposal, manufacturing and packaging—make up 50 per cent of total food system emissions (Garnett 2011). The adoption of refrigeration, transport and processing technologies that are more efficient and rely on renewable energy sources, combined with better waste management via better inventory control, reduced packaging and modification of portion sizes, will significantly reduce emissions (Garnett 2014).

Reducing food miles

Due to increasing urbanisation and loss of **peri-urban agriculture**, the distance food needs to travel from where it is grown to where it is consumed is increasing. Transporting food over these distances also requires inputs into keeping the food safe (through refrigeration or other mechanisms) and maintaining quality, requiring additional packaging. One of the strategies for reducing greenhouse gas emissions post-production is to reduce this distance by utilising more local food networks. This approach, however, is too simplistic and fails to take into consideration other energy inputs that may increase the overall production of greenhouse gas emissions. Life-cycle energy assessment (Steduto et al. 2018) is now increasingly used to map the energy and carbon footprint of various food items.

Life-cycle assessment (LCA) is a systematic process to evaluate the environmental burdens and impacts associated with a product, process or activity by identifying and quantifying energy and materials used and wastes released to the environment. The assessment includes the entire life cycle of the product, process or activity, including:

- extracting, growing and processing raw materials
- manufacturing
- transportation and distribution
- use, re-use, maintenance
- recycling
- disposal.

An LCA covers all the stages of food production including the following six steps: farm inputs, agricultural stage, production, distribution, use and waste management (Dijkman et al. 2018). The LCA is very country-specific, relying on articulation of local horticultural and animal husbandry practices. For some food products the greenhouse gas emissions generated on a farm are much greater than the emissions associated with processing and transport

and so miles travelled makes little impact. For example, in Europe intensive farming of tomatoes in heated greenhouses throughout the year generates high greenhouse gas emissions, so much so that 'locally' produced tomatoes could be less environmentally friendly than field-grown tomatoes that had to be transported longer distances (Theurl et al. 2014).

Reducing consumption of ultra-processed foods

Ultra-processed foods are typically those that have undergone a high degree of processing and packaging and are typically foods that are energy-dense but nutrient-poor (see Chapter 19). Such foods contribute significantly to poor eating patterns and result in higher rates of overweight, obesity and chronic conditions. There is a known health benefit from reducing consumption of these foods but what has been less explicit is the environmental impacts (Friel et al. 2013). Consumption of ultra-processed foods contributes up to 39 per cent of total food-related life-cycle energy use, 35 per cent of water use and 33 per cent of food-related greenhouse gas emissions (Hadjikakou 2017). The priority for households in order to reduce environmental impact would be to reduce consumption of alcohol, carbonated beverages, processed meats, baked goods and confectionery (Hadjikakou 2017; Hyland et al. 2017).

Reducing food waste

One-third of world food production is lost or wasted along the food supply chain (FAO 2011) (see Chapter 6 on microbial spoilage). Food waste can be defined as 'any food, and inedible parts of food, removed from the food supply chain to be recovered or disposed (including composted, crops ploughed in/not harvested, anaerobic digestion, bio-energy production, incineration, disposal to sewer, landfill or discarded to sea)' (Food Use for Social Innovation by Optimising Waste Prevention Strategies [FUSIONS] 2014). Contributions to food waste are extensive across the food system and include post-harvest losses, food processing and retail losses and consumer food waste (Table 26.2).

The cost of food waste is often neglected in nutritional economics. However, it is being

Table 26.2: Categorisation of food waste

Agricultural production	Losses due to mechanical damage or spillage during harvest, or due to death (during breeding)
Post-harvest handling and storage	Losses due to spillage and degradation during handling, storage and transportation between farm and distribution points; for animals this would include death during transport to slaughter, or degradation after landing (e.g. fish, eggs)
Processing	Losses due to spillage, degradation during processing, e.g. juice production, canning, peeling, slicing, trimming (e.g. meat) or due to process interruptions
Distribution	Losses and waste in the market system, e.g. wholesale markets, supermarkets, retailers
Consumption	Losses and waste during consumption both within and outside (e.g. restaurants, hospitals) the household

Source: Gustavsson et al. (2011)

increasingly recognised at all levels from farm to post-plate (Huang 2010). It is estimated that 19,000 kJ/day of food are harvested for every person on the planet but only 8000 kJ are consumed, representing lost energy in the system (Cooper et al. 2018). Food waste post-harvest is usually described as food loss. In high-income countries the greatest potential for reducing food waste along the supply chain is with retailers, food services and consumers (Parfitt et al. 2010), although reducing the impact of cosmetic specifications set by retailers will also significantly reduce waste at the farm-gate. For example, in Far North Queensland 10–30 per cent of the banana crop is discarded on farm; of this, 78 per cent is due to cosmetic imperfections. This equates to 37,000 tonnes per annum and represents a loss of 137 billion kilojoules (White et al. 2011). In 2016, the Australian government committed to a National Food Waste strategy, linking it to UN Sustainable Development Goal 12, for sustainable consumption and production patterns. The strategy identifies the need to effectively manage food waste across the food supply chain, including:

- increasing agricultural efficiency
- changes to food ordering, transport and storage practices
- effective and sustainable packaging
- partnerships between food and grocery retailers and charitable food relief agencies (see Chapter 27)
- household education and community initiatives
- incentives and investment in alternative treatment technologies and landfill disposal
- creating value from waste.

NUTRITION PRACTICE

Environmental sustainability is increasingly recognised as an important consideration in the development of food-based dietary guidelines that underpin nutrition advice for citizens. A review of the diets consumed in nine middle-income and 28 high-income countries indicated that animal products accounted for 22 per cent, 65 per cent and 70 per cent of greenhouse gas emissions in low-middle, upper-middle and high-income countries respectively. Brazil and Australia had over 200 per cent higher emissions than the average in their income group due to high intakes of grass-fed meat linked to elevated methane production (Behrens et al. 2017). In countries like China there is growing recognition that increases in meat and cooking oil consumption have led to a reduction in nutritional quality of Chinese diets, as well as negative environmental consequences (He et al. 2018).

Shifting from the average diet consumed to nationally recommended diets reduced greenhouse gas emissions, due mainly to recommended decreases in meat consumption and increases in fruit, vegetable and grains (Behrens et al. 2017). However, other modelling indicates that current dietary guidelines do not go far enough to meet long-term climate change impacts or to meet the Sustainable Development Goals (Ritchie et al. 2018). So, while consuming a diet that is in line with national recommendations would improve the sustainability of diets, some countries are also utilising the dietary guidelines as an important policy tool to further reduce the environmental impact of food consumption, Table 26.3 provides

Table 26.3: Dietary guidelines from four countries incorporating sustainability principles

Source/Country	Environmentally effective food choices (Sweden), 2009	Sustainable shopping basket (Germany), 1990s–2013	Guidelines for a healthy diet: the ecological perspective (The Netherlands), 2011	Qatar National Dietary Guidelines, 2014
Prime concerns	Pro-health and environment to reduce climate change	To integrate advice from many sources for daily food shopping	Linking gains in public health nutrition to lower ecological impact	To integrate principles of sustainability
Actual advice	Eat less meat, replace it with vegetarian meals; choose local meats or organic if possible	Follow the food pyramid	Move to a less animal-based more plant-based diet—this is the key advice	Emphasise a plant-based diet including vegetables, fruit, whole grain cereals, legumes
	Eat fish 2–3 times per week from sustainable sources	Eat less meat and fish but savour them	Lower energy intake and eat fewer snacks	Reduce leftovers and waste
	Eat fruit, vegetables, berries: a good rule of thumb is to choose seasonal, local and preferably organic products	Follow 5 a day on fruit and vegetables	Eat 2 portions of fish a week but from sustainable sources	When available consume locally and regionally produced foods
	Choose locally grown potatoes and cereals rather than rice	Eat seasonally and regionally as your first choice	Reduce food waste	Choose fresh, homemade foods over highly processed foods and fast foods
	Choose pesticide-free or organic when possible	Eat organic products		Conserve water in food preparation
	Choose rapeseed oil rather than palm oil fats	Choose fair trade products		Follow the recommendations of the Qatar DGs

Source: Adapted from Lang (2016)

examples from four countries—Sweden, Germany, the Netherlands and Qatar—that have integrated sustainability into dietary guidelines.

Australian dietary guidelines have been identified as being poorly aligned with greenhouse gas mitigation requirements (Ritchie et al. 2018). In 2003, the Australian Dietary Guidelines included an appendix that highlighted the need for a focus on sustainability. In 2011, consideration was given to incorporating sustainability and an appendix to the main guidelines, 'Australian Dietary Guidelines through an Environmental Lens', was released. However, the NHMRC indicated that while sustainability was not a new concept, it was complex and that there were numerous gaps in evidence which precluded their inclusion (Johnson 2015). The inclusion of sustainability was strongly opposed by farmers and indicates once again that dietary guidelines are highly political documents that balance a number of agendas, not just those around diet and health (Nestle 2013).

The Lancet has published a framework for a healthy reference diet that simultaneously is healthful for humans, ensures food security in order to feed a global population and is environmentally sustainable (Willett et al. 2019) (see the 'Planetary health diet' box in Chapter 33). One of the ongoing challenges will be how to factor in the impact of climate change and alteration in planetary health on calculations related to diet and the global burden of disease (GBD). The GBD will need to consider developing additional health-related metrics such as biodiversity, climate change and ecosystem failure. The guidance for individuals regarding eating a sustainable diet are numerous and diverse as they need to take into consideration local values and cultural norms. There are, however, some recurring themes.

Strategy 1: Eat more plants, eat less meat

Eating a more plant-based diet is now considered to be one of the key strategies for improving sustainability. Raising animals for consumption is inherently less efficient that relying on plants; this is because more energy is lost as you move up the chain. For example, most animals are intensively farmed and rely on grain—this grain could be used for human consumption. When looking at a mixed diet, a vegetarian diet uses 2.9 times less water, 2.5 times less primary energy, 13 times less fertiliser and 1.4 times less pesticides than a non-vegetarian diet (Marlow et al. 2009).

Based on these data, a more sustainable diet is one that contains less meat. There are four strategies that could be employed to achieve this.

1. Go completely vegetarian—if you do this you need to remember to follow the principles of ensuring good quality protein.
2. Go 'flexitarian', which means at least halving the meat you eat.
3. Have meat-free days in a week.
4. Eat meat from smaller rather than larger animals, e.g. chicken or rabbit rather than beef.

Strategy 2: Eat locally and in season

Local eating has emerged as an alternative food system, one way to disrupt the large-scale, multinational food system that dominates the industrialised world. Local eating manifests as eating food that is only grown in the local area or region so that food miles are reduced (to lessen environmental impact), social relationships are built and, economically, money stays in the area. The original concept was designed to reduce food miles—that is, to reduce the distance travelled between where food was grown and where it was consumed. Practically, this manifests as shopping at farmer's markets, utilising community-supported agriculture, frequenting restaurants that have local suppliers and only eating foods in season.

'Local' has now been transformed to a more 'place-based' approach. This means that the concept of local is fluid and contextual and should be considered on the basis of a range of factors, including diet diversity (Cleveland et al. 2015). In Australia, for example, eating locally as defined by a 160-kilometre radius would, in some areas, drastically reduce diet diversity, especially given the penetration of industrialised monoculture farming. One conceptualisation of eating locally would be choosing foods grown and produced in Australia. In 2016, consumer advocates

IS THE 'REDUCE MEAT CONSUMPTION' MESSAGE TOO SIMPLE?

Reducing meat consumption would need to take into consideration the likely impacts on nutrient intake and more holistic diet changes need to be made to compensate for those changes (Meybeck & Gitz 2017). Modelling undertaken in the Netherlands indicated that replacing all meat and dairy lowered environmental impacts by 40 per cent but intakes of zinc, thiamin, vitamins A and B and calcium were sub-optimal. Replacing 30 per cent of meat and dairy reduced environmental impacts by 14 per cent without compromising nutritional intake (Seves et al. 2017). The recent EAT–*Lancet* Commission Report indicates that 0–58 g of meat a day is required (Willett et al. 2019). The planetary health diet is 'flexitarian'; that is, largely plant-based but can optionally include modest amounts of fish, meat and dairy.

WHAT ABOUT SEAFOOD?

Seafood is recognised as an important component of healthy diets, contributing vital fatty acids and protein. However, the sustainability of both wild fish capture and aquaculture have been called into question, due to overfishing and poor practices. There is a delicate balance in promoting fish consumption for health within a sustainability framework. Sourcing fish from wild stocks that are considered sustainable and focusing on underutilised species is a priority (Farmery et al. 2017). The Australian Marine Conservation Society and the Forest & Bird in New Zealand both produce online sustainable seafood guides if you are interested in knowing more.

- What might be the most appropriate message at the population level for guiding sustainable diet intakes?
- Thinking about your family and friends, what message would appeal to them? Why?
- What would be your advice around seafood?
- How could you 'sell' insects as a suitable protein source?

successfully argued for clearer labelling of food items so that now foods are labelled:

- Grown in Australia—all ingredients are grown in Australia.
- Produced in Australia—for food where all the ingredients were grown and all major processing was undertaken in Australia.
- Made in Australia—for food where the ingredients come from Australia or overseas and major processing has been done in Australia. (Department of Industry, Innovation and Science 2018)

While there is a clear mandate to eat within your locale, what is our responsibility as a citizen of a high-income country? Should we be purchasing food products from lower-income countries to assist in generating sustainable livelihoods? In order to ensure social and environmental sustainability, regardless of the origin of the food, some questions that could be asked are as follows.

- Are farmers given a fair price for their product? Fair trade coffee is an example of a product in which fair trade principles are used to ensure that farmers in some of the world's most impoverished areas receive a fair price.
- Are farmers able to use seeds they have saved themselves or do they need to purchase seed stock every year? Large multinational seed

FINDING OUT MORE ABOUT DIET AND SUSTAINABILITY

If you are interested in diet and sustainability then there are a number of books that may be of interest:

Francis Moore Lappé's *Diet for a Small Planet* was one of the first to identify the impact of meat eating. This has been followed more recently by Anna Lappé's *Diet for a Hot Planet*:

- Moore Lappé, F., 1971, *Diet for a Small Planet*, New York, NY: Ballantine
- Lappé, A., 2010, *Diet for a Hot Planet*, New York, NY: Bloomsbury.

Michael Pollan has written a number of books exploring food, diet and meals:

- Pollan, M., 2006, *The Omnivore's Dilemma: A natural history of four meals*, London: Penguin
- Pollan, M., 2008, *In Defense of Food: An eater's manifesto*, London: Penguin.

Other options include:

- Patel, R., 2008, *Stuffed and Starved: The hidden battle for the world food system*, New York, NY: Melville House
- Mason, P. & Lang, T., 2017, *Sustainable Diets: How ecological nutrition can transform consumption and the food system*, London: Routledge.

WHAT FOODS ARE YOU EATING THAT MAY BE ETHICALLY COMPROMISED?

Keep a food diary for a week.

- Identify which foods you are eating that could have ethical dilemmas associated with their consumption.
- What similar but ethically defensible products could you be consuming?

- Are labourers who are involved in the growing, harvesting or processing fairly treated? The production of cocoa in West Africa relies heavily on slave child labour. The demand for cocoa to feed the appetite for cheap chocolate in industrialised countries has driven down prices. This creates a situation where farmers need to reduce their overheads, including labour costs.
- Are animals or their by-products humanely grown or harvested? Eggs are an example of an animal by-product that can potentially be harvested inhumanely. Caged eggs are produced by chickens with minimal space and were banned in the UK in 2012. There are controversies, however, with some animal welfare activists arguing that large flocks of 'free-range' chickens can be as stressed as those that are caged (Scrinis et al. 2017).
- Are local environments and ecological systems maintained in order to grow or harvest the food item? Intensive production of palm oil (a fat commonly used in processed food products and cosmetics) has resulted in deforestation of rainforests in Malaysia, lost habitat for animal species (e.g. the orangutan) and dispossession of Indigenous peoples.
- Are foods sourced from sustainable wild sources or, if not, from environmentally sound farming practices? Many of the world's wild fish stocks have been overharvested and need to be protected.

companies have patented genetically modified seeds that farmers must purchase every year. These seeds include corn, soy and canola. Genetic modification contributes to the homogeneity of crops, reducing biodiversity. Requiring farmers to purchase seed annually reduces opportunities for sustainable livelihoods, especially among small-scale farmers.

Strategy 3: Follow the dietary guidelines

One of the key contributors to climate change and poor sustainability is the production and consumption of ultra-processed foods (foods produced by industrialised methods and ingredients). Most of these foods are also produced by multinationals who, as 'big' food companies, are potentially engaging in unethical practices in order to drive consumption (Clapp & Scrinis 2017; Monteiro et al. 2018). A key strategy is to decrease consumption of energy-dense/nutrient-poor foods and follow the dietary guidelines (Willett et al. 2019).

Strategy 4: Reduce your food waste

Home food waste is thought to contribute to approximately 30 per cent of all food waste across the supply chain (Aschemann-Witzel et al. 2015). Estimates in Australia indicate that Australians throw away approximately 3.1 tonnes of food each year, with a further 2.2 tonnes thrown away by commercial and industry sectors (Department of Environment and Energy 2017). State governments and local councils are investing in 'Love Food Hate Waste' campaigns to reduce household food waste. Many of these campaigns feature challenges you can undertake to reduce your food waste, including:

- working out how much food you are throwing away
- buying nothing new—use what you have in the freezer, pantry and fridge
- storing food to reduce food waste
- cooking to reduce waste
- learning to use leftovers
- starting to compost.

SUMMARY

- Sustainability is a complex concept requiring the intersection of environmental, economic and social dimensions.
- Sustainability within the food and nutrition context encompasses the entire food system from production to consumption and post-consumption to waste.
- Sustainability needs to ensure that both the health of humans and the health of the environment are maintained, and in fact one is not possible without the other. This has been described as an ecological approach to nutrition—the idea that nutrition, human and agricultural productivity and environmental sustainability are interlinked.
- Sustainable diets are those with low environmental impacts; they are protective and respectful of biodiversity and ecosystems, culturally acceptable, accessible, economically fair and affordable, and nutritionally adequate, safe and healthy.
- There are a number of threats to sustainable diets. Climate change will potentially impact on the ability to grow food and on where food can be grown. One of the biggest contributors to climate change is agricultural practices.
- Agricultural practices threaten sustainability through poor land management, use of pesticides and herbicides, and loss of biodiversity. Post-production practices contribute to greenhouse emissions through excessive food miles, overconsumption of ultra-processed foods and increased food waste across the food system.
- Economic measures have contributed greatly to the sustainability of the food system but need to be viewed with caution. Trade liberalisation has the potential to create equity but can also increase access to energy-dense/nutrient-poor foods.

- As nutrition professionals we have a responsibility to ensure dietary advice is in line with sustainable practice. Many dietary guidelines are incorporating sustainability as a core tenet.
- As a food citizen, you can explore the sustainability of your own diet; eat locally and in season; follow the dietary guidelines; and reduce your food waste.

KEY TERMS

Biodiversity sinks: places where biodiversity proliferates; that is, they have extremely high numbers of species. An example would be the Amazonian rainforest.

Fallow: in cultivation, inactive; a piece of land normally used for food production should be left with no crops for a season to enable its fertility to recover.

No-till cultivation: a way of growing crops without disturbing the soil through tillage. It increases retention of organic matter and improves nutrient cycling.

Oil crisis: in the 1970s oil production peaked and began to decline. The crisis occurred when major industrial countries faced significant shortages and elevated prices. Supplies were interrupted by major conflicts occurring in the Middle East. As a result, economic growth slowed. This was the first realisation that oil production may not be able to meet ongoing demands.

Peri-urban agriculture: agriculture that takes place on the edge of urban areas—that is, within or outside cities.

Productionist: a phase of agriculture in which there was a commitment to intensive, industrially driven agriculture supported by governments to encourage increased outputs.

Vector-borne disease: any disease transmitted by a living being, such as an insect vector to a vertebrate host—for example, malaria, Lyme disease, Japanese encephalitis.

REFERENCES

Aschemann-Witzel, J., de Hooge, I., Amani, P., Bech-Larsen, T. & Oostindjer, M., 2015, 'Consumer-related food waste: Causes and potential for action', *Sustainability,* 7(6): 6457–77, doi:10.3390/su7066457

Australian Government, Bureau of Meterology & CSIRO, 2016, *State of the Climate 2016*, <www.bom.gov.au/state-of-the-climate/State-of-the-Climate-2016.pdf>, accessed 25 February 2018

Australian Organic Ltd, 2017, *Australian Organic Market Report 2017*, <https://user-cprcmgz.cld.bz/AOMR-2017-Web-File-Download/4>, accessed 22 February 2019

Behrens, P., Kiefte-de Jong, J.C., Bosker, T., Rodrigues, J.F.D., de Koning, A. & Tukker, A., 2017, 'Evaluating the environmental impacts of dietary recommendations', *Proceedings of the National Academy of Sciences,* 114(51): 13412–17, doi:10.1073/pnas.1711889114

Béné, C., Oosterveer, P., Lamotte, L., Brouwer, I.D., de Haan, S. et al., 2019, 'When food systems meet sustainability: Current narratives and implications for actions', *World Development,* 113: 116–30, doi:10.1016/j.worlddev.2018.08.011

Berry, E.M., Dernini, S., Burlingame, B., Meybeck, A. & Conforti, P., 2015, 'Food security and sustainability: Can one live without the other?', *Public Health Nutrition,* 18(13): 2293–302, doi:10.1017/S136898001500021X

Betts, R.A., Alfieri, L., Bradshaw, C., Caesar, J., Feyen, L. et al., 2018, 'Changes in climate extremes, fresh water availability and vulnerability to food insecurity projected at 1.5°C and 2°C global warming with a higher-resolution global climate model', *Philosophical Transactions of the Royal Society A: Mathematical, Physical and Engineering Sciences,* 376(2119): 20160452, doi:10.1098/rsta.2016.0452

Brantsaeter, A.L., Ydersbond, T.A., Hoppin, J.A., Haugen, M. & Meltzer, H.M., 2017, 'Organic food in the diet: Exposure and health implications', *Annual Review of Public Health, 38*(1): 295–313, doi:10.1146/annurev-publhealth-031816-044437

Burlingame, B., Dernini, S. & Nutrition and Consumer Protection Division FAO, 2010, *Sustainable Diets and Biodiversity*, <www.fao.org/docrep/016/i3004e/i3004e.pdf>, accessed 23 February 2018

Chappell, M.J. & LaValle, L.A., 2011, 'Food security and biodiversity: Can we have both? An agroecological analysis', *Agriculture and Human Values, 28*(1): 3–26, doi:10.1007/s10460-009-9251-4

Clapp, J. & Scrinis, G., 2017, 'Big food, nutritionism, and corporate power', *Globalization, 14*(4): 578–95, doi:10.1 080/14747731.2016.1239806

Cleveland, D.A., Carruth, A. & Mazaroli, D.N., 2015, 'Operationalizing local food: Goals, actions, and indicators for alternative food systems', *Agriculture and Human Values, 32*(2): 281–97, doi:10.1007/s10460-014-9556-9

Commonwealth of Australia, 2017, *Australia: State of the environment 2016*, <https://soe.environment.gov.au/>, accessed 10 March 2017

Cooper, K.A., Quested, T.E., Lanctuit, H., Zimmermann, D., Espinoza-Orias, N. & Roulin, A., 2018, 'Nutrition in the bin: A nutritional and environmental assessment of food wasted in the UK', *Frontiers in Nutrition, 5*: 19, doi:10.3389/fnut.2018.00019

Cordell, D., Drangert, J. & White, S., 2009, 'The story of phosphorus: Global food security and food for thought', *Global Environmental Change—Human and Policy Dimensions, 19*(2): 292–305, doi:10.1016/j.gloenvcha.2008.10.009

Declerck, F.A.J., Fanzo, J., Palm, C. & Remans, R., 2011, 'Ecological approaches to human nutrition', *Food and Nutrition Bulletin, 32*(1 suppl. 1): S41–S50, doi:10.1177/15648265110321s106

Department of Environment and Energy, 2017, *Working Together to Reduce Food Waste in Australia*, <www.environment.gov.au/protection/waste-resource-recovery/publications/food-waste-factsheet#footnote>, accessed 12 December 2018

Department of Industry, Innovation and Science, 2018, *Country of Origin Food Labels*, <www.industry.gov.au/regulation-and-standards/country-of-origin-food-labels>, accessed 16 December 2018

Dijkman, T.J., Basset-Mens, C., Antón, A. & Núñez, M., 2018, 'LCA of food and agriculture', in M. Hauschild, R. Rosenbaum & S. Olsen (eds), *Life Cycle Assessment*, Cham: Springer, pp. 723–54

Elser, J. & Bennett, E., 2011, 'A broken biogeochemical cycle', *Nature, 478*: 29–31, doi:10.1038/478029a

Fanzo, J., Davis, C., McLaren, R. & Choufani, J., 2018, 'The effect of climate change across food systems: Implications for nutrition outcomes', *Global Food Security, 18*: 12–19, doi:10.1016/j.gfs.2018.06.001

FAO, 2011, *Global Food Losses and Food Waste: Extent, causes, and prevention*, Düsseldorf, Germany: <www.fao.org/docrep/014/mb060e/mb060e.pdf>, accessed 23 February 2018

—— 2014, *The Water–Energy–Food Nexus: A new approach in support of food security and sustainable agriculture*, <www.fao.org/3/a-bl496e.pdf>, accessed 22 February 2019

—— 2018, *State of Food and Nutrition Security in the World 2018: Building climate resilience for food and nutrition security*, <www.fao.org/3/I9553EN/i9553en.pdf>, accessed 15 December 2018

Farmery, A.K., Gardner, C., Jennings, S., Green, B.S. & Watson, R.A., 2017, 'Assessing the inclusion of seafood in the sustainable diet literature', *Fish and Fisheries, 18*(3): 607–18, doi:10.1111/faf.12205

Food Use for Social Innovation by Optimising Waste Prevention Strategies (FUSIONS), 2014, *FUSIONS Definitional Framework for Food Waste: Full report*, <www.eu-fusions.org/phocadownload/Publications/FUSIONS%20 Definitional%20Framework%20for%20Food%20Waste%202014.pdf>, accessed 18 February 2018

Friel, S., Barosh, L.J. & Lawrence, M., 2013, 'Towards healthy and sustainable food consumption: An Australian case study', *Public Health Nutrition, 17*(5): 1156–66, doi:10.1017/S1368980013001523

Friel, S. & Ford, L., 2015, 'Systems, food security and human health', *Food Security, 7*(2): 437–51, doi:10.1007/s12571-015-0433-1

Garnett, T., 2011, 'Where are the best opportunities for reducing greenhouse gas emissions in the food system (including the food chain)?', *Food Policy, 36*: S23–S32, doi:10.1016/j.foodpol.2010.10.010

—— 2014, 'Three perspectives on sustainable food security: Efficiency, demand restraint, food system transformation. What role for life cycle assessment?', *Journal of Cleaner Production, 73*: 10–18, doi:10.1016/j.jclepro.2013.07.045

Gunasekera, D., Kim, Y., Tulloh, C. & Ford, M., 2007, *Climate Change Impacts on Australian Agriculture*, <http://data.daff.gov.au/data/warehouse/pe_abarebrs99001405/ac07.4.4_climate.pdf>, accessed 18 February 2018

Gussow, J.D. & Clancy, K.L., 1986, 'Dietary guidelines for sustainability', *Journal of Nutrition Education & Behavior*, *18*(1): 1–5, doi:10.1016/S0022-3182(86)80255-2

Gustavsson, J., Cederberg, C., Sonesson, U., van Otterdijk, R. & Meybeck, A., 2011, *Global Food Losses and Food Waste: Extent, causes and prevention*, Rome: FAO

Hadjikakou, M., 2017, 'Trimming the excess: Environmental impacts of discretionary food consumption in Australia', *Ecological Economics, 131*: 119–28, doi:10.1016/j.ecolecon.2016.08.006

Hansen, T., Sørensen, M.I. & Eriksen, M.-L.R., 2018, 'How the interplay between consumer motivations and values influences organic food identity and behavior', *Food Policy, 74*: 39–52, doi:10.1016/j.foodpol.2017.11.003

He, P., Baiocchi, G., Hubacek, K., Feng, K. & Yu, Y., 2018, 'The environmental impacts of rapidly changing diets and their nutritional quality in China', *Nature Sustainability, 1*(3): 122–7, doi:10.1038/s41893-018-0035-y

Horne, J., 2018, 'Water security in Australia', in World Water Council (ed.), *Global Water Security: Lessons learnt and long-term implications*, Singapore: Springer, pp. 21–52

Huang, S.T.-Y., 2010, 'A recycling index for food and health security: Urban Taipei', *Asia Pacific Journal of Clinical Nutrition, 19*(3): 402–11, doi:10.6133/apjcn.2010.19.3.15

Hyland, J.J., McCarthy, M.B., Henchion, M. & McCarthy, S.N., 2017, 'Dietary emissions patterns and their effect on the overall climatic impact of food consumption', *International Journal of Food Science & Technology, 52*(12): 2505–12, doi:10.1111/ijfs.13419

International Federation of Organic Agriculture Movements, 2014, *The IFOAM NORMS for Organic Production and Processing*, Bonn: IFOAM

IPCC, 2018, *Global Warming of 1.5°C*, <www.ipcc.ch/sr15/>, accessed 15 December 2018

Johnson, H., 2015, 'Eating for health and the environment: Australian regulatory responses for dietary change', *QUT Law Review, 15*(2): 122–39, doi:10.5204/qutlr.v15i2.587

Johnston, J.L., Fanzo, J.C. & Cogill, B., 2014, 'Understanding sustainable diets: A descriptive analysis of the determinants and processes that influence diets and their impact on health, food security, and environmental sustainability', *Advances in Nutrition, 5*(4): 418–29, doi:10.3945/an.113.005553

Khoury, C.K., Bjorkman, A.D., Dempewolf, H., Ramirez-Villegas, J., Guarino, L. et al., 2014, 'Increasing homogeneity in global food supplies and the implications for food security', *Proceedings of the National Academy of Sciences, 111*(11): 4001–6, doi:10.1073/pnas.1313490111

Kingsbury, D., 2015, 'The role of resources in the resolution of the Western Sahara issue', *Global Change, Peace & Security, 27*(3): 253–62, doi:10.1080/14781158.2015.1084615

Kluser, S. & United Nations Environment Programme, 2010, *Global Honey Bee Colony Disorders and Other Threats to Insect Pollinators*, New York, NY: UNEP

Lairon, D., 2012, 'Biodiversity and sustainable nutrition with a food-based approach', in B. Burlingame & S. Dernini (eds), *Sustainable Diets and Biodiversity: Directions and solutions for policy, research and action*, Rome: FAO, pp. 30–5

Lang, T., 2016, *Re-fashioning Food Systems with Sustainable Diet Guidelines: Towards a SDG2 Strategy*, <https://friendsoftheearth.uk/sites/default/files/downloads/Sustainable_diets_January_2016_final.pdf>, accessed 16 December 2018

Lappé, A., 2010, *Diet for a Hot Planet: The climate crisis at the end of your fork and what you can do about it*, New York, NY: Bloomsbury Publishing

Lee, M.-S., Huang, Y.-C., Su, H.-H., Lee, M.-Z. & Wahlqvist, M.L., 2011, 'A simple food quality index predicts mortality in elderly Taiwanese', *Journal of Nutrition, Health & Aging, 15*(10): 815–21, doi:10.1007/s12603-011-0081-x

Marlow, H.J., Hayes, W.K., Soret, S., Carter, R.L., Schwab, E.R. & Sabate, J., 2009, 'Diet and the environment: Does what you eat matter?', *American Journal of Clinical Nutrition, 89*(5): 1699S–703S, doi:10.3945/ajcn.2009.26736Z

Mason, P. & Lang, T., 2017, *Sustainable Diets: How ecological nutrition can transform consumption and the food system*, London: Routledge

Meybeck, A. & Gitz, V., 2017, 'Sustainable diets within sustainable food systems', *Proceedings of the Nutrition Society, 76*(1): 1–11, doi:10.1017/S0029665116000653

Mihelcic, J.R., Fry, L.M. & Shaw, R., 2011, 'Global potential of phosphorus recovery from human urine and feces', *Chemosphere, 84*(6): 832–9, doi:10.1016/j.chemosphere.2011.02.046

Monteiro, C.A., Cannon, G., Moubarac, J.-C., Levy, R.B., Louzada, M.L.C. & Jaime, P.C., 2018, 'The UN Decade of Nutrition, the NOVA food classification and the trouble with ultra-processing', *Public Health Nutrition, 21*(1): 5–17, doi:10.1017/S1368980017000234

Moore Lappé, F., 1971, *Diet for a Small Planet*, New York, NY: Ballantine

Motta, E.V., Raymann, K. & Moran, N.A., 2018, 'Glyphosate perturbs the gut microbiota of honey bees', *Proceedings of the National Academy of Sciences, 115*(41): 10305–10, doi:10.1073/pnas.1803880115

Müller, D.B., Vogel, C., Bai, Y. & Vorholt, J.A., 2016, 'The plant microbiota: Systems-level insights and perspectives', *Annual Review of Genetics, 50*: 211–34, doi:10.1146/annurev-genet-120215-034952

Nestle, M., 2013, *Food Politics: How the food industry influences nutrition and health*, Berkeley, CA: University of California Press

Parfitt, J., Barthel, M. & Macnaughton, S., 2010, 'Food waste within food supply chains: Quantification and potential for change to 2050', *Philosophical Transactions of the Royal Society B: Biological Sciences, 365*(1554): 3065–81, doi:10.1098/rstb.2010.0126

Patel, R., 2008, *Stuffed and Starved: The hidden battle for the world food system*, New York, NY: Melville House

Pollan, M., 2006, *The Omnivore's Dilemma: A natural history of four meals*, London: Penguin

—— 2008, *In Defense of Food: An eater's manifesto*, London: Penguin

Quintana, C., 2014, *Family Farming: Feeding the world, caring for the earth*, <www.astc.org/astc-dimensions/family-farming-feeding-the-world-caring-for-the-earth/>, accessed 20 May 2019

Richards, R.A., Hunt, J.R., Kirkegaard, J.A. & Passioura, J.B., 2014, 'Yield improvement and adaptation of wheat to water-limited environments in Australia: A case study', *Crop and Pasture Science, 65*(7): 676–89, doi:10.1071/CP13426

Ritchie, H., Reay, D.S. & Higgins, P., 2018, 'The impact of global dietary guidelines on climate change', *Global Environmental Change, 49*: 46–55, doi:10.1016/j.gloenvcha.2018.02.005

Rockström, J., Bai, X. & deVries, B., 2018, 'Global sustainability: The challenge ahead', *Global Sustainability, 1*: e6, doi:10.1017/sus.2018.8

Sandilyan, S., 2017, 'Decline in honey bee population in southern India: Role of disposable paper cups', *Journal of Zoological and Bioscience Research, 1*(3), <https://journalzbr.com/index.php/jzbr/article/view/21>, accessed 20 May 2019

Scrinis, G., Parker, C. & Carey, R., 2017, 'The caged chicken or the free-range egg? The regulatory and market dynamics of layer-hen welfare in the UK, Australia and the USA', *Journal of Agricultural and Environmental Ethics, 30*(6): 783–808, doi:10.1007/s10806-017-9699-y

Sen, A., 2000, *Social Exclusion: Concept, application, and scrutiny* <www.adb.org/sites/default/files/publication/29778/social-exclusion.pdf>, accessed 22 February 2019

Seves, S.M., Verkaik-Kloosterman, J., Biesbroek, S. & Temme, E.H.M., 2017, 'Are more environmentally sustainable diets with less meat and dairy nutritionally adequate?', *Public Health Nutrition, 20*(11): 2050–62, doi:10.1017/S1368980017000763

Sonnino, R., Moragues Faus, A. & Maggio, A., 2014, 'Sustainable food security: An emerging research and policy agenda', *International Journal of Sociology of Agriculture and Food, 21*(1): 173–88, <www.ijsaf.org/archive/21/1/sonnino.pdf>, accessed 14 December 2018

Steduto, P., Schultz, B., Unver, O., Ota, S., Vallee, D. et al., 2018, 'Food security by optimal use of water: Synthesis of the 6th and 7th World Water Forums and developments since then', *Irrigation and Drainage, 67*(3): 327–44, doi:10.1002/ird.2215

Theurl, M.C., Haberl, H., Erb, K.-H. & Lindenthal, T., 2014, 'Contrasted greenhouse gas emissions from local versus long-range tomato production', *Agronomy for Sustainable Development, 34*(3): 593–602, doi:10.1007/s13593-013-0171-8

United Nations, 1987, *Report of the World Commission on Environment and Development: Our Common Future—Brundtland Report*, <https://sswm.info/sites/default/files/reference_attachments/UN%20WCED%201987%20Brundtland%20Report.pdf>, accessed 20 May 2019

—— 2015, *High Level Task Force on Global Food and Nutrition Security*, <www.un.org/en/issues/food/taskforce/wg3.shtml>, accessed 14 December 2018

—— 2017, *World Population Prospects*, <https://esa.un.org/unpd/wpp/publications/Files/WPP2017_KeyFindings.pdf>, accessed 15 December 2018

Vanham, D., Comero, S., Gawlik, B.M. & Bidoglio, G., 2018, 'The water footprint of different diets within European sub-national geographical entities', *Nature Sustainability, 1*(9): 518–25, doi:10.1038/s41893-018-0133-x

Vinnerås, B., Hedenkvist, M., Nordin, A. & Wilhelmson, A., 2009, 'Peepoo bag: Self-sanitising single use biodegradable toilet', *Water Science and Technology, 59*(9): 1743–9, doi:10.2166/wst.2009.184

Wahlqvist, M.L., 2014, 'Ecosystem health disorders: Changing perspectives in clinical medicine and nutrition', *Asia Pacific Journal of Clinical Nutrition, 23*(1): 1–15, doi:10.6133/apjcn.2014.23.1.20

Watts, N., Adger, W.N., Ayeb-Karlsson, S., Bai, Y., Byass, P. et al., 2017, 'The *Lancet* Countdown: Tracking progress on health and climate change', *Lancet, 389*(10074): 1151–64, doi:10.1016/S0140-6736(16)32124-9

Weber, O., Delince, J., Duan, Y., Maene, L., McDaniels, T. et al., 2014, 'Trade and finance as cross-cutting issues in the global phosphate and fertilizer market', in R.W. Scholz, A.H. Roy, F.S. Brand, D. Hellums & A.E. Ulrich (eds), *Sustainable Phosphorus Management: A global transdisciplinary roadmap*, New York, NY: Springer, pp. 275–99

White, A., Gallegos, D. & Hundloe, T., 2011, 'The impact of fresh produce specifications on the Australian food and nutrition system: A case study of the north Queensland banana industry', *Public Health Nutrition, 14*(8): 1489–95, doi:10.1017/S1368980010003046

Willett, W., Rockström, J., Loken, B., Springmann, M., Lang, T. et al., 2019, 'Food in the Anthropocene: The EAT–Lancet Commission on healthy diets from sustainable food systems', *Lancet, 393*(10170): 447–92, doi:10.1016/S0140-6736(18)31788-4

{CHAPTER 27}
SOCIAL AND CULTURAL INFLUENCES ON FOOD AND NUTRITION

Danielle Gallegos

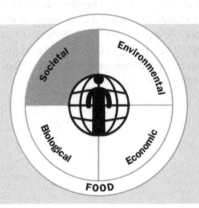

OBJECTIVES

- List the elements of food choice.
- Identify the social determinants of health and their impact on food choices and nutrition.
- Explain the social and cultural influences on food choices and consumption.
- Analyse the impact of social and cultural influences on your own food intake.

INTRODUCTION

One of the criticisms of nutrition as a science is that it has been preoccupied with 'post-swallowing' aspects—largely focusing on the biology, physiology, biochemistry, and pathology of too many or too few nutrients (Crotty 1995). This has been referred to as 'nutritionism'—where nutrients and their role are taken out of context, decoupled from the 'foods, dietary patterns and broader social contexts in which they are embedded' (Scrinis 2013, p. 6). This chapter considers these broader social and cultural perspectives as they relate to food choice and nutritional status.

FOOD CHOICE

Food choice is recognised as a complex area that integrates biological, environmental, economic and social systems. Food choice is defined as people's thoughts, feelings and actions related to food and eating. It is conceptualised as multilevel, contextual, dynamic and diverse (Sobal et al. 2014). The Food Choice Process Model provides a description of this concept; Figure 27.1 and Table 27.1 outline the key elements of the model.

SOCIAL DETERMINANTS

Social determinants are defined as the 'upstream' social and economic factors that influence health and disease of individuals and populations. The WHO defines them as the conditions in which people are born, grow, work, live and age as influenced by a range of systems—economic, developmental, social and political (WHO 2017).

A social determinants approach provides an irrefutable link between social disadvantage and

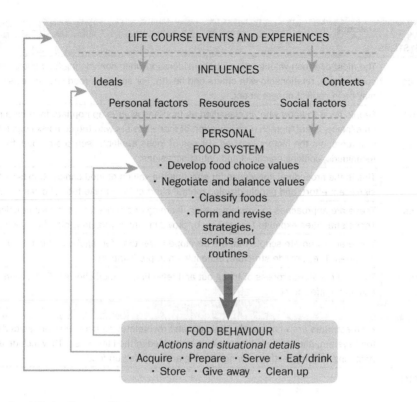

Figure 27.1: The Food Choice Process Model

Source: Sobal & Bisogni (2009). Reproduced by permission of Oxford University Press

Table 27.1: Elements of the Food Choice Process Model

Element	Description
LIFE-COURSE EVENTS AND EXPERIENCES	
Life-course	This is how people experience food choice across time and within the context of life-stages and life events. For example, food choices will be different for a single person and for someone also feeding a child.
INFLUENCES	
Ideals	Ideas that are collectively constructed; they are the values and norms that provide expectations and reference points that are learned through socialisation within a particular culture. For example, what individuals consume for breakfast will differ across cultures.
Personal factors	These are a person's needs, preferences and capabilities related to how they manage food and eating. These include a wide range of factors, among them physiological conditions and health characteristics, medications, taste sensitivity, gender, allergies, personality, age, internalised roles people play and personal food identities.
Resources	These are assets that can be used in food choice. They include financial resources, time, available equipment.
Social factors	People consider others when they eat, and these others can modify where, when, how, how much and what they consume.
Contexts	These incorporate the settings in which people live. The physical environment (climate, transportation), food system and media/marketing are included in this element.

Element	Description
PERSONAL FOOD SYSTEMS	
Constructing and managing food choice values	The most common values taken into consideration when considering food choice are taste, price, convenience, relationship with others and health. For any given food choice decision these values may be in conflict or agreement.
Classifying foods and situations	People need to know what is classified as food and what is appropriate food for a particular time/place/event/person. Classification of foods assists with the complex cognitive processes that represent the factors involved in types of foods available, sources of food, food preparation techniques, cooking practices and eating occasions.
Constructing and enacting scripts	This is the procedural knowledge for enacting the values of food choice. Choosing food requires significant effort, and people develop mental short cuts to make food choices more efficient.
Developing strategies and tactics	These are approaches to problem-solving, learning or discovery that involve practical methods. These strategies expedite food choice by providing underlying principles for making decisions.
Establishing and performing routines	These are elaborate scripts that are developed over time for regular and established food choice activities. They provide structure, schedules and predictability.
Monitoring and revision	This is a constant process of trying out and reflecting on food choices. This occurs particularly across the life-course.
FOOD ACTIVITIES	
Food activities	Food activities are what people think, do, and reel related to food. They are guided by the personal food system, shaped by influences and embedded in the life-course. They include acquiring, preparing, serving, eating, storing, sharing and cleaning up food.

Source: Bisogni et al. (2016)

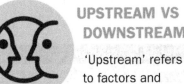

UPSTREAM VS DOWNSTREAM

'Upstream' refers to factors and interventions that address the root cause of a health issue for many people. The contrast is with 'downstream', which is working to solve an issue for a person. Read the following article in the *Medical Journal of Australia* by medical student Victoria Smith on the differences between upstream and downstream. Reflect on what you would do in a similar situation. What are the upstream approaches?

- Smith, V.C., 2015, 'Upstream or downstream?', *Medical Journal of Australia*, 202(10): 412–13.

health outcomes, with not only between-country differences but also within-country differences. This acknowledges that disadvantage is not absolute but, rather, relative. That is, how disadvantaged you are relative to other members of your society has a greater impact on health than your absolute level of disadvantage. It is proposed that the mechanisms of health inequalities arise from social contexts leading to social stratification, resulting in differential exposures to heath damaging conditions and, in turn, to differential susceptibilities and vulnerabilities resulting in differential consequences (Diderichsen et al. 2001). The social context includes the structure of society and social relations that assign an individual to a particular social position and will vary depending on economic and industrial structures. Based on this, the WHO has developed a conceptual framework outlining the influence of the social determinants on health (Figure 27.2).

The more disadvantaged are more likely to have higher rates of morbidity and mortality from most major causes of disease; they are also more likely to

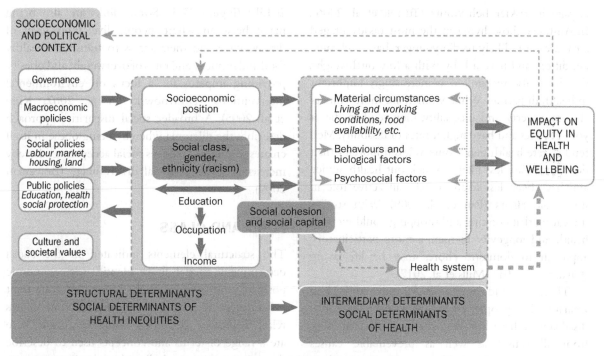

Figure 27.2: Conceptual framework for action on the social determinants of health

Source: Reprinted from Solar & Irwin (2010)

OUTCOMES OF THE SOCIAL DETERMINANTS OF HEALTH IN AUSTRALIA

- The 20 per cent of Australians living in the lowest socioeconomic areas in 2014–15 were 1.6 times as likely as the 20 per cent living in the highest socioeconomic areas to have at least two chronic health conditions, such as heart disease and diabetes (AIHW 2016).
- Australians living in the lowest socioeconomic areas lived about three years less than those living in the highest socioeconomic areas in 2009–2011 (AIHW 2016).
- If all Australians had the same death rates as people living in the highest socioeconomic areas in 2009–2011, overall mortality rates would have reduced by 13 per cent—and there would have been 54,000 fewer deaths (AIHW 2016).
- Mothers in the lowest socioeconomic areas were 30 per cent more likely to have a low birthweight baby than mothers in the highest socioeconomic areas in 2013 (AIHW 2016).
- An Aboriginal man can expect to live 10.8 years less than his non-Indigenous counterpart (ABS 2013).

engage in riskier behaviours (Turrell et al. 2006). In Australia, those living in the most disadvantaged areas are more likely to die younger, have a chronic condition, and have a baby with a low birthweight. Gender is also recognised as increasingly important in health disparities. While women are more vulnerable to poverty and inequality, men tend to die at younger ages and have higher rates of disability. Men tend to rate health behaviours as less important than do women, are less likely to seek out health advice and have been less likely to take an active role in household affairs (Pan et al. 2009). With studies indicating that cooking and shopping could increase health and longevity in men, a more participatory approach to domestic chores may be life-saving (Chang et al. 2011; Mills et al. 2017).

There are indications in Australia and New Zealand that people with higher levels of social disadvantage have higher death rates and morbidity from all causes as well as preventable causes (figures 27.3 and 27.4). They are also more likely to be overweight/obese, smoke more, have fewer or no daily serves of fruit and exercise less (ABS 2015b) (Figure 27.5). Strong links are also being made between where people live, their level of disadvantage and their access to transport, healthy food and services, and rates of overweight and obesity, providing impetus for a focus on environmental interventions (Drewnowski et al. 2007; King et al. 2005). A broader social disparities approach describes the dilemma whereby being obese in itself creates stigma and reduces social acceptance, thereby increasing levels of social disadvantage (Braveman 2009).

FOOD AND CLASS

The structural elements indicated in the social determinants model above identify socioeconomic position and social/cultural values as important influencers on health. Some of these influencers relate to income and others to opportunities. There are a range of terms and concepts used to describe these influencers, including low income, poverty, deprivation, disadvantage and class. These descriptors are described in more detail below.

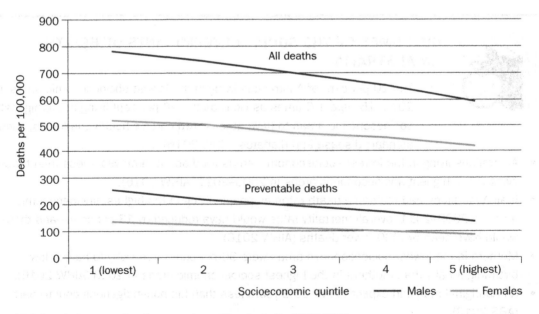

Figure 27.3: Deaths by sex and socioeconomic position, Australia, 2009–2011

Source: AIHW (2014)

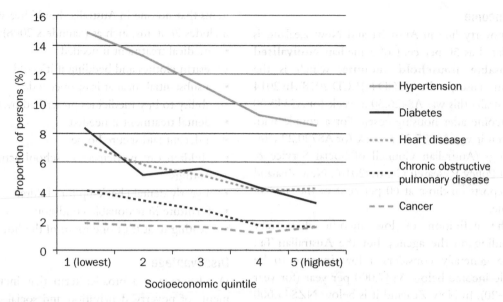

Figure 27.4: Long-term health conditions by socioeconomic status (proportion of persons %)

Source: Developed from ABS (2015b)

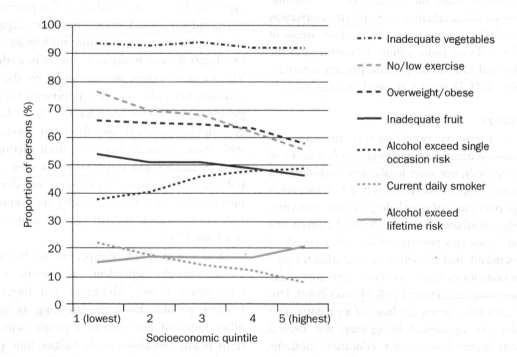

Figure 27.5: Health risk factors by socioeconomic status (proportion of persons %)

Source: Developed from ABS (2015b)

Low income

The poverty line in Australia and New Zealand is calculated as 50 per cent of a median **equivalised disposable household income**, which is the definition used by the OECD (OECD 2018). In 2014 in Australia this was A$426.30 a week (or A$343.00 for income after housing costs). For a couple with children it was A$895.22 a week (or A$720.22 after housing) (Australian Council of Social Service & Social Policy Research Centre 2016). New Zealand also reports on those at 60 per cent of the median income.

The definition of low income does vary depending on the agency but the Australian Tax Office generally considers a low income to be taxable income below A$37,000 per year (for year 2019–20). In New Zealand it is below NZ$44,000 (about A$40,500) (New Zealand Inland Revenue 2018).

In Australia and New Zealand the discussion is about relative poverty, where those on lower incomes are not able to maintain a standard of living comparable to those on higher incomes. Absolute poverty is where there is significant deprivation and insufficient means to sustain the basic needs of life. This will vary from country to country but the international standard for extreme poverty is earning less than US$1.25 per day (United Nations 2017).

Deprivation

Measuring poverty using income measures has limitations, as income does not necessarily reflect low living standards, nor does it take into consideration health and social connections. While low income is an important cause of poor living, it is not necessarily the only contributor (Saunders 2008). An alternative approach measures poverty within a framework of living standards that takes into consideration the prevailing community standards about what constitutes the basic necessities (Saunders & Naidoo 2018). This list of necessities forms the basis of an income that provides a living wage. A living wage will allow a family to secure food, shelter, education, clothing, health care, transport and other aspects of modern living (Werner & Lim 2015). This list of necessities—

items that no one in Australia should live without—includes 26 items, such as (Saunders 2008):

- medical treatment if needed
- warm clothes and bedding if it's cold
- a substantial meal at least once a day
- ability to buy medicines prescribed by a doctor
- dental treatment if needed
- a decent and secure home
- children can participate in school activities and outings
- a yearly dental check-up for children
- furniture in reasonable condition
- heating in at least one room of the house.

Disadvantage

Disadvantage is a broader term that includes elements of poverty, deprivation and social exclusion. Social exclusion is typically defined as the lack of access to resources and the lack of personal skills to access available resources to allow a person to fully participate in social and economic life (Caniglia et al. 2010). The concept takes into consideration Sen's capability framework, which states that poverty exists when individuals lack certain minimum capabilities which in turn can translate into inadequate income or education, poor health or a sense of powerlessness. The focus, therefore, should not be on the means of living but rather on the opportunities a person possesses (Sen 2000) (see Chapter 25). In Australia, geographical location contributes to disadvantage, with those living further away from metropolitan areas in remote and very remote locations having reduced access to resources. This has been developed into an index called the Accessibility and Remoteness Index of Australia (ABS 2018) (see 'Remoteness' box in Chapter 24).

Those most at risk of experiencing disadvantage include people dependent on income support, unemployed people, Aboriginal and Torres Strait Islander peoples, those experiencing racism and other forms of discrimination, people with long-term health conditions or disabilities, lone parents, people with low levels of educational attainment and public housing tenants (McLachlan et al. 2013).

Class

Social class is increasingly recognised as not just being about the type of work you do but more an interplay between economic, social and cultural capital (Bourdieu 1984). These elements work to stratify society into groups which share similar backgrounds, social connections and tastes. Social class is a well-recognised factor in dietary differences within a society. These differences are related to the types of foods accessible and available as well as the preferences of different groups. Social class also relates to how being overweight or obese is perceived. Bourdieu (1984) argues that food as a component of *habitus* maintains social distinctions through the control and production of bodily practices that are a part of everyday life. This means that food provides a means by which social classes can distinguish themselves not only in the types of foods that are chosen but in the approach to food and eating.

The increased availability of cheap, easily accessible poor-quality foods in disadvantaged areas creates a normative culture of unhealthy diets. In so doing it polarises high-value (healthier food choices) for the rich and low-value foods (less healthy food choices) for the poor (Dowler & O'Connor 2012). This phenomenon is what Bourdieu described as the 'taste of freedom' versus the 'taste of necessity'. Those experiencing hardship appreciate the functional value of cultural objects and practices. In the case of food, the taste of necessity results in the consumption of cheaper, more filling foods that then become the norm. Changing the quality of food is a recognised strategy for food-insecure households

DEFINITION OF ECONOMIC, CULTURAL AND SOCIAL CAPITAL

Economic capital: comprises material assets that can be converted into wealth and income. In terms of health, economic capital is the material resources that are used to acquire or maintain better health (Pinxten & Lievens 2014).

Cultural capital: the knowledge, skills and behaviours allowing social mobility; knowing the 'right' things. This comes in three forms:
- embodied—knowledge, skills and information we accumulate over time through socialisation and education, e.g. table manners
- objectified—the material objects we possess or seek to acquire that signify our economic class; for example, meat in some societies has cultural capital as it signifies wealth
- institutionalised—these include ranks and titles, related to educational attainment (e.g. doctor) or role (e.g. mother). (Bourdieu 1984)

Social capital: the contacts and connections that allow people to draw on their social networks and enable the building of trust that lead to coordination and cooperation for mutual benefit. Social capital is about bonding similar people and bridging diverse people underpinned by repaying in kind what another has done for us (norms of reciprocity) (Field 2016).

Habitus: the manifestation of class through the development of tastes for particular cultural forms. Preferences that feel individual are actually socially produced and express and recreate social class (Bourdieu 1984).

(see section 'Household food security', below). In order to reduce the risk of hunger, energy-dense foods that are cheaper per kilojoule are consumed in higher quantities and consumption of fruits and vegetables, which are less energy-dense and more costly per kilojoule, is decreased (Brimblecombe & O'Dea 2009; Drewnowski & Darmon 2005).

The taste of freedom, on the other hand, means that form can be valued over function and those without the urgency to put food on the table can become concerned with, for example:

- ethical food choices (eating organic, eating 'local') (Shugart 2014; Zimmerman 2015)
- eclectic food choices (eating a broad range of cultural foods) (Beagan et al. 2015)
- aesthetic food choices (gaining pleasure in preparing, cooking and eating) (Beagan et al. 2015)
- differentiating food choices (to distinguish yourself from others) (Palma et al. 2017).

Class, culture and weight perception

Body weight has become an outward manifestation of *habitus*, such that class socialisation results in the privileging of, in high-income countries, thinness as the ideal. For high-income countries this fits with the neoliberal approach—thinness is the epitome of control and personal responsibility; obesity is linked to the opposite. Maintaining fashionably lean and fit figures for men and women involves a conscious or unconscious effort by high-income groups to symbolically define health. Such outward bodily displays are indicators of cultural capital—time and income to expend on maintaining this ideal body shape through physical activity and healthy eating. Campos and colleagues (2006) argue that the increased weight of the population is perceived as a sign of increasing moral laxity, driving the ideological individual responsibility approach and alleviating responsibility for structural change, although there are indications that the spread of environments that facilitate obesity is potentially making these class distinctions more difficult to maintain (McLaren 2007).

The association between body weight and cultural capital varies in countries where food is less available. In such countries being overweight or obese is an indicator of wealth, prosperity and, for women, fertility (Monteiro et al. 2004; Xiao et al. 2013). In Fiji, for example, large bodies are considered more aesthetically pleasing and people are encouraged to eat through mottoes such as 'kana, mo urouro' or 'eat, so you will become fat' (Becker 2004). For countries experiencing the nutrition transition the situation is more complex. In China, for example, women of higher socioeconomic status are more concerned about physical appearance, internalising slimness as an indicator of beauty and good health. While a larger body size in men has been associated with prosperity, wealth and power, male members of the middle class are perhaps more aware of the health complications and are aspiring to a different weight status (Bonnefond & Clément 2014).

Household food security

Food insecurity is a global issue that encompasses all aspects of the food system and is linked with poverty (see chapters 4 and 26 for a discussion of food security at the global and national level). At a national level, the poorest countries are most at risk and, within countries, those with the least access to economic, educational or agricultural resources are the ones who experience higher levels of household food insecurity (Wahlqvist et al. 2012). In high-income countries this is relative and those living in poverty, on low incomes or with disadvantage are most at risk of food insecurity (Friel & Baker 2009; Wahlqvist et al. 2009).

Table 27.2 provides a summary of the prevalence of food insecurity among high-income countries and then within particular groups in Australia and New Zealand. Recently the FAO has used an eight-item standard tool to collect data on food insecurity (FAO 2016). Those most at risk of food insecurity in high-income countries include those: on low incomes or experiencing financial stress; with a disability; who are or are at risk of being homeless; or who are refugees or asylum seekers (Gallegos et al. 2017). The outcomes of food insecurity can be physical impairment, decreased capacity to learn or work, poorer child development outcomes, nutritional inadequacies, and

Table 27.2: Prevalence of food insecurity in high-income countries

Country	Year	Prevalence and severity	Tool of measurement	Notes
USA (Coleman-Jensen et al. 2017)	2016	12.3% food insecure, 4.9% very low food security.	USDA Food Security Survey Module—18 questions	National data collected annually
Canada (Health Canada 2017)	2011–2012	8.4% food insecure, 5.8% moderate and 2.6% severe.	USDA Food Security Survey Module—18 questions	National data collected biannually
UK	Not measured			
New Zealand (Parnell et al. 2011)	2008–2009	34% moderately food secure, 7% low food security. 14% of households report running out of food often.	Series of 8 questions	National data collected on an ad hoc basis
Australia (ABS 2015a)	2011–2012	4% Aboriginal and/or Torres Strait Islander households, 22% food insecure with 31% in remote areas with two-thirds of these (21%) going without food.	Single question	National data collected on an ad hoc basis

WHAT IS THE ROLE OF FOOD BANKS IN ALLEVIATING FOOD INSECURITY?

Food banks have arisen as alternative food systems for those who are food-insecure in countries such as the USA, UK, Canada and Australia. Some of these rely on donations from the retail food sector or on fresh food that has been rescued. In Australia, these organisations are represented by FoodBank, Second Bite and Oz Harvest.

Read the following book:

- Riches, G., 2018, *Food Bank Nations: Poverty, corporate charity and the right to food*, London: Routledge.

Think about the following questions and write a 500–1000-word opinion piece for your local newspaper:

- How do food banks fit with a human rights approach to food security?
- What systems are being realigned to create the food bank system?
- What is your opinion of the value of food banks in alleviating food security?
- What could be alternative approaches to alleviating food insecurity?

higher rates of depressive illness, social isolation or exclusion. In high-income countries, there is a link with obesity, especially in women, and increased risk of chronic conditions (Kaur et al. 2015; Leung et al. 2014; Ramsey et al. 2012; Ramsey et al. 2011).

The international data using the standardised tool from the FAO for the countries listed in Table 27.2 indicate prevalence rates for food insecurity of between 8 per cent and 10.6 per cent (FAO 2016). Australia had the highest prevalence.

Strategies used by food insecure households

Many households are not necessarily hungry but still worry about where their next meal will come from and may not be able to access foods that promote and maintain health. Even anxiety about where the next meal is coming from can have detrimental effects on child development outcomes (Shankar et al. 2017). Children in most food insecure households are protected for as long as possible from going hungry. Children going hungry is the most severe form of food insecurity. Figure 27.6 shows the steps that occur before children go hungry.

The typical pattern is that households will change purchasing and cooking practices in order to save money, then will compromise diet quality to make the food budget go further; adults will limit the size of their meals or skip meals; and finally, when this fails, children have their meals limited. Households tend to use emergency food relief only when all other options are exhausted. In some cases, food consumption for the working adult in the household may be protected if this will maximise productivity and maintain an income. Often in households the food budget is the only flexible budget item and so other financial commitments (housing, energy, water, child care, education) will be prioritised over food (Gallegos 2016). This often

means developing strategies to reduce food costs and extend consumption further such as:

- buying in bulk
- identifying where to shop and shopping at different stores based on price
- purchasing different items based on pay cycles
- prioritising food items based on children's needs and preferences
- buying canned or frozen foods over fresh
- using foods beyond their expiry dates
- removing spoiled areas and insects to extend usability
- cooking dishes that are cheap and filling
- maximising food intake from external sources (visiting family)
- pooling limited food resources in order to feed larger numbers
- staggering mealtimes in order to facilitate food consumption for certain members of the household (Nielsen et al. 2015; Rose 2011; Wiig & Smith 2009).

There is growing evidence that families experiencing food insecurity have an understanding of healthy eating but that external conditions mean that they need to prioritise quantity and satiety over quality (Garthwaite et al. 2015). This will often mean

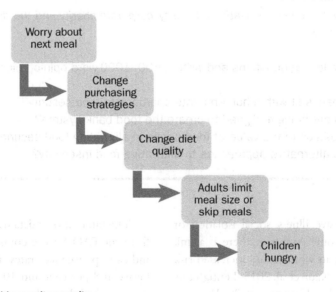

Figure 27.6: Levels of food insecurity severity

purchasing energy-dense/nutrient-poor foods. One of the paradoxes of food insecurity in households in high-income countries is that adults, especially women, may be overweight or obese. This is thought to be a result of the overconsumption of energy-dense/nutrient-poor foods when they are available.

FOOD AND GENDER

Gender inequality has been linked to poverty, hunger and poor health. Women in both high- and low-income countries play an important role in food production and preparation. Feeding households requires both visible and invisible work as food and meals are planned, organised, procured, prepared and cleaned away (Delormier et al. 2009). In developed, industrialised and transitioning countries this work is largely carried out by women. Cooking as caring becomes an outward manifestation of gender in which 'a woman conducts herself as recognizably womanly' (DeVault 1994, p. 118). Men's cooking practice has previously been constructed as being optional—related to 'helping out' or as leisure and self-realisation rather than a domestic duty (van Hooff 2011). There is, however, purportedly a growing involvement of men 'doing cooking' related to a growing sense of gender equality where the sharing of domestic tasks is more evenly distributed (Neuman et al. 2017). While qualitative and quantitative studies in Australia suggest there is a more equal distribution of cooking between men and women in younger couple households, time-use data indicate that the bulk of this work is still undertaken by women (ABS 2008) (see Table 27.3).

There is an established beneficial association between cooking (and shopping) and life expectancy,

COMPARE THE COST OF COOKING

Investigate the full cost of three commonly consumed types of meals:

1. home-cooked from scratch
2. cooked at home from convenience foods (e.g. frozen meals)
3. fast food.

In your calculation, factor in the following costs:

- ingredients
- energy
- transport
- time for planning, preparation, cooking, cleaning up.

Use the minimum wage for adults in Australia/New Zealand to calculate the time costs (in 2018 this was A$18.29 in Australia; in 2017, $NZ 16.50 in New Zealand).

- Reflect on how long it takes for each meal.
- If you were working shifts, what would be the easiest option?
- If you were working more than 40 hours a week, what would be the easiest option?

Table 27.3: Time spent on food and drink preparation, clean-up and child care

Activity	1992		1997		2006	
	Men	Women	Men	Women	Men	Women
	Hours:minutes per week					
Time spent in paid employment	26:37	12:48	27:00	13:30	28:12	14:35
Food and drink preparation and clean-up	2:48	8:29	3:03	8:05	3:38	8:05

Source: ABS (2008)

with a gender difference where women benefited from cooking more than men; and men from shopping more than women (Chen et al. 2012; Erlich et al. 2012)

For those couples who are working either part-time or full-time, women are spending three times longer on food preparation and clean-up (ABS 2008). However, despite the focus on food and cooking in the media, overall individuals and families appear to be spending less time preparing food. In Australia and elsewhere, food and cooking skills have been removed as part of the primary and secondary school curricula to be replaced with food technology and more scientific subjects (Worsley et al. 2016). Time poverty among individuals who are working in paid and unpaid employment for longer hours has meant an increasing trend of out-sourced food provisioning.

Food, nutrition and gender in low-income countries

Women play an integral role in food production and their contribution to the food and economic security of their families, communities and countries is significant. The FAO (2011) and the World Bank (World Bank 2011) both state that closing the gender gap in agriculture is essential to increase agricultural productivity, thereby reducing food insecurity and ultimately hunger. Women on average make up 43 per cent of the agricultural labour force in low-income countries and account for an estimated two-thirds of the world's 600 million poor livestock keepers (FAO 2018). In these same countries women produce 60–80 per cent of the food crops and are more likely to spend their income on the wellbeing of their families, including medical treatment, education and more nutritious foods (Bunch & Mehra 2008; World Bank et al. 2008). However, women hold less than 20 per cent of the land in all the main developing regions of the world (FAO 2011).

Without the involvement of women and without an understanding of the influences of other members of the household, there is a risk that interventions to improve nutritional status in low-income countries will fail to take into consideration the limitations and experiences of everyday life. There are several key areas to consider.

- Resource allocation within households: men and women within households do not necessarily make decisions together, they may not pool resources or have the same preferences. When women control the resources, children have improved education, health and nutritional outcomes.
- Women with higher status relative to men have better nutritional status and greater control over household resources, fewer time constraints, better access to information and health services, better mental health and self-confidence, and higher self-esteem.
- Women who are empowered receive a larger share of the benefits of household resources, including nutritious food. However, this may not necessarily translate into improved nutritional status, as empowered women may be exerting greater effort in agricultural activities and while they have greater diet diversity they also have increased energy requirements (Malapit & Quisumbing 2015).
- Land ownership is one key element in women's empowerment—being able to access, control and own assets such as land, labour, finance and social capital enhances productivity (Mishra & Sam 2016). However, the situation is complex even when women control the assets: the ensuing income can be used to purchase more assets which are controlled by men—so the benefits do not necessarily flow to all members of the household (Roy et al. 2015).

OTHER ELEMENTS OF CULTURE

Cuisines

How foods are acquired, prepared and eaten, and what people believe and understand about these activities, define a cuisine. A cuisine provides a framework within which people choose food. This means that not all of those who adhere to a particular cuisine follow the same diet—indeed, within a food culture or cuisine there is significant variation. Adherence to particular food traditions is affected by the reality of everyday life. Any meal may be influenced by the particularities of the day, place or group of people. The person responsible for cooking may arrive home late, there may be guests present for the meal, or children may require something to eat that is quicker to prepare than the usual meal. These everyday occurrences may mean meals are different from the 'ideal' several times a week or more. The realities of a particular meal are also influenced by the experiences and preferences of an individual. It may be influenced by social class, religious beliefs or whether it is a festive occasion. Variations also occur depending on the stage of life.

This means that care needs to be taken when using cuisines to describe what a particular group might eat. One of the key features of cuisine as a product of culture is that it is constantly changing. Health workers should not, therefore, stereotype individual or family choices based on ethnicity but rather use cuisine as a general guide only. A culturally competent practitioner would use the cuisine framework to understand the possible scope of choices to guide further questioning or research (see Chapter 2).

A cuisine is a set of socially situated food behaviours incorporating four main elements:

1 a set of basic foods
2 distinctive cooking techniques
3 flavour principles
4 a set of rules or code of etiquette.

Basic foods

The basic foods that characterise a cuisine are selected by any group from the range available. What influences that selection is complex and includes environmental factors such as climate, ease of production or availability, palatability, nutritional costs and benefits, and social and religious beliefs (Rozin 1982). The selected foods produce varying flavours, aromas, textures and appearances—all basic aspects of the human eating experience. Basic foods can be divided into core or staples and accessory or 'fringe' foods. The staples are what provide the caloric bulk, while the fringe foods give the staple food taste. 'Fringe foods' help you eat more staples; the staple tastes better with the 'fringe' and the 'fringe' by itself is less

appetising than if combined with the staple (Mintz 1994). In defining Italian cuisine, for example, the basic foods are the staples wheat, corn and rice, the dominance of which depends on which part of Italy you are from. In the south, you will more likely consume wheat as bread and pasta, while in the north you would be more likely to consume wheat as bread, corn as polenta, and rice. The 'fringe' foods are the olive, in particular olive oil, and tomatoes.

Cooking techniques

Converting basic foods from a raw to a cooked state is another feature distinguishing cuisines. Cooking in this instance refers not just to the application of heat but to all the ways in which food can be transformed. A food such as chicken may be common to many cuisines, but it can be prepared in characteristic ways by being cut into large pieces, bite-sized pieces, baked, fried, stewed or smoked. The development of particular cooking techniques in different parts of the world may be an indication of how some groups use scarce energy resources. The selection of cooking techniques, then, as well as the interpretation of how those techniques are to be performed, determines what makes a cuisine distinctive (Rozin 1983).

Flavour principles

Each cuisine also has a distinctive way of flavouring food, and this taste defines the dish. Flavourings are also used as 'group markers' to distinguish cuisines from each other. Care must be taken when using these flavour principles, as regional and personal variations can be extensive and there is a risk of overgeneralisation. Table 27.4 provides examples of flavour principles

Codes of etiquette

Each cuisine has a set of rules that govern what, when and how it is eaten. Over time a vast array of behaviours has been constructed to be socially acceptable around mealtimes. These may incorporate the number of meals to be eaten each day, the times these meals are eaten, the utensils used to eat them (fingers, chopsticks, cutlery) and where they are to be eaten (some cultures eat on the floor, while others

Table 27.4: Flavour principles

Region	Flavours
Southern Italy and France	Olive oil–garlic–parsley and/or anchovy with one variant of tomato added to these, and another where basil replaces parsley
Northern Italy	Wine, vinegar and garlic
China (general)	Soy sauce, rice wine, ginger root
China (north)	Soy sauce, rice wine, ginger root, soybean paste (miso), and/or garlic, and/or sesame oil
Szechuan (west central China)	Soy sauce, rice wine, ginger root, hot pepper and/or sweet–sour
Canton (southern China)	Soy sauce, rice wine, ginger root, garlic and/or stock, and/or fermented black beans

Source: Rozin (1982)

use a table). There may be codes about whether women eat with men, or whether children can eat with adults (Belasco 2008).

Religious practices and food intake

Food can be used in a variety of different ways as an expression of individual and collective identity.

Food can also be an expression of religious ritual and spiritual practice. As an outward expression of spirituality, food does not necessarily need to be linked to a particular religious faith. For example, in many Australian families food is used at Easter and Christmas to celebrate family but the links to Christianity are no longer necessarily relevant. Religions exert a strong influence on food habits through food laws that require the avoidance of certain foods and the consumption of others in celebration. Fasting is a practice common in some religions and is an expression of mastery over physical desires and of piety. The adherence to these practices will vary for each individual and will be dependent on a range of factors including orthodoxy, age and migration. So again the general tenets are useful to explore generalities but as a nutrition professional never make assumptions about practices at the individual level. Table 27.5 provides a summary of some of the practices of major religions. It includes some of the terminology commonly used and geographical areas where the religion is commonly practised. These geographical areas are important as they will further influence the types of food consumed.

Table 27.5: Food practices and terminology associated with major world religions

Religion	Relevant terminology	Geographical areas	Major celebrations/ festivals	Common practices
Baha'i		Originated in Iran.	Naw-Ruz (Baha'i New Year). There are ten holy days that mark anniversaries of the births, declarations and deaths of the founder.	No food rules, prohibitions or food rituals. Food is, however, involved in health and healing. Fasting is considered a spiritual duty and the main fasting season lasts 19 days and begins on the first day of the last month of the Baha'i year which is 2–20 March in the Western calendar. Alcohol is strictly prohibited. Friday is the Baha'i day of rest.
Buddhism		The largest Buddhist populations are in China, Japan, Thailand, Bhutan and Cambodia.	Buddhist festivals vary between countries, regions and cultures.	Some people who practise Buddhism may be vegetarian. Avoiding meat is said to strengthen compassion. For some sects meat is consumed; other sects may avoid meat as well as strong-smelling plant foods such as onion, garlic, chives, shallot and leek. Alcohol is discouraged but not forbidden. There may be days during the year when fasting may take place. Some lay Buddhists may forgo meat on full moon days, which is seen as a form of fasting.

Religion	Relevant terminology	Geographical areas	Major celebrations/ festivals	Common practices
Christianity	Three main forms: Roman Catholic Eastern Orthodox Protestant	Global religion, 78 countries have >90% of population identifying as Christian.	Food marks the celebration of the majority of the sacraments: baptism, marriage and death. Food is also used to celebrate Easter (the death of Jesus) and Christmas (marking the birth of Jesus).	Food is considered important in Christianity for bodily and spiritual health, and in expressing fellowship and charity. The central sacrament of Christianity is celebrated as a shared meal and is known as Holy Communion. Due to the diversity of practices few food rules have been retained over time. Fasting is still practised, especially in the Eastern Orthodox tradition; over half the days of the year are designated as fast days. Lent and Advent were typically times when people gave up meat and other highly valued foods such as olive oil and wine. For Catholics historically Fridays were meat-free days but this practice is not currently common.
Hinduism	Prasada—food offered to and sanctified by the gods Farfar—foods permitted during fasting	Approximately 15% of the world's population identify as Hindu, and 93% of Hindus live in India, with additional populations in Bali, Bangladesh, the Caribbean, Fiji, Nepal, Mauritius, Sri Lanka.	Religious holidays and celebrations vary between regions, countries and ethnic groups. Diwali—festival of lights may involve exchanging boxes of sweets, dried fruits and nuts.	Taboo foods include beef or items containing beef. Some who practise Hinduism may be vegetarian. Strict Hindus may also not eat 'hot' foods such as carrots, onions, eggplants, chilli, ginger, dates, eggs, meat, fish, tea, honey and brown sugar. Consumption of alcohol is not prohibited but moderation is recommended. Fasting is a common practice and may take three forms: 1. self-control 2. atonement for sins 3. asking or thanking a deity. Many Hindus may also adhere to **Ayurvedic** principles.
Islam	Halal—food that has been prepared according to Muslim law Haram—foods that are strictly forbidden	Wide diaspora. Distinct cuisines over which Islam is layered; for example, Malaysia, Indonesia, Pakistan, Bosnia–Herzegovina, Kosovo, Turkey, Jordan, Libya, Iraq, Saudi Arabia, UAE. There are three branches of Islam: 1. Shi'ite 2. Sunni 3. Sufi.	Ramadan—the month of fasting. Eid el Fitr—the celebration that marks the end of Ramadan.	Haram foods include blood, alcohol, meat or any products from a forbidden animal, including pigs and any carnivorous animals or birds of prey, meat or any products of an animal which has not been slaughtered in the correct manner in the name of Allah. Hospitality and sharing food as a means of creating common bonds is a central tenet of Islam and it is important to accept any food offered. Fasting is one of the five pillars of Islam and is considered an important religious duty. The major obligatory fast is the month-long Ramadan during which no food or drink can be consumed between sunrise and sunset. The fast is typically broken with dates and water. Fasting is prohibited on five days of the year.

Religion	Relevant terminology	Geographical areas	Major celebrations/festivals	Common practices
Jehovah's Witness				Cannot consume blood. They thus cannot eat raw meat, extremely rare meat, or dishes made out of blood products, such as black pudding, blood soup or blood sausage.
Judaism	Kosher—food that has been prepared according to *kashrut* or Judaic law Trefa—foods not fit to consume Shabbat—Sabbath or day of rest	Wide diaspora. Distinct Jewish cuisines emerged from areas in Eastern Europe (Ashkenazi) and from Turkey/Greece (Sephardic). Also distinct cuisines from Syria, Yemen, Latin America. The centre of Jewish faith is located in Israel.	Shabbat is the day of rest and begins just before sunset on Friday and continues until an hour after sunset on Saturday. Passover: the first night of Passover sees the ritual Seder meal performed in all observant Jewish homes. Yom Kippur (Day of Atonement). Hanukkah (Festival of Lights) is the Winter Festival and historically not a major festival. However, its proximity to Christmas means that it is an opportunity to exchange gifts.	Taboo foods include pork, rabbit, fish without fins or scales (includes shellfish, eels, catfish), horse, frog. Milk products and meat should not be eaten in the same meal together. A kosher household will have at least two sets of pots, pans and dishes: one for meat and one for dairy and may have two kitchens. No blood can be consumed—the blood is salted or cooked out. For observant Jews no work, including food preparation, can take place on the Sabbath. Fasting ordained by the Bible occurs on Yom Kippur
Seventh Day Adventist		A Christian religion founded in the mid-19th century.		The Seventh Day Adventists have a concern for the health of the body and so commend a vegetarian diet and adherence to the laws of kashrut outlined in the Old Testament. About one-third are ovo-lacto vegetarian; 10% are vegan and 10% are pescatarians. Avoid stimulants such as caffeine and alcohol.

Source: Fieldhouse (2017); Gallegos & Perry (1995)

DEVELOPING A MENU TAKING INTO CONSIDERATION RELIGIOUS AND CULTURAL PRACTICES

You have been asked to develop a menu for a multicultural childcare centre—there are children from India, Vietnam, China, Pakistan and Malaysia.

- Write a list of all the possible religious and cultural considerations that you may need to consider.
- Develop a list of meals that would potentially meet these cultural variations.

FOOD AND MIGRATION

One of the significant influences on food habits and dietary patterns is migration. Such population shifts result in exchanges of culinary and dietary techniques and preferences. Food habits will change when new foods are locally produced or, conversely, local foods are sold outside the community; when new foods become available commercially; or when people move to a new locality or when a community receives immigrants. Australia is described as the most multicultural country in the world, with one in four Australians born overseas and over 300 languages spoken at home, and 11.5 per cent of individuals not speaking English well or at all. This diversity is also reflected in New Zealand, where one in four New Zealanders were also born overseas (ABS 2017; Stats NZ 2017). In culturally pluralistic immigrant societies such as Australia, New Zealand, the USA and Canada, individual foods as well as combinations of foods, cooking techniques and other food practices have all been influenced by waves of migration. Immediately after World War 2, the influence of Greece and Italy was felt; more recently, the Asianisation of the Australian food supply can be described with the increase in the diversity of vegetables, fruits, grains (rice), legumes and condiments (Wahlqvist 2002; 2016).

Australia and New Zealand accept migrants and refugees. There are important differences between these categories. Migrants make a conscious choice. They are able to explore which country they would like to move to, seek education and employment opportunities. They can plan their travel, take their belongings and say goodbye to those around them. They are also able to return at any time. Refugees are forced to leave their country because they are at risk of or have experienced persecution. Most have to leave behind their homes, possessions and families and some may have experienced trauma. They have no choice about where they will be settled and are unable to return unless the situation that forced them to leave improves.

The settlement of migrants and refugees in a new country does not follow a single pattern. 'Successful' settlement has been described in terms of integration—that is, the ability to participate fully in economic, social, cultural and political activities—and this is certainly the goal of the Australian and New Zealand governments (Valtonen 2004). Previous Australian policy was proactive in supporting assimilation, the 'melting pot' analogy whereby the customs, behaviours and the national or collective identity of the host country are adopted. Acculturation, on the other hand, is more multidimensional and describes the cultural modification of an individual, group, or community by adapting to or borrowing traits from another culture. Key to this definition is that the contact between two groups results in changes in both groups. Adaptation of food habits and dietary patterns vary significantly depending on the trajectory of acculturation—that is, maintenance of culture or seeking out contact with those outside your group.

Changes to food habits on migration are variable; some elements are resistant to change and others are more mutable. International and Australian studies have indicated that breakfast and lunch have changed but more 'traditional' meals are retained for 'the major meal at dinner, which has higher emotional attachment' (Lee et al. 1999, p. 1089). Migrants may continue to consume foods strongly tied to identity, and dietary change will involve foods that play a less central role (Koctürk-Runefors 1991). A recent investigation of South Asian Surinamese living in the Netherlands found that staple food consumption was stable irrespective of acculturation strategy, while intake of accessory foods such as fruit varied (Raza et al. 2016). Australian examples of similar patterns are found with elderly Greek-born Australians who increased energy consumption when they first arrived but maintained a Mediterranean diet, including legumes, which reduced their all-cause and cardiovascular disease mortality despite the presence of risk factors (Kouris-Blazos & Itsiopoulos 2014). Notable, too, were food consumption patterns among Somali and Sudanese migrants who maintained the structure of their diets according to their country of birth but increased 'accessory' foods such as instant noodles, crisps and pizza. Breakfast was the most common meal to change (Burns 2004; Renzaho & Burns 2006).

SUMMARY

- Food choice is complex and involves the intersection of a number of personal, collective and environmental factors. It will depend on your stage in the life-course, your personal values and skills as well as the foods available to choose from.
- Among the biggest influences on food choice and nutritional status are social determinants. Social determinants are the conditions in which people are born, grow, work, live and age as influenced by a range of systems—economic, developmental, social and political. Those with unfavourable social determinants generally have poorer health and nutritional outcomes.
- The social determinants can be described in a variety of ways and are typically classified based on income, with incomes below a designated poverty line indicative of poor outcomes. However, income is not the only determinant. As a result, deprivation, disadvantage and class are also used to describe the influence of social determinants. These are usually more multifactorial than income alone.
- Class describes not only socioeconomic status but tends to also group individuals with similar tastes. Weight perception can be class-based, with some groups of individuals valuing high weight as symbols of status and others favouring thinness.
- Household food insecurity is more likely to occur in households experiencing some level of disadvantage. It is associated with poor outcomes in children and adults.

KEY TERMS

Ayurvedic: relating to Ayurveda, a dietary classification system that aims to maintain health through balance. Diet is one of the eight branches of Ayurvedic medicine. The body's life force is maintained by eating the right food, which means matching the characteristics of the food with the needs of the individual body. All substances, whether food or people, have qualities which come in ten dichotomous pairs: hot/cold, heavy/light, liquid/viscous, oily/dry, soft/hard, cloudy/clear, rough/slimy, stable/mobile, subtle/gross, sharp/dull.

Equivalised disposable household income: the total income of a household, after tax and other deductions, that is available for spending or saving, divided by the number of household members.

ACKNOWLEDGEMENTS

This chapter has been substantially changed from previous versions but acknowledgement must be made to Pat Crotty. Pat Crotty wrote the original version of this chapter and I would like to acknowledge Pat as Australia's first critical social nutritionist.

REFERENCES

ABS, 2008, *How Australians Use Their Time, 2006*, <www.abs.gov.au/AUSSTATS/abs@.nsf/DetailsPage/6530.02009-10?OpenDocument>, accessed 21 May 2017

—— 2013, *Life Tables for Aboriginal and Torres Strait Islanders, 2010–2012*, <www.abs.gov.au/AUSSTATS/abs@.nsf/DetailsPage/3302.0.55.0032010-2012?OpenDocument>, accessed 22 February 2019

—— 2015a, *Australian Aboriginal and Torres Strait Islander Health Survey: Nutrition results—food and nutrients, 2012–13*, <www.abs.gov.au/ausstats/abs@.nsf/mf/4727.0.55.005>, accessed 24 February 2019

—— 2015b, *Health Survey—First results 2014–2015*, <www.abs.gov.au/AUSSTATS/abs@.nsf/DetailsPage/4364.0.55.0012014-15?OpenDocument>, accessed 23 February 2019

—— 2017, *Census Reveals a Fast Changing, Culturally Diverse Nation*, <www.abs.gov.au/ausstats/abs@.nsf/lookup/Media%20Release3>, accessed 18 December 2018

—— 2018, *The Australian Statistical Geography Standard (ASGS) Remoteness Structure*, <www.abs.gov.au/websitedbs/d3310114.nsf/home/remoteness+structure>, accessed 15 May 2018

AIHW, 2014, *Mortality Inequalities in Australia 2009–2011*, <www.aihw.gov.au/reports/social-determinants/mortality-inequalities-in-australia-2009-11/contents/table-of-contents>, accessed 18 February 2018

—— 2016, *Australia's Health 2016*, <www.aihw.gov.au/australias-health/2016/>, accessed 18 February 2018

Australian Council of Social Service & Social Policy Research Centre, 2016, *Poverty in Australia 2016*, <www.acoss.org.au/wp-content/uploads/2016/10/Poverty-in-Australia-2016.pdf>, accessed 24 February 2019

Beagan, B.L., Power, E.M. & Chapman, G.E., 2015, '"Eating isn't just swallowing food": Food practices in the context of social class trajectory', *Canadian Food Studies, 2*(1): 75–98, doi:10.15353/cfs-rcea.v2i1.50

Becker, A.E., 2004, 'Television, disordered eating and young women in Fiji: Negotiating body image and identity during rapid social change', *Culture, Medicine and Psychiatry, 28*: 533–59, doi:10.1007/s11013-004-1067-5

Belasco, W., 2008, *Food: The key concepts*, Oxford: Berg

Bisogni, C., Bostic, S., Sobal, J. & Jastran, M., 2016, 'Food literacy and food choice', in H. Vidgen (ed.), *Food Literacy: Key concepts for health and education*, Oxon: Routledge, pp. 102–17

Bonnefond, C. & Clément, M., 2014, 'Social class and body weight among Chinese urban adults: The role of the middle classes in the nutrition transition', *Social Science & Medicine, 112*: 22–9, doi:10.1016/j.socscimed.2014.04.021

Bourdieu, P., 1984, *Distinction: A social critique of the judgement of taste*, Cambridge: Harvard University Press

Braveman, P., 2009, 'A health disparities perspective on obesity research', *Preventing Chronic Disease: Public Health Research, Practice, and Policy, 6*(3): A91, <www.cdc.gov/pcd/issues/2009/jul/pdf/09_0012.pdf>, accessed 16 September 2009

Brimblecombe, J.K. & O'Dea, K., 2009, 'The role of energy cost in food choices for an Aboriginal population in northern Australia', *Medical Journal of Australia, 190*(10): 549–51, doi:10.5694/j.1326-5377.2009.tb02560.x

Bunch, S. & Mehra, R., 2008, *Women Help Solve Hunger: Why is the world still waiting?*, <www.icrw.org/wp-content/uploads/2016/10/Women-Help-Solve-Hunger.pdf>, accessed 24 February 2019

Burns, C., 2004, 'Effect of migration on food habits of Somali women living as refugees in Australia', *Ecology of Food and Nutrition, 43*(3): 213–29, doi:10.1080/03670240490447541

Campos, P., Saguy, A., Ernsberger, P., Oliver, E. & Gaesser, G., 2006, 'The epidemiology of overweight and obesity: Public health crisis or moral panic?', *International Journal of Epidemiology, 35*(1): 55–60, doi:10.1093/ije/dyi254

Caniglia, F., Bourke, P. & Whiley, A.P., 2010, *A Scan of Disadvantage in Queensland 2010: From analysis to innovation in place-based practice*, <https://apo.org.au/node/22421>, accessed 23 February 2019

Chang, Y.-H., Chen, R.C.-Y., Wahlqvist, M.L. & Lee, M.-S., 2011, 'Frequent shopping by men and women increases survival in the older Taiwanese population', *Journal of Epidemiology & Community Health, 66*(7): e20, doi:10.1136/jech.2010.126698

Chen, R.C., Lee, M.S., Chang, Y.H. & Wahlqvist, M.L., 2012, 'Cooking frequency may enhance survival in Taiwanese elderly', *Public Health Nutrition, 15*(7): 1142–9, doi:10.1017/s136898001200136x

Coleman-Jensen, A., Rabbitt, M.P., Gregory, C.A. & Singh, A., 2017, *Household Food Insecurity in the United States in 2016*, <www.ers.usda.gov/webdocs/publications/84973/err-237.pdf>, accessed 22 February 2019

Crotty, P., 1995, *Good Nutrition: Fact and fashion in dietary advice*, Sydney: Allen & Unwin

Delormier, T., Frohlich, K.L. & Potvin, L., 2009, 'Food and eating as social practice: Understanding eating patterns as social phenomena and implications for public health', *Sociology of Health & Illness, 31*(2): 215–28, doi:10.1111/j.1467-9566.2008.01128.x

DeVault, M.L., 1994, *Feeding the Family: The social organization of caring as gendered work*, Chicago, IL: University of Chicago Press

Diderichsen, F., Evans, T. & Whitehead, M., 2001, 'The social basis of disparities in health', in T. Evans, M. Whitehead, F. Diderichsen, A. Bhuiya & M. Wirth, *Challenging Inequities in Health: From ethics to action*, New York, NY: Oxford University Press, pp. 12–23

Dowler, E.A. & O'Connor, D., 2012, 'Rights-based approaches to addressing food poverty and food insecurity in Ireland and UK', *Social Science & Medicine, 74*(1): 44–51, doi:10.1016/j.socscimed.2011.08.036

Drewnowski, A. & Darmon, N., 2005, 'The economics of obesity: Dietary energy density and energy cost', *American Journal of Clinical Nutrition, 82*(1): 265S–73S, doi:10.1093/ajcn/82.1.265S

Drewnowski, A., Rehm, C.D. & Solet, D., 2007, 'Disparities in obesity rates: Analysis by ZIP code area', *Social Science & Medicine, 65*: 2458–63, doi:10.1016/j.socscimed.2007.07.001

Erlich, R., Yngve, A. & Wahlqvist, M.L., 2012, 'Cooking as a healthy behaviour', *Public Health Nutrition, 15*(7): 1139–40, doi:10.1017/S1368980012002662

FAO, 2011, *State of Food and Agriculture: Women in agriculture—Closing the gender gap for development*, <www.fao.org/docrep/013/i2050e/i2050e.pdf>, accessed 22 February 2019

—— 2016, *Voices of the Hungry: Methods for assessing comparable rates of food insecurity experienced by adults throughout the world*, <www.fao.org/3/a-i4830e.pdf>, accessed 22 February 2019

—— 2018, *FAOSTAT*, <www.fao.org/faostat/en/#home>, accessed 17 December 2018

Field, J., 2016, *Social Capital*, London: Routledge

Fieldhouse, P., 2017, *Food, Feasts, and Faith: An encyclopedia of food culture in world religions*, Santa Barbara, CA: ABC-CLIO, LLC

Friel, S. & Baker, P.I., 2009, 'Equity, food security and health equity in the Asia Pacific region', *Asia Pacific Journal of Clinical Nutrition, 18*(4): 620–32, doi:10.6133/apjcn.2009.18.4.23

Gallegos, D., 2016, 'The nexus between food literacy, food security and disadvantage', in H. Vidgen (ed.), *Food Literacy: Key concepts for health and education*, London: Routledge, pp. 134–50

Gallegos, D., Booth, S., Kleve, S., McKechnie, R. & Lindberg, R., 2017, 'Food insecurity in Australian households: From charity to entitlement', in J. Germov & L. Williams (eds), *A Sociology of Food and Nutrition: The social appetite* (4th edn), Oxford: Oxford University Press, pp. 55–74

Gallegos, D.L. & Perry, E.A., 1995, *A World of Food: A manual to assist in the provision of culturally appropriate meals for older people*, Canberra: Commonwealth Dept of Human Services and Health

Garthwaite, K.A., Collins, P.J. & Bambra, C., 2015, 'Food for thought: An ethnographic study of negotiating ill health and food insecurity in a UK foodbank', *Social Science & Medicine, 132*: 38–44, doi:10.1016/j.socscimed.2015.03.019

Health Canada, 2017, *Household Food Insecurity in Canada Statistics and Graphics (2011 to 2012)*, <www.canada.ca/en/health-canada/services/nutrition-science-research/food-security/household-food-security-statistics-2011-2012.html?wbdisable=true>, accessed 15 May 2018

Kaur, J., Lamb, M.M. & Ogden, C.L., 2015, 'The association between food insecurity and obesity in children: The National Health and Nutrition Examination Survey', *Journal of the Academy of Nutrition and Dietetics, 115*(5): 751–8, doi:10.1016/j.jand.2015.01.003

King, T., Kavanagh, A.M., Jolley, D., Turrell, G. & Crawford, D., 2005, 'Weight and place: A multilevel cross-sectional survey of area-level social disadvantage and overweight/obesity in Australia', *International Journal of Obesity, 30*: 281–7, doi:10.1038/sj.ijo.0803176

Koctürk-Runefors, T., 1991, 'A model for adaptation to a new food pattern: The case of immigrants', in E.L. Fürst, R. Prättälä, M. Ekström, L. Holm & U. Kjærnes (eds), *Palatable Worlds: Sociocultural food studies*, Oslo: Solum Norvag, pp. 185–92

Kouris-Blazos, A. & Itsiopoulos, C., 2014, 'Low all-cause mortality despite high cardiovascular risk in elderly Greek-born Australians: Attenuating potential of diet?', *Asia Pacific Journal of Clinical Nutrition, 23*(4): 532–44, doi:10.6133/apjcn.2014.23.4.16

Lee, S.-K., Sobal, J. & Frongillo, E.A., 1999, 'Acculturation and dietary practices among Korean Americans', *Journal of the American Dietetic Association, 99*(9): 1084–9, doi:10.1016/S0002-8223(99)00258-8

Leung, C.W., Epel, E.S., Ritchie, L.D., Crawford, P.B. & Laraia, B.A., 2014, 'Food insecurity is inversely associated with diet quality of lower-income adults', *Journal of the Academy of Nutrition and Dietetics, 114*(12): 1943–53, e1942, doi:10.1016/j.jand.2014.06.353

McLachlan, R., Gilfillan, G. & Gordon, J., 2013, *Deep and Persistent Disadvantage in Australia: Productivity Commission staff working paper*, <www.pc.gov.au/research/completed/deep-persistent-disadvantage/deep-persistent-disadvantage.pdf>, accessed 24 February 2019

McLaren, L., 2007, 'Socioeconomic status and obesity', *Epidemiology Review, 29*(1): 29–48, doi:10.1093/epirev/mxm001

Malapit, H.J.L. & Quisumbing, A.R., 2015, 'What dimensions of women's empowerment in agriculture matter for nutrition in Ghana?', *Food Policy, 52*: 54–63, doi:10.1016/j.foodpol.2015.02.003

Mills, S., White, M., Brown, H., Wrieden, W., Kwasnicka, D. et al., 2017, 'Health and social determinants and outcomes of home cooking: A systematic review of observational studies', *Appetite, 111*: 116–34, doi:10.1016/j.appet.2016.12.022

Mintz, S., 1994, 'Eating and being: What food means', in B. Harris-White & S.R. Hoffenberg (eds), *Food: Multidisciplinary perspectives,* London: Blackwell, pp. 102–15

Mishra, K. & Sam, A.G., 2016, 'Does women's land ownership promote their empowerment? Empirical evidence from Nepal', *World Development, 78*: 360–71, doi:10.1016/j.worlddev.2015.10.003

Monteiro, C.A., Moura, E.C., Conde, W.L. & Popkin, B.M., 2004, 'Socioeconomic status and obesity in adult populations of developing countries: A review', *Bulletin of the World Health Organization, 82*(12): 940–6, doi:10.1017/S0042-96862004001200011

Neuman, N., Gottzén, L. & Fjellström, C., 2017, 'Narratives of progress: Cooking and gender equality among Swedish men', *Journal of Gender Studies, 26*(2): 151–63, doi:10.1080/09589236.2015.1090306

New Zealand Inland Revenue, 2018, *Individual Income Earner,* <www.ird.govt.nz/income-tax-individual/tax-credits/ietc/>, accessed 15 May 2018

Nielsen, A., Lund, T.B. & Holm, L., 2015, 'The taste of "the end of the month" and how to avoid it: Coping with restrained food budgets in a Scandinavian welfare state context', *Social Policy and Society, 14*(3): 429–42, doi:10.1017/S1474746415000056

OECD, 2018, *Poverty Rate (Indicator),* <https://data.oecd.org/inequality/poverty-rate.htm>, accessed 20 February 2019

Palma, M.A., Ness, M.L. & Anderson, D.P., 2017, 'Fashionable food: A latent class analysis of social status in food purchases', *Applied Economics, 49*(3): 238–50, doi:10.1080/00036846.2016.1194965

Pan, W.-H., Hsieh, Y.-T. & Wahlqvist, M.L., 2009, 'Gender-specific roles and needs in food-health security', *Asia Pacific Journal of Clinical Nutrition, 18*(4): 642–6, doi:10.6133/apjcn.2009.18.4.26

Parnell, W., Wilson, N., Thomson, C., Mackay, S. & Stefanogiannis, N., 2011, *A Focus on Nutrition: Key findings of the 2008/09 New Zealand Adult Nutrition Survey,* <www.health.govt.nz/publication/focus-nutrition-key-findings-2008-09-nz-adult-nutrition-survey>, accessed 18 February 2018

Pinxten, W. & Lievens, J., 2014, 'The importance of economic, social and cultural capital in understanding health inequalities: Using a Bourdieu-based approach in research on physical and mental health perceptions', *Sociology of Health & Illness, 36*(7): 1095–110, doi:10.1111/1467-9566.12154

Ramsey, R., Giskes, K., Gavin, T. & Gallegos, D., 2012, 'Food insecurity among adults residing in disadvantaged urban areas: Potential health and dietary consequences', *Public Health Nutrition 15*: 227–37, doi:10.1017/S1368980011001996

Ramsey, R., Giskes, K., Turrell, G. & Gallegos, D., 2011, 'Food insecurity among Australian children: Potential determinants, health and developmental consequences', *Journal of Child Health Care, 15*(4): 401–16, doi:10.1177/1367493511423854

Raza, Q., Nicolaou, M., Snijder, M.B., Stronks, K. & Seidell, J.C., 2016, 'Dietary acculturation among the South-Asian Surinamese population in the Netherlands: The HELIUS study', *Public Health Nutrition, 20*(11): 1–10, doi:10.1017/S1368980016000914

Renzaho, A.M.N. & Burns, C., 2006, 'Post-migration food habits of sub-Saharan African migrants in Victoria: A cross-sectional study', *Nutrition & Dietetics, 63*(2): 91–102, doi:10.1111/j.1747-0080.2006.00055.x

Riches, G., 2018, *Food Bank Nations: Poverty, corporate charity and the right to food,* London: Routledge

Rose, D.J., 2011, 'Captive audience? Strategies for acquiring food in two Detroit neighborhoods', *Qualitative Health Research, 21*(5): 642–51, doi:10.1177/1049732310387159

Roy, S., Ara, J., Das, N. & Quisumbing, A.R., 2015, '"Flypaper effects" in transfers targeted to women: Evidence from BRAC's "Targeting the Ultra Poor" program in Bangladesh', *Journal of Development Economics, 117*: 1–19, doi:10.1016/j.jdeveco.2015.06.004

Rozin, E., 1982, 'The structure of cuisine', in L.M. Barker (ed.), *The Psycho–biology of Human Food Selection,* Westport, CT: AVI Publishing, pp. 189–203

—— 1983, *Ethnic Cuisine: The flavor principle cookbook,* Brattleboro, VT: Stephen Greene Press

Saunders, P., 2008, 'Measuring wellbeing using non-monetary indicators', *Family Matters, 78*: 8–17, <https://aifs.gov.au/publications/family-matters/issue-78/measuring-wellbeing-using-non-monetary-indicators>, accessed 20 May 2019

Saunders, P. & Naidoo, Y., 2018, 'Mapping the Australian poverty profile: A multidimensional deprivation approach', *Australian Economic Review, 51*(3): 336–50, doi:10.1111/1467-8462.12266

Scrinis, G., 2013, *Nutritionism: The science and politics of dietary advice,* New York, NY: Columbia University Press

Sen, A., 2000, *Social Exclusion: Concept, application, and scrutiny* <www.adb.org/sites/default/files/publication/29778/social-exclusion.pdf>, accessed 22 February 2019

Shankar, P., Chung, R. & Frank, D.A., 2017, 'Association of food insecurity with children's behavioral, emotional, and academic outcomes: A systematic review', *Journal of Developmental & Behavioral Pediatrics, 38*(2): 135–50, doi:10.1097/DBP.0000000000000383

Shugart, H.A., 2014, 'Food fixations', *Food, Culture & Society, 17*(2): 261–81, doi:10.2752/1751744 14X13871910531665

Smith, V.C., 2015, 'Upstream or downstream?', *Medical Journal of Australia, 202*(10): 412–13, doi:10.5694/mja15.00718

Sobal, J. & Bisogni, C.A., 2009, 'Constructing food choice decisions', *Annals of Behavioral Medicine, 38*(suppl. 1): s37–s46, doi:10.1007/s12160-009-9124-5

Sobal, J., Bisogni, C.A. & Jastran, M., 2014, 'Food choice is multifaceted, contextual, dynamic, multilevel, integrated, and diverse', *Mind, Brain, and Education, 8*(1): 6–12, doi:10.1111/mbe.12044

Solar, O. & Irwin, A., 2010, 'A conceptual framework for action on the social determinants of health', Geneva: World Health Organization, <www.who.int/sdhconference/resources/Conceptualframeworkforactionon SDH_eng.pdf>, accessed 12 July 2019

Stats NZ, 2017, *National Ethnic Population Projections: 2013 (Base)—2038 (Update)*, <www.stats.govt.nz/information-releases/national-ethnic-population-projections-2013base2038-update>, accessed 18 December 2018

Turrell, G., Stanley, L., de Looper, M. & Oldenburg, B., 2006, *Health Inequalities in Australia: Morbidity, health behaviours, risk factors and health service use*, <www.aihw.gov.au/reports/australias-health/health-inequalities-australia/contents/table-of-contents>, accessed 24 February 2019

United Nations, 2017, *Sustainable Development Goals: Poverty*, <www.un.org/sustainabledevelopment/poverty/>, accessed 22 February 2019

Valtonen, K., 2004, 'From the margin to the mainstream: Conceptualizing refugee settlement processes', *Journal of Refugee Studies, 17*(1): 70–96, doi:10.1093/jrs/17.1.70

van Hooff, J.H., 2011, 'Rationalising inequality: Heterosexual couples' explanations and justifications for the division of housework along traditionally gendered lines', *Journal of Gender Studies, 20*(1): 19–30, doi:10.108 0/09589236.2011.542016

Wahlqvist, M.L., 2002, 'Asian migration to Australia: Food and health consequences', *Asia Pacific Journal of Clinical Nutrition, 11*(Suppl.): S562–S568, doi:10.1046/j.1440-6047.11.supp3.13.x

—— 2016, 'Future food', *Asia Pacific Journal of Clinical Nutrition, 25*(4): 706–15, doi:10.6133/apjcn.092016.01

Wahlqvist, M.L., Keatinge, J., Butler, C., Friel, S., McKay, J. et al., 2009, 'A Food in Health Security (FIHS) platform in the Asia-Pacific Region: The way forward', *Asia Pacific Journal of Clinical Nutrition, 18*(4): 688–702, doi:10.6133/apjcn.2009.18.4.34

Wahlqvist, M.L., McKay, J., Chang, Y.-C. & Chiu, Y.-W., 2012, 'Rethinking the food security debate in Asia: Some missing ecological and health dimensions and solutions', *Food Security, 4*(4): 657–70, doi:10.1007/s12571-012-0211-2

Werner, A. & Lim, M., 2015, 'The ethics of the living wage: A review and research agenda', *Journal of Business Ethics, 137*(3): 1–15, doi:10.1007/s10551-015-2562-z

WHO, 2017, *Social Determinants of Health*, <www.who.int/social_determinants/en/>, accessed 23 March 2017

Wiig, K. & Smith, C., 2009, 'The art of grocery shopping on a food stamp budget: Factors influencing the food choices of low-income women as they try to make ends meet', *Public Health Nutrition, 12*(10): 1726–34, doi:10.1017/S1368980008004102

World Bank, 2011, *World Development Report 2012: Gender equality and development*, <https://openknowledge.worldbank.org/handle/10986/4391>, accessed 22 February 2019

World Bank, FAO & IFAD, 2008, *Gender in Agriculture Sourcebook: Agriculture and rural development*, <http://documents.worldbank.org/curated/en/799571468340869508/pdf/461620PUB0Box3101OFFICIAL0USE 0ONLY1.pdf>, accessed 24 February 2019

Worsley, A., Wang, W.C., Yeatman, H., Byrne, S. & Wijayaratne, P., 2016, 'Does school health and home economics education influence adults' food knowledge?', *Health Promotion International, 31*(4): 925–35, doi:10.1093/heapro/dav078

Xiao, Y., Zhao, N., Wang, H., Zhang, J., He, Q. et al., 2013, 'Association between socioeconomic status and obesity in a Chinese adult population', *BMC Public Health, 13*(1): 355, doi:10.1186/1471-2458-13-355

Zimmerman, H., 2015, 'Caring for the middle class soul', *Food, Culture & Society, 18*(1): 31–50, doi:10.2752/1751 74415X14101814953729

{CHAPTER 28}
UNDERSTANDING FOOD AND NUTRITION FOR INDIGENOUS PEOPLES

Danielle Gallegos, Leisa McCarthy and Christina McKerchar

OBJECTIVES

- Outline the role Indigenous peoples have in maintaining food systems.
- Identify the impact of colonisation on Indigenous health including the role of trauma and racism.
- List key nutritional issues for Indigenous peoples, in particular Australian Aboriginal and Torres Strait Islander and Māori populations.

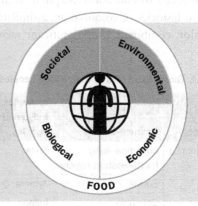

INTRODUCTION

The primary component of defining as **Indigenous** is self-identification and acceptance and belonging to a group with a shared world view that humans are integral to the world but are part of a seamless relationship with nature (land, seas, air, animals, plants) (Cunningham & Stanley 2003). The controversy around definitions of indigeneity is not one for Indigenous peoples, who have very clear definitions about who they are—it is for governments who fail to recognise political sovereignty of different nations within a nation.

The definition refers to groups of people who have historical continuity with and occupation of land before invasion and colonisation. This is accompanied by distinct social, cultural, economic and political systems as well as distinct language,

religious and cultural beliefs (Gracey & King 2009). From a food perspective, Indigenous peoples retain knowledge of the land and of food resources that are rooted in historical continuity (Turner et al. 2013). Food provides the link between country, identity, culture and health. Having access to and use of Indigenous food resources to increase diet quality works towards making local food resources sources of pride, pleasure and responsibility, thereby ensuring local determination (Kuhnlein et al. 2006). Indigenous food resources are more important in that they provide a spiritual connection to the land and act as medicine for **healing** the spirit as well as overall health and wellness.

There are 370 million Indigenous peoples globally in about 90 countries, making up 5 per cent of the world's population (World Bank 2018).

Table 28.1 provides some examples of Indigenous peoples across different continents. Indigenous peoples in many situations share the experience of being minority populations, overshadowed by a more demographically significant and economically prosperous majority. The health of Indigenous peoples is linked with their ecosystems and the complexities of their social and economic circumstances (Kuhnlein et al. 2006). While only being 5 per cent of the global population, Indigenous populations make up 15 per cent of the extreme poor (World Bank 2018) and continue to suffer disproportionately from poverty, marginalisation, poor health, poor housing and poor access to education (Stephens et al. 2005). Prolonged histories of colonisation, assimilation and exploitation combined with significant racism and discrimination and a neglect of human rights have created alarming health disparities.

Some Indigenous communities maintain their isolation from the prevailing culture, while others appear to move between the ancestral and prevailing cultures while maintaining a sense of Indigenous identity. However, for some Indigenous peoples living without any trace of their ancestral culture is a reality, and not necessarily a choice. Many Indigenous groups have elements of both their 'traditional' culture and the current prevailing cultural norms. The urbanisation of traditional ways of living typically means a reduction in access to hunting, fishing, herding, gathering and production on lands that have been subsumed and repurposed. Reduced consumption of traditional foods and increased consumption of readily available energy-dense and nutrient-poor foods, combined with elevated risk of poverty, increases the risk of nutritionally related

Table 28.1: Global examples of Indigenous peoples

Continent	Country–Locality	Examples of Indigenous peoples
South America	Argentina–Jujuy (north-western region)	Kolla
	Bolivia	Aymara, Quechua
	Colombia	Ingano
	Peru	Awajún
North America	Canada–Nanavut (Arctic Circle)	Inuit
Pacific Island	Micronesia	Pohnpei
Asia	India—Andhra Pradesh	Adivasi
	Thailand	Karen
	Thailand, Laos, Burma, Vietnam	Hmong
	Japan—Hokkaido	Ainu
Africa	Nigeria—southeastern region	Igbo
	Kenya	Maasai
	Tanzania	Hadza, Sandawe
	Zambia	Twa
	South Sudan	Nuer, Dinka, Acholi
Northern Europe	Northern Norway, Sweden, Finland	Sami

WHAT'S IN A NAME?

Indigenous peoples are geographically diverse populations known in different parts of the world by different terms including: native peoples, tribes, tribal groups, autochthonous peoples, aboriginal peoples, First Nations or Founding Nations. In Australia, 'Aboriginal and Torres Strait Islander peoples' is the preferred term, used in full and capitalised. When referring to individual people who identify as Aboriginal or Torres Strait Islander their language group is preferred—for example: Budjalung woman, Jane Smith (Creative Spirits 2018). Māori are the tangata whenua, the Indigenous people, of New Zealand.

chronic conditions (Damman et al. 2008). In most countries across the world, Indigenous peoples have a higher prevalence of low birthweight infants, infant mortality, maternal death, wasting and stunting and chronic conditions compared to the non-Indigenous population (Anderson et al. 2016).

Internationally, Indigenous peoples are facing:
- an increase in land conflicts, such as the loss of rangelands for the Maasai in Tanzania through the expansion of national parks; loss of land undermines economic security, health and wellbeing, sociocultural cohesion and human dignity
- ongoing racism and discrimination
- an escalation of violence—for example, in Nepal 150,000 Indigenous people have been forcibly evicted since 2017 for a national road expansion project
- ongoing poor health outcomes
- substance misuse as an outcome of trauma, including intergenerational trauma

- the effects of climate change as it disrupts ways of living and livelihoods (International Work Group for Indigenous Affairs 2018).

INDIGENOUS PEOPLES' HUMAN RIGHTS

Indigenous peoples often suffer from discrimination and racism due to institutionalisation of unfair policies, practices and behaviours that do not sufficiently represent Indigenous peoples' interests, cultures and ways of living. Countries have dual obligations towards Indigenous peoples: to ensure non-discrimination, and to safeguard their special right to live according to their distinct cultural identities. The United Nations Declaration on the Rights of Indigenous Peoples was adopted by the General Assembly in 2007 (Australia, Canada, the USA and New Zealand voted against its adoption but by 2016 had all endorsed the declaration). The declaration is a non-binding statement on how

---

WHAT IS 'TRADITIONAL' FOOD?

Traditional food refers to what was consumed historically. A 'traditional food system' is used to identify all food specific to a particular culture where availability is from local natural resources and is culturally accepted. It includes the sociocultural meanings, acquisition and processing techniques, and nutritional consequences.

Food and the ways of acquiring and using foods are always changing. For example, if you are discussing a 'traditional' Italian diet, to what would you be referring? If you go back to Roman times that would, near Rome, have included olives, wheat and grapes (Santich 1995). However, after the discovery of the New World and the spread of corn, potatoes and tomatoes, the Italian diet underwent a renaissance. For Indigenous peoples a 'traditional' diet may be what was eaten prior to any contact with others; alternatively, 'traditional' could mean the post-colonial diet. Traditional diets (that is, diets that were common prior to colonisation and/or industrialisation) for Indigenous peoples are linked to better health. Recently, it was identified that in the Northern Territory traditional foods are being consumed regularly and need to be taken into consideration (Ferguson et al. 2017). However, care needs to be taken when recommending traditional diets as a way forward for improving health. Does everybody have a shared understanding of what 'traditional' means? Do not assume that all Indigenous peoples will want to move to a traditional diet—it will depend on an individual's level of interaction and alignment with their cultural ancestry as well as the availability of traditional foods.

Indigenous peoples should be treated. The major themes covered include: self-determination; rights of Indigenous peoples to protect their culture (language, dress, food, media, and religion); rights to specific governance and economic development; and land rights. The full document can be located on the United Nations or Australian Human Rights Commission websites (Australian Human Rights Commission 2018; United Nations 2008).

INDIGENOUS PEOPLES—CUSTODIANS OF BIODIVERSITY

Indigenous peoples play a significant role internationally as stewards of ecosystems that include the land, waterways, animals, plants and microorganisms. Maintaining these ecosystems is, due to strong spiritual connections, integral to community and individual wellbeing (Figure 28.1).

INDIGENOUS HUMAN RIGHTS IN AUSTRALIA AND NEW ZEALAND

A special rapporteur is an independent expert who is under a mandate from the United Nations to report, monitor, advise and publicly report on human rights issues. There are currently 43 thematic and 14 country-specific rapporteurs. The thematic rapporteurs cover:

- education
- food
- internally displaced people
- poverty
- racism
- slavery
- arbitrary detention/enforced or involuntary disappearances
- disabilities
- freedom of expression
- violence against women.

The Special Rapporteur on the Rights of Indigenous Peoples visited Australia in 2010 and 2017 and New Zealand in 2011.

- Visit the following website <www.ohchr.org/EN/Issues/IPeoples/SRIndigenousPeoples/Pages/SRIPeoplesIndex.aspx> and read the Special Rapporteur's analysis of the situation (United Nations Human Rights Office of the High Commissioner 2018).
- Have a look at the materials located on the website of the International Work Group for Indigenous Affairs (IWGA) <www.iwgia.org/en/>.
- Use the web to search for organisations mentioned in the report.
- From an ethical perspective what do you think is the best approach for Australia and New Zealand to take to ensure the rights of Indigenous peoples?
- For the full *Declaration on the Rights of Indigenous Peoples* visit the United Nations or Australian Human Rights Commission websites (Australian Human Rights Commission 2018; United Nations 2008).

Indigenous communities are responsible for the development and use of plant varieties and animal breeds that have traits that have permitted adaptation to local environments and climates. They conserve and use domestic and wild species, sustainably ensuring ongoing food security (Turner et al. 2013). Tapping into Indigenous ecological understandings, conservation practices and resource management goals will be imperative to maintain food security in light of climate change and environmental devastation.

AUSTRALIAN FIRST NATION PEOPLES: ABORIGINAL AND TORRES STRAIT ISLANDER PEOPLES

The impact of history

Little is known about the cultural and social life of Aboriginal and Torres Strait Islander populations prior to the colonisation of Australia, beginning with the arrival of the First Fleet in 1788. The pre-settlement Indigenous peoples have been described as pre-agriculturalists with no domesticated animals

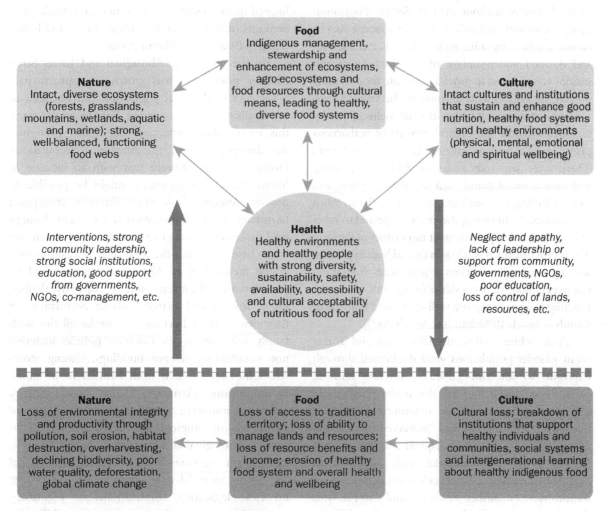

Figure 28.1: Indigenous food systems and wellbeing

Source: Turner, Plotkin & Kuhnlein (2013). Reproduced with permission

apart from native dogs (Gracey 2000). The fact that the communities at the time did not have any perceptible cultivation of crops or animal husbandry formed the basis of Britain's claim of *terra nullius*, meaning 'land that belongs to no one'. This single notion gave rise to years of exploitation and discrimination, and it was not until the *Mabo* decision in 1992 that the judgment was reversed.

While it is true that Australian Aboriginal and Torres Strait Islander peoples were among the most successful hunter-gatherer groups on one of the driest continents in the world, there are indications of a high degree of sophistication in the management of land and system of food sharing to ensure the exploitation of food sources without their depletion. Population groups were semi-nomadic, following seasonal cues to ensure access to ripening fruit and seeds. An intricate and detailed understanding of the flora, fauna and seasons was required to provide adequate food to meet nutritional requirements for most of the year. There is evidence of the use of fire to increase yields of starchy seeds, to promote the cyclical growth of herbaceous plants and to manage grazing kangaroos in forests. There were also indications of deliberate planting and cultivation of plants such as tuberous yams, and various fruiting trees and grasses (Pascoe 2014). From all accounts, the hunter-gatherer diet appeared to meet basic nutritional requirements at most times of the year. The diet as described was low in fat and high in protein, and met most micronutrient requirements. It required the expenditure of a considerable amount of energy, resulting in lean, strong and well-nourished individuals (Smith & Smith 1999; Smith & Smith 2003).

Upon white settlement Aboriginal and Torres Strait Islander populations were decimated through exposure to infectious diseases, forcible removal of lands and massacre. After this initial phase, there was some concern that the remaining population needed to be preserved and 'protected'. Expansion of pastoral leases forced Aboriginal and Torres Strait Islander people off traditional lands and curtailed nomadic movements. Reserves known as missions or stations were established to civilise and control, with the ultimate aim of isolating Aboriginal and Torres Strait Islander peoples to enable them to 'die out'

(Rowse 2002). Work was generally exchanged for food. Groups living on cattle stations and missions managed on rations, making traditional sources of food less important except for recreational purposes. In some cases, sourcing traditional foods was not an option and there was a total dependency on the foods provided by the stations. The removal of children from stations and the undermining of the rights of Aboriginal adults to parent their children meant that the passing on of oral histories relating to the knowledge and collection of foods was no longer possible (Foley 2005). The rations on most cattle stations consisted of beef, flour, sugar (with tea used as the vehicle) and tobacco. There were limited quantities of powdered milk, and inadequate amounts of fruit, vegetables, milk, cheese and butter (Kouris-Blazos & Wahlqvist 2000).

By the 1950s, the Aboriginal and Torres Strait Islander population had grown to approximately 1 per cent of the total population and was seen to be stabilising, if not increasing. For the government, this meant that 'protection' had failed to ensure the disappearance of the Aboriginal populations. However, it was thought that with an increase in 'mixed-blood Aborigines', it might be possible to destroy Aboriginal identity through absorption (Armitage 1995). Assimilation was enacted through dual processes of incentives and coercion. Incentives were based around the granting of exemptions, which meant that an Aboriginal person could be considered a full citizen—able to vote, buy alcohol, move around and marry without permission—if they denied their heritage and broke all ties with family and community. Coercive policies included not maintaining reserve buildings, closing stores and removing children from families to be raised in institutions (Armitage 1995). Social security payments, industrial awards, wage regulations and conditions of employment all had provision to exclude Aboriginal and Torres Strait Islander people. Mainstream agencies even excluded Aboriginal and Torres Strait Islander people when there were no clear legislative, constitutional or regulatory reasons for doing so, claiming that responsibility for Aboriginal individuals or communities did not lie with them (Dixon & Scheurell 1995). Having been forcibly removed from their lands, and placed under the 'protection' of the government and church, where food and in some cases an income were provided, the situation was now that the reserve infrastructure was taken away and, with it, food provision and the capacity to collect native foods.

In the 1960s there was a resurgence of Indigenous activism, provoked by increasing frustration at the inability to protect traditional lands and inspired by the civil rights movement in the United States. In 1966, the poor working conditions and low wages of Indigenous pastoral workers prompted the Wave Hill strike, which eventually led to legal establishment of equal wages. The result was that, without a cheap labour pool, pastoralists moved to mechanise stock management and employ European stockmen, sacking Indigenous workers on a large scale. The pressure to remove Aboriginal and Torres Strait Islander peoples from the land increased (Dixon & Scheurell 1995). The 1967 referendum saw 90 per cent of the Australian population voting to include Aboriginal and Torres Strait Islander people in the Census count and to give the Commonwealth government (rather than state governments) power to make specific laws in respect of Indigenous people. While the referendum had little effect politically for the Aboriginal and Torres Strait Islander populations, it was a pivotal moment in history, heralding a move towards empowerment and self-determination (Attwood & Markus 2007).

Unlike other Indigenous peoples in colonised countries such as the Māori in New Zealand, the Native Indian/Alaskan peoples in the USA and other First Nations people elsewhere, Australian Aboriginal and Torres Strait Islander peoples did not enter into any formal treaties. The Treaty of Waitangi, for example, recognised there were peoples living in New Zealand and that they had rights. Colonisation was by negotiation rather than by a declaration of *terra nullius* (Belgrave et al. 2005). It was not until 1992, almost 200 years after the arrival of the British, and after ten years of applications by Eddie Mabo, that the High Court recognised *terra nullius* as invalid in Australia and decreed that the common law of Australia would recognise native title.

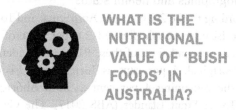

WHAT IS THE NUTRITIONAL VALUE OF 'BUSH FOODS' IN AUSTRALIA?

Native, traditional or bush foods in Australia are considered nutritious. Using a variety of sources, including food tables, peer-reviewed literature, government and non-government websites, develop a list of animal- and plant-based bush foods and their nutrition profiles. Determine which macro- and micronutrients you may want to include. Compare the nutritional value to a commonly available alternative in the supermarket.

The recognition of native title legally allows Aboriginal and Torres Strait Islander peoples to live on an area; access the area for traditional purposes; visit and protect important places and sites; hunt, fish and gather food and other traditional resources; and teach law and custom on country (Australian Native Title Tribunal 1996). The granting of native title is more significant in that it recognises that the social, economic and health situation of Australian Indigenous peoples is linked to the impact of dispossession and removal from traditional lands. More recently there has been increased action calling for changes to the Australian Constitution and a treaty. The Uluru Statement in 2017 asks for constitutional recognition through a First Nations voice in the Constitution. This would be a constitutionally enshrined representative body to guarantee Indigenous peoples will always have a say when the Australian parliament makes laws and policies about them. A stronger political voice for Aboriginal and Torres Strait Islander Australians is not a new idea, having been raised since at least the 1920s with the aim of encouraging self-determination and empowerment (Referendum Council 2017).

Demographics and health status

According to the 2016 census, Aboriginal and Torres Strait Islander people formed 2.8 per cent of the Australian population; of these 91 per cent identify as Aboriginal, 5 per cent as Torres Strait Islander and the remaining 4 per cent as both Aboriginal and Torres Strait Islander (ABS 2017). The Census provides the most accessible data for estimating Aboriginal and Torres Strait Islander populations. There are, however, significant challenges to using these data for such a purpose. These challenges are due to different understandings of 'household', geographical distributions, reporting of births and deaths, and high mobility between areas (Taylor & Biddle 2008). Recognition should also be given to the fact that the generic term 'Aboriginal and Torres Strait Islander' conflates an estimated 250 different language groups and significant cultural diversity.

The poor health of Aboriginal and Torres Strait Islander people demonstrates the powerful impact of determinants that are often out of the control of individuals and frequently not within the jurisdiction of the health sector. Specific social determinants connected to the poor health of Australian and Torres Strait Islander communities include colonisation, racism, poverty, unemployment, lack of education and training, lack of access to appropriate health services, low incomes and lack of housing infrastructure (Campbell et al. 2007). Trauma (historical and current) as a direct result of colonisation and collective experience has had the effect of disempowering Indigenous societies; it has 'fostered community dysfunction, disrupted child-rearing, compromised individual wellbeing and degraded physiological processes' that have continued into the present (Kirmayer et al. 2014). The causal pathways for the impact of historical trauma are outlined in Figure 28.2.

This pathway has been described across the generations for Australian Aboriginal and Torres Strait Islander peoples. This was derived from experiences in South America and has been mapped to the Australian experience but is equally applicable in New Zealand, Canada and the USA (Table 28.2).

Racism can cause reduced or unequal access to health, employment and health resources; increased exposure to risk factors associated with ill-health; racially motivated physical assault; stress; and negative reactions such as smoking, alcohol and drug use, all of which contribute to mental and physical ill-health (Zubrick et al. 2004).

Despite the presence of first-class health systems in highly industrialised countries such as Australia, New Zealand, Canada and the United States, key health indicators show that Indigenous peoples are suffering a far greater percentage of the disease burden than non-Indigenous populations (Anderson et al. 2016; Freemantle et al. 2014). Among these 'first world' countries, it is the Australian Aboriginal and Torres Strait Islander populations that are suffering the most (Hill et al. 2007). Australian Aboriginal and Torres Strait Islander populations have a lower adult life expectancy (ten years lower), a younger median age (23 years versus 38 years) and higher infant mortality rates (6.2 deaths per 1000 births versus 3.5) than non-Indigenous Australians (ABS 2016). The 'Close the Gap' campaign refers to efforts to reduce the difference between Aboriginal and Torres Strait Islander life expectancy and that of other Australians. A ten-year review of the strategy by the Australian Human Rights Commission indicated that the strategy had failed due to lack of funding and commitment (Close the Gap Campaign Steering Committee for Indigenous Equality 2018). The largest contributor to both poor infant and child outcomes and the lower life expectancy (primarily due to the higher prevalence of chronic conditions) is nutrition. However, since the demise of the National Aboriginal and Torres Strait Islander Nutrition Strategy and Action Plan 2000–10 (Strategic Inter–Governmental Nutrition Alliance 2001), and despite the acknowledgement of the role of nutrition in the recent Close the Gap progress report, there is no coordinated, funded action plan to address food and nutrition for Aboriginal and Torres Strait Islander populations.

Key areas for nutrition action for Aboriginal and Torres Strait Islander populations are outlined in Table 28.3. Many of these issues have an underlying

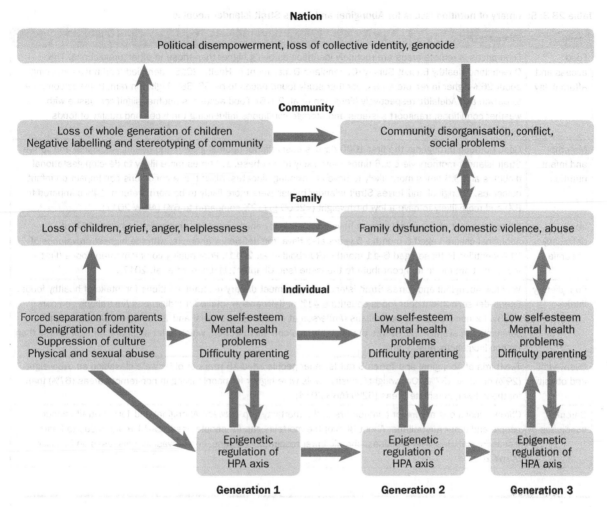

Figure 28.2: Transgenerational transmission of trauma

Source: Kirmayer, Gone & Moses (2014). Reprinted by permission of SAGE Publications, Ltd.

Table 28.2: Intergenerational transmission of trauma

Generation 1	Conquered males were killed, imprisoned, enslaved or in some way deprived of the ability to provide for their families.
Generation 2	Many men misused alcohol and/or drugs to cope with the resultant loss of cultural identity and self-esteem. The trauma was exacerbated by being removed to or forced to remain on reservations or in missions.
Generation 3	Increased prevalence of spousal abuse and other forms of personal and domestic violence. The breakdown in the family unit that accompanied this violence required the removal of children from families, often into unsuitable environments. The situation of mothers was not improved.
Generation 4	Trauma is re-enacted and directed at spouse and child. The family unit and societal norms of acceptable behaviour are seriously challenged.
Generation 5	The cycle of violence is repeated and compounded, increasingly severe violence and increasing societal distress.

Source: Atkinson et al. (2010)

Table 28.3: Summary of nutrition issues for Aboriginal and Torres Strait Islander peoples

Issue	Summary
Food access and affordability	Food prices in remote areas are routinely identified as being higher than those in other jurisdictions. The Queensland Healthy Basket Survey (Queensland Department of Health 2015) identified food prices as being about 26% higher in remote areas; another study found prices to be 60–68% higher in remote areas compared to Darwin and Adelaide respectively (Ferguson et al. 2016). Food access is another significant issue with weather conditions, transport systems and storage conditions influencing the types and quality of foods available in remote areas.
Maternal and infant nutrition	Good nutrition throughout the first 1000 days is essential for optimal growth and health. Aboriginal and Torres Strait Islander mothers were 1.6 times more likely to be obese, 1.3 times more likely to develop gestational diabetes and 3.6 times more likely to have pre-existing diabetes. All of these conditions can impact on infant outcomes. Aboriginal and Torres Strait Islander babies were more likely to be born preterm (14% compared to 8%) and more likely to have a low birthweight (<2500 g) (12% compared to 6%) (AIHW 2017).
Iron deficiency anaemia	Fifteen per cent of Aboriginal women have iron deficiency anaemia during pregnancy and up to 25% of Aboriginal children aged 6 months–5 years also have iron deficiency anaemia, with the highest prevalence of 31% identified in those aged 6–11 months (Rumbold et al. 2011). Poor quality complementary foods (first foods) that are low in iron contribute to the issue (see Chapter 21) (Leonard et al. 2017).
Poor dietary intake	Very few Aboriginal and Torres Strait Islander people meet dietary recommendations for intake of healthy foods. Energy-dense/nutrient-poor foods constitute 41% of daily energy intake for Indigenous Australians compared to 35% for non-Indigenous Australians (Anderson et al. 2016). Aboriginal and Torres Strait Islander adults consumed on average 2.1 serves of vegetable and one serve of fruit, which, after adjusting for age, is less than for non-Indigenous Australians.
Overweight and obesity	Two-thirds of Aboriginal and Torres Strait Islander people aged 15 years or older were classified as overweight (29%) or obese (37%). Overweight/obesity levels were higher for people living in non-remote areas (67%) than for those living in remote areas (62%) (ABS 2014).
Chronic conditions	Chronic conditions are major contributors to the mortality gap between Aboriginal and Torres Strait Islander people and other Australians. About 80% of the mortality gap for people aged 35–74 years is due to heart diseases, diabetes, liver diseases, chronic lower respiratory disease, cerebrovascular diseases and cancer (AIHW 2011).

ABORIGINAL AND TORRES STRAIT ISLANDER DEFINITION OF HEALTH

The accepted definition of health from an Aboriginal and Torres Strait Islander perspective has been described by the National Aboriginal Community Controlled Health Organisation as:

not just the physical well-being of an individual but ... the social, emotional and cultural well-being of the whole Community in which each individual is able to achieve their full potential as a human being thereby bringing about the total well-being of their Community. It is a whole of life view and includes the cyclical concept of life–death–life. (NACCHO 2018)

The Indigenous concept of health is broad, embracing community, family and individual, and including physical, spiritual, mental, environmental, social and emotional aspects. Health encompasses not only the physical body but also the spiritual world and the land.

Part of this concept of health is the link to 'country', an interdependent relationship between Aboriginal and Torres Strait Islander peoples and their ancestral lands and seas. Country consists of people, animals, plants, **Dreamings**, earth, soil, minerals, water and air. The dual effects of being forcibly removed from country, as well as the environmental degradation of remote areas due to declining land management practices, weeds, wildfires and introduced animals, impacts on health in a way that is not taken into consideration in a Western healthcare system (Burgess et al. 2005). Caring for country has been linked directly to better health outcomes, including lower prevalence of obesity and chronic disease (Burgess et al. 2005).

COMMUNICATING WITH ABORIGINAL AND TORRES STRAIT ISLANDER PEOPLES

Everyone has a different way of communicating but there are some aspects that are culturally derived. These tips are not definitive for all people and should be used as a guide only.

1. English may not be the first language. Many Aboriginal and Torres Strait Islander people do not speak English as a first language. Some also speak a different dialect of English. If this is the case:
   - avoid jargon and complex words
   - explain why you need to ask questions
   - use pictures, videos and other visual ways to explain complex concepts
   - ask for assistance from local Aboriginal and Torres Strait Islander staff.
2. Concept of time. Most Western cultures view time as sequential but for other cultures this may not be the case. Often family commitments will take precedence over appointments or meetings. Flexible appointment times may need to be provided. Take time to build rapport and relationships and try not to rush explanations.
3. Silence. Extended periods of silence in conversations with Aboriginal and Torres Strait Islander people are considered the norm. Silence is used to show respect or consensus. Silence should not be taken as lack of understanding or agreement. Provide adequate time and seek clarification if you are unsure.
4. Eye contact. For many Aboriginal and Torres Strait Islander people avoidance of eye contact is a sign of respect. Making direct eye contact may be considered rude, disrespectful or aggressive. Follow the other person's lead and modify eye contact accordingly.
5. Titles. In Aboriginal and Torres Strait Islander culture the titles 'aunty' and 'uncle' are used as a sign of respect. Only address people with these titles if approval has been given or a positive relationship exists.
6. Questioning. In Aboriginal and Torres Strait Islander cultures, direct questioning may lead to misunderstanding and may make it difficult to obtain information. Use a roundabout way of questioning, such as making a statement rather than asking a question.
7. The use of 'yes'. Sometimes people may say yes or have a tendency to agree with questions when they don't understand, do not want to answer, because they feel uncomfortable or because they want the conversation to end. Building rapport, understanding non-verbal cues and reading and understanding verbal cues are integral to communication.

basis in environmental and social issues that need to be addressed upstream. These include ensuring an adequate income, improved food availability and access, housing infrastructure, reduced overcrowding and improved educational opportunities.

NEW ZEALAND FIRST NATIONS PEOPLES: MĀORI

> Te ngahuru tikotikoiere
> Ko Poutu-te-rangi te mātahi o te tau
> Te putunga o te hinu, e tama!
>
> Hence the bounteous harvest time
> When the star Poutu-te-rangi brings forth the
> first-fruits of the year
> And the calabashes overflow with game fat, O Son!
> (Ngata & Jones 2005)

The final lines of this traditional oriori or lullaby from the east coast of the North Island celebrate the autumn harvest. The song is sung to assure a child they will be nourished and it describes the many foods available to a child and especially narrates the origins of kumara. The lyrics highlight that a safe and abundant food supply has always been an important issue for Māori and food remains intrinsic to Māori wellbeing and identity today.

The ancestors of Māori were the first humans to discover New Zealand, around AD 1300 (Anderson et al. 2014). They found an environment very different to their Eastern Polynesian island homelands. Early food sources included easy sources of protein, such as the flightless moa and seals (Anderson et al. 2014) Fishing practices were adapted to deal with larger, rougher harbours rather than settled lagoons (Durie 1998). Several varieties of fish and shellfish were eaten, and people would work together to make communal resources such as nets. Archaeological evidence shows extensive gardens and kumara (sweet potato), hue (gourds), uwhi (yams) and taro were cultivated (Roskruge 2007). The seeds of these species had been brought from Polynesia and innovative practices were developed to grow these in New Zealand's colder climate.

The edible plants of New Zealand forests were identified and food sources included fern roots (aruhe), shoots (pikopiko), many varieties of berries, and mushrooms (Roskruge 2007). Ti kouka (cabbage tree) leaves were eaten and young plants' roots became sweet when cooked to produce a food known as kouru (Roskruge 2007). The edible foods from rivers and lakes included tuna (eels) as well as freshwater crayfish (koura) and mussels (kakahi). The juvenile species of native fish were eaten in a food known as inanga (whitebait).

Systems were developed to manage food resources sustainably, such as placing restrictions on taking food at certain times of the year (Durie 1998). The year was divided into a calendar based on the moon cycle, and certain foods were harvested at each time to take advantage of the seasonal abundance. Food was preserved through a variety of methods (e.g. dried, or smoked) so that it would be available out of season (Anderson 1998). Huahua was the name given to birds preserved in their own fat and stored in calabashes and they were highly prized. Food resources were shared collectively, and the right to harvest food in certain areas was determined through ancestry (Anderson et al. 2014). Food was traded between peoples living in different localities, and areas of New Zealand were well-known for a specific kind of food. For example, the islands of Te Ara a Kiwa (Foveaux Strait) were known for the bird titi (sooty shearwater) (Anderson 1998).

The arrival of Europeans in New Zealand post-1769 increased the variety of food sources available to Māori. Particularly significant was the potato, which facilitated year-long settlement in the southern parts of New Zealand, and trade in the northern parts (Anderson 1998; Anderson et al. 2014). Farm animals, especially pigs, were also traded for European goods. At the time, commodities such as sugar, flour, alcohol and tobacco were introduced to Māori. Prior to 1860, Māori communities used their extensive land resources to produce food and participate in the settler economy. The early settlement of Auckland, for example, relied on produce from the Waikato and Northland (O'Malley 2016). Some Iwi (the Māori word for tribe) exported their food as far as Australia and several owned resources such as shipping vessels or flour-mills. After 1860 Māori participation in the economy diminished, as the settler government asserted its power and alienated Māori from their land. A variety of methods were used such as unjust land purchases, war and subsequent land confiscation, or the individualisation of land titles via land court processes (Anderson et al. 2014; O'Malley 2016). This system, as well as freeing up land for European settlement, was also a deliberate attempt to break down the communal structure of Māori society.

The loss of land left Māori communities impoverished and Māori health and life expectancy dramatically declined (Reid & Cram 2005). This decline was arrested around the turn of the 19th century through the work of Māori doctors utilising public health methods to improve the health of Māori communities (Durie 1998; Lange 1999). In the early 1900s Māori communities were largely rural, and many still practised communal gardening or fishing activities (Roskruge 2007). Rapid urbanisation following World War 2 resulted in many Māori families becoming city-based in urban centres such as Auckland or Wellington (Pool 1991). Māori were encouraged into work in manufacturing and labouring industries, and New Zealand's education system actively discouraged Māori from academic pursuits (Theodore et al. 2015). Food patterns changed to reflect the food available in retail outlets in cities.

Demographics and health

After 1984, New Zealand governments successively introduced a raft of economic restructuring that negatively impacted on Māori. Māori were more likely to work in industries impacted by the restructuring so unemployment levels rose, peaking at 27.3 per cent in 1992 (Poata-Smith 2013). In 1991 social security benefit entitlements were also reduced, leading to many Māori families experiencing economic hardship. Food bank use rose in New Zealand in this period. In 2013, 23.5 per cent of the Māori population lived in the most socioeconomically deprived areas of New Zealand, compared with 6.8 per cent of non-Māori (MOH 2015b). The 1997, 2002 and 2008/09 National Nutrition Surveys reported Māori experiencing a greater burden of food insecurity than non-Māori New Zealanders (MOH 2003b, 2010; Russell et al. 1999). In 2008–2009, only one-third (33.3 per cent) of Māori females reported living in households that were fully food secure, and half (48.3 per cent) reported they experienced moderate food security. That is, they responded positively to the statement ('I/we can afford to eat properly') but also to statements such as 'food runs out due to a lack of money', or they reported experiencing stress because of not having enough money for food (Parnell et al. 2011). Of concern were the 18.4 per cent of Māori females who reported living in households of low food security, in that they needed to rely on others for food or money for food, or they reported using special food grants or food banks (Parnell et al. 2011). In 2010 and 2011, Regional Public Health in Wellington calculated that families living on low incomes in their region needed to spend 43–89 per cent of their income after rent to purchase food that would provide a basic healthy diet in line with New Zealand nutrition guidelines.

Today, Māori experience a higher burden of nutrition-related disease than other New Zealanders. Specifically, rates of obesity, heart disease and diabetes are higher for Māori than non-Māori (MOH 2015b; Parnell et al. 2011). Children's obesity is also of concern. These rates are related to the higher socioeconomic deprivation experienced by Māori; for example, 20 per cent of children in New Zealand living in socioeconomically deprived areas are obese compared to 4 per cent living in the least deprived areas. There is also evidence Māori are more likely to experience racial discrimination than non-Māori, and this impacts on a wide range of risk factors for health (MOH 2015b).

Today, approximately one in seven people living in New Zealand identify as belonging to the Māori ethnic group (598,605 in 2013). In the 1990s, the growth of Māori health organisations led to the establishment of many nutrition programs specifically tailored to Māori communities. Examples include programs developed by Māori dietitians Hiki Pihema and Makuini McKerchar and others (Pihema 1989;

Tunks, Moewaka-Barnes, Dacey & Pardoe-Ropata 1998). These programs were evaluated as effective for Māori communities because they were informed by a Māori world view and used Māori staff who were able to work with their communities (Tunks, Moewaka-Barnes, Dacey & Pardoe-Ropata 1998; Tunks, Moewaka-Barnes, Dacey, Porima, et al. 1998). Māori health providers also partnered with research institutions to build the evidence base for community interventions. The Ngati and healthy diabetes intervention program on the east coast of New Zealand is one example where Ngati Porou Hauora worked with the University of Otago (Tipene-Leach et al. 2013). This intervention—featuring community-responsive health promotion, monitoring of high-risk individuals and a structural approach to adapt the local environment—was successful in improving the health of the community in relation to diabetes, specifically insulin resistance (Coppell et al. 2009).

The government of New Zealand has responded to Māori nutrition-related issues through a variety of policies. The most comprehensive national strategy relating to nutrition, Healthy Eating–Healthy Action (Oranga Kai–Oranga Pumau), was launched in 2003 (MOH 2003a). This ambitious strategy was informed by the **Ottawa Charter** and focused on environmental changes in school, community and workplace settings. This policy was significant in that it recognised the principles of the Treaty of Waitangi and actively involved Māori in its development and implementation. The policy supported Māori communities to develop their own strategies, and several developed their own healthy personal behaviour programs (HEHA Strategy Evaluation Consortium 2009; Lakes District Health Board 2010). Funding for this program was cut in 2011 and the program abandoned following a change of government in 2008. Since 2008, the government's approach to nutrition and obesity prevention

---

INDIVIDUALISTIC VERSUS COLLECTIVIST CULTURES

Collectivism is a social pattern consisting of closely linked individuals who see themselves as parts of one or more collectives (family, co-workers, tribe, nation). They are willing to give priority to the goals of these collectives over their own personal goals. They are interdependent. Individualism is a social pattern that consists of loosely linked individuals who view themselves as independent of collectives. They are motivated by their own preferences and needs and give priority to personal goals. They are independent.

Here are some examples of individualistic (I) versus collective (C) cultural behaviours. Which ones do you relate to more?

- Group harmony is more important than your own personal opinion (C).
- You are expected to speak up and state your opinion even if that is contrary to those of the group (I).
- A man marries a woman his parents disapprove of (I).
- A woman marries a man her parents have hand-picked (C).
- A waiter brings one menu for four people and gives it to the 'senior' member of the group, who orders the same food for all (C).
- Each member of a group orders a different meal at a restaurant (I).
- An older woman scolds a mother she does not know because she thinks the mother has not wrapped her child warmly enough (C).
- A worker does not mention to his supervisor that his father has just died (I).

has focused on educating people to make better choices and be 'self-managing', rather than policies that emphasise a broader environmental focus (Ministry of Health 2015a). This approach has been questioned by Māori and public health academics, as it is unlikely to reduce the disparities in nutrition experienced by Māori (Theodore et al. 2015). They have instead advocated for the New Zealand government to create healthier food environments by addressing the cost and availability of healthy and unhealthy foods, limiting unhealthy food marketing and reducing the socioeconomic disparities that drive current health inequities, including obesity (Theodore et al. 2015).

Māori also recognise the importance of the environment in relation to health and food (Durie 1999; Panelli & Tipa 2009). Customary food gathering sites and practices are named **mahinga kai** (Pehi et al. 2009).

The loss of mahinga kai sites due to environmental degradation has long been the focus of protest by Iwi (McKerchar et al. 2015). Early examples include disputes between Māori and pastoralists over the water levels of the Wairarapa lakes in the 1880s (Wairau 2002) or, around 1913, Māori leader Whina Cooper leading her first protest at the age of 18 over the draining of mudflats that had traditionally been a source of seafood for the Iwi (King 1983). Since 1985, Iwi have been able to go to the Waitangi Tribunal to seek redress for Crown breaches of the Treaty of Waitangi. Many early claims were to do with the environmental pollution of food sources— for example, the Kaituna River claim by Ngati Pikiao (Waitangi Tribunal 2016). As Iwi and the Crown have worked through the claims process, there are increasing examples of Māori participation in the management of local waterways such as the Waikato River, the Te Arawa lakes in Rotorua and

the Whanganui River (Bennett 2010). There are also several examples from the South Island of work by the local Iwi to improve the health of waterways in order to improve mahinga kai (Pauling 2010). However, the struggle to protect the environment remains ongoing, with recent examples of Iwi in Taranaki or on the east coast protesting the possible environmental degradation of the seabed through mining (sand or oil) (Radio New Zealand 2011, 2016). Climate change poses new threats to Iwi based in coastal communities and to food security more generally (Jones et al. 2014).

The above examples highlight that, for Indigenous peoples, the 'right to food' is tied closely to broader political determinants of health (Damman et al. 2008; United Nations 2008). There are recent initiatives by Māori communities to reclaim **food sovereignty** or a sense of control over local food systems. For example, in Christchurch, Māori woman Jade Temepara started a social enterprise called Kakano Café which is based on food grown and gathered locally, with an emphasis on using traditional ingredients (Te Runanga o Ngai Tahu 2016). Dr Taima Moeke-Pickering carried out research with Māori involved in gardening and food gathering initiatives, and the importance of reviving practices of growing, preparing and obtaining Māori foods was emphasised by participants as a medium for passing on traditional knowledge and improving food security and health (Moeke-Pickering et al. 2015).

To summarise, current Māori health status in relation to food and nutrition is largely an outcome of historical factors that have shaped the socio-economic and environmental determinants of health for Māori today. While there are significant challenges faced by Māori, there are also many examples from history of the ability to overcome these.

SUMMARY

- Indigenous peoples refers to groups of people who self-identify and have a historical continuity with and occupation of land prior to invasion and colonisation. Indigenous peoples make up 5 per cent of the world's populations but 15 per cent of the extreme poor.
- Most Indigenous peoples globally have shared histories of exploitation, discrimination and the neglect of human rights, resulting in a disproportionate number suffering from poverty, marginalisation, poor health, poor housing and poor access to education.
- The abuse of the human rights of Indigenous peoples has prompted the United Nations to issue a Declaration on the Rights of Indigenous Peoples. The declaration is non-binding but is a statement of aspiration on how Indigenous peoples should be treated.
- Food is an integral component of Indigenous culture, spirituality and health as it provides a tangible link between country (land), identity, spirituality, culture and health.
- Australian Aboriginal and Torres Strait Islander peoples have inhabited the lands and islands of what is now called Australia for millennia. They were, prior to colonisation (or invasion), predominantly hunter-gatherers with some evidence of cultivation and herding. The diet was low in fat, high in protein and met most micronutrient requirements.
- Since colonisation there has been a systematic, politically endorsed annihilation of the Aboriginal and Torres Strait Islander and Māori peoples and ways of life. This has resulted in the breakdown of social structures, intergenerational trauma and ongoing physical and mental health issues. Loss of land undermines economic security, health and wellbeing, sociocultural cohesion and human dignity.
- Australian and New Zealand Indigenous peoples suffer a higher burden of disease from chronic conditions and mental health issues. This has led in Australia to the Closing the Gap campaign, which refers to reducing the ten-year gap in age at death that exists between Aboriginal and non-Aboriginal people.
- The focus on improving nutritional status for Aboriginal, Torres Strait Islander and Māori peoples has been limited in both Australia and New Zealand. The ongoing focus on promoting individual responsibility is not likely to work for collectivist cultures.

KEY TERMS

Dreaming: a world view that provides an explanation of creation, a set of plans for all living forms and a set of rules for living.

Food sovereignty: the ability of Indigenous peoples to continue to grow, gather or hunt traditional foods. It promotes everyone's right to access culturally appropriate and nutritious food grown and distributed in ethical and ecologically sound ways.

Healing: within an Indigenous context, healing works towards reclaiming balance and harmony between the physical, psychological, social, cultural and spiritual dimensions of health (Mackean 2009). This healing is not necessarily related to the individual. As a kin–based society, individuals are defined first by their relationships—they are not seen as autonomous (McDonald 2006). Healing may not necessarily be a matter of privacy or confidentiality; rather, it is a community witnessing that requires group consultations and the involvement of kin (McDonald 2006).

Indigenous: Within Australia and internationally, when referring to First Peoples, the word 'Indigenous' is capitalised. For example, within the Australian context reference is made to Indigenous Australians.

Mahinga Kai: Māori term for food gathering or cultivation sites. Kai is Māori for food.

Ottawa Charter: a health promotion framework developed in 1986 to guide interventions. It has three basic strategies: advocate, enable and mediate; and six areas for priority action: build healthy public policy, create supportive environments, strengthen community actions, develop personal skills, reorient health services, move into the future.

Terra nullius: Latin for 'nobody's land'; legal term for land that is unoccupied or uninhabited. It was used in the colonisation of Australia to deny Aboriginal and Torres Strait Islander sovereignty.

REFERENCES

ABS, 2014, *Australian Aboriginal and Torres Strait Islander Health Survey: Updated results, 2012–13*, <www.abs.gov.au/ausstats/abs@.nsf/mf/4727.0.55.006>, accessed 19 December 2018

—— 2016, *Causes of Death, Australia 2014*, <www.abs.gov.au/ausstats/abs@.nsf/Lookup/by%20Subject/3303.0~2014~Main%20Features~Infant%20Mortality~10023>, accessed 18 December 2018

—— 2017, *Census: Aboriginal and Torres Strait Islander Population*, <www.abs.gov.au/ausstats/abs@.nsf/Media RealesesByCatalogue/02D50FAA9987D6B7CA25814800087E03?OpenDocument>, accessed 18 December 2018

AIHW, 2011, *Contribution of Chronic Disease to the Gap in Adult Mortality Between Aboriginal and Torres Strait Islander and Other Australians*, <www.aihw.gov.au/getmedia/79b73a27-c970-47f0-931b-32d7badade40/12304.pdf.aspx?inline=true>, accessed 18 February 2018

—— 2017, *Australia's Mothers and Babies 2015—In brief*, <www.aihw.gov.au/getmedia/728e7dc2-ced6-47b7-addd-befc9d95af2d/aihw-per-91-inbrief.pdf.aspx?inline=true>, accessed 24 February 2019

Anderson, A., 1998, *The Welcome of Strangers: An ethnohistory of southern Maori A.D. 1650–1850*, Otago: University of Otago Press

Anderson, A., Binney, J. & Harris, A., 2014, *Tangata Whenua: An illustrated history*, Wellington: Bridget Williams Books.

Anderson, I., Robson, B., Connolly, M., Al-Yaman, F., Bjertness, E. et al., 2016, 'Indigenous and tribal peoples' health (The *Lancet*–Lowitja Institute Global Collaboration): A population study', *Lancet, 388*(10040): 131–57, doi:10.1016/S0140-6736(16)00345-7

Armitage, A., 1995, *Comparing the Policy of Aboriginal Assimilation: Australia, Canada and New Zealand*, Vancouver: UBC Press

Atkinson, J., Nelson, J. & Atkinson, C., 2010, 'Trauma, transgenerational transfer and effects on community wellbeing', in N. Purdie, P. Dudgeon & R. Walker (eds), *Working Together: Aboriginal and Torres Strait Islander mental health and wellbeing principles and practice*, Canberra: Australian Council of Educational Research, pp. 135–44

Attwood, B. & Markus, A., 2007, *The 1967 Referendum: Race, power, and the Australian Constitution*, Canberra: Australian Aboriginal Studies Press

Australian Human Rights Commission, 2018, *United Nations Declaration on the Rights of Indigenous Peoples*, <www.humanrights.gov.au/publications/un-declaration-rights-indigenous-peoples-1>, accessed 18 December 2018

Australian Native Title Tribunal, 1996, *What is Native Title?*, <www.nntt.gov.au/News-and-Publications/latest-news/Pages/What_is_native_title_27_September_1996.aspx>, accessed 18 December 2018

Belgrave, M., Kawharu, M. & Williams, D.V., 2005, *Waitangi Revisited: Perspectives on the Treaty of Waitangi*, Melbourne: Oxford University Press

Bennett, A., 2010, 'Uncharted waters—Recent settlements as new spaces for enhancing Māori participation in fresh-water management and decision making', in R. Selby, P. Moore & M. Mulholland (eds), *Māori and the Environment: Kaitiaki*, Wellington: Huia Publishers, pp. 175–84

Burgess, C.P., Johnston, F.H., Bowman, D.M. & Whitehead, P.J., 2005, 'Healthy country: Healthy people? Exploring the health benefits of Indigenous natural resource management', *Australian and New Zealand Journal of Public Health, 29*(2): 117–22, doi:10.1111/j.1467-842X.2005.tb00060.x

Campbell, D., Pyett, P., McCarthy, L., Whiteside, M. & Tsey, K., 2007, 'Community development and empowerment: A review of interventions to improve Aboriginal health', in I. Anderson, F. Baum & M. Bentley (eds), *Beyond Bandaids: Exploring the underlying social determinants of Aboriginal health*: Cooperative Research Centre for Aboriginal Health, pp. 165–80

Close the Gap Campaign Steering Committee for Indigenous Equality, 2018, *A Ten-year Review: The Closing the Gap strategy and recommendations for reset*, <www.humanrights.gov.au/social_justice/health/index.html> and <www.oxfam.org.au/closethegap>, accessed 22 February 2019

Coppell, K.J., Tipene-Leach, D.C., Pahau, H.L., Williams, S.M., Abel, S. et al., 2009, 'Two-year results from a community-wide diabetes prevention intervention in a high risk Indigenous community: The Ngati and Healthy project', *Diabetes Research and Clinical Practice, 85*(2): 220–7, doi:10.1016/j.diabres.2009.05.009

Creative Spirits, 2018, *How to Name Aboriginal People?*, <www.creativespirits.info/aboriginalculture/people/how-to-name-aboriginal-people>, accessed 16 December 2018

Cunningham, C. & Stanley, F., 2003, 'Indigenous by definition, experience, or world view', *BMJ, 327*(7412): 403–4, doi:10.1136/bmj.327.7412.403

Damman, S., Eide, W.B. & Kuhnlein, H.V., 2008, 'Indigenous peoples' nutrition transition in a right to food perspective', *Food Policy, 33*(2): 135–55, doi:10.1016/j.foodpol.2007.08.002

Dixon, J. & Scheurell, R.P., 1995, *Social Welfare for Indigenous Peoples*, New York, NY: Routledge

Durie, M., 1998, *Whaiora Māori Health Development*, Auckland: Oxford University Press

—— 1999, *Te Pae Māhutonga: A model for Māori health promotion*, paper presented at the Health Promotion Forum of New Zealand

Ferguson, M., Brown, C., Georga, C., Miles, E., Wilson, A. & Brimblecombe, J., 2017, 'Traditional food availability and consumption in remote Aboriginal communities in the Northern Territory, Australia', *Australian and New Zealand Journal of Public Health, 41*(3): 294–8, doi:10.1111/1753-6405.12664

Ferguson, M., O'Dea, K., Chatfield, M., Moodie, M., Altman, J. & Brimblecombe, J., 2016, 'The comparative cost of food and beverages at remote Indigenous communities, Northern Territory, Australia', *Australian and New Zealand Journal of Public Health, 40*(Suppl. 1): S21–S26, doi:10.1111/1753-6405.12370

Foley, W., 2005, 'Tradition and change in urban indigenous food practices', *Postcolonial Studies, 8*(1): 25–44, doi:10.1080/13688790500134356

Freemantle, J., Ring, I., Arambula Solomon, T.G., Gachupin, F.C., Smylie, J. et al., 2014, 'Indigenous mortality (revealed): The invisible illuminated', *American Journal of Public Health, 105*(4): 644–52, doi:10.2105/AJPH.2014.301994

Gracey, M., 2000, 'Historical, cultural, political, and social influences on dietary patterns and nutrition in Australian Aboriginal children', *American Journal of Clinical Nutrition, 72*(5): 1361s–7s, doi:10.1093/ajcn/72.5.1361s

Gracey, M. & King, M., 2009, 'Indigenous health part 1: Determinants and disease patterns', *Lancet, 374*(9683): 65–75, doi:10.1016/S0140-6736(09)60914-4

HEHA Strategy Evaluation Consortium, 2009, *Healthy Eating—Healthy Action: Oranga Kai—Oranga Pumau strategy evaluation: Interim report*, <http://weightmanagement.hiirc.org.nz/page/21622/healthy-eating-healthy-action-oranga-kai/?tab=138&contentType=194>, accessed 18 February 2018

Hill, K., Barker, B. & Vos, T., 2007, 'Excess Indigenous mortality: Are Indigenous Australians more severely disadvantaged than other Indigenous populations?', *International Journal of Epidemiology, 36*(3): 580–9, doi:10.1093/ije/dym011

International Work Group for Indigenous Affairs, 2018, *The Indigenous World 2018*, <www.iwgia.org/en/resources/publications/305-books/3327-the-indigenous-world-2018>, accessed 22 February 2019

Jones, R., Bennett, H., Keating, G. & Blaiklock, A., 2014, 'Climate change and the right to health for Māori in Aotearoa/New Zealand', *Health and Human Rights Journal, 16*(1): 54–68, <www.jstor.org/stable/10.2307/healhumarigh.16.1.54>, accessed 22 February 2019

King, M., 1983, *Whina: A biography of Whina Cooper*, London: Hodder & Stoughton

Kirmayer, L.J., Gone, J.P. & Moses, J., 2014, 'Rethinking historical trauma', *Transcultural Psychiatry, 51*(3): 299–319, doi:10.1177/1363461514536358

Kouris-Blazos, A. & Wahlqvist, M., 2000, 'Indigenous Australian food culture on cattle stations prior to the 1960s and food intake of older Aborigines in a community studied in 1988', *Asia Pacific Journal of Clinical Nutrition, 9*(3): 224–31, doi:10.1046/j.1440–6047.2000.00189.x

Kuhnlein, H., Erasmus, B., Creed-Kanashiro, H., Englberger, L., Okeke, C. et al., 2006, 'Indigenous peoples' food systems for health: Finding interventions that work', *Public Health Nutrition, 9*(8): 1013–19, doi:10.1017/PHN2006987

Lakes District Health Board, 2010, *Heha Maori at Lakes District Health Board: A special journey*, <www.lakesdhb.govt.nz/Article.aspx?ID=3028>, accessed 24 February 2019

Lange, R., 1999, *May the People Live: A history of Maori health development 1900–1920*, Auckland: Auckland University Press

Leonard, D., Aquino, D., Hadgraft, N., Thompson, F. & Marley, J.V., 2017, 'Poor nutrition from first foods: A cross-sectional study of complementary feeding of infants and young children in six remote Aboriginal communities across northern Australia', *Nutrition & Dietetics, 74*(5): 436–45, doi:10.1111/1747-0080.12386

McDonald, H., 2006, 'East Kimberley concepts of health and illness: A contribution to intercultural health programs in northern Australia', *Australian Aboriginal Studies, 2*: 86, <https://search.informit.com.au/fullText;dn=429992484938647;res=IELAPA>, accessed 22 February 2019

Mackean, T., 2009, 'A healed and healthy country: Understanding healing for Indigenous Australians', *Medical Journal of Australia, 190*(10): 522–3, doi:10.5694/j.1326-5377.2009.tb02545.x

McKerchar, C., Bowers, S., Heta, C., Signal, L. & Matoe, L., 2015, 'Enhancing Māori food security using traditional kai', *Global Health Promotion, 22*(3): 15–24, doi:10.1177/1757975914543573

MOH, 2003a, *Healthy Eating—Healthy Action: Oranga Kai—Oranga Pumau*, <www.health.govt.nz/publication/healthy-eating-healthy-action-oranga-kai-oranga-pumau-strategic-framework>, accessed 24 February 2019

—— 2003b, *NZ Food, NZ Children: Key results of the 2002 National Children's Nutrition Survey*, <www.health.govt.nz/publication/nz-food-nz-children>, accessed 24 February 2019

—— 2010, *2008/09 Adult Nutrition Survey*, <www.moh.govt.nz/moh.nsf/indexmh/dataandstatistics-survey-nutrition>, accessed 1 September 2010

—— 2015a, *Childhood Obesity Plan*, <www.Health.Govt.Nz/our-work/diseases-and-conditions/obesity/childhood-obesity-plan>, accessed 20 August 2017

—— 2015b, *Tatau Kahukura: Māori Health Chart Book 2015* (3rd edn), Wellington: Ministry of Health

Moeke-Pickering, T., Heitia, M., Heitia, S., Karapu, R. & Cote-Meek, S., 2015, 'Understanding Māori food security and food sovereignty issues in Whakatāne', *MAI Journal, 4*(1): 29–42, <http://www.journal.mai.ac.nz/sites/default/files/MAIJrnl_V4Iss1_Pickering.pdf>, accessed 22 February 2019

NACCHO, 2018, *Aboriginal Health*, <www.naccho.org.au/about/aboriginal-health/definitions/>, accessed 18 December 2018

Ngata, A.T. & Jones, P.T.H., 2005, *Ngā Mōteatea: He maramara rere nō nga waka maha*, Auckland: Auckland University Press

O'Malley, V., 2016, *The Great War for New Zealand Waikato 1800–2000*, Wellington: Bridget Williams Books

Panelli, R. & Tipa, G., 2009, 'Beyond foodscapes: Considering geographies of Indigenous well-being', *Health & Place, 15*(2): 455–65, doi:10.1016/j.healthplace.2008.08.005

Parnell, W., Wilson, N., Thomson, C., Mackay, S. & Stefanogiannis, N., 2011, *A Focus on Nutrition: Key findings of the 2008/09 New Zealand Adult Nutrition Survey*, <www.health.govt.nz/publication/focus-nutrition-key-findings-2008-09-nz-adult-nutrition-survey>, accessed 18 February 2018

Pascoe, B., 2014, *Dark Emu Black Seeds: Agriculture or accident?*, Broome: Magabala Books

Pauling, C., 2010, 'Ngā wai pounamu: The state of South Island waterways, a ngai tahu perspective', in R. Selby, P. Moore & M. Mulholland (eds), *Māori and the Environment: Kaitiaki*, Wellington: Huia Publishers, pp. 141–54

Pehi, P., Kanawa, L., Lambert, S. & Allen, W., 2009, *The Restitution of Marae and Communities Through Mahinga Kai: Building the management of Maori customary fisheries'*, Auckland: Nga Pae o te Maramatanga and Otago University

Pihema, H., 1989, 'Food and nutrition education: Education for Maori people', *Proceedings of the Nutrition Society of New Zealand, 14*: 137–42, <https://natlib.govt.nz/records/20708987>, accessed 17 July 2019

Poata-Smith, E.T.A., 2013, 'Inequality and Maori', in M. Rashbrooke (ed.), *Inequality: A New Zealand crisis,* Wellington: Bridget Williams Books, pp. 148–58

Pool, I., 1991, *Te Iwi Māori: A New Zealand population past, present and projected,* Auckland: Auckland University Press

Queensland Department of Health, 2015, *Healthy Food Basket Access Survey 2014,* <www.health.qld.gov.au/research-reports/reports/public-health/food-nutrition/access/overview>, accessed 12 December 2018

Radio New Zealand, 2011, 'Hundreds attend oil exploration protests', <www.Radionz.Co.Nz/news/national/73404/hundreds-attend-oil-exploration-protests>, accessed 17 July 2019

—— 2016, 'Seabed mining plan draws 6000 opponents', <www.Radionz.Co.Nz/news/national/313707/seabed-mining-plan-draws-6000-opponents>, accessed 17 July 2019

Referendum Council, 2017, *Uluru Statement from the Heart,* <www.referendumcouncil.org.au/sites/default/files/2017-05/Uluru_Statement_From_The_Heart_0.PDF>, accessed 18 December 2018

Reid, P. & Cram, F., 2005, 'Connecting health, people and country in Aotearoa New Zealand', in K. Dew & P. Davis (eds), *Health and Society in Aotearoa New Zealand,* Melbourne: Oxford University Press

Roskruge, N., 2007, 'Hokia Ki Te Whenua' (Doctor of Philosophy), Massey University, Auckland, NZ, <https://mro.massey.ac.nz/handle/10179/1725>, accessed 24 February 2019

Rowse, T., 2002, *White Flour, White Power: From rations to citizenship in Central Australia,* Cambridge: Cambridge University Press

Rumbold, A.R., Bailie, R.S., Si, D., Dowden, M.C., Kennedy, C.M. et al., 2011, 'Delivery of maternal health care in Indigenous primary care services: Baseline data for an ongoing quality improvement initiative', *BMC Pregnancy and Childbirth, 11*(1): 16, doi:10.1186/1471-2393-11-16

Russell, D.G., Parnell, W., Wilson, N., Faed, J., Ferguson, E., Herbison, P. et al, 1999, *New Zealand Food: New Zealand People—Key results of the 1997 National Nutrition Survey,* Wellington: Ministry of Health

Santich, B., 1995, *The Original Mediterranean Cuisine: Medieval recipes for today,* Mile End: Wakefield Press

Smith, P.A. & Smith, R.M., 1999, 'Diets in transition: Hunter-gatherer to station diet and station diet to the self-select store diet', *Human Ecology, 27*(1): 115–33, doi:10.1023/A:1018709401639

Smith, R. & Smith, P.A., 2003, 'An assessment of the composition and nutrient content of an Australian Aboriginal hunter-gatherer diet', *Australian Aboriginal Studies, 2*: 39–51, <https://search.informit.com.au/fullText;dn=446408132617121;res=IELAPA>, accessed 24 February 2019

Stephens, C., Nettleton, C., Porter, J., Willis, R. & Clark, S., 2005, 'Indigenous peoples' health: Why are they behind everyone, everywhere?', *Lancet, 366*(9479): 10–13, doi:10.1016/S0140-6736(05)66801-8

Strategic Inter-Governmental Nutrition Alliance, 2001, *National Aboriginal and Torres Strait Islander Nutrition Strategy and Action Plan 2000–2010,* <www.health.gov.au/internet/main/publishing.nsf/Content/health-pubhlth-strateg-food-nphp.htm>, accessed 24 February 2019

Taylor, J. & Biddle, N., 2008, *Locations of Indigenous Population Change: What can we say?,* <http://caepr.cass.anu.edu.au/sites/default/files/docs/CAEPRWP43_0.pdf>, accessed 24 February 2018

Te Runanga o Ngai Tahu, 2016, *Cafe and Cookery School Opens,* <http://ngaitahu.Iwi.Nz/our_stories/cafe-and-cookery-school-opens/>, accessed 18 December 2018

Theodore, R., McLean, R. & TeMorenga, L., 2015, 'Challenges to addressing obesity for Māori in Aotearoa/New Zealand', *Australian and New Zealand Journal of Public Health, 39*(2): 509–12, doi:10.1111/1753-6405.12418

Tipene-Leach, D.C., Coppell, K.J., Abel, S., Pāhau, H.L.R., Ehau, T. & Mann, J.I., 2013, 'Ngāti and healthy: Translating diabetes prevention evidence into community action', *Ethnicity & Health, 18*(4): 402–14, doi:10.1080/13557858.2012.754406

Tunks, M., Moewaka-Barnes, H., Dacey, B. & Pardoe-Ropata, J., 1998, *Te Taro o Te Ora—Outcome evaluation report,* Auckland: Ministry of Maori Development

Tunks, M., Moewaka-Barnes, H., Dacey, B., Porima, L. & Porima, H., 1998, *Kai o Te Hauora—Outcome evaluation report,* Auckland: Whariki, Alcohol and Public Health Research Unit, University of Auckland

Turner, N.J., Plotkin, M. & Kuhnlein, H.V., 2013, 'Global environmental challenges to the integrity of Indigenous Peoples' food systems', in H.V. Kuhnlein, B. Erasmus, D. Spigelski & B. Burlingame (eds), *Indigenous Peoples' Food Systems & Wellbeing,* Rome: FAO, pp. 23–38

United Nations, 2008, *United Nations Declaration on the Rights of Indigenous Peoples,* <www.un.org/esa/socdev/unpfii/documents/DRIPS_en.pdf>, accessed 18 December 2018

United Nations Human Rights Office of the High Commissioner, 2018, *Special Rapporteur on the Rights of Indigenous Peoples,* <www.ohchr.org/EN/Issues/IPeoples/SRIndigenousPeoples/Pages/SRIPeoplesIndex.aspx>, accessed 18 December 2018

Wairau, W., 2002, *Wairarapa Maori Ki Pouakani Research Report* Wellington: <https://forms.justice.govt.nz/search/Documents/WT/wt_DOC_94241226/Wai%20863%2C%20A029.pdf>, accessed 24 February 2019

Waitangi Tribunal, 2016, *Background to the Kaituna Claim,* <https://waitangitribunal.govt.nz/publications-and-resources/school-resources/waitangi-tribunal-and-kaituna-river-claim/background-to-the-kaituna-claim/>, accessed 24 February 2019

World Bank, 2018, 'Indigenous Peoples', <www.worldbank.org/en/topic/indigenouspeoples>, accessed 22 May 2018

Zubrick, S.R., Dudgeon, P., Gee, G., Glaskin, B., Kelly, K. et al., 2004, 'Social determinants of Aboriginal and Torres Strait Islander social and emotional wellbeing', in P. Dudgeon, H. Milroy & R. Walker (eds), *Working Together: Aboriginal and Torres Strait Islander mental health and wellbeing—Principles and practice,* Perth: Kulunga Aboriginal Research Development Unit, Telethon Kids Institute, pp. 75–90

{CHAPTER 29}
INTERNATIONAL NUTRITION AND HEALTH

Mark L. Wahlqvist

OBJECTIVES

- Describe a systems approach to international nutrition governance and solution development.
- Identify the key governmental and civil society agencies and organisations which address international nutrition and health problems.
- Summarise international nutrition issues and the impact of economic development.
- Recognise the elements of survival or emergency nutrition.

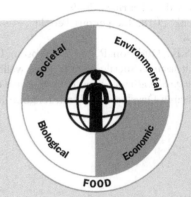

INTRODUCTION

Historically, local and international nutritional problems have been considered as principally those of food or nutrient intake inadequacy, of microbial or contaminant food-borne illness, and of increased nutritional needs in times of situational stress, or illness. However, the complexity of nutritionally related disorders and disease has become more evident with the interplay of demographic, socioeconomic, food system and environmental change, especially since colonisation, the Industrial Revolution in the 1700s and now ecological degradation and climate change. Much of this change is *borderless*, affecting peoples whose home-base has become less recognisable or who are on the move for many reasons, such as displaced persons, migrants or occasional travellers. Thus, as important as locality is for nutritional wellbeing, an international view, understanding and management of food and health is necessary and becoming more so.

The mix of nutritional problems is usually complex for reasons of locality, culture and ethnicity, demography, gender, governance, socioeconomic development, biology, health care, food, education, and other systems. For this reason, it is an analytic and problem-solving advantage not to be locked in to a particular nutritional point of view and to use systems thinking when conceptualising solutions (see Chapter 2). These actions are occurring at all levels of government, from local jurisdictions (e.g. village or local government) to state level (covering of regional areas) to national and, ultimately, international efforts. All of these efforts need to be coordinated to increase effectiveness.

This chapter reviews the governance of nutrition internationally, identifying the key agencies and systems involved. It then explores the nutrition issues that are impacted by economic development. Finally, it provides a brief introduction to the role of nutrition in emergency situations including natural disasters (drought, tsunamis) and conflict (feeding displaced people).

THE ORGANISATIONAL FRAMEWORK

Maintaining food security—and therefore the health of individuals and populations—in terms of both quantity and quality of food is an international endeavour. Technology is ensuring that the movement of people and information, as well as access to food and health care, is now much faster and more efficient. Technology is also ensuring improved access to health. However, while mobilising people and products across countries is now effective and efficient, sometimes moving food a short distance from where it is grown to market can be impossible. Australia is a good example of this conundrum. As a net exporter of food we are able to fly fresh food to a multitude of countries but are unable to supply remote Indigenous communities with fresh food year-round. It is encouraging that, in spite of conflict and climate change, some communities continue to improve their nutritional situation by means which we need to better understand and transfer to those who are in greater need (FAO et al. 2017; Hetherington et al. 2017; Rogers et al. 2012) (see Chapter 4).

Food is political. It requires vested interests from governments and industry around what and how food is grown, manufactured and traded. Such interests have led to famine, the degradation of environments and to the proliferation of ultra-processed foods. Yet feeding people to ensure health is a basic human right. In recognition of this, a collective of international, relatively apolitical organisations is involved in attempting to provide a coordinated effort to address food and nutrition issues. These are underpinned by the Sustainable Development Goals (see also chapters 4 and 26). In seeking solutions to growing dysnutrition and eco-health failures, there are a number of core principles for action.

Sound governance

In the most demanding environmental and economic circumstances, well-managed if limited food and health system resources can mitigate nutritionally related health problems (Oniang'o & Allotey 1999; Wahlqvist et al. 2009).

Societal cohesion—especially and essentially women and literacy

A consistent feature of community and household nutrition development initiatives is that women are actively involved and that they are literate (International Women's Development Agency (IWDA) 2018; Olney et al. 2013). The communication, organisational, entrepreneurial and caring capacities of women may be enhanced by availability of education, home gardens and digital technologies along with other means (Curry et al. 2016; Mehra & Rojas 2008). This links to the SDG regarding improving the education of women.

Ecological integrity

The health-promoting role of public open spaces and the ecosystems which they encompass is now acknowledged (Mitchell & Popham 2008) (see Chapter 31). As the greater part of the world's population is urbanised, how food and health systems interconnect across the rural–urban divide will be of paramount ecological importance (Wahlqvist 2014; Wolch et al. 2014). For example, how will people and crops both withstand the more extreme heat in cities and manage flood potential where hardened surfaces prevent water from soaking and nourishing the soil? Ecological integrity will be eroded in many ways by climate change.

Public and clinical health

The need for emphasis on and deployment of resources in public health to serve greater population numbers, to prevent suffering and premature death, and to take account of the planet, is evident. This strategy can embrace entire food, health and other systems. The more clinical approach can be diagnostic and therapeutic of system disorder, but in general will be less accessible, costlier and have greater intrinsic risk. For example, adequate public open space and food gardens offering physical and social activity, along with biodiverse foods, can reduce the risk of obesity and diabetes, along with their complications and associated premature mortality; the absence of these problems represents major savings in the clinical sector.

KEY INTERNATIONAL ORGANISATIONS

There are several key agencies involved in food and nutrition internationally. The United Nations has a suite of organisations, funds and programs that are intergovernmental and have a global jurisdiction. It is funded through mandatory payments from each member country and via voluntary contributions. The majority of funds support humanitarian and development assistance. For example, the mandatory contributions assist in funding the World Health Organization and voluntary payments support programs such as the World Food Programme

(WFP). The UN agencies are all focused on ensuring that human rights are upheld. These organisations are outlined in Table 29.1. In addition to the United Nations **intergovernmental organisations (IGOs)** there are a range of other non-government and philanthropic organisations that have a role.

EXAMPLES OF INTERNATIONAL GOVERNANCE

There are numerous examples of international governance and policy harmonisation in the area of nutrition—for example, the food-based dietary guidelines outlined in Chapter 19. The Sustainable Development Goals, the United Nations Decade of Action on Nutrition and Scaled Up Nutrition (SUN) are three more examples.

Sustainable Development Goals

The Sustainable Development Goals (SDGs) underpin sustainable food systems (see Chapter 4)

UNDERSTANDING INTERNATIONAL NON-GOVERNMENT NUTRITION ORGANISATIONS

There are a range of international organisations that work in the food and nutrition space. Using the skills you learned in Chapter 3, investigate a range of organisations and evaluate their websites for:

- mission, vision and activities
- funding sources
- conflicts of interest
- evidence-base of information uploaded.

Summarise each organisation and make an evaluation of its legitimacy and credibility. You can find your own organisations in addition to the ones listed below:
- Global Alliance for Improved Nutrition
- Greenpeace
- International Food Policy Research Institute
- CGIAR (formerly the Consultative Group for International Agricultural Research)
- Sight and Life
- One Thousand Days
- Food Tank
- Bill & Melinda Gates Foundation.

Table 29.1: International organisations with a food and nutrition remit

Organisation	Location of headquarters	Focus	Description	Website
Food and Agriculture Organization (FAO)	Rome	Food, agriculture and nutrition	IGO. Goal is to achieve worldwide food security. 194 member states (as of 2019). The focus is on eliminating hunger, food insecurity and malnutrition, building more productive and sustainable agriculture, forestry and fisheries, reducing rural poverty, increasing resilient livelihoods and enabling sustainable food systems.	www.fao.org
United Nations Human Rights Council (UNHRC)	Geneva	Humanitarian	IGO. The UNHRC is the guardian of the rights of refugees. It provides international protection for displaced peoples.	www.unhcr.org
United Nations Children's Fund (UNICEF)	New York City	Children's health, wellbeing and safety	IGO. UNICEF is also a registered charity. UNICEF upholds the rights of the child. Food and nutrition programs focus on immunisation, nutrition monitoring, malnutrition alleviation, breastfeeding promotion, emergency feeding, water, sanitation and hygiene.	www.unicef.org
United Nations Educational, Scientific, and Cultural Organization (UNESCO)	Paris	Education and culture	IGO. UNESCO seeks to build peace through mutual understanding and international cooperation in education, culture and science. There is a focus on Indigenous knowledges and on protecting food cultures more broadly. For example kimchi making, the French meal, and Nsima (the culinary tradition of Malawi) are all listed as intangible cultural heritage elements.	https://en.unesco.org
World Health Organization (WHO)	Geneva	Health	IGO. The WHO works towards achieving the highest possible standard of health by providing leadership, setting norms and standards, developing ethical and evidence-based policy, providing technical support and monitoring the health situation.	www.who.int
World Food Programme (WFP)	Rome	Emergency food relief	IGO. The WFP works with the most vulnerable populations to provide emergency food relief during emergencies, cash-based transfers where food is available but unaffordable, and technical support to facilitate the design and implementation of in-country strategies for alleviating food insecurity.	www.wfp.org
International Fund for Agricultural Development (IFAD)	Rome	Agriculture	IGO. IFAD focuses on sustainable rural development by increasing the productive capacity of poor rural people, increasing their benefits from market participation and strengthening environmental sustainability and climate resilience.	www.ifad.org
United Nations Environment Programme (UNEP)	Nairobi	Environment	IGO. The UNEP provides leadership on the global environmental agenda and the implementation of the environmental dimension for sustainable development.	www.unenvironment.org
United Nations Development Programme (UNDP)	New York City	Poverty	IGO. The UNDP has as its mission the eradication of poverty, and the building of livelihoods by building resilience to shocks and crises. It is responsible for the Sustainable Development Goals.	www.undp.org
United Nations System Standing Committee on Nutrition (UNSCN)		Nutrition	The UNSCN is a platform where UN agencies can have open discussions on nutrition strategies and initiatives. It functions as knowledge exchange and acts to harmonise food and nutrition policy across UN agencies. The FAO, IFAD, UNICEF, the WFP and the WHO, all of which have an explicit nutrition mandate, are members.	www.unscn.org

and sustainable food and nutrition practice (see Chapter 26). The SDGs are a set of targets that aim to address global challenges such as poverty, injustice and environmental degradation by 2030 (United Nations 2018). The 17 goals are listed in Table 29.2.

United Nations Decade of Action on Nutrition (2016–2025)

The delivery of sustainable and nutritious food to all people is the primary focus of effective food systems, thus collaborative, international action to address drivers of food system changes are necessary. Nutrition has been and will continue to be a central health, economic and sustainable development challenge for every country. It is widely recognised that nutrition challenges are complex and their solutions require strong and sustained political leadership. The UN Decade of Action on Nutrition provides an opportunity for achieving nutrition impact towards eradicating hunger and preventing all forms of malnutrition worldwide. The common vision for global action was defined by ten commitments

(Table 29.3) of the Rome Declaration on Nutrition in 2014, and they coincided with the release of the SDGs. Based on the commitments of the Rome Declaration on Nutrition, UN member states are to act across six pillars (Table 29.3) for nutrition actions.

In this context, UN member states are to set commitments for action. Obviously these commitments are country-specific, as they need to reflect national priorities and depend on each country's nutrition situation, and food and health systems. Strategies should be action-oriented and require commitments which have been designated 'SMART' (Table 29.4). SMART is a good acronym to remember whether you are developing goals and objectives for international, national, local or personal action. SMART is commonly used in developing evaluation frameworks.

Table 29.2: The UN's Sustainable Development Goals

1	End Poverty*
2	Zero Hunger*
3	Good Health and Wellbeing*
4	Quality Education*
5	Gender Equality*
6	Clean Water and Sanitation*
7	Affordable and Clean Energy*
8	Decent Work and Economic Growth*
9	Industry, Innovation and Infrastructure*
10	Reduced Inequalities*
11	Sustainable Cities and Communities*
12	Responsible Production and Consumption*
13	Climate Action*
14	Life Below Water*
15	Life on Land*
16	Peace, Justice and Strong Institutions*
17	Partnerships for the Goals

Note: * Direct link to food and nutrition

Source: United Nations (2018)

Table 29.3: Ten commitments and six pillars for the Decade of Action on Nutrition

Ten commitments
- Eradicate hunger and prevent all forms of malnutrition.
- Increase investments for effective interventions and actions to improve people's diets and nutrition.
- Enhance sustainable food systems.
- Raise the profile of nutrition with national strategies and align national resources accordingly.
- Strengthen human and institutional capacities to improve nutrition.
- Strengthen and facilitate contributions and action by all stakeholders.
- Ensure healthy diets throughout the life-course.
- Create enabling environment for making informed choices.
- Implement these ten commitments through the Framework for Action.
- Integrate the Declaration's vision and commitments into the post-2015 development agenda process.

Six pillars
- Sustainable food systems for healthy diets
- Aligned healthy systems providing universal coverage of essential nutrition actions
- Social protection and nutrition education
- Trade and investment for improved nutrition
- Enabling food and breastfeeding environments
- Review, strengthen and promote nutrition governance and accountability

Source: WHO (2018b)

SUSTAINABILITY REQUIRES SYSTEMS THINKING

To understand sustainability requires systems thinking (see Chapter 2). The UN Sustainable Development Goals (SDGs) are simplified versions to help everybody understand the dimensions of sustainability. Currently the SDGs have not been fully integrated with each other and systems thinking will be required to join up the different elements (Development Initiatives 2017). Forum for the Future, which is a non-government organisation facilitating sustainability through collaborations, has identified three levels of operation (Draper 2018):

Level 1—Joined up efforts on individual goals
The first step is to identify the system and the interlinkages, who holds the power and resources that work for or against change. Understanding the details means that the most powerful opportunities for significant change can take place. By working together the work can be complementary and synergistic.

Level 2—A network of goals
What are the interrelationships across the goals? How can we understand the different drivers and root causes of a number of different goals regionally, nationally and globally? Which goals work together to deliver a change in a system, and how do we make the most of those combinations? Mapping the activities around the individual goals will speed up progress but we also need to look across the goals at possible synergies.

Level 3—Figuring out the how
If today's systems were working, there would be no need for the SDGs. How we tackle the SDGs is as important as what needs to happen. This means an inclusive approach, revealing the assumptions that are made to enable people to take control of their own destiny.

With a colleague, brainstorm two of the SDGs and identify what systems are involved in each of these.
- What might be the synergies between them?
- How will gains in one assist with gains in the second?

Table 29.4: What does 'SMART' mean?

S = Specific	Refers to a specific action and indicates who is responsible for achieving it.
M = Measurable	Includes an indicator to enable measuring progress and achieving the commitment.
A = Achievable	Refers to a realistic context based on level of progress achieved in the past.
R = Relevant	Reflects the situation, the priorities of the locality and the challenges it faces.
T = Time-bound	The key milestones are met within a realistic timeframe for achievement.

Source: WHO & FAO (2018)

Scaling Up Nutrition (SUN)

SUN is a global collaboration for action and invest-ment to improve maternal and child nutrition. The collaborative process has evolved into a movement that is both stimulated and reinforced by political interest in nutrition among leaders of governments and development partners. Priorities and plans are established with supports from different stakeholders, including civil society, private sectors or business enterprises, academic and research institutions, development agencies, UN specialised agencies (FAO, UNICEF, WFP and WHO), nutrition-specific collaboration organisations of the UN—the Standing Committee on Nutrition (SCN) and Renewed Efforts Against Child Hunger (REACH)—and the World Bank. The vision of the SUN Movement is:

> By 2030, a world free from malnutrition in all its forms. Led by governments, supported by organisations and individuals—collective action ensures every child, adolescent, mother and family can realise their right to food and nutrition, reach their full potential and shape sustainable and prosperous societies. (Scaling Up Nutrition 2018)

Since the launch of the SUN Movement in 2010, over 60 countries and states have committed to scaling up nutrition with support from hundreds of actors or stakeholders. The SUN Movement has progressed tremendously in creating space to mobilise global support to scale up nutrition at country-level, enabling governments and their supporters to deliver better impact.

THE IMPACT OF ECONOMIC DEVELOPMENT ON NUTRITION

While there has been a focus on major and rapid changes in food habits, nutritional and health status with industrialisation and economic development, a broad spectrum of nutritionally related health problems is becoming universally entrenched. Thus, what was once seen as a conjunction of under- and overnutrition, the '**triple burden**' of nutritionally related disease in transitional economies is now more complex at all stages of economic development. This means food and physical activity energy imbalances with food component deficiencies and excesses in various combinations. The more extensive expression of complex nutritional status has been particularly evident with the appearance of global climate change and crises in energy (fuels), water, food prices and affordability, and finance, concomitant with growing food insecurity.

The nutrition transition is a term used to describe the shifts associated with economic development characterised by increased urbanisation and industrialisation (technological changes, food processing, mass media), epidemiological changes (decreased infant mortality and increased ageing populations) and dietary changes that include increased consumption of meat, fats and sugars (Popkin 2006). There are undoubtedly health benefits associated with the transition, but also disadvantages. The changes manifest as decreases in infectious (communicable) disease and increases in non-communicable disease. Pattern 1 describes the Palaeolithic/hunter-gatherer phase characterised by low fertility and low life expectancy; pattern 2 is the emergence of settlements and famine, where there is high fertility, high infant and maternal mortality and low life expectancy. Patterns 3, 4 and 5 are illustrated in Figure 29.1.

Most of the risks for premature mortality, especially hypertension, and for disability-adjusted life expectancy, especially early-life nutrition, are nutritionally dependent, irrespective of economic development, as shown in figures 29.2 and 29.3 (see colour section). Lower middle-income and middle-income countries (for example, India, Vietnam, Brazil) are typically transitioning between patterns 3 and 4, while many high-income countries would be experiencing pattern 5. Stunting and micronutrient deficiencies are associated with countries where incomes are lowest. With increasing income, stunting decreases, micronutrient deficiencies are less prevalent and obesity emerges and becomes dominant.

Internationally, an ecohealth approach to nutrition and health issues could be systemised according to the headings given in Table 29.5. Many of these issues

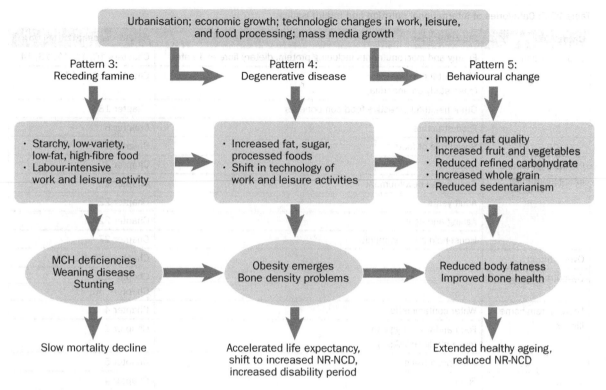

Figure 29.1: The nutrition transition

Notes: MCH = maternal and child health; NR-NCD = nutritionally related non-communicable disease

Source: Popkin (2006). Reproduced by permission of The American Society of Nutrition

are discussed elsewhere in the textbook. Case studies for particular issues are described below. These link with the goals of the international IGOs.

Anaemia

It is not surprising that when the food system fails a wide range of food components are not available. These include various micronutrients, both vitamins and minerals. Some of these are more commonly recognised and likely to have functional and clinical consequences. Depending on locality and population, the focus may be on the fat-soluble vitamins A and D, the water-soluble vitamins B-1 (thiamin), B-2 (riboflavin), B-3 (niacin), B-6 (pyridoxine), B-9 (folic acid), B-12 (cobalamin) and vitamin C (ascorbic acid). Of the minerals, iron, calcium, magnesium, zinc, copper, iodine and selenium are of most interest internationally. The three micronutrients on which there has been a particular focus internationally—

due to their impact across the life-course and, in particular, on maternal and child health—are iron, vitamin A and iodine.

Anaemia, which is most commonly attributable to iron deficiency, can impair health and wellbeing in women and increase the risk of maternal and neonatal adverse outcomes (see Chapter 17). It is reported that over half a billion women of reproductive age worldwide were anaemic, with half of these cases due to iron deficiency (WHO 2015). The most likely cause of iron deficiency anaemia is intestinal iron loss due to intestinal helminthiasis with hookworm (which also causes loss of zinc). Supplementation with iron is complicated in areas where malaria and tuberculosis are endemic. Single or isolated iron supplementation can impair immune function. For example, there was increased infant mortality when iron supplementation was given in a malarious area in Africa (Sazawal et al. 2006), perhaps because

Table 29.5: Categories of international nutrition and health issues

Categories	Subcategories	Reference chapter
Undernutrition	Energy and macronutrients including protein, dietary fibre and water	Chapters 10, 11, 12, 13, 14
	Micronutrients (case study on anaemia)	Chapters 16 and 17
	Other healthful bioactive food components	Chapter 18
	Food structure	Chapter 8
	Social role of food	Chapter 27
Pre-conception and intergenerational	Maternal	Chapter 20
	Growth and development	Chapter 21
	Adult years	Chapter 22
	Ageing and aged	Chapter 22
	Household and community	Chapter 27
Overnutrition		Chapters 31, 32, 33
Dysnutrition		Chapter 22 Chapters 30, 31
Food system-borne illness	Water contamination	Chapter 4
	Food and water hygiene (case study on WASH)	Chapter 6
	Food processing	Chapter 5
Waste	Food	Chapter 4 Chapter 26
	Packaging	Chapter 5
Environmental degradation	(case study on contamination)	Chapter 26 Chapter 31

rapid erythropoiesis increases larger red blood cell **reticulocyte** counts, favourable for malarial parasite invasion. As a consequence, in malarious areas, iron intake is increased with food-based methods like biofortification (HarvestPlus 2019) in conjunction with malarial management programs. An advantage of food-based approaches is that food provides a delivery matrix which modulates digestive absorption. A 50 per cent reduction of anaemia in women of reproduction age by 2025 is one of the WHO global nutrition targets 2025 (see the section 'Key elements for a favourable international health situation' in this chapter).

Water, sanitation and hygiene (WASH)

One of the most commonly experienced international health problems is diarrhoeal disease. It is intimately associated with malnutrition, since each increases the risk of the other in a vicious cycle. Together, these problems account for most of child mortality globally. It is estimated that lack of sanitation contributes to about 700,000 child deaths due to diarrhoea every year, mainly in low-income countries (Bhutta et al. 2013). Affordable and sustainable access to WASH is a key public health issue in international development, and is one of the focuses of the SDGs. Access to WASH includes safe water, adequate sanitation and hygiene education (UNICEF 2018). This can reduce illness and death, and also reduce poverty and improve socioeconomic development. Lack of WASH facilities can prevent students from attending school, impose an unusual burden on women and reduce work productivity. Several international development agencies assert that attention to WASH can also improve health, life expectancy, student learning, gender equality and other important issues of international development.

Diarrhoeal disease is an example of the close connection between nutritional status and the body's defence or immune system. This applies at all ages, but especially where either the food system is compromised or the immune system is weakened. In some situations, such as influenza, the virus can become more pathogenic where its host is malnourished—in the case of influenza, deficient in the essential element selenium. The case of influenza can be an international ecological problem where birds or poultry share the same exposures to the virus. Nutritional problems are commonly community-wide and a shared responsibility is needed for their control.

Environmental pollution and contamination

Environmental pollution and contamination is a growing problem for international nutrition and health. Examples of potential contaminants with far-reaching consequences are microplastics with endocrine-disruptor properties. The global contamination of sea and land—and the food and water supply dependent on them—with plastic has become

an endemic problem. One of the constituents of microplastics is phthalates, which are added to plastics to increase their flexibility and durability. These substances have potential anti-androgenic or **androgen–disruptor** effects. There is evidence that the high consumption of these substances via food from fast-food outlets, restaurants and cafeterias has challenged the reproductive status of the younger generation in the USA (Varshavsky et al. 2018) (Figure 29.4). The nutritional benefits of fish are being compromised because of almost universal contamination by microplastic (Galloway & Lewis 2016; Thompson et al. 2009).

EMERGENCY OR SURVIVAL NUTRITION

Situations occur when normal supplies of food and drink are unavailable, and some **emergency** supply must be arranged. Food aid is of global importance for millions of people in the short to medium term, but longer-term approaches to survival and wellbeing require sustainable food systems.

Short-term measures

In low-income countries, feeding programs aimed at saving lives are often needed in times of famine, war

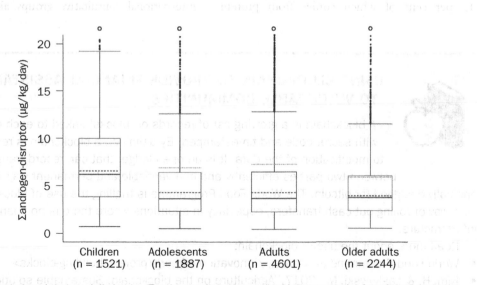

Figure 29.4: Cumulative phthalate daily intake (Σandrogen-disruptor, μg/kg/day) among the American population in NHANES, 2005–2014

Source: Varshavsky, Morello-Frosch, Woodruff & Zota (2018). Reproduced with permission from Elsevier

or other natural or human-made disaster. The main aims are the provision of energy and the correction of dehydration. Energy needs to be provided in a form that is digestible and culturally acceptable to those in need. Intense refeeding for severely malnourished individuals has to be undertaken with care, as severe electrolyte imbalances may occur and themselves cause death (Armer & White 2014; Friedli et al. 2017; Ralib et al. 2018).

For short-term management of severe acute malnutrition, it may be possible to use foods referred to as 'ready-to-use therapeutic foods' (RTUF). This approach can markedly improve outlook for morbidity and mortality to a significant extent. Plumpy'nut is an example of a peanut-based RTUF. Increasingly, attempts are being made to utilise local ingredients and labour to make RTUFs in order to provide income and livelihoods for local communities (Choudhury et al. 2018).

In addition to RTUFs to treat acute malnutrition, the World Food Programme delivers rations in times of emergency and to displaced persons. Typically, the emergency relief provided includes a combination of cereals, pulses, vegetable oil (fortified with vitamins A and D), nutrient-enriched flour, sugar and iodised salt. These rations are designed to provide 8800 kJ (10–12 per cent of which comes from protein and 17 per cent from fat) and micronutrients such as vitamin A, iron, iodine and zinc. These can be accompanied by cash transfers sent via mobile phones to enable recipients to purchase fresh food from local traders (if they exist).

Long-term measures

The causes of undernutrition are varied and, as such, any measures to improve the situation require a comprehensive assessment of a whole range of issues. Poverty is often associated with poor education, overpopulation, poor sanitation, poor medical services and poor agricultural practices. Climate change and natural disasters have become the greatest of threats to food and water security requiring concerted efforts at all levels from local to international. In many countries, the overriding issue is often the need for peace, a change in political will, improved economic growth, improved health and education facilities, and an emphasis on creating sustainable agriculture. Specific measures to treat severe deficiencies of iron, vitamin A and iodine are also needed in a number of countries as an immediate measure to reduce the severe impact of deficiency diseases. Progress has been made with vitamin A and iodine, but there is a need for governments, international consultative groups, aid agencies and,

---

USING BLOCKCHAIN TO PROVIDE FINANCIAL ASSISTANCE TO VULNERABLE COMMUNITIES

A blockchain is a growing list of records or 'blocks' linked to each other with secret code and timestamped. By definition a blockchain is resistant to modification of the data. It is an open ledger that can record transactions between two parties efficiently and in a verifiable and permanent way. It was originally designed for bitcoin. The World Food Programme is trialling the use of blockchain as a way of rolling out cash transfers, especially in situations where there is no financial infrastructure.

Read more about the use of blockchain:

- World Food Programme at <https://innovation.wfp.org/project/building-blocks>
- Kim, H. & Laskowski, M., 2017, 'Agriculture on the blockchain: Sustainable solutions for food, farmers, and financing', available at <https://ssrn.com/abstract=3028164>.

increasingly, the private sector to work together in looking for innovative approaches (Darnton-Hill et al. 2006). Poverty eradication and zero hunger by 2030 are Goals 1 and 2 of the UN Sustainable Development Goals.

KEY ELEMENTS FOR A FAVOURABLE INTERNATIONAL HEALTH SITUATION

Successful implementation of actions during the UN Decade of Nutrition (2016–2025) is intended to enable the world to achieve the six global nutrition targets and the nine global nutritionally related non-communicable disease targets.

The global nutrition targets 2025 (WHO 2017) to improve maternal, infant and young child nutrition include:

- 40 per cent global reduction in the number of stunted children under five
- 50 per cent reduction of anaemia in women of reproductive age
- 30 per cent reduction of low birthweight
- no increase in childhood overweight
- increased rate of exclusive breastfeeding in the first six months to at least 50 per cent
- reduction of childhood wasting to less than 5 per cent.

The voluntary global targets 2025 (WHO 2018a) for non-communicable diseases include:

- 25 per cent relative reduction in risk of premature mortality from cardiovascular diseases, cancer, diabetes, or chronic respiratory diseases
- at least 10 per cent relative reduction in the harmful use of alcohol, as appropriate, within the national context
- 10 per cent relative reduction in prevalence of insufficient physical activity
- 30 per cent relative reduction in mean population intake of salt/sodium
- 30 per cent relative reduction in prevalence of current tobacco use in persons aged 15 years or older
- 25 per cent relative reduction in the prevalence of raised blood pressure, or contain the prevalence

of raised blood pressure, according to national circumstances

- halt the rise in diabetes and obesity
- at least 50 per cent of eligible people receive drug therapy and counselling (including glycaemic control) to prevent heart attacks and strokes
- 80 per cent availability of the affordable basic technologies and essential medicines, including generics, required to treat major non-communicable diseases in both public and private facilities.

In order for these targets to be reached, a number of key elements and structures need to be put in place. These are outlined in Figure 29.5.

- **Restrict population size**
  A global population in excess of nine billion by 2050 is anticipated, with the increase mainly occurring in Asia and Sub-Saharan Africa (Lutz & KC 2010). Increasing population size will place mounting pressure on global food and water security because the world has limited ability to provide healthful and environmentally sustainable diets for its people. Restriction of population size could be achieved through concerted family planning and literacy.

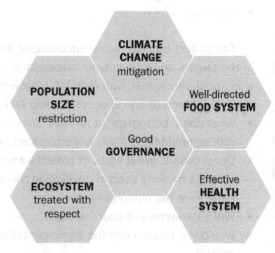

Figure 29.5: Key elements for a favourable international nutrition situation

- **Climate change minimisation and mitigation**

  This will require ecosystem conservation in the face of rampant and accelerating destruction; renewable energy and the cessation of fossil fuel usage, especially in the food system; decreased consumerism, materialism and waste; and socio-economic advancement without net environmental cost.

- **Treat nature and ecosystem with respect (maintenance of healthful ecosystem)**

- **Accessible, affordable and effective nutritionally oriented health systems available to all**

  These will require universal preventive approaches and clinical care.

- **Well-directed agriculture and food system**

  With shrinkage of arable land, contamination of ocean water and disappearance of ground water, there will be insufficient water—and, therefore, food—from most rivers of the world, notably those emanating from the Tibetan plateau and

---

CASE STUDY—THE MILLENNIUM VILLAGES PROJECT IN AFRICA

Initiated in 2005, the Millennium Villages Project was a ten-year, multisector, rural development demonstration project which was intended to evaluate the capacity of the **Millennium Development Goals (MDGs)** to effect change through targeted local intervention. It was designed to be a 'bottom-up' approach to lift villages out of poverty. The project is an example of how a coordinated effort across a range of areas can achieve significant improvements in health, education, development and poverty reduction. The project was based around a number of key principles, including:

- community empowerment
- evidence-based projects combined with local knowledge
- self-sustaining outcomes
- low cost.

The project has had some encouraging outcomes, with favourable results against one-third of the targets and all outcome indices improved. The investments in agriculture and health were most impressive, with modest improvements in nutrition (Mitchell et al. 2018).

Search the web and in peer-reviewed and grey literature for the Millennium Villages Project.

- What does 'bottom-up', 'top-down' and 'inside-out' mean with respect to working with communities? If you are interested, read more about Assets Based Community Development. What sorts of projects were implemented as part of the project? How was systems thinking used in developing these projects to ensure synergies across areas? What were the outcomes?
- Write a summary of your findings.
- Would you recommend the implementation of the Millennium Villages Project in other areas?

supplying fresh water to over 45 per cent of the world's population. It is predicted that 75 per cent of the world's population will face freshwater scarcity by 2050 (Lovelle 2016).

- **Effective governance of the commons for livelihoods**

  Elinor Ostrom, Nobel laureate in Economics, has shown that people will manage 'the Commons'—such as public open space, foods, water and education—if it is in the collective interest to do so, and provided that sanctions apply to those who do not cooperate (Ostrom 2015). This can contribute to a basic livelihood including food, shelter, clothing, education, health care, transport and communication for all.

In order to be able to reverse the current situation, the 2018 Global Nutrition Report (Scaling Up Nutrition 2018) identified five key steps.

1 Break down silos between all forms of malnutrition and develop comprehensive programs.
2 Prioritise and invest in the data needed and the capacity to use them.
3 Scale up and diversify financing of nutrition (but be mindful of conflicts of interest).
4 Focus on healthy diets to drive better nutrition for everyone.
5 Improve the targets and commitments that are driving stakeholders.

SUMMARY

- International health is very dependent on food security in all its respects: safety, sufficiency (the supply chain and affordability), satisfactoriness (acceptability and nutritional value) and sustainability. Food insecurity is a present and future threat throughout the world as a result of poor governance, socioeconomic inequity, climate change and conflict.
- International nutritional status is complex in its origins with biomedical, ecological, sociocultural and economic determinants and manifestations intergenerationally, in food excess, deficiency and quality. Undernutrition, overnutrition and dysnutrition belie more basic problems in nutritional biology, the environment and socioeconomics.
- International agencies, principally the UN system, play a defining role in ameliorating nutritionally related health problems.
- The Sustainability Development Goals (SDGs), which succeeded the Millennium Development Goals (MDGs), provide a collective international approach to nutritionally related health problems.

KEY TERMS

Androgen-disruptor: an environmental chemical that has anti-androgenic properties. It interferes with the biosynthesis, metabolism or action of endogenous androgens, which are a group of hormones, such as testosterone, that regulates the development of sex characteristics. Examples of androgen-disruptors include phthalates and bisphenol A (BPA), both of which are used in the manufacturing process of plastics.

Emergency: emergencies are 'urgent situations in which there is clear evidence that an event, or series of events, has occurred which causes human suffering or imminently threatens lives or livelihoods, and which the government concerned has not the means to remedy; and it is a demonstrably abnormal event, or series of events, which produces dislocation in the life of a community on an exceptional scale' (World Food Programme 2019).

Intergovernmental organisation (IGO): an organisation composed of sovereign states established by treaty or other agreement.

Millennium Development Goals (MDGs): a collection of eight international development goals that all 189 UN member states in 2000 committed to help achieve, in combating poverty, hunger, disease, illiteracy, environmental degradation and discrimination against women by the year 2015. A post-2015 agenda, comprising seventeen Sustainable Development Goals (SDGs), took their place and sets out to be reached by 2030. Integrated and indivisible, SDGs build on the achievements of the MDGs but are broader, deeper and far more ambitious in scope.

Reticulocytes: red blood cells that are immature or are not yet fully developed.

Triple burden (of disease): refers to a situation where malnutrition is expressed as undernutrition (endemic wasting, stunting) and overnutrition (obesity and related disorders) and micronutrient deficiencies. This is a limited description of what is more often a 'spectrum of nutritionally related disorders and diseases', perhaps better embraced by a more general descriptor like 'dysnutrition'.

REFERENCES

Armer, S. & White, R., 2014, 'Enteral nutrition', in J. Gandy (ed.), *Manual of Dietetic Practice* (5th edn), West Sussex: John Wiley & Sons, pp. 344–56

Bhutta, Z.A., Das, J.K., Walker, N., Rizvi, A., Campbell, H. et al., 2013, 'Interventions to address deaths from childhood pneumonia and diarrhoea equitably: What works and at what cost?', *The Lancet, 381*(9875): 1417–29, doi:10.1016/S0140-6736(13)60648-0

Choudhury, N., Ahmed, T., Hossain, M.I., Islam, M.M., Sarker, S.A. et al., 2018, 'Ready-to-Use Therapeutic Food made from locally available food ingredients is well accepted by children having severe acute malnutrition in Bangladesh', *Food and Nutrition Bulletin, 39*(1): 116–26, doi:10.1177/0379572117743929

Curry, G.N., Dumu, E. & Koczberski, G., 2016, 'Bridging the digital divide: Everyday use of mobile phones among market sellers in Papua New Guinea', in M.E. Robertson (ed.), *Communicating, Networking: Interacting,* Cham: Springer, pp. 39–52

Darnton-Hill, I., Bloem, M.W. & Chopra, M., 2006, 'Achieving the Millennium Development Goals through mainstreaming nutrition: Speaking with one voice', *Public Health Nutrition, 9*(5): 537–9, doi:10.1079/PHN2006965

Development Initiatives, 2017, *Global Nutrition Report 2017: Nourishing the SDGs,* <https://globalnutritionreport.org/documents/2/Report_2017.pdf>, accessed 22 December 2018

Draper, S., 2018, 'Systems thinking: Unlocking the Sustainable Development Goals', <www.forumforthefuture.org/blog/systems-thinking-unlocking-the-sustainable-development-goals>, accessed 29 May 2019

FAO, IFAD, UNICEF, WFP & WHO, 2017, *The State of Food Security and Nutrition in the World 2017: Building resilience for peace and food security,* <www.fao.org/3/a-I7695e.pdf>, accessed 22 December 2018

Friedli, N., Stanga, Z., Sobotka, L., Culkin, A., Kondrup, J. et al., 2017, 'Revisiting the refeeding syndrome: Results of a systematic review', *Nutrition, 35*: 151–60, doi:10.1016/j.nut.2016.05.016

Galloway, T.S. & Lewis, C.N., 2016, 'Marine microplastics spell big problems for future generations', *Proceedings of the National Academy of Sciences, 113*(9): 2331–3, doi:10.1073/pnas.1600715113

Global Burden of Disease Collaborative Network, 2018, *Global Burden of Disease Study 2017 (GBD 2017): Results,* <http://ghdx.healthdata.org/gbd-results-tool>, accessed 27 January 2019

HarvestPlus, 2019, *Biofortification: The nutrition revolution is now,* <www.harvestplus.org/biofortification-nutrition-revolution-now>, accessed 15 January 2019

Hetherington, J.B., Wiethoelter, A.K., Negin, J. & Mor, S.M., 2017, 'Livestock ownership, animal source foods and child nutritional outcomes in seven rural village clusters in Sub-Saharan Africa', *Agriculture & Food Security, 6*(1): 9, doi:10.1186/s40066-016-0079-z

International Women's Development Agency (IWDA), 2018, *Women's Leadership,* <https://iwda.org.au/what-we-do/womens-leadership/>, accessed 25 December 2018

Kim, H. & Laskowski, M., 2017, 'Agriculture on the blockchain: Sustainable solutions for food, farmers, and financing', *SSRN, December,* doi:10.2139/ssrn.3028164

Lovelle, M., 2016, *Tibet: A major source of Asia's rivers,* <www.futuredirections.org.au/publication/tibet-a-major-source-of-asias-rivers/>, accessed 22 December 2018

Lutz, W. & KC, S., 2010, 'Dimensions of global population projections: What do we know about future population trends and structures?', *Philosophical Transactions of the Royal Society B: Biological Sciences, 365*(1554): 2779–91, doi:10.1098/rstb.2010.0133

Mehra, R. & Rojas, M.H., 2008, *Women, Food Security and Agriculture in a Global Marketplace,* <www.icrw.org/wp-content/uploads/2016/10/A-Significant-Shift-Women-Food-Security-and-Agriculture-in-a-Global-Marketplace.pdf>, accessed 22 December 2018

Mitchell, R. & Popham, F., 2008, 'Effect of exposure to natural environment on health inequalities: An observational population study', *Lancet, 372*(9650): 1655–60, doi:10.1016/S0140-6736(08)61689-X

Mitchell, S., Gelman, A., Ross, R., Chen, J., Bari, S. et al., 2018, 'The Millennium Villages Project: A retrospective, observational, endline evaluation', *Lancet Global Health, 6*(5): e500–13, doi:10.1016/S2214-109X(18)30065-2

Olney, D.K., Vicheka, S., Kro, M., Chakriya, C., Kroeun, H. et al., 2013, 'Using program impact pathways to understand and improve program delivery, utilization, and potential for impact of Helen Keller International's homestead food production program in Cambodia', *Food and Nutrition Bulletin, 34*(2): 169–84, doi:10.1177/156482651303400206

Oniang'o, R. & Allotey, J., 1999, 'Food safety and the role of government', in A. Ogunrinade, R. Oniang'o & J.D. May (eds), *Not by Bread Alone: Food security and governance in Africa,* Witwatersrand: Witwatersrand University Press/Toda Institute for Global Peace and Policy Research, pp. 264–97

Ostrom, E., 2015, *Governing the Commons: The evolution of institutions for collective action,* Cambridge: Cambridge University Press

Popkin, B.M., 2006, 'Global nutrition dynamics: The world is shifting rapidly toward a diet linked with noncommunicable diseases', *American Journal of Clinical Nutrition, 84*(2): 289–98, doi:10.1093/ajcn/84.2.289

Ralib, A.M., Nor, M. & Basri, M., 2018, 'Refeeding hypophosphataemia after enteral nutrition in a Malaysian intensive care unit: Risk factors and outcome', *Asia Pacific Journal of Clinical Nutrition, 27*(2): 329–35, doi:10.6133/apjcn.062017.09

Rogers, P.P., Jalal, K.F. & Boyd, J.A., 2012, *An Introduction to Sustainable Development,* London: Earthscan

Sazawal, S., Black, R.E., Ramsan, M., Chwaya, H.M., Stoltzfus, R.J. et al., 2006, 'Effects of routine prophylactic supplementation with iron and folic acid on admission to hospital and mortality in preschool children in a high malaria transmission setting: Community-based, randomised, placebo-controlled trial', *Lancet, 367*(9505): 133–43, doi:10.1016/S0140-6736(06)67962-2

Scaling Up Nutrition, 2018, *The 2018 Global Nutrition Report: Shining a light to spur action on nutrition,* <https://scalingupnutrition.org/news/the-2018-global-nutrition-report-shining-a-light-to-spur-action-on-nutrition/>, accessed 15 January 2019

Thompson, R.C., Moore, C.J., Vom Saal, F.S. & Swan, S.H., 2009, 'Plastics, the environment and human health: Current consensus and future trends', *Philosophical Transactions of the Royal Society B: Biological Sciences, 364*(1526): 2153–66, doi:10.1098/rstb.2009.0053

UNICEF, 2018, *Water, Sanitation and Hygiene,* <www.unicef.org/wash/>, accessed 15 January 2019

United Nations, 2018, *Sustainable Development Goals,* <www.un.org/sustainabledevelopment/sustainable-development-goals/>, accessed 16 December 2018

Varshavsky, J.R., Morello-Frosch, R., Woodruff, T.J. & Zota, A.R., 2018, 'Dietary sources of cumulative phthalates exposure among the US general population in NHANES 2005–2014', *Environment International, 115*: 417–29, doi:10.1016/j.envint.2018.02.029

Wahlqvist, M.L., 2014, 'Ecosystem health disorders: Changing perspectives in clinical medicine and nutrition', *Asia Pacific Journal of Clinical Nutrition, 23*(1): 1–15, doi:10.6133/apjcn.2014.23.1.20

Wahlqvist, M.L., Keatinge, J.D.H., Butler, C.D., Friel, S., McKay, J. et al., 2009, 'A Food in Health Security (FIHS) platform in the Asia-Pacific Region: The way forward', *Asia Pacific Journal of Clinical Nutrition, 18*(4): 688–702, doi:10.6133/apjcn.2009.18.4.34

WHO, 2015, *The Global Prevalence of Anaemia in 2011,* <www.who.int/nutrition/publications/micronutrients/global_prevalence_anaemia_2011/en/>, accessed 22 December 2018

—— 2017, *Global nutrition monitoring framework: Operational guidance for tracking progress in meeting targets for 2025,* <www.who.int/nutrition/publications/operational-guidance-GNMF-indicators/en/>, accessed 22 December 2018

—— 2018a, *Global Action Plan for the Prevention and Control of Noncommunicable Diseases 2013–2020,* <www.who.int/nmh/events/ncd_action_plan/en/>, accessed 22 December 2018

—— 2018b, *United Nations Decade of Action on Nutrition 2016–2025,* <www.who.int/nutrition/decade-of-action/en/>, accessed 22 December 2018

WHO & FAO, 2018, *Driving Commitment for Nutrition within the UN Decade of Action on Nutrition: Policy brief,* <www.who.int/nutrition/publications/decade-of-action-commitment-policybrief/en/>, accessed 16 December 2018

Wolch, J.R., Byrne, J. & Newell, J.P., 2014, 'Urban green space, public health, and environmental justice: The challenge of making cities "just green enough"', *Landscape and Urban Planning, 125*: 234–44, doi:10.1016/j.landurbplan.2014.01.017

World Food Programme, 2019, *Emergency Relief,* <www1.wfp.org/emergency-relief>, accessed 15 January 2019

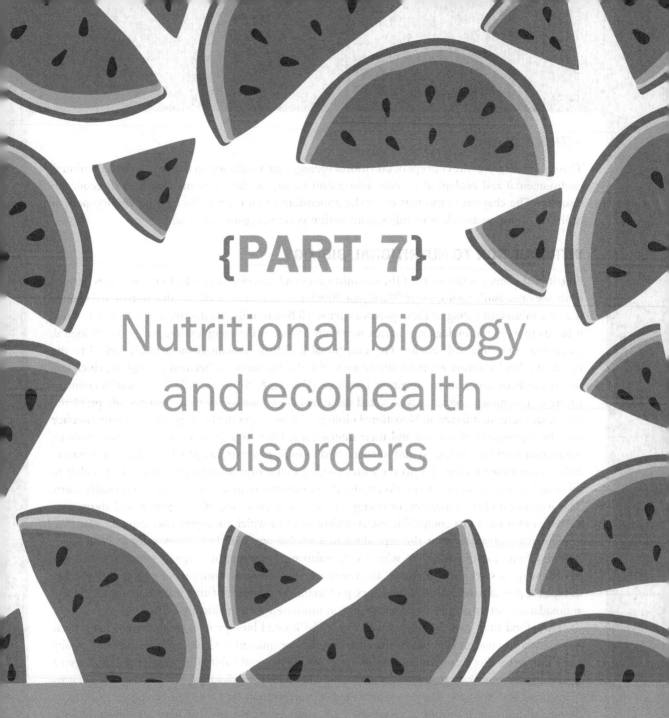

{PART 7}

Nutritional biology and ecohealth disorders

INTRODUCTION

This section explores the concept of nutritional biology and its reliance on the broader social, cultural, environmental and ecological systems. Disruption to any of these systems may lead to ecohealth disorders. The chapters in this part cover the dimensions of nutritional biology, the development of ecohealth disorders and their manifestations within systems, organs and mind.

INTRODUCTION TO NUTRITIONAL BIOLOGY

Nutritional science is the study of the assimilation of and function dependent on molecules derived from any organism's environment (Wahlqvist 2006). This definition indicates that nutritional science requires an understanding of these processes across all forms of life. As discussed in Chapter 1, while it has its roots in the biological sciences, nutrition science is the complex integration of biological, social and environmental systems. The nutritional health of humans is inextricably linked to the health of other life forms and their interactions with the environment (termed ecological principles); this is the basis for modern nutritional science (Döring & Ströhle 2015). The multidisciplinary nature of nutritional science is well suited to contribute to the solution of everyday-life problems, which are often multifactorial. Nutritional biology acknowledges the biology-environment interface and the importance of systems and their interactions. There is a complex, dynamic and evolving interaction between, diet, food and nutrient within biological systems (Raubenheimer & Simpson 2016). Nutritional biology has to do with enabling living organisms to perform tasks peculiar to them and their ecosystem. These tasks require the conversion of mass into energy in a utilisable form. The acquisition of the substrates for energy production requires mobility, digestion and absorption, excretion of waste and a compatible social environment in which these processes can take place.

The living organism must also reproduce in a reliable way with little if any error in its genome, acquired from parents as DNA with its cumulative expression of parental exposures, and the environment as several microbiomes. To reproduce with minimal damage and maintain the ability to repair injury and defend from predators, protectants in the form of anti-inflammatory agents and antioxidants must be acquired or formed and an immune system maintained.

Thus, food must serve a range of functions. The limited biology of humans cannot meet these needs without consuming a biodiverse diet in sufficient quantities. Other creatures usually require a less biodiverse diet than humans but have a narrower range of habitats in which they can survive. A great risk to humans is that, in ranging far and wide with their dietary resilience, they may destroy many or most of the ecosystems on which they depend without realising their ecological limitations. Given the limits of food bioactive component density, humans need to have a sufficiently large energy throughput to achieve this without accumulating excess energy stores as fat, best achieved by enough physical activity).

The dietary needs of humans require engagement with an ecosystem locally or through transfer from elsewhere of foods capable of provision of the same needs (Wahlqvist et al. 2012). More than that, there is no clear interface between people and their environment, of which they are an integral part through microbiomic, bioregulatory, security and social connectedness (Wahlqvist et al. 2014). This connectedness is represented by environmental determinants of genomic expression, sensory inputs and societal arrangements, all of which have nutritional features. Humans are socioecological creatures.

The following fields of nutritional biology (Figure 7.A) illustrate the adaptability to changing nutrition environments or the specific modification of food environment by organisms, and its biological consequences in the sense of coevolution of nature and culture:

- homeostasis
- nutritional energetics
- nutrient–gene interactions
- microbiomics
- gut physiology (digestion and absorption) (see Part 3)
- sensory nutrition
- nutritional modulation of inflammation.

A key feature of nutritional biology is that, through its several dimensions, it supports homeostasis, the provision of energy and food component diversity, genetic regulation and expression, microbiomic and sensory connectedness, and inflammatory processes and immunity which allow responses to injury and insult. Each dimension is in part a product of food intake patterns and gut physiology. Chapter 30 describes each of these elements.

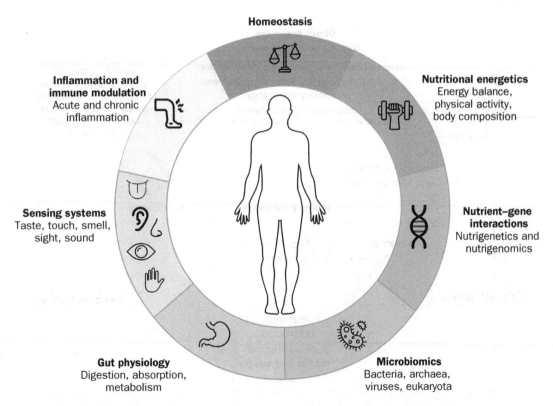

Figure 7.A: Fields of nutritional biology

575

INTRODUCTION TO ECOHEALTH DISORDERS

An ecosystems or ecohealth approach to human health is a strategy designed to shift our thinking from the traditional, unidimensional biomedical approach towards a new transdisciplinary and integrated approach (Lang & Heasman 2004; Wahlqvist 2016; Wahlqvist & Specht 1998). It makes use of the conceptual construct of an ecosystem to examine the complex and myriad factors influencing human health concerns, and seeks ways to improve human health and wellbeing through sustainable management of all components of the environment (Wahlqvist 2018). The health of individuals, as well as that of communities, is inextricably linked to the health of biophysical, social and economic environments, and all ought to be considered in tandem (see Chapter 1 for definitions of econutrition). Underpinning the shift towards more econutritional thinking about health was the significant body of evidence for food intake patterns as a basis for ill-health and the opportunities for clinical application. The pathways to ecohealth disorders are illustrated in Figure 7.B and are described in Chapter 31.

The results of disruption to the biological process via direct and indirect pathways and the resultant ecohealth disorders are discussed in more depth in Chapters 32, 33 and 34. Chapter 32 discusses disruption to systems (endocrine, immune, neoplastic, gastrointestinal), organs (heart and blood vessels, muscles, bones, teeth and gums) and mental health (cognitive, mood and emotions and stress).

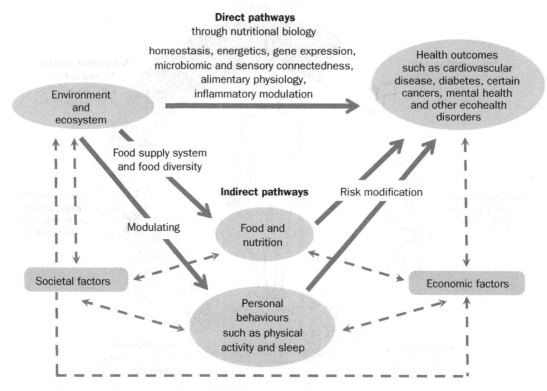

Figure 7.B: Environmental pathways to health: econutrition and ecohealth

576

REFERENCES

Döring, F. & Ströhle, A., 2015, 'Nutritional biology: A neglected basic discipline of nutritional science', *Genes & Nutrition, 10*(6): 55, doi:10.1007/s12263-015-0505-z

Lang, T. & Heasman, M., 2004, *Food Wars: The global battle for mouths, minds and markets*, London: Earthscan

Raubenheimer, D. & Simpson, S.J., 2016, 'Nutritional ecology and human health', *Annual Review of Nutrition, 36*(1): 603–26, doi:10.1146/annurev-nutr-071715-051118

Wahlqvist, M.L., 2006, 'Towards a new generation of international nutrition science and scientist: The importance of Africa and its capacity', *Journal of Nutrition, 136*(4): 1048–9, doi:10.1093/jn/136.4.1048

—— 2016, 'Ecosystem dependence of healthy localities, food and people', *Annals of Nutrition and Metabolism, 69*: 75–8, doi:10.1159/000449143

—— 2018, 'Nutrition science and future earth: Current nutritional policy dilemmas', in T. Beer, J. Li & K. Alverson (eds), *Global Change and Future Earth: The geoscience perspective,* Cambridge: Cambridge University Press, pp. 209–22

Wahlqvist, M.L. & Specht, R.L., 1998, 'Food variety and biodiversity: Econutrition', *Asia Pacific Journal of Clinical Nutrition, 7*(3/4): 314–19, <http://apjcn.nhri.org.tw/server/APJCN/7/3/4/314.pdf>, accessed 4 January 2019

Wahlqvist, M.L., Huang, L.-Y., Lee, M.-S., Chiang, P.-H., Chang, Y.-H. & Tsao, A.P., 2014, 'Dietary quality of elders and children is interdependent in Taiwanese communities: A NAHSIT mapping study', *Ecology of Food and Nutrition, 53*(1): 81–97, doi:10.1080/03670244.2013.772512

Wahlqvist, M.L., McKay, J., Chang, Y.-C. & Chiu, Y.-W., 2012, 'Rethinking the food security debate in Asia: Some missing ecological and health dimensions and solutions', *Food Security, 4*(4): 657–70, doi:10.1007/s12571-012-0211-2

{CHAPTER 30}
NUTRITIONAL BIOLOGY

Mark L. Wahlqvist and Naiyana Wattanapenpaiboon

OBJECTIVES

- Describe homeostasis.
- Describe the components and mechanics of energy balance.
- Explain the factors associated with nutrient–gene interactions.
- Recognise the importance of microbiomes and their relevance to health.
- Appreciate the importance of sensory nutrition in human health.
- Discuss how inflammation is an intrinsic part of nutrition biology and provides for repair and maintenance.

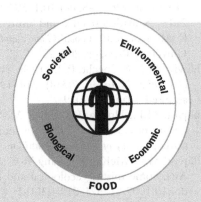

HOMEOSTASIS

The maintenance of the body's internal environment within narrow physiological limits against external and internal challenges, including those from food intake and usage, is referred to as 'homeostasis'.

Homeostasis depends on a range of settings or optima that allow survival and reproduction. These are the product of a complex array of sensing and feedback mechanisms, which include:

- body temperature regulation as a way to dissipate heat generated from energy metabolism
- regulation by and of genes or **gene analogues** (DNA, RNA and other replicating nucleotides, even proteins as in prions)
- **bioenergetics** (ATP and **adenosine monophosphate-activated protein kinase (AMPK)** for cellular energy status; glucose transporter membrane proteins)
- body water (aquaporins for water movement in and out of cells and osmolarity)
- gas transport (oxygen, carbon dioxide, hydrogen, methane, nitrogen)
- ionic concentrations of monovalent (sodium, potassium, chloride) and divalent (calcium, magnesium, zinc, phosphate) cations and anions and their interrelationships
- enzyme kinetics (substrate and product)
- intercellular communication (locally produced metabolites and cytokines)

- inter-organ regulation (endocrinological and hormones; microbiomes)
- system reflexes (cardiovascular, neurological—especially the autonomic nervous system—respiratory, gastrointestinal, renal, hepatic)
- storage, synthesis, detoxification (hepatic functions, bone, bone marrow)
- nutrient and substrate assimilation (liver, biliary system, pancreas, gut microbiome)
- defence and repair (**integumentary**, epithelial, interstitial, lymphoid, **haemopoietic**, microbiomic systems).

Key risks to cellular, organ and systems function arise if the ranges of pH (acid–base balance), electrolyte concentrations, blood glucose, transport proteins (such as albumin with calcium, zinc, free fatty acids, various polyphenolics, steroids and pharmaceuticals), lipoproteins (with lipids as fuels and for membrane structure; carotenoids, vitamers of vitamin E), other protein carriers (like retinol-binding protein and ferritin), hormones, blood cells (red, white and platelets) and many more items are not physiologically optimal and thus not compatible with health.

As metabolic processes are intimately intertwined with food intake, the main contributors to homeostasis are nutritionally related, principally through intake (or inputs), utilisation/turnover and storage (Table 30.1).

Many homeostatic systems in the body, including the metabolic, immune, central nervous, cardiovascular, digestive and reproductive systems, are regulated by the hypothalamic-pituitary-adrenal axis. It integrates physical and psychosocial influences in order to allow the body to adapt effectively to the environment.

Acid–base balance

The proper balance between the acids and alkalis (or bases) in body fluids is crucial for the normal physiology of the body and cellular metabolism. Acid–base imbalance occurs when the blood pH shifts out of the normal range for any reason. The body is geared to keep the body fluids mildly alkaline, at a pH 7.35–7.45 for extracellular fluid (ECF) and about 7.1 for intracellular fluid, and avoid acidosis. This is because the alkalinity is essential for muscle, heart and nerve cells. The body normally responds very effectively to perturbations in acid or base production, with the chemical buffers, the respiratory system, and the renal system.

The most abundant chemical buffer in the ECF consists of a solution of carbonic acid and the bicarbonate salt. When there is an excess of alkaline OH^- ions in the solution, carbonic acid partially neutralises them by forming bicarbonate ion and water. Similarly, an excess of acid H^+ ions is partially neutralised by the bicarbonate component of the buffer solution to form carbonic acid, which is a relatively weaker acid. Other mechanisms include excretion of carbon dioxide (CO_2) by the lungs (about 13,000 mmol/day), which in a way removes carbonic acid (volatile acid); and, by the kidneys, excretion of non-volatile acids, such as lactate, phosphate, sulphate and acetoacetate, or regeneration of alkali bicarbonate (Figure 30.1).

Table 30.1: Examples of nutritionally related contributors to homeostasis

Intake	Endocrine control of appetite: leptin and ghrelin Thirst: hydration and water
Utilisation/turnover in normal bodily functions	Acid–base balance: intracellular and extracellular buffer systems to maintain optimal pH Endocrine control of blood calcium: vitamin D, parathyroid hormone and calcitonin Body temperature regulation
Storage	Bone: calcium, phosphate, magnesium, zinc Liver: folate, vitamin B-12, iron Muscles: proteins and amino acids Adipose tissue: fat as energy and essential fatty acids, fat-soluble vitamins

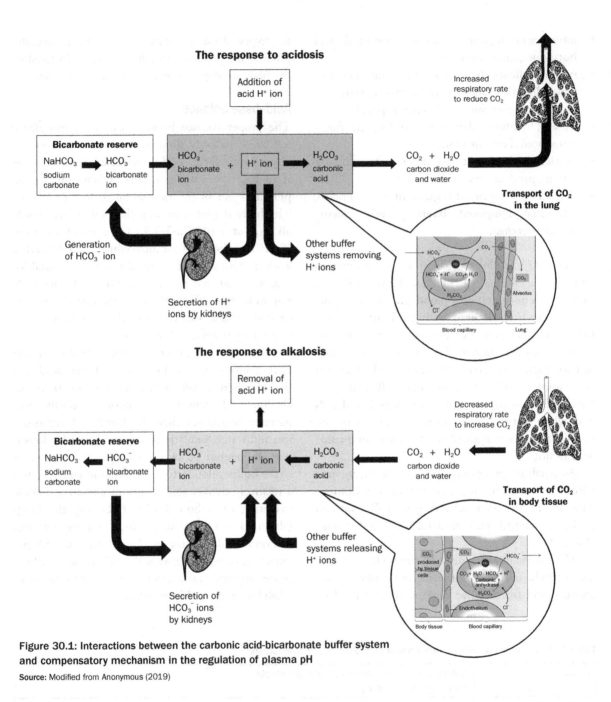

Figure 30.1: Interactions between the carbonic acid-bicarbonate buffer system and compensatory mechanism in the regulation of plasma pH

Source: Modified from Anonymous (2019)

The molar concentration ratio of a weak acid to a weak base determines the pH of buffer solutions. The higher the weak acid, the lower the pH and vice versa. The carbonic acid-bicarbonate ratio in ECF is such that the pH is 7.4. From a biological point of view, the ratio is dependent on the action of carbonic anhydrase enzymes in different locations, particularly the red blood cells on the passage through the tissues, notably lungs and kidneys.

The major challenge to hydrogen ion homeostasis is metabolic. This challenge is greater with exercise and the production of lactic acid, and in fasting with the production of ketone bodies (aceto-acetate, β-hydroxybutyrate and acetone). Ketone bodies are also produced in insulin deficiency and with alcohol excess. Metabolic processes generate both volatile and non-volatile acids. Volatile acid (carbonic acid) is removed through respiration as carbon dioxide, while non-volatile acids are excreted by the kidneys and are the result of incomplete digestion of the macronutrients. The three commonly reported sources of endogenous acid production are the metabolism of sulphur amino acids (methionine and cysteine), the metabolism or ingestion of organic acids, and the metabolism of phosphate esters or dietary phosphoproteins.

It is recommended that the terms 'acidosis' and 'alkalosis' be used with either 'respiratory' (indicating a change in the partial pressure of carbon dioxide), or 'metabolic' (indicating a change in the bicarbonate concentration of the ECF). Metabolic acidosis is usually associated with impaired renal acid excretion, respiratory acidosis with a reduced respiratory rate causing carbon dioxide retention. Metabolic alkalosis is uncommon, while respiratory alkalosis from hyperventilation is quite common.

Cations and anions

Monovalent cations, notably sodium and potassium, serve cellular functions like those of water distribution or hydration and osmolarity, **membrane potential**, energy transporters, enzyme activity and communication channels. These functions are coordinated by hormonal, cardioregulatory, autonomic nervous system and other pathways. Divalent cations and anions, especially calcium, magnesium, phosphate, zinc and copper, complement the monovalent functions, but with a different hormonal architecture (see Chapter 17).

There appears to be a link between acid–base balance and certain metal ions. For example, the carbonic anhydrase enzymes are one of more than 300 zinc metallo-enzymes. The carbonic anhydrase enzymes play an important role in maintaining acid–base balance in blood and other tissues (Figure 30.1), by converting carbon dioxide and water to bicarbonate and hydrogen ions, and vice versa, and

in helping transport carbon dioxide out of tissues. Other zinc metallo-enzymes are those involved in reproduction, cell turnover (DNA and RNA polymerase), and vision (retinol dehydrogenase, which is also alcohol dehydrogenase) (McCall et al. 2000).

Glucose homeostasis

Maintaining blood glucose concentrations within narrow limits (4–7 mmol/L) is critical for organ function; otherwise the rapid development of hypoglycaemia (low blood glucose) can lead to widespread organ dysfunction with sympathetic nervous system activation and impaired brain function and loss of consciousness. Hyperglycaemia (high blood glucose), where insulin is deficient or tissues are insulin-resistant, is also associated with organ dysfunction, including that of the brain, resulting in drowsiness and loss of consciousness. Added to this, the **hyperosmolar hyperglycaemic state (HHS)** leads to polyuria (increased urination) and polydipsia (difficult-to-quench thirst), with its own functional consequences. In health, when not eating, and during sleep, blood glucose is maintained by hepatic gluconeogenesis. Similar events happen during physical activity, when more fuel from circulating glucose, free fatty acids and triglyceride is required by muscle and heart.

Regulation of retinol-binding protein

Vitamin A intake, whether preformed as retinol or provitamin A as carotenoids, is notoriously variable from day to day, week to week or over even longer timeframes. Yet it is required every day for a range of essential functions, especially vision and immune function. Too much at once, however, can have toxic effects on bones. The homeostatic mechanisms in place include a shared digestive biology with lipids (as vitamin A is fat-soluble), hepatic storage, and a blood transport system based on retinol-binding protein which keeps tissue exposure within safe limits.

Vitamin B-12 and folate

With variations in intake, and in order that our internal environment is sufficiently stable for its functions to be realised and damage avoided, homeostatic mechanisms must operate. They do so with remarkable resilience due to intensive sensing, complex feedback loops, and integrated mechanisms. Vitamins B-12 and folate provide examples of this resilience.

When replete, vitamin B-12 stores in the liver can last for about five years. This is both reassuring and of concern. It is reassuring because such a critical nutrient for fetal development, cell turnover, haemopoiesis and neurological function is held in reserve, provided the diet has been plentiful at some time in the past. Conversely, it is of concern, because the ultimate source of vitamin B-12 is microbiological or dependent on animal-derived foods. This means that people who consume very hygienic foods to avoid risks of contamination or people who are vegan (consuming only plant-derived foods) will be deficient in vitamin B-12, but such deficiency may not become evident for a long time while liver stores are drawn down. If this were to occur during pregnancy or lactation, the baby would suffer.

Similarly, liver stores, when replete with folic acid, will last about three months. If a mother-to-be is well-nourished, the fetus would be relatively protected against folic acid deficiency during the critical first trimester, even without further dietary intake. Of course, this is not to be recommended given that, for some women, folic acid requirements are more difficult to meet and neural tube defects in the offspring are a risk.

NUTRITIONAL ENERGETICS

When food energy intake equals energy expenditure, energy balance is achieved (see Chapter 13). Most people maintain a close balance of total energy intake with energy output through basal metabolic rate and physical activity. However, even a slight imbalance in the energy balance equation, if maintained over a long period, can result in significant weight loss or weight gain. When there is net energy surplus or positive balance, the body stores extra food as fats; a net energy deficit or negative balance results in weight loss as the body draws on stored fat to provide energy for work.

Energy metabolism in the fasted state is dependent on the duration of the fast, the type of meal ingested before the fast, and available body energy stores. Energy metabolism in the fed state is mediated by the cephalic phase (see Chapter 9) response to a meal, meal size, meal type, structure and consistency, meal composition and the metabolic processes required to digest, absorb and store the ingested energy. Both energy intake and body energy stores affect activity or exercise-related energy expenditure. Human beings, especially adults, do not maintain energy balance from one day to the next but do so over a period of several days, with energy intake playing a stronger role in this regulatory process. In conditions where energy intake and expenditure are relatively steady, there may still be variations in body composition and fatness. If we wish to find out what contributes to the varying degree of body fatness, we need to explore the circumstances in play at that time. For example, bursts of physical activity may deplete hepatic and muscle glycogen stores—which are associated with considerable water and potassium—so that weight decreases; the opposite occurs with repletion of glycogen stores with intake of a carbohydrate load. During periods of growth, energy intake needs to exceed expenditure. In addition, people can undergo little weight change as physical activity changes by altering fat and muscle stores.

Overall energy throughput comprises consumption and expenditure, through basal metabolism, various forms of exertion, physical and mental (the brain is very energy-requiring), and thermogenesis by 'energy inefficiency' and brown or beige fat metabolism. The long history of evolution is that we have retained cellular mechanisms to sense and restore energy equilibrium. Energy is stored in mammalian systems as energy-rich macromolecules such as glycogen, triglycerides and proteins, or in covalent chemical bonds, the most prevalent and efficient being nucleoside triphosphates, principally ATP (see Chapter 13).

The dephosphorylation or hydrolysis of ATP to ADP and AMP (adenosine monophosphate) yields energy for cellular metabolism, principally through involvement of membrane ions. In turn,

WHAT ARE BROWN AND BEIGE FATS?

In some mammals, including humans, a special kind of adipose tissue, called brown fat, burns the energy obtained from food and produces heat without the animal having to expend any effort, through a process called non-shivering thermogenesis. The ability of brown fat to generate heat (thermogenesis) comes from a protein called 'thermogenin' or 'uncoupling protein 1' often referred to as UCP1, present in the mitochondria in the brown fat cells. It was once thought that, in humans, only babies had brown fat. The thermogenetic function of brown fat is activated when the body is exposed to the cold; therefore, it is vital for regulating body temperature in babies who are unable to shiver to keep warm.

However, in 2009, several studies reported that functional brown fat was present in small amounts in adults, around the neck and shoulder blades and around the spinal cord (Cypess et al. 2009). They also found that people with a lower BMI tended to have more brown fat. It is suggested that being obese is somehow associated with a decline in brown fat, and leanness could be secondary to having greater amounts of active brown fat. It is estimated that 50 g of brown fat burns about 2000 kJ, which is equivalent to one hour of aerobic exercise.

In 2012, another kind of fat, called beige fat, was identified (Wu et al. 2012). Beige fat has a different origin to brown fat, but it contains the same all-important protein, UCP1. Beige fat is dispersed in white fat cells (hence the name 'beige' for 'brown in white') and, interestingly, it was shown in animal studies that with cold exposure or certain hormones, this energy-burning beige variety can be transformed into white fat. It was also shown that the white-to-beige conversion of fat cells, or the activation of UCP1 protein, can be suppressed by the gene 'Regulator of Calcineurin 1' (RCAN1), thereby resulting in the systemic down-regulation of energy expenditure. It is suggested that RCAN1-mediated suppression of the adaptive energy expenditure process, especially in the context of abundant food resources, may contribute to the growing epidemic of obesity (Rotter et al. 2018).

In animal and human studies, a number of bioactive food compounds have been reported to promote energy dissipation, by activating the thermogenetic function of brown fat cells and/or promoting the browning of white fat cells, or even by up-regulating brown or beige adipogenesis. These bioactive compounds include capsaicin in chillies, and a range of polyphenols, such as quercetin in onion, apple berries and buckwheat; isoflavones in soy products; resveratrol in red wine and red cabbage; flavan-3-ol in green tea, dark chocolate and berries; curcumin in turmeric; and gallic acid in red wine, tea and some berries (Mele et al. 2017).

The question as to whether we can manipulate the RCAN1 gene expression, or whether we can make use of the energy-burning protein UCP1, either by upregulating it or delivering it to cells, has been an important line of inquiry in research into weight management and the treatment of obesity (or excessive accumulation of white fat). Activation of brown/beige fat cells improves glucose homeostasis and insulin sensitivity in humans and may play an important role in bone health and bone density, and even brain health. These findings open up a whole new set of potential therapeutic uses of foods, agents or natural bioactive food compounds that enhance the activation of brown/beige fat cells.

the AMP-activated protein kinase (AMPK) enzyme senses the AMP:ATP ratio and interacts accordingly with a wide range of metabolic pathways. In this way, AMPK-mediated phosphorylation regulates energy metabolism. This is a phenomenon involving all tissues, including the brain (therefore affecting appetite), the endocrine system, skeletal muscle (and movement), cardiac muscle, liver and cholesterol synthesis, pancreas and insulin, adipose tissue and its adipokines, and more. It is possible, therefore, for AMPK indirectly to sense external events like eating and physical activity.

Impaired energy regulation may be located in AMPK activation as in the commonly encountered 'metabolic syndrome', a precursor of diabetes. It features increased abdominal fat stores, nocturnal hepatic gluconeogenesis with fasting hyperglycaemia, hypertriglyceridaemia with greater triglyceride blood transport, each indicative of energy dysregulation, and low serum concentrations of high-density lipoprotein, along with hypertension (Alberti et al. 2005). Metformin, a medication used in the management of diabetes, activates AMPK enzyme and minimises these metabolic abnormalities (López et al. 2016). It also appears to reduce the risk of diabetes-related cancers (Lee et al. 2011) and neurodegeneration (Wahlqvist et al. 2012).

It should be acknowledged that the efficiency of energy utilisation may vary according to physical activity, body composition, with certain foods and food patterns, with climate and with health and illness. Physical activity interacts with a range of dietary, environmental and social factors to impact energy balance, and these are discussed in the next section.

Physical activity and sedentary behaviour

Being physically active and limiting sedentary behaviour is important for health and wellbeing. Regular physical activity has many health benefits and plays an important role in promoting healthy weight. It can help prevent heart disease, type 2 diabetes and some cancers, and also improve psychological wellbeing. The Australian Government Department of Health (2017) has defined 'physical activity' as an activity that gets our body moving, makes breathing become quicker and the heart beat faster, and 'sedentary behaviour' as sitting or lying down, except when sleeping. The word 'sedentary' comes from the Latin *sedere*, meaning 'to sit', and the term 'sedentary behaviour' is generally used to describe a distinct class of behaviours characterised

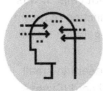

ENERGY BALANCE

Very few of us eat the same amount of food every day. Some days we eat more; this could be because of the types of food available, special occasions, when we are out of routine (for example, travelling) or for psychological reasons. Some days we may eat less.

How do you adjust for a few days' energy imbalance (over- or undereating)? Some examples include:

- eating differently on weekdays compared to weekends
- eating differently at different meals
- observing fast days
- undertaking additional physical activity.

One way of adjusting energy intake that has been popularised is the 5:2 fasting diet. In this way of eating you eat as you normally would for five days of the week; then, for two days, you limit your intake to about 2000 kJ. Intermittent fasting has been linked to weight loss, reduced insulin resistance and a range of other benefits. Does it work?

1. Review the latest scientific papers on intermittent fasting. What are the key benefits? What are the drawbacks?
2. To whom would you recommend this way of eating? To whom would you not recommend this way of eating?

primarily by sitting or lying. It is important to note that being sedentary and being physically inactive are two different things. A person can be sufficiently active and still be considered sedentary if they spend a large amount of their day sitting or lying down at work, at home, for travel, for study or during their leisure time.

Numerous lines of evidence have shown that a higher level of habitual physical activity is associated with less body fat, and that highly active people are much less likely to be obese. Almost all activities of daily living and working involve less energy expenditure than was the case one or two generations ago. Reduced physical activity affects body composition as well; lean muscle tissue decreases in mass and this reduces resting metabolic rate, thus further reducing total energy expenditure. Both duration and intensity of physical activity are important when considering the health benefits.

Physical activity duration

Physical activity taken as short sessions at intervals throughout the day (for example, three sessions of ten minutes) is as effective as that taken in one longer session. While **cardiorespiratory fitness** might be achieved in only three to four aerobic sessions weekly, weight control is best assisted by daily physical activity. Slow and prolonged physical activity utilises a higher proportion of fat to carbohydrate than more vigorous aerobic physical activity. In addition, 'personal behaviour-based' activity is just as effective, or more so, than 'planned' exercise classes when it comes to losing body fat. In the personal behaviour approach, individuals are encouraged to look for opportunities to accumulate several short bouts of physical activity over the course of the day instead of planning for and participating in one major exercise session. The former leads to an increased (and the latter can actually lead to a decreased) energy expenditure (Paoli et al. 2012).

For most individuals, physical activity alone has a comparatively minor effect on existing overweight and it is much more effective to combine physical activity with a modest restriction of food energy with an increase in dietary protein, especially if resistance

training is being undertaken. Restricting food intake without accompanying physical activity leads to a loss of lean tissue as well as fat, since body protein also functions as a glucose reserve. By stimulating muscle development, physical activity helps to maintain muscle mass, thus resulting in preferential loss of fat. It is important to differentiate between change in weight and change in body fat. The overweight individual who begins regular physical activity may maintain (or even gain) muscle while losing body fat, and the result is a gain in health benefits, such as blood pressure and insulin sensitivity, with only a small reduction in body weight. It is the internal abdominal fat that constitutes most risk, and it is this fat that is more readily mobilised and used with regular physical activity, resulting in a reduction in abdominal girth. Abdominal girth, rather than total body weight or fat, is a more sensitive indicator of health risk (see Chapter 23).

Physical activity intensity

Intensity level of physical activity refers to the extent to which the activity is being performed or the magnitude of the effort required to perform an activity or exercise; it can be regarded as 'how hard a person works to do the activity'. The intensity of different forms of physical activity varies between people depending on an individual's previous physical activity experience and their relative fitness level. There are several ways to measure the level of intensity of our activities. The intensity of physical activities is commonly expressed as metabolic equivalent, or MET, which is the ratio of a person's working metabolic rate relative to their resting metabolic rate. By convention, one MET is equivalent to the consumption of 3.5 mL of oxygen per kilogram body weight per minute, and is roughly equivalent to energy expenditure of 1 kcal/kg/hour, or the energy cost of sitting quietly. It is estimated that, compared with sitting quietly, a person's energy consumption is three to six times higher when being moderately active (3–6 METs) and more than six times higher when being vigorously active (>6 METs). Moderate-intensity physical activity requires a moderate amount of effort and noticeably accelerates the heart rate, while vigorous-intensity physical activity requires a large amount of effort and causes rapid breathing and a substantial increase in heart rate. The World Health Organization (2010) recommends that adults participate in 150 minutes of moderate-intensity physical activity each week. Examples of moderate-intensity and vigorous-intensity physical activity are shown in Table 30.2.

Strong evidence indicates that a sedentary way of life contributes to many preventable causes of death, and excessive time spent watching a screen (such as television, computer monitor or mobile device) is linked to negative health consequences. In adults, a greater amount of time spent in sedentary behaviour is consistently associated with higher risk for overweight or obesity, high blood pressure, type 2 diabetes, metabolic syndrome and site-specific cancers, including colon, endometrial and ovarian. There is also a reasonable level of evidence to suggest that sedentary behaviour during childhood and adolescence is a strong predictor of obesity during adulthood (Hesketh et al. 2005). Movements such

as fidgeting, moderate arm movements or swinging the legs may be sufficient to alleviate some adverse metabolic consequences of sitting. A systemic review and meta-analysis of sixteen prospective cohort studies involving more than one million individuals suggests that high levels of moderate-intensity physical activity (about 60–75 minutes per day) could eliminate the increased risk of death associated with high sitting time; however, this high activity level appears to attenuate, but not eliminate, the increased risk associated with high TV-viewing time (Ekelund et al. 2016). Therefore it is important to be physically active if long periods of sitting time each day, such as for work or transport, are unavoidable.

These aspects of physical activity have been combined to inform Australia's Physical Activity and Sedentary Behaviour Guidelines (Table 30.3). These outline the minimum levels of physical activity required for health benefits in general, and also for healthy development in infants, and include ways to incorporate physical activity and minimise sedentary behaviour.

Table 30.2: Examples of activities with various levels of intensity

Level of intensity	Example of activities
Light intensity (approximately <3 METs)	Sleeping (0.9 MET) Watching television (1.0 MET) Desk work (1.8 METs) Walking <4 km/hour (2.9 METs)
Moderate intensity (approximately 3–6 METs)	Brisk walking ≥4 km/hour (3.0 METs) Cycling <16 km/hour (4.0 METs) Recreational swimming (4.0 METs) Social tennis Golfing Ballroom dancing General gardening Housework and domestic chores Walking domestic animals Active involvement in games and sports with children Carrying or moving moderate loads <20 kg
Vigorous intensity (approximately >6 METs)	Race walking, jogging or running (8–10 METs) Briskly walking or climbing up a hill Fast swimming Aerobic dancing Fast cycling ≥16 km/hour Heavy gardening (continuous digging or hoeing) Carrying or moving heavy loads >20 kg

Table 30.3: Australia's Physical Activity and Sedentary Behaviour Guidelines

Age range	Physical Activity Recommendations	Sedentary Behaviour Recommendations
Birth to 5 years	• For healthy development in infants (birth to one year), physical activity, particularly supervised floor-based play in safe environments, should be encouraged from birth. • Toddlers (1–3 years) and preschoolers (3–5 years) should be physically active every day for at least three hours, spread throughout the day.	• Children under 2 years of age should not spend any time watching television or using other electronic media (DVDs, computer and other electronic games). • For children 2–5 years of age, sitting and watching television and the use of other electronic media* should be limited to less than one hour per day. • Infants, toddlers and preschoolers (all children birth to 5 years) should not be sedentary, restrained, or kept inactive, for more than one hour at a time, with the exception of sleeping.
5–12 years	• Accumulate at least 60 minutes of moderate to vigorous-intensity physical activity every day. • Include a variety of aerobic activities, including some vigorous-intensity activity. • Engage in activities that strengthen muscle and bone at least three days per week. • Achieve additional health benefits, children should engage in more activity—up to several hours per day.	• Limit use of electronic media for entertainment (e.g. television, seated electronic games and computer use) to no more than two hours a day. Break up long periods of sitting as often as possible.
13–17 years	• Accumulate at least 60 minutes of moderate to vigorous-intensity physical activity every day. • Include a variety of aerobic activities, including some vigorous-intensity activity. • Engage in activities that strengthen muscle and bone at least three days per week. • Achieve additional health benefits, young people should engage in more activity—up to several hours per day.	• Limit use of electronic media for entertainment[†] to no more than two hours a day. • Break up long periods of sitting as often as possible.
18–64 years	• Doing any physical activity is better than doing none. If you currently do no physical activity, start by doing some and gradually build up to the recommended amount. • Be active on most, preferably all, days every week. • Accumulate 150–300 minutes (2.5–5 hours) of moderate-intensity physical activity or 75–150 minutes (1.25–2.5 hours) of vigorous-intensity physical activity, or an equivalent combination of both moderate and vigorous activities, each week. • Do muscle-strengthening activities on at least 2 days each week.	• Minimise the amount of time spent in prolonged sitting. • Break up long periods of sitting as often as possible.
65 years and older	• Do some form of physical activity, no matter what your age, weight, health problems or abilities. • Be active every day in as many ways as possible, doing a range of physical activities that incorporate fitness, strength, balance and flexibility. • Accumulate at least 30 minutes of moderate-intensity physical activity on most, preferably all, days. • For those who have stopped physical activity, or who are starting a new physical activity—to start at a level that is easily manageable and gradually build up the recommended amount, type and frequency of activity. • For those who continue to enjoy a lifetime of vigorous physical activity—to carry on doing so in a manner suited to their capability into later life, provided recommended safety procedures and guidelines are adhered to.	• (No recommendation)

Notes: * Other electronic media include DVDs, computer and other electronic games; † Electronic media for entertainment, such as television, seated electronic games and computer use

Source: Australian Government (2017)

Benefits of being physically active
Food intake and energy balance

Physical activity naturally increases energy expenditure and can influence total food intake in ways which make intake more likely to match needs. One reason for this is that physical activity can help regulate eating behaviour via endocrine mediators such as insulin, leptin and ghrelin. The emotional state following physical activity might influence food intake or choice after stress exposure (for example, by reducing the intake of high energy sweet or salty foods). If there is a reduction or no compensatory increase in stress-induced food intake after physical activity, this could have a beneficial influence on overall energy balance in these stressful situations.

Another important contribution physical activity makes to energy balance is to maintain or increase skeletal muscle mass, whose bulk and strength are major determinants of resting and active energy metabolism. Thus, being physically active is beneficial in both obesity prevention and treatment, especially in the development of childhood obesity (see also the section 'Heart and blood vessels' in Chapter 33).

Obesity-associated gene expression

Decline in daily physical activity is thought to be a key contributor to the global obesity epidemic. However, it appears that changes in adiposity in response to environmental influences are genetically determined. In 2007, certain variants of the fat mass- and obesity-associated FTO gene were identified as the first robust obesity-susceptibility locus in genome-wide association studies (Frayling et al. 2007; Scuteri et al. 2007). Adults with a copy of the FTO variant had a 20–30 per cent higher risk of becoming obese than people without the variant. After the discovery of FTO, several studies reported that its obesity-increasing effect may be attenuated in individuals who are physically active.

In one study, researchers re-analysed data from 45 previous studies involving more than 200,000 adults to measure the interaction between the obesity risk variant of the FTO gene, physical activity and BMI. About three-quarters of the study participants were physically active—that is, they did at least 30 minutes of physical activity, such as walking the dog or pulling weeds, five days a week. It was found that people with the variant who were not physically active had a 30 per cent increased risk, whereas those who did physical activity had a 22 per cent

---

THE GENETICS OF OBESITY

Read the following review of obesity genetics:
- Albuquerque, D., Stice, E., Rodríguez-López, R., Manco, L. & Nóbrega, C., 2015, 'Current review of genetics of human obesity: From molecular mechanisms to an evolutionary perspective', *Molecular Genetics and Genomics*, 290(4): 1191–221.

- Identify the three different types of genetic obesity and their characteristics.
- Investigate further the clinical signs and management of syndromic obesity. See, for example, Geets et al. (2019).
- What are some of the genetic variations for common obesity?
- This review has explored individual approaches to obesity management. With a partner or group, discuss what your response would be to a politician who wanted to abandon public health measures such as reformulating products or changing obesogenic environments. Is it all in the genes?

increased risk (Kilpeläinen et al. 2011). Similar results were reported in another study, namely that physical activity can reduce the weight-gaining effects of the strongest known genetic risk factor for obesity, the obesity risk variant of the FTO gene, by about 30 per cent (Graff et al. 2017).

Body composition and body fat distribution

Regular physical activity has modest effects on reducing body weight, with substantially greater effects on improving body composition. However, physical activity can vary in intensity, and different intensities may have different associations with body fat and distribution. Moderate or vigorous physical activity may be associated with increases in lean mass, and with changes in body fat distribution (Deere et al. 2012; Ekelund et al. 2011). Physical activity in sufficient amounts can lead to substantial decreases in body weight, total body fat and visceral fat. Evidence now supports the conclusion that more physical activity can lead to additional benefits. In addition, there are a number of important risk factors for **cardiometabolic syndrome** that are more favourably affected by moderate-intensity than by vigorous-intensity physical activity. Furthermore, physical activity training-induced changes in mitochondrial oxidative capacity in skeletal muscle appear to improve insulin action by reducing the accumulation of incompletely oxidised fatty acids in muscle (Slentz et al. 2009).

ENERGY BALANCE IN REAL LIFE

Use the checklist below to see if you are meeting your physical activity requirements. Are you:

- matching your energy intake to your energy needs?
- using a combination of not being sedentary and undertaking regular physical activity on most if not all days of the week?
- accumulating 150–300 minutes (20–40 minutes a day) of moderate-intensity physical activity (like gardening, cycling, swimming) over the week?
- doing muscle-strengthening activities at least two days a week?

Eating just 650 kJ (or 150 kcal) more than you burn each day can lead to a gain of five kilograms over twelve months. If you don't want this weight gain to happen, or you want to lose the extra weight, you can either reduce your energy in or increase your energy out. Doing both is the best way to achieve and maintain a healthy body weight.

Examples of ways to cut down your 'energy in' include:

- drink water instead of a sugary or alcoholic beverage
- avoid potato chips or fries, or order a salad without dressing
- eat a boiled or poached egg instead of fried eggs
- ask for grilled rather than fried fish
- cut the fat spread on your bread.

Are there any other ways you could reduce your energy in?

Examples of ways to burn 650 kJ ('energy out') in just 30 minutes (for a 70 kg person):

- walk briskly for three kilometres
- do garden work (raking leaves, digging, etc.)
- go for a bike ride or swim
- dance with your family or friends.

Reduced mortality and extended life expectancy

The dose–response relationship between physical activity time and mortality benefits has been demonstrated in a prospective cohort study of over 400,000 adults (Wen et al. 2011). The results of this study suggest that a minimum of fifteen minutes a day of moderate-intensity physical activity might be of benefit to adults in all age groups, including those with CVD risks. Every additional fifteen minutes of daily physical activity beyond the minimum could further reduce all-cause mortality by 4 per cent and all-cancer mortality by 1 per cent (Wen et al. 2011).

NUTRIENT–GENE INTERACTIONS

Traditionally, nutrition research has assumed that all similar individuals have the same nutritional requirements. Increasingly, however, it is being recognised that there are individual needs and preferences driven by genetic and cultural factors. Although the average response to a dietary intervention can be predicted for groups of individuals, the specific response for each individual in a group can vary dramatically. The nutritional requirements are not optimised for genetic subgroups, which may differ critically, for example, in the activity of transport proteins for a micronutrient and/or enzymes that require that micronutrient as a cofactor. These inter-individual differences may be partially engrained in an individual's genetic make-up. The science that pursues the identification of informative genetic variants responsible for these gene–diet interactions—or, put simply, the science of the effect of genetic variation on dietary response—is known as '**nutrigenetics**' (Fenech et al. 2011). The discovery of interactions between diet and genetic variants has led to intense research and debate about the effectiveness of personalised nutrition as a more suitable tool for the prevention of chronic diseases than the traditional one-size-fits-all recommendations (Konstantinidou et al. 2014).

Genetic variation across the human genome is recognised as increasingly complex. Single nucleotide polymorphisms are the most common form of sequence variation in the human genome, but variants, which appear to be much more widespread than previously expected, may be a great source of genetic variation. Nucleotide repeats, insertions and deletions are other types of variations that could also modify an individual's response to diet. Genetic polymorphisms are normally found in at least 1 per cent of the population, but common polymorphisms can occur in up to 40–50 per cent of the population. Genetic polymorphisms may have no consequence, or they may have significant effects on the structure or function of the gene product. The genomic information allows us to acquire new knowledge aimed at a better understanding of nutrient–gene interactions depending on the genotype. Different experimental approaches are used to identify genetic variants that modify the effects of dietary factors or influence food preferences.

While genes are critical for determining function, certain nutrients can modify the extent to which different genes are expressed and thereby modulate whether individuals attain the potential established by their genetic background. The ability of diet to affect the flow of genetic information can occur at multiple sites of regulation. Diet can affect the expression levels of genes by acting on transcription factors or by causing epigenetic changes, such as methylating DNA. The expression of genetic formation can be altered by nutrients at the level of gene regulation, signal transduction and through alterations of chromatin structure and protein function. '**Nutrigenomics**' initially referred to the study of the role of nutrients and bioactive food compounds in the expression of an individual's genetic make-up (Figure 30.2). This definition has been broadened to encompass nutritional factors that protect the genome from damage (Fenech et al. 2011). Ultimately, nutrigenomics is concerned with the impact of dietary components on the genome, the proteome (the sum total of all proteins), and the metabolome (the sum of all metabolites).

There are three identified principles underpinning the science of nutrigenetics and nutrigenomics (Fenech et al. 2011).

1. The inherited genome varies widely among ethnic groups and individuals, and this affects nutrient bioavailability and metabolism.

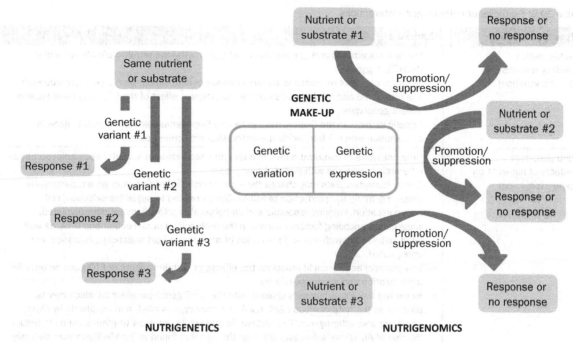

Figure 30.2: How genes interact with certain nutrients or substrates

2. There are great differences in food/nutrient availability and food choices depending on people's cultural, economic, geographical and taste perception differences.

3. Gene expression and genome stability can be affected by malnutrition (deficiency or excess) itself. Genome stability can affect mutations at the gene sequence or chromosomal level which may result in an abnormal gene dosage and gene expression so leading to adverse phenotypes at various stages of life.

Another important aspect of nutrient–gene interaction studies with the potential for both intra- and transgenerational effects is 'epigenetics', which refers to the processes that regulate how and when certain genes are expressed or silenced over time (see Chapter 1). The mechanisms that allow nutritional epigenetics to operate include methylation of DNA strands and **histones** modifications. Certain foods have greater capacity to do this, such as those with components that provide methyl groups (e.g. choline or methionine). Note that these modifications do not change the

DNA sequence but, instead, affect how cells 'read' genes. Epigenetic processes have a strong influence on normal growth and development, and may be deregulated in certain diseases such as cancer. Diet on its own, or by interaction with other environmental factors, can cause epigenetic changes that may turn certain genes on or off. Epigenetic silencing of genes that would normally protect against a disease could make people more susceptible to developing that disease later in life (Jang & Serra 2014; Pembrey 2002; Simopoulos 2010). See examples of nutrient–gene interactions in Table 30.4.

The findings of the Barker theory are now familiar—that is, that maternal nutrition is critical for fetal development, birthweight, placental dimensions and gene expression, all of which can affect the health of the child into adulthood and later life (Barker 2012). Barker's theory states that a baby's nourishment before birth and during infancy 'programs' the development of risk factors for obesity, CVD and diabetes (see also chapters 20–22). Furthermore, subsequent studies have found that even brief periods of famine or plenty in the lives of

Table 30.4: Examples of nutrient–gene interactions

Type of interaction	Example
Nutrigenetics (dietary response to genetic variation)	• Folate requirements and specific variant of 5,10-methylene tetrahydrofolate reductase (MTHFR) enzyme. • Serum cholesterol response to dietary cholesterol is apolipoprotein E genotype-dependent. • The role of n-6 and n-3 fatty acids on the atherogenic effect of the 5-lipoxygenase enzyme variant genotypes. • Genetic variants in the 5-lipogenase gene and 5-lipogenase-activating protein gene in combination with n-6 fatty acids are associated with breast cancer risk.
Nutrigenomics (effects of nutrients on gene expression)	• Different types of carbohydrates can alter gene expression in subcutaneous adipose tissue differently in persons with metabolic syndrome. • Energy-restricted diets may change the expression of adipose tissue genes, particularly those regulating the production of PUFAs. Genes related to signal transduction, cell communication, immune response and carbohydrate metabolism are downregulated, while genes encoding factors involved in the metabolism of nucleotide and DNA, as well as in cellular biosynthesis and regulation of protein and lipid metabolic processes, are upregulated. • Low physical activity could modulate the effects of certain variants of FTO gene on body fat accumulation and insulin sensitivity. • Increased risk for Alzheimer's disease with the ApoE genotypic allele ε4 which may be present as the heterozygous ε2ε4, ε3ε4 and homozygous ε4ε4, and modifiable by diets which are also atherogenic. The problem is that we do not know whether such diets reduce the risk of Alzheimer's disease, although the patterns found in the Mediterranean diet may do so.
Epigenetics (processes that regulate how and when certain genes are turned on and off	• In the development of some cancers, an epigenetic change that silences a tumour suppressor gene, which keeps the growth of the cell in check, could lead to uncontrolled cellular growth. Or another epigenetic change that 'turns off' genes that help repair damaged DNA, may lead to an increase in DNA damage, which in turn, increases cancer risk.

Source: Simopoulos (2010)

grandparents and parents, or of smoking at puberty, predicted health and life expectancy in descendants (Bygren et al. 2001; Wahlqvist et al. 2015). These observations provided the population evidence for epigenetics, where intergenerational effects of genome modulation can be seen. Moreover, they provide evidence for much more rapid evolutionary change than we thought, and of the importance of today's food systems for future generations.

Nutrigenetic and nutrigenomic approaches of disease and disorder prevention and treatments

It is speculated that better health outcomes can be achieved if nutritional requirements are customised for each individual, taking into consideration both inherited and acquired genetic characteristics depending on life-stage, dietary preferences and health status. Advances in nutrigenomics and nutrigenetics have been seen with the use of

animal models and systems biology approaches to explore interactions with gene pathways; however, extrapolation to humans and clinical implementation is not widespread at present. Despite this, advances in nutrigenomic and nutrigenetic research will make it increasingly possible to move towards a more personalised nutrition approach for optimal health and disease prevention (Konstantinidou et al. 2014).

In addition to providing a more rational basis for giving personalised dietary advice, the knowledge gained by applying genomic information to nutrition research will also improve the quality of evidence used for making population-based dietary recommendations. Discoveries made in the field of nutrigenomics should translate into more effective dietary strategies to improve overall health by identifying unique targets for prevention. The sequencing of an individual's genome has stimulated interest in the field of personalised—and what is

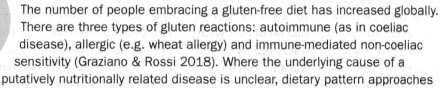

GLUTEN REACTIONS

The number of people embracing a gluten-free diet has increased globally. There are three types of gluten reactions: autoimmune (as in coeliac disease), allergic (e.g. wheat allergy) and immune-mediated non-coeliac sensitivity (Graziano & Rossi 2018). Where the underlying cause of a putatively nutritionally related disease is unclear, dietary pattern approaches with minimal risk are preferred to those that are food component-specific. The global increase in removing gluten from diets has increased the risk of nutrition deficiencies and can limit social engagement and quality of life (Lerner et al. 2018).

Coeliac disease has a genetic component but environmental factors are strongly implicated and involve nutrigenic and epigenetic pathways (see Barisani 2019). Coinciding with the increased incidence of coeliac disease has been increased use within the food industry of isolated transglutaminase enzymes from microbiological sources to modify the functionality of proteins in food products. Microbial transglutaminase enzymes are used for multiple purposes, such as to improve the texture and volume of foods in commercially baked goods; to improve the texture, appearance, hardness and shelf life of meat; to increase the hardness of fish products; to improve the quality and texture of milk and dairy products; and to improve the texture and elasticity of confectionery (Lerner & Torsten 2018).

Endogenous human tissue transglutaminase enzyme is believed to be the **autoantigen** of coeliac disease. Therefore, it has been hypothesised that using microbial transglutaminase enzymes in food processing poses a risk to gluten-sensitive populations, and that this may in part be responsible for the surge in the incidence of the disease.

The application of nutrigenomics to 'personalised nutrition' may be particularly beneficial in these conditions, where gut mucosal sensitivity to gluten has been established and its avoidance is therapeutically effective. This has been demonstrated in clinical trials where the risks of avoidance of gluten-containing foods are determined, minimised and weighed up against the benefits. However, if changes in the food system are primarily responsible for the increasing incidence and prevalence, should the emphasis not be on regulation of the food system? Such an emphasis would still be consistent with the best available clinical or personal management of those exhibiting the gluten-induced pathologies. The changing pattern of this disorder in the population might be a reflection of disconnectedness between the food and health systems.

increasingly referred to as 'precision'—medicine. Not only does the replication and validation of nutrigenetic studies often remain necessary, but the single nutrient (or other bioactive food component), **single nucleotide polymorphism (SNP)** involved requires a more contextual approach involving several factors, dietary, environmental and social, along with an evaluation of overall health benefit (Simopoulos 2010).

MICROBIOMICS

It has been known for some time that the human body is inhabited by trillions of microorganisms, primarily bacteria in the gut, outnumbering human cells by ten to one; however, because of their small size, they make up only about 1–3 per cent of the body's mass. In healthy individuals, these microbes live most of the time in harmony with their human hosts, providing essential functions for human health and survival. Human microbiota can include bacteria, archaea, unicellular eukaryotes and viruses. Some of them are even known to be pathogens, but, in normal circumstances, they cause no disease. What seems to happen with gut **microbiomes**—and presumably others that occupy skin, the reproductive tract, the lactating breast, and the respiratory tract— is that biodiversity allows a set of functions to be operative; these are more likely to support health if the microbiome in question is more diverse. This diversity, at least in the gut, may be influenced by diet (David et al. 2014). Microbiome projects have been launched worldwide in an attempt to understand the roles that these microorganisms play and their impacts on human health. Even the definition of the human microbiome has been complicated by confusion about terminology; for example, 'microbiota' (the microbial populations associated with humans) and 'microbiome' (the catalogue of these microbes and their genes) are often used interchangeably.

The Human Microbiome Project (https://hmpdacc.org/hmp/), established in 2008, is one such project. This project has analysed nearly 5000 specimens from 129 men and 113 women, revealing a high degree of variation in the microbial make-up for a given body site (gastrointestinal tract, mouth, nasal cavity, skin and vagina), not only in type but also in abundance (Human Microbiome Project Consortium et al. 2012; Huttenhower et al. 2012). Much of this diversity is unexplained, although host genetics, early microbial exposure, diet, environment and personal behaviours are all implicated. Cataloguing the necessary and sufficient sets of microbiome features that support health, and identifying the normal ranges of these features in healthy populations, is essential if microbial configurations are implicated in disease and require manipulation. Nevertheless, it seems that microbiomic functions are the key driver for microbiomic population characteristics, best served by diversity, rather than the other way around.

The distribution of microbial metabolic activities matters more than the species of microbes providing them. For example, in the healthy gut, a population of bacteria always exists to help with fat digestion, but the bacterial species carrying out this function may not be the same. These microbes contribute to normal, healthy human physiology. However, diseases such as bacteraemia or sepsis, pneumonia and peritonitis can occur if the microbe numbers grow beyond their typical ranges (e.g. due to a compromised immune system), or if microbes populate, through poor hygiene or injury, areas of the body normally not colonised or sterile, such as the blood, lower respiratory tract or abdominal cavity. When one or more bacterial species are affected, such as when a person is sick or takes antibiotics, the species make-up of the microbiome may shift substantially; however, the microbiome will return to a state of equilibrium, even if the previous composition of microbe types does not.

Dynamic interactions between human microbiota and the environment

In humans, the first microbial colonisation occurs in the gastrointestinal tract of an infant. The earliest colonisers are usually facultative anaerobic bacteria, those that can grow without oxygen, such as enterobacteria, streptococci and staphylococci; later colonisers tend to be obligate anaerobes, which are destroyed by exposure to oxygen, e.g. bifidobacteria, clostridia and bacteroides. The mode of childbirth strongly influences the microbiota that an infant begins to acquire (Yang et al. 2016). Immediately or about twenty minutes after birth, the microbiota of vaginally delivered infants resembles that of their mother's vagina, while infants delivered via caesarean section harbour microbial communities typically found on human skin. At age 3–6 weeks, bifidobacteria appear to be predominant in exclusively breastfed infants, whereas formula-fed infants have more diverse microbiota with lower numbers of bifidobacteria. The acquisition of microbiota continues over the first few years of life. By the end of the first year after birth, when the infant has already started to eat the same foods as the adults, their gut microbiota begins to resemble that of an adult (Yang et al. 2016) (see Chapter 21 for a discussion on breastmilk as personalised medicine).

In healthy individuals, microbial colonies living on or in the body are normally benign (doing no harm) or beneficial. These microbes are considered to be non-pathogenic, and either commensal or mutualistic. Table 30.5 provides a list of organs with microbiota. These microorganisms carry out a series of necessary functions, and work in tandem with the host's defences and the immune system in the gut and skin to protect against pathogen colonisation and invasion (Conrad & Vlassov 2015). They can prevent the growth of harmful pathogens by altering pH, consuming nutrients required for pathogen survival and secreting toxins that inhibit growth of pathogens.

The interaction between the human microbiota and the environment is dynamic, with human microbes flowing freely onto touched surfaces. Each dietary change can lead to changes in the gut microbiota, and microbial community structures differ depending on diets. When the adult diet is introduced to the infant, genes in the microbiome associated with vitamin biosynthesis and poly-saccharide digestion become enriched. It has been demonstrated that short-term consumption of diets composed entirely of animal or plant products can alter microbial community structure, reflecting trade-offs between the protein and carbohydrate fermentation; such responses to altered diets thus allows the diversity of human dietary patterns (David et al. 2014).

The establishment of a 'healthy' relationship early in life appears to be crucial to maintaining intestinal homeostasis (Gonçalves et al. 2018). While we do not yet have a clear understanding of what constitutes a 'healthy' colonic microbiota, many studies have identified particular bacterial species that are

Table 30.5: Predominant bacteria on the surface of various organs or location in human adults

Organ or location	Predominant bacteria
Skin	*Corynebacterium*, *Propionibacterium* and *Staphylococcus*
Eye (conjunctiva)	*Pseudomonas*, *Propionibacterium*, *Bradyrhizobium* and *Corynbacterium*
Ear	*Pseudomonas*, *Streptococcus* and *Fusobacterium*
Nose (nasal membranes)	*Staphylococcus* and *Corynebacterium*
Oral cavity (mouth and throat)	*Streptococcus*
Throat (pharynx)	*Streptococcus*, *Neisseria*, gram-negative rods and cocci
Lung	*Pseudomonas*, *Streptococcus*, *Prevotella*, *Fusobacterium* and *Veillonella*
Gastrointestinal tract	
– Stomach	*Helicobacter pylori*
– Small intestine	*Streptococci*, *Staphylococci* and **lactic acid bacteria** such as *Lactobacillus*, *Enterococcus* and *Bifidobacterium*
– Colon	*Bacteriodes*, *Clostridium* and lactic acid bacteria such as *Lactobacillus*, *Enterococcus* and *Bifidobacterium*
Urogenital tract	
– Anterior urethra	*Staphylococcus*, *Corynebacterium* and enterics
– Vagina	Lactic acid bacteria (during child-bearing years)
Placenta	*Escherichia coli*, Firmicutes, Tenericutes, Proteobacteria, Bacteriodetes and Fusobacteria (In aggregate, the placenta profiles are most akin to the non-pregnant human oral microbiome.)
Breastmilk	*Weisella*, *Leuconostoc*, *Staphylococcus*, *Streptococcus* and *Lactococcus* (In 1- and 6-month milk samples, the typical inhabitants of the oral cavity increase significantly.)

Source: Conrad & Vlassov (2015)

associated with a healthy microbiota. The bacterial species residing within the mucous layer of the colon may affect whether host cellular homeostasis is maintained. This could occur through either direct contact with host cells, or through indirect

THE MICROBIOME

The microbiome has been described as a complex ecosystem. There are within- and between-species interactions internally, as well as complex interfaces with environmental and food systems. The way we build our environment increases or decreases our contact with microbial organisms, affecting colonisation. Individual foods will have their own microbial network, and where the food is grown and how it is processed will impact on that network.

In a group or with a partner, brainstorm all the factors that interconnect to impact on your microbiome. Start from when you were a baby and move to the present day. Think not only about your biological system but also the environmental and food systems with which you are in contact. You may need to do some research to find out what these factors may be. Remember the first step for systems thinking is unpacking all the interconnections.

Some non-food related factors that may influence the microbiome include:

- hygiene, including living with animals
- infection
- inflammation
- antibiotics and medications
- physical activity
- stress
- sleep.

communication via bacterial metabolites. In addition, the genetic diversity within the gut microbiota appears to allow the digestion of compounds via metabolic pathways which are not explicitly coded for the human genome, and therefore greatly increases the ability of humans to extract energy from diverse diets (Rowland et al. 2018).

Gut microbiota and human health

The human gut microbiota (GM) has the largest numbers of microbes—estimated to be trillions—and the greatest number of species of the human body. The number, type and function of microbes vary along the length of the gastrointestinal tract. Most are found in the colon, which has a rich nutrient environment serving as a preferred site for intestinal microbial colonisation (Conrad & Vlassov 2015).

Studies in humans and animal models have highlighted the key role that diet plays in shaping gut microbial ecology, and how the GM enables the digestion of substrates inaccessible to our own human enzymes. At the same time, the GM exerts its role through several integrated pathways, including the host immune system, responses to the environment (including diet) and their genome (Quigley 2013).

Increasing attention is being directed towards the GM, its role in metabolic health and its overall metabolic capacity. Carbohydrates and proteins that escape digestion in the small intestine constitute the major substrates at the disposal of the GM. Undigested food components, as well as endogenous compounds such as digestive enzymes and shed epithelial cells and associated mucus, enter the colon and become available for anaerobic fermentation by the colonic microbiota. Fermentation of these substrates results in the production of a range of metabolites, including short-chain fatty acids (SCFAs) such as acetic, propionic and butyric acids, branched-chain fatty acids, ammonia, amines, phenolic compounds, and gases, including hydrogen, methane and hydrogen sulphide (Maukonen & Saarela 2014). It is estimated that up to 95 per cent of microbiota-produced SCFAs are readily absorbed by the colonocytes for use as energy substrates, and act as signalling molecules involved in systemic lipid metabolism and glucose/insulin regulation. Furthermore, the SCFAs produced by the GM have been reported to exert anti-inflammatory properties, such as leukocyte recruitment, leukocyte chemotaxis and chemokine production. However, only a few studies confirm the modulation of immune function by these SCFAs (Morrison & Preston 2016). In animal models, it is shown that the GM can affect innate immunity, resulting in increased susceptibility to allergic inflammation. Early-life microbial exposure seems critical for the establishment of tolerance to mucosal innate immune cells and subsequent protection from the inflammation later in life (Olszak et al. 2012).

In addition, the GM is involved in the production of vitamins, the activation or inactivation of bio-active food components such as isoflavonoids and plant lignans, the conversion of **prodrugs** to their bioactive forms, and the transformation of bile acids and xenobiotics (Rowland et al. 2018). Bacterial conversion of these compounds results in a wide variety of metabolites that are in close contact with the host's cells, and these metabolites can affect the metabolic phenotype of the host. Collectively, the microbiota exert a fundamental influence on systemic metabolism and immunity, and healthy GM are largely responsible for the overall health of the host (Quigley 2013).

Gut microbiota and the mucosal immunity system

Due to the high selectivity of the gut environment, only microbes that are able to establish a 'dialogue' with the host can inhabit the gastrointestinal tract; the others are eliminated by the combined action of the host's immune system and the resident microbes (Conrad & Vlassov 2015). With the trillions of microbes that inhabit the gastrointestinal tract, there is a need for a balance between tolerance to commensals and a robust protective response against pathogens, to avoid unnecessary immune responses against otherwise harmless bacteria. The GM appears to be essential for maintaining homeostasis of the mucosal immune system. The mechanisms by which the immune system maintains this critical balance remain unclear. One of the possible pathways is

through the secretion of SCFA butyric acid in large amounts by commensal bacteria (Gonçalves et al. 2018). This fatty acid appears to be able to suppress the function or response of intestinal macrophages, and this then enables the host to maintain tolerance to the intestinal microbiota (Chang et al. 2014). This process must operate within the context of a dynamic equilibrium of microbial diversity that rapidly fluctuates in response to an environment of ingested dietary materials. Research has begun to unravel the chemical 'language' of host–commensal interactions, and to decipher how specific microbial metabolites affect different host cell types.

Factors affecting the gut microbiota

The host's age, gender, genetics, ethnicity, medications, disorders or diseases and diet can affect the composition of the human GM. As previously mentioned, bacterial colonisation of the infant gastrointestinal tract is influenced by a number of factors, including mode of delivery, prematurity, type of feeding (breastfeeding or formula feeding) and antibiotic treatment (Yang et al. 2016). Twins, especially monozygotic twins, tend to have similar inter-individual faecal microbiota. The GM of preterm infants is less diverse than that of full-term babies. The GM evolves with age. Changes in diet and physical activity, salivary function, digestion and slower intestinal transit time can affect the GM of ageing people. The GM of the elderly has been reported to be relatively stable and, compared with that of younger adults, more diverse and with greater inter-individual variation (Rodríguez et al. 2015).

Successful colonisation of a species acquired from the environment may depend on the ability to utilise differential nutrient sources, perform chemical sensing, and coordinate gene expression in favourable ways. Two important external factors affecting the GM are dietary components and antibiotic use. Due to its dynamic nature, the GM could potentially be manipulated via dietary changes and administration of either antibiotics or probiotics to, respectively, decrease or increase microbial numbers and diversity. It is likely that substantial microbiota adaptation has accompanied

GENE TRANSFER

It has been demonstrated that gene transfer may occur within and from outside the GM. In Japan, where consumption of seaweeds or marine algae is high, a gut bacterium, *Bacteroides phebeius*, can acquire genes coding for carbohydrate-active enzymes and associated proteins from marine bacteria, enabling it to utilise polysaccharides from marine algae. These algae are not readily fermentable by GM established with Western diets (Hehemann et al. 2010).

Read the following articles and discuss the possibilities of bacterial populations susceptible to antibiotics becoming resistant through the transfer and expression of resistance genes from other strains.

- Hehemann, J.-H. et al., 2010, 'Transfer of carbohydrate-active enzymes from marine bacteria to Japanese gut microbiota', *Nature*, 464(7290), 908–12
- Huddleston, J.R., 2014, 'Horizontal gene transfer in the human gastro-intestinal tract: Potential spread of antibiotic resistance genes', *Infection and Drug Resistance*, 7, 167–76.

the dietary changes that have occurred throughout human history.

The impact of habitual diet on GM has been studied for decades. Carbohydrates are mainly fermented in the proximal colon, whereas the fermentation of proteins takes place mainly in the distal colon. Apparently, carbohydrate metabolism is more favourable to the host than protein metabolism; some of the end products of amino acid metabolism may be deleterious to the host, such as ammonia, amines and phenol compounds (Maukonen & Saarela 2014). It has been suggested that the GM may metabolise dietary fats, convert primary bile acids into secondary bile acids and impact on the enterohepatic circulation of bile acids and fat absorption from the small intestine. The metabolic output of the microbial community, however, depends not only on available dietary components, but also on the gut environment, with the pH having an important effect on the growth and composition of GM. It is worth noting the production of SCFAs by intestinal bacteria and the absorption of the SCFAs through colonic epithelial cells alters the pH of colon, which in turn affects the composition and population of GM (David et al. 2014). Changes to normal diet or, more specifically, changes in the type and amount of non-digestible carbohydrates in the human diet influence both the metabolic products formed in the lower regions of the gastrointestinal tract and levels of bacterial populations in faeces (Maukonen & Saarela 2014).

Manipulation of gut microbiota: probiotics, prebiotics and synbiotics

There has been interest in being able to manipulate or modulate the composition of GM for health benefits. This may be achieved through the targeted use of dietary supplementation, such as probiotics, prebiotics and synbiotics.

Probiotics

Derived from a Greek word meaning 'for life', the term 'probiotics' is used to define 'live micro-organisms that, when administered in adequate amounts, confer a health benefit on the host' (Hill et al. 2014) by improving microbial balance. Probiotics are bacteria that help maintain a healthy gut by reducing the number of harmful bacteria that reside in the intestine, such as pathogenic *Escherichia coli* and *Clostridia* spp., by increasing the sizes of populations of friendly bacteria, which ferment carbohydrates and have reduced proteolytic activity. Probiotics are also important for a healthy immune system, for optimal absorption of nutrients and for the production of vitamin K. Consumption of probiotics has been associated with several health-related benefits, including immune function enhancement, reducing symptoms of irritable bowel syndrome, improved lactose intolerance and, possibly, reduced risk of colon cancer (Kerry et al. 2018; Suez et al. 2019).

Probiotics are found in yoghurts and fermented milk. They are also added to infant formula and are available as dietary supplements. Probiotic products may contain either a single strain or a mixture of two or more strains. The most common types of probiotics are *Bifidobacterium* and *Lactobacillus* spp. Probiotic effects are very strain-specific and cannot be generalised. A single strain may exhibit different benefits when used individually and in combination. The benefits of a probiotic formulation also differ with the patient groups. Limited studies have shown greater efficacy with multi-strain probiotics.

The most common side effect of consuming probiotics is gastrointestinal distress, such as bloating. Serious adverse effects are rare; however, those with compromised immunity, such as elderly people, newborns, and pregnant women, could be at higher risk of potential probiotic infection.

Prebiotics

A prebiotic is defined as 'a substrate that is selectively utilised by host microorganisms conferring a health benefit' (Gibson et al. 2017). The principal concept associated with this definition is that the prebiotic has a selective effect on the microbiota that results in an improvement in health of the host. Typically, prebiotics are carbohydrates that pass through the body undigested until they reach the colon; they include dietary fibre, resistant starch, oligosaccharides and other non-absorbed sugars. In the colon, the carbohydrates are fermented, which leads to increased bowel function and the production of beneficial SCFAs. The carbohydrates also become an important fuel source for the healthy bacteria in the gut, helping them to grow in numbers. The composition of GM modified by prebiotics can lead to the predominance of some potentially health-promoting bacteria, especially (but not exclusively) *Lactobacillus* and *Bifidobacterium* (Gibson et al. 2017).

Prebiotics have been added to many foods, including breakfast cereals, bread, spreads, drinks and yoghurt. Common prebiotics in use include inulin (which is naturally found in garlic, asparagus, onions, leeks and artichokes), fructo-oligosaccharides and galacto-oligosaccharides (Pandey et al. 2015). Research has demonstrated several potential health benefits of prebiotics, such as increased bowel movement frequency and reduced episodes of constipation, particularly in children and the elderly; relief from inflammation and other symptoms associated with functional bowel disorder; and reduction of colorectal cancer risk. They are also implicated in reducing risk of developing osteoporosis, obesity and diabetes, although more research is needed to confirm these claims (Kerry et al. 2018).

It is worth noting that the immediate addition of substantial quantities of prebiotics, especially oligosaccharides, to the diet may result in an increase in fermentation, leading to increased gas production, bloating or bowel movement. Until the GM is gradually established to rehabilitate or restore intestinal bacteria, nutrient absorption may be impaired and colonic transit time temporarily increased with an immediate addition of higher prebiotic intake (Marteau & Seksik 2004).

Synbiotics

To get the most benefit from probiotics, it is crucial that live microorganisms survive the passage through the digestive tract in large numbers to reach the bowel. Since not all the health benefits can be conferred by individual types of microorganisms, it is also advisable to consume a variety of probiotics. One practical way of managing GM is the use of synbiotics, in which probiotics and prebiotics work together in a synergistic way to improve the survival of the probiotic organisms because the prebiotic or its specific substrate is readily available for fermentation. While using prebiotics and probiotics in combination is often described as synbiotic, the FAO recommends that the term 'synbiotic' be used

MICROBIOTA-TARGETED THERAPIES: IS IT A FUTURE DIRECTION?

A healthy human state must represent in part homeostasis between the host and the microbiota. Several disorders or diseases seem characterised by a disruption of this homeostasis, a state known as dysbiosis. A future in which new diagnostics and therapies enable the management of our microbiota to treat and prevent these disorders or diseases is under development.

Read the following articles and any additional material you can find:

- Haiser, H.J. & Turnbaugh, P.J., 2012, 'Is it time for a metagenomic basis of therapeutics?' *Science*, 336(6086), 1253–55
- Lemon, K.P. et al., 2012, 'Microbiota-targeted therapies: An ecological perspective, *Science Translational Medicine*, 4(137), 137rv5.

Discuss two of the challenges for the development of microbiota-targeted therapies. One will be whether and which microbiotal profile or function change would be causal for a disorder or disease. Another will be the need to understand how microbiota-targeted therapies work, as we currently expect for drug development.

only if the net health benefit is synergistic (Pineiro et al. 2008).

Can microbiota manipulate the host's behaviour?

While commensal gastrointestinal microorganisms can extract nutrients from the food, they do require specific nutrients to thrive. Dynamically responding to environmental conditions, the microbiome responds to nutritional changes, including fasting and malnutrition. In fact, early GM development is particularly important in children, whose microbiota shifts as they grow and change diet (Bergström et al. 2014). Microbiota remodelling by antibiotic therapy improved survival of children with severe acute malnutrition (Subramanian et al. 2014; Trehan et al. 2013).

It is essential for microbes (including pathogens) to acquire resources if they are to colonise the competitive environment of the human gastro-intestinal tract. The inherent colonisation resistance and competitive environment of the mammalian intestine must be overcome. In healthy individuals, competition for both nutrients and attachment sites makes pathogenic microbes, such as *Clostridium difficile*, less likely to colonise the gut and become a burden to the host (Faust et al. 2015; Guarner & Malagelada 2003).

The GM can interact with the host through a variety of processes. Analysis of metabolites shows a range of small molecules produced in the microbiome which mimic or act as neurosignallers or neurotransmitters, and through many pathways the GM can affect distal organs directly or indirectly. These pathways include the trimethylamine/trimethylamine N-oxide pathway, SCFAs pathway, and primary and secondary bile acid pathways (Ma & Li 2018). Some of these molecules appear to interact with other endocrine hormones, including ghrelin, leptin, glucagon-like peptide 1, and peptide YY. Others are reported to stimulate the parasympathetic nervous system, thereby impacting glucose homeostasis and other metabolic processes linked to development of metabolic syndrome (Clemmensen et al. 2017).

SENSORY NUTRITION

There are five generally acknowledged sensory inputs: sight, sound, smell, taste and touch. Each provides information about food, food systems and their biological, social, economic and ecological consequences. The processes involved are complex and synergistic, involving any combination of the five (Spence 2015). The biological pathways between the sensory nutritional inputs and a state of wellbeing with minimal disability include microbiomes and multiple homeostatic mechanisms in a diverse range of organs and tissues, including the brain, heart, vasculature, liver, lungs, lymphoid, bone marrow, kidneys, bone and muscle. The interaction of these sensory, microbiomic and homeostatic processes influences functions like mobility, cognition, inflammation, immunity, reproduction and mindfulness. An example of such a pathway is the way in which we gather information about foodstuffs by sight, touch, smell, taste and sound (as we crunch and chew) with remarkable potential for discrimination (e.g. among cheeses, apples and wines) (Wahlqvist 2016). This is dependent on prior learning and the representation of the collective database in the brain, especially the amygdala and hippocampus, as 'food memory' (Nishijo & Ono 1992). However, it is precarious and can be erased, for example, by the co-ingestion of excess salt.

It is, therefore, understandable that the most comprehensive and reinforced sensory nutritional input will be one where there is intimate contact with nature, rich in its embodiment of the sources of sensory information. We can expect that, as we become more remote from nature, so our nutritional status will change, and not just through a deficiency of certain nutrients, as important as they may be. We can also be at risk of broader sensory nutritional deprivation. That said, it is difficult to separate the food from non-food system contributions to nutritional wellbeing in situations like walking and gardening. There is a growing recognition and appreciation of the functional significance of landscapes to health. The industrialisation of and change to once familiar places is creating a sense of loss. There are counterparts in the dispossession of the territorial intimacy of Indigenous peoples (Louv 2011). Similarly, open public space, community and urban gardens, with food-producing and climate change mitigation potential, contribute sensory inputs to nutritional status (Hale et al. 2011); green space may overcome the contribution of socioeconomic disadvantage to all-cause and cardiovascular mortality (Figure 30.3) (Mitchell & Popham 2008). This understanding strengthens the case for the inclusion of sensory science in nutritional biology.

Sight

It is not just being able to see food grow but also the appearance of food, the eating ambience and the presentation—by way of colour, plate size and design, eating aids and more—that affect nutritional outcomes. Plate size, for example, is relevant to how we perceive serving sizes—as too little or too much—or to what we serve ourselves, e.g. from other dishes in a buffet, smorgasbord, or Chinese-style table with common dishes. Progressive size increases in drinking vessels, bowls and plates have contributed to overeating (Kairey et al. 2018). Conversely, pre-arranged food trays can help limit excess for the overweight, reduce food waste and ensure adequacy for marginally nourished elders (Lorenz & Langen 2018; Wu et al. 2018). While blemishes on food may signify damage and risk, much food is discarded unnecessarily because of scarring and shape. Educational programs to reduce this wastefulness of 'ugly food' are making headway (de Hooge et al. 2017).

Sound

Food consumers and purveyors have long chosen and traded in food based partly on its sound when chewed, e.g. crackling, crunching or popping (Duizer 2001). Even 'mouthfeel', which is a key feature of food palatability, depends partly on characteristics like crunchiness; the sound of food contributes to a multisensory experience that contributes to food preference (Stokes et al. 2013; Wahlqvist 2016). The structural and compositional basis of the sound may have nutritional relevance by way of taste alteration

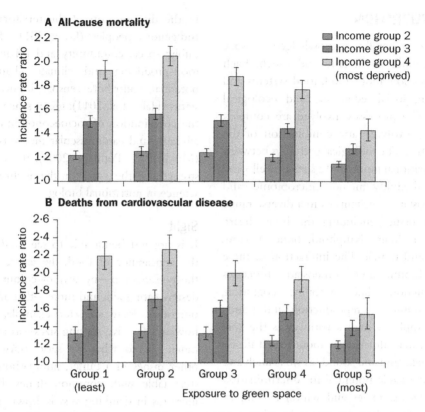

Note: Participants were grouped according to their income-deprivation quartiles and their exposure to green space. Incidence rate ratios in income-deprivation quartiles 2–4 are presented with the income-deprivation quartile 1 (least deprived or highest income) as the reference group (ratio = 1). Error bars indicate 95% CIs.

Figure 30.3: Effect of exposure to green space on all-cause and cardiovascular mortality rates

Source: Mitchell & Popham (2008). Reproduced with permission from Elsevier

and propensity to under- or overeat; energy and nutrient density; bioavailability; and chewability.

Smell

The olfactory bulb above the nose is replete with receptors so numerous that we have the potential ability to distinguish thousands of different compounds (Zozulya et al. 2001). We are unlikely ever to avail ourselves of this capacity, but it does indicate how much sensory nutritional input we could achieve, and how much we increasingly miss as our environments become less natural, more regularised for living, working and travelling, and more challenged by environmental contaminants.

More than that, these so-called olfactory receptors are widely distributed outside of the olfactory system in many different tissues throughout the body, and

they are involved in a variety of functions such as the modulation of cell–cell recognition, migration, proliferation and cell death cycle (Maßberg & Hatt 2018). For example, they are found in the brain, involved in cognition and memory; muscle; testis, affecting male reproduction; prostate gland; pancreas; kidney; cardiovascular system and more. These receptors also respond to endogenously produced metabolites so that there is cross-over between sensing the external and internal environments. This signifies that olfaction presumably plays a role in sorting and selecting chemicals that are appropriate modulators of our physiology and risk factors for disordered health. Olfaction creates a close intimacy with our environment, which we perceive in part as food or beverage. Its loss has substantial health consequences (Schiffman 1983).

Taste

There are at least five tastes—sweet, bitter, salt, sour and **umami**—represented on the tongue. In Asian food cultures, there is generally a greater preference for umami as a taste, which may discourage the intake of energy-dense foods (Gabriel et al. 2018). Umami is activated by the amino acid glutamate and ribonucleotides, including inosinate and guanylate, found notably in fermented soy products, but also in tomatoes, fish, mushrooms, seaweed, cheese and onions among others (Table 30.6). Important modulators of taste receptors include caffeine, which may explain some food and beverage preferences such as those for tea, coffee and caffeinated sugary soft drinks and associated food intakes. With age, taste sensitivity or thresholds generally change (Schiffman & Graham 2000). Mammalian olfactory and taste spectra expose us to a wide, environmentally biodiverse range of foods.

Like olfactory receptors, taste receptors are found beyond the mouth, notably in the gut, brain, and reproductive tract (Janssen & Depoortere 2013). In animal models, the microbiota may have a role to play in the gut, the activity of taste receptors and appetite (Fetissov 2016). It has been shown that preference for bitter taste is a factor affecting spermatogenesis,

meaning that how a father eats can affect his offspring (Avau & Depoortere 2016). It is likely that many other associations of food chemistry and intergenerational health will be discovered in time.

Touch

At the most obvious level, we touch our food. This is clear when people shop and check food purchases by sight and touch. Touch also contributes to food memory (Nishijo & Ono 1992). Depending on food culture, convenience or preference, we may distance ourselves from the food we eat with chopsticks or cutlery. For most of the human experience we ate with our fingers, and this still takes place in many cultures. In many parts of Africa and India, for example, hands are still used to convey food from plate to mouth. These practices are surrounded by strict protocols—for example, only using the right hand.

NUTRITIONAL MODULATION OF INFLAMMATION

For us to keep in good health we need to be able to repair ourselves after injury, infection and other challenges to our biology. Mechanical damage and insult recognised by our immune system initiates

Table 30.6: List of foods rich in umami substances

Umami substances	Foods rich in umami substances
Glutamate	Tomatoes
	Onions
	Seaweed
	Broccoli
	Peas
	White asparagus
	Cheese
	Mushrooms
	Beets
Inosinate	Sardines
	Poultry
	Pork
	Beef
Guanylate	Dried porcini
	Dried shiitake
	Dried morels

Source: Umami Information Center (2017)

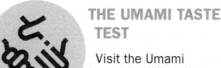

THE UMAMI TASTE TEST

Visit the Umami Information Center Website (www.umamiinfo.com/).

Make a list of foods rich in umami substances that you are not familiar with. Choose the three foods with the highest levels of umami and take a taste test. Reflect on the taste, find a person from a different cultural background to yourself and compare your notes on taste preferences.

acute inflammatory responses involved in restoration of health when these events occur. There is capillary damage and leakage with swelling, pain, heat and redness. Inflammation involves the accumulation of cells and **exudates** in irritated tissues that allows protection from further damage. Products of inflammation that contribute to these effects include eicosanoids, cytokines, reactive oxygen species and adhesion molecules. Inflammation may be protracted if the injury or insult continues, and many, if not most, chronic disorders and diseases are characterised by continuing inflammation with further damage. These are regarded as chronic inflammatory diseases, such as some forms of arthritis, bowel disease, skin disease and autoimmune diseases.

We also recognise that metabolic diseases, such as obesity and diabetes, CVD like coronary heart disease, degenerative diseases such as those of the brain, bone and joints, and **neoplastic** disease, also have inflammatory features (Pan et al. 2010)

(Figure 30.4). These are discussed in more detail in the following chapters on ecohealth disruptors.

Some biodiverse and plant-based dietary patterns, like those observed around the Mediterranean Sea, dampen inflammation, which may partly explain their health-protective properties (Wahlqvist et al. 2005). Support for this phenomenon is provided by the extensive list of natural food and medicinal products known to be associated with inflammatory modulation (Yuan et al. 2006). Prostaglandins and leukotrienes derived from long-chain n-3 fatty acids from animals (e.g. fish, eggs, lean meat, insects), but not from shorter-chain n-3 fatty acids from plants (e.g. flaxseed, purslane) are established anti-inflammatory agents (Calder 2006); the phytonutrients in plants may be more relevant (Table 30.7; see also Chapter 8). Since the GM are known to alter inflammatory responses, it is probable that dietary patterns may affect inflammation by this route (Maslowski et al. 2009).

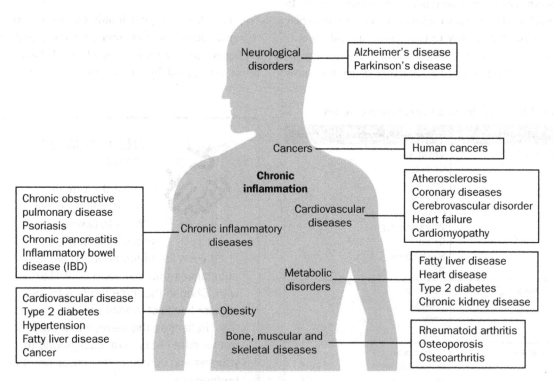

Figure 30.4: Disorders or diseases that are closely linked to chronic inflammation

Source: Pan et al. (2010). Reproduced by permission of the Royal Society of Chemistry

Table 30.7: List of natural compounds in food with anti-inflammatory properties

Compound	Type of compound	Main source
Curcumin	Polyphenol	Root of turmeric (*Curcuma longa*)
Cucurbitacins	Triterpenes	Bitter principles of the Cucurbitaceae plants
1,8-cineole	Monoterpene oxide	Essential oils from eucalyptus, sage, rosemary, psidium/guava leaves
Bromelain	Proteolytic enzyme	Flesh and stem of pineapple
Flavones, flavanones, catechins and anthocyanins	Flavonoids	Widely distributed in plants: fruits, vegetables, grains, bark, roots, stems, flowers, tea and wine
Saponin	Glycosides	Tea leaves

Source: Yuan et al. (2006)

SUMMARY

- Human nutritional biology can be understood as an ecologically and societally dependent transfer of mass and natural elements into a living, reproducing organism dependent on and capable of connectedness with others as part of an animate and inanimate world.
- Food systems support this biology and provide for the transfer of energy and various elements, molecules and bioactive compounds and effective homeostatic mechanisms.
- The adaptability of the human body to changing food or nutrition environments, and its biological consequences, can be demonstrated as part of nutritional biology.
- The human body maintains homeostasis, or a stable, relatively constant internal environment, through various mechanisms, including acid–base balance, electrolyte balance, hormonal control of blood glucose and acquisition of certain nutrients.
- The balance of total energy intake and energy output can be achieved by limiting energy intake to no greater than the required level, and a combination of engaging in regular physical activity and not being sedentary.
- Research on nutrient–genetic interactions, such as nutrigenetics, nutrigenomics and epigenetics, aims to determine the effectiveness of personalised nutrition as a more suitable tool for the prevention of chronic diseases than the traditional one-size-fits-all recommendations.
- Microbiota living in harmony with their human host can provide essential functions of health and survival of the host; however, commensal or mutualistic microbiota can become pathogenic if the host resistance mechanisms fail, either through some other infection process or through immunodeficiency.
- The composition (type and amount) of gut microbiota can be manipulated using probiotics, prebiotics or synbiotics.
- Sensory inputs—sight, sound, smell, taste and touch—play an important role in survival and a state of general wellbeing and minimal disability.
- Inflammatory processes are involved in many metabolic disorders or diseases, such as heart disease, diabetes, degenerative and neoplastic diseases.
- Managing injury, insult and chronic disease involves inflammatory processes, which can be optimised by dietary patterns. Human biological advantage and vulnerability provide evidence for an ultimate interrelationship between humans and the ecosystem.

KEY TERMS

Adenosine monophosphate-activated protein kinase (AMPK): a conserved fuel-sensing enzyme present in all mammalian cells. It plays a key role in regulating the cellular energy homeostasis. AMPK is activated in response to stresses that deplete cellular ATP supplies, such as glucose deprivation or hypoxia, or increase energy expenditure, such as muscle contraction during physical activities. When activated, AMPK stimulates energy-generating processes, such as glucose uptake and fatty acid oxidation, and turns off energy-consuming processes, such as protein and lipid synthesis, to restore energy balance.

Autoantigen: an antigen that is not recognised as a normal bodily constituent by the immune system resulting in a stimulation of autoantibody production, as in an autoimmune reaction.

Bioenergetics: the energy transformation process of cells, such as the production and utilisation of adenosine triphosphate (ATP).

Cardiometabolic syndrome: a combination of metabolic disorders or risk factors which include hyperlipidaemia, hypertension, abdominal fatness, insulin resistance and impaired glucose tolerance.

Cardiorespiratory fitness: the ability of the circulatory and respiratory systems to supply oxygen to skeletal muscles during prolonged physical activity. Cardiorespiratory fitness is mainly increased by aerobic endurance activities and in some less-fit populations a small benefit can be achieved by muscular strength activities.

Exudate: a fluid rich in protein and cells that leaks out with inflammation.

Gene analogues: compounds or substances that differ in structure but are similar in function to the general genetic materials such as DNA and RNA.

Haemopoietic: relating to the production of blood cells and platelets, which occurs in the bone marrow.

Histones: a group of proteins that help compact or condense DNA strands, which enables the compacted DNA to fit inside the nucleus. The positive charges of histones allow them to link with DNA, which is negatively charged. Some histones act as spools for the thread-like DNA to wrap around.

Hyperosmolar hyperglycaemic state: a complication of diabetes. It involves extremely high blood glucose concentrations, resulting in high osmotic concentrations without the presence of ketones, and an extreme dehydration.

Integumentary system: the set of organs that forms the external covering of the body and protects it from various kinds of damage, such as loss of water, abrasion, chemical assault and radiation damage. The system includes the skin, hairs, nails and exocrine glands, such as sweat and sebaceous glands.

Lactic acid bacteria: usually found in decomposing plants and milk products, the bacteria produce lactic acid as the major metabolic end product of carbohydrate fermentation.

Membrane potential: the difference in electric potential caused by the disparities in concentration of ions across the cell membrane. Changes in membrane potentials give cells the ability to send electrical signals, which carry messages or information, to other cells.

Microbiome: the combined genetic material of microorganisms in a particular environment; this can be, for example, in the soil or in parts of the body (gut, lung, skin). It is an ecological community of commensal, mutualistic and pathogenic microorganisms that share our body space. Commensal means the microorganisms do not offer any benefit or cause any harm to their host;

mutualistic is where the microorganisms offer some benefits to the host; and pathogenic means the microorganisms can cause some harm to the host (Lederberg & McCray 2001).

Neoplastic: the abnormal growth of tissue as in tumours and cancers.

Nutrigenetics: the field of nutrigenetics recognises the effect of genetic variation on dietary response.

Nutrigenomics: covers the effect of nutrients on gene expression.

Prodrug: a compound that is usually pharmacologically inactive, and, after administration, is metabolised into an active form of drug in the body.

Single nucleotide polymorphism (SNP): pronounced 'snip', the most common type of genetic variation among people. Each SNP represents a difference in a nucleotide, which is a single DNA building block, and is present to some appreciable degree within a population. SNPs occur normally throughout a person's DNA, and most of them have no effect on health or development; however, some of these genetic variations have proven to be very important in human health.

Umami: a Japanese term describing a savoury taste that is a characteristic of cooked meats and broths. The term 'umami' was recognised in 1985 as the scientific term to describe the taste of umami substances, glutamates and nucleotides inosinate and guanylate.

REFERENCES

Alberti, K.G.M., Zimmet, P. & Shaw, J., 2005, 'The metabolic syndrome: A new worldwide definition', *Lancet* 366(9491): 1059–62, doi:10.1016/S0140-6736(05)67402-8

Albuquerque, D., Stice, E., Rodríguez-López, R., Manco, L. & Nóbrega, C., 2015, 'Current review of genetics of human obesity: From molecular mechanisms to an evolutionary perspective', *Molecular Genetics and Genomics*, 290(4): 1191–221, doi:10.1007/s00438-015-1015-9

Anonymous, 2019, 'Carbonic acid bicarbonate buffer system', <https://back-ground2.blogspot.com/2019/01/carbonic-acid-bicarbonate-buffer-system.html>, accessed 4 January 2019

Australian Government, 2017, *Physical Activity and Sedentary Behaviour*, <www.health.gov.au/internet/main/publishing.nsf/Content/pasb>, accessed 4 January 2019

Avau, B. & Depoortere, I., 2016, 'The bitter truth about bitter taste receptors: Beyond sensing bitter in the oral cavity', *Acta Physiologica, 216*(4): 407–20, doi:10.1111/apha.12621

Barisani, D., 2019, 'miRNAs and their role in the pathogenesis of celiac disease: A review', in V.B. Patel & V.R. Preedy (eds), *Handbook of Nutrition, Diet, and Epigenetics*, Cham: Springer International Publishing, pp. 1079–99

Barker, D.J.P., 2012, 'Developmental origins of chronic disease', *Public Health Nutrition, 126*(3): 185–9, doi:10.1016/j.puhe.2011.11.014

Bergström, A., Skov, T.H., Bahl, M.I., Roager, H.M., Christensen, L.B. et al., 2014, 'Establishment of intestinal microbiota during early life: A longitudinal, explorative study of a large cohort of Danish infants', *Applied and Environmental Microbiology, 80*(9): 2889–900, doi:10.1128/AEM.00342-14

Bygren, L.O., Kaati, G. & Edvinsson, S., 2001, 'Longevity determined by paternal ancestors' nutrition during their slow growth period', *Acta Biotheoretica, 49*(1): 53–9, doi:10.1023/A:1010241825519

Calder, P.C., 2006, 'n-3 Polyunsaturated fatty acids, inflammation, and inflammatory diseases', *American Journal of Clinical Nutrition, 83*(6): 1505S–19S, doi:10.1093/ajcn/83.6.1505S

Chang, P.V., Hao, L., Offermanns, S. & Medzhitov, R., 2014, 'The microbial metabolite butyrate regulates intestinal macrophage function via histone deacetylase inhibition', *Proceedings of the National Academy of Sciences, 111*(6): 2247–52, doi:10.1073/pnas.1322269111

Clemmensen, C., Müller, T.D., Woods, S.C., Berthoud, H.-R., Seeley, R.J. & Tschöp, M.H., 2017, 'Gut–brain cross-talk in metabolic control', *Cell, 168*(5): 758–74, doi:10.1016/j.cell.2017.01.025

Conrad, R. & Vlassov, A.V., 2015, 'The human microbiota: Composition, functions, and therapeutic potential', *Medical Science Review, 2*: 92–103, doi:10.12659/MSRev.895154

Cypess, A.M., Lehman, S., Williams, G., Tal, I., Rodman, D. et al., 2009, 'Identification and importance of brown adipose tissue in adult humans', *New England Journal of Medicine, 360*(15): 1509–17, doi:10.1056/NEJMoa0810780

David, L.A., Maurice, C.F., Carmody, R.N., Gootenberg, D.B., Button, J.E. et al., 2014, 'Diet rapidly and reproducibly alters the human gut microbiome', *Nature, 505*(7484): 559–63, doi:10.1038/nature12820

de Hooge, I.E., Oostindjer, M., Aschemann-Witzel, J., Normann, A., Loose, S.M. & Almli, V.L., 2017, 'This apple is too ugly for me! Consumer preferences for suboptimal food products in the supermarket and at home', *Food Quality and Preference, 56*: 80–92, doi:10.1016/j.foodqual.2016.09.012

Deere, K., Sayers, A., Davey Smith, G., Rittweger, J. & Tobias, J.H., 2012, 'High impact activity is related to lean but not fat mass: Findings from a population-based study in adolescents', *International Journal of Epidemiology, 41*(4): 1124–31, doi:10.1093/ije/dys073

Duizer, L., 2001, 'A review of acoustic research for studying the sensory perception of crisp, crunchy and crackly textures', *Trends in Food Science & Technology, 12*(1): 17–24, doi:10.1016/S0924-2244(01)00050-4

Ekelund, U., Besson, H., Luan, J.a., May, A.M., Sharp, S.J. et al., 2011, 'Physical activity and gain in abdominal adiposity and body weight: Prospective cohort study in 288,498 men and women', *American Journal of Clinical Nutrition, 93*(4): 826–35, doi:10.3945/ajcn.110.006593

Ekelund, U., Steene-Johannessen, J., Brown, W.J., Fagerland, M.W., Owen, N. et al., 2016, 'Does physical activity attenuate, or even eliminate, the detrimental association of sitting time with mortality? A harmonised meta-analysis of data from more than 1 million men and women', *Lancet 388*(10051): 1302–10, doi:10.1016/S0140-6736(16)30370-1

Faust, K., Lahti, L., Gonze, D., De Vos, W.M. & Raes, J., 2015, 'Metagenomics meets time series analysis: Unraveling microbial community dynamics', *Current Opinion in Microbiology, 25*: 56–66, doi:10.1016/j.mib.2015.04.004

Fenech, M., El-Sohemy, A., Cahill, L., Ferguson, L.R., French, T.-A.C. et al., 2011, 'Nutrigenetics and nutrigenomics: Viewpoints on the current status and applications in nutrition research and practice', *Lifestyle Genomics, 4*(2): 69–89, doi:10.1159/000327772

Fetissov, S.O., 2016, 'Role of the gut microbiota in host appetite control: Bacterial growth to animal feeding behaviour', *Nature Reviews Endocrinology, 13*: 11, doi:10.1038/nrendo.2016.150

Frayling, T.M., Timpson, N.J., Weedon, M.N., Zeggini, E., Freathy, R.M. et al., 2007, 'A common variant in the FTO gene is associated with body mass index and predisposes to childhood and adult obesity', *Science, 316*(5826): 889–94, doi:10.1126/science.1141634

Gabriel, A.S., Ninomiya, K. & Uneyama, H., 2018, 'The role of the Japanese traditional diet in healthy and sustainable dietary patterns around the world', *Nutrients, 10*(2): 173, doi:10.3390/nu10020173

Geets, E., Meuwissen, M.E.C. & Van Hul, W., 2019, 'Clinical, molecular genetics and therapeutic aspects of syndromic obesity', *Clinical Genetics, 95*(1): 23–40, doi:10.1111/cge.13367

Gibson, G.R., Hutkins, R., Sanders, M.E., Prescott, S.L., Reimer, R.A. et al., 2017, 'Expert consensus document: The International Scientific Association for Probiotics and Prebiotics (ISAPP) consensus statement on the definition and scope of prebiotics', *Nature Reviews Gastroenterology & Hepatology, 14*: 491–502, doi:10.1038/nrgastro.2017.75

Gonçalves, P., Di Santo, J.P. & Araújo, J.R., 2018, 'A cross-talk between microbiota-derived short-chain fatty acids and the host mucosal immune system regulates intestinal homeostasis and inflammatory bowel disease', *Inflammatory Bowel Diseases, 24*(3): 558–72, doi:10.1093/ibd/izx029

Graff, M., Scott, R.A., Justice, A.E., Young, K.L., Feitosa, M.F. et al., 2017, 'Genome-wide physical activity interactions in adiposity: A meta-analysis of 200,452 adults', *PLoS Genetics, 13*(4): e1006528, doi:10.1371/journal.pgen.1006528

Graziano, M. & Rossi, M., 2018, 'An update on the cutaneous manifestations of coeliac disease and non-coeliac gluten sensitivity', *International Reviews of Immunology, 37*(6): 291–300, doi:10.1080/08830185.2018.1533008

Guarner, F. & Malagelada, J.-R., 2003, 'Gut flora in health and disease', *Lancet, 361*(9356): 512–19, doi:10.1016/S0140-6736(03)12489-0

Haiser, H.J. & Turnbaugh, P.J., 2012, 'Is it time for a metagenomic basis of therapeutics?', *Science, 336*(6086): 1253–5, doi:10.1126/science.1224396

Hale, J., Knapp, C., Bardwell, L., Buchenau, M., Marshall, J. et al., 2011, 'Connecting food environments and health through the relational nature of aesthetics: Gaining insight through the community gardening experience', *Social Science & Medicine, 72*(11): 1853–63, doi:10.1016/j.socscimed.2011.03.044

Hehemann, J.-H., Correc, G., Barbeyron, T., Helbert, W., Czjzek, M. & Michel, G., 2010, 'Transfer of carbohydrate-active enzymes from marine bacteria to Japanese gut microbiota', *Nature, 464*(7290): 908–12, doi:10.1038/nature08937

Hesketh, K., Waters, E., Green, J., Salmon, L. & Williams, J., 2005, 'Healthy eating, activity and obesity prevention: A qualitative study of parent and child perceptions in Australia', *Health Promotion International, 20*(1): 19–26, doi:10.1093/heapro/dah503

Hill, C., Guarner, F., Reid, G., Gibson, G.R., Merenstein, D.J. et al., 2014, 'Expert consensus document: The International Scientific Association for Probiotics and Prebiotics consensus statement on the scope and appropriate use of the term probiotic', *Nature Reviews Gastroenterology & Hepatology, 11*(8): 506–14, doi:10.1038/nrgastro.2014.66

Huddleston, J.R., 2014, 'Horizontal gene transfer in the human gastrointestinal tract: Potential spread of antibiotic resistance genes', *Infection and Drug Resistance, 7*: 167–76, doi:10.2147/IDR.S48820

Human Microbiome Project Consortium, Methé, B.A., Nelson, K.E., Pop, M., Creasy, H.H. et al., 2012, 'A framework for human microbiome research', *Nature, 486*(7402): 215–21, doi:10.1038/nature11209

Huttenhower, C., Gevers, D., Knight, R., Abubucker, S., Badger, J.H. et al., 2012, 'Structure, function and diversity of the healthy human microbiome', *Nature, 486*(7402): 207–14, doi:10.1038/nature11234

Jang, H. & Serra, C., 2014, 'Nutrition, epigenetics, and diseases', *Clinical Nutrition Research, 3*(1): 1–8, doi:10.7762/cnr.2014.3.1.1

Janssen, S. & Depoortere, I., 2013, 'Nutrient sensing in the gut: New roads to therapeutics?', *Trends in Endocrinology & Metabolism, 24*(2): 92–100, doi:10.1016/j.tem.2012.11.006

Kairey, L., Matvienko-Sikar, K., Kelly, C., McKinley, M., O'Connor, E. et al., 2018, 'Plating up appropriate portion sizes for children: A systematic review of parental food and beverage portioning practices', *Obesity Reviews, 19*(12): 1667–78, doi:10.1111/obr.12727

Kerry, R.G., Patra, J.K., Gouda, S., Park, Y., Shin, H.-S. & Das, G., 2018, 'Benefaction of probiotics for human health: A review', *Journal of Food and Drug Analysis, 26*(3): 927–39, doi:10.1016/j.jfda.2018.01.002

Kilpeläinen, T.O., Qi, L., Brage, S., Sharp, S.J., Sonestedt, E. et al., 2011, 'Physical activity attenuates the influence of FTO variants on obesity risk: A meta-analysis of 218,166 adults and 19,268 children', *PLoS Medicine, 8*(11): e1001116, doi:10.1371/journal.pmed.1001116

Konstantinidou, V., Daimiel, L. & Ordovás, J.M., 2014, 'Personalized nutrition and cardiovascular disease prevention: From Framingham to PREDIMED', *Advances in Nutrition: An International Review Journal, 5*(3): 368S–71S, doi:10.3945/an.113.005686

Lederberg, J. & McCray, A.T., 2001, 'Ome SweetOmics: A genealogical treasury of words', *The Scientist, 15*(7): 8, <www.the-scientist.com/commentary/ome-sweet-omics---a-genealogical-treasury-of-words-54889>, accessed 4 January 2019

Lee, M.-S., Hsu, C.-C., Wahlqvist, M.L., Tsai, H.-N., Chang, Y.-H. & Huang, Y.-C., 2011, 'Type 2 diabetes increases and metformin reduces total, colorectal, liver and pancreatic cancer incidences in Taiwanese: A representative population prospective cohort study of 800,000 individuals', *BMC Cancer, 11*(1): 20, doi:10.1186/1471-2407-11-20

Lemon, K.P., Armitage, G.C., Relman, D.A. & Fischbach, M.A., 2012, 'Microbiota-targeted therapies: An ecological perspective', *Science Translational Medicine, 4*(137): 137rv135, doi:10.1126/scitranslmed.3004183

Lerner, A., Ramesh, A. & Matthias, T., 2018, 'Going gluten free in non-celiac autoimmune diseases: The missing ingredient', *Expert Review of Clinical Immunology, 14*(11): 873–5, doi:10.1080/1744666X.2018.1524757

Lerner, A. & Torsten, M., 2018, 'Microbial transglutaminase: A new potential player in celiac disease', *Clinical Immunology, 199*: 37–43, doi:10.1016/j.clim.2018.12.008

López, M., Nogueiras, R., Tena-Sempere, M. & Diéguez, C., 2016, 'Hypothalamic AMPK: A canonical regulator of whole-body energy balance', *Nature Reviews Endocrinology, 12*: 421–32, doi:10.1038/nrendo.2016.67

Lorenz, B.A. & Langen, N., 2018, 'Determinants of how individuals choose, eat and waste: Providing common ground to enhance sustainable food consumption out-of-home', *International Journal of Consumer Studies, 42*(1): 35–75, doi:10.1111/ijcs.12392

Louv, R., 2011, *The Nature Principle: Reconnecting with life in a virtual age*, Chapel Hill NC: Algonquin Books of Chapel Hill

Ma, J. & Li, H., 2018, 'The role of gut microbiota in atherosclerosis and hypertension', *Frontiers in Pharmacology, 9*: 1082, doi:10.3389/fphar.2018.01082

McCall, K.A., Huang, C.-c. & Fierke, C.A., 2000, 'Function and mechanism of zinc metalloenzymes', *Journal of Nutrition, 130*(5): 1437S–46S, doi:10.1093/jn/130.5.1437S

Marteau, P. & Seksik, P., 2004, 'Tolerance of probiotics and prebiotics', *Journal of Clinical Gastroenterology, 38*: S67–9, doi:10.1097/01.mcg.0000128929.37156.a7

Maslowski, K.M., Vieira, A.T., Ng, A., Kranich, J., Sierro, F. et al., 2009, 'Regulation of inflammatory responses by gut microbiota and chemoattractant receptor GPR43', *Nature, 461*(7268): 1282-6, doi:10.1038/nature08530

Maßberg, D. & Hatt, H., 2018, 'Human olfactory receptors: Novel cellular functions outside of the nose', *Physiological Reviews, 98*(3): 1739–63, doi:10.1152/physrev.00013.2017

Maukonen, J. & Saarela, M., 2014, 'Human gut microbiota: Does diet matter?', *Proceedings of the Nutrition Society, 74*(1): 23–36, doi:10.1017/S0029665114000688

Mele, L., Bidault, G., Mena, P., Crozier, A., Brighenti, F. et al., 2017, 'Dietary (poly) phenols, brown adipose tissue activation, and energy expenditure: A narrative review', *Advances in Nutrition, 8*(5): 694–704, doi:10.3945/an.117.015792

Mitchell, R. & Popham, F., 2008, 'Effect of exposure to natural environment on health inequalities: An observational population study', *Lancet, 372*(9650): 1655–60, doi:10.1016/S0140-6736(08)61689-X

Morrison, D.J. & Preston, T., 2016, 'Formation of short chain fatty acids by the gut microbiota and their impact on human metabolism', *Gut Microbes, 7*(3): 189–200, doi:10.1080/19490976.2015.1134082

Nishijo, H. & Ono, T., 1992, 'Food memory: Neuronal involvement in food recognition', *Asia Pacific Journal of Clinical Nutrition, 1*(1): 3–12, <http://apjcn.nhri.org.tw/server/APJCN/1/1/3.htm>, accessed 4 January 2019

Olszak, T., An, D., Zeissig, S., Vera, M.P., Richter, J. et al., 2012, 'Microbial exposure during early life has persistent effects on natural killer T cell function', *Science, 336*(6080): 489–93, doi:10.1126/science.1219328

Pan, M.-H., Lai, C.-S. & Ho, C.-T., 2010, 'Anti-inflammatory activity of natural dietary flavonoids', *Food & Function, 1*(1): 15–31, doi:10.1039/C0FO00103A

Pandey, K.R., Naik, S.R. & Vakil, B.V., 2015, 'Probiotics, prebiotics and synbiotics: A review', *Journal of Food Science and Technology, 52*(12): 7577–87, doi:10.1007/s13197-015-1921-1

Paoli, A., Moro, T., Marcolin, G., Neri, M., Bianco, A. et al., 2012, 'High-intensity interval resistance training (HIRT) influences resting energy expenditure and respiratory ratio in non-dieting individuals', *Journal of Translational Medicine, 10*(1): 237, doi:10.1186/1479-5876-10-237

Pembrey, M.E., 2002, 'Time to take epigenetic inheritance seriously', *European Journal of Human Genetics, 10*(11): 669–71, doi:10.1038/sj.ejhg.5200901

Pineiro, M., Asp, N.-G., Reid, G., Macfarlane, S., Morelli, L. & et al., 2008, 'FAO Technical meeting on prebiotics', *Journal of Clinical Gastroenterology, 42*(Suppl. 3): S156–159, doi:10.1097/MCG.0b013e31817f184e

Quigley, E.M.M., 2013, 'Gut bacteria in health and disease', *Gastroenterology & Hepatology, 9*(9): 560–9, <www.ncbi.nlm.nih.gov/pmc/articles/PMC3983973/pdf/GH-09-560.pdf>, accessed 4 January 2019

Rodríguez, J.M., Murphy, K., Stanton, C., Ross, R.P., Kober, O.I. et al., 2015, 'The composition of the gut microbiota throughout life, with an emphasis on early life', *Microbial Ecology in Health and Disease, 26*: 26050, <www.tandfonline.com/doi/full/10.3402/mehd.v26.26050>, accessed 4 January 2019

Rotter, D., Peiris, H., Grinsfelder, D.B., Martin, A.M., Burchfield, J. et al., 2018, 'Regulator of Calcineurin 1 helps coordinate whole-body metabolism and thermogenesis', *EMBO Reports, 19*(12): e44706, doi:10.15252/embr.201744706

Rowland, I., Gibson, G., Heinken, A., Scott, K., Swann, J. et al., 2018, 'Gut microbiota functions: Metabolism of nutrients and other food components', *European Journal of Nutrition, 57*(1): 1–24, doi:10.1007/s00394-017-1445-8

Schiffman, S. & Graham, B., 2000, 'Taste and smell perception affect appetite and immunity in the elderly', *European Journal of Clinical Nutrition, 54*(Suppl. 3): S54, doi:10.1038/sj.ejcn.1601026

Schiffman, S.S., 1983, 'Taste and smell in disease', *New England Journal of Medicine, 308*(22): 1337–43, doi:10.1056/NEJM198306023082207

Scuteri, A., Sanna, S., Chen, W.-M., Uda, M., Albai, G. et al., 2007, 'Genome-wide association scan shows genetic variants in the FTO gene are associated with obesity-related traits', *PLoS Genetics, 3*(7): e115, doi:10.1371/journal.pgen.0030115

Simopoulos, A.P., 2010, 'Nutrigenetics/nutrigenomics', *Annual Review of Public Health, 31*: 53–68, doi:10.1146/annurev.publhealth.031809.130844

Slentz, C.A., Houmard, J.A. & Kraus, W.E., 2009, 'Exercise, abdominal obesity, skeletal muscle, and metabolic risk: Evidence for a dose response', *Obesity, 17*(Suppl. 3): S27–S33, doi:10.1038/oby.2009.385

Spence, C., 2015, 'Multisensory flavor perception', *Cell, 161*(1): 24–35, doi:10.1016/j.cell.2015.03.007

Stokes, J.R., Boehm, M.W. & Baier, S.K., 2013, 'Oral processing, texture and mouthfeel: From rheology to tribology and beyond', *Current Opinion in Colloid & Interface Science, 18*(4): 349–59, doi:10.1016/j.cocis.2013.04.010

Subramanian, S., Huq, S., Yatsunenko, T., Haque, R., Mahfuz, M. et al., 2014, 'Persistent gut microbiota immaturity in malnourished Bangladeshi children', *Nature, 510*(7505): 417–21, doi:10.1038/nature13421

Suez, J., Zmora, N., Segal, E. and Elinav, E., 2019. 'The pros, cons, and many unknowns of probiotics', *Nature Medicine, 25*: 716–29, doi:10.1038/s41591-019-0439-x

Trehan, I., Goldbach, H.S., LaGrone, L.N., Meuli, G.J., Wang, R.J. et al., 2013, 'Antibiotics as part of the management of severe acute malnutrition', *New England Journal of Medicine, 368*: 425–35, doi:10.1056/NEJMoa1202851

Umami Information Center, 2017, 'Umami rich ingredients', <www.umamiinfo.com/>, accessed 7 January 2019

Wahlqvist, M.L., 2016, 'Food structure is critical for optimal health', *Food & Function, 7*(3): 1245–50, doi:10.1039/C5FO01285F

Wahlqvist, M.L., Darmadi-Blackberry, I., Kouris-Blazos, A., Jolley, D., Steen, B. & Horie, Y., 2005, 'Does diet matter for survival in long-lived cultures?', *Asia Pacific Journal of Clinical Nutrition, 14*(1): 2–6, doi:10.2254/0964-7058.14.1.0164

Wahlqvist, M.L., Krawetz, S.A., Rizzo, N.S., Dominguez-Bello, M.G., Szymanski, L.M. et al., 2015, 'Early-life influences on obesity: From preconception to adolescence', *Annals of the New York Academy of Sciences, 1347*(1): 1–28, doi:10.1111/nyas.12778

Wahlqvist, M.L., Lee, M.-S., Chuang, S.-Y., Hsu, C.-C., Tsai, H.-N. et al., 2012, 'Increased risk of affective disorders in type 2 diabetes is minimized by sulfonylurea and metformin combination: A population-based cohort study', *BMC Medicine, 10*(1): 150, doi:10.1186/1741-7015-10-150

Wen, C.P., Wai, J.P.M., Tsai, M.K., Yang, Y.C., Cheng, T.Y.D. et al., 2011, 'Minimum amount of physical activity for reduced mortality and extended life expectancy: A prospective cohort study', *Lancet, 378*(9798): 1244–53, doi:10.1016/S0140-6736(11)60749-6

WHO, 2010, *Global Recommendations on Physical Activity for Health*, <www.who.int/dietphysicalactivity/factsheet_recommendations/en/>, accessed 4 January 2019

Wu, J., Boström, P., Sparks, L.M., Ye, L., Choi, J.H. et al., 2012, 'Beige adipocytes are a distinct type of thermogenic fat cell in mouse and human', *Cell, 150*(2): 366–76, doi:10.1016/j.cell.2012.05.016

Wu, S.-Y., Hsu, L.-L., Hsu, C.-C., Hsieh, T.-J., Su, S.-C. et al., 2018, 'Dietary education with customised dishware and food supplements can reduce frailty and improve mental well-being in elderly people: A single-blind randomized controlled study', *Asia Pacific Journal of Clinical Nutrition, 27*(5): 1018–30, doi:10.6133/apjcn.032018.02

Yang, I., Corwin, E.J., Brennan, P.A., Jordan, S., Murphy, J.R. & Dunlop, A., 2016, 'The infant microbiome: Implications for infant health and neurocognitive development', *Nursing Research, 65*(1): 76–88, doi:10.1097/NNR.0000000000000133

Yuan, G., Wahlqvist, M.L., He, G., Yang, M. & Li, D., 2006, 'Natural products and anti-inflammatory activity', *Asia Pacific Journal of Clinical Nutrition, 15*(2): 143–52, <http://apjcn.nhri.org.tw/server/APJCN/15/2/143.pdf>, accessed 4 January 2019

Zozulya, S., Echeverri, F. & Nguyen, T., 2001, 'The human olfactory receptor repertoire', *Genome Biology, 2*(6): research0018.1–0018.12, doi:10.1186/gb-2001-2-6-research0018

{CHAPTER 31}
ECOHEALTH DISORDERS

Mark L. Wahlqvist and Naiyana Wattanapenpaiboon

OBJECTIVES

- Describe the link between food, nutrition and some disorders or diseases related to ecohealth.
- Identify beneficial dietary patterns, foods and nutrients.
- Apply the evidence to reduce risks or improve health outcomes.

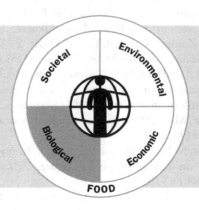

CHANGING PERSPECTIVES OF DIET AND HEALTH

Nutrients are essential for life; we cannot live without intake of the essential nutrients in the short to medium term. That patients who cannot eat can be sustained by way of **enteral** or parenteral feeding for these durations does not mean that this is optimal or commensurate with the life expectancy experienced by the population at large. Dependency on these feeding methods requires an understanding of what, in food-based oral feeding, is essential. In practice, a measure of less than optimal but acceptable health, for limited periods of time, can be achieved short of the more desirable oral route and with incomplete knowledge of food and food component essentiality. Beyond the basic nutritional elements that have been known to account for health disruptions, disorders and disease for centuries, other nutritional factors are required. They include several health-protective bioactive compounds, many of

them from plants (phytonutrients) and others from animals (zoonutrients) or fungi (phyconutrients) or the microbiota in our gut, on our skin, and in our respiratory or reproductive tracts. Their essentiality on a one-by-one basis is arguable, but collectively or with complementarity between each other and other nutrients they do confer a health advantage. Yet this advantage can be rapidly or slowly gained or lost in ways that involve the concerted action of both dietary patterns and the microbiota.

The most successful way to achieve the spectrum of bioactive elements and compounds required for human biology, given that we are omnivorous with a plant food bias for optimal health, is for food intake to be characterised by diversity (see Chapter 8). This also dilutes potential adverse food components and contaminants. However, there does need to be a sufficient energy throughput, allowed by being physically active enough, to gain the health-protective bioactive adequacy that diversity can provide. Studies demonstrating the value of dietary patterns over individual foods or nutrients generally find that the patterns represent dietary diversity.

A number of potentially adverse health outcomes are mitigated by dietary patterns, especially those which are biologically varied and reflect ecosystem integrity. The evidence is not only that dietary diversity is a preferred way of eating for health, but that it is also an index of food security (Hoddinott & Yohannes 2002). Yet most of the world's population have little choice but to depend on a single staple, which is a precarious food habit. It is worth knowing, however, that even diverse cultivars of a staple like rice, wheat, maize and/or potatoes can provide enhanced food security in the event of pestilence or adverse weather conditions (see Chapter 26). The principal rationale for the biofortification of staples with micronutrients is to reduce the nutritional adversity evident with food monoculture. This does not diminish the parallel efforts to develop mixed farming and diverse home gardens. It is, moreover, an unfortunate reality that increased food production, whether in emerging economies or many advanced economies, falls short of meeting the dietary quality that is required for health and which could be met by dietary diversity and attention to supportive ecosystems.

Food is the primary source of nutrients needed to sustain life, promote health and normal growth and development, and assure human productivity. While sustainability is now generally accepted as key to the future of our food supply, we cannot afford to ignore the nutritional content of food either. Poor diet remains a significant factor in many diseases, from diabetes to cancer. Large-scale, industrial food production has led to a loss of much of the nutritional value of the food we eat today. Where high yields, uniformity and profit are the main objective in food production, nutritional value is not a priority. Modern methods of food production no longer meet the broad health needs of the consumer; increasing reliance on industrial food production to meet our needs is not sufficient for our health, or the health of our environment.

ECOHEALTH DISORDERS

Since the 1960s, rapid expansion in several relevant scientific fields, in particular the amount of population-based epidemiological evidence, has helped to clarify the role of diet in preventing and controlling morbidity and premature mortality resulting from **non-communicable diseases** (NCDs), also referred to as chronic diseases. Some dietary components that increase the probability of these diseases, and interventions to modify their impact, have been identified.

While the term 'chronic disease/condition' or 'non-communicable disease' says nothing or little about **aetiology** or pathogenesis, there is logic in 'econutritional disease' or 'ecohealth disorder' as an alternative descriptor when the major importance of food, physical activity and the required 'environmental buffer zones' to minimise the risk of known and emerging transmissible pathogens is considered. Even dependence on substances like tobacco and alcohol is less likely where the environment itself provides fulfilling and less stressful experiences.

The physiology and disorders of all body systems are recognised as nutritionally responsive (Figure 31.1). The mechanism of these disorders was thought to be principally metabolic, hormonal or gut-related. With better understanding, it is now recognised that some of the mechanisms could be gene and genomic expression, inflammatory or immunological, degenerative (ageing or age-related or both) or sociobehavioural (Wahlqvist & Lee 2006).

The Australian Institute of Health and Welfare reported that the five diseases or injuries with the highest burden among Australians in 2011 were cancer, cardiovascular disease, mental (and substance use) disorders, musculoskeletal disorders, and injuries; altogether, they accounted for about 67 per cent of the total burden (Figure 31.2, see colour section) (see Chapter 24 for a discussion on burden of disease). The leading causes of this disease pattern included tobacco use, overweight and obesity, high alcohol consumption, physical inactivity and high blood pressure.

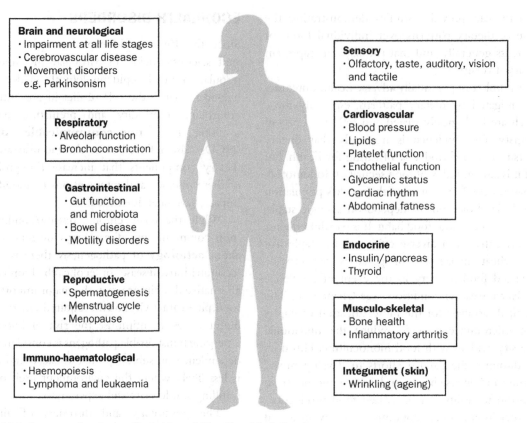

Figure 31.1: Organs and systems affected by nutritionally related disorders
Source: Modified from Wahlqvist & Lee (2006)

'Ecological disruptive disorders' might be a useful way of systematising ecohealth disorders, which could take into account those disorders with a recognisable connection (or disconnection) to locality (Table 31.1). An example would be how the internal combustion engine as a basis of transport requiring fossil fuels has changed our propensity towards obesity (Figure 31.3).

Table 31.1: Functional connectedness with the environment and ecological disruptive disorders

Type of environment	Examples of connectedness
Animate environment	Genomic convergence and cooperativity
	Biorhythms
	Energy throughput and regulation
	Locomotion
	Sensory inputs
	Hormonal and other homeostatic mechanisms
	Microbiomic pathways
	Other immune processes
	Food systems
Inanimate environment	From geochemistry to appreciation of spatial characteristics, aesthetics, seasons and weather

Source: Wahlqvist (2014)

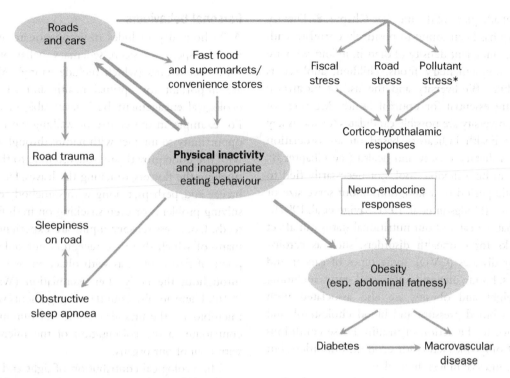

Note: * Pollutant stress, e.g. xeno-estrogens, such as pesticide residues

Figure 31.3: Illustration of fundamental and intermediate causes of ecologically and nutritionally related disease: the example of eating, activity, cars and the road

Source: Wahlqvist (2014). Reproduced with permission

SELECTED FACTORS RELATING TO ECOHEALTH DISORDERS

Socioeconomic development and rapid changes in diets and personal behaviours impact the health and nutritional status of populations. As standards of living have improved, food availability has expanded and become more diversified, and access to services has increased, so also have inappropriate dietary patterns, decreased physical activity and substance abuse (like that of tobacco and alcohol) emerged, with a corresponding increase in diet-related 'chronic disease', especially among the disadvantaged (WHO 2017).

The relationships between wellbeing and a closeness to nature or environment are complex. A good indicator of these relationships is sensory function and the physiology other than the sensory

organs (see also Chapter 30). When it comes to food, this appreciation involves sight, smell, taste, texture or touch, and sound as we eat (Spence 2015). How and what we eat, however, could affect us in ways well beyond the nutrient physiology. It is now evident that receptor mechanisms similar to those of taste receptors are used by organ systems other than taste buds in the oral cavity. These so-called taste receptors are also present in the nasal cavity, the trachea, stomach, and the upper part of the small intestine, reproductive system and elsewhere (Finger & Kinnamon 2011).

Diet and its biodiversity

Dietary diversity is often defined as the number of certain food groups consumed by an individual or family. Many studies conducted on people of different age groups show that an increase in individual dietary diversity is related to increased nutrient adequacy of the diet (see Chapter 8). Dietary diversity has been found to positively correlate with the micronutrient density of diets in infants who are given complementary foods, children, adolescents and adults. Biodiversity and the use of biodiverse foods are essential for optimal health. Measures of dietary diversity are possible candidates for use as key positive health indicators, based on an association between dietary variety and health (see Chapter 8). They can be a flexible tool, not necessarily tied to a specific period or assumptions about serve size or frequency (Hodgson et al. 1991; Savige et al. 1997).

What we eat and our nutritional status can affect the risks for ecohealth disorders, such as cardio-vascular diseases (CVD), some types of cancer and diabetes. Foods, diet and nutritional status, including overweight and obesity, are also associated with elevated blood pressure and blood cholesterol, and resistance to the action of insulin. These conditions are not only risk factors for ecohealth disorders, but major causes of illness themselves.

Consuming predominantly plant-based diets reduces the risk of developing obesity, diabetes, CVD and some forms of cancer. Plant-based diets are high in vegetables and fruits, whole grains, pulses, nuts and seeds, and have only modest amounts of meat and dairy (see Chapter 26). These diets help to achieve and maintain a healthy weight, reduce blood pressure, and are rich in sources of dietary fibre. Fruits and vegetables independently contribute to preventing CVD (see Chapter 8). It is likely that particular vegetables and fruits, including cruciferous vegetables such as cabbage and broccoli, and many fruits or vegetables that are rich in folate, also protect from cancers of the colon and rectum, mouth, pharynx, larynx and oesophagus. Eating red and processed meat increases risk of developing colorectal cancer. Saturated fat and trans fats increase blood cholesterol and CVD risk. Higher sodium or salt intake is a major risk factor for elevated blood pressure and CVD, and probably stomach cancer. Diets high in meat and dairy also increase blood pressure. Diets high in energy-dense, highly processed foods and refined starches and/or sugary beverages contribute to overweight and obesity.

Personal behaviours

A 24-hour day includes disproportionate amounts of time spent on sleep, sedentary behaviours and active behaviours (which include eating). All three are important for optimal health and all require ecological engagement, be it favourable or adverse. For example, in the course of walking we have the opportunity to interact with nature through contact with the undergrowth and soil, listening to the birds, smelling the flowers, touching the leaves, feeling the breeze and, perhaps, talking with somebody else and solving problems or even snacking on fresh fruits or seeds. Countless sensory inputs are experienced, for many of which there are receptors not only at the point of first contact as with olfaction or taste, but throughout the body after assimilation (Wahlqvist 2016). There are also countless engagements with the microbiota of the air, soil and other surroundings that contribute to the colonisation of the microbiome within all of our organs.

The ecological contribution of light and dark is another ecological health consideration. The synchrony of daylight or sunlight with the times for eating contributes to health; evidence suggests that there is a **circadian** (night and day) gut microbiomic rhythm (see Figure 31.4 for the interplay between the gut microbiota and the circadian clock). It is better for most food consumption to occur earlier rather than later in the day (Asher & Sassone-Corsi 2015; Panda 2018), and not when we should be sleeping, insofar as energy regulation and the risk of it being disordered is concerned (Gabel et al. 2018).

PHYSICAL ACTIVITY

Physical inactivity accounts for more than five million premature deaths each year, making it one of the most important contributors to the global burden of disease. An analysis of burden of disease worldwide in 2012 (Lee et al. 2012) revealed that elimination of physical inactivity could increase the life expectancy of the world's population by 0.7 years. Physical activity is prominently featured in the 2013–2020 WHO Global Action Plan for the Prevention and Control of Non-Communicable

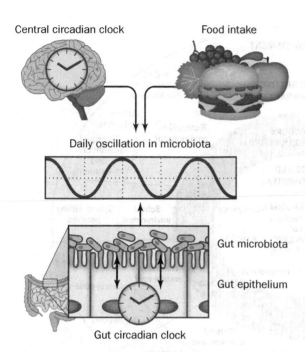

Central circadian clock

Food intake

Daily oscillation in microbiota

Gut microbiota

Gut epithelium

Gut circadian clock

Figure 31.4: Interplay between the gut microbiota and gut circadian clock

Source: Asher & Sassone-Corsi (2015). Reprinted with permission from Elsevier

Diseases, and also in the targets and indicators within a global monitoring framework for NCDs (WHO 2013). Nearly one-third of adults are inactive worldwide, and there is growing evidence on the relationships and determinants of physical activity and effective interventions to increase it. Many countries, including the United States, United Kingdom, Brazil, Colombia, Australia, and India, have implemented national public health plans with specific objectives that support and encourage physical activity. However, substantial gaps in the evidence remain, especially related to interventions in low- and middle-income countries and interventions at a scale beyond the community level.

Australia's Physical Activity and Sedentary Behaviour Guidelines, produced by the Australian Government Department of Health, suggest the minimum levels of physical activity required for health benefits, and ways to incorporate physical activity and minimise sedentary behaviour in everyday life (see Chapter 30).

Barriers to being physically active

Physical inactivity is a complex and multifactorial behaviour and its determinants vary across countries. These determinants include individual factors, such as age and gender, as well as environmental, geopolitical and economic factors. Health-related and psychosocial factors, such as the presence of a chronic disease or poor **self-efficacy**, can affect the ability to engage in regular physical activity. A high crime rate, dense traffic and the absence of parks or footpaths can discourage people from exercising outdoors.

Physical activity can be influenced by the combination and interaction of a range of diverse factors at the individual, social, environmental, governance and global levels (Bauman et al. 2012; Sallis et al. 2006). This multilevel model of physical activity influences is ecological, because it includes interrelations between individuals and their social and physical environments (Figure 31.5). While variables within individuals, such as psychological and biological factors, and interpersonal variables are widely studied, environmental, policy, and global variables are less reported.

A comprehensive review of research in adults suggests that environmental attributes of physical activity include recreation facilities and locations, transportation environments and aesthetics, while consistent relationships are reported in young people between physical activity and specific domains of transport and leisure activity (Bauman et al. 2012). Environmental changes can be achieved through population-wide changes to governance and policy. However, policy decisions are sometimes made outside the health sector; partnerships between sectors are needed to influence physical environments at all levels of development to make them more supportive of physical activity behaviours.

Built environment

Physical activity is related to the physical or built environment. The term 'built environment' is used to refer to places, spaces or man-made surroundings that provide the setting for human activity, and

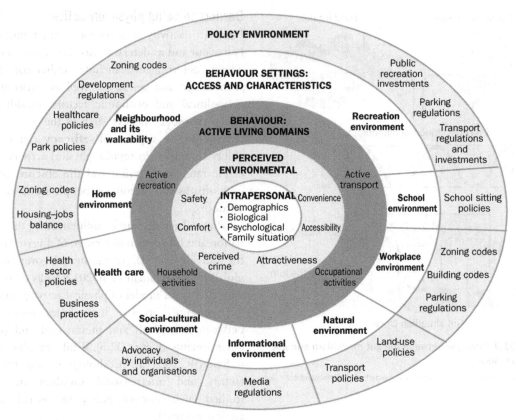

Figure 31.5: Ecological model of the determinants of physical activity

Source: Adapted from Sallis et al. (2006). Reproduced with permission of Annual Reviews via Copyright Clearance Center

these include buildings, parks and transportation systems. The presence and conditions of paths, traffic flow, cleanliness and maintenance of public spaces, perceptions of safety and community security, zoning and land-use mix, and population density also form part of the built environment. The environment can be built to support personal behaviour with characteristics of improved physical and mental health. Built environments that are specifically designed to improve physical activity have been shown to be linked to higher rates of physical activity, which in turn favourably affects health (Carlson et al. 2012). Access to healthy food, such as proximity to grocery stores and community gardens, is also considered a part of the built environment. Improved access to markets or, in low-income neighbourhoods, the presence of a local grocery store has been shown to be correlated with lowered

risk for overweight or obesity (Chiang et al. 2011). Community gardens appear to have positive social and psychological impacts that lead to lower levels of stress and hypertension, and an improved sense of wellness, affecting the overall health of the individual and the community.

Numerous studies at the individual and population levels have reported that health benefits are related to contact with public open space, especially green spaces (Lee & Maheswaran 2011). Indeed, urban green spaces provide opportunities for contact with the natural environment. Accessibility of public open space influences not just the likelihood of physical activity being undertaken but also its frequency. Public open spaces thus may help facilitate active personal behaviours in the urban setting. The benefits of public open spaces also include positive restorative effects on mental health by alleviating stress and anxiety, and improving mood; and facilitation of social interactions, which could help reduce social isolation and lead to greater personal resilience and wellbeing. The latter benefit seems to be particularly important for elderly populations (Sugiyama & Thompson 2008). An Australian study was the first to demonstrate an increase in pleasure associated with being in a landscaped garden for people with dementia (Cox et al. 2004).

Public health research has expanded the definition of built environment to include walkability and bikeability. Walkability refers to safety, pathway construction, and areas in which to walk, while bikeability refers to access to safe biking through multiple bike paths and bike lanes. Neighbourhoods with more walkability tend to have not only increased physical activity, but also lower rates of obesity and depression, higher social capital and less alcohol abuse. The perception of the built environment may also be an important factor in people's behaviour. The perception of a walkable neighbourhood—one that is perceived to have good footpaths and connectivity—is associated with higher rates of physical activity (Renalds et al. 2010). Hence, adapting existing neighbourhoods and building new ones with walkability or bikeability in mind can structure society's way to better health.

SLEEP

It has been shown that we can benefit, in relation to decreased ecohealth disorder risk, from having optimal sleep duration (7–8 hours), moderate to vigorous physical activity such as brisk walking, swimming and hard labour work, and even light-intensity physical activity or personal behaviours, such as doing household chores or leisurely walking. Conversely, long periods of sedentary behaviour—sitting/lying with low energy expenditure—and too short or too long sleep duration can be associated with increased CVD risk.

Habitual sleep duration among adults shows considerable variance within and between individuals. Research findings on the effects of sleep restriction on behavioural and physiological functions suggest that adequate sleep duration of 7–8 hours per day is of importance. Many epidemiological studies have found that both relatively long sleepers (eight hours or more per day) and relatively short sleepers (less than seven hours per day) had increased risks of all-cause mortality (Jike et al. 2018; Khan et al. 2018). Research has found that reduced sleep time can alter a range of physiological indices. While the clinical significance of these findings in healthy adults is unknown, the indices affected by reduced sleep time are apparently related to health outcomes. Sleep deprivation can cause a range of neurobehavioral deficits, including lapses of attention, slowed working memory, reduced cognitive throughput, depressed mood, anxiety and continuous thinking about negative events.

Researchers speculate that there are several ways chronic sleep deprivation might lead to weight gain, either by increasing how much food people eat or decreasing the energy that they burn. The amount of sleep is a determinant of weight status, and sleep security is increasingly recognised as being as vital to child development as food security (Pattinson et al. 2018). Sleep deprivation could increase hunger by increasing the appetite-stimulating hormone ghrelin and lowering the satiety-inducing hormone leptin, resulting in an increased appetite—especially for foods rich in fat and carbohydrates. In addition, sleep deprivation simply affords more waking time in which to eat, and prompts people to choose less healthy diets, such as snacking, eating out and irregular meal patterns. The human circadian rhythm is a critical determinant of sleep, and one of the major determinants of human circadian rhythms is exposure to bright light. Extensive evidence suggests that spending time outdoors may result in improved sleep because of increased exposure to sunlight (Campbell et al. 1993). Conversely, exposure to artificial light—in particular, blue light from devices such as mobile phones, televisions and other screens—may disrupt sleeping duration and pattern (Sampasa-Kanyinga et al. 2018; Shechter et al. 2018). It has also been demonstrated that food diversity can offset the adverse effect of poor sleep on mortality, at least among men (Huang et al. 2013).

BIOLOGICAL COMPETENCIES OF HUMANS

To some extent there can be synergy between traditional and envisaged socioecological approaches to nutritionally related health. These are evident from emerging biological developments and technologies for integrins, integrons, exosomes and exposomes, which are themselves integrational. These several biological competencies, which may be available in both the **prokaryotic** microbiomes and **eukaryotic** genome, should allow a greater connectedness between people and the environment than previously recognised (see Chapter 30). These biological developments may require access to extensive personal data and societal metadata. In that event, new ethical and equity questions will arise. The optimal approach, therefore, might be to focus our appreciation and management of the food and health relationship on our personal, intergenerational and community ecology in a sustainable, controllable and affordable way.

A genetic and cellular counter to the rather reductionist approach embedded in nutrigenomics is the recognition of exosomes, or vesicles containing proteins and the 'cargo' of messenger RNAs and microRNAs. Exosomes can deliver their cargo RNA molecules from one cell to another, and this could explain the role of exosomes in cell-to-cell signalling and biological effects. Exosomes appear to bundle much metabolic and nutritional information together in cells and export it to other body sites, and may even transfer the information intergenerationally and between species (Johnstone 2006; Vlassov et al. 2012). For example, exosomes in milk from lactating animals of one species can survive digestion and then be taken up by animals of another species, and this could result in an alteration of gene expression species (Lonnerdal et al. 2015). Human breastmilk also contains exosomes. This provides breastmilk with a mechanism to regulate immune and gut function and for person-to-person transfer of genetic material other than by reproduction (Admyre et al. 2007; Kosaka et al. 2010) (see also Chapter 20). It is a paradigm shift in our understanding of lactation and nutrition, and of what can and cannot be imitated by breastmilk substitutes at present.

In the case of exposome, it is defined as being 'composed of every exposure to which an individual is subjected from conception to death' (Wild 2012). The exposome would require measurement of exposures over time across the life-course of an individual. This exposome concept aligns with the quest for a more ecological approach to health, including that which is nutritionally dependent.

CLINICAL NUTRITION IN A CHANGING WORLD

In general, basic elements of effective clinical practice include:
* ascertainment of patient needs, reasons for health-seeking behaviour and health beliefs
* ability to establish a diagnosis or define the problem
* recognition of multifactorial basis of health problems and of their recent, medium-term and remote determinants
* awareness of the epidemiology of the problem—its geography, ethnicity, age and gender, relationships, frequency of occurrence, transmissibility or transferability, time course, consequences
* management plans that take into account patient perceptions and biomedical and sociocultural realities, are communicated and supported by the patient and their carers, and are cost–benefit–risk-effective in the short and long term
* an ethical framework.

The argument is made in this chapter that a deeper understanding of how food affects health requires a more socioecological view. In turn, this should allow diagnoses which enable more effective management of the disorders and diseases attributable to these relationships. This might be more challenging, given its complexity and multidisciplinary approach, but it offers wider and more sustainable health, societal and environmental benefits (Solomons 2002). It is likely to need a new kind of health workforce. Nevertheless, these basic elements of effective clinical practice ought to remain the same, with 'diagnosis' followed by a 'management plan' and then monitoring and evaluation. This aligns with the Nutrition Care Process outlined in Chapter 23.

The socioecological diagnostic process needs to be advanced alongside the familiar diagnostic criteria. These are currently benchmarked by ICD (International Classification of Diseases) or DSM (Diagnostic and Statistical Manual of Mental Disorders) criteria and resourced accordingly. The ICD classification, which is managed by the World Health Organization, underpins the coding required by most electronic health records in healthcare facilities. The Academy of Nutrition and Dietetics has also developed the Nutrition Care Process Terminology, which provides a consistent way of diagnosing nutrition disorders (Academy of Nutrition and Dietetics 2018). See Table 31.2 for current classifications of nutritional disorders.

The question is how the emergence of 'personalised nutrition' and 'precision medicine' (see Chapter 30) of the nutritional kind relates to what might be regarded as 'socioecological

Table 31.2: International Classification of Diseases (11th Revision, ICD-11) of nutritional disorders

Type of nutritional disorders	Diagnostic code	
Undernutrition	5B54	Underweight in adults
	5B55	Vitamin A deficiency
	5B56	Vitamin C deficiency
	5B57	Vitamin D deficiency
	5B58	Vitamin E deficiency
	5B59	Vitamin K deficiency
	5B5A	Vitamin B-1 deficiency
	5B5B	Vitamin B-2 deficiency
	5B5C	Vitamin B-3 deficiency
	5B5D	Vitamin B-6 deficiency
	5B5E	Folate deficiency
	5B5F	Vitamin B-12 deficiency
	5B5G	Biotin deficiency
	5B5H	Pantothenic acid deficiency
	5B5J	Choline deficiency
	5B5K	Mineral deficiencies
	Sequelae of malnutrition and certain specified nutritional deficiencies:	
	5B60	Sequelae of protein energy malnutrition
	5B61	Sequelae of vitamin A deficiency
	5B62	Sequelae of vitamin C deficiency
	5B63	Sequelae of rickets
	5B6Y	Other specified sequelae of malnutrition and certain specified nutritional deficiencies
	5B6Z	Sequelae of malnutrition and certain specified nutritional deficiencies, unspecified
	5B70	Essential fatty acid deficiency
	5B71	Protein deficiency
	5B7Y	Other specified undernutrition
Overweight, obesity or specific nutrient excesses	Overweight or obesity:	
	5B80	Overweight or localised adiposity
	5B81	Obesity
	Certain specified nutrient excesses:	
	5C1Y	Other specified overweight, obesity or specific nutrient excesses
	5C1Z	Overweight, obesity or specific nutrient excesses, unspecified

Source: WHO (2018)

PRECISION MEDICINE

Precision medicine (also sometimes termed or considered a feature of personalised medicine) is an approach in medical practice that uses specific information about the genetic predisposition and environment of an individual to tailor prevention, diagnosis, treatments and prognosis of a disorder or disease, to that person. When this approach is used in clinical nutritional practice, the terms 'personalised nutrition' or 'precision nutrition' are sometimes used. The concept is in reality not new, since health (and nutrition) care practice has always been directed to the individual, tempered by public health (including nutrition), in the most targeted way possible. However, a substantial shift towards patient ownership of a digitised, password-protected, medical record is under way and may generate a more cooperative, integrated, reliable, relevant and mobile approach to health (and nutrition) care. The changing conceptualisation of food and health, irrespective of its place on the genetic–behavioural–environmental spectrum of pathogenesis and management, has the potential to be relegated to a place or position where it is more relevant or advantageous.

The notion that precision or personalised nutrition, which allows for individual differences, should operate in the general, apparently healthy, population rather than within the clinical realm includes problematic assumptions, namely:

1. That optimising individual health comes with limited if any change in cost–risk–benefit ratios.
2. That a reductionist **Mendelian randomisation**, single nucleotide polymorphisms or epigenetics approach to health is applied without bio-socioecological context.
3. That early detection, risk management and prevention are simple strategies for health advancement.
4. That clinical diagnosis and management can operate widely and be internet-based, with little professional involvement.
5. That this activity has unique ethical and equity needs. For example, if fish is universally contaminated with microplastic, how does this affect the fish–health link? What could be done about it collectively rather than personally? How are cost and supply affected? Does benefit still exceed risk? And who gets what is safest and most beneficial to eat?

Stratified medicine or nutrition and health could be more reflective of these concerns, as proposed by the European Patients' Academy (EUPATI 2017). However, this approach endeavours to categorise people with a range of genotypes or single nucleotide polymorphisms by some form of phenotype so that their commonalities allow efficiencies in nutritional or other approaches to health, rather than adopting a more resource-intensive individualised approach. **Stratified nutrition** would fall somewhere between public health and clinical nutrition.

diagnostic criteria'. There is growing interest in how people might use digital technology and artificial intelligence systems to evaluate their own health and its management, with or without a healthcare practitioner. In relation to food and health, this appears attractive and has the potential to counter the increasing remoteness of food systems from the individual. Coupled with a greater appreciation of how food affects genomic expression, a future can be imagined for 'personalised nutrition' and for approaches that might be more precise (Ordovas et al. 2018). However, the socioecological complexity of nutrition and health makes it unlikely that, for apparently healthy individuals, narrow and precise approaches to food and nutrient intake for greater health will have an acceptable cost–risk–benefit ratio. Nonetheless, once a nutritionally related disorder or disease occurs, the benefit of personalised, rather than public, and precise, rather than general, approaches may exceed the risk.

Any of these approaches could be 'personalised', as should all health care. The question is where personalisation sits in the scheme of a 'cost–risk–benefit' analysis. Presumably, and in accordance with the basic ethical principle of autonomy, the more personalised the nutritional health plan the more the consumer or patient will be an undirected decision-maker. 'Precision medicine and nutrition' may be considered using nutrigenomic or immunonutritional techniques. These tend to move management in a very particular, unifactorial and reductionist direction, in situations where the need for intervention is pressing on account of the severity or urgency of the disorder. In these circumstances, there is a corresponding shift in the 'cost–risk–benefit' analysis.

SUMMARY

- Where and how we live in relation to a changing environment may be changing who we are and our health. This may warrant a conceptual shift in the understanding of the relationships between the food and health systems.
- These relationships may be multiple and involve our energy equilibrium, sensory faculties, biorhythms, locomotive capacity, defence and immune functions, hormonal, homeostatic and regulatory integrity, and our orientation and appreciation of our place in the natural and virtual world.
- Categorising many of the predominant diseases as ecohealth disorders takes into consideration disruptions to broad interactions between individuals and their environments for food, physical activity, sleep and mental health.
- Personal behaviours—including selecting a diverse diet, undertaking regular physical activity, accessing green spaces and optimising sleep duration and pattern—are known to contribute to the prevention of ecohealth disorders.
- Since we presently prevent, diagnose and manage nutritionally related health problems using criteria and classifications like ICD and DSM, a deeper understanding of these problems' origins and the corresponding potential for solutions to them requires that emerging and current conceptualisations operate in parallel or in conjunction with each other.

KEY TERMS

Aetiology: refers to the study to determine the origin or cause(s) of a disease or illness. The term 'pathogenesis' of a disease describes how the disease occurs and develops, i.e. the mechanism that leads to the diseased state.

Circadian: refers to rhythmic biological activities or functions recurring at approximately 24-hour intervals. Circadian rhythm (or circadian clock) is an internal biological clock that regulates sleeping and feeding patterns.

Enteral feeding: refers to a method of feeding that uses the gastrointestinal tract to deliver part or all of energy and nutrients. When the gastrointestinal tract cannot be used, parenteral feeding delivers energy and nutrients through a vein; if it provides the only source of nutrients, it is called total parenteral nutrition.

Eukaryotic: relating to eukaryotes, single-celled organisms that evolved from the more primitive prokaryotes and contain a nucleus and other organelles.

Mendelian randomisation: a method in observation studies that examines the putative causal effect(s) of modifiable risk factors on a disease, using genetic variants as natural experiments.

Non-communicable (or chronic) disease (NCD): a disease that is by definition non-infectious and non-transmissible among people. NCDs are usually of long duration and slow progression, hence the term 'chronic'. Examples of NCDs include cardiovascular diseases, cancers, chronic respiratory diseases and diabetes.

Prokaryotic: relating to prokaryotes, single-celled organisms that lack membrane-bound compartments (called organelles) such as nucleus, mitochondria and endoplasmic reticulum. Without a nucleus, prokaryotes are primitive in nature.

Self-efficacy: a term used in health behaviour theory. It refers to an individual's belief in their ability to achieve goals. It is determined by a range of factors including positive reinforcement, ability to access information and personal coping strategies (Bandura 1982).

Stratified medicine: an approach that sorts a population or patients, using genetic or other biomarker information, into subgroups based on their risk of disease or response to therapy, so that medication and treatment management can be tailored. This approach is also used in stratified nutrition for clinical diagnosis and management of metabolic disorders/diseases.

REFERENCES

Academy of Nutrition and Dietetics, 2018, *eNCPT*, <www.ncpro.org/>, accessed 7 January 2019

Admyre, C., Johansson, S.M., Qazi, K.R., Filén, J.-J., Lahesmaa, R. et al., 2007, 'Exosomes with immune modulatory features are present in human breast milk', *Journal of Immunology, 179*(3): 1969–78, doi:10.4049/jimmunol.179.3.1969

AIHW, 2016, *Australian Burden of Disease Study: Impact and Causes of Illness and Death in Australia, 2011*, <www.aihw.gov.au/getmedia/d4df9251-c4b6-452f-a877-8370b6124219/19663.pdf.aspx?inline=true>, accessed 7 January 2019

Asher, G. & Sassone-Corsi, P., 2015, 'Time for food: The intimate interplay between nutrition, metabolism, and the circadian clock', *Cell, 161*(1): 84–92, doi:10.1016/j.cell.2015.03.015

Bandura, A., 1982, 'Self-efficacy mechanism in human agency', *American Psychologist, 37*(2):122–47, doi:10.1037/0003-066X.37.2.122

Bauman, A.E., Reis, R.S., Sallis, J.F., Wells, J.C., Loos, R.J. et al., 2012, 'Correlates of physical activity: Why are some people physically active and others not?', *Lancet, 380*(9838): 258–71, doi:10.1016/S0140-6736(12)60735-1

Campbell, S.S., Dawson, D. & Anderson, M.W., 1993, 'Alleviation of sleep maintenance insomnia with timed exposure to bright light', *Journal of the American Geriatrics Society, 41*(8): 829–36, doi:10.1111/j.1532-5415.1993.tb06179.x

Carlson, C., Aytur, S., Gardner, K. & Rogers, S., 2012, 'Complexity in built environment, health, and destination walking: A neighborhood-scale analysis', *Journal of Urban Health, 89*(2): 270–84, doi:10.1007/s11524-011-9652-8

Chiang, P.-H., Wahlqvist, M.L., Lee, M.-S., Huang, L.-Y., Chen, H.-H. & Huang, S.T.-Y., 2011, 'Fast-food outlets and walkability in school neighbourhoods predict fatness in boys and height in girls: A Taiwanese population study', *Public Health Nutrition, 14*(9): 1601–9, doi:10.1017/S1368980011001042

Cox, H., Burns, I. & Savage, S., 2004, 'Multisensory environments for leisure: Promoting well-being in nursing home residents with dementia', *Journal of Gerontological Nursing, 30*(2): 37–45, doi:10.3928/0098-9134-20040201-08

European Patients' Academy (EUPATI), 2017, *Stratified Versus Personalised Medicine*, <www.eupati.eu/personalised-medicine/stratified-versus-personalised-medicine/>, accessed 7 January 2019

Finger, T.E. & Kinnamon, S.C., 2011, 'Taste isn't just for taste buds anymore', *F1000 Biology Reports, 3*: 20, doi:10.3410/B3-20

Gabel, K., Hoddy, K.K., Haggerty, N., Song, J., Kroeger, C.M. et al., 2018, 'Effects of 8-hour time restricted feeding on body weight and metabolic disease risk factors in obese adults: A pilot study', *Nutrition and Healthy Aging, 4*(4): 345–53, doi:10.3233/NHA-170036

Hoddinott, J. & Yohannes, Y., 2002, *Dietary Diversity as a Food Security Indicator*, <http://ebrary.ifpri.org/cdm/ref/collection/p15738coll2/id/81672>, accessed 7 January 2019

Hodgson, J., Hage, B., Wahlqvist, M., Kouris-Blazos, A. & Lo, C., 1991, 'Development of two food variety scores as measures for the prediction of health outcomes', *Proceedings of Nutrition Society of Australia, 16*: 62–5, <http://211.76.170.15/server/MarkWpapers/abstracts/A203.pdf>, accessed 7 January 2019

Huang, Y.-C., Wahlqvist, M.L. & Lee, M.-S., 2013, 'Sleep quality in the survival of elderly Taiwanese: Roles for dietary diversity and pyridoxine in men and women', *Journal of the American College of Nutrition, 32*(6): 417–27, doi:10.1080/07315724.2013.848158

Jike, M., Itani, O., Watanabe, N., Buysse, D.J. & Kaneita, Y., 2018, 'Long sleep duration and health outcomes: A systematic review, meta-analysis and meta-regression', *Sleep Medicine Reviews, 39*: 25–36, doi:10.1016/j.smrv.2017.06.011

Johnstone, R.M., 2006, 'Exosomes biological significance: A concise review', *Blood Cells, Molecules, and Diseases, 36*(2): 315–21, doi:10.1016/j.bcmd.2005.12.001

Khan, H., Kella, D., Kunutsor, S.K., Savonen, K. & Laukkanen, J.A., 2018, 'Sleep duration and risk of fatal coronary heart disease, sudden cardiac death, cancer death, and all-cause mortality', *American Journal of Medicine, 131*(12): 1499–505, doi:10.1016/j.amjmed.2018.07.010

Kosaka, N., Izumi, H., Sekine, K. & Ochiya, T., 2010, 'microRNA as a new immune-regulatory agent in breast milk', *Silence, 1*(1): 7, doi:10.1186/1758-907X-1-7

Lee, A.C. & Maheswaran, R., 2011, 'The health benefits of urban green spaces: A review of the evidence', *Journal of Public Health, 33*(2): 212–22, doi:10.1093/pubmed/fdq068

Lee, I.-M., Shiroma, E.J., Lobelo, F., Puska, P., Blair, S.N. et al., 2012, 'Effect of physical inactivity on major non-communicable diseases worldwide: An analysis of burden of disease and life expectancy', *Lancet, 380*(9838): 219–29, doi:10.1016/S0140-6736(12)61031-9

Lonnerdal, B., Du, X., Liao, Y. & Li, J., 2015, 'Human milk exosomes resist digestion in vitro and are internalized by human intestinal cells', *FASEB Journal, 29*(1_suppl): 121–3, doi:10.1096/fasebj.29.1_supplement.121.3

Ordovas, J.M., Ferguson, L.R., Tai, E.S. & Mathers, J.C., 2018, 'Personalised nutrition and health', *BMJ, 361*: k2173, doi:10.1136/bmj.k2173

Panda, S., 2018, '*The Circadian Code: Lose weight, supercharge your energy, and transform your health from morning to midnight*', New York, NY: Rodale Books

Pattinson, C.L., Smith, S.S., Staton, S.L., Trost, S.G. & Thorpe, K.J., 2018, 'Investigating the association between sleep parameters and the weight status of children: Night sleep duration matters', *Sleep Health*, 4(2): 147–53, doi:10.1016/j.sleh.2017.12.009

Renalds, A., Smith, T.H. & Hale, P.J., 2010, 'A systematic review of built environment and health', *Family & Community Health*, 33(1): 68–78, doi:10.1097/FCH.0b013e3181c4e2e5

Sallis, J.F., Cervero, R.B., Ascher, W., Henderson, K.A., Kraft, M.K. & Kerr, J., 2006, 'An ecological approach to creating active living communities', *Annual Review of Public Health*, 27: 297–322, doi:10.1146/annurev. publhealth.27.021405.102100

Sampasa-Kanyinga, H., Hamilton, H.A. & Chaput, J.-P., 2018, 'Use of social media is associated with short sleep duration in a dose–response manner in students aged 11 to 20 years', *Acta Paediatrica*, 107(4): 694–700, doi:10.1111/apa.14210

Savige, G.S., Hsu-Hage, B. & Wahlqvist, M.L., 1997, 'Food variety as nutritional therapy', *Current Therapeutics, March*: 57–67, <http://211.76.170.15/server/MarkWpapers/Papers/Papers%201997/P226.pdf>, accessed 7 January 2019

Shechter, A., Kim, E.W., St-Onge, M.-P. & Westwood, A.J., 2018, 'Blocking nocturnal blue light for insomnia: A randomized controlled trial', *Journal of Psychiatric Research*, 96: 196–202, doi:10.1016/j.jpsychires.2017.10.015

Solomons, N.W., 2002, 'Ethical consequences for professionals from the globalization of food, nutrition and health', *Asia Pacific Journal of Clinical Nutrition*, 11: S653–S665, doi:10.1046/j.1440-6047.11.supp3.14.x

Spence, C., 2015, 'Multisensory flavor perception', *Cell*, 161(1): 24–35, doi:10.1016/j.cell.2015.03.007

Sugiyama, T. & Thompson, C.W., 2008, 'Associations between characteristics of neighbourhood open space and older people's walking', *Urban Forestry & Urban Greening*, 7(1): 41–51, doi:10.1016/j.ufug.2007.12.002

Vlassov, A.V., Magdaleno, S., Setterquist, R. & Conrad, R., 2012, 'Exosomes: Current knowledge of their composition, biological functions, and diagnostic and therapeutic potentials', *Biochimica et Biophysica Acta (BBA)—General Subjects*, 1820(7): 940–8, doi:10.1016/j.bbagen.2012.03.017

Wahlqvist, M.L., 2014, 'Ecosystem health disorders: Changing perspectives in clinical medicine and nutrition', *Asia Pacific Journal of Clinical Nutrition*, 23(1): 1–15, doi:10.6133/apjcn.2014.23.1.20

—— 2016, 'Ecosystem dependence of healthy localities, food and people', *Annals of Nutrition and Metabolism*, 69: 75–8, doi:10.1159/000449143

Wahlqvist, M.L. & Lee, M., 2006, 'Nutrition in health care practice', *Journal of Medical Sciences* 26(5): 157–64, <http://jms.ndmctsgh.edu.tw/2605157.pdf>, accessed 7 January 2019

WHO, 2013, *Global Action Plan for the Prevention and Control of NCDs 2013–2020*, <www.who.int/nmh/events/ncd_action_plan/en/>, accessed 7 January 2019

—— 2017, *World Health Statistics 2017: Monitoring health for the SDGs, Sustainable Development Goals'*, <www.who.int/gho/publications/world_health_statistics/2017/en/ >, accessed 7 January 2019

—— 2018, *ICD-11 for Mortality and Morbidity Statistics*, <https://icd.who.int/browse11/l-m/en#/http://id.who.int/icd/entity/1671987290>, accessed 7 January 2019

Wild, C.P., 2012, 'The exposome: From concept to utility', *International Journal of Epidemiology*, 41(1): 24–32, doi:10.1093/ije/dyr236

{CHAPTER 32}
DISORDERED SYSTEM FUNCTIONS

Mark L. Wahlqvist and Naiyana Wattanapenpaiboon

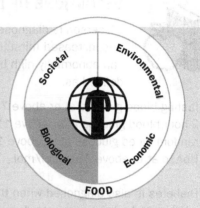

OBJECTIVES

- Describe how systems which connect between bodily functions may depend on, be influenced by and be disrupted by nutritional factors.
- Identify nutritional and environmental factors in the risk profile for certain ecohealth disorders as a result of dysfunctional nutritional biological systems.
- Examine how the function of 'internal' systems (endocrine and immune) and that of the cells (cellular kinetics) are incomplete without 'external' inputs (from the natural world).
- Explore the interactions, whether adverse, aberrant or favourable, between nutritional factors and immune function.
- Explain the importance of hormonal and microbiomic connections as vulnerable to nutritional disturbance.
- Recognise common disorders of these systems to envisage food and nutritional approaches for their management.

INTRODUCTION

The physiology of most, if not all, human body systems are nutritionally responsive, and the body can adapt itself to changing nutrition environments, as discussed in Chapter 30. The mechanisms of adaptation include restoring homeostasis, varying gene expression, or modulating the inflammatory process. These capabilities, however, have limits, and when the thresholds are reached, the nutritional biological systems and/or organs can become dys-

functional, resulting in a disorder or subsequently a disease (see Figure 31.1 in Chapter 31). This chapter focuses on the body systems, dysfunctionalities of which lead to the major burden of disease worldwide.

ENDOCRINE SYSTEM

Diabetes mellitus

Diabetes mellitus is a disorder of blood glucose regulation characterised by a failure to maintain the blood glucose concentration in the normal range (Cypess et al. 2009). Type 1 diabetes (T1DM), known as insulin-dependent diabetes, is associated with an absolute deficiency of insulin, usually resulting from autoimmune destruction of the β-cells of the pancreas. Type 2 diabetes (T2DM), known as non-insulin-dependent diabetes, accounts for most cases of diabetes worldwide. This type of diabetes develops when the production of insulin is insufficient to overcome the underlying abnormality of increased resistance to its action (insulin resistance). The early stages of T2DM are characterised by overproduction of insulin, and, as the disease progresses, the insulin concentration may fall as a result of failure of the insulin-producing β-cells of the pancreas. Some 1–2 per cent of diabetes cases

---

DEFINITIONS OF DIABETES MELLITUS

A person is diagnosed with diabetes if they have symptoms of diabetes such as increased thirst, urination, tiredness and unexplained weight loss, and an abnormally high blood glucose concentration (IDF 2017b; WHO 2006), defined as:

- fasting blood glucose at or above 7.0 mmol/L, or
- 2-hour blood glucose at or above 11.0 mmol/L after ingestion of 75 g of glucose load, or
- random blood glucose at or above 11.0 mmol/L in symptomatic patient, or
- HbA1c at or above 48 mmol/mol.

Diabetes is also diagnosed when there have been no symptoms but two abnormally high blood glucose tests on separate days.

There are three main types of diabetes:

1. **Type 1 diabetes (T1DM)** is caused by an absolute deficiency in insulin production in genetically susceptible individuals.
2. **Type 2 diabetes (T2DM)** involves insulin resistance and relative insulin deficiency, rather than an absolute insulin deficiency as seen in T1DM. Even though there are important predisposing genetic factors in T2DM, their expression is almost entirely dependent on environmental and personal behavioural circumstances, notably environmental contaminants, sociocultural situation, emotional stress, physical inactivity and diet.
3. **Gestational diabetes (GDM)** is a form of diabetes that is diagnosed when higher than normal blood glucose first appears during pregnancy. It may be intergenerationally recurrent.

Most people with T1DM and many with T2DM have diabetes symptoms. Some may have signs such as the slow healing of wounds, or persistent or unusually recurrent infections. Many people with T2DM have no symptoms at all, even though tissue damage is under way.

Pre-diabetes (or intermediate hyperglycaemia) conditions

A person can have no signs or symptoms but have a pre-diabetes condition in which blood glucose concentrations are higher than normal, but not high enough to be diagnosed as diabetes. There are two pre-diabetes conditions.

- Impaired fasting glucose (IFG) is where blood glucose is escalated in the fasting state but not enough to be regarded as diabetes.

- Impaired glucose tolerance (Steegers-Theunissen et al. 2013) is where blood glucose is higher than normal on a **glucose challenge**, but not high enough to be regarded as diabetes.

It is possible to have both of these conditions at the same time.

Research suggests that diabetes can be classified into five distinct types based on six variables; BMI, age and **HbA1c** at diagnosis, the presence of glutamic acid decarboxylase autoantibodies (GADA), homoeostatic estimates of β-cell function, and insulin resistance. Of nearly 15,000 newly diagnosed T2DM patients, five distinct clusters of the patients with differing disease progression and risk of diabetes complications have been identified (Ahlqvist et al. 2018). (The presence of GADA suggests an autoimmune reaction leading to subclinical β-cell damage and impaired insulin secretion. It is the most commonly used predictive marker for T1DM. However, the absence of GADA does not necessarily indicate that the patient does not have T1DM.)

Cluster 1: Severe autoimmune diabetes: characterised by early-onset disease, relatively low BMI, poor metabolic control, insulin deficiency and presence of GADA.

Cluster 2: Severe insulin-deficient diabetes: similar to Cluster 1, but GADA is absent. Patients in this cluster are currently classified as T2DM as they do not have an autoimmune disease. They tend to have a higher risk of blindness.

Cluster 3: Severe insulin-resistant diabetes: characterised by insulin resistance and high BMI. Patients in this cluster have the greatest risk of kidney disease.

Cluster 4: Mild obesity-related diabetes: characterised by obesity but not by insulin resistance.

Cluster 5: Mild age-related diabetes: similar to Cluster 4, but being older than those in other clusters.

This refined classification could eventually help to tailor and target early treatment to patients who would benefit most.

Explore the current available guidelines for the treatment and management of diabetes. Using T2DM, compare and contrast the guidelines. What is similar and what is different? Explain the differences based on where the guidelines are coming from or how old they are.

Look at guidelines from the following sources:

- The World Health Organization—Definition and Diagnosis of Diabetes Mellitus and Intermediate Hyperglycaemia
- The International Diabetes Federation—Recommendations for Managing Type 2 Diabetes in Primary Care
- The Royal Australian College of General Practitioners and Diabetes Australia—General Practice Management of Type 2 Diabetes 2016–2018
- New Zealand Ministry of Health—Guidance on the Management of Type 2 Diabetes 2011 (New Zealand Guidelines Group 2011).

are secondary to drug treatments or other disorders or diseases, such as inflammation and damage of the pancreas, or increased production of hormones whose action is antagonistic to insulin.

Although there are genetic predispositions to T2DM, they may have existed for generations without being expressed (Prasad & Groop 2015). Environmental factors during life, *in utero*, or affecting our ancestors have allowed these genetic predispositions to be expressed (see Chapter 30). Problems with energy regulation and insulin sensitivity are the primary underlying determinants of diabetes and its precursors. Precursor situations include (a) impaired fasting glucose (IFG), (b) impaired glucose tolerance (IGT), and (c) gestational diabetes. Resistance to the action of insulin, which is an important underlying abnormality in T2DM, is also associated with a range of additional clinical and metabolic abnormalities that are often seen in association with T2DM, IGT and IFG, but may also occur with normal blood glucose levels.

Diabetes prevalence and incidence have increased globally, particularly in association with economic transition. According to the International Diabetes Federation (2017a), in 2017 one in eleven adults had diabetes, and one in two adults with diabetes was undiagnosed. Worldwide, the number of cases has reached 425 million, predicted to nearly double by 2045 (Figure 32.1, see colour section), with most new cases expected in China and India. T2DM was once a disease of the middle-aged and elderly but now affects all age groups, including adolescents and children.

There is no single cause of T2DM, but major changes in dietary patterns towards foods which are highly processed, energy-dense, and minimally biodiverse, together with physical inactivity, emotional stress and environmental contamination, are factors. Higher stress levels, short sleep duration and disruptions to circadian rhythms have all been implicated in the development of insulin resistance (Javeed & Matveyenko 2018; Reutrakul & Van Cauter 2018).

Many studies, mostly in low-income countries, suggest that intrauterine growth retardation and low birthweight are associated with the development of insulin resistance (Stern et al. 2000). In countries where there has been chronic undernutrition, insulin resistance may have been selectively advantageous in terms of surviving famine. However, as energy intake has increased and behaviours become more sedentary, insulin resistance and the consequent risk of T2DM have been enhanced. The risk of T2DM in later life is further increased, especially when rapid catch-up growth occurs in infancy and childhood. It is likely that maternal, even paternal and grandparental, nutrition affects gene programming and expression, via epigenetics, so that offspring and descendants are more susceptible to diabetes where there is a food surfeit and limited energy expenditure (Barker et al. 1993; Pembrey et al. 2006) (see Chapter 20).

Gestational diabetes (GDM)

During pregnancy, hormones from the placenta can cause a build-up of glucose in the mother's body because these hormones block the action of insulin, and lead to an increased demand for insulin to keep blood glucose level normal. If the pancreas is unable to produce the additional insulin needed at this time, the mother develops GDM. It is estimated that 12–14 per cent of pregnant women will develop GDM, and this usually occurs around the 24th to 28th week of pregnancy. It is therefore recommended that pregnant women be tested for GDM, using an oral glucose tolerance test, during this period of their pregnancy, except those who already have diabetes (Australian Diabetes in Pregnancy Society 2014). Achieving optimal weight gain for mother and fetus during pregnancy is an increasing challenge, as the population at large is experiencing difficulty in this respect. In most women, their blood glucose becomes normal after giving birth.

For pregnant women who have some form of diabetes, the dietary recommendations include those suggested for all pregnancies. In addition, they should carefully distribute the glycaemic load throughout the day to avoid episodes of hypoglycaemia. Regular snacks between meals and a bedtime snack can help avoid overnight hypoglycaemia with associated ketone body formation, a risk to the fetus.

Diabetes complications

Diabetes is associated with a range of problems, including those directly related to blood glucose, and to macrovascular and microvascular complications (involving large and small blood vessels respectively). Nerves may be affected due either to damage to the nerves themselves or to the problems with small and large blood vessels. Microvascular complications can affect the retina of the eye and the vessels in the kidney. Long-term complications of diabetes (Table 32.1) develop gradually and, eventually, may be disabling or even life-threatening.

Atherosclerotic cardiovascular disease (CVD) and its complications are by far the most common cause of death in diabetes. While the causes of the accelerated atherosclerosis in diabetes are unclear, it is speculated that it may involve dyslipidaemia, hypertension, high insulin, vessel wall abnormalities, impaired chemical release from endothelial cells, and alterations in haemostasis. The lipid abnormalities seen in poorly controlled T1DM improve when glucose control is improved. Hypertension plays an important role in **microangiopathy**, especially diabetic nephropathy; improved control of blood

pressure can reduce the onset and progression of retinopathy and nephropathy.

People at risk of and with diabetes may have a range of problems with brain health, including cognitive impairment, **Parkinson's disease** and **affective disorders** (unipolar and bipolar depression), diseases in which neurodegeneration plays a role (Hsu et al. 2011; Wahlqvist, Lee, Chuang, et al. 2012). Thus, the improvement of dietary patterns, in the direction of diabetes prevention and management, should decrease the burden of **neurodegeneration** (Jacka et al. 2011; Wahlqvist, Lee, Hsu, et al. 2012). Risks for not only dementia, but also Parkinson's disease and affective disorders (major and minor depression) are increased in diabetes (Wahlqvist, Lee, Chuang, et al. 2012; Wahlqvist, Lee, Hsu, et al. 2012) (Figure 32.2).

Prevention of type 2 diabetes

Modification of personal behaviours is the cornerstone of both prevention and treatment of T2DM. It has been demonstrated that self-management (weight reduction and regular moderate physical activity) can prevent or delay the onset of T2DM (Colberg et al. 2016; IDF 2017b). Many patients

Table 32.1: Possible complications of diabetes

Complication	Symptoms or mechanisms
Cardiovascular disease	• Increased risk of various cardiovascular problems, including coronary artery disease with chest pain (angina), heart attack, stroke and atherosclerosis.
Nerve damage (neuropathy)	• Excess glucose can injure the walls of capillaries that nourish the nerves, especially in the legs. This can cause tingling, numbness, burning or pain that usually begins at the tips of the toes or fingers and gradually spreads upward. If untreated, this can lead to a loss of sensation in the affected limbs. • Nerve damage in the feet or poor blood flow to the feet increases the risk of various foot complications. Cuts and blisters can develop serious infections, which often heal poorly. These infections may ultimately require toe, foot or leg amputation. • Damage to the nerves related to digestion can cause problems with nausea, vomiting, diarrhoea or constipation. • Neurodegeneration of the central nervous system contributing to cognitive impairment, dementia, Parkinson's disease and affective disorders (unipolar and bipolar depression). • For men, it may lead to erectile dysfunction.
Kidney damage (nephropathy)	• Excess glucose can damage the glomeruli (tiny blood vessel clusters that filter waste from the blood) in the kidneys and severe damage can lead to kidney failure or irreversible end-stage kidney disease, which may require dialysis or a kidney transplant.
Eye damage (retinopathy)	• The blood vessels of the retina can be damaged, potentially leading to blindness. Diabetes also increases the risk of other serious vision conditions, such as cataracts and glaucoma.

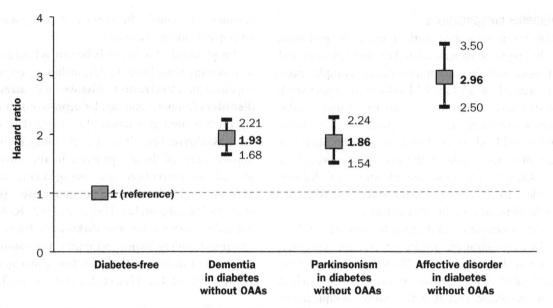

Note: Subjects were matched by gender and by year and month of birth. OAAs = oral anti-hyperglycaemic agents

Figure 32.2: Increased risk of neurodegenerative and affective disorders in type 2 diabetes
Source: Developed from Wahlqvist, Lee, Chuang, et al. (2012); Wahlqvist, Lee, Hsu, et al. (2012)

with T2DM are overweight (BMI 25.0–29.9) or obese (BMI >30); however, waist circumference or waist-to-hip ratio, both of which reflect **abdominal visceral adiposity**, are more powerful determinants of subsequent risk of T2DM than BMI. Abdominal adiposity is an important determinant of insulin resistance, which is the underlying abnormality in most cases of T2DM. Weight loss can improve insulin sensitivity and can reduce the risk of progression from IGT to T2DM (Tuomilehto et al. 2001). The changes required to reduce the risk of developing diabetes at the population level are, however, unlikely to be achieved without major environmental changes to facilitate suitable choices by individuals.

The general nutritional principles for the prevention of T2DM include (American Diabetes Association 2018; Ley et al. 2014; Wahlqvist & O'Brien 1993):

1. Avoiding overfatness, especially around the abdomen, by regular moderate physical activity (a minimum of 150 minutes per week).
2. Reducing overall energy intake, in particular by reducing total fat intake.
3. Having a wide variety of foods, especially plant foods, to provide different natural colours and dietary fibre types.
4. Having fish regularly. Whatever the controversy over fish oil, the whole fish has several nutritional advantages as a source of n-3 fatty acids, vitamin D and calcium and protein.
5. Having alcohol in moderation and preferably with food to minimise its impact on blood levels and tissues like the pancreas.
6. Avoiding having too much food at once, spreading intake over the day.
7. Using foods with a low glycaemic index (GI) (see Chapter 12), provided they are not associated with fats, such as:
   – wholegrain rather than wholemeal (and wholemeal rather than white flour)
   – legumes/lentils
   – low glycaemic fruit.
8. Minimising sodium (salt) intake in favour of potassium.

Some individuals are at greater risk of T2DM due to genetic reasons, or have a predisposition to diabetes because of some other disease or treatment (e.g. disease of the pancreas, which produces insulin, or administration of steroids, which antagonise the insulin action).

Treatment of diabetes mellitus

Diabetes Australia recommends that people with diabetes follow the Australian Dietary Guidelines (Diabetes Australia 2015), which promote healthy eating patterns, with an emphasis on a range of nutrient-dense foods in appropriate portion sizes. In addition, patients with diabetes are encouraged to seek advice on medical nutrition therapy to take into consideration individual variations and comorbidities if they exist (RACGP 2016).

The nutritional goals for all types of diabetes include the following (American Diabetes Association 2018; RACGP 2016; Wahlqvist & O'Brien 1993):

1. Weight control by reducing weight and in particular abdominal fat by 5–10 per cent.
2. Managing elevated blood glucose so as to reduce its damaging effects on tissues like the eye, kidneys, nervous system and arteries.
3. Keeping blood lipids (cholesterol, triglycerides, HDL cholesterol) as normal as possible, because these, when abnormal, also increase the risk of damaging the large and distributing arteries supplying heart, brain, lower limbs and kidneys, by way of the process of atherosclerosis.
4. Reducing the damaging effects on tissues by any other mechanism, such as oxidation.
5. Improving the action of available insulin by:
   – minimising abdominal fatness
   – improving the action of the insulin receptor in cell membranes, possibly by altering its fatty acid composition in the direction of PUFAs
   – improving the action of insulin in the cell, especially by reducing the amount of circulating free fatty acids or increasing their utilisation by ways that do not interfere with glucose metabolism—physical activity and reducing body fatness are important.

Dietary components
Macronutrients

There is no ideal percentage of energy intake from carbohydrate, protein or fat for individuals with diabetes; most authorities, however, agree that individuals with diabetes should consume carbohydrates to about 50–60 per cent of daily energy intake, and that this should comprise largely unrefined or complex carbohydrate. Historically, people with diabetes were advised to exclude sucrose from their diet. Nevertheless, research reveals that the use of sucrose as a sweetener in small amounts does not have a deleterious effect on glycaemic control, provided energy intake is maintained at a constant level. However, since weight control is usually an important goal of the dietary therapy of T2DM, consumption of unnecessary nutrients or 'empty' calories in the form of sucrose should be avoided. Naturally occurring fructose in fruits seems to have a better effect on glycaemic control compared to sucrose or starch, if consumption is not excessive. Consuming low GI foods that are rich in fibre and other important nutrients, and substituting foods with lower glycaemic load for those with higher load, should be encouraged for the prevention and management of diabetes (see Chapter 12). Those requiring insulin therapy or some forms of oral medication may require more even carbohydrate intakes throughout the day, timed with insulin delivery and/or physical activity, to prevent hypoglycaemia.

Replacing saturated fatty acids (SFAs) with unsaturated fats (MUFAs and PUFAs) can enhance insulin sensitivity and improve glucose tolerance. However, when total fat intake is high (greater than 37 per cent of total energy), changing the quality of dietary fat appears to have little effect. Dietary protein may play a role in the regulation of glucose metabolism and an excess may accelerate the development of kidney complications. As for the general population, it is recommended that the diet contain about 10–20 per cent of energy intake from protein, less than 10 per cent from SFAs and about 10 per cent from PUFAs, including n-3 PUFAs from fish and plant products. To achieve adequate intake of dietary fibre, regular consumption of wholegrain cereals, legumes, fruits and vegetables is also recommended.

The gut microbiome has been implicated in the pathogenesis of both T1DM and T2DM diabetes and research is continuing on the relationship between the microbiome, insulin resistance and the dietary factors that can influence these (Aydin et al. 2018; Zheng et al. 2018).

Micronutrients

While there is insufficient evidence to support the claim that vitamin E reduces the risk of developing T2DM, it is speculated that vitamin E and other antioxidants may protect against diabetes complications such as coronary heart disease and retinopathy by reducing free radical damage of proteins and lipids. Other antioxidants include vitamin C and lycopene and are present in fruits, vegetables and grains. Research suggests chromium may improve glucose tolerance because it forms part of the 'glucose tolerance factor', which promotes efficient insulin function. Chromium is a mineral found in brewer's yeast, egg yolk, cheese, and whole wheat products. However, its protective effect against the development of T2DM is inconclusive. Both T1DM and T2DM patients exhibit low levels of zinc in the blood, although the underlying causes in some patients have not been identified conclusively.

Advanced glycation end products

Advanced glycation end products (AGEs), also known as glycotoxins, are formed when sugar reacts in a non-enzymatic way with free amino groups of proteins and lipids or nucleic acids, resulting in the cross-linking of the glycated proteins. This occurs both endogenously (in the body) or exogenously (outside the body such as in food). AGEs are naturally present in uncooked animal-derived foods, and additionally can be formed by the Maillard reaction, in which certain foods exposed to high heat are browned, such as bread (crust) and meat (grilled, roasted, seared, fried or baked) (see the Maillard reaction, Chapter 5). The products of this reaction add a desirable colour and taste to foods. It is estimated that about 10 per cent of ingested AGEs enter the circulation, and about one-third is excreted within three days of ingestion. Impairment in AGE excretion appears to be associated with diabetes. High dietary intake of AGEs accelerates the produc-

tion of endogenous AGEs and increases circulating AGEs (Uribarri et al. 2010). The formation of AGEs is a part of normal metabolism in humans, but they can become harmful if AGEs are excessively high in the circulation and tissues. AGEs promote oxidative stress and inflammation by binding with cell surface receptors or cross-linking with body proteins, causing the reduction of tissue elasticity and impediment of cellular functions. AGEs have been identified as having a pathogenic role in the development and progression of diabetic nephropathy and vascular complications (Vlassara et al. 2002). Thus, caution is warranted with regard to the potential effects of a high blood glucose on AGE formation and increased risk of diabetes complications.

Type 2 diabetes in children and adolescents

There is an increasing incidence of T2DM among children and adolescents worldwide. This followed an increase both in the prevalence and the degree of obesity in children and adolescents in many populations. Furthermore, offspring of women with diabetes during pregnancy (including GDM) are often large and heavy at birth, tend to develop obesity in childhood and are at high risk of developing T2DM at an early age.

Puberty plays a major role in the development of T2DM in children. Increased growth hormone secretion during puberty is believed to be responsible for increased insulin resistance. After puberty, basal and stimulated insulin responses decline. Given this knowledge, it is not surprising that the peak age at presentation of T2DM in children coincides with the usual age of mid-puberty.

Children and adolescents with T2DM have a higher risk of diabetes complications compared to adults with diabetes. Accordingly, developing T2DM at a younger age is also associated with a much higher risk of long-term CVD than for those who develop diabetes in middle age. Young people with T2DM also appear to be at a much higher risk of developing complications than those with T1DM.

Both T1DM and T2DM are lifelong conditions requiring adherence to specific dietary and physical activity regimens. Achieving patient adherence to

TYPE 2 DIABETES CASE STUDY

Mrs Phillips has just been diagnosed with T2DM. She is 47 years old, 170 cm tall and weighs 85 kg. She takes the dog for a walk every day for about 20 minutes. Her diet history is listed below.

- What would be the primary goals for major changes in personal behaviour?
- What foods would you recommend Mrs Phillips change in her diet? What substitutions or changes to her dietary pattern would be recommended? Provide a rationale for your choice.

Breakfast

2 slices of white toast with butter and honey
1 banana
Glass of fruit juice drink

Morning tea

Café latte with one sugar
Piece of cake

Lunch

Nil

Afternoon tea

Chocolate bar

Evening meal

2 glasses of white wine
About 150 g meat served with potatoes and one other vegetable
Fish (battered) and chips on Friday nights
Ice cream or custard with canned fruit

the diet is a constant challenge for both patients and healthcare professionals (Dunkley et al. 2014). A trial of behaviour modification is recommended with a review of glycaemic control (self-monitoring of blood glucose and HbA1c) before medications are considered. Simplifying the dietary instructions improves patient adherence, while explaining the rationale for the diet and individualising meal plans that take into account a patient's usual eating habits, personal behaviours and cultural background have been shown to be essential components of any dietary education. Group education has been shown to be more effective (Galaviz et al. 2018). In addition, a range of technologies, including mobile phone apps, are being explored to enhance adherence to changes in personal behaviours (Lunde et al. 2018). Most of the recommended guidelines for treatment in children with T2DM are extrapolated from experience gained in adults. However, careful management so growth is not disrupted needs to be taken into consideration and managed. Initial management of obese children and adolescents with T2DM should consist of behaviour modification strategies, such as reducing energy–dense food choice and sedentary behaviour while increasing physical activity.

The financial and societal consequences of the increasing prevalence and incidence of T2DM epidemic are substantial and demand, in addition to individual management, a public health response. Emphasis has been placed upon preventive behaviours and early detection. Prevention of T2DM means prevention of obesity in childhood. As prevention should start very early in life, perhaps even before birth, a population and community approach for prevention of obesity in childhood (Bell et al. 2008; Bleich et al. 2013; Sacher et al. 2010), and hence T2DM in childhood and adolescence, will require changes to the environment as well as social and cultural practices (Borys et al. 2013).

THYROID DISORDERS

Thyroid disorders are a medical condition that affects the function of the thyroid gland, and are usually diagnosed using blood concentrations of thyroid stimulating hormone (TSH), and thyroid hormones triiodothyronine (T3) and thyroxine (T4). TSH stimulates iodine uptake by the thyroid and synthesis of T3 and T4, and its levels are determined by a classic negative feedback system in which high levels of T3 and T4 suppress the production of TSH, and low levels of T3 and T4 increase the production of TSH. Elevation of TSH is the first warning sign of hypothyroid disorders, telling us that thyroid hormone production is inadequate, while suppressed TSH levels can point to excessive thyroid hormone production (hyperthyroidism).

The TSH reference range for adults cited by many laboratories is 0.5–4.0 mU/L. This has been lowered due to evidence of an increased risk of developing hypothyroidism at lower levels of TSH (Australian Thyroid Foundation 2018; Garber et al. 2012). Identifying thyroid dysfunction (Table 32.2) early enables clinicians to reduce the risk of progression to overt hypothyroidism—this could be as simple as correcting nutritional deficiencies and using dietary treatment.

Nutrition plays an important role in the function of the thyroid gland, and impaired function may easily be corrected with food and short-term supplementation, thus negating the need for thyroxine

therapy. If a patient is diagnosed with autoimmune hypothyroid disease, it is still important to determine the extent to which their nutritional status has affected their thyroid function, because correcting any deficiencies may result in a reduced dose of replacement thyroxine due to improved production of T4 by the thyroid gland and better conversion of T4 from the medication to T3 in the body. Iodine and selenium deficiency can increase the production of autoantibodies to peroxidase enzyme in the thyroid.

Iodine and thyroid function

The relationship between iodine and thyroid function is complex. Iodine is required by the body to form thyroid hormone and, in moderate deficiency, the thyroid gland enlarges to increase its capacity to absorb iodine, hence forming a goitre. Goitre can be caused by an iodine deficiency, by eating foods that contain substances causing goitre (goitrogens), or by other disorders that interfere with thyroid hormone production; however, in many cases, the cause of goitre cannot be determined (see also 'Iodine' in Chapter 17).

Failure of the thyroid gland to function adequately can result in reduced levels of thyroid hormone in the body (a condition called hypothyroidism), and failure of the pituitary gland or hypothalamus

Table 32.2: Thyroid conditions

Hyperthyroidism	A condition in which an overactive thyroid gland excessively produces thyroid hormones. Hyperthyroidism can accelerate the body's metabolism, and its common symptoms include excessive sweating, rapid or irregular heartbeat, nervousness or irritability, muscle weakness, fatigue, sleep problems, heat intolerance, diarrhoea, menstrual disturbances, increased appetite, and sudden weight loss.
Thyrotoxicosis	The condition that occurs due to excessive thyroid hormone of any cause; it is not necessarily due to excessive production by the thyroid gland.
Hypothyroidism	A condition in which the thyroid gland is underactive and fails to produce enough thyroid hormones. This causes the person's metabolism to slow down leading to symptoms, such as poor ability to tolerate cold, fatigue, dry skin, muscle cramps, menstrual irregularities, hair loss, constipation, depression and weight gain. Congenital iodine deficiency syndrome (also known as cretinism) is a type of hypothyroidism that occurs at birth and results in stunted physical growth, impaired mental function, deaf mutism and disorders of gait. Severe hypothyroidism is called myxoedema and can cause dwarfism and impaired mental function.
Graves' disease	An autoimmune disease that causes the thyroid gland to produce too much thyroid hormone. It is often the underlying cause of hyperthyroidism.
Hashimoto's disease	An autoimmune disease in which the thyroid gland is gradually destroyed. Inflammation from Hashimoto's disease, also known as chronic lymphocytic thyroiditis, often leads to hypothyroidism.

to properly stimulate the thyroid gland can cause a condition known as secondary hypothyroidism. Goitre and hypothyroidism is usually seen with iodine intakes of less than 50 µg/day, and congenital iodine deficiency syndrome in children can occur with intakes of less than 30 µg/day in the mother. Both may be exacerbated by coexisting selenium and zinc deficiency and/or consumption of goitrogens (Hetzel 2000). Goitre may be reversible by treatment with iodine administration. Nevertheless, iodine deficiency does not always cause goitre but may simply manifest as hypothyroidism. Australia has been identified as mildly iodine deficient, and this has been identified as a common cause for primary hypothyroidism; however, low vitamin A, zinc, selenium, iron and possibly vitamin D can also contribute. In recognition of this deficiency, there is mandatory fortification of salt used in breadmaking in Australia (see Chapter 17).

Other nutrients and thyroid function
Vitamin A and zinc
Vitamin A plays a role in thyroid function by assisting with the uptake of iodine into the thyroid gland, with the incorporation of iodine into thyroglobulin, the induction of the enzyme activity in the liver and thyroid which helps convert T4 to T3 and by helping T3 bind to receptors on cells. Vitamin A deficiency can therefore contribute to iodine deficiency. Zinc is a cofactor for the enzymes involved in T4 and T3 production. Low zinc status can reduce T4 and T3 levels by 30 per cent and reduce the activity of the liver deiodinase enzyme by 67 per cent, suggesting that zinc deficiency may affect the metabolism of thyroid hormones. On the other hand, an underactive thyroid can result in a zinc deficiency because thyroid hormones increase intestinal and renal absorption of zinc.

To complicate matters, both zinc deficiency and thyroid disorders can lead to vitamin A deficiency, because enzymes in the brush border of the intestine require zinc and T4 to convert β-carotene in plant food to vitamin A. Additionally, zinc is needed to mobilise vitamin A from the liver. Increasing the intake of vitamin A and zinc through diet (or supplementation,

if concentrations in blood are found to be low) may help correct thyroid function and associated symptoms such as reduced taste and smell.

Selenium
Selenium deficiency can worsen the effects of a coexisting iodine deficiency because selenium is a component of enzymes that catalyse the conversion of inactive T4 to active T3, and it is also required in other enzymes involved in the assimilation of iodine. Selenium deficiency can be measured in the serum or by assessing the ratio of T4 to T3, which should be three to one. A higher ratio suggests reduced conversion of T4 to T3 due to inadequate selenium.

Both Australia and New Zealand have soils with some of the lowest selenium concentrations in the world (Thomson 2004), and yet to date there are no reports of blood selenium levels in Australia. In certain countries with severe selenium deficiency, there is a higher incidence of thyroiditis due to a decreased activity of selenium-dependent glutathione peroxidase activity within the thyroid. Selenium deficiency may lower glutathione peroxidase activity in the thyroid gland, resulting in increased hydrogen peroxide production and cytotoxicity.

Researchers have suggested that people who are deficient in both selenium and iodine should not take selenium supplements without first receiving iodine or thyroid hormone supplementation. This is because iodine deficiency must be corrected first to enable the thyroid to respond to selenium supplementation. There is no evidence that selenium supplementation can help people with hypothyroidism who are not selenium-deficient (assessed with a blood test).

Other dietary factors
Iron is needed for the production of T3 and T4, and it helps absorb iodine from the gut. Therefore, an adequate intake of iron is important. Interestingly, an underactive thyroid will reduce the absorption of iron, which explains why this condition is often associated with anaemia. Gluten sensitivity and coeliac disease can increase the risk of developing autoimmune hypothyroidism or hyperthyroidism. Patients with these conditions should be screened for

coeliac disease because avoiding gluten may reduce the progress of these conditions.

Hypothyroidism and the thyroid medication used to treat it can increase blood glucose levels by decreasing insulin function, thus increasing the risk of diabetes. Hypothyroidism can also increase the risk of heart disease through elevated cholesterol and triglycerides. It is therefore advisable to avoid refined starchy foods, sugar-dense foods and foods high in saturated fat. Poor fatty acid conversion has been reported in hypothyroidism, probably contributing to the symptoms of dry skin and hair.

IMMUNE SYSTEM

Poor immunity and malnutrition, mainly protein energy undernutrition, increase the risk of infectious diseases. Malnutrition was first linked to poor immune status in epidemiological studies and from historical accounts of famines and pestilence. Malnutrition is known to make the consequences of infectious diseases more serious but also creates nutritional disturbances (Scrimshaw et al. 1959).

The immune system and inflammatory processes have also been found to be involved in the development of so-called chronic diseases (which can actually develop and manifest quickly) such as obesity, diabetes, cancer and CVDs. Nutritional approaches that improve immune function and modulate inflammation can alter the course of these chronic diseases (see chapters 30 and 31). However, allergies and autoimmune diseases such as rheumatoid arthritis are examples of hyperactive or misdirected immune reactions and inflammation, and are potentially amenable to diet. (See also 'Nutritional modulation of inflammation' in Chapter 30.)

Effects of nutrition on the immune system

Immune function can be impaired by not only deficiencies of various nutrients, but also by imbalances of nutrients, as with leucine excess and iron excess, and with changes in n–3 and n–6 essential fatty acid ratios. Phytonutrients, notably flavonoids and other polyphenolic compounds, are recognised as immunomodulatory (Figure 32.3).

THE HUMAN IMMUNE SYSTEM IN A NUTSHELL

The innate (inherited) immune system is non-specific and does not confer long-lasting immunity against **pathogens**. The innate immune system is the dominant system of host defence in most organisms. The innate response includes physical barriers (e.g. skin), chemical barriers (e.g. tears, complement system) and the participation of cells such as macrophages, neutrophils, dendritic cells, natural killer cells and microbicide molecules such as nitric oxide (NO) and the superoxide anion (O_2^-).

The adaptive immune system is **antigen**-specific and requires the recognition of specific 'non-self' antigens during a process called antigen presentation. The adaptive immune response mainly involves T lymphocytes T (CD4$^+$ and CD8$^+$), B lymphocytes and their products, cytokines and antibodies respectively. It can be divided into a **humoral immune response** (mediated by antibodies) and a **cell-mediated immune response** (cell-mediated, such as T lymphocytes and macrophages). Antigen specificity allows for the generation of responses tailored to specific pathogens or pathogen-infected cells. The ability to mount these tailored responses is maintained in the body by 'memory cells', and these specific memory cells are used to quickly eliminate pathogens that infect the body more than once.

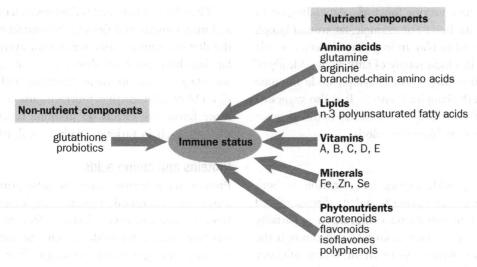

Figure 32.3: Food factors affecting immune status

Energy intake
Undernutrition

Protein energy malnutrition, or PEM (Pembrey et al. 2006), is a major cause of immunodeficiency, and can clinically manifest as marasmus, which is a severe form of general undernutrition or starvation, or kwashiorkor, which is caused by protein deficiency (see also Chapter 10). The immunologic manifestations of PEM are broad and include lymphoid tissue atrophy, decreases in lymphocyte numbers, and abnormally low cell-mediated and humoral immune responses. PEM is characterised by impairment of the complement system of cell-mediated immunity, of cytokine production by macrophages, and of phagocytic function by monocytes and leucocytes (neutrophilic granulocytes). Consequently, PEM is associated with a high incidence of morbidity and mortality from infections, which are usually accompanied by other nutrient deficits.

Moderate energy restriction

Defining the sources of energy is important, since fatty acids, particularly n-6 and n-3, provide functions other than energy, such as being precursors of eicosanoids, which are signalling molecules, while certain amino acids, such as glutamine, are energy sources for lymphocytes and macrophages.

Energy restriction, often practised by people trying to lose weight, may increase the risk of immune dysfunction if the foods selected are not nutrient-dense. Therefore, the alleged benefits of energy restriction should be evaluated with caution.

Overnutrition

Although it is still unclear, there are indications that obesity may lead to immune dysfunction. Part of the problem may be the pathogenesis of obesity, with physical inactivity and the use of foods of low nutrient and phytonutrient density. The balance of energy intake relative to expenditure partially determines body weight and composition, which in turn influence immune characteristics. Leanness has been associated with resistance to tumours and infection.

Adipose tissue is an immunity organ because it produces a range of hormones, and some of these hormones interact with the immune systems and are hence referred to as adipokines (adipose-derived cytokines). Tumour necrosis factor (TNF)-α, one of the adipokines, are pro-inflammatory, and can be produced widely in the body.

Fat can have varying functions, depending on its location in the body. For example, fat around lymph nodes is found to play an important interactive role with them in a local supply of fatty acids—ideally of a composition that enhances lymph node immune function in the lymphatic system. It is also suggested that local fat may play a role in the body's defence against infections like tuberculosis.

Lipids

Fatty acids provide energy, and function as both cell membrane components and mediators of cell signalling. Cell membrane composition is partially dependent on the fatty acids taken in through the diet; therefore dietary fats are an important influence on cell function, especially cells involved in immune function. Eicosanoids, which are derived from 20-carbon PUFAs (arachidonic acid, C20:4 n–6, and EPA, C20:5 n–3), are involved in cell signalling, inflammation, immunity, reproduction, blood flow and temperature regulation. The 2-series eicosanoids, derived from n–6 linoleic acid, include prostaglandin E2 and thromboxane A2 (in platelet membranes promote platelet aggregation) and leukotriene B4 (in neutrophils promote inflammation). The 3-series eicosanoids, which are derived from n–3 linolenic acid and have opposing actions to the 2-series eicosanoids, include thromboxane A3 and prostaglandin I3 (in platelet membranes, which inhibits platelet aggregation) and leukotriene B5 (in neutrophils, which inhibits inflammation).

Replacing n–6 fatty acid rich vegetable oils (sunflower, safflower, corn) with n–3 fatty acid rich oils (canola, fish) has been one of the approaches attempting to attenuate a number of inflammatory states and immune-mediated diseases, such as autoimmune diseases and multiple sclerosis. Many of the anti-inflammatory and anti-aggregatory (i.e. non-clumping of platelets) properties attributed to n–3 fatty acids are believed to be due to them replacing arachidonic acid (derived from n–6 fatty acids) in membrane phospholipids, which in turn leads to more anti-inflammatory 3-series eicosanoids to be produced. Therefore, the ratio of n–6 to n–3 fatty acids in the diet is important.

The effect of saturated (of different chain lengths) and monounsaturated fats and the total fat content of the diet on immune function is controversial. Low-fat diets have not been shown to be unequivocally advantageous for immune function, and shorter-chain SFAs with less than fourteen carbons may have more favourable effects on immune function than the longer-chain varieties (Yoshida et al. 1999).

Proteins and amino acids

Protein malnutrition leads to sub-optimal tissue repair and decreased resistance to infections and tumours, and can have selective effects on immune function. Emerging evidence on the amino acids arginine and glutamine point to their potential uses in food supplementation to enhance wound healing, increase resistance to tumour formation and infections, and improve immune function in aged and immunocompromised persons.

Glutamine

Glutamine is the most abundant amino acid in the blood and in the body's free amino acid pool. There are large intracellular stores of glutamine in skeletal muscle, and it is also synthesised by the lungs. Lymphocytes and macrophages use the amino acid glutamine as a source of energy. Infection and inflammation release glutamine from skeletal muscles, and there is evidence that it may play a role in regulating leukocyte metabolism. Glutamine is also used for the synthesis of DNA nucleic acids (purine and pyrimidine). Therefore, a deficiency in glutamine stores, which can occur with the loss of muscle mass or through poor food intake, is likely to lead to poor immune responses. Dietary sources of glutamine include meat, eggs, wheat and soy beans.

Arginine

Arginine, a non-essential amino acid important to the urea cycle, assists in the synthesis of other amino acids and of polyamines, urea and nitric oxide. Arginine is important for cell-mediated immunity; exogenous sources are often required during sepsis. A product of arginine metabolism, nitric oxide, induces blood vessel dilation and influences leukocyte-endothelial cell adhesion. Growth hormone receptors are widespread in the immune system and it is suspected that arginine triggers the release of growth hormone, which in turn increases the cytotoxic activities of macrophages, natural killer cells, cytotoxic T cells and neutrophils (Yoshida et al. 1999). Good sources of arginine include nuts and fish.

Nucleic acids

Preformed purines and pyrimidines in the diet appear to enhance a number of cell-mediated immunologic mechanisms. For example, they appear to increase the activity of natural killer cells. Foods containing substantial quantities of purines include anchovies, sardines, shellfish, fish, meat, offal, wine, lentils, dried beans and peas, asparagus, spinach, cauliflower, mushrooms, wheat germ and bran.

Micronutrients and phytonutrients

Table 32.3 summarises the effects of certain vitamins, minerals and phytonutrients on the immune system.

The nexus between malnutrition and the immune system

Any form of malnutrition can impair immune status through the various arms of the immune system—innate and adaptive, cellular and humoral. For example, protein or zinc deficiency could impair the ability of **epithelial tissues** to repair an injury, and may therefore allow invasion by infective organisms. With deficiencies of protein and several water-soluble vitamins, antibody responses are suppressed. In PEM, the reduced production of secretory immunoglobulin A from epithelial or mucosal surfaces presents problems of susceptibility to infection in the ears, eyes and gastrointestinal tract.

Malnutrition, particularly undernutrition, whatever the cause, predisposes the individual to infection and to other health problems where the integrity of the immune system is vital. This means that individuals in the following groups are at risk of immune dysfunction.

* Where there is food shortage and food insecurity, as with poverty and famine (Lukito et al. 1994).
* In those who make poor food choices in the presence of an adequate food supply—this may include people who lack access to suitable transportation and readily available nutritious foods or those with poor budgeting or cooking skills or inadequate storage facilities.
* In those who cannot eat enough or whose nutritional needs are increased.
* In the immunosuppressed, whether:
  – for medical reasons, such as through use of steroids as in rheumatoid arthritis, asthma, or chronic inflammatory bowel disease or with transplant patients
  – through HIV (Human Immunodeficiency Virus) positivity and AIDS (Acquired Immunodeficiency Syndrome)
  – through declining immune function with age, although not all of this decline is inevitable (see Chapter 22) (Lukito et al. 1994).

Table 32.3: List of vitamins, minerals and phytonutrients and their effects on immune function

Nutrient	Effects and possible mechanisms
Vitamin A	• Vitamin A deficiency results in a reduced number of leucocytes, reduced circulating levels of complements and antibodies, impaired T cell functions and decreased resistance to immunogenic tumours.
B vitamins	• Vitamin B-6 (pyridoxine) and biotin deficiencies impair both cell-mediated and humoral immunity. • Vitamin B-12 (cyanocobalamin) and folate deficiency depress phagocytosis and T cell function. • Inadequate intakes of pantothenic acid, thiamin or riboflavin commonly lead to decreased antibody responses.
Vitamin C	• Immunologic problems associated with vitamin C deficiency include decreases in resistance to infections and cancer, skin allograft rejection, decreased wound repair and enhanced antibody responses and phagocyte function. Research does not support the use of mega-doses of vitamin C (>1 g/day) to prevent common colds, but low doses may reduce the incidence and duration of symptoms.

Nutrient	Effects and possible mechanisms
Vitamin D	• Vitamin D both stimulates and inhibits immune responses for several reasons, one being its influence on mineral metabolism. It also functions as a hormone, whose active form 1,25-OH vitamin D, is produced in macrophages. • Vitamin D plays a crucial role in the function of human T lymphocytes, where it and its receptors are necessary for cell multiplication. Receptors for vitamin D can be found on the surface of lymphocytes and phagocytes. It can activate innate responses (phagocytosis) and inhibit an acquired immune response (antibodies). • Vitamin D can stimulate differentiation of monocytes and macrophages and reduce tumour growth. The immunosuppression it promotes may be important in the reported modulation of autoimmune diseases and tumorigenesis.
Vitamin E	• Deficiency of vitamin E leads to depressed leucocyte proliferation, phagocytosis, low antibody levels and decreased tumour resistance, while natural killer cell cytotoxicity is either unchanged or enhanced. Vitamin E supplementation has its greatest effect on cell-mediated immunity by reducing the synthesis of the pro-inflammatory 2-series eicosanoids (prostaglandin E2). • High intakes have been found to increase resistance to infections among the elderly.
Copper	• Copper deficiency is associated with increased susceptibility to infections by decreasing phagocyte functions, decreasing T cell numbers and activities, increasing B cell numbers and lowering interleukin production. • Excess copper intake can decrease immune function because of its involvement in complement function, cell membrane integrity, immunoglobulin structure, copper–zinc dismutase and interactions with iron.
Selenium	• Chronic selenium deficiency decreases resistance to infection by reducing antibody synthesis, cytotoxicity, cytokine secretion and lymphocyte proliferation. • Selenium and vitamin E are essential components of glutathione peroxidase, an antioxidant enzyme that prevents peroxidation of lipids in cell membranes. Lowered antibody production caused by selenium deficiency can be reversed by vitamin E supplementation. Limiting the potential for lipid peroxidation during immune and inflammatory processes is important to prevent autoxidation as well as damage to surrounding tissue.
Iron	• Microbial infection can be associated with increased iron storage. At the same time, infection (and inflammation) can increase blood concentration of the storage iron ferritin, an acute phase reactant, even though plasma iron itself may be low. This response limits iron availability for microbial agents and promotes the antimicrobial and antitumour effects of nitric oxide, a locally produced blood vessel hormone. Chronic inflammation seen in various disease states (for example, arthritis) is also associated with low serum iron concentrations and increased iron stores, known as 'anaemia of chronic disease'. • Iron deficiency appears to both stimulate and inhibit most parameters of immune function. This may be related to its involvement in folate metabolism, mitochondrial energy production and metallo-enzymes, such as nitric oxide synthase, catalase. Excessive iron intake and storage may increase susceptibility to some infections. Thus, optimal iron nutrition needs to be addressed in relation to the body's overall defence systems.
Zinc	• The immunologic consequences of zinc deficiency are T cell defects, including reductions in T cell numbers and responsiveness and T cell help towards antibody production. Zinc deficiency in older people is likely to be an important contributor to proneness to infection, in particular respiratory infection, especially pneumonia.
Phytonutrients	• β-carotene directly protects cells from oxidation and promotes lymphocyte proliferation, T cell functions, cytokine production and cell-mediated toxicity—for example, natural killer cell cytotoxicity. However, carotenoids can exhibit pro-oxidant as well as antioxidant activity, and their record in attenuating chronic disease is not consistent, especially when taken as a supplement. • Polyphenolic compounds in plants are more potent antioxidants than vitamins A, C and E. Antioxidants assist in preventing the oxidation of fatty acids in cell membranes, especially of the different lymphocyte subsets. In this respect, they assist in the regulation of the immune system, especially cell-mediated immunity, because reactive oxygen can stimulate inflammation via T cells as seen in rheumatic diseases and autoimmune disorders such as allergies.

A vicious cycle between malnutrition and infection is shown in Figure 32.4. While it is possible for this cycle to be interrupted at any point, the most threatening health problems in this cycle are the advent of anorexia (lack of appetite and inability to eat) and diarrhoea, which may limit the ability to provide nutritional support to the immunocompromised. Failure to recognise or anticipate the development of hospital malnutrition can allow the needless presence of nutritionally related immunodeficiency and proneness to infection, with increased hospital morbidity and mortality.

Disordered energy regulation with overfatness as well as wasting is also associated with immune dysfunction and inflammatory disorders. In the presence of obesity, lean mass can be reduced, a condition known as sarcopenic obesity (see Chapter 22). The metabolic, immune system and inflammatory disorders in this situation are associated with premature mortality.

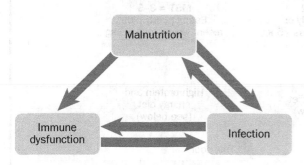

Figure 32.4: The malnutrition and infection cycle

Personal behaviours and immune responses
Sleep and immunity

There is strong evidence that sleep enhances immune defence, in agreement with the old wisdom that 'sleep helps healing'. Sleep can affect a wide variety of immune functions, including the numbers of specific leukocyte subsets in circulating blood, the cell-specific production of cytokines and further immune cell functions. Its effect is, however, selective, influencing some components of the immune system but not others. Sleep appears to preferentially promote the pro-inflammatory cytokine production, which is important for the mounting of adaptive immune responses, and this action might primarily affect less differentiated immune cells (Tobaldini et al. 2018). This supportive role of sleep in the initiation of an adaptive immune response can eventually lead to the long-term maintenance of the antigenic memory, a function hallmarking the immune system.

Physical activity and immunity

It is evident that regular practice of exercise has health benefits; however, from the immunological point of view, the duration and intensity of the activity performed should be considered for exercise programs to obtain the best results. Physical activity of moderate intensity stimulates a protective response against infections caused by intracellular micro-organisms. Conversely, high-intensity activities tend to promote anti-inflammatory responses, presumably to decrease damage in muscular tissue resulting from

---

HOSPITAL MALNUTRITION

In Australia, malnutrition in hospitals is at around 30 per cent. Malnutrition increases with length of stay, age and certain diagnoses (for example, chronic obstructive pulmonary disease and cancer). As a result, hospitals now routinely screen for malnutrition on admission (Agarwal et al. 2012).

There are a number of screening tools that are used, including the Nutrition Risk Screening 2002, the Malnutrition Universal Screening Tool and the Malnutrition Screening Tool (MST). The MST was developed and validated by Australian dietitians (Ferguson et al. 1999). The tool and the algorithm for action are shown in Figure 32.5.

Malnutrition Screening Tool (MST)

1. Have you/the patient lost weight recently without trying?		*Applies to the last six months*
No	0	
Unsure	2	*If unsure, ask if they suspect they have lost weight,*
Yes, how much (kg)?		*e.g. clothes are looser*
1–5	1	
6–10	2	
11–15	3	
>15	4	
Don't know	2	
2. Have you/the patient been eating poorly because of a decreased appetite?		*For example, less than three-quarters of usual intake; may also be eating poorly due to chewing and swallowing problems*
No	0	
Yes	1	
TOTAL SCORE		*Of weight loss and appetite questions*

Source: Based on Ferguson et al. (1999)

Malnutrition Action Flowchart

What is your patient's malnutrition risk?
Malnutrition Screening Tool Score:

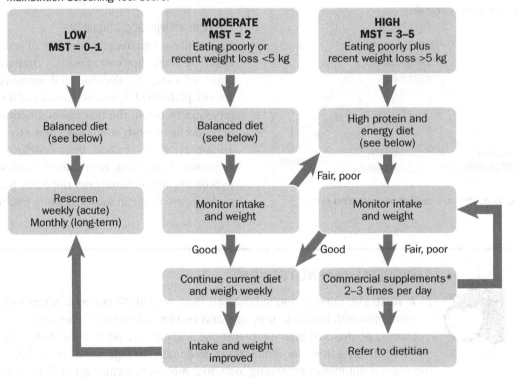

Note: * Commercial supplements with additional vitamins and minerals are recommended if poor variety/volume of foods/fluids is being consumed.

Figure 32.5: Algorithm for action on malnutrition screening in hospitals

Source: M. Banks © 2018, <www.health.qld.gov.au/__data/assets/pdf_file/0015/143502/hphe_maf.pdf>. Reproduced with permission

inflammation, and this may result in an increase of susceptibility to infections (Terra et al. 2012).

NEOPLASTIC DISEASE

Cell division, or cell multiplication, is a normal event that allows the development or regeneration of tissue. Cancer or neoplastic disease could occur when the factors controlling the cell division or its expected death (apoptosis) are no longer operative, leading to a variety of uncontrolled tissue proliferation or overgrowth of defective cells (called aberrant cells). It is normal for defective cells to be produced occasionally; this might be because of an occurrence of genetic mutation which can result from exposure to certain chemicals, radiation or viruses. In the normal situation, the body's defence system may get rid of aberrant cells if there are not too many.

The process by which normal cells transform into aberrant cells and progress to a neoplastic disease or cancer (called oncogenesis) is the result of complex interactions involving diet, nutrition, physical activity and other personal behaviour, environmental and host factors (Figure 32.6). The interaction between the host metabolic state and dietary, nutritional, physical activity and other environmental exposures over the whole life-course is critical to protection from, or susceptibility to, cancer development. Theoretically, nutritional factors could influence the development of neoplastic disease by affecting mutation, through the defence system or by regulation of cell death.

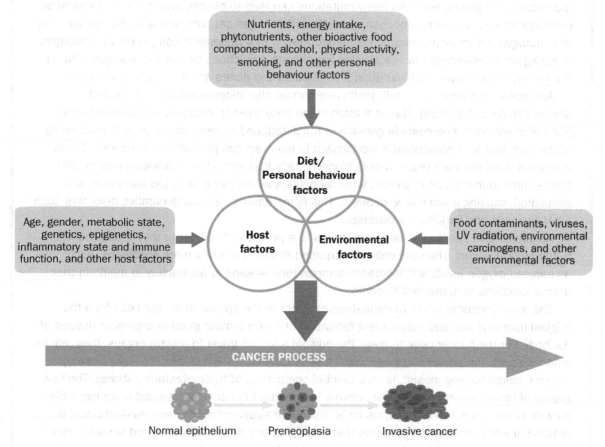

Figure 32.6: Interactions between diet/personal behaviour, environmental and host factors can affect the cancer process
Source: Modified from WCRF & AICR (2018)

CONVERSATIONS ABOUT CANCER: UNDERSTANDING TERMINOLOGY

'Cancer' is the term used to refer to a variety of uncontrolled tissue proliferations. 'Oncology' is the name given to the branch of medicine that deals with the diagnosis and treatment of cancers. The term 'malignant tumour' is also used to describe the cancerous mass due to its propensity to grow uncontrollably, to metastasise (or spread) to surrounding tissues, and possibly spread to distant tissues. In contrast, these properties are not found in a 'benign tumour'.

'Neoplasia' and 'neoplastic disease' are less emotive terms than 'cancer' to describe disorders of tissue proliferation.

A carcinogen is a biological, chemical or physical agent or process that promotes the formation of cancer (called carcinogenesis) by altering cellular metabolism or damaging DNA directly in cells, which interferes with normal biological processes.

A mutagen is a biological, chemical or physical agent or process that causes the permanent alteration of genetic elements (called mutation), and increases the frequency of mutations from the natural background level. As many mutations can lead to cancer, mutagens are likely to be carcinogens, but not always necessarily so. An antimutagen can interfere with the mutagenicity of a mutagen, either by preventing the transformation of a mutagenic compound into mutagen, or acting as a desmutagen by inactivating the chemical reactions before the mutagen attacks the genes, or by stopping the mutation process after the genes are damaged by mutagens.

Apoptosis, or programmed cell death, is a normal physiological process of cell self-destruction (or cell suicide). This is a method the body uses to eliminate old, unnecessary and abnormal cells. Apoptosis is genetically regulated, and is required for smooth functioning of the body and as a homeostatic mechanism to maintain cell populations in tissues. When apoptosis does not work properly or is blocked, cells that should be eliminated may persist and become immortal, as in cancer. When apoptosis works overly well, too many cells are eliminated, causing grave tissue damage. This is the case in neurodegenerative disorders such as Alzheimer's and Parkinson's diseases.

As opposed to apoptosis, 'necrosis' refers to a process of cell death that is detrimental to the body. It occurs when the cells are exposed to toxins or to extreme conditions, such as reduced oxygen levels and increased temperature, leading to an inability to maintain their normal functions and, eventually, death.

The term 'metastasis' (or to metastasise) refers to the spread of cancer cells from the original (primary) site and subsequent formation of a new tumour in other organs or tissues of the body. For the cancer cells to leave the original site and travel to distant organs, they require blood vessels. The process through which new blood vessels are formed from pre-existing vessels, called 'angiogenesis', is an essential component of the metastatic pathway. The new growth of blood vessels or vascular network is important because the spread of cancer cells, as well as the proliferation, depends on an adequate supply of oxygen and nutrients, and the removal of waste products. It appears that the higher the density of new blood vessels within a tumour, the higher is the risk of metastasis of that tumour.

Carcinogenesis and the influence of nutrition

Carcinogenesis refers to the biological processes that underpin the development and progression of cancer. What we eat can play a role in various steps of carcinogenesis (Figure 32.7). Food may contain mutagens, like aflatoxins produced by moulds, or nitrosamines produced from food nitrites, or nitrates present naturally and added to food, and so initiate cancer. It is estimated that dietary factors account for about 30 per cent of cancers in industrialised countries, making diet second only to tobacco smoking as a preventable cause of cancer (WHO 2003). Food and beverages may promote cancer or inhibit cancer or slow down growth or metastases. Certain food components, such as genistein from soy products, have anti-angiogenic properties, which reduce the formation of new blood vessels, a process known as angiogenesis that is required for tumour growth. Apoptosis, another mechanism for inhibiting tumour growth, may also be achieved by quercetin,

a polypholic compound present in onion, apple and berries.

There are a number of antimutagens in foods. Some bioactive compounds, such as vanillin from the vanilla plant and cinnamaldehyde from cinnamon, may be bio-antimutagens, which reduce DNA damage caused by mutagens, and some, such as the peptide glutathione and vitamin E, are desmutagens, which inactivate mutagens.

Nutritional risk factors for certain cancers

The mechanisms by which food and food components influence the development of cancer are still not understood in detail. However, it is becoming clear that a number of factors in food, not only those described as nutrients, are important. For example, all those factors that alter immune status may, in turn, affect the risk of cancer. The immunodeficiency associated with ageing, with HIV positivity and with transplantation of organs where immunosuppression is required increases the risk of cancer.

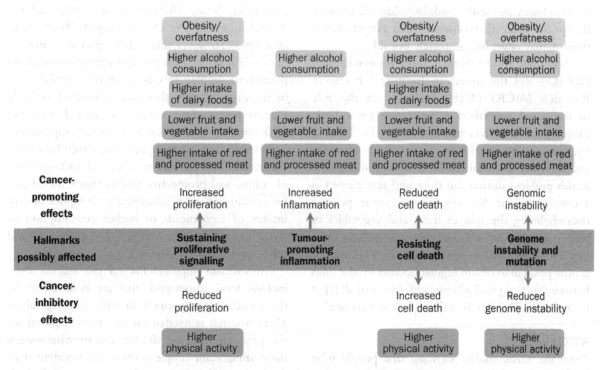

Figure 32.7: Potential impact of diet, nutrition and physical activity in altering susceptibility to cancer

Source: Developed from WCRF & AICR (2018)

The case for nutritional risk factors for cancer is derived from several lines of evidence. These could be experimental in animals; observational in humans at one point in time or over extended periods of time; or intervention. No one research type provides enough conclusive results, even with intervention studies where situational or food cultural relevance needs to be taken into account. But as the evidence increases, so dietary change can be made with more confidence. Any changes also ought to favourably affect total health, morbidity and mortality, and not just be related to cancer.

Fruits and vegetables

Higher consumption of fruits and especially vegetables is related to a reduced risk of cancers at many sites. For prostate cancer, a lower risk has been observed with the higher intake of tomato products, the primary source of the non-provitamin A carotenoid lycopene. The constituents in fruit and vegetables responsible for the reduced cancer risks are not known, although the myriad phytonutrients in these foods are clearly candidates. Identification of the specific protective constituents, or a combination thereof, may never be completely possible.

According to the World Cancer Research Fund (WCRF) and the American Institute for Cancer Research (AICR) (2018), evidence on the role of fruits and vegetables as protective for colonic cancer is not convincing. This may be because energy imbalance reflected in physical inactivity and increased body fatness became a greater public health problem during this time, and was viewed as a convincing risk for large bowel cancer, perhaps overwhelming the role of fruits and vegetables in protection. But there remain protective roles for these foods in other cancers as well as in other diseases. It is now possible to obtain regular updates on the links between diet, physical activity and cancer of all types from the WCRF/AICR website (www.wcrf.org/).

Antioxidants

From the many studies showing that people who have more fruit and vegetables in their diet are less likely to get cancer, researchers have queried whether an above-average intake of vitamins in supplement form could confer similar protection. Experimental research has also shown that very high levels of antioxidants can provide a degree of protection against free radical damage that leads to cancer. Antioxidant vitamins including vitamins A, C, E and β-carotene were considered the obvious choices to simulate the properties of fruit and vegetables, even though it could well have been other nutrients or phytonutrients in plant food. The shortcomings of these results are that people were fed only one or two antioxidants in an attempt to get that effect. Not enough is known about the full composition of the antioxidant defence system to state that significant protection is provided by one or two antioxidants.

In the 1980s–1990s, a number of randomised intervention trials were conducted in an attempt to assess the efficacy of these antioxidant vitamins, particularly β-carotene, as preventive agents for cancer. Examples of these trials include the Beta-Carotene and Retinol Efficacy Trial (Omenn et al. 1996), the Alpha-Tocopherol Beta-Carotene Cancer Prevention Study (Albanes et al. 1995) and the Australian Polyp Prevention Project (MacLennan et al. 1995). However, these trials reported an increase in cancer at several sites among participants receiving β-carotene supplements. Some of these trials had to be terminated before they were scheduled to finish. Due to these findings, caution is required in the use of β-carotene in isolation as a nutrient supplement or food ingredient. More promising results have been reported from systemic reviews and meta-analyses of cohort and prospective studies that reduced risk for certain cancers is associated with higher dietary intakes of carotenoids or higher consumption of fruits and vegetables containing carotenoids and other oxidants (see Chapter 18).

Antioxidant supplements on the market even include food compounds that are believed to be the bioactive components in fruit and vegetables. More research is needed on the doses required for the protection against disease, and to what extent these antioxidant supplements could interfere with the body's self-defence mechanisms, some of which require oxidation processes. Since we do not know exactly what in plant foods confers protection against cancer, it is safer to consume large amounts and a wide variety of plant foods instead of currently available antioxidant supplements (see Chapter 18).

Dietary fibre and refined carbohydrates

Cereal fibre has been shown in several studies to protect against colon cancer. In the Australian Polyp Prevention Project, a combination of low-fat and wheat bran-supplemented diets (providing 11.5 g fibre/ day) was associated with fewer new large adenomas over the four years of study (MacLennan et al. 1995). A study from the Arizona Cancer Center involving 1429 men and women aged 40–80 years who had recently had an **adenoma** removed from the bowel was unable to show that taking a fibre supplement (13.5 g fibre/day) would prevent the recurrence of adenomas. In fact, multiple adenomas were more common in the high-fibre group (Alberts et al. 2000). The different results obtained in these two studies may be explained by the types of fibre supplements used. In the Australian study, an unrefined wheat bran was used as a dietary fibre source; this was probably also higher in protective phytoestrogens, vitamin E, B-6 and folate. The American study used a more processed/refined fibre supplement. Furthermore, fibre intake does not appear to account for the reduced risk of colon cancer through consumption of fruits and vegetables, and evidence supporting higher consumption of cereal fibre alone to reduce risk of colon cancer is not strong.

A meta-analysis of evidence indicates that eating too many refined cereal products can increase the risk of cancer and in particular stomach cancer (Xu et al. 2018). The Seven Countries Study has followed the eating patterns of over 12,000 men for almost 30 years (Jansen et al. 1999). This study has shown a decreased risk of stomach cancer with a high fruit and vegetable intake. High grain intakes were associated with low intakes of fruit and vegetables—so people with a high intake of grains may have other dietary characteristics that increase their risk.

Bioactive food components

The protective effect of traditional soy-based foods, like tofu (bean curd), has raised the possibility that the weakly oestrogenic factors they contain, like genistein, may be responsible for this protection. Such compounds may compete with the body's own oestrogens (endogenous oestrogen) and reduce possible adverse effects, but may also work in other ways since they may be antioxidant, immuno-modulatory or anti-angiogenic.

Salicylates, related to acetyl salicylic acid (aspirin) may be protective against certain gastrointestinal tract cancers and in particular large bowel cancer (Elwood et al. 2009), possibly through effects on cell membranes. Salicylate-rich foods include grapes, dates, cherries, and herbs such as thyme, oregano, cinnamon and mints. Some people are sensitive to salicylates and therefore may need to be moderate in their intake of these foods. They are likely to be able to achieve a higher intake from foods taken in several small amounts on different occasions rather than as medication.

Experimental studies provide strong evidence for cancer prevention (especially skin cancer) by black and green tea and its constituent polyphenols, but evidence from epidemiologic and clinical studies on humans is inconclusive. However, consumption of very hot tea may be a risk for oesophageal cancer.

Fat quality and meat

A strong correlation between fat consumption and rates of cancers of the breast, colon, prostate and endometrium has been observed in the comparisons among countries. However, these correlations are limited to animal, not vegetable, fat (Willett 2000). For colon cancer, the apparently stronger association with red meat than with fat in several cohort studies needs further confirmation. Evidence suggests that this might be explained by factors in red meat other than simply its fat content (e.g. haem iron, carcinogens generated during cooking). This issue has major practical implications, as many food guides around the world support daily consumption of red meat as long as it is lean.

Energy balance, growth rate and body size

The role of energy intake in carcinogenesis is complex. There has been a popularised view, derived mainly from animal studies, which has argued that energy restriction may decrease cancer risk and increase longevity. Most of these studies are flawed insofar as extrapolation to humans is concerned, either because they are conducted from early life with excessive early mortality, or because they do not account for energy expenditure, and therefore energy balance, reflected in body fatness and/or its distribution. Where the full energy equation is available, increased energy throughput (for example, higher energy intakes with no increase in body fatness) has been associated with decreased cancer risk and/or increased life expectancy. Increased energy intake (and possibly its frequency) is, in its own right, associated with increased cancer risk at several sites. Again, the quality of extra food intake seems important. The Zutphen prospective study in the Netherlands reported that increased energy intake, which included relatively more plant-derived food and fish, was associated with lower cancer and total mortality over ten years (Kromhout et al. 1982).

Positive energy balance can contribute to higher growth rates in children, resulting in taller and fatter body size. Several studies have shown that greater height is associated with increased risk of breast, colon and other cancers. Rapid growth rates prior to puberty play an important role in determining future risk of breast and probably other cancers. Early menarche is a well-established risk factor for breast cancer. Positive energy balance and overfatness in adult life contribute to cancers of the endometrium, gall bladder and colon. A review in 2018 identified that adult obesity is causally related to cancer risk at various anatomic sites including oesophagus, colon and rectum, liver, pancreas, kidney, breast (in postmenopausal women), ovary and thyroid gland (Colditz & Peterson 2018). For breast cancer, there is a reduced risk with greater adiposity prior to menopause; the reverse is true after menopause. The various ways in which overfatness might increase cancer risk are shown in Figure 32.8 (see colour section).

Food preservation and cooking

Intake of meat and fish may increase certain cancers because of the way they are preserved or cooked (for example, curing, smoking, salting, charring during grilling or barbecuing). Several carcinogenic N-nitroso compounds (nitrosamines or nitrosamides) are formed in the meat during the curing process, in the reaction between nitrite used in the preserving process and the degradation products of amino acids.

Other carcinogenic substances, including heterocyclic amines and polycyclic aromatic hydrocarbons (PAHs), can be produced if meat is cooked over an open flame, at high temperatures, and charred or 'well done'. Cooking muscle meats such as beef, pork, poultry and fish at high temperatures can generate heterocyclic amines, which are formed in the reaction of amino acids and creatine (a chemical found in muscles). PAHs are a group of over 100 different chemicals formed when organic substances like meat are burnt incompletely. Grilling and barbecuing meat, fish or other foods with intense heat over a direct flame results in fat dropping on the hot fire; this produces PAHs that stick to the surface of food. Home smoking of foods also results in addition of PAHs to the food. Occasional consumption of home-smoked foods does not appear to be associated with any known harmful effects, however, and commercially produced smoked foods from big companies probably do not contain enough harmful chemicals to worry about.

Vitamin C can prevent the conversion of dietary nitrite and nitrate (in cured meats) to the carcinogenic nitrosamines in the stomach; the nitrosamine pathway for human cancer remains unproven. Protective effects of fruit and vegetables against cancer could be partly due to their vitamin C content, but research has shown that allium foods (onions and garlic) are also protective. It seems that the active compound could be diallyl sulphide, which has been shown to increase the activity of glutathione S-transferase, an enzyme that is involved in the detoxification of carcinogens.

Prebiotics and probiotics

The consumption of milk has been shown to reduce the incidence of human stomach cancers induced by alkylating agents, while human subjects and experimental animals receiving dietary supplements of *Lactobacillus acidophilus* (found in yoghurt) had significantly lower levels of faecal enzymes that are associated with colon carcinogenesis. It is proposed that in the intestine probiotic bacteria, mainly lacto-bacilli and bifidobacteria, may bind, block or remove carcinogens; inhibit bacteria which directly or indirectly convert procarcinogens to carcinogens by enzyme activity; activate the host's immune system to act against tumours; reduce the intestinal pH, thereby altering microbial activity, solubility of bile acids and mucus secretion; and alter colonic motility and transit time.

Recommendations for cancer prevention

The Third Expert Report of the WCRF/AICR included eight general recommendations and two special recommendations for cancer prevention (WCRF & AICR 2018). These are outlined in Table 32.4. These recommendations are designed to be used as the basis of action and to inform policy, not only to reduce the incidence of cancer in general, but also, to some extent, to prevent other non-communicable diseases. They represent an integrated pattern of behaviours that can be considered as an overall 'package' and they are culturally relevant throughout the world.

Table 32.4: WCRF/AICR cancer prevention recommendations

Aspects—Recommendations	Description
Body weight—Be a healthy weight	Keep body weight within the healthy range and avoid weight gain (measured as body weight or waist circumference) in adult life. The healthy range of BMI for adults is 18.5–24.9 kg/m². The healthy range for BMI during childhood varies with age. Follow the WHO recommendations for waist circumferences.
Physical activity—Be physically active	Be at least moderately physically active as part of everyday life—walk more and sit less. Moderate physical activity increases heart rate to 60–75% of its maximum.
Plant foods—Eat a diet rich in whole grains, vegetables, fruit and beans	Make whole grains, vegetables, fruit, and pulses (legumes) such as beans and lentils a major part of your usual daily diet.
Foods and drinks that promote weight gain—Limit consumption of 'fast foods' and other processed foods high in fat, starches or sugars	'Fast foods' are readily available convenience foods that tend to be energy-dense and are often consumed frequently and in large portions. Limiting these foods helps control energy intake and maintain a healthy body weight.
Animal foods—Limit consumption of red and processed meat	Limit consumption to no more than about three portions (350–500 grams)/week of cooked weight of red meat such as beef, pork and lamb. Eat little, if any, processed meat.
Sugar-sweetened drinks—Limit consumption of sugar-sweetened drinks	Drink mostly water and unsweetened drinks.
Alcoholic drinks—Limit alcohol consumption	For cancer prevention, it is best not to drink alcohol.
Dietary supplements—Do not use supplements for cancer prevention	Aim to meet nutritional needs through diet alone.
Breastfeeding (special recommendation)—For mothers: breastfeed the baby if possible	Breastfeeding is good for both mother and baby. WHO recommends infants are exclusively breastfed for six months, and then up to two years of age or beyond alongside appropriate complementary foods.
Cancer survivors (special recommendation)—After a cancer diagnosis: follow the recommendations if possible	Cancer survivors are people who have been diagnosed with cancer, including those who have recovered from the disease. All cancer survivors should receive nutritional care and guidance on physical activity from trained professionals.

Source: Adapted from WCRF & AICR (2018)

Nutritional management of patients with cancer

The management of patients with cancer is a different proposition to the prevention of cancer. The neoplasms themselves, as well as the treatments (radiation and chemotherapy), can result in significant side effects that can limit food intake. These include but are not limited to wasting (known as cachexia), nausea, vomiting, dry mouth, sticky mouth, sore mouth and tongue, bowel obstruction, diarrhoea or constipation, and inability to swallow. As a result, foods of increased energy density and potentially altered texture need to be provided. This may even require an increased intake of certain fats. Other foods may be needed to reduce the problems of nausea—a reason for using ginger-based food or beverages since ginger is known to possess these properties. Finding palatable foods can be a major challenge. Many people with cancer are highly vulnerable to practising non-evidence-based food and dietary practices. In some cases there is no harm in undertaking these practices; in others these can delay medical treatment or be generally detrimental to health.

There is uncertainty about what provision of energy or nutrient surplus might do for certain tumours. There are ongoing trials to review the impact of periodic fasting (with and without energy restriction) on increasing the efficacy of chemotherapy but these need to be viewed with some caution (Brandhorst & Longo 2016). There is also the possibility that growth factors and growth inhibitors in food may play a role in tumour modulation. Sometimes the major value of nutrition support is to allow the successful use of other therapies, such as chemotherapy or radiotherapy. In some cases, food and nutrition support is **palliative**.

Harmonisation with other health recommendations

The WCRF/AICR report took into account an evidence-based review of many other dietary recommendations, including those to do with disadvantaged undernourished populations, breast-feeding guidelines, international, regional and national FBDGs (food-based dietary guidelines and those to do with particular health outcomes like

CURES FOR CANCER

A number of cures for cancer have been proposed over the years that have a dietary basis. Using your skills in searching the peer-reviewed literature, find the evidence to support or refute three of the following cancer cures. Write a one-page summary or develop an infographic that could be used on a website to inform the public about the use of three of these items as a cancer cure:

- apricot kernels
- pureed asparagus
- carrot juice
- Gerson therapy (injections of liver extracts)
- coffee enemas or other gastrointestinal cleansing methods
- turmeric
- grape seed extract
- energy restriction (fasting).

A good place to start for some background information would be:

- the Cancer Council iheard website (https://iheard.com.au, Cancer Council 2018)
- the Practice-based Evidence in Nutrition (PEN) database. (Check to see if your university library has access to this database. This database also provides evidence summaries for medical nutrition therapy for various treatments of cancer and its treatment side effects.)

obesity, diabetes, heart disease, and dental health). It devoted a major part of the review to evidence for the prevention of overfatness and obesity, total and abdominal, when it was recognised how important a risk for cancer it had rapidly become.

To improve the prospects for impact, the WCRF/AICR in 2018 identified at least eight groups of actors, including policy-makers and decision-takers at all levels, from global and national to local. The common feature of successful policy is concerted action led by governments with the support of actors across all sectors in society, all working in the public interest (Figure 32.9).

All actor groups have an opportunity, and in many cases a responsibility, to make decisions with a view to their impact on public health. The impact of policies and actions depends on successful, mutually reinforcing interactions among all actor groups. However, the development, adoption and implementation of policies to promote health are often strongly opposed by industry or other actors, such as government agencies concerned with trade. Ultimately the highest level of government must play a role in mandating and supporting a joint and coordinated action for a successful impact on public health (WCRF & AICR 2018).

PATHOLOGIES WITH ALTERED GUT MICROBIOTA

A symbiotic relationship between gut microbiota (GM) and the host (human body) has been recognised for decades. Through its metabolites and enzymatic arsenal, the microbiota influences host metabolism, extracts energy from the diet and contributes to the normal development of the immune system and to tissue inflammation (see Chapter 30). There is growing evidence that the disruption of the homeostasis between the host (human body) and the GM, the state called dysbiosis, is associated with the pathogenesis of disorders and diseases ranging from obesity, diabetes, heart disease, inflammatory bowel disease, rheumatoid arthritis and asthma through to cancer (Claesson et al. 2012; Keeney et al. 2014). GM interacts with the host immunity at multiple levels, and, because of the complexity and reciprocity of the interactions, it is debated whether dysbiosis could be the cause or the result of the pathology (Buttó & Haller 2016). Furthermore, research suggests that disruption of GM may trigger epigenetic deregulation of transcription, which can be observed in chronic metabolic diseases (Devaux & Raoult 2018).

Alterations of the composition of the GM may occur upon exposure to antibiotics, drugs or radiation, infections, and nutritional changes. Asthma and inflammatory bowel diseases have both been found to be directly affected by the interactions between the GM and host immunity (Carding et al. 2015; Selber-Hnatiw et al. 2017). In addition

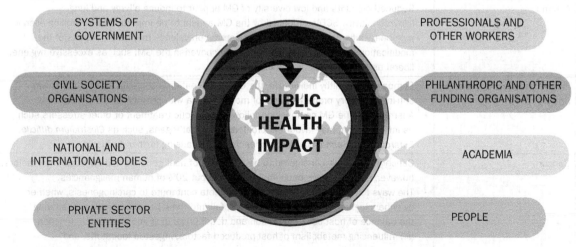

Figure 32.9: Concerted action for public health impact

Source: WCRF & AICR (2018)

to alterations in microbiota composition, metabolic products of microbiota can contribute to the development of disorders or diseases (see Table 32.5). As in the case of colorectal cancer, the products of interaction between diet and the microbiome, rather than dysbiosis, may be the most important factor. High–protein diets are believed to result in the production of carcinogenic metabolites from GM that may result in the induction of neoplasia in the colonic epithelium.

Table 32.5: Example of disorders and diseases associated with gut microbiota dysbiosis

Disorder/Disease	Features
Cardiovascular disease	• Certain bacterial metabolites, such as trimethylamine-N-oxide (TMAO) which is synthesised from choline/carnitine, are potentially associated with CVD risk by accelerating atherosclerosis.
Obesity	• SCFAs produced by GM from the anaerobic fermentation process of undigested dietary carbohydrates contribute to energy. SCFAs produced by the GM may also cause satiety, resulting in reduced food intake, through the secretion and gene expression of satiety or anorexigenic hormones. • Within the GM, Bacteroidetes and Firmicutes in particular, may modulate the expression of taste receptors, affect the gut–brain vagal communication, and influence the release of toxins and neurotransmitters. GM actively participates in bile acid activation, metabolism and regulation, and thus, to some extent, provides help in lipid absorption.
Diabetes	• Disruption of the maternal GM during gestation or that of the offspring during early infant development, may promote a pro-inflammatory environment leading to the development of autoimmunity and metabolic disturbance, which could contribute to the development of type 1 diabetes. • In animal models, changes to the GM can improve glycaemic control by altering the expression of hepatic and intestinal genes involved in inflammation and metabolism, and by changing the hormonal, inflammatory and metabolic status of the host.
Asthma	• Reduced amounts and low diversity of GM appear to induce allergy and lung hypersensitivity. SCFAs produced by the GM appear to be important in controlling allergic pulmonary inflammation. Increases in asthma prevalence may be the results of the modifications of personal behaviours that impoverish the GM, such as excessive hygiene, liberal use of antibiotics and a high-fat diet.
Inflammatory bowel disease (IBD)	• Compared to healthy individuals, the GM of IBD patients contains fewer bacteria with anti-inflammatory properties and/or more bacteria with pro-inflammatory properties. • Aberration of the GM composition following antibiotic treatment or other stressors such as inflammation, may favour the proliferation of pathogens, such as *Clostridium difficile*, *Enterococcus*, *Salmonella* and *Escherichia* spp., causing further dysbiosis.
Cancer	• Cancer is generally considered to be a disease of host genetics and environmental factors; however, microbes have been implicated in about 20% of human malignancies. • The ways in which microbes and the microbiota contribute to carcinogenesis, whether by enhancing or diminishing a host's risk, fall into three broad categories: (i) altering the balance of host cell proliferation and death (ii) guiding immune system function (iii) influencing metabolism of host-produced factors, ingested foodstuffs, and pharmaceuticals.

Sources: Byrne et al. (2015); Chu et al. (2016); McNeil (1984); Membrez et al. (2008); Paun & Danska (2016); Selber-Hnatiw et al. (2017)

SUMMARY

- Food (including food systems), nutrition and personal behaviours can influence normal functions of many systems in the human body.
- Diabetes is increasingly common globally, particularly with economic transition. Type 2 diabetes is associated with increased body fatness, sedentariness, emotional stress and environmental contamination with endocrine disruptors. To prevent type 2 diabetes and treat all forms of diabetes, food biodiversity and low glycaemic foods that are generally minimally processed and include seeds like grains, nuts and legumes, are preferred.
- Hypothyroidism can also be caused by nutritional deficiencies. However, it can be exacerbated by coexisting iron, selenium, zinc, vitamin A and vitamin D deficiency (often caused by the hypothyroidism, and which in turn affect iodine uptake). A less common cause is eating goitrogens that affect thyroid function.
- Both primary and secondary malnutrition can impair immune status and predispose the individual to infections and other health problems, including diseases of affluence or age like heart disease and cancer. Immune dysfunction can occur in the presence of an adequate or excessive energy intake where there are also subclinical micronutrient deficiencies.
- Immune dysfunction is more common in certain 'at-risk' groups—for example, where there are food shortages and food insecurity; where poor food choices are made (often in the presence of an adequate food supply); where there is loss of appetite or increased nutritional needs; or in the immunosuppressed.
- The evidence that nutrition plays a role in the development of many cancers is strong. The mechanisms are increasingly understood, and involve cancer events of protection or inhibition and of progression and growth control.
- Adequate intakes of plant foods, especially pulses (legumes), fruit and vegetables, play an important role in cancer prevention at various sites. On the other hand, food factors like processed meats, quality of dietary fat, food preservation with salt, and cooking techniques by way of barbecuing and grilling can increase cancer risk.
- There is convincing evidence that physical activity throughout life, a diet oriented towards a variety of plant foods, and the avoidance of high intakes of animal fats, salt, sugary drinks, alcohol and processed or overcooked meat will reduce cancer risk.
- There is increasing evidence that a wide range of contemporary health problems can be better understood by taking human microbiomes into account. This justifies a more ecological approach to nutritional disorders than previously acknowledged.

KEY TERMS

Abdominal visceral adiposity: body fat that is stored in the abdominal cavity and wrapped around major organs, including the liver, pancreas and kidneys. Abnormally high deposition of visceral fat, known as visceral or central obesity or abdominal overfatness is associated with increased risks of CVD, diabetes and several malignancies including prostate, breast and colorectal cancers.

Adenoma: a benign tumour of epithelial tissue in a glandular organ ('adeno' in Greek means 'gland') such as thyroid, prostate and adrenal glands, or of epithelial tissue in non-glandular areas but expressing glandular characteristics. If adenomas become malignant, they are called adenocarcinomas.

Affective disorders: also referred to as mood disorders—psychiatric syndromes characterised by significant disturbances in mood. Two separate categories of affective disorders are recognised: (i) major depressive or unipolar disorder for patients who have experienced the feelings of sadness or hopelessness, and (ii) bipolar disorder for those who have experienced both depressive episodes and periods of mania.

Antigens: chemicals, toxins and microorganisms that are foreign to the body and induce an immune response, especially the production of antibodies, which are proteins made by white blood cells to destroy or neutralise specific antigens.

Cell-mediated (or cellular) immune response: characterised by the activation of phagocytes, antigen-specific cytotoxic T-cells, and the release of various cytokines in response to antigens. It is responsible for detecting and destroying intracellular pathogens, e.g. cells infected with bacteria or viruses, and it does not involve antibodies.

Epithelial tissues: the thin layer of tissues that cover the outer surfaces of organs and blood vessels, and the inner surfaces of cavities in many internal organs.

Glucose challenge: a test used to determine whether the body has difficulty metabolising sugar or carbohydrate. In the most commonly performed version of the test, an oral glucose tolerance test, a standard dose of glucose is orally taken and blood glucose is measured two hours later.

HbA1c: refers to glycated haemoglobin, which develops when haemoglobin combines with glucose in the blood. Measurement of HbA1c can be used to reflect average blood glucose over the preceding period of 10–12 weeks, and is therefore a useful gauge of blood glucose control.

Humoral immune response: mediated by antibodies that are produced by plasma B cells against specific antigens or pathogens that are circulating in the lymph or blood or outside the infected cells. The antibodies will bind to the antigens, neutralising them or causing dissolution or destruction of cells, or phagocytosis. Its aspects involving antibodies are often called antibody-mediated immunity.

Microangiopathy: a disease of the small blood vessels (capillaries) where the walls become thick and weak and they leak protein, slowing the flow of blood.

Neurodegeneration: refers to the progressive loss of structure or function of nerve cells in the brain. Neurodegenerative diseases are incurable and can cause problems with muscle movements or mental functioning. Examples of neurodegenerative diseases include Alzheimer's disease and Parkinson's disease.

Palliative: means managing symptoms to improve quality of life, rather than providing a cure. It is often used to describe the situation at end of life.

Parkinson's disease: a neurodegenerative disorder resulting from damage to the nerve cells in a specific area of the brain that produces dopamine, which is a chemical vital for the smooth control of muscles and movement. The cause of Parkinson's remains largely unknown; the disease itself is not fatal, but its complications can be serious.

Pathogen: a microorganism, such as bacteria, fungi and viruses, that can cause infection or disease.

ACKNOWLEDGEMENT

This chapter has been modified and updated from those written by Antigone Kouris-Blazos, Gayle S. Savige and Mark L. Wahlqvist, which appeared in the third edition of *Food and Nutrition*.

REFERENCES

Agarwal, E., Ferguson, M., Banks, M., Bauer, J., Capra, S. & Isenring, E., 2012, 'Nutritional status and dietary intake of acute care patients: Results from the Nutrition Care Day Survey 2010', *Clinical Nutrition, 31*(1): 41–7, doi:10.1016/j.clnu.2011.08.002

Ahlqvist, E., Storm, P., Käräjämäki, A., Martinell, M., Dorkhan, M. et al., 2018, 'Novel subgroups of adult-onset diabetes and their association with outcomes: A data-driven cluster analysis of six variables', *Lancet Diabetes & Endocrinology, 6*(5): 361–9, doi:10.1016/S2213-8587(18)30051-2

Albanes, D., Heinonen, O.P., Huttunen, J.K., Taylor, P.R., Virtamo, J. et al., 1995, 'Effects of alpha-tocopherol and beta-carotene supplements on cancer incidence in the Alpha-Tocopherol Beta-Carotene Cancer Prevention Study', *American Journal of Clinical Nutrition, 62*(6): 1427S–30S, doi:10.1093/ajcn/62.6.1427S

Alberts, D.S., Martínez, M.E., Roe, D.J., Guillén-Rodríguez, J.M., Marshall, J.R. et al., 2000, 'Lack of effect of a high-fiber cereal supplement on the recurrence of colorectal adenomas', *New England Journal of Medicine, 342*(16): 1156–62, doi:10.1056/NEJM200004203421602

American Diabetes Association, 2018, 'Prevention or delay of type 2 diabetes: Standards of medical care in diabetes—2018', *Diabetes Care, 41*(Suppl. 1): S51–4, doi:10.2337/dc18-S005

Australian Diabetes in Pregnancy Society, 2014, *ADIPS Consensus Guidelines for the Testing and Diagnosis of Hyperglycaemia in Pregnancy in Australia and New Zealand*, <www.adips.org/downloads/2014ADIPSGDMGu idelinesV18.11.2014_000.pdf>, accessed 14 January 2019

Australian Thyroid Foundation, 2018, *Do I Have a Thyroid Disorder?*, <www.thyroidfoundation.org.au/page/24/i-suspect-i-have-a-thyroid-disorder-what-do-i-do>, accessed 14 January 2019

Aydin, Ö., Nieuwdorp, M. & Gerdes, V., 2018, 'The gut microbiome as a target for the treatment of type 2 diabetes', *Current Diabetes Reports, 18*(8): 55, doi:10.1007/s11892-018-1020-6

Barker, D.J., Hales, C.N., Fall, C., Osmond, C., Phipps, K. & Clark, P., 1993, 'Type 2 (non-insulin-dependent) diabetes mellitus, hypertension and hyperlipidaemia (syndrome X): Relation to reduced fetal growth', *Diabetologia, 36*(1): 62–7, doi:10.1007/BF00399095

Bell, A.C., Simmons, A., Sanigorski, A.M., Kremer, P.J. & Swinburn, B.A., 2008, 'Preventing childhood obesity: The sentinel site for obesity prevention in Victoria, Australia', *Health Promotion International, 23*(4): 328–36, doi:10.1093/heapro/dan025

Bleich, S.N., Segal, J., Wu, Y., Wilson, R. & Wang, Y., 2013, 'Systematic review of community-based childhood obesity prevention studies', *Pediatrics, 132*(1): e201–10, doi:10.1542/peds.2013-0886

Borys, J., Valdeyron, L., Levy, E., Vinck, J., Edell, D. et al., 2013, 'EPODE—a model for reducing the incidence of obesity and weight-related comorbidities', *European Endocrinology, 9*(2): 116–20, doi:10.17925/EE.2013.09.02.116

Brandhorst, S. & Longo, V.D., 2016, 'Fasting and caloric restriction in cancer prevention and treatment', in T. Cramer & C.A. Schmitt (eds), *Metabolism in Cancer*, Cham: Springer, pp. 241–66

Buttó, L.F. & Haller, D., 2016, 'Dysbiosis in intestinal inflammation: Cause or consequence', *International Journal of Medical Microbiology, 306*(5): 302–9, doi:10.1016/j.ijmm.2016.02.010

Byrne, C., Chambers, E., Morrison, D. & Frost, G., 2015, 'The role of short chain fatty acids in appetite regulation and energy homeostasis', *International Journal of Obesity, 39*(9): 1331–8, doi:10.1038/ijo.2015.84

Cancer Council, 2018, *iheard*, <https://iheard.com.au/>, accessed 14 January 2019

Carding, S., Verbeke, K., Vipond, D.T., Corfe, B.M. & Owen, L.J., 2015, 'Dysbiosis of the gut microbiota in disease', *Microbial Ecology in Health and Disease, 26*(1): 26191, <www.tandfonline.com/doi/full/10.3402/mehd.v26.26191%40zmeh20.2015.26.issue-s2>, accessed 14 January 2019

Chu, H., Khosravi, A., Kusumawardhani, I.P., Kwon, A.H.K., Vasconcelos, A.C. et al., 2016, 'Gene-microbiota interactions contribute to the pathogenesis of inflammatory bowel disease', *Science, 352*(6289): 1116–20, doi:10.1126/science.aad9948

Claesson, M.J., Jeffery, I.B., Conde, S., Power, S.E., O'Connor, E.M. et al., 2012, 'Gut microbiota composition correlates with diet and health in the elderly', *Nature, 488*: 178–84, doi:10.1038/nature11319

Colberg, S.R., Sigal, R.J., Yardley, J.E., Riddell, M.C., Dunstan, D.W. et al., 2016, 'Physical activity/exercise and diabetes: A position statement of the American Diabetes Association', *Diabetes Care, 39*(11): 2065–79, doi:10.2337/dc16-1728

Colditz, G.A. & Peterson, L.L., 2018, 'Obesity and cancer: Evidence, impact, and future directions', *Clinical Chemistry, 64*(1): 154–62, doi:10.1373/clinchem.2017.277376

Cypess, A.M., Lehman, S., Williams, G., Tal, I., Rodman, D. et al., 2009, 'Identification and importance of brown adipose tissue in adult humans', *New England Journal of Medicine, 360*(15): 1509–17, doi:10.1056/NEJMoa0810780

Devaux, C.A. & Raoult, D., 2018, 'The microbiological memory, an epigenetic regulator governing the balance between good health and metabolic disorders', *Frontiers in Microbiology, 9*: 1379, doi:10.3389/fmicb.2018.01379

Diabetes Australia, 2015, *What Should I Eat?*, <www.diabetesaustralia.com.au/what-should-i-eat>, accessed 14 January 2019

Dunkley, A.J., Bodicoat, D.H., Greaves, C.J., Russell, C., Yates, T. et al., 2014, 'Diabetes prevention in the real world: Effectiveness of pragmatic lifestyle interventions for the prevention of type 2 diabetes and of the impact of adherence to guideline recommendations: A systematic review and meta-analysis', *Diabetes Care, 37*(4): 922–33, doi:10.2337/dc13-2195

Elwood, P.C., Gallagher, A.M., Duthie, G.G., Mur, L.A. & Morgan, G., 2009. 'Aspirin, salicylates, and cancer', *Lancet, 373*(9671): 1301–9, doi:10.1016/S0140-6736(09)60243-9

Ferguson, M., Capra, S., Bauer, J. & Banks, M., 1999, 'Development of a valid and reliable malnutrition screening tool for adult acute hospital patients', *Nutrition, 15*(6): 458–64, doi:10.1016/S0899-9007(99)00084-2

Galaviz, K.I., Weber, M.B., Straus, A., Haw, J.S., Narayan, K.V. & Ali, M.K., 2018, 'Global diabetes prevention interventions: A systematic review and network meta-analysis of the real-world impact on incidence, weight, and glucose', *Diabetes Care, 41*(7): 1526–34, doi:10.2337/dc17-2222

Garber, J.R., Cobin, R.H., Gharib, H., Hennessey, J.V., Klein, I. et al., 2012, 'Clinical practice guidelines for hypothyroidism in adults: Cosponsored by the American Association of Clinical Endocrinologists and the American Thyroid Association', *Thyroid, 22*(12): 1200–35, doi:10.1089/thy.2012.0205

Hanahan, D. & Weinberg, R.A., 2011, 'Hallmarks of cancer: The next generation', *Cell, 144*(5): 646–74, doi:10.1016/j.cell.2011.02.013

Hetzel, B.S., 2000, 'Iodine-deficiency disorder', in J.S. Garrow, W.P.T. James & A. Ralph (eds), *Human Nutrition and Dietetics*, London: Churchill Livingstone, pp. 621–40

Hsu, C.-C., Wahlqvist, M.L., Lee, M.-S. & Tsai, H.-N., 2011, 'Incidence of dementia is increased in type 2 diabetes and reduced by the use of sulfonylureas and metformin', *Journal of Alzheimer's Disease, 24*(3): 485–93, doi:10.3233/JAD-2011-101524

IDF, 2017a, *IDF Diabetes Atlas, 8th Ed*, <www.diabetesatlas.org/resources/2017-atlas.html >, accessed 1 April 2018
—— 2017b, *Recommendations for Managing Type 2 Diabetes in Primary Care*, <www.idf.org/managing-type2-diabetes>, accessed 14 January 2019

Jacka, F.N., Mykletun, A., Berk, M., Bjelland, I. & Tell, G.S., 2011, 'The association between habitual diet quality and the common mental disorders in community-dwelling adults: The Hordaland Health study', *Psychosomatic Medicine, 73*(6): 483–90, doi:10.1097/PSY.0b013e318222831a

Jansen, M.C., Bueno-de-Mesquita, H.B., Räsänen, L., Fidanza, F., Menotti, A. et al., 1999, 'Consumption of plant foods and stomach cancer mortality in the seven countries study: Is grain consumption a risk factor?', *Nutrition and Cancer, 34*(1): 49–55, doi:10.1207/S15327914NC340107

Javeed, N. & Matveyenko, A.V., 2018, 'Circadian etiology of type 2 diabetes mellitus', *Physiology, 33*(2): 138–50, doi:10.1152/physiol.00003.2018

Keeney, K.M., Yurist-Doutsch, S., Arrieta, M.-C. & Finlay, B.B., 2014, 'Effects of antibiotics on human microbiota and subsequent disease', *Annual Review of Microbiology, 68*: 21735, doi:10.1146/annurev-micro-091313-103456

Kromhout, D., Bosschieter, E. & Coulander, C.D.L., 1982, 'Dietary fibre and 10-year mortality from coronary heart disease, cancer, and all causes: The Zutphen Study', *Lancet, 320*(8297): 518–22, doi:10.1016/S0140-6736(82)90600-6

Ley, S.H., Hamdy, O., Mohan, V. & Hu, F.B., 2014, 'Prevention and management of type 2 diabetes: Dietary components and nutritional strategies', *Lancet, 383*(9933): 1999–2007, doi:10.1016/S0140-6736(14)60613-9

Lukito, W., Boyce, N.W. & Chandra, R.K., 1994, 'Nutrition and immunity', in M.L. Wahlqvist & J.S. Vobecky (eds), *Medical Practice of Preventive Nutrition*, London: Smith-Gordon, pp. 27–51

Lunde, P., Nilsson, B.B., Bergland, A., Kværner, K.J. & Bye, A., 2018, 'The effectiveness of smartphone apps for lifestyle improvement in noncommunicable diseases: Systematic review and meta-analyses', *Journal of Medical Internet Research, 20*(5): e162, doi:10.2196/jmir.9751

MacLennan, R., Macrae, F., Bain, C., Battistutta, D., Chapuis, P. et al., 1995, 'Randomized trial of intake of fat, fiber, and beta carotene to prevent colorectal adenomas', *Journal of the National Cancer Institute, 87*(23): 1760–6, doi:10.1093/jnci/87.23.1760

McNeil, N., 1984, 'The contribution of the large intestine to energy supplies in man', *American Journal of Clinical Nutrition, 39*(2): 338–42, doi:10.1093/ajcn/39.2.338

Membrez, M., Blancher, F., Jaquet, M., Bibiloni, R., Cani, P.D. et al., 2008, 'Gut microbiota modulation with norfloxacin and ampicillin enhances glucose tolerance in mice', *FASEB Journal, 22*(7): 2416–26, doi:10.1096/fj.07-102723

New Zealand Guidelines Group, 2011, *New Zealand Guidelines Group, Guidance on the Management of Type 2 Diabetes 2011*, <www.moh.govt.nz/NoteBook/nbbooks.nsf/0/60306295DECB0BC6CC257A4F000FC0CB/$file/NZGG-management-of-type-2-diabetes-web.pdf>, accessed 14 January 2019

Omenn, G.S., Goodman, G.E., Thornquist, M.D., Balmes, J., Cullen, M.R. et al., 1996, 'Effects of a combination of beta carotene and vitamin A on lung cancer and cardiovascular disease', *New England Journal of Medicine, 334*(18): 1150–5, doi:10.1056/NEJM199605023341802

Paun, A. & Danska, J.S., 2016, 'Modulation of type 1 and type 2 diabetes risk by the intestinal microbiome', *Pediatric Diabetes, 17*(7): 469–77, doi:10.1111/pedi.12424

Pembrey, M.E., Bygren, L.O., Kaati, G., Edvinsson, S., Northstone, K. et al., 2006, 'Sex-specific, male-line trans-generational responses in humans', *European Journal of Human Genetics, 14*(2): 159–66, doi:10.1038/sj.ejhg.5201538

Prasad, R.B. & Groop, L., 2015, 'Genetics of type 2 diabetes: Pitfalls and possibilities', *Genes, 6*(1): 87–123, doi:10.3390/genes6010087

RACGP, 2016, *General Practice Management of Type 2 Diabetes: 2016–18*, <https://static.diabetesaustralia.com.au/s/fileassets/diabetes-australia/5d3298b2-abf3-487e-9d5e-0558566fc242.pdf>, accessed 14 January 2019

Reutrakul, S. & Van Cauter, E., 2018, 'Sleep influences on obesity, insulin resistance, and risk of type 2 diabetes', *Metabolism, 84*: 56–66, doi:10.1016/j.metabol.2018.02.010

Sacher, P.M., Kolotourou, M., Chadwick, P.M., Cole, T.J., Lawson, M.S. et al., 2010, 'Randomized controlled trial of the MEND program: A family-based community intervention for childhood obesity', *Obesity, 18*(S1): S62–8, doi:10.1038/oby.2009.433

Scrimshaw, N.S., Taylor, C.E. & Gordon, J.E., 1959, 'Interactions of nutrition and infection', *American Journal of Medical Sciences, 237*(3): 367–403, <www.cabdirect.org/cabdirect/abstract/19592703595>, accessed 14 January 2019

Selber-Hnatiw, S., Rukundo, B., Ahmadi, M., Akoubi, H., Al-Bizri, H. et al., 2017, 'Human gut microbiota: Toward an ecology of disease', *Frontiers in Microbiology, 8*: 1265, doi:10.3389/fmicb.2017.01265

Steegers-Theunissen, R.P.M., Twigt, J., Pestinger, V. & Sinclair, K.D., 2013, 'The periconceptional period, reproduction and long-term health of offspring: The importance of one-carbon metabolism', *Human Reproduction Update, 19*(6): 640–55, doi:10.1093/humupd/dmt041

Stern, M.P., Bartley, M., Duggirala, R. & Bradshaw, B., 2000, 'Birth weight and the metabolic syndrome: Thrifty phenotype or thrifty genotype?', *Diabetes/Metabolism Research and Reviews, 16*(2): 88–93, doi:10.1002/(SICI)1520-7560(200003/04)16:2<88::AID-DMRR81>3.0.CO;2-M

Terra, R., Silva, S.A.G.d., Pinto, V.S. & Dutra, P.M.L., 2012, 'Effect of exercise on immune system: Response, adaptation and cell signaling', *Revista Brasileira de Medicina do Esporte, 18*(3): 208–14, doi:10.1590/S1517-86922012000300015

Thomson, C.D., 2004, 'Selenium and iodine intakes and status in New Zealand and Australia', *British Journal of Nutrition, 91*(5): 661–72, doi:10.1079/BJN20041110

Tobaldini, E., Fiorelli, E.M., Solbiati, M., Costantino, G., Nobili, L. & Montano, N., 2018, 'Short sleep duration and cardiometabolic risk: From pathophysiology to clinical evidence', *Nature Reviews Cardiology, 16*(4): 213–24, doi:10.1038/s41569-018-0109-6

Tuomilehto, J., Lindström, J., Eriksson, J.G., Valle, T.T., Hämäläinen, H. et al., 2001, 'Prevention of type 2 diabetes mellitus by changes in lifestyle among subjects with impaired glucose tolerance', *New England Journal of Medicine, 344*(18): 1343–50, doi:10.1056/NEJM200105033441801

Uribarri, J., Woodruff, S., Goodman, S., Cai, W., Chen, X. et al., 2010, 'Advanced glycation end products in foods and a practical guide to their reduction in the diet', *Journal of the American Dietetic Association, 110*(6): 911–16. e912, doi:10.1016/j.jada.2010.03.018

Vlassara, H., Cai, W., Crandall, J., Goldberg, T., Oberstein, R. et al., 2002, 'Inflammatory mediators are induced by dietary glycotoxins, a major risk factor for diabetic angiopathy', *Proceedings of the National Academy of Sciences, 99*(24): 15596–601, doi:10.1073/pnas.242407999

Wahlqvist, M.L., Lee, M.-S., Chuang, S.-Y., Hsu, C.-C., Tsai, H.-N. et al., 2012, 'Increased risk of affective disorders in type 2 diabetes is minimized by sulfonylurea and metformin combination: A population-based cohort study', *BMC Medicine, 10*(1): 150, doi:10.1186/1741-7015-10-150

Wahlqvist, M.L., Lee, M.-S., Hsu, C.-C., Chuang, S.-Y., Lee, J.-T. & Tsai, H.-N., 2012, 'Metformin-inclusive sulfonylurea therapy reduces the risk of Parkinson's disease occurring with Type 2 diabetes in a Taiwanese population cohort', *Parkinsonism & Related Disorders, 18*(6): 753–8, doi:10.1016/j.parkreldis.2012.03.010

Wahlqvist, M.L. & O'Brien, R., 1993, 'Clinical nutrition of diabetes', *Asia Pacific Journal of Clinical Nutrition, 2*: 149–150, <http://apjcn.nhri.org.tw/server/apjcn/2/3/149.htm>, accessed 14 January 2019

WCRF & AICR, 2018, *Food, Nutrition, Physical Activity, and Cancer: A global perspective*, <www.wcrf.org/dietandcancer/about>, accessed 14 January 2019

WHO, 2003, *Diet, Nutrition and the Prevention Of Chronic Diseases. Report of the Joint WHO/FAO Expert Consultation*, <www.who.int/dietphysicalactivity/publications/trs916/summary/en/>, accessed 14 January 2019

—— 2006, *Definition and Diagnosis of Diabetes Mellitus and Intermediate Hyperglycemia. Report of a WHO/IDF Consultation*, <www.who.int/diabetes/publications/Definition%20and%20diagnosis%20of%20diabetes_new. pdf>, accessed 14 January 2019

Willett, W.C., 2000, 'Diet and cancer', *Oncologist 5*(5): 393–404, doi:10.1634/theoncologist.5-5-393

Xu, Y., Yang, J., Du, L., Li, K. & Zhou, Y., 2018, 'Association of whole grain, refined grain, and cereal consumption with gastric cancer risk: A meta-analysis of observational studies', *Food Science & Nutrition, 7*(1): 256–65, doi:10.1002/fsn3.878

Yoshida, S.H., Keen, C.L., Ansar, A.A. & Gershwin, M.E., 1999, 'Nutrition and the immune system', in M.E. Shils, J.A. Olsen, M. Shike & A. Katherine-Ros (eds), *Modern Nutrition in Health and Disease* (9th edn), Baltimore MD: Lipincott, Williams and Wilkins, pp. 725–50

Zheng, P., Li, Z. & Zhou, Z., 2018, 'Gut microbiome in type 1 diabetes: A comprehensive review', *Diabetes/Metabolism Research and Reviews, 34*(7): e3043, doi:10.1002/dmrr.3043

{CHAPTER 33}
DISORDERED ORGAN FUNCTIONS

Mark L. Wahlqvist and Naiyana Wattanapenpaiboon

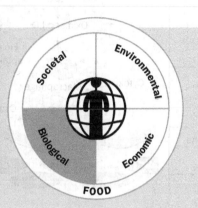

OBJECTIVES

- Define organs, their structures, functions, nutritional requirements and related disorders.
- Identify dietary factors which influence the development of atherosclerosis and its impact on organs through disordered blood flow.
- Explore the interactions, whether adverse, aberrant or favourable, between nutritional and environmental factors affecting bone health.
- Explain how nutritional and non-nutritional factors contribute to disordered function, structure or health of muscles, teeth and gums by reference to nutritional biology and ecohealth concepts in general.

INTRODUCTION

Apart from body systems, nutrients are part of the structure or play a role in bodily functions of many organs. This chapter focuses on the organs, the functions of which could be influenced by excessive or inadequate nutritional and personal behaviour factors.

THE HEART AND BLOOD VESSELS

Cardiovascular disease (CVD) refers to a group of diseases that involve the heart and/or blood vessels, and these diseases appear to arise from the same or similar mechanisms. The most common types of CVD in Australia are coronary artery disease,

stroke and heart failure/cardiomyopathy, and less common forms include rheumatic and congenital heart disease.

CVD is commonly related to atherosclerosis, which is chronic inflammatory disease of large and medium-sized arteries causing a disruption of the homeostasis between the endothelium and smooth muscle cells of blood vessels. Atherosclerosis is characterised by endothelial dysfunction, vascular inflammation and accumulation of lipids, cholesterol, calcium and cellular debris in the innermost layer of blood vessel wall (Figure 33.1). Atherosclerotic disease occurs via a number of independent but interrelated mechanisms that combine to produce the overall effect of the disease.

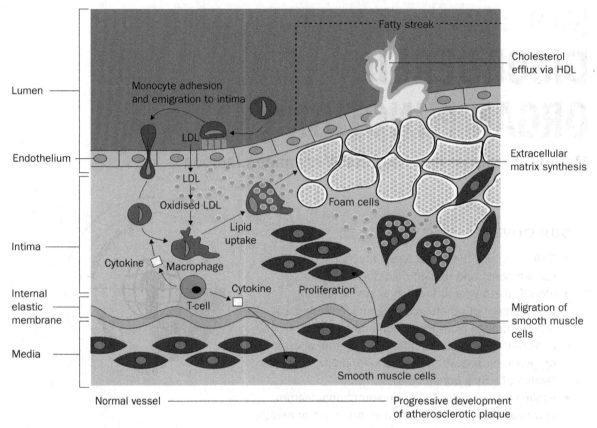

Note: LDL = low-density lipoproteins; HDL = high-density lipoproteins

Figure 33.1: Formation of atherosclerotic plaque

Source: Adapted from Rafieian-Kopaei et al. (2014)

Diet

The role of nutrition in the initiation, progression, and reversal of cardiovascular disease (CVD) is well established, and a heart–healthy diet has long been a focal point in prevention and treatment of CVD. Intakes of a number of nutrients have been associated with blood lipids, and there has been much interest in various bioactive compounds in food that favourably influence platelet aggregation, susceptibility of low-density lipoproteins (LDL) to oxidation, cholesterol synthesis, plasma lipoprotein status and/or other CVD risk factors. As our knowledge base has expanded, it has become evident that nutrition affects the heart and blood vessels in a multitude of ways by targeting important risk factors. For example, possible mechanisms or pathways by which fruit and vegetable intake could influence CVD risk have been elucidated (Figure 33.2). Moreover, although our understanding of the mechanisms by which diet affects CVD has increased, there still are many lines of inquiry that remain to be resolved.

A shift towards more urbanised ways of living as well as increased industrialisation in most countries has resulted in marked changes in diet and personal behaviours, such as physical activity and sleep pattern (see Chapter 29). Diet becomes more energy-dense and higher in fat, and personal behaviours trend towards being more sedentary. The combination of nutrition and personal behaviour modifications has proven beneficial in reducing cardiovascular disease risk (Table 33.1).

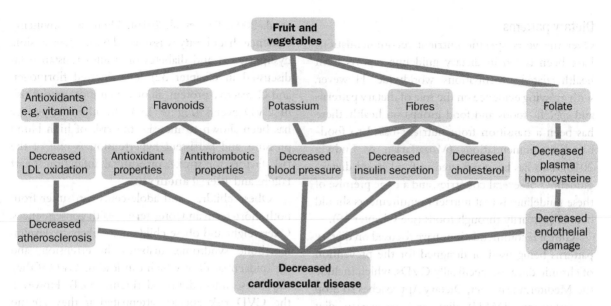

Figure 33.2: Possible mechanisms of fruit and vegetable consumption and cardiovascular disease

Source: Adapted from European Heart Network (2011)

Table 33.1: Strength of evidence on dietary and personal behaviour factors associated with cardiovascular disease risk

Strength of evidence	Risk modification	Dietary and personal behaviour factors
Convincing evidence	Decreased risk	• Fruits and vegetables • Potassium • Fish and fish oils (EPA and DHA) • Linoleic acid • Low to moderate alcohol intake • Regular physical activity
	Increased risk	• High sodium intake • Trans fats • Myristic and palmitic acids • High alcohol intake (for stroke) • Overweight and obesity
	No relationship	• Vitamin E supplementation
Probable evidence	Decreased risk	• Wholegrain cereals • Dietary fibre • α-linolenic acid • Oleic acid • Folate • Plant sterols
	Increased risk	• Dietary cholesterol
	No relationship	• Stearic acid
Possible evidence	Decreased risk	• Flavonoids • Soy products
	Increased risk	• Fats rich in lauric acid • β-carotene supplements
Insufficient evidence	Decreased risk	• Calcium, magnesium, vitamin C
	Increased risk	• Carbohydrates, iron

Sources: European Heart Network (2011); Piepoli et al. (2016); Richter et al. (2017); WHO (2003)

Dietary patterns

Over the years, specific nutrient recommendations have been issued in dietary guideline reports from health-related organisations worldwide. However, with growing evidence on the role of dietary patterns and specific foods and food groups on health, there has been a transition from nutrient-based to food-based recommendations (Mozaffarian & Ludwig 2010). This has been reflected in food-based dietary guidelines of several countries, and a basic premise of these guidelines is that nutrient requirements should be met primarily through foods (see Chapter 19).

Global recommendations have focused on dietary patterns being used or designed for the prevention of chronic diseases, specifically CVDs, which include the Mediterranean diet, Dietary Approaches to Stop Hypertension (DASH) diet, and vegetarian diet (Table 33.2). Moreover the EAT–Lancet Commission on Healthy Diets from Sustainable Food Systems has identified a 'planetary health diet' (see 'The planetary health diet' box and Chapter 26).

OBESITY AND PERSONAL BEHAVIOURS

CVD morbidity and mortality have been shown to increase in overweight people, particularly with abdominal obesity (Calle et al. 1999; Dagenais et al. 2005; Fan et al. 2016). There is convincing evidence that obesity is associated with hypertension, dyslipidaemia and diabetes or insulin resistance (as discussed in Chapter 32), and elevated fibrinogen and C-reactive protein, all of which increase the risk of CVD events (Figure 33.3). In addition, obesity has been shown to increase the risk of high blood pressure, and persistent hypertension is one of the risk factors for stroke, myocardial infarction, heart failure and arterial **aneurysm**.

Obese children and adolescents can suffer from both short-term and long-term health consequences. Overweight and obese children are likely to develop metabolic syndrome, diabetes, hypertension, and dyslipidaemia, all of which can lead to CVD, if they stay obese into adulthood (Figure 33.4). However, the CVD risk appears attenuated if they are no longer obese as adults (Juonala et al. 2011).

As with the prevention of diabetes described in Chapter 31, at least 150 minutes of moderate-intensity physical activity per week and adequate sleep duration (that is neither too short nor too long) will reduce the risk of CVD (Jike et al. 2018).

A Joint WHO/FAO Expert Consultation published in 2003 a technical report on Diet, Nutrition and the Prevention of Chronic Diseases which provides general diet recommendations for the

Table 33.2: Dietary patterns for the prevention of cardiovascular disease

Dietary pattern	Composition/Emphasis
MEDITERRANEAN This dietary pattern is plant-based diverse and tends to be high in MUFAs and low in SFAs.	• To increase fruits, vegetables (especially root vegetables), whole grains, legumes, nuts, seeds and olive oil. • Low to moderate consumption of wine, fish, poultry and dairy products. • To reduce red meats.
DIETARY APPROACHES TO STOP HYPERTENSION (DASH)	• To emphasise fruits, vegetables and low-fat dairy products. • To incorporate whole grains, fish, nuts and poultry. • To reduce red meats, sweets and sugar, sweetened beverages.
VEGETARIAN 'Vegetarian' is a broadly encompassing term used for various categories: vegans (strictly no animal products); ovo-lacto vegetarians (no meat or fish); ovo vegetarians (no meat, fish, or dairy products); lacto vegetarians (no meat, fish, or eggs).	• To emphasise fruits, vegetables, whole grains, legumes, nuts, seeds, and soy foods. • To include little or no animal products.

Sources: Schulze et al. (2018); US Department of Health and Human Services & US Department of Agriculture (2015)

THE PLANETARY HEALTH DIET

The 'planetary health diet' has been developed by a team of more than 30 scientists from across the globe, as part of the EAT–Lancet Commission on Healthy Diets From Sustainable Food Systems, to reach a scientific consensus that defines a healthy and sustainable diet, a diet that encompasses human health and environmental sustainability (Willett et al. 2019).

Their report titled 'Food in the Anthropocene' outlines ranges of intakes for food groups to ensure human health and planetary boundaries for food production to ensure a 'stable Earth system'.

With the aim of feeding more people while maintaining sustainable food production, the planetary health diet suggests that we should eat less red meat and sugar, more fruit and vegetables, and much more nuts, seeds and pulses (see Figure 33.5, colour section).

It builds on a growing emphasis on plant-based diets in national and international dietary guidelines. However, some recommendations need more context and greater emphasis, such as local support for ecologically sensitive food production and nature-engaging healthy habits (Foyer et al. 2016). Ethical and equity nutritional dilemmas are emerging, however, where desirable foodstuffs like fish and seafood are contaminated with microplastic and fermented dairy products add to the dependency on ruminant animals which add to the methane load on the atmosphere (Wahlqvist 2016). These can be prioritised through means such as novel green technology.

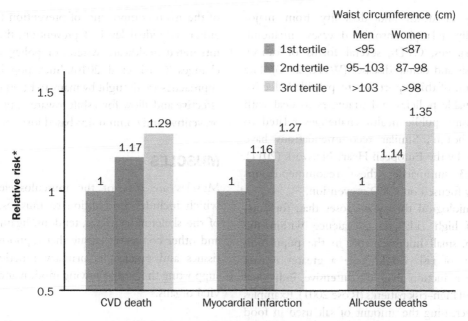

Note: * Adjusted for age, sex, body mass index, cardiovascular disease, diabetes, HDL cholesterol and total cholesterol

Figure 33.3: Abdominal obesity and increased risk of cardiovascular events—results from the HOPE Study

Source: Developed from Calle et al. (1999); Dagenais et al. (2005); Fan et al. (2016)

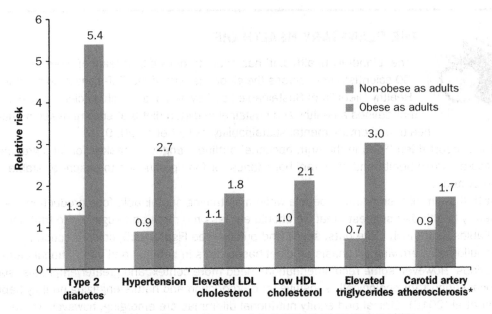

Notes: 'Reference group' (relative risk = 1) = subjects with a normal body mass index in childhood and non-obese as adults;
* Carotid artery atherosclerosis indicated by increased thickness of the carotid artery

Figure 33.4: Cardiovascular risk outcomes in adulthood among overweight or obese in childhood (23-year follow-up of 6328 children)

Source: Developed from Juonala et al. (2011)

prevention of death and disability from major nutritionally related chronic diseases, including obesity, diabetes, CVDs, several forms of cancer, osteoporosis and dental diseases (WHO 2003). The primary aim of this report was to provide 'effective and sustainable policies and strategies to deal with the increasing public health challenges related to diet and health'. Similar recommendations have been made by the European Heart Network (2011). Table 33.3 summarises these recommendations specifically focused on CVD prevention.

Epidemiological theory proposes that, for conditions of high risk and prevalence within the population, small improvements in the population distribution of risk would have a greater impact on disease reduction than the intensive, individual treatment of high-risk patients (Rose 2001). Examples include decreasing the amount of salt used in food processing, removing certain fats from the food chain, or having a smoke-free environment. Public-health responses may utilise several combinations

of the main components of prevention that include either individual level of prevention, the use of an integrated healthcare system, or policy and societal changes (Gersh et al. 2010). Such population-based approaches are thought by many to be especially cost-effective and allow for a shift towards a more primary, preventive and community-based form of health care.

MUSCLES

Muscles are part of the musculoskeletal system, which includes, in addition to muscles, the bones of the skeleton, cartilage, tendons, ligaments, joints, and other connective tissue that supports and binds tissues and organs. Its primary functions include supporting the body, allowing motion and protecting vital organs.

Sarcopenia

Sarcopenia (literally deficiency of muscle mass) is a direct cause of the age-related decrease in muscle

Table 33.3: Recommendations for preventing cardiovascular disease by the Joint WHO/FAO Expert Consultation and the European Heart Network

Component and justification	WHO/FAO Expert Consultation recommendations	European Heart Network's intermediate population goal	How to achieve
Dietary fat intake (mg/day or % of daily energy intake) Justification: Adverse effects on blood lipids, thrombosis, blood pressure, endothelial function, arrhythmogenesis and inflammation	Total fat 15–30% PUFAs 6–10% – n-6 PUFAs 5–8% – n-3 PUFAs 1–2% SFAs less than 10% TFAs less than 1%	Total fat less than 30% PUFAs 6–11% – α-linolenic acid 1–2% – n-3 PUFAs 250–500 mg/day MUFAs 8–13% SFAs less than 10% TFAs less than 1%	• Limiting intake of fat from dairy and meat sources. • Avoiding use of hydrogenated oils and fats in cooking and manufacture of food products. • Using appropriate edible vegetable oils in small amounts. • Ensuring a regular intake of fish (1–2 times/week) or plant sources of α-linolenic acid. • Eating nuts with appropriate fatty acid profiles (see Chapter 8). • Avoiding use of frying methods in food preparation practices.
Fruits and vegetables Justification: Variety of phytonutrients, potassium and fibre	400–500 g/day	More than 400 g/day	• Daily consumption of fresh fruit and vegetables (including berries, green leafy and cruciferous vegetables, legumes) in an adequate quantity.
Sodium/salt Justification: Effects on blood pressure	Less than 5 g/day salt Less than 70 mmol or 1.7 g/day of sodium	Less than 5 g/day salt	• Minimising sodium intake from additives, preservatives and other dietary sources.
Potassium Justification: Protective against stroke and cardiac arrhythmias	Potassium 70–80 mmol/day		• Adequate daily consumption of fruits and vegetables.
Total carbohydrates		More than 55%	
Added sugars		Less than 10%	• Reducing consumption of sugar-sweetened drinks as much as possible.
Dietary fibre Justification: Protective against coronary heart disease and used in diet to lower blood pressure		More than 20 g/day non-starch polysaccharide (more than 1.6 g/day non-starch polysaccharide/MJ energy)	• Adequate daily consumption of fruits, vegetables and wholegrain cereals.
Alcohol Justification: CVD and other health risks outweigh the protective effects of regular low to moderate consumption of alcohol against coronary heart disease.			• Generally not recommended.
Physical activity Justification: Recommended amount is sufficient to raise cardiorespiratory fitness	At least 30 minutes of at least moderate-intensity physical activity on most days of the week	150 minutes/week of at least moderate intensity physical activity	
Body mass index		Average BMI of less than 23 for adults	

Notes: MUFAs = monounsaturated fatty acids; PUFAs = polyunsaturated fatty acids; SFAs = saturated fatty acids; TFAs = trans fatty acids

Sources: European Heart Network (2011); WHO (2003)

REDUCING SODIUM AND TRANS FATS IN THE FOOD SUPPLY

In Australia the Commonwealth Department of Health has established the Food and Health Dialogue (Australian Government 2016). This collaboration between the health sector and food industry has set targets for reducing consumption of risk-associated nutrients via a voluntary reformulation program. Search the literature (both peer-reviewed and grey literature) for what you can find on reformulation generally and the Food and Health Dialogue specifically.

Think about and discuss the following:
- Which foods are included and which are excluded?
- Are there any population groups who may be missing out on this initiative?
- Why is the program voluntary and not mandatory?
- How successful is a population-wide approach compared to an individual approach in reducing consumption of these nutrients?

HEART DISEASE CASE STUDY: WHAT WOULD BE YOUR ADVICE?

Mr Crow has just experienced his first bout of angina and his doctor has suggested he needs to change his diet. Look at the following basic diet history and identify the foods that need to change and what the alternatives could be. Think about what needs to be swapped but also what may need to be added.

What other risk factors does Mr Crow have for CVD? What additional information do you need for a full risk profile?

Mr Crow is 56 years old and has worked as a labourer his whole life. Apart from work, Mr Crow does no additional physical activity and he has recently given up smoking. He lives at home with his wife. He is 180 cm tall and weighs 110 kg. His diet history is as follows.

Breakfast:
3 slices of white toast with butter and 3 fried eggs

Morning tea:
Iced coffee with milk
Scone with jam and cream

Lunch:
Meat pie or sausage roll

Dinner:
Sausages or steak or fried chicken
Mashed potato
Carrots or peas
Ice cream with chocolate sauce
2 cans of beer

strength. Evidence suggests that skeletal muscle mass and strength start to decline in a linear fashion as early as the age of 40, and up to 50 per cent of mass is lost by the age of 80. The decline in muscle strength is responsible for much of the disability and frailty in older adults. People with sarcopenia are at increased risk of injurious falls, leading to lack of mobility and independence (see also Chapter 22).

The cause of sarcopenia is multifactorial; contributory factors include nutritional status, inflammatory pathway activation, reduction in neuromuscular junctions and declines in hormones important in muscle mass maintenance, such as IGF-1, oestrogen and testosterone (Farshidfar et al. 2015) (see Figure 22.4 in Chapter 22). Nutritional factors that contribute to sarcopenia include an inadequate intake of energy or protein, which may be due to poor food intake and/or disease.

Lack of exercise is thought to be a risk factor for sarcopenia, as inactivity or immobilisation can lead to muscle wasting. However, even highly trained athletes can experience sarcopenia (Faulkner et al. 2007). On the other hand, evidence indicates short-term resistance exercise could increase the ability and capacity of skeletal muscle to synthesise proteins (Yarasheski 2003). A systematic review in 2018 also revealed that multicomponent exercise training in older adults can improve physical performance and muscular strength (Liao et al. 2018).

MANAGEMENT OF SARCOPENIA

A body of evidence supports the notion that nutrition plays an important role both in the prevention and management of sarcopenia. The importance of dietary patterns that provide sufficient intakes of protein, vitamin D, long-chain polyunsaturated fatty acids, antioxidant nutrients (selenium, vitamins C and E) and phytonutrients (such as carotenoids and polyphenols) has been emphasised as essential in preventing or managing sarcopenia. Interestingly, the benefits of antioxidant supplementation for these purposes are uncertain.

Read the following two review articles and describe the key strategies for the prevention and management of sarcopenia.
- Dhillon, R.J. and Hasni, S., 2017, 'Pathogenesis and management of sarcopenia', *Clinics in Geriatric Medicine*, 33(1): 17–26
- Robinson, S.M. et al., 2017, 'Does nutrition play a role in the prevention and management of sarcopenia?', *Clinical Nutrition*, 37: 1121–32.

BONES

Bone is the skeletal portion of the musculoskeletal system. In addition to supporting the structure of the body, bone protects the brain, heart and other organs from injury and allows us to move. It also serves as the main storage system for calcium, phosphorus and compounds essential for maintaining an optimal pH balance, and contains the bone marrow, which is the critical component of the **haematopoietic** system.

Bone homeostasis involves multiple but co-ordinated cellular and molecular events. Bone remodelling or bone turnover is a dynamic process throughout life; it is the process where new bone tissue is formed (bone formation) and mature bone tissue is removed from the skeleton (bone resorption) into blood plasma. The constant bone reshaping process principally involves two specialised types of bone cells: **osteoblasts** and **osteoclasts**. During human growth, the turnover is biased towards bone formation, with bone resorption occurring at a slower rate. The amount of bone mass can keep growing until around age 30. At that point, bones have reached their maximum strength and density, known as peak bone mass. Bone mass then stabilises until bone density in women falls dramatically in the years following menopause; in men, the decline is more gradual after about age 50. Bones can become sufficiently brittle to be easily fractured, a condition known as osteoporosis.

The deterioration of the body with age makes individuals, particularly the elderly, susceptible to and affected by poor bone health. Disorders like osteoporosis and osteomalacia can increase the risk of hip fractures and other life-changing secondary symptoms (see Chapter 22).

Osteomalacia and rickets

Osteomalacia is a condition in which the bones are weakened and fragile due to bone decalcification, potentially leading to hip fractures. Osteomalacia in children, known as rickets, is characterised by stunted growth and deformity of the leg bones. Rickets in children and osteomalacia in adults are nutritionally related bone disorders that are mainly caused by insufficient exposure to sunlight and uncompensated for by the dietary intake of vitamin D (see Chapter 16). Some defects in vitamin D metabolism or action can lead to impaired bone matrix mineralisation. Renal diseases and phosphate depletion are also among the major causes of osteomalacia.

Osteoporosis

The clinical significance of osteoporosis, which is characterised by an absolute decrease in bone mass, lies in the fractures that mostly occur at the spine, wrist and hip, although many fractures at other sites are also associated with a low bone mass independently of age and should be considered to be osteoporotic. The WHO (2007) defines osteoporosis based on bone mineral density (BMD) (Table 33.4).

The most widely validated technique to measure BMD is dual energy x-ray absorptiometry (DXA) (see Chapter 23). A T-score is a standardised score used to compare BMD to average values for young adult reference populations. Although the reference standard for the description of osteoporosis is **femoral neck** BMD, other central sites, such as lumbar spine, hip and forearm, can be used for diagnosis in clinical practice.

Osteoporosis is a major cause of fractures and debilitation in post-menopausal women and the elderly and constitutes an important public health problem. Although it affects individuals of all races and ethnicities, and both genders, women are at highest risk because their skeletons are smaller than those of men and because of the accelerated bone loss that accompanies menopause. The adverse effect of osteoporotic fractures on quality of life is substantial, and increases with increasing age and number of fractures. In terms of hospital costs, the burden of osteoporotic fractures in women exceeds those attributable to breast cancer, myocardial infarction or stroke.

While primary osteoporosis is a result of ageing and post-menopausal oestrogen deficiency, secondary osteoporosis may be caused by numerous medications and disorders. It is worth noting that a history of a fragility fracture is consistent with a diagnosis of osteoporosis, independently of BMD. Evidence indicates that osteoporosis is easier to prevent than to treat. The prevention of osteoporosis and osteoporosis-related fractures may best be achieved by initiating appropriate healthy behaviours early in life and continuing them throughout life. Healthy

Table 33.4: Categories for diagnosis of osteoporosis based on bone mineral density at the femoral neck

Classification	Bone mineral density*	T-score
Normal	Within 1 SD of the mean	−1.0 and above
Osteopenia (low bone mass)	Between 1 and 2.5 SD below the mean	Between −1.0 and −2.5
Osteoporosis	2.5 SD or more below the mean	−2.5 and below
Severe osteoporosis	2.5 SD or more below the mean with history of one or more fractures	−2.5 and below with history of one or more fractures

Notes: * Bone mineral density in comparison with the mean level for a young adult reference population; SD = standard deviation

Source: WHO (2007)

practices—including the adequate consumption of most nutrients, regular physical activities and other healthy behaviours—contribute to greater bone mineral measurements and optimal peak bone mass. Adequate intakes of calcium and vitamin D, as well as regular exercise (both weight-bearing such as walking, running and activities against gravity, and resistance exercises such as calisthenics and those involving weights) are critical to the development and maintenance of healthy bones throughout the life-cycle.

Nutritional factors affecting bone health

Bone mass is the result of the interplay of three factors: heredity, exercise and nutrition (Heaney 1987). Nutrition, particularly calcium intake, may be permissive relative to the other two factors, because it is necessary for the achievement of peak bone mass; however, it is not in itself a limiting factor. Low calcium intake is associated with low bone density, but dietary calcium by itself does not seem to alter the rate of bone loss. It is estimated that about 70 per cent of the variance in bone parameters is genetically determined. Other important factors in the protection against osteoporosis include consuming enough dietary calcium during childhood and adolescence to ensure maximum bone growth; maintenance of adequate intakes of calcium through-out adult life; engaging in regular exercise; and, in the case of women, hormone replacement therapy after menopause. Nutritional factors affecting bone health are listed in Table 33.5.

Non-nutritional factors affecting bone health

Several non-nutritional factors can affect bone health and the risk for osteoporosis.

Genetic make-up

The genetic component in bone density is well-documented in several twin and mother–daughter studies. It is estimated that heredity explains about 70–80 per cent of variation in bone mass or density by early adulthood in all ethnic groups. It is suggested that there is a strong genetic component in peak bone mass, and possibly also in post-menopausal bone status.

Menstrual status

Menstrual status is a major determinant of osteoporosis risk in women. Acceleration of bone loss coincides with the menopause, either natural or surgical, at which time the ovaries stop producing oestrogen. Early menarche is believed to be associated with a higher peak bone mass in young women, but little is known about its effect on later bone status. On the other hand, it is very widely accepted that early menopause predisposes to osteoporosis.

Body weight

Traditionally, it was believed that osteoporosis is one condition where being overweight acts as a beneficial factor. However, it appears that thinness is a risk factor for osteoporosis, not that obesity is protective.

Lack of physical activity

Physical activity, especially of a vigorous weight-bearing nature, promotes bone formation. Stresses from muscle contraction and maintaining the body in an upright position against the pull of gravity stimulate osteoblast function. Maintenance of healthy bone requires exposure to weight-bearing pressures.

Medications

A number of medications contribute to osteoporosis, either by interfering with calcium absorption or by actively promoting calcium loss from bone. Steroids, for example, affect vitamin D metabolism and can lead to bone loss. Excessive amounts of exogenous thyroid hormone, even in very low amounts, can promote loss of bone mass over a period of time.

Alcohol and tobacco consumption

Cigarette smoking and alcohol consumption are risk factors for developing osteoporosis, probably because of toxic effects on osteoblasts. Excessive alcohol directly impairs bone formation or the replacement of resorbed cavities with new bone, but social drinking is reported to actually improve bone density. Smoking has been implicated in osteoporosis because there is a direct relationship between smoking and decreased bone density. However, it is difficult to

Table 33.5: Examples of nutritional factors affecting bone health

Nutrient	Effects and/or mechanisms
Calcium	• The adequate consumption of calcium, in conjunction with vitamin D, in early life will optimise peak bone mass, and adequate intakes of these two nutrients should continue throughout the remainder of life to help maintain bone mass. • Those with a lifetime history of adequate calcium intake are less susceptible to osteoporosis at advanced ages. • The requirement of calcium to maintain the optimal bone health varies at the different stages of the life-cycle beyond infancy. The demand for calcium during the peripubertal period is probably greater than at any other period of the life-cycle. Although the level of calcium intake has little effect on age-related bone loss in either men or women, it has an impressive effect on hip fractures. • There is a threshold with calcium. If intake is sufficient, above threshold it will not be significantly related to bone density. Intake below threshold is significantly related.
Sodium	• High salt intake is a well-recognised risk factor for osteoporosis because it increases urinary calcium excretion. • Evidence suggests that excessive sodium intake might accelerate bone turnover, particularly bone resorption.
Vitamin D	• 1,25-OH vitamin D stimulates intestinal absorption of calcium. • Age-associated changes in several aspects of vitamin D synthesis, absorption and metabolism may be deleterious to bone health. • Vitamin D also plays a role in preventing rickets in children and osteomalacia in adults.
Vitamin K	• Vitamin K is an essential cofactor in the conversion process of γ-carboxyglutamic acid (Gla), also known as osteocalcin or bone Gla protein, and accounts for up to 15% of the non-collagenous bone. • Dietary vitamin K intake is positively related to BMD, and may be protective against fractures (Pearson 2007). • Vitamin K is required to sustain maximal formation of osteocalcin and other vitamin K-dependent proteins, and therefore adequate vitamin K status is necessary throughout the lifespan.
Dietary acid load	• Acid normally impairs cell function, including that of osteoblasts, but it has an unusual stimulatory effect on osteoclasts. • High dietary acid load may be detrimental to bone, and calcium intake could counteract the adverse effect of dietary acid load on bone health. • Dietary patterns high in fruits and vegetables, which are rich sources of potassium, have a beneficial effect on BMD. Any beneficial effect of potassium on bone may relate to the accompanying bicarbonate precursors.
Phytonutrients	• Phytoestrogenic compounds might exert oestrogenic effect on bone in a similar manner to endogenous oestrogens. Certain isoflavones in soy have been shown to reduce bone resorption. Supplementation, either with isolated soy protein that contains mainly isoflavones or with isoflavone tablets, can inhibit bone resorption and stimulate bone formation.
Other nutritional factors	• Oxalates, which are present in high concentration in spinach, bind calcium in an insoluble form and decrease absorption. • Phytate (unless broken down by food phytase as with bread leavened with yeast) also reduces calcium availability. • Large amounts of dietary fibre can interfere with calcium bioavailability. • Diets high in fat reduce the bioavailability of calcium. • Large doses of zinc supplementation or mega-doses of vitamin A can lower calcium bioavailability. • Caffeine and phosphates found in soft drinks are known to increase urinary calcium excretion as related to prostaglandin synthesis. • Boron at levels obtainable from fruits and vegetables interacts with magnesium intake and changes endogenous oestrogen status.

DIETARY ACID LOAD

'Dietary acid load' is the term used to describe the difference between endogenously produced acid and base/alkali during the combustion of foods. Dietary protein is a primary contributor to dietary acid load, mainly through the metabolism of methionine and cysteine to sulfuric acid. Plant foods generate base-forming constituents, primarily in the form of bicarbonate. The calculation of dietary acid load from dietary constituents includes both the acid- and the base-generating capacity of the entire diet. Western diets tend to have high dietary acid load because of their high animal protein.

A diet rich in acidogenic foods, such as meat, fish and cheese, but low in alkaline foods, such as fruit and vegetables, can induce endogenous acid production. The acid-forming and base-forming properties of a food cannot be judged from the actual acidity of the food itself. Organic acids like citric, oxalic, malic, tartaric and benzoic acids from fruit are processed in the upper stomach so that their net effect on body acid–base balance is more likely to be alkaline. High dietary acid load is associated with type 2 diabetes and CVD, as well as with adverse effects on bone health.

Read the following articles.

- Kiefte-de Jong, J.C. et al., 2017, 'Diet-dependent acid load and type 2 diabetes: Pooled results from three prospective cohort studies', *Diabetologia*, 60(2): 270–9
- Mazidi, M., Mikhailidis, D.P. & Banach, M., 2018, 'Higher dietary acid load is associated with higher likelihood of peripheral arterial disease among American adults', *Journal of Diabetes and its Complications*, 32(6): 565–9
- Park, Y.-M.M. et al., 2019, 'Higher diet-dependent acid load is associated with risk of breast cancer: Findings from the sister study', *International Journal of Cancer*, 144(8): 1834–43.

Answer the following questions.

- What foods contribute to higher dietary acid load?
- What are net endogenous acid production (NEAP) and potential renal acid load (PRAL)? How are they measured?
- What factors does the PRAL take into consideration that could impact on the overall dietary acid load?
- What are the potential confounders to take into consideration when exploring the association between dietary acid load and the development of disease?
- What is the take-home message from these articles regarding consumption of foods to reduce dietary acid load?

determine whether a decrease in bone density is due to smoking itself or to other risk factors common among smokers. In addition, research on the effects of smoking suggests that smoking increases the fracture risk and also has a negative impact on bone healing after fracture.

It is difficult to determine the worldwide incidence and prevalence of osteoporosis because of problems with definition and diagnosis. The most useful way of comparing osteoporosis prevalence between populations is to use fracture rates in older people. Table 33.6 summarises the strength of evidence on risk factors for osteoporotic fracture, which is considered to be the end-point outcome of osteoporosis.

Adequate dietary vitamin D intake appears to be a key factor in the prevention of post-menopausal bone loss. In addition, vitamin D deficiency can lead to decreased muscle strength and consequent increased risk of falling, thus increasing the risk of hip fracture (Karpouzos et al. 2017). However, research has repeatedly found that calcium, vitamin D, or combined calcium and vitamin D supplementation, while producing limited improvement in bone density, does not seem to confer any protective effect against fractures (Kahwati et al. 2018; Zhao et al. 2017); hence, the routine use of such supplementation is not supported by these research findings. Nevertheless, the NHMRC recommends adults aged 70 and over take 1300 mg/day of calcium for bone health and prevention of fractures (see chapters 17 and 22). Calcium and vitamin D supplementation may benefit older people living in residential aged care facilities, who are likely to have osteoporosis because of their poorer mobility, infrequent sun exposure and, perhaps, poorer diet (Duque et al. 2016).

Table 33.6: Strength of evidence on dietary factors associated with osteoporotic fractures

Strength of evidence	Risk modification	Dietary factors
Convincing evidence (in older people)	Decreased risk	Vitamin D Calcium Physical activity
	Increased risk	High alcohol intake Low body weight
Probable evidence (in older people)*	No relationship	Fluoride (at levels used to fluoridate water supplies)
Possible evidence	Decreased risk	Fruits and vegetables Moderate alcohol intake Soy products
	Increased risk	High sodium intake High protein intake* Low protein intake (in older people)
	No relationship	Phosphorus

Notes: *A meta-analysis in 2017 indicated no relationship between higher protein intake and decreased risk of osteoporotic fracture (Shams-White et al. 2017)

Source: Modified from Karpouzos et al. (2017); WHO (2003)

TEETH AND GUMS

Oral health is often viewed in isolation from the rest of the body and from general health. Dental diseases, although not life-threatening, have a detrimental effect on quality of life in childhood through to old age, having an impact on self-esteem, eating ability, nutrition and health. Despite being associated with a low mortality rate, the cost of treating dental diseases exceeds the cost of treating many other chronic diet-related diseases, including CVD, cancer and osteoporosis. In addition to being costly to treat, dental diseases cause unnecessary pain and anxiety, and eventually may lead to loss of teeth, which in turn impairs chewing function. Chewing ability allows eating a nutritious diet, the enjoyment of food, the confidence to socialise and the quality of life. Chewing function is associated with nutritional status, food selection, body composition and muscle strength in elderly populations (Semba et al. 2006). Compromised chewing ability could put the elderly at a greater mortality risk, especially in those with metabolic syndrome (Lee et al. 2010); hence, favourable oral health is associated with less CVD.

Dental caries

Minerals in the hard tissues of the teeth (enamel, dentine and cementum) are constantly undergoing processes of demineralisation and remineralisation. The demineralisation is caused by organic acids formed by bacteria in dental plaque through the anaerobic metabolism of sugars derived from diet. Saliva is saturated with calcium and phosphate at pH 7, which promotes remineralisation. When the demineralisation rate is faster than the remineralisation, net mineral loss occurs and leads to tooth decay or dental caries.

Dental caries are a major cause of tooth loss. Diet and nutrition have a direct influence on the progression of tooth decay, a communicable but preventable oral disease. Certain foods, including milk, cheese, unrefined plant foods and tea, contain factors that protect against dental caries. Milk and cheese contain calcium, phosphate and casein, all of which have anticariogenic properties. Unrefined plant foods contain phosphates and phytate, both of which are **cariostatic**. Consumption of these foods also stimulates the salivary flow, which in turn helps neutralise dental plaque acids, thus preventing dental caries development. Esters in honey, cocoa factor in chocolate, and glycyrrhizinic acid in liquorice have cariostatic properties, but the foods containing them remain **cariogenic** because of their high content of sugars (Moynihan 2000).

The cariogenic, cariostatic and anticariogenic properties of diet are primarily determined by the physical form of food (liquid, solid or sticky, slowly dissolving), nutrient composition (frequency and amount of sugar and other fermentable carbohydrates), ability to stimulate saliva, sequence of food in the meal and combinations of foods. Tooth erosion is associated with frequent consumption of acidic foods and beverages. In low-income countries, undernutrition coupled with a high intake of sugars may exacerbate the risk of caries. Erosion of the teeth due to frequent regurgitation of highly acidic stomach contents is a common finding in eating disorders such as anorexia nervosa and bulimia nervosa. Gastroesophageal reflux can also weaken tooth integrity and increase caries risk. Poor oral health

behaviour appears to be a risk indicator for high urinary sodium excretion (Han et al. 2018).

Fluoride undoubtedly protects against dental caries. Dietary fluoride principally comes from drinking water (see Chapter 17), and ingested fluoride is incorporated into enamel during tooth formation, increasing the resistance of the tooth to decay. Fluoride also repairs the damage caused by acids produced by plaque bacteria, but it does not remove the cause of caries, which is dietary sugars. Optimum exposure to fluoride and a reduction in sugar intake have an additive effect on caries prevention. Exposure to fluoride is largely responsible for an overall reduction in caries, but it does not eliminate dental caries altogether (WHO 2003).

Periodontal disease

Periodontal disease, comprising gingivitis and periodontitis, is an oral infectious disease involving inflammation and loss of bone and the supporting tissue of the teeth. The global burden of periodontal disease increased by 43 per cent from 2001 to 2016, with over 750 million people suffering from the disease (Tonetti et al. 2017). Although the pathogenesis of periodontal disease involves bacteria and the host response to these bacteria, there are local, systemic and behavioural factors that influence the severity and progression of the disease. Poor oral hygiene is the most important risk factor in the development of periodontal disease. Severe vitamin C deficiency can cause scurvy-related periodontitis. Higher serum 25-OH vitamin D is associated with a lower rate of periodontal attachment loss in adults over the age of 50 years. Some evidence suggests that periodontal disease progresses more rapidly in undernourished populations. Furthermore, malnutrition can intensify the severity of oral infections, and may eventually progress into life-threatening diseases. This emphasises the importance of diet in maintaining an adequate immune response.

Periodontal disease has been linked with a number of conditions, such as CVD, stroke and diabetes, all likely through systemic inflammatory pathways. It has been reported that those with periodontitis have increased risk of CVD (Yu et al. 2015). In addition,

COULD THE DISRUPTION OF THE ORAL MICROBIOME LEAD TO CVD AND DIABETES?

The oral cavity is inhabited by a highly diverse microbiota consisting of over 600 bacterial species. Due to its position, the composition of the oral microbiota is influenced by various factors including personal hygiene, diet and smoking. Pathogenic oral bacteria can contribute to the development of periodontal diseases such as periodontitis and gingivitis. Epidemiological studies have found that the presence of periodontal diseases is associated with coronary heart disease and diabetes.

Explore the peer-reviewed literature to answer the following question.

- What could be possible explanations for the link between the dysbiosis of oral microbiota and the development of metabolic syndrome and increased risk of CVD and diabetes? Develop a short article for the media to explain the relationship.

periodontal disease appears to be a risk factor for future cardiovascular and cerebrovascular events (Kaur & Sahota 2018).

Epidemiological and clinical research has found that periodontal disease is a risk factor for the development of rheumatoid arthritis, and changes in the oral microbiota could contribute to systemic inflammation and arthritis (Scher et al. 2014). Furthermore, it has been shown that periodontal disease is associated with adverse pregnancy outcomes, such as preterm birth, pre-eclampsia, preterm pre-labour rupture of the membranes and pregnancy loss; however, treatment of periodontal disease during pregnancy is unlikely to prevent or reduce the risk of preterm birth or low birthweight, or maternal morbidity and mortality (Daalderop et al. 2018; Iheozor-Ejiofor et al. 2017).

SUMMARY

- A biodiverse diet combined with regular physical activity while being socially active in ecologically favourable conditions is relatively organ-protective.
- A plant-based dietary pattern with biologically varied sources of dietary fats and other food components characterised by fruit, nuts and vegetables can aid prevention and management of CVD. Being less sedentary and more physically active is associated with better heart and blood vessel, muscle and bone health.
- A diet with little biodiversity, poor vitamin D status and excess sodium, genetic factors, menstrual status, low physical activity, limited exposure to sunlight, cigarette smoking, excessive alcohol consumption and certain medications are all risk factors for developing osteoporosis.
- A good diet is essential for the development and maintenance of healthy teeth, and healthy teeth in turn are important in enabling the consumption of a varied and healthy diet throughout the life-course.

- Dental caries and periodontal disease each contribute to tooth loss and chewing difficulty throughout life; oral hygiene, a relatively unrefined diet and, probably, an optimal fluoride intake reduce the risk of tooth loss and chewing disability.
- Dietary patterns favourable to one organ are, in general, favourable to others. Exceptions which require particular attention are (a) iodine and thyroid and iodine deficiency disorders, and (b) protein intake and quality to which the kidney is susceptible, but where lower intakes are possible with high-quality protein—a conclusion supported by studies in vegetarians and where fish consumption is preferred.

KEY TERMS

Aneurysm: a weak spot in an artery that bulges out, causing a bubble or balloon. They can occur in any artery and commonly occur in the heart (aortic), brain or in the aorta within the abdomen.

Cariogenic: contributing to tooth decay. Anticariogenic compounds or foods promote and protect remineralisation.

Cariostatic: preventing or retarding the formation and progression of dental caries.

Femoral neck: a short section of the femur (thigh bone) that joins the long shaft of the bone to the ball-like protrusion that fits into the hip socket. The femoral neck has a larger percentage of soft bone than the rest of the femur, making it more vulnerable to fracturing.

Haematopoietic: relating to the bodily system of organs and tissues involved in the production of cellular blood components, such as red and white blood cells. The system includes the bone marrow, spleen, thymus and lymph nodes.

Osteoblasts: cells that synthesise the organic matrix of bone in the bone-formation process.

Osteoclasts: cells that break down bone tissues by secreting acid and collagenase enzyme in the bone resorption process.

REFERENCES

Australian Government, 2016, *Food and Health Dialogue,* <www.health.gov.au/internet/main/publishing.nsf/Content/fhd>, accessed 22 January 2019

Calle, E.E., Thun, M.J., Petrelli, J.M., Rodriguez, C. & Heath Jr, C.W., 1999, 'Body-mass index and mortality in a prospective cohort of US adults', *New England Journal of Medicine, 341*(15): 1097–105, doi:10.1056/NEJM199910073411501

Daalderop, L., Wieland, B., Tomsin, K., Reyes, L., Kramer, B. et al., 2018, 'Periodontal disease and pregnancy outcomes: Overview of systematic reviews', *JDR Clinical & Translational Research, 3*(1): 10–27, doi:10.1177/2380084417731097

Dagenais, G.R., Yi, Q., Mann, J.F., Bosch, J., Pogue, J. et al., 2005, 'Prognostic impact of body weight and abdominal obesity in women and men with cardiovascular disease', *American Heart Journal, 149*(1): 54–60, doi:10.1016/j.ahj.2004.07.009

Dhillon, R.J. & Hasni, S., 2017, 'Pathogenesis and management of sarcopenia', *Clinics in Geriatric Medicine, 33*(1): 17–26, doi:10.1016/j.cger.2016.08.002

Duque, G., Lord, S.R., Mak, J., Ganda, K., Close, J.J.T. et al., 2016, 'Treatment of osteoporosis in Australian residential aged care facilities: Update on consensus recommendations for fracture prevention', *Journal of the American Medical Directors Association, 17*(9): 852–9, doi:10.1016/j.jamda.2016.05.011

European Heart Network, 2011, *Diet, Physical Activity and Cardiovascular Disease Prevention in Europe*, <www.ehnheart.org/publications-and-papers/publications/521:diet-physical-activity-and-cardiovascular-disease-prevention.html>, accessed 22 January 2019

Fan, H., Li, X., Zheng, L., Chen, X., Wu, H. et al., 2016, 'Abdominal obesity is strongly associated with cardiovascular disease and its risk factors in elderly and very elderly community-dwelling Chinese', *Scientific Reports, 6*: 21521, doi:10.1038/srep21521

Farshidfar, F., Shulgina, V. & Myrie, S.B., 2015, 'Nutritional supplements and administration considerations for sarcopenia in older adults', *Nutrition and Aging, 3*: 147–70, doi:10.3233/NUA-150057

Faulkner, J.A., Larkin, L.M., Claflin, D.R. & Brooks, S.V., 2007, 'Age-related changes in the structure and function of skeletal muscles', *Clinical and Experimental Pharmacology and Physiology, 34*(11): 1091–6, doi:10.1111/j.1440-1681.2007.04752.x

Foyer, C.H., Lam, H.-M., Nguyen, H.T., Siddique, K.H., Varshney, R.K. et al., 2016, 'Neglecting legumes has compromised human health and sustainable food production', *Nature Plants, 2*(8): 16112, doi:10.1038/nplants.2016.112

Gersh, B.J., Sliwa, K., Mayosi, B.M. & Yusuf, S., 2010, 'The epidemic of cardiovascular disease in the developing world: Global implications', *European Heart Journal, 31*(6): 642–8, doi:10.1093/eurheartj/ehq030

Han, K., Kim, N., Ko, Y., Park, Y.-G. & Park, J.-B., 2018, 'Oral health behavior as a risk factor for high urinary sodium among Korean women', *Asia Pacific Journal of Clinical Nutrition, 27*(3): 671-80, doi:10.6133/apjcn.012018.01

Heaney, R.P., 1987, 'The role of nutrition in prevention and management of osteoporosis', *Clinical Obstetrics and Gynecology, 30*(4): 833–46, doi: 10.1097/00003081-198712000-00007

Iheozor-Ejiofor, Z., Middleton, P., Esposito, M. & Glenny, A.M., 2017, 'Treating periodontal disease for preventing adverse birth outcomes in pregnant women', *Cochrane Database of Systematic Reviews, 6*:1–84, doi:10.1002/14651858.CD005297.pub3

Jike, M., Itani, O., Watanabe, N., Buysse, D.J. & Kaneita, Y., 2018, 'Long sleep duration and health outcomes: A systematic review, meta-analysis and meta-regression', *Sleep Medicine Reviews, 39*: 25–36, doi:10.1016/j.smrv.2017.06.011

Juonala, M., Magnussen, C.G., Berenson, G.S., Venn, A., Burns, T.L. et al., 2011, 'Childhood adiposity, adult adiposity, and cardiovascular risk factors', *New England Journal of Medicine, 365*(20): 1876–85, doi:10.1056/NEJMoa1010112

Kahwati, L.C., Weber, R.P., Pan, H., Gourlay, M., LeBlanc, E. et al., 2018, 'Vitamin D, calcium, or combined supplementation for the primary prevention of fractures in community-dwelling adults: Evidence report and systematic review for the US Preventive Services Task Force', *JAMA, 319*(15): 1600–12, doi:10.1001/jama.2017.21640

Karpouzos, A., Diamantis, E., Farmaki, P., Savvanis, S. & Troupis, T., 2017, 'Nutritional aspects of bone health and fracture healing', *Journal of Osteoporosis, 2017*(4218472): 1–10, doi:10.1155/2017/4218472

Kaur, M. & Sahota, J.K., 2018, 'Co-relation between periodontitis and cardiovascular disorders: A review', *Journal of Advanced Medical and Dental Sciences Research, 6*(4): 46–9, doi:10.21276/jamdsr

Kiefte-de Jong, J.C., Li, Y., Chen, M., Curhan, G.C., Mattei, J. et al., 2017, 'Diet-dependent acid load and type 2 diabetes: Pooled results from three prospective cohort studies', *Diabetologia, 60*(2): 270–9, doi:10.1007/s00125-016-4153-7

Lee, M.S., Huang, Y.C. & Wahlqvist, M.L., 2010, 'Chewing ability in conjunction with food intake and energy status in later life affects survival in Taiwanese with the metabolic syndrome', *Journal of the American Geriatrics Society, 58*(6): 1072–80, doi:10.1111/j.1532-5415.2010.02870.x

Liao, C.-D., Lee, P.-H., Hsiao, D.-J., Huang, S.-W., Tsauo, J.-Y. et al., 2018, 'Effects of protein supplementation combined with exercise intervention on frailty indices, body composition, and physical function in frail older adults', *Nutrients, 10*(12): 1916, doi:10.3390/nu10121916

Mazidi, M., Mikhailidis, D.P. & Banach, M., 2018, 'Higher dietary acid load is associated with higher likelihood of peripheral arterial disease among American adults', *Journal of Diabetes and its Complications, 32*(6): 565–9, doi:10.1016/j.jdiacomp.2018.03.001

Moynihan, P., 2000, 'Foods and factors that protect against dental caries', *Nutrition Bulletin, 25*(4): 281–6, doi:10.1046/j.1467-3010.2000.00033.x

Mozaffarian, D. & Ludwig, D.S., 2010, 'Dietary guidelines in the 21st century: A time for food', *JAMA, 304*(6): 681–2, doi:10.1001/jama.2010.1116

Park, Y.-M.M., Steck, S.E., Fung, T.T., Merchant, A.T., Elizabeth Hodgson, M. et al., 2019, 'Higher diet-dependent acid load is associated with risk of breast cancer: Findings from the sister study', *International Journal of Cancer, 144*(8): 1834–43, doi:10.1002/ijc.31889

Pearson, D.A., 2007, 'Bone health and osteoporosis: the role of vitamin K and potential antagonism by anticoagulants', *Nutrition in Clinical Practice, 22*(5): 517–44, doi:10.1177/0115426507022005517

Piepoli, M.F., Hoes, A.W., Agewall, S., Albus, C., Brotons, C. et al., 2016, '2016 European guidelines on cardiovascular disease prevention in clinical practice', *European Heart Journal, 37*(29): 2315–81, doi:10.1093/eurheartj/ehw106

Rafieian-Kopaei, M., Setorki, M., Doudi, M., Baradaran, A. & Nasri, H., 2014, 'Atherosclerosis: Process, indicators, risk factors and new hopes', *International Journal of Preventive Medicine, 5*(8): 927–46, <https://core.ac.uk/download/pdf/143841435.pdf>, accessed 22 January 2019

Richter, C., Skulas-Ray, A. & Kris-Etherton, P., 2017, 'The role of diet in the prevention and treatment of cardiovascular disease', in A.M. Coulston, C.J. Boushey, M. Ferruzzi & L. Delahanty (eds), *Nutrition in the Prevention and Treatment of Disease* (4th edn), Oxford: Elsevier, pp. 595–623

Robinson, S.M., Reginster, J.Y., Rizzoli, R., Shaw, S.C., Kanis, J.A. et al., 2017, 'Does nutrition play a role in the prevention and management of sarcopenia?', *Clinical Nutrition, 37*: 1121–32, doi:10.1016/j.clnu.2017.08.016

Rose, G., 2001, 'Sick individuals and sick populations', *International Journal of Epidemiology, 30*(3): 427–32, doi:10.1093/ije/30.3.427

Scher, J.U., Bretz, W.A., & Abramson, S.B., 2014, 'Periodontal disease and subgingival microbiota as contributors for rheumatoid arthritis pathogenesis: Modifiable risk factors?', *Current Opinion in Theumatology, 26*(4), 424–9, doi:10.1097/BOR.0000000000000076

Schulze, M.B., Martínez-González, M.A., Fung, T.T., Lichtenstein, A.H. & Forouhi, N.G., 2018, 'Food based dietary patterns and chronic disease prevention', *BMJ, 361*: K2396, doi:10.1136/bmj.k2396

Semba, R., Blaum, C., Bartali, B. & Xue, Q., 2006, 'Denture use, malnutrition, frailty, and mortality among older women living in the community', *Journal of Nutrition, Health & Aging, 10*(2): 161–7, <www.ncbi.nlm.nih.gov/pubmed/16554954>, accessed 22 January 2019

Shams-White, M.M., Chung, M., Du, M., Fu, Z., Insogna, K.L. et al., 2017, 'Dietary protein and bone health: A systematic review and meta-analysis from the National Osteoporosis Foundation', *American Journal of Clinical Nutrition, 105*(6): 1528–43, doi:10.3945/ajcn.116.145110

Tonetti, M.S., Jepsen, S., Jin, L. & Otomo-Corgel, J., 2017, 'Impact of the global burden of periodontal diseases on health, nutrition and wellbeing of mankind: A call for global action', *Journal of Clinical Periodontology, 44*(5): 456–62, doi:10.1111/jcpe.12732

US Department of Health and Human Services & US Department of Agriculture, 2015, *2015—2020 Dietary Guidelines for Americans,* <https://health.gov/dietaryguidelines/2015/guidelines/>, accessed 22 January 2019

Wahlqvist, M.L., 2016, 'Future food', *Asia Pacific Journal of Clinical Nutrition, 25*(4): 706–15, doi:10.6133/apjcn.092016.01

WHO, 2003, *Diet, Nutrition and the Prevention of Chronic Diseases. Report of the Joint WHO/FAO Expert Consultation,* <www.who.int/dietphysicalactivity/publications/trs916/summary/en/>, accessed 22 January 2019

—— 2007, *WHO Scientific Group on the Assessment of Osteoporosis at the Primary Health Care Level, Brussels 5–7 May 2004,* <www.who.int/chp/topics/Osteoporosis.pdf>, accessed 22 January 2019

Willett, W., Rockström, J., Loken, B., Springmann, M., Lang, T. et al., 2019, 'Food in the Anthropocene: The EAT–Lancet Commission on healthy diets from sustainable food systems', *Lancet, 393*(10170): 447–92, doi:10.1016/S0140-6736(18)31788-4

Yarasheski, K.E., 2003, 'Exercise, aging, and muscle protein metabolism', *Journals of Gerontology Series A: Biological Sciences and Medical Sciences, 58*(10): M918–22, doi:10.1093/gerona/58.10.M918

Yu, Y.H., Chasman, D.I., Buring, J.E., Rose, L. & Ridker, P.M., 2015, 'Cardiovascular risks associated with incident and prevalent periodontal disease', *Journal of Clinical Periodontology, 42*(1): 21–8, doi:10.1111/jcpe.12335

Zhao, J.-G., Zeng, X.-T., Wang, J. & Liu, L., 2017, 'Association between calcium or vitamin d supplementation and fracture incidence in community-dwelling older adults: A systematic review and meta-analysis', *JAMA, 318*(24): 2466–82, doi:10.1001/jama.2017.19344

{CHAPTER 34}
MENTAL HEALTH DISORDERS

Mark L. Wahlqvist and Naiyana Wattanapenpaiboon

OBJECTIVES

- Explore the effects of food and food patterns on cognitive function.
- Recognise the relationship between diet and psychological outcomes.
- Identify the impact of stress on eating behaviours.
- Discuss how the mind can be affected by food.

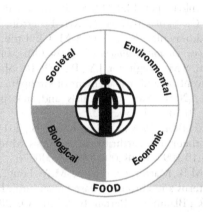

INTRODUCTION

The human brain has high energy and nutrient needs. Intakes of energy and several different nutrients affect levels of neurotransmitters in the brain, and therefore have an impact on mental health. For proper physiological and psychological functioning, the human brain and nervous system require specific dietary nutrients, such as essential fatty acids, amino acids, vitamins and minerals. Changes in energy or nutrient intake can alter both brain chemistry and the functioning of nerves in the brain. Deficiencies or excesses of certain vitamins or minerals can damage nerves in the brain, causing changes in memory, limiting problem-solving ability and impairing brain function. Often, deficiencies of multiple nutrients, rather than a single nutrient, are responsible for changes in brain functioning.

There is evidence that people who eat more fruit and vegetables have better mental health (Conner et al. 2017; Jacka et al. 2011, 2017). Deficiency of certain micronutrients can result in changes in mental function that precede overt deficiency diseases. Individuals suffering from various mental disorders, such as **attention deficit hyperactivity disorder** and **bipolar disorder**, as well as stress, have shown significant improvement in their symptoms, including improved or stabilised mood, following supplementation with vitamins and minerals (Rucklidge et al. 2011). Even healthy individuals exhibited improved mental functioning and mood following this supplementation (Kennedy et al. 2010). Thus, it is likely that mood symptoms are associated with nutrient inadequacy.

COGNITIVE FUNCTION

Age-associated cognitive decline has many aspects and stages. At its earliest and least consequential, minor memory impairment may be experienced, while at the other extreme **dementia** can be personally and socially devastating. The central nervous system requires a constant supply of glucose, and adequate brain function and maintenance depend on almost all essential nutrients. There are candidate food-based strategies that may minimise cognitive impairment.

There is little evidence that the macronutrient profile of the diet alters the risk for cognitive impairment, except that glycaemic load and insulin resistance may affect glucose handling in the brain. n-3 fatty acids contribute to **neuronal plasticity** and integrity, so they could enhance learning and cognition. Neuroprotection may be provided by vitamins B-6, folate and B-12; conversely, zinc may have adverse effects in vulnerable individuals, as in the elderly. Those nutrients that lower serum homocysteine may decrease the risk of cognitive impairment, and these may include n-3 fatty acids (de Jager et al. 2012; Huang et al. 2010; Luchtman & Song 2013; Tassoni et al. 2008; Wang et al. 2018). Foods containing the carotenoids lutein and zeaxanthin, such as marigold flowers, corn, eggs and goji (wolfberries), may also be neuroprotective (Bovier et al. 2014). Owing to its anti-inflammatory properties, a polyphenolic compound in turmeric called curcumin could enhance cognitive function (Lee et al. 2014). Dietary diversity may enhance survival by improving cognitive function in a variety of ways (Chen et al. 2011). Regular physical activity improves cognition with advancing years.

ALZHEIMER'S DISEASE

Alzheimer's disease (AD) is a premature neuro-degenerative disease of the brain which has now become a leading cause of morbidity among older people and of premature death globally (see Chapter 22). The underlying contributions to AD and interventions are outlined in Figure 34.1.

A high prevalence of AD is associated with low fish consumption (Morris et al. 2003) as well as with high dietary fat and total energy intakes. n-3 fatty acids are important in the structural components of neurones and play a role in the formation of

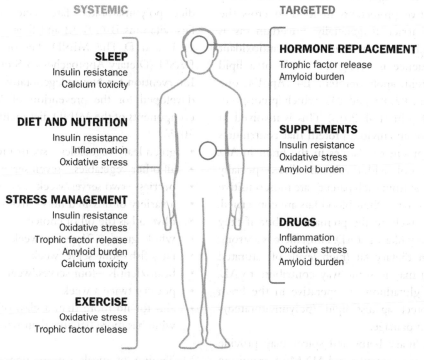

Figure 34.1: Modalities of Alzheimer's disease prevention

Source: © 2018 Schelke, Attia, Palenchar, Kaplan, Mureb et al. (2018), <www.frontiersin.org/articles/10.3389/fnagi.2018.00096/full>. Creative Commons Attribution License (CC BY) 4.0.

neurotransmitters; therefore, the consumption of fish, which is a valuable source of n-3 fatty acids, may be favourable for brain function. However, a review in 2018 indicates that supplementation with n-3 fatty acids may be beneficial with disease onset or in mild AD but not in those with severe cognitive dysfunction (Canhada et al. 2018). Vitamin D and folic acid could affect memory function in later life because they may exert an influence on brain protein synthesis. Vitamin K2, or menaquinones, appears to modulate the calcium balance in cells and cell proliferation in tissues such as the brain. It is thought that it may be important for brain function and could help protect against AD. Excessive ingestion of dietary aluminium is no longer believed to cause AD; however zinc supplements may increase the development of AD.

Free radicals are believed to be involved in the ageing processes in the brain that lead to memory impairment. Experimental evidence suggests that antioxidants, such as vitamin E, may play a role in brain ageing and possibly the prevention of progressive cognitive impairment. However, the ability of these putative protectants in food to cross the blood–brain barrier is generally uncertain, as is the relative advantage of oxidant and antioxidant activities. Evidence is strong for a role of a lipid transport protein, apolipoprotein E4 (ApoE4, one of three alleles, ε2, ε3 and ε4), which predisposes people to AD (Liu et al. 2013). This is involved in the transport of an amyloid protein that contributes to the development of plaques in the brain in AD. Interestingly, people with the ApoE4 allele, especially ε4/ε4 (one gene from each parent), are most sensitive to dietary fat as far as their blood fats are concerned. They are also likely to die prematurely but, if they survive, will very likely get AD. Thus, there is a strong possibility that dietary fat (high levels of saturated and trans fats) may in some way contribute to AD. Furthermore, glutathione is operative in the brain and may protect against lipid (polyunsaturated)-mediated brain damage.

Certain culinary herbs and spices may provide protection against dementia and AD. Most promising are turmeric (Lee et al. 2014; Mishra & Palanivelu 2008) and cinnamon (Wahlqvist et al. 2016), which appear to improve working memory. The mechanism(s) of this property is uncertain, but could involve mitochondrial function and energy regulation, or neurotransmission and protein-folding disorders. Herbal compounds, such as *Ginkgo biloba* extract, have received attention as a cognitive enhancer, but the mechanism of action, if any, in the central nervous system is poorly understood; there may be a synergistic action of three ginkgo constituents, the flavonoids, terpenoids and organic acids.

Dietary and eating patterns

In contrast to intake of specific nutrients, emerging evidence suggests that dietary patterns, particularly Mediterranean diet and the Dietary Approaches to Stop Hypertension (DASH) diet, may be important for cognitive health (Smith & Blumenthal 2016; van de Rest et al. 2015). Both diets are associated with lower rates of dementia, and the DASH diet and energy restriction diet may improve cognitive functioning.

Protective factors include a Mediterranean diet, polyunsaturated fatty acids and fish-related fats, vitamins B-6, B-12 and folate, and vitamins A, C, E and D. The MIND diet or Mediterranean-DASH (Dietary Approaches to Stop Hypertension) Intervention for Neurodegenerative Delay has been developed for the prevention of AD. The dietary components of the MIND diet include (Morris et al. 2015):

- green leafy vegetables—six or more serves/week
- all other vegetables—seven serves/week
- berries—two serves/week
- a variety of unsalted nuts—five serves/week
- olive oil as the oil of choice
- whole grains—21 serves/week
- fatty fish—one serve/week
- beans/lentils—four serves/week
- poultry twice a week
- aim for no more than a glass of wine daily; red wine has more benefits than white.

Timing of meals can influence the effects of food on cognitive behaviour. Experimental evidence suggests that skipping breakfast, which may decrease

WHAT ARE THE KEY NUTRITION CHANGES TO PREVENT DEMENTIA?

Review this chapter and the relevant peer-reviewed literature to answer the following questions.

- In Australia and New Zealand, what are the key nutrition changes that need to occur in order to prevent dementia?
- How affordable are these changes for those on low incomes?
- What do you think are the key barriers to implementation?
- Is fortification of bread with folate and iodine making a contribution?
- Are there any other measures that should be taken?

the overall availability of glucose to the brain, can lead to temporary impairment of cognitive performance. It is generally accepted that missing breakfast will adversely impact on cognition and, in particular, on the earlier cognitive processes, such as early decoding in working memory (Benton & Parker 1998; González-Garrido et al. 2019). Afternoon snacks may also have positive effects on cognitive performance.

There is evidence that periodontal disease and the oral microbiota associated with it, particularly *Porphyromonas gingivalis*, increases the risk of AD and is found in the brains of such patients (Dominy et al. 2019; Singhrao et al. 2015). Thus, dental hygiene may also help to prevent dementia.

Possible relationship(s) of food with the 'mind'?

The mind is said to comprise cognitive functions like consciousness, thought, memory, judgement, perception and communication (Pinker 1999). It is therefore dependent on brain function; much more than that, however, the mind enables us to have an

identity and to be mentally connected to others and our environment. Study of the mind is the province of biologists, philosophers, ecologists and others, who have generally struggled with the question of how integrated the mind is with the body, and how socioecologically dependent it is. The mind requires consciousness and awareness—which could, and at best should, embrace all aspects of nature and the environment, including health and food systems (Williams 2017) (see also Chapter 30). Inasmuch as the mind reflects brain health and function, it depends on multiple sensory and other informational inputs, in some measure processed by the gut microbiome (Cryan & O'Mahony 2011; Ghaisas et al. 2016).

Nutritional biology allows for how organs other than the brain could be integral to our mind. These organs include the highly innervated gut connected to the brain, together with its microbiome; our sensory input apparatus; and the musculoskeletal system that moves us within and between environments. Should the underpinning nutritional biology be dysfunctional, our mind and the mental health dependent on it may suffer and our quality of life with it.

By analogy with the health of the body, mental health (or mental fitness) can be metaphorically referred to as a state of health of the mind or the way we think and feel, our mood and capacity for learning. Good mental health and a favourable state of mind depend not only on the absence of neuropsychological illness, such as dementia, depression and anxiety, but also on our socioecological connections. Mechanistically, nutritional biology, which encompasses homeostasis, energetics, gene interactions, microbiomics, gut physiology, sensory nutrition, and the modulation of inflammation, can be brought to bear on how the mind may be influenced by food systems.

MOOD AND EMOTIONS

The most common link between food and mood is the daily cue that hunger provides for food ingestion. Unmet hunger is globally the most pervasive human disorder, usually dependent on poverty, socioeconomic inequity, natural disaster or conflict (see chapters 26 and 27). Where access to food is not limiting, food intake patterns may still contribute to neuropsychological disorder. Higher consumption of fruit and vegetables is correlated with several more favourable psychological outcomes, including less depression and anxiety, greater happiness, higher life

satisfaction, being more energetic and greater social–emotional wellbeing (Conner et al. 2017).

The relationship between sleep, mood and food is complex and not fully elucidated, although it is almost certainly bidirectional and probably a vicious circle (Opie et al. 2015). Most commonly, if a person is deprived of sleep, they tend to become more irritable, angry, more prone to stress, and less energised throughout the day; disordered eating tends to follow. Even partial sleep deprivation has a significant effect on mood; feeling more stress, anger, sadness and mental exhaustion have been reported. Restricted sleep time affects many different aspects of waking cognitive performance, but especially behavioural alertness. Sleep deprivation increases behavioural lapses during performance, which are assumed to reflect **microsleep**s. The converse, where food intake disrupts circadian (day–night) rhythm, can instigate or exacerbate sleep and mood disorders (Huang et al. 2011; Opie et al. 2015) (see also the section 'Sleep' in Chapter 31).

DEPRESSION

Depression is a leading contributor to disease burden and a major contributor to disability, with a global prevalence of 4 per cent in men and 7 per cent in women (Steel et al. 2014; Vos et al. 2017). Weight loss and weight gain are both associated with depression. Weight gain and obesity in depression can be mediated by emotional eating (Chiang et al. 2013; van Strien et al. 2016), while weight loss is associated with loss of appetite and loss of interest in surroundings and social relationships. Typically, anorexia is manifested by loss of interest in eating and its associated pleasure. The risk of being depressed is rising rapidly; the reasons for this are unknown, although many hypotheses have been proposed. These include the increasing prevalence of obesity and chronic conditions, and increased screen time disrupting circadian rhythms, sleep patterns and diet. It has been suggested that dietary factors could account for some of the variation in prevalence of major depression between countries.

A 2018 review of dietary indices and depression

SLEEP, FOOD AND MOOD

Keep a seven-day diary noting down your mood at least three times a day (you can go on the internet to find a wide range of diaries). Your mood could be one of those listed in Table 34.1. Also note the number of hours sleep you had, any other activities and what you had been eating. Make a particular note of your mood after physical activity, meditation, a big meal, or any period of fasting.

Table 34.1: Adjectives for moods

Positive expression	Negative expression
Joyful	Sad
Happy	Lonely
Relaxed	Depressed
Silly	Insecure
Content	Numb
Great	Sick
Productive	Tired
Energetic	Lazy
Active	Unmotivated
Motivated	Bored
Alive	Dull
Average	Uneventful
Normal	Angry
Good	Anxious
	Frustrated
	Annoyed
	Grumpy

Reflect on how food and physical activity alter your moods.

has shown that the Mediterranean dietary pattern and a lower Dietary Inflammatory Index score (see below) are associated with lower depression incidence (Lassale et al. 2018). Evidence suggests that there are abnormalities of fatty acid and eicosanoid metabolism in depression. In a transnational ecological study of about 170,000 people, a strong relationship was found between apparently high fish consumption and lower prevalence of depression (Hibbeln & Salem 1995) (Figure 34.2).

In terms of fatty acids, the most consistent observations link depression to low blood concentrations of both n–3 and n–6 PUFAs. One particularly striking observation is that plasma concentrations of total long-chain PUFAs are strongly positively related to cerebrospinal fluid 5-hydroxyindolactic acid, the main metabolite of serotonin, which is a neurotransmitter involved in mood control. Fish consumption is associated with high self-reported

mental health status (Silvers & Scott 2007). Moreover, a higher concentration of DHA in breastmilk and greater seafood consumption can both predict lower prevalence of postpartum depression (Hibbeln 2002). These studies therefore emphasise the importance of long-chain PUFAs (both n–3 and n–6) in modulation of mood.

It is of interest that depression is associated with a wide range of other diseases where development may partly be affected by fatty acid requirements and metabolism, including CVD, diabetes, multiple sclerosis, cancer and osteoporosis. Chronic excessive alcohol consumption depletes DHA from the membranes of neurones, and may contribute to the secondary depression seen with alcohol excess. DHA deficiency may be associated with susceptibility to multiple sclerosis, and with the high incidence of depression in patients with multiple sclerosis (Hibbeln & Salem 1995). Some of the interactions

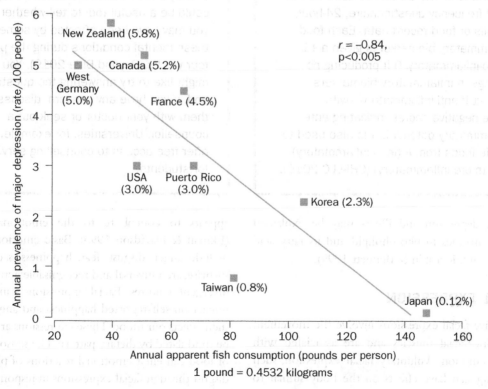

Figure 34.2: Transnational comparison of fish consumption and prevalence of depression

Source: Hibbeln (1998). Reproduced with permission from Elsevier

THE DIETARY INFLAMMATORY INDEX (DII)

The DII is a validated measure of the inflammatory potential of a diet (Hébert et al. 2019). There is evidence that inflammation plays a pivotal role in the development of depression and that people with a confirmed depression diagnosis have elevated inflammatory markers such as C-reactive protein, interleukin-6 and tumour necrosis factor (Köhler et al. 2017; Köhler et al. 2018; Shivappa et al. 2018). The development of the DII, described by Shivappa and colleagues (2013), included 45 food and nutrient parameters. The DII can be used with a food frequency questionnaire, 24-hour recalls or food record data. Each food inflammatory biomarker is given a +1 if pro-inflammatory, 0 if producing no change in inflammatory biomarkers and −1 if anti-inflammatory—with more negative scores indicating anti-inflammatory potential. It is also used to grade foods from A (less inflammatory) to F (more inflammatory) (CHI-LLC 2019).

HAVE YOU EXPERIENCED DEPRESSION AND/OR ANXIETY?

Beyond Blue (www.beyondblue.org.au) is an independent organisation working with various community organisations to address issues associated with depression, anxiety, suicide and other related mental disorders (Beyond Blue 2019). The Black Dog Institute (www.blackdoginstitute.org.au) is another organisation committed to understanding, preventing and treating mental illness (Black Dog Institute 2019).

The 'Anxiety and depression checklist' (www.beyondblue.org.au/the-facts/anxiety-and-depression-checklist-k10) could be a useful tool to tell whether you may have been affected by some of these mental conditions during the past four weeks (Beyond Blue 2019). You might like to try answering the questions and, if you have any concern, discuss them with your doctor or seek out a counsellor. Universities, for example, offer free access to counselling services for students.

between depression and illness may be explained by abnormalities in phospholipid and its fatty acid metabolism (Horrobin & Bennett 1999).

FACIAL EXPRESSION

Distinctive facial expressions involve the movement of specific facial muscles and are associated with specific emotions. Voluntary facial expression, such as smiling, can have effects on the body similar to those resulting from the actual emotion, such as happiness; sensory feedback from the expression appears to contribute to the emotional feeling (Ekman & Davidson 1993). Basic emotions, which include anger, disgust, fear, happiness, sadness and surprise, are universal and recognisable across widely divergent cultures. Facial expressions can have an impact on self-reported happiness and anger, which then affects our mood. These expressions are likely to be modulated by dietary pattern. The sensory aspects of food can elicit emotional reactions of pleasure or disgust through facial expressions in response to taste and smell stimulation (Steiner 1979).

Environmental factors, including food, are

believed to play a role in the development and function of our facial features and structure (González-José et al. 2005). Chewing is one way in which this occurs (Grünheid et al. 2009). Thus, directly and indirectly through how we feel, our diet can affect facial expression in subtle and complex ways—and this can begin even *in utero* (Mennella et al. 2001).

STRESS

Stress has been implicated as a primary trigger of overeating. The hormonal pathway that controls the endocrine response to stress is the hypothalamic–pituitary–adrenal (HPA) axis. Increased serum cortisol concentrations, which is an outcome of stress-induced activation of the HPA system, is often used as an indicator of stress. Cortisol secretion has been implicated as a potential mediator for increased energy intake in humans (Roberts 2008). Higher basal cortisol concentrations, as the result of excessive HPA responses to stress, have been observed in women with eating disorders, such as anorexia nervosa, bulimia nervosa and binge-eating disorder.

Stress is associated with both psychological and biological adaptation. Chronic stress, however, impairs adaptation and may consequently lead to illness. Stress may affect health not only through its direct biological effects but also through changes in health behaviours, one of which is food choice. Research suggests that stress may compromise the health of susceptible individuals through deleterious stress-related changes in food choice (Oliver et al.

2000). Individuals with a BMI on the higher side of 'healthy' are reported to be more vulnerable to gain weight under chronic stress, compared to those with lower BMI (Roberts 2008). It is possible that restrained eaters are particularly vulnerable to adverse effects of stress on health, through influences on food intake (Wardle et al. 2000). Stress can also increase snacking behaviour, and food choice is shifted from meal-type foods, such as meat, fish, fruit and vegetables, towards snack-type foods (Oliver & Wardle 1999). Overconsumption of these 'comfort foods', which are high in fat and carbohydrate, may be stimulated by cortisol in response to stress and can result in abdominal obesity. Persistently elevated levels of cortisol can promote insulin resistance, and in turn activate abdominal fat storage.

Experimental studies have demonstrated that psychological stress causes oxidative damage by reducing DNA repair and inhibiting radiation-induced apoptosis in human blood cells. Oxidative stress may persist during psychological stress and may increase the propensity of a pathological development damage (Møller et al. 1996). Research suggests that phytonutrients, such as carotenoids, flavonoids and organic sulphides, have the potential to modulate stress. β-carotene is reported to suppress the secretion of corticotropin-releasing hormone, subsequently inhibiting the stimulation of adrenaline and noradrenaline secretion. In addition, the gut microbiota has been implicated in a variety of stress-related conditions, including anxiety and depression, through the gut–brain axis (Farzi et al. 2018; Foster & Neufeld 2013; Foster et al. 2017; Liew et al. 2015).

STRESS AND THE STRESS CASCADE

Stress causes disruptions in homeostasis and leads to the activation of two systems, the hypothalamic–pituitary–adrenal (HPA) axis and the sympathetic nervous system (SNS) (Figure 34.3). Stressor-induced activation of the HPA axis and the SNS results in a series of neural and endocrine adaptations known as the stress response or stress cascade. The stress cascade is responsible for allowing the body to make the physiological and metabolic changes required to cope with the demands of a homeostatic challenge.

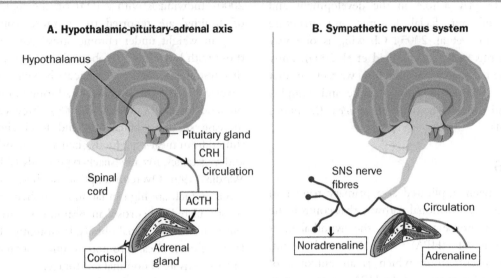

A. Hypothalamic-pituitary-adrenal axis

Hypothalamus

Pituitary gland

CRH

Circulation

Spinal cord

ACTH

Cortisol

Adrenal gland

B. Sympathetic nervous system

SNS nerve fibres

Circulation

Noradrenaline

Adrenaline

Notes: CRH = corticotropin-releasing hormone; ACTH = adrenocorticotropic hormone

Figure 34.3: The hypothalamic–pituitary–adrenal (HPA) axis, sympathetic nervous system (SNS) and stress

The HPA axis comprises three organs—the hypothalamus, pituitary gland and adrenal glands—and the feedback interactions among the glands, hormones and parts of the brain. During times of stress, the ultimate result of its activation is to increase blood cortisol. Cortisol has an important role in releasing glucose into the bloodstream in order to facilitate the 'flight or fight' response.

The activation process of HPA axis is initiated by the hypothalamic release of corticotropin-releasing hormone (CRH), also known as corticotropin-releasing factor. CRH binds to its receptors on the anterior pituitary gland, causing it to release adrenocorticotropic hormone (ACTH). The ACTH in turn binds to receptors on the adrenal cortex, resulting in the release of cortisol.

Another important hormone released by the pituitary gland along with ACTH is β-endorphin, a morphine-like hormone. ACTH and β-endorphin are similar in structure and are released together in response to CRH stimulation by the hypothalamus. Endorphins are thought to be important in reducing pain during times of stress.

In response to stressors, CRH and ACTH are released in short pulses, each of which causes a sustained release of cortisol from the adrenal cortex, which could last for several hours after encountering the stressor. At a certain blood concentration of cortisol, this protection is ostensibly achieved and the cortisol exerts negative feedback to the hypothalamic release of CRH and to the pituitary release of ACTH. At this point, systemic homeostasis returns. Positive and negative feedback occurs to ensure that cortisol production stays within certain bounds, depending on the requirements and stress levels in that particular situation. The HPA axis has been reported to be involved in a number of mental health disorders, including mood disorders and affective disorders (unipolar and bipolar).

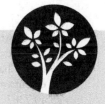

SUMMARY

- Although a number of food components are candidates for neuroprotection, their ability to do so effectively and safely is likely to be dependent on a background biodiverse diet and being physically active.
- Mental health is a growing concern in ageing populations and is becoming a major contributor to the burden of disease and mortality and healthcare system viability.
- Stress could compromise the health of susceptible individuals through deleterious stress-related changes in food choice.
- A healthy state of mind requires a functional brain and a connectedness with nature as a provider of food and health.
- The optimisation of the association between mind, brain and environment (including its food and health systems) could allow communities to achieve more favourable socioeconomic outcomes.

KEY TERMS

Attention deficit hyperactivity disorder (ADHD): is the most commonly diagnosed mental disorder in children. Children with ADHD may have difficulty concentrating or paying attention, or be unable to control their impulses and hyperactive (constantly restless and fidgeting).

Bipolar disorder: a mental disorder with strong changes in mood and energy. It is associated with episodes of mood swings ranging from depression lows to manic highs. Its causes are not clearly understood, but it is believed that both genetic and environmental factors play a role.

Dementia: a general term that describes a group of symptoms associated with a decline in mental ability severe enough to affect a person's thinking, behaviour and ability to perform everyday tasks. Memory loss or having problems with short-term memory is the most recognised example. Dementia is not a normal part of ageing; most people with dementia are older, but not all older people have dementia (see Chapter 22).

Microsleep: a fleeting, uncontrollable, brief episode of sleep or drowsiness which can last for a single fraction of a second or up to several seconds. During a microsleep an individual fails to respond to some arbitrary sensory input and have a brief lapse in consciousness.

Neuronal plasticity: the ability of the brain to change its structure and/or function in response to alterations in its environment. This allows new nerve connections to be formed throughout life, or the nerve cells in the brain to adjust their activities in response to new situations, or to compensate for injury.

REFERENCES

Benton, D. & Parker, P.Y., 1998, 'Breakfast, blood glucose, and cognition', *American Journal of Clinical Nutrition, 67*(4): 772S–8S, doi:10.1093/ajcn/67.4.772S

Beyond Blue, 2019, *Beyond Blue,* <www.beyondblue.org.au/>, accessed 9 January 2019

Black Dog Insitute, 2019, *Black Dog Institute,* <www.blackdoginstitute.org.au/>, accessed 9 January 2019

Bovier, E.R., Renzi, L.M. & Hammond, B.R., 2014, 'A double-blind, placebo-controlled study on the effects of lutein and zeaxanthin on neural processing speed and efficiency', *PLoS One, 9*(9): e108178, doi:10.1371/journal.pone.0108178

Canhada, S., Castro, K., Perry, I.S. & Luft, V.C., 2018, 'Omega-3 fatty acids supplementation in Alzheimer's disease: A systematic review', *Nutritional Neuroscience, 21*(8): 529–38, doi:10.1080/1028415X.2017.1321813

Chen, R.-Y., Chang, Y.-H., Lee, M.-S. & Wahlqvist, M.L., 2011, 'Dietary quality may enhance survival related to cognitive impairment in Taiwanese elderly', *Food & Nutrition Research, 55*(1): 7387, doi:10.3402/fnr. v55i0.7387

Chiang, P.-H., Huang, L.-Y., Lo, Y.-T., Lee, M.-S. & Wahlqvist, M.L., 2013, 'Bidirectionality and gender differences in emotional disturbance associations with obesity among Taiwanese schoolchildren', *Research in Developmental Disabilities, 34*(10): 3504–16, doi:10.1016/j.ridd.2013.06.023

CHI-LLC, 2019, *Overview of the Dietary Inflammatory Index,* <http://chi-llc.net/about/dii-scale/>, accessed 9 January 2019

Conner, T.S., Brookie, K.L., Carr, A.C., Mainvil, L.A. & Vissers, M.C., 2017, 'Let them eat fruit! The effect of fruit and vegetable consumption on psychological well-being in young adults: A randomized controlled trial', *PloS One, 12*(2): e0171206, doi:10.1371/journal.pone.0171206

Cryan, J.F. & O'Mahony, S.M., 2011, 'The microbiome-gut-brain axis: From bowel to behavior', *Neurogastroenterology & Motility, 23*(3): 187–92, doi:10.1111/j.1365-2982.2010.01664.x

de Jager, C.A., Oulhaj, A., Jacoby, R., Refsum, H. & Smith, A.D., 2012, 'Cognitive and clinical outcomes of homocysteine-lowering B-vitamin treatment in mild cognitive impairment: A randomized controlled trial', *International Journal of Geriatric Psychiatry, 27*(6): 592–600, doi:10.1002/gps.2758

Dominy, S.S., Lynch, C., Ermini, F., Benedyk, M., Marczyk, A. et al., 2019, 'Porphyromonas gingivalis in Alzheimer's disease brains: Evidence for disease causation and treatment with small-molecule inhibitors', *Science Advances, 5*(1): eaau3333, doi:10.1126/sciadv.aau3333

Ekman, P. & Davidson, R.J., 1993, 'Voluntary smiling changes regional brain activity', *Psychological Science, 4*(5): 342–5, doi:10.1111/j.1467-9280.1993.tb00576.x

Farzi, A., Hassan, A.M., Zenz, G. & Holzer, P., 2018, 'Diabesity and mood disorders: Multiple links through the microbiota–gut–brain axis', *Molecular Aspects of Medicine, 66*: 80-93, doi:10.1016/j.mam.2018.11.003

Foster, J.A. & Neufeld, K.-A.M., 2013, 'Gut–brain axis: how the microbiome influences anxiety and depression', *Trends in Neurosciences, 36*(5): 305–12, doi:10.1016/j.tins.2013.01.005

Foster, J.A., Rinaman, L. & Cryan, J.F., 2017, 'Stress & the gut–brain axis: Regulation by the microbiome', *Neurobiology of Stress, 7*: 124–36, doi:10.1016/j.ynstr.2017.03.001

Ghaisas, S., Maher, J. & Kanthasamy, A., 2016, 'Gut microbiome in health and disease: Linking the microbiome–gut–brain axis and environmental factors in the pathogenesis of systemic and neurodegenerative diseases', *Pharmacology & Therapeutics, 158*: 52–62, doi:10.1016/j.pharmthera.2015.11.012

González-Garrido, A.A., Brofman-Epelbaum, J.J., Gómez-Velázquez, F.R., Balart-Sánchez, S.A. & Ramos-Loyo, J., 2019, 'Skipping breakfast affects the early steps of cognitive processing: An event-related brain potentials study', *Journal of Psychophysiology, 33*(2): 109–18, doi:10.1027/0269-8803/a000214

González-José, R., Ramírez-Rozzi, F., Sardi, M., Martínez-Abadías, N., Hernández, M. & Pucciarelli, H.M., 2005, 'Functional-cranial approach to the influence of economic strategy on skull morphology', *American Journal of Physical Anthropology, 128*(4): 757–71, doi:10.1002/ajpa.20161

Grünheid, T., Langenbach, G.E., Korfage, J.A., Zentner, A. & Van Eijden, T.M., 2009, 'The adaptive response of jaw muscles to varying functional demands', *European Journal of Orthodontics, 31*(6): 596–612, doi:10.1093/ejo/cjp093

Hébert, J.R., Shivappa, N., Wirth, M.D., Hussey, J.R. & Hurley, T.G., 2019. 'The Dietary Inflammatory Index (DII): Lessons learned, improvements made, and future directions', *Advances in Nutrition, 10*(2): 185-95, doi: 10.1093/advances/nmy071

Hibbeln, J.R., 1998, 'Fish consumption and major depression', *Lancet, 351*(9110): 1213, doi:10.1016/S0140-6736(05)79168-6

—— 2002, 'Seafood consumption, the DHA content of mothers' milk and prevalence rates of postpartum depression: A cross-national, ecological analysis', *Journal of Affective Disorders, 69*(1–3): 15–29, doi:10.1016/S0165-0327(01)00374-3

Hibbeln, J.R. & Salem, J.N., 1995, 'Dietary polyunsaturated fatty acids and depression: When cholesterol does not satisfy', *American Journal of Clinical Nutrition, 62*(1): 1–9, doi:10.1093/ajcn/62.1.1

Horrobin, D. & Bennett, C., 1999, 'Depression and bipolar disorder: Relationships to impaired fatty acid and phospholipid metabolism and to diabetes, cardiovascular disease, immunological abnormalities, cancer, ageing and osteoporosis—possible candidate genes', *Prostaglandins, Leukotrienes and Essential Fatty Acids (PLEFA)*, *60*(4): 217–34, doi:10.1054/plef.1999.0037

Huang, T., Wahlqvist, M.L. & Li, D., 2010, 'Docosahexaenoic acid decreases plasma homocysteine via regulating enzyme activity and mRNA expression involved in methionine metabolism', *Nutrition*, *26*(1): 112–19, doi:10.1016/j.nut.2009.05.015

Huang, W., Ramsey, K.M., Marcheva, B. & Bass, J., 2011, 'Circadian rhythms, sleep, and metabolism', *Journal of Clinical Investigation*, *121*(6): 2133–41, doi:10.1172/JCI46043

Jacka, F.N., Mykletun, A., Berk, M., Bjelland, I. & Tell, G.S., 2011, 'The association between habitual diet quality and the common mental disorders in community-dwelling adults: The Hordaland Health study', *Psychosomatic Medicine*, *73*(6): 483–90, doi:10.1097/PSY.0b013e318222831a

Jacka, F.N., O'Neil, A., Opie, R., Itsiopoulos, C., Cotton, S. et al., 2017, 'A randomised controlled trial of dietary improvement for adults with major depression (the "SMILES" trial)', *BMC Medicine*, *15*(1): 23, doi:10.1186/s12916-017-0791-y

Kennedy, D.O., Veasey, R., Watson, A., Dodd, F., Jones, E. et al., 2010, 'Effects of high-dose B vitamin complex with vitamin C and minerals on subjective mood and performance in healthy males', *Psychopharmacology*, *211*(1): 55–68, doi:10.1007/s00213-010-1870-3

Köhler, C.A., Freitas, T.H., Maes, M., de Andrade, N.Q., Liu, C.S. et al., 2017, 'Peripheral cytokine and chemokine alterations in depression: A meta-analysis of 82 studies', *Acta Psychiatrica Scandinavica*, *135*(5): 373–87, doi:10.1111/acps.12698

Köhler, C.A., Freitas, T.H., Stubbs, B., Maes, M., Solmi, M. et al., 2018, 'Peripheral alterations in cytokine and chemokine levels after antidepressant drug treatment for major depressive disorder: Systematic review and meta-analysis', *Molecular Neurobiology*, *55*(5): 4195–206, doi:10.1111/acps.12698

Lassale, C., Batty, G.D., Baghdadli, A., Jacka, F., Sánchez-Villegas, A. et al., 2018, 'Healthy dietary indices and risk of depressive outcomes: A systematic review and meta-analysis of observational studies', *Molecular Psychiatry*, *2018*: 1–22, doi:10.1038/s41380-018-0237-8

Lee, M.-S., Wahlqvist, M.L., Chou, Y.-C., Fang, W.-H., Lee, J.-T. et al., 2014, 'Turmeric improves post-prandial working memory in pre-diabetes independent of insulin', *Asia Pacific Journal of Clinical Nutrition*, *23*(4): 581–91, doi:10.6133/apjcn.2014.23.4.24

Liew, W.-P.-P., Ong, J.-S., Gan, C.-Y., Yahaya, S., Khoo, B.-Y. & Liong, M.-T., 2015, 'Gut microbiome and stress', in M.-T. Liong (ed.), *Beneficial Microorganisms in Medical and Health Applications*, Cham: Springer, pp. 223–55

Liu, C.-C., Kanekiyo, T., Xu, H. & Bu, G., 2013, 'Apolipoprotein E and Alzheimer disease: Risk, mechanisms, and therapy', *Nature Reviews. Neurology*, *9*(2): 106–18, doi:10.1038/nrneurol.2012.263

Luchtman, D.W. & Song, C., 2013, 'Cognitive enhancement by omega-3 fatty acids from child-hood to old age: Findings from animal and clinical studies', *Neuropharmacology*, *64*: 550–65, doi:10.1016/j.neuropharm.2012.07.019

Mennella, J.A., Jagnow, C.P. & Beauchamp, G.K., 2001, 'Prenatal and postnatal flavor learning by human infants', *Pediatrics*, *107*(6): e88, doi:10.1542/peds.107.6.e88

Mishra, S. & Palanivelu, K., 2008, 'The effect of curcumin (turmeric) on Alzheimer's disease: An overview', *Annals of Indian Academy of Neurology*, *11*(1): 13-9, doi:10.4103/0972-2327.40220

Møller, P., Wallin, H. & Knudsen, L.E., 1996, 'Oxidative stress associated with exercise, psychological stress and life-style factors', *Chemico-Biological Interactions*, *102*(1): 17–36, doi:10.1016/0009-2797(96)03729-5

Morris, M.C., Evans, D.A., Bienias, J.L., Tangney, C.C., Bennett, D.A. et al., 2003, 'Consumption of fish and n-3 fatty acids and risk of incident Alzheimer disease', *Archives of Neurology*, *60*(7): 940–6, doi:10.1001/archneur.60.7.940

Morris, M.C., Tangney, C.C., Wang, Y., Sacks, F.M., Bennett, D.A. & Aggarwal, N.T., 2015, 'MIND diet associated with reduced incidence of Alzheimer's disease', *Alzheimer's & Dementia*, *11*(9): 1007–14, doi:10.1016/j.jalz.2014.11.009

Oliver, G. & Wardle, J., 1999, 'Perceived effects of stress on food choice', *Physiology & Behavior*, *66*(3): 511–5, doi:10.1016/S0031-9384(98)00322-9

Oliver, G., Wardle, J. & Gibson, E.L., 2000, 'Stress and food choice: A laboratory study', *Psychosomatic Medicine, 62*(6): 853–65, doi:10.1097/00006842-200011000-00016

Opie, R.S., O'Neil, A., Itsiopoulos, C. & Jacka, F.N., 2015, 'The impact of whole-of-diet interventions on depression and anxiety: A systematic review of randomised controlled trials', *Public Health Nutrition, 18*(11): 2074–93, doi:10.1017/S1368980014002614

Pinker, S., 1999, 'How the mind works', *Annals of the New York Academy of Sciences, 882*(1): 119–27, doi:10.1111/j.1749-6632.1999.tb08538.x

Roberts, C., 2008, 'The effects of stress on food choice, mood and bodyweight in healthy women', *Nutrition Bulletin, 33*(1): 33–9, doi:10.1111/j.1467-3010.2007.00666.x

Rucklidge, J., Taylor, M. & Whitehead, K., 2011, 'Effect of micronutrients on behavior and mood in adults with ADHD: Evidence from an 8-week open label trial with natural extension', *Journal of Attention Disorders, 15*(1): 79–91, doi:10.1177/1087054709356173

Schelke, M.W., Attia, P., Palenchar, D., Kaplan, B., Mureb, M. et al., 2018, 'Mechanisms of risk reduction in the clinical practice of Alzheimer's disease prevention', *Frontiers in Aging Neuroscience, 10*: 96, doi:10.3389/fnagi.2018.00096

Shivappa, N., Hébert, J.R., Veronese, N., Caruso, M.G., Notarnicola, M. et al., 2018, 'The relationship between the dietary inflammatory index (DII®) and incident depressive symptoms: A longitudinal cohort study', *Journal of Affective Disorders, 235*: 39–44, doi:10.1016/j.jad.2018.04.014

Shivappa, N., Steck, S.E., Hurley, T.G., Hussey, J.R. & Hébert, J.R., 2013, 'Designing and developing a literature-derived, population-based dietary inflammatory index', *Public Health Nutrition, 17*(8): 1689–96, doi:10.1017/S1368980013002115

Silvers, K.M. & Scott, K.M., 2007, 'Fish consumption and self-reported physical and mental health status', *Public Health Nutrition, 5*(3): 427–31, doi:10.1079/PHN2001308

Singhrao, S.K., Harding, A., Poole, S., Kesavalu, L. and Crean, S., 2015, '*Porphyromonas gingivalis* periodontal infection and its putative links with Alzheimer's disease', *Mediators of Inflammation, 2015*, doi: 10.1155/2015/137357

Smith, P. & Blumenthal, J., 2016, 'Dietary factors and cognitive decline', *Journal of Prevention of Alzheimer's Disease, 3*(1): 53-64, doi:10.14283/jpad.2015.71

Steel, Z., Marnane, C., Iranpour, C., Chey, T., Jackson, J.W. et al., 2014, 'The global prevalence of common mental disorders: A systematic review and meta-analysis 1980–2013', *International Journal of Epidemiology, 43*(2): 476–93, doi:10.1093/ije/dyu038

Steiner, J.E., 1979, 'Human facial expressions in response to taste and smell stimulation', *Advances in Child Development and Behavior, 13*(5): 257–95, doi:10.1016/S0065-2407(08)60349-3

Tassoni, D., Kaur, G., Weisinger, R.S. & Sinclair, A.J., 2008, 'The role of eicosanoids in the brain', *Asia Pacific Journal of Clinical Nutrition, 17*(S1): 220–8, doi:10.6133/apjcn.2008.17.s1.53

van de Rest, O., Berendsen, A.A., Haveman-Nies, A. & de Groot, L.C., 2015, 'Dietary patterns, cognitive decline, and dementia: A systematic review', *Advances in Nutrition, 6*(2): 154–68, doi:10.3945/an.114.007617

van Strien, T., Konttinen, H., Homberg, J.R., Engels, R.C.M.E. & Winkens, L.H.H., 2016, 'Emotional eating as a mediator between depression and weight gain', *Appetite, 100*: 216–24, doi:10.1016/j.appet.2016.02.034

Vos, T., Abajobir, A.A., Abate, K.H., Abbafati, C., Abbas, K.M. et al., 2017, 'Global, regional, and national incidence, prevalence, and years lived with disability for 328 diseases and injuries for 195 countries, 1990–2016: A systematic analysis for the Global Burden of Disease Study 2016', *Lancet, 390*(10100): 1211–59, doi:10.1016/S0140-6736(17)32154-2

Wahlqvist, M.L., Lee, M.-S., Lee, J.-T., Hsu, C.-C., Chou, Y.-C. et al., 2016, 'Cinnamon users with prediabetes have a better fasting working memory: A cross-sectional function study', *Nutrition Research, 36*(4): 305–10, doi:10.1016/j.nutres.2015.12.005

Wang, D., Sun, X., Yan, J., Ren, B., Cao, B. et al., 2018, 'Alterations of eicosanoids and related mediators in patients with schizophrenia', *Journal of Psychiatric Research, 102*: 168–78, doi:10.1016/j.jpsychires.2018.04.002

Wardle, J., Steptoe, A., Oliver, G. & Lipsey, Z., 2000, 'Stress, dietary restraint and food intake', *Journal of Psychosomatic Research, 48*(2): 195–202, doi:10.1016/S0022-3999(00)00076-3

Williams, F., 2017, *The Nature Fix: Why nature makes us happier, healthier, and more creative*, New York, NY: W.W. Norton & Company

{CHAPTER 35}
FOOD AND HEALTH: LIFELONG LEARNING AND ACTION

Mark L. Wahlqvist

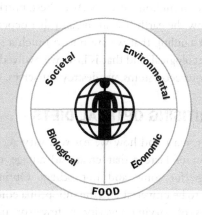

CONCEPTUALISATION

The scope of food and nutrition science and practice is wide and deep, inclusive of several disciplines and providing opportunities for application in many fields of endeavour.

This edition of *Food and Nutrition* subscribes to the view that the dimensions of food and nutrition include the biological, environmental, societal and economic; each of these is undergoing paradigm shifts, identified chapter by chapter as quadrants of a circle. These dimensions are interactive and synergistic, as are the factors that support them and, in turn, their personal and planetary health outcomes.

The evidence for action is observational and experimental, and forever subject to challenge and review for its coherence and utility. Predictive models assessed for benefit, risk and cost are underutilised in evidence-gathering for food systems and individual

and ecosystem health. As with all things, the only certainty is uncertainty.

As scholars and practitioners of the food and nutrition compendium of knowledge, skills and attitudes, we are expected—and expect of ourselves—to develop it and use it to the best of our ability. This is a part of nutritional ethics. These ethics operate in ways which address questions of food and health equity, in a planet ecologically sustainable and favourable to our wellbeing, and to which our autonomy must be sensitive (Solomons 2002; Wahlqvist 2018; Wahlqvist et al. 2009 & 2012).

ECOLOGICAL CREATURES

The nature of nutritional biology and its ecological dependence is one of the most dynamic and conceptually challenging areas of food and nutrition science (see Chapter 30). Think of how the interface between us and the environment is blurred; even changes in our oral microbiome can affect our brain (Claesson et al. 2012; Dominy et al. 2019; Foster & Neufeld 2013; Foster et al. 2017). There are countless examples of food–biology–health connections yet to be explored. It is remarkable that what we know presently can be put to our benefit with low apparent risk, if somewhat narrow advantage. Perhaps we do not recognise or measure the wider and longer consequences of what we do. It is salutary to remember how short our tenure of some 200,000 years has been as a recognisable part of earth's systems, when other forms of life have histories measured in millions of years. At its best, nutrition is about how the earth sustains us, and that depends on us understanding that we are not so much a species, but are ecological, and that is how we evolved. If we destroy our ecosystems, we destroy ourselves.

PRIORITISING OPTIMAL DIETS

Whether, what and how we eat will vary according to a host of factors that create advantage or disadvantage for some and not others. Optima are unlikely to be universal, and the suboptima constitute problems of varying severity. A few—or many—may suffer dysnutrition (disordered nutrition), requiring individualised (clinical) or population-wide (public health) solutions. Yet different food patterns—a Mediterranean, Scandinavian, Japanese or pluralistically cultural Australian diet—may have similar health or planetary outcomes, at least insofar as comparability of wellness and longevity are concerned (Darmadi-Blackberry et al. 2004; Wahlqvist et al. 2005; Wahlqvist & Lee 2007). But this comparability is modulated notably by ethnicity and locality. It is food intake biodiversity, and some food categories such as legumes, that provide the comparability. This is a background against which we might establish priorities for food and nutrition action plans.

A perennial difficulty is the pressure to commodify the perceived characteristics of favourable dietary patterns, often for commercial reasons, and, in the process, lose health-enhancing properties.

Biodiversity as a health optimiser is difficult to emulate without its connection to nature, although it can operate in a range of cultural formats as indicated earlier. The proliferation of salty, fatty, sugary diets is the most pervasive example of profit-taking through appetite satisfaction with scant regard to health. Yet food staples to meet energy requirements, such as grains or tuberous vegetables, are almost universal across food cultural settings to avoid undernutrition of the energy deficiency kind. If we are physically active, and eat enough of these in relatively intact form, together with plentiful fruits, legumes and other vegetables, we will remain nutritionally healthy. Problems arise when there are continuing or new threats to our food systems—climate change in particular. There will be efforts to address these problems through food simulation technologies, but these efforts may have difficulty in meeting our more fundamental ecosocial nutritional needs. Examples include an array of extruded and 3-D printed foods (Wahlqvist 2016) (see Chapter 5).

PROBLEM IDENTIFICATION AND SOLVING

The food and nutrition problems that we identify may have their origins outside our usual frame of reference. For example, child obesity is least likely to be genetic in the Mendelian sense, and more likely to be a phenotype with contributors including intergenerational factors, intrauterine factors, child rearing, child abuse, cultural, growth and development, town planning, recreational facilities, educational access, school environs, environmental contamination, personal behaviour, childhood illness and its management (as with antibiotics affecting the gut microbiome) and climate change, among others. Moreover, the understanding of its pathogenesis will evolve, change and be subject to our peculiar vantage point (Chiang et al. 2013; Chiang et al. 2011; Hesketh et al. 2005; Wahlqvist et al. 2015). Given the complexity and multifactoriality of pathogenesis, the most successful approaches to child obesity prevention have been where the entire community cooperates to solve the problem (Bell et al. 2008;

Bleich et al. 2013; Borys et al. 2013; Sacher et al. 2010). Unfortunately, body compositional disorders are increasing globally and inexorably regardless, requiring greater understanding and innovation. The child obesity experience informs how other challenging food security and nutritionally related health problems might be addressed. Historical and contextual analysis can be instructive. The trajectories of the major nutritionally related health disorders we see today have taken off with the Industrial Revolution, population explosion, use of fossil fuels and the internal combustion engine, development and excessive use of antibiotics and the advent of plastic, with no or little evaluation of their medium- to long-term consequences. Of course, this is circumstantial and not an argument for causality. But as the environmental determinants of health, including those to do with food systems, become clearer, it may be possible for the generation that studies this book to mitigate the threats to the planet that sustains us and our ecology.

From the relevant chapters of *Food and Nutrition*, a priority list of pressing food and nutrition problems might be compiled. It would include:

- climate change
- energy flows in the food and health systems
- biodiversity, econutrition and the agreed commons (what we must share)
- population characteristics, hearth (family and food) and displacement
- personal behaviours
- microbiomics and integrated ecobiology
- food security and future food
- disaster nutrition and preparedness
- future health—dynamic prospects.

Solving problems more often comes with inspiration, but the process can be promoted with regularised protocols and repertoires when not *de novo* or spontaneously creative and innovative. The areas to be addressed can be systematised by way of one's responsibilities, whether personal (clinical, precision) or population-wide (public health).

Often, in food and nutrition science, we need evidence that is integrative and multifactorial rather than reductionist and unifactorial. This is where modelling and monitoring outcomes with research-in-progress methods can be invaluable (Wahlqvist et al. 1999). Time and resources are of the essence in addressing the escalation of food-related insecurity and disorders, largely on account of overpopulation and climate change. Only a small part of this challenge can be tackled in timely fashion and by the understanding we get from randomised and blinded clinical trials (Wahlqvist et al. 2008).

Case studies play an important role in clinical nutrition problem definition and logically derived solutions (Wahlqvist 2013). Natural experiments are among the most instructive pieces of evidence. Good examples of this are where the food supply of communities or countries has changed inadvertently, as with the reduction in ischaemic heart disease in Poland after more liberal imports of fresh fruit and vegetables (Zatonski et al. 1998); the loss and recovery of food habits and health patterns by migrants and refugees; or the recognition of inter-generational epigenetics in northern Sweden through local record-keeping of weather, harvests, food security and health (Bygren et al. 2001; Jang & Serra 2014; Pembrey 2002). We can expect more revelations of how food and health systems interact as metadata is interrogated in relation to incidental perturbations and planned interventions, a process under way through sites like the 'Dr Foster Unit' at Imperial College London (www.imperial.ac.uk/dr-foster-unit).

PERSONAL AND CAREER DEVELOPMENT

Food and Nutrition encourages its users to develop a toolkit as they learn. This can contribute knowledge and skills and develop the attitudes required not only in a career involving food and nutrition science, but also as a framework for continuing nutrition education and lifelong engagement in the field for personal, family and societal benefit.

There is little doubt that a different workforce will be required to enable access to the increasingly vulnerable local and global food, water, energy and health systems for the billions who need them. It is hoped that the global population will stabilise by around 2050, allowing the earth's ecosystems, which provide us with inestimable services, to progressively recover. This book endeavours to alert readers to this prospect and provide some of the tools needed for the new workforce.

LIVELIHOODS, SURVIVAL, INTERGENERATIONALISM

This book's authors desire its readers, their networks and the world-at-large to achieve adequate and sustainable livelihoods (see chapters 25 and 26). Food, environmental and health security, with good governance, are integral to livelihoods for the community at large, now and in the future. Thus, the food and health sciences can and must assume an intergenerational outlook.

Intergenerationalism depends on extensive interaction between nutritionally sensitive multidimensional systems; in this way, phenotypes may be transmitted by genetic and non-genetic pathways that are integrally ecological and especially dependent on microorganisms (Devaux & Raoult 2018). Our microbiomes represent much of our personal ecology; information for our survival from generation to generation; interconnections within and between us and nature; and resilience when exposed to unfamiliar or threatening agents. We are just beginning to appreciate how connected we are and how important that is for our health and wellbeing. Food habits themselves also provide for interconnectedness with families and communities—the social beyond the nutrientisation so evident in much of the nutrition discourse, to its detriment (Wahlqvist et al. 2014). It is an aspiration of the authors that the future of nutrition in human and planetary affairs will go beyond the paucity of nutrients to food, food habits, food systems, food security, optimal health and sustainable livelihoods. At all times, the food and health policy we promote or choose will need to be contextual, taking into account benefit, risk and cost, no less with personalisation or the desirability of precision, as evidence and case studies show (Joshi et al. 2019).

REFERENCES

Bell, A.C., Simmons, A., Sanigorski, A.M., Kremer, P.J. & Swinburn, B.A., 2008, 'Preventing childhood obesity: The sentinel site for obesity prevention in Victoria, Australia', *Health Promotion International, 23*(4): 328–36, doi:10.1093/heapro/dan025

Bleich, S.N., Segal, J., Wu, Y., Wilson, R. & Wang, Y., 2013, 'Systematic review of community-based childhood obesity prevention studies', *Pediatrics, 132*(1): e201–10, doi:10.1542/peds.2013-0886

Borys, J.,Valdeyron, L., Levy, E.,Vinck, J., Edell, D. et al., 2013, 'EPODE–a model for reducing the incidence of obesity and weight-related comorbidities', *European Endocrinology, 9*(2): 116–20, doi:10.17925/EE.2013.09.02.116

Bygren, L.O., Kaati, G. & Edvinsson, S., 2001, 'Longevity determined by paternal ancestors' nutrition during their slow growth period', *Acta Biotheoretica, 49*(1): 53–9, doi:10.1023/A:1010241825519

Chiang, P.-H., Huang, L.-Y., Lo,Y.-T., Lee, M.-S. & Wahlqvist, M.L., 2013, 'Bidirectionality and gender differences in emotional disturbance associations with obesity among Taiwanese schoolchildren', *Research in Developmental Disabilities, 34*(10): 3504–16, doi:10.1016/j.ridd.2013.06.023

Chiang, P.-H., Wahlqvist, M.L., Lee, M.-S., Huang, L.-Y., Chen, H.-H. & Huang, S.T.-Y., 2011, 'Fast-food outlets and walkability in school neighbourhoods predict fatness in boys and height in girls: A Taiwanese population study', *Public Health Nutrition, 14*(9): 1601–9, doi:10.1017/S1368980011001042

Claesson, M.J., Jeffery, I.B., Conde, S., Power, S.E., O'Connor, E.M. et al., 2012, 'Gut microbiota composition correlates with diet and health in the elderly', *Nature, 488*: 178–84, doi:10.1038/nature11319

Darmadi-Blackberry, I., Wahlqvist, M.L., Kouris-Blazos, A., Steen, B., Lukito, W. et al., 2004, 'Legumes: The most important dietary predictor of survival in older people of different ethnicities', *Asia Pacific Journal of Clinical Nutrition, 13*(2): 217–20, <http://apjcn.nhri.org.tw/server/APJCN/13/2/217.pdf>, accessed 9 January 2019

Devaux, C.A. & Raoult, D., 2018, 'The microbiological memory, an epigenetic regulator governing the balance between good health and metabolic disorders', *Frontiers in Microbiology, 9*: 1379, doi:10.3389/fmicb.2018.01379

Dominy, S.S., Lynch, C., Ermini, F., Benedyk, M., Marczyk, A. et al., 2019, 'Porphyromonas gingivalis in Alzheimer's disease brains: Evidence for disease causation and treatment with small-molecule inhibitors', *Science Advances,* 5(1): eaau3333, doi:10.1126/sciadv.aau3333

Foster, J.A. & Neufeld, K.-A.M., 2013, 'Gut–brain axis: How the microbiome influences anxiety and depression', *Trends in Neurosciences, 36*(5): 305–12, doi:10.1016/j.tins.2013.01.005

Foster, J.A., Rinaman, L. & Cryan, J.F., 2017, 'Stress & the gut–brain axis: Regulation by the microbiome', *Neurobiology of Stress,* 7: 124–36, doi:10.1016/j.ynstr.2017.03.001

Hesketh, K., Waters, E., Green, J., Salmon, L. & Williams, J., 2005, 'Healthy eating, activity and obesity prevention: A qualitative study of parent and child perceptions in Australia', *Health Promotion International, 20*(1): 19–26, doi:10.1093/heapro/dah503

Jang, H. & Serra, C., 2014, 'Nutrition, epigenetics, and diseases', *Clinical Nutrition Research, 3*(1): 1–8, doi:10.7762/cnr.2014.3.1.1

Joshi, P.A., Smith, J., Vale, S. & Campbell, D.E., 2019, 'The Australasian Society of Clinical Immunology and Allergy infant feeding for allergy prevention guidelines', *Medical Journal of Australia, 210*: 89–93, doi:10.5694/mja2.12102

Pembrey, M.E., 2002, 'Time to take epigenetic inheritance seriously', *European Journal of Human Genetics, 10*(11): 669–71, doi:10.1038/sj.ejhg.5200901

Sacher, P.M., Kolotourou, M., Chadwick, P.M., Cole, T.J., Lawson, M.S. et al., 2010, 'Randomized controlled trial of the MEND program: A family-based community intervention for childhood obesity', *Obesity, 18*(S1): S62–8, doi:10.1038/oby.2009.433

Solomons, N.W., 2002, 'Ethical consequences for professionals from the globalization of food, nutrition and health', *Asia Pacific Journal of Clinical Nutrition,* 11: S653–65, doi:10.1046/j.1440-6047.11.supp3.14.x

Wahlqvist, M.L., 2013, 'Case studies and evidence based nutrition', *Asia Pacific Journal of Clinical Nutrition, 22*(4): 664–6, doi:10.6133/apjcn.2013.22.4.22

—— 2016, 'Future food', *Asia Pacific Journal of Clinical Nutrition,* 25(4): 706–15, doi:10.6133/apjcn.092016.01

—— 2018, 'Nutrition science and future earth: Current nutritional policy dilemmas', in T. Beer, J. Li & K. Alverson (eds), *Global Change and Future Earth: The geoscience perspective,* Cambridge: Cambridge University Press, pp. 209–22

Wahlqvist, M.L., Darmadi-Blackberry, I., Kouris-Blazos, A., Jolley, D., Steen, B. & Horie, Y., 2005, 'Does diet matter for survival in long-lived cultures?', *Asia Pacific Journal of Clinical Nutrition, 14*(1): 2–6, <http://apjcn.nhri.org.tw/server/APJCN/14/1/2.pdf>, accessed 9 January 2019

Wahlqvist, M.L., Hsu-Hage, B.H.H. & Lukito, W., 1999, 'Clinical trials in nutrition', *Asia Pacific Journal of Clinical Nutrition, 8*(3): 231–41, doi:10.1046/j.1440-6047.1999.00120.x

Wahlqvist, M.L., Huang, L.-Y., Lee, M.-S., Chiang, P.-H., Chang, Y.-H. & Tsao, A.P., 2014, 'Dietary quality of elders and children is interdependent in Taiwanese communities: A NAHSIT mapping study', *Ecology of Food and Nutrition, 53*(1): 81–97, doi:10.1080/03670244.2013.772512

Wahlqvist, M.L., Keatinge, J.D.H., Butler, C.D., Friel, S., McKay, J. et al., 2009, 'A Food in Health Security (FIHS) platform in the Asia-Pacific Region: The way forward', *Asia Pacific Journal of Clinical Nutrition, 18*(4): 688–702, doi:10.6133/apjcn.2009.18.4.34

Wahlqvist, M.L., Krawetz, S.A., Rizzo, N.S., Dominguez-Bello, M.G., Szymanski, L.M. et al., 2015, 'Early-life influences on obesity: From preconception to adolescence', *Annals of the New York Academy of Sciences, 1347*(1): 1–28, doi:10.1111/nyas.12778

Wahlqvist, M.L., Lee, M.-S., Lau, J., Kuo, K.N., Huang, C.-j. et al., 2008, 'The opportunities and challenges of evidence-based nutrition (EBN) in the Asia Pacific region: Clinical practice and policy-setting', *Asia Pacific Journal of Clinical Nutrition, 17*(1): 2–7, doi:10.6133/apjcn.2008.17.1.01

Wahlqvist, M.L. & Lee, M.S., 2007, 'Regional food culture and development', *Asia Pacific Journal of Clinical Nutrition, 16*(Suppl 1): 2–7, doi:10.6133/apjcn.2007.16.s1.02

Wahlqvist, M.L., McKay, J., Chang, Y.-C. & Chiu, Y.-W., 2012, 'Rethinking the food security debate in Asia: Some missing ecological and health dimensions and solutions', *Food Security, 4*(4): 657–70, doi:10.1007/s12571-012-0211-2

Zatonski, W.A., McMichael, A.J. & Powles, J.W., 1998, 'Ecological study of reasons for sharp decline in mortality from ischaemic heart disease in Poland since 1991', *BMJ, 316*(7137): 1047–51, doi:10.1136/bmj.316.7137.1047

ACRONYMNS AND ABBREVIATIONS

gram	g
milligram	mg
microgram	μg
nanogram	ng
litre	L
millilitre	mL
joule	J
kilojoule	kJ
megajoule	MJ
calorie	cal
kilocalorie	kcal
kilogray	kGy
millimole	mmol
milliosmole	mOsm
osmole	Osm

α-TE	α-tocopherol equivalent
AAS	amino acid score
ABCDE	anthropometry, biochemistry, clinical assessment, dietary assessment, environmental and social assessment
ABS	Australian Bureau of Statistics
ACTH	adrenocorticotropic hormone
AD	Alzheimer's disease
ADH	alcohol dehydrogenase
ADHD	attention deficit hyperactivity disorder
ADI	Acceptable Daily Intake
ADP	adenosine diphosphate
AGE	advanced glycation end product
AI	adequate intake
AICR	American Institute for Cancer Research
AIDS	acquired immunodeficiency syndrome
AIHW	Australian Institute of Health and Welfare
ALA	α-linolenic acid
AMDR	acceptable macronutrient distribution range
AMP	adenosine monophosphate
AMPK	adenosine monophosphate-activated protein kinase
ANZFA	Australia New Zealand Food Authority
APVMA	Australian Pesticides and Veterinary Medicines Authority

ARC	Australian Research Council
ARIA	Accessibility and Remoteness Index of Australia
ATDS	Australian Total Diet Study
ATP	adenosine triphosphate
AUSNUT	AUStralian Food and NUTrient Database
aw/Aw	water activity
BAC	blood alcohol content
BMD	bone mineral density
BMI	body mass index
BMR	basal metabolic rate
CARS	credibility, accuracy, reasonability, support
CDC	(US) Centers for Disease Control and Prevention
CI	confidence interval
CoA	coenzyme A
CRH	corticotropin-releasing hormone
CVD	cardiovascular disease
DALYs	disability-adjusted life years
DASH	Dietary Approaches to Stop Hypertension
DEXA	dual energy x-ray absorptiometry
DFE	dietary folate equivalents
DHA	docosahexaenoic acid
DIAAS	Digestible Indispensable Amino Acid Score
DNA	deoxyribonucleic acid
DP	degree of polymerisation
DSM	Diagnostic and Statistical Manual of Mental Disorders
EAA	essential amino acid
EAR	Estimated Average Requirement
ECF	extracellular fluid
EFA	essential fatty acid
EPA	eicosapentaenoic acid
EPIC	European Prospective Investigation into Cancer and Nutrition
FAD	flavin adenine dinucleotide
FAO	Food and Agriculture Organization
FAS	fetal alcohol syndrome
FBDG	food-based dietary guidelines
FFM	fat-free mass
FFQ	food frequency questionnaire
FHILL	Food Habits in Later Life
FODMAP	fermentable oligo-, di- and monosaccharides and polyols
FRAIL	Fatigue, Resistance, Ambulation, Illnesses and Loss of Weight (scale)
FSANZ	Food Standards Australia New Zealand
GADA	glutamic acid decarboxylase autoantibodies
GBD	global burden of disease
GDM	gestational diabetes
GDP	gross domestic product

GHG	greenhouse gas
GI	glycaemic index
GL	glycaemic load
Gla	γ-carboxyglutamate
Glu	glutamate
GM	genetically modified; gut microbiota
GMP	good manufacturing practice
HA	hypoallergenic
HACCP	Hazard Analysis and Critical Control Points
HANI	Healthy Ageing Nutrition Index
HBGV	health–based guidance value
HDDS	Household Dietary Diversity Score
HHC	health harmful commodities
HIV	human immunodeficiency virus
HOPE	Heart Outcomes Prevention Evaluation
HPA	hypothalamic–pituitary–adrenal
HPLC	high-performance liquid chromatography
IBD	inflammatory bowel disease
IBS	irritable bowel syndrome
ICD	International Classification of Diseases
ICF	intracellular fluids
ICN2	Second International Conference on Nutrition
IDD	iodine deficiency disorders
IDF	International Diabetes Federation
IFAD	International Fund for Agricultural Development
IFG	impaired fasting glucose
IgE	immunoglobulin E
IGO	intergovernmental organisation
IGT	impaired glucose tolerance
ISFR	Implementation Subcommittee for Food Regulation
JECFA	Joint FAO/WHO Expert Committee on Food Additives
LA	linoleic acid
LCA	life-cycle assessment
LDL	low–density lipoproteins
MAIF	Marketing in Australia of Infant Formula
MAMA	mid-arm muscle area
MAMC	mid-arm muscle circumference
MAP	modified atmosphere packaging
MDG	Millennium Development Goal
MEOS	microsomal ethanol oxidising system
MeSH	Medical Subject Headings
MET	metabolic equivalent
MIND	Mediterranean-DASH Intervention for Neurodegenerative Delay
ML	maximum level
MPI	Ministry of Primary Industries

MPL	maximum permitted levels
MRL	maximum residue limit
mRNA	messenger RNA
MST	Malnutrition Screening Tool
MUAC	mid-upper arm circumference
MUFA	monounsaturated fatty acid
MUST	Malnutrition Universal Screening Tool
NCD	non-communicable disease
NDNS	National Diet and Nutrition Survey
NE	niacin equivalent
NFA	National Food Authority
NGO	non-profit organisation
NHANES	National Health and Nutrition Examination Survey
NHMRC	National Health and Medical Research Council
NRS	National Residue Survey
NRV	nutrient reference value
NSAID	non-steroidal anti-inflammatory drug
NSP	non-starch polysaccharides
OECD	Organisation for Economic Co-operation and Development
PA	physical activity
PAH	polycyclic aromatic hydrocarbons
PE	price elasticity
PED	protein-energy dysnutrition
PEM	protein-energy malnutrition
PEN	Practice-based Evidence in Nutrition
PGA	pteroyl glutamic acid
PG-SGA	Patient-Generated Subjective Global Assessment
PKU	phenylketonuria
PLP	pyridoxal 5'-phosphate
PTH	parathyroid hormone
PUFA	polyunsaturated fatty acid
PVC	polyvinyl chloride
RAE	retinol activity equivalence
RBP	retinol-binding protein
RCAN1	regulator of calcineurin 1
RCT	randomised controlled trial
RDI	Recommended Dietary Intake
RE	retinol equivalent
REACH	Renewed Efforts Against Child Hunger and undernutrition
REE	resting energy expenditure
RNA	ribonucleic acid
ROS	reactive oxygen species
RS	resistant starch
RTUF	ready-to-use therapeutic foods
SCFA	short-chain fatty acid

SD	standard deviation
SDG	Sustainable Development Goal
SDT	suggested dietary target
SEM	socioecological model
SFA	saturated fatty acid
SGA	Subjective Global Assessment
SMART	specific, measurable, achievable, relevant, time-bound
SNP	single nucleotide polymorphism
SNS	sympathetic nervous system
SSB	sugar-sweetened beverage
SUN	Scaling Up Nutrition
SWOT	strengths, weaknesses, opportunities and threats
T1DM	type 1 diabetes mellitus
T2DM	type 2 diabetes mellitus
TCA	tricarboxylic acid
TFA	trans fatty acid
TMA	trimethylamine
TMAO	trimethylamine-N-oxide
TSH	thyroid stimulating hormone
UCP1	uncoupling protein 1
UHT	ultra-heat treatment
UK	United Kingdom
UL	upper limit
UN	United Nations
UNDP	United Nations Development Programme
UNEP	United Nations Environment Programme
UNESCO	United Nations Educational, Scientific and Cultural Organization
UNHRC	United Nations Human Rights Council
UNICEF	United Nations Children's Fund
UNSCN	United Nations System Standing Committee on Nutrition
UNU	United Nations University
US	United States
USDA	US Department of Agriculture
UV	ultra-violet
VARK	visua/auditory/kinetic
vCJD	variant Creutzfeldt-Jakob disease
WASH	water, sanitation and hygiene
WCRF	World Cancer Research Fund
WFP	World Food Programme
WHO	World Health Organization
WHR	waist-to-hip ratio
WKS	Wernicke-Korsakoff syndrome
WTO	World Trade Organization
YLD	Years Lost due to Disability
YLL	Years of Life Lost

INDEX

Entries are filed word-by-word. Numbers, letters and Greek letters that precede the names of chemicals are ignored in filing. For example, α-linolenic acid is filed under linolenic acid. Page numbers in **bold** indicate the major treatment of a topic. Page numbers in *italics* refer to figures.

as a food group, 145
in the food supply, 201–4
health benefits and risks, 163–4, 649
for infants, 374
as nutrients, *141*
nutritional qualities, 163
oxidation of, 236
for people with diabetes, 633
recommended intake, 200, 202, 667
satiety effect caused by, *179*
sources of, 153, 161, 163
storage of in the liver, 259
see also fatty acids
fatty acids
abnormalities of in depression, 685
as an energy source for the body, 175, 199
biological roles of, 199, *199*
essential fatty acids, 199, 202, 206, 306, 437, 621
esters of, 119
fatty acid content of selected foods, 201
functions of, 639–40
in glycolipids, 195
influence on cell function, 640
intake of and body weight, 199
nomenclature, 196–7
oxidation of, 199
role in feeling of satiety, 178
structure of common fatty acids, *196*, 196–9
in triglycerides, 195
see also saturated fatty acids; trans fatty acids; unsaturated fatty acids
fatty liver disease, 251, *604*
favism-causing compounds, 111
FBDGs, 323, **325–38**, 501–6, 652, 664
feedback loops, 29
feeding, of infants *see* infant nutrition
female fertility, 349–50, *350*
femoral neck, 670, 677
fennel seeds, 153
fermentation, 79, 90
fermented beverages, 79
fermented foods, 79, 140, 145, 281
fermented milks, 160
ferroportin, 303, 308
ferritin, 303–5, 436, 579, 642
ferroproteins, 292
fertilisers, 64, 498
fertility, nutritional influences on, 349–50, *349–50*
Fetal Alcohol Spectrum Disorder, 359
fetal alcohol syndrome, 252, 254
fetal growth, 240, 360
fetal life, *345*
FFAs, *196*
FFM, 372, *372*, 389
fibre *see* dietary fibre
fibrinogen, 664
fight or flight response, 688
Fiji, 475, 520
firming agents, 86
first foods, 381–2

First Nations, 536
fish
consumption of, 157, 681, 685, *685*
contamination with microplastic, 565, 665
cultural significance, 157
description of, 156
effect on sperm cell membrane, 349
as a food group, 144
health benefits and risks, 114, 157, 203
low fish consumption and Alzheimer's, 681
low fish consumption and depression, 685, *685*
mercury in, 114, 361
natural toxicants in, 112
nutritional qualities, 157
for people with diabetes, 632
pH range, 124
protein in, 191
recommended intake, 203, 373
as a source of n-3 fatty acids, 163, 201, 203, 682
as a source of selenium, 307
fish farming, 157
fish oil, 163, 203
fish poisoning, 112
Five Keys to Safer Food program (WHO), 135–6
flatus factors, 152, 214
flatus gas, 175
flavan-3-ols, 315, 583
flavanones, 312, 315, 605
flavin adenine dinucleotide, 280
flavin mononucleotide, 280
flavones, 312, 315, 605
flavonoids
anti-inflammatory properties, 605
biological properties, 312, *313*
in chocolate, 166
in ginkgo biloba extract, 682
as immunomodulators, 638
in parsley, 155
potential to modulate stress, 687
range and structural complexity, 314–15
in tea, 165
flavonols, 312, 315
flavour enhancers, 86
flavour principles, 525
flaxseed, 153, 604
flaxseed oil, 163
flexitarian diet, 503–4
flood irrigation, 64, 72
flour, 75, 77–8, 150, 213, 282, 357
fluid loss, in older adults, 412
fluid requirements, in older adults, 401
fluoride, 112, 289–90, 300–1, 675
fluorinated gases, 493
fluorine, 292, 300
fluorosis, 301
foaming agents, 86
FODMAPs, 147, 217
folate
absorption of, 404

bioavailability of, 282
in the blood, 436
as coenzymes, 277
compounds comprising, 281
deficiency of, 251, 258, 277, 282–3, 305, 411, 437–8, 444, 621, 641
diagnostic benchmarks for deficiency, 621
in dietary modelling, 325
difficulty of measuring, 282
in DNA synthesis, 258
fortification of food with, 118
functions of, 277
gene interactions, 592
homeostasis of, 581–2
intake by children, 383
intake by older adults, 405
neuroprotection provided by, 681
nutrient reference values, 277
during pregnancy, 356–7
recommended dietary intake, 277, 283
requirements in older adults, 401
sources of, 148, 157, 161, 277, 281
storage of, 579
synthesis of, 176
toxicity of, 277
folic acid
bioavailability of, 282
chemical structure, *274*
deficiency of, 306
effect on maturity of oocytes, 350
fortification of food with, 88, 118
influence on brain protein synthesis, 682
possible health risks, 281
protection against heart disease, 36
sources of, 36, 155
unmetabolised folic acid, 281
'follow-on formulas', 381
food
categorisation of into groups, 140
classification of, 514
as a commodity, 472
consumer behaviour, 66–8, 477–81, 512–13, *513*, 519–20
ecological approach to, 3
expenditure on, 67, 471, *472*
food group mind map, *143*
in the human environment, 6
influence of migration on, 529
potentially hazardous foods, 132–3
relation to social class, 519–20
transit time through the gut, 176
use of food crops for biofuel, 472
variety of food groups, 142, 144–5
see also carbohydrates; eating patterns; fats; food additives; food safety; food security; functional foods; minerals; nutrients; proteins; vitamins
food activities, 514
food additives, 85–7, 103, 105, 108, 111–13, 118
food aid, 565–7
food allergens, 114–15, 117
food allergies, 161, 185, 376, 386, 389–90